CARDIOVASCULAR NURSING PRACTICE:
A COMPREHENSIVE RESOURCE MANUAL AND STUDY GUIDE FOR CLINICAL NURSES

Carol Jacobson, RN, MN

Karen Marzlin, RN, C, BSN, CCRN, CMC

Cynthia Webner, RN, C, BSN, CCRN, CMC

Cardiovascular Nursing Practice: A Comprehensive Resource Manual and Study Guide for Clinical Nurses

Published by:

Cardiovascular Nursing Education Associates
3324 SW 172nd St.
Burien, WA 98166
www.cardionursing.com

Copyright 2007, Cardiovascular Nursing Education Associates. All rights reserved.

No part of this publication may be reproduced or transmitted in any form or by any means, electronic or mechanical, including photocopying, recording or any information storage and retrieval system, without permission in writing from the authors. For permission, write to Cardiovascular Nursing Education Associates, 3324 SW 172nd St., Burien, WA 98166.

Copies of this book can be obtained by writing to Cardiovascular Nursing Education Associates, 3324 SW 172nd St., Burien, WA 98166; or at www.cardionursing.com.

Notice:

Every effort has been made to assure the accuracy of information presented and to describe accepted and current practice. Health care is a rapidly changing field, and new research and clinical experience may prompt changes in practice, including drug and device therapy, that are different from what is presented in this text. Care has been taken to confirm the accuracy of drug information presented, including indications, dosages, and side effects. Readers are advised to check the package insert and the most current information available for each drug to verify correct dosage and for added warnings and precautions. Neither the publisher nor the authors assumes any liability for injury and/or damage to persons or property due to application of the information presented in this book.

Cover design by Nitro Graphics, Grand Junction, CO (www.nitrographics.biz).

International Standard Book Number 978-0-9785045-0-2.

Printed in United States of America.

Dedication from Carol Jacobson

To all the nurses who continue to pursue excellence in patient care every day and who have inspired me to continue teaching and to write this book. And to my wonderful husband Mike, for putting up with me while I did it.

To Karen and Cindy, my partners and colleagues who have motivated me and worked tirelessly to make this book happen.

Dedication from Karen Marzlin and Cynthia Webner

To Carol, our friend and colleague, who shares our passion of teaching. We have been blessed with this partnership and look forward to our future endeavors.

To our friend and colleague Rhonda, who has consistently shared our vision for Raising the Bar throughout every step of our professional journey.

To our parents – Rodney and Nancy, Judy and Jack, and Larry and Waneta – for their continual support.

To Ron and Nathan who really know and appreciate what it takes to write a Comprehensive Resource Manual. Thanks for pulling some extra weight. Nathan – it has been a special joy to share so many milestones with you. We look forward to many future celebrations.

To God – The reason for everything.

PREFACE FROM THE AUTHORS

As educators, the three of us have been asked by nurses when we were going to write a book that matches our approach to teaching. Our teaching style focuses on an understanding of concepts that can be easily applied in clinical practice. This book was born from the need expressed by nurses across the country for a user-friendly resource that would help them learn and grow in the field of cardiovascular nursing practice and also prepare them for cardiovascular certification. Although this book is an excellent tool for nurses preparing to sit for a certification examination, it is much more than a study guide, hence the title *Comprehensive Resource Manual AND Study Guide*. This book is primarily for clinical nurses working with patients in all types of clinical settings: intensive care, telemetry units, step-down units, emergency departments, chest pain centers, cardiac and interventional radiology laboratories, physician offices and clinics, and in cardiac rehabilitation and home health care. It is a useful resource for educators in hospitals as well as schools of nursing, and for clinical nurse specialists who are responsible for teaching and supporting clinical nursing staff. The major focus is on cardiovascular nursing practice; however, there are chapters that address non-cardiac issues in the cardiac patient, such as pulmonary and renal disorders, electrolyte imbalances, and sepsis.

Some of the features of this book that make it user friendly for clinical nurses include:
- ♡ Size 12 font for easier reading.
- ♡ Full page layout instead of columns of text.
- ♡ Many illustrations to help explain concepts discussed in the text.
- ♡ A combination of prose and bulleted text instead of outline format.
- ♡ Linking Knowledge to Practice sections to help apply knowledge from the text to bedside practice.
- ♡ Self-assessment questions, practice rhythm strips and ECGs at the end of chapters to test your understanding of the concepts presented in the chapter.
- ♡ A glossary of terms and an abbreviation list for quick reference.

Certification
There is a number of certification examinations from which to choose if you are interested in cardiovascular certification. Certification examinations should be accredited by one of the two major accreditation bodies listed below:
- ♡ American Board of Nursing Specialties (ABNS)
- ♡ National Commission for Certifying Agencies (NCCA)

Listed below are some accredited organizations, their certification examinations, and contact information:
- ♡ American Nurses Credentialing Center (www.nursingworld.org/ancc/)
  - ♦ Cardiac/Vascular Nurse Certification
- ♡ American Association of Critical Care Nurses Certification Corporation (www.AACN.org)
  - ♦ CCRN – Certified Critical-Care Registered Nurse
  - ♦ PCCN – Progressive Care Certified Nurse
  - ♦ CMC – Cardiac Medicine Certification (subspecialty exam)
  - ♦ CSC – Cardiac Surgery Certification (subspecialty exam)

If you are considering another examination, ask the sponsoring organization about their accreditation by one of the recognized accreditation bodies.

ABOUT CARDIOVASCULAR NURSING EDUCATION ASSOCIATES (CNEA)

CNEA was established in 2005 when three top nursing educators joined to offer cardiovascular nursing continuing education and certification review courses for nurses who were engaged in advancing their knowledge of cardiovascular nursing practice. Carol Jacobson, Karen Marzlin, and Cindy Webner met at a cardiovascular nursing conference where they were each scheduled to speak. The three quickly discovered that they shared a passion for teaching and for helping the learner to really understand and apply information rather than just memorizing facts. They also share a commitment to helping nurses apply knowledge in the clinical setting for the provision of excellent patient care. The focus of CNEA is to empower nurses to link knowledge to clinical practice for the purpose of improving patient outcomes.

CNEA offers preparation courses for certification as well as continuing education programs on a variety of cardiovascular and critical care topics. All programs can be customized for hospitals and nursing organizations. Visit our website at **www.cardionursing.com** for specific information about our cardiovascular nursing courses and for information on how to bring these courses to your area.

ABOUT THE AUTHORS

Carol Jacobson RN, MN received her BSN from the University of Colorado and her MN from the University of Washington. She has over 30 years of experience in critical care nursing; including staff nurse, manager of a coronary care unit, manager of a cardiac cath lab, and as a critical care clinical nurse specialist. Most of her career was spent practicing cardiovascular nursing at Swedish Medical Center in Seattle, WA. She held the CCRN certification for over 20 years while in active clinical practice. In 1991 she received the Excellence in Critical Care Education Award from the American Association of Critical Care Nurses. In 1993 she started her own business, Quality Education Services in Seattle, through which she continues to offer high-quality programs for nurses. She has been on the clinical faculty at the University of Washington School of Nursing since 1979 and continues in that capacity today. She currently works at Childrens Hospital and Regional Medical Center scanning holter monitors for the Heart Center.

Carol is the author of several chapters in the Cardiac Nursing textbook (Lippincott) and has written chapters in several other books. She is the author of AACN's Bedside Monitoring Protocol and a contributer to the AACN Procedure Manual for Critical Care. She is currently the editor for the ECG Challenges column in AACN Advanced Critical Care. Carol is especially known for her humorous and common-sense approach to teaching difficult topics and making them understandable. She specializes in cardiac topics such as arrhythmias, 12-lead ECG interpretation, hemodynamic monitoring, pacemakers, and cardiovascular drugs and is a frequently requested speaker at conferences across the country and at AACN's National Teaching Institute.

Karen M. Marzlin BSN, RN,C, CCRN, CMC and **Cynthia L. Webner BSN, RN,C, CCRN. CMC**
Karen's clinical focus has been the care of the medical cardiac patient. She has practiced in a variety of settings and roles including coronary intensive care, cardiac stress testing, ambulatory cardiac care, heart failure tele-management, and cardiac risk factor modification counseling. Karen dedicated 10 years of her nursing career to the management and administration of the cardiac catherization and electrophysiology labs, non invasive diagnostic testing areas, and the cardiac rehabilitation department within a cardiovascular service line. As a speaker for PESI Healthcare, Karen teaches Cardiac Emergenics at many locations througout the country.

During Cindy's 27 years of nursing practice, she has cared for the cardiovascular patient as a staff nurse, educator, manager and administrator. Cindy has worked in a variety of clinical settings including the coronary care unit, coronary care step-down unit and cardiothoracic ICU. Cindy also has administrative experience in the management of inpatient medical and surgical cardiac nursing services including the design and

Cardiovascular Nursing Practice: A Comprehensive Resource Manual and Study Guide for Clinical Nurses

development of a chest pain observation unit. Cindy is on the speakers bureau for PESI Healthcare and teaches Cardiac Diagnostics and Interventions which is offered in multiple locations across the country.

Karen and Cindy are co-owners in Key Choice, a nursing consulting and education business with the primary goal of raisng the bar for excellence in nursing practice. They are known for their passion for excellence and their dynamic and creative teaching strategies, which they utilize when providing a variety of eduational programs for nurses and other healthcare professionals. Karen and Cindy co-authored *Cardiovascular Nursing* published by Western Schools in 2005. In addition, they have presented at several national meetings including featured preconference workshops at the last three AACN National Teaching Institutes. Karen and Cindy completed their legal nurse consulting degrees from Kaplan College, Boca Raton, Florida, their bachelor of science degrees from Walsh University, Canton, Ohio, and are currently completing their masters of science degrees in nursing education through Duquesne University in Pittsburgh, Pennsylvania. Karen and Cindy maintain a current clinical practice in an acute care medical cardiac unit that consists of 56 universal beds. In this universal bed unit, they provide care for a wide variety of ICU and step down patients, including patients with acute coronary syndrome, heart failure, and arrhythmia disturbances. They also provide care for patients in a 6-bed chest pain observation unit where chest pain differentiation and 12-lead ECG interpretation are the primary aspects of care.

ACKNOWLEDGMENTS

This book is the result of the efforts of several people other than the authors, each of whom has made a great contribution to the success of this project. A big thank you to our nurse reviewers, who read each chapter and gave honest and constructive feedback about content and style:

Karen Chirumbolo RN, MSN, APRN, BC
Education Specialist
Cardiovascular Surgical Intensive Care Unit / Cardiovascular Operating Room
Aultman Health Foundation
Canton, OH

Rhonda K. Fleischman, MSN, RN, CNS, CCRN
Clinical Education Specialist
Cardiac Care Unit
Aultman Health Foundation
Canton, OH

Suzanne A. Meader, MN, ARNP, ACNP, ANP, CCRN
Cardiovascular Nurse Practitioner
Overlake Hospital, Bellevue WA

We would also like to thank our editors for their hard work and much needed help in getting this book into printable form:

Layout Editor: **Diane Thornton**
　　　　　　Desktop Publishing Specialist
　　　　　　Westwood, MA

Copy Editor: **Carolyn Embree**
　　　　　　Instructor of Language and Literature
　　　　　　Walsh University
　　　　　　North Canton, OH

And thank you to **Karl Almgren** and **Christina VanDahm** at Nitro Graphics for the beautiful cover design and for help with some of the illustrations, and to **Katie M. Petty,** Kent State University, marketing and advertising major, for many illustrations used in the book.

TABLE OF CONTENTS

Preface v

About the Authors vi

Acknowledgments vii

Figures and Tables ....

Chapter 1: Cardiovascular Anatomy and Physiology...1

    Introduction 1

    Basic Cardiac Anatomy 1

    Circulatory System...4

    Cardiac Cycle 7

    Coronary Circulation 9

    Cardiac Action Potential 11

    Contractile Properties of Cardiac Muscle 14

    Cardiac Conduction System..16

    Hemodynamic Principles 17

    The Cardiopulmonary Circuit and Delivery of Oxygen 19

    Neurological Control of the Heart and Blood Pressure.....................................21

    Regulation of Fluid Balance 25

    Test Your Knowledge 30

    Answers 32

    References 33

Chapter 2: Cardiovascular Assessment 35

    Introduction 35

    Health History 35

    Physical Assessment 42

    Test Your Knowledge 62

    Answers 65

    References 65

Chapter 3: Oxygenation and Pulmonary Physiology 67

    Overview 67

    Pulmonary Physiology 71

    Oxygen Therapy and Mechanical Ventilation 89

    Acid-Base Balance 103

    Let's Practice – ABG Analysis on Room Air 107

    Test Your Knowledge 108

    Practice ABG Answers..113

    Answers 113

    References 113

Chapter 4: Hemodynamics/Shock States/Intra-Aortic Balloon Pump Therapy 115

    Hemodynamic Concepts 115

    Invasive Hemodynamic Monitoring...127

Cardiovascular Nursing Practice: A Comprehensive Resource Manual and Study Guide for Clinical Nurses

Altered Hemodynamic States: Valvular Heart Disease 145

Altered Hemodynamic States: Tamponade 146

Altered Hemodynamic States: Shock States 147

Intra-Aortic Balloon Pumping 157

Test Your Knowledge 166

Answers 173

References 173

Chapter 5: Cardiac Arrhythmias **177**

Basics of Rhythm Interpretation 177

Rhythms Originating in the Sinus Node 181

Rhythms Originating in the Atria 184

Supraventricular Tachycardia (SVT) 189

Rhythms Originating in the AV Junction 192

Rhythms Originating in the Ventricles 193

AV Blocks 199

Asystole 205

Bundle Branch Block 206

Differential Diagnosis of Wide QRS Beats and Tachycardias 208

Accessory Pathway Conduction..215

Practice Strips 217

Practice Strip Answers 221

References 221

Chapter 6: 12 Lead Electrocardiography **225**

Introduction 225

Anatomy of a 12 Lead ECG 226

Normal and Abnormal ECG Waveforms and Intervals 227

ECG Leads..230

Normal Cardiac Depolarization 232

The 12 Views of the Heart 233

Frontal Plane Axis 235

Bundle Branch Block..234

Fascicular Blocks (Hemiblocks) 247

Chamber Enlargement 250

Preexcitation Syndromes 256

Ischemia, Injury and Infarction 259

Locating the Infarction on the 12 Lead ECG 264

Myocardial Ischemia Versus Non-ST Elevation Myocardial Infarction 271

Ischemia and MI Practice 272

Practice Strip Answers 281

References 282

Cardiovascular Nursing Practice: A Comprehensive Resource Manual and Study Guide for Clinical Nurses

Chapter 7: Risk Factors and Prevention of Coronary Artery Disease 285

Outline 285

Overview 285

Nonmodifiable Risk Factors 286

Tobacco Use 287

Hypertension 291

Dyslipidemia 297

Diabetes Mellitus 307

Obesity 308

Metabolic Syndrome 309

Physical Inactivity 310

Stress and Other Psychosocial Risk Factors 311

Alcohol 311

Emerging Risk Factors 311

Other Issues in Risk Factor Modification 313

Conclusion 315

Test Your Knowledge 315

Answers 319

References 319

Chapter 8: Acute Coronary Syndrome 325

Introduction 325

Pathophysiology of Coronary Artery Disease 326

Clinical Signs and Symptoms of Coronary Artery Disease 327

Classification and Special Features of Angina Pectoris 328

Diagnosis of Coronary Artery Disease 329

Cardiac Catheterization 332

Cardiac Ischemia 333

Treatment Options for Stable Angina 333

Acute Coronary Syndrome Overview 335

ST Segment Elevation MI 338

Non-ST-Segment Elevation MI 355

Special Considerations 357

Long Term Management of ACS 358

Test Your Knowledge 366

Answers 370

References 370

Chapter 9: Heart Failure 373

Introduction 373

Clinical Presentation 374

Etiology 375

Initial Evaluation 375

Classifications of Heart Failure 376

Cardiovascular Nursing Practice: A Comprehensive Resource Manual and Study Guide for Clinical Nurses

Neurohormonal Responses in Heart Failure 380

Ongoing Assessment in Heart Failure Management 384

Treatment Goals 386

Pharmacological Treatment of Heart Failure 388

Nonpharmacological Treatment Strategies for Heart Failure 394

Special Issues in Heart Failure 396

Patient Education 401

Conclusion 404

Test Your Knowledge 405

Answers 408

References 408

Chapter 10: Cardiomyopathy 413

Introduction 413

Dilated Cardiomyopathy 415

Restrictive Cardiomyopathy 424

Hypertrophic Cardiomyopathy 430

Arrhythmogenic Cardiomyopathy 442

Test Your Knowledge 445

Answers 447

References 447

Chapter 11: Valve Disease 451

Normal Valve Function 451

Aortic Valve Disease 453

Mitral Valve Disease 478

Test Your Knowledge 498

Answers 501

References 501

Chapter 12: Inflammatory Cardiovascular Diseases: Diseases Involving the Pericardium, Myocardium and Endocardium 505

Pericardial Disease 505

Myocarditis 522

Endocardial Disease 524

Test Your Knowledge 534

Answers 537

References 538

Chapter 13: Peripheral Arterial Disease and Ischemic Stroke 543

Peripheral Arterial Disease Overview 543

Lower Extremity PAD 543

Renal Artery Disease 557

Diseases of the Aorta: Aneurysms 562

Diseases of the Aorta: Dissections 568

Carotid Disease and Ischemic Stroke 572

Cardiovascular Nursing Practice: A Comprehensive Resource Manual and Study Guide for Clinical Nurses

Test Your Knowledge 584

Answers 586

References 587

Chapter 14: Cardiovascular Drugs 590

Physiologic Basis of Cardiovascular Drug Therapy 590

Pharmacologic Manipulation of Cardiac Output..................................594

Pharmacologic Manipulation of O_2 Supply and Demand 595

ACE Inhibitors 598

Angiotensin Receptor Blockers (ARB) 601

Aldosterone Blockers 602

Beta Blockers 603

Calcium Channel Blockers 607

Diuretics 610

Sympathomimetic Drugs 612

Inotropes..612

Vasopressors..617

Vasodilators 619

Antithrombotic Drugs 624

Antiarrhythmic Drugs 640

Drugs Used for Heart Rate and Rhythm Control 643

Anti-Lipid Drugs 653

Test Your Knowledge 655

Answers 660

References 660

Chapter 15: Cardiac Catheterization and Interventional Cardiology 663

Diagnostic Cardiac Catheterization 663

Percutaneous Coronary Interventional Procedures 668

Test Your Knowledge 682

Answers 685

References 686

Chapter 16: Open Heart Surgery and Coronary Artery Bypass Grafting (CABG) 689

Overview 689

Preoperative Care 690

Traditional CABG 694

Intraoperative Patient Management Issues 701

Complications of Cardiopulmonary Bypass 706

Alternatives to Traditional CABG 708

Graft Material in CABG 711

Postoperative Care 713

Postoperative Complications 727

Special Patients Populations 734

Post-Discharge Care..736

xiii

Cardiovascular Nursing Practice: A Comprehensive Resource Manual and Study Guide for Clinical Nurses

Test Your Knowledge 737
  Answers 741
  References 741

Chapter 17: Electrical Management of Arrhythmias 745
  Defibrillation 745
  Cardioversion 746
  Pacemakers...749
  Dual Chamber Pacemakers 763
  Biventricular Pacing...774
  Single Chamber Pacing Terminology 777
  Dual Chamber Pacemaker Terminology 779
  Implantable Cardioverter Defibrillators (ICD) 780
  Electrophysiology Studies and Radiofrequency Catheter Ablation for Arrhythmias 787
  Practice Strips 796
  References 803

Chapter 18: Non Cardiac Issues in the Cardiac Patient 805
  Pulmonary Pathophysiology 805
  Electrolyte Abnormalities 827
  Renal Issues in Cardiac and Critical Care 844
  Sepsis 862
  Conclusion 869
  Test Your Knowledge 869
  Answers 874
  References 874

Glossary 879
Abbreviations 907
Index 911

FIGURES AND TABLES

Chapter 1

Figure 1.1: Location of the heart in the chest cavity 1

Figure 1.2: 1

Figure 1.3: Layers of the heart 2

Figure 1.4: Cardiac valves 3

Figure 1.5: AV valve showing the papillary muscles and chordae tendineae 3

Figure 1.6: Closed aortic valve (left); Open aortic valve (right) 4

Figure 1.7: Layers of the arterial wall 5

Figure 1.8: One-way vein valves 6

Figure 1.9: Arterial trunk of normal circulation 6

Figure 1.10: Blood flow through the heart 7

Figure 1.11: Early ventricular diastole. Passive ventricular filling phase. Cardiac diastole 8

Figure 1.12: Atrial systole. Late ventricular diastole. Active ventricular filling 8

Figure 1.13: Isovolumic contraction – ventricular systole 8

Figure 1.14: Ventricular systole 9

Figure 1.15: Aortic recoil 9

Figure 1.16: Perfusion of the coronary arteries 9

Figure 1.17 The coronary arteries..10

Table 1.1: Coronary Artery Supply...11

Figure 1.18: A. Action potential of a Purkinje fiber. Atrial and ventricular muscle cell APs are similar
B. Action potential of a sinus node cell. AV node AP is similar....................................12

Figure 1.19: Phases of the action potential (0, 1, 2, 3, 4) and absolute and
relative refractory period 14

Figure 1.20: Sarcomere...15

Figure 1.21: Transverse tubule-sarcoplasmic reticulum system..15

Figure 1.22: Cardiac conduction system 16

Figure 1.23: Components of cardiac output 17

Table 1.2: Key Definitions Relating to Cardiac Output 17

Figure 1.24: Schematic of the cardiopulmonary circuit..20

Figure 1.25: Capillary network...20

Table 1.3: Adrenergic Receptor Location and Response 22

Figure 1.26:...23

Figure 1.27:...24

Figure 1.28: Distribution of body fluid 26

Figure 1.29: Diffusion..26

Figure 1.30: Osmosis 27

Chapter 2

Figure 2.1: Numeric pain scale...36

Table 2.1: Assessment for Cardiac Perfusion and Pulmonary Congestion 43

Figure 2.2: Assessment of JVD 47

Figure 2.3: Cardiac cycle 50

Figure 2.4: Auscultatory sites 50

Figure 2.5: Normal S1 and S2 52

Figure 2.6: S1, S2, and S3 53

Figure 2.7: S4, S1, and S2 53

Figure 2.8: Early ventricular systole and late ventricular diastole 54

Figure 2.9: Summation gallop 54

Figure 2.10: Drawing demonstrating turbulence of flow 55

Figure 2.11: Murmur configuration for aortic or pulmonic stenosis 56

Figure 2.12: Murmur configuration for tricuspid and mitral regurgitation 57

Figure 2.13: Murmur configuration for aortic or pulmonic regurgitation 58

Figure 2.14: Murmur configuration for tricuspid stenosis 58

Figure 2.15: Murmur configuration for mitral stenosis 58

Figure 2.16: Configuration of pulsus alternans 61

Figure 2.17: Configuration of bisferiens pulse..61

Table 2.2: Clinical Differentiation of Arterial and Venous Disease 61

Chapter 3

Figure 3.1: Conducting airwaysof the respiratory system 69

Table 3.1: Lung volumes 70

Figure 3.2: Alveoli surrounded by pulmonary capillaries 75

Figure 3.3: Zones of distribution of perfusion 76

Figure 3.4: Diffusion of oxygen across the alveoli capillary membrane 78

Figure 3.5: Gas exchange at the alveolar capillary membrane 79

Figure 3.6: Increased V/Q ratio 81

Figure 3.7: Decreased V/Q ratio..81

Figure 3.8: Oxyhemoglobin dissociation curve 83

Figure 3.9: Shift to the right mnemonic...84

Table 3.2: Relationship Between Delivery and Reserve 87

Figure 3.10: Continuous positive airway pressure 92

Figure 3.11: Assist control ventilation 92

Figure 3.12: Peak inspiratory and plateau pressures 96

Figure 3.13: Auto PEEP 97

Table 3.3: Classification of Neuromuscular Blocking Agents 99

Figure 3.14: Peripheral nerve stimulator 100

Figure 3.15: Endotracheal tube location...101

Chapter 4

Figure 4.1: Cardiac output 115

Figure 4.2: Preload 116

Figure 4.3: Left ventricular preload 116

Figure 4.4: Relationship between volume and pressure...117

Figure 4.5: Afterload...119

Figure 4.6: Left ventricular function curve 123

Figure 4.7: Impact of altering preload on left ventricular function 124

Figure 4.8: Improved contractile performance 124

Figure 4.9: Impact of afterload reduction on left ventricular function 124

Table 4.1: Relationship between delivery and reserve 126

Figure 4.10: Basic PA catheter 127

Figure 4.11: PA catheter in proper position with proximal port in right atrium and distal port in a branch of the pulmonary artery..128

Figure 4.12: Pulmonary artery pressure monitoring system 128

Figure 4.13: Marking of phlebostatic axis 130

Figure 4.14: Normal square wave test 131

Figure 4.15: Poor frequency and underdamped system 131

Figure 4.16: Overdamped system 132

Figure 4.17: RA waveform 133

Figure 4.18: RV waveform 133

Figure 4.19: Diastolic pressure increase compared to RV diastolic pressure 134

Figure 4.20: Pulmonary artery occlusive pressure (PAOP) 134

Figure 4.21: Transition of PA pressure to PAOP pressure 134

Figure 4.22: PAOP waveform 135

Figure 4.23: Example of correct measurement of an RA tracing 136

Figure 4.24: Large *a* waves...136

Figure 4.25: Rhythm change from sinus to atrial fibrillation and the change in the RA pressure tracing 137

Figure 4.26: Large *v* waves 137

Figure 4.27: Impact of respiratory cycle on hemodynamic pressure waveforms 138

Figure 4.28: PA to PAOP Tracing...138

Figure 4.29: Correct reading of a Pa pressure tracing on a ventilated patient. 139

Table 4.2: Potential complications of PA catheters 141

Table 4.3: Normal hemodynamic values 143

Figure 4.30: Normal arterial waveform 144

Table 4.4: Classification of Shock 149

Table 4.5: Hemodynamic Profile in Hypovolemic Shock 150

Table 4.6: Clinical Findings Associated with Progressive Loss of Blood 151

Table 4.7: Colloids 152

Table 4.8: Hemodynamic Profile in Cardiogenic Shock 154

Table 4.9: Hemodynamic Profile of Distributive Shock 155

Figure 4.31: Intra-aortic balloon pump (IABP) placement 157

Figure 4.32: Intra-aortic balloon pump inflation and deflation...159

Figure 4.33: Timing assessment points 160

Figure 4.34: Correct inflation timing 162

Figure 4.35: Early inflation prior to valve closure 162

Figure 4.36: Late inflation 162

Figure 4.37: Early deflation 163

Cardiovascular Nursing Practice: A Comprehensive Resource Manual and Study Guide for Clinical Nurses

Figure 4.38: Late deflation 163

Figure 4.39: Balloon pressure waveform 164

Figure 4.40: Low plateau pressure 164

Figure 4.41: Poor autmentation 164

Figure 4.42: Elevated baseline 164

Figure 4.43: Baseline of balloon pressure waveform 165

Figure 4.44: Square plateau and high pressure 165

Chapter 5

Figure 5.1: Cardiac conduction system 177

Figure 5.2: Waves and intervals of cardiac cycle 178

Figure 5.3: Standard intervals on ECG paper...180

Figure 5.4: AV nodal passive SVTs 190

Figure 5.5: AV nodal active SVTs 190

Figure 5.6: Rhythms in AV junction 192

Figure 5.7: Second degree AV block 200

Table 5.1: AV blocks 204

Figure 5.8: Normal conduction in V_1 and V_6 206

Figure 5.9: RBBB 206

Figure 5.10: LBBB 207

Figure 5.11: Causes of wide QRS complex 208

Table 5.2: Normal Conduction and Bundle Branch Block Conduction........208

Figure 5.12: Effect of refractory periods and cycle length on conduction ...209

Figure 5.13: Right bundle branch morphology 211

Figure 5.14: Left bundle branch block pattern 212

Figure 5.15: Ventricular depolarization 213

Figure 5.16: Accessory pathway conduction 215

Chapter 6

Figure 6.1: Normal ECG 226

Figure 6.2: ECG paper 226

Figure 6.3: How ECG leads record 230

Figure 6.4: Placement of recording electrodes...231

Figure 6.5: Frontal plane leads recording electrical activity 231

Figure 6.6: Precordial chest leads: V_1-V_6 232

Figure 6.7: Mean QRS axis 232

Figure 6.8: Normal sequence of depolarization 233

Figure 6.9: Position of precordial leads 234

Figure 6.10: Hexaxial reference system 235

Figure 6.11: Definitions of QRS axis 235

Figure 6.12: QRS axis..236

Figure 6.13: QRS axis determination 237

Figure 6.14: QRS axis determination 238

Figure 6.15: QRS axis determination 239

xviii

Cardiovascular Nursing Practice: A Comprehensive Resource Manual and Study Guide for Clinical Nurses

Figure 6.16: QRS axis determination 240

Figure 6.17: Normal ventricular depolarization 243

Figure 6.18: Electrical forces in blocked right bundle branch 244

Figure 6.19: Electrical forces in blocked left bundle branch 245

Figure 6.20: Normal intraventricular conduction system...247

Figure 6.21: Normal left ventricular activation through both fascicles 247

Figure 6.22: Left anterior fascicular block (LAFB)..248

Figure 6.23: Left posterior fascicular block (LPFB) 249

Figure 6.24: Normal P wave..250

Figure 6.25: Right atrial enlargement (RAE) (P pulmonale)..250

Figure 6.26: Left antrial enlargement (LAE) (P mitrale)..251

Figure 6.27: Normal and abnormal P waves in atrial enlargement 251

Figure 6.28: ST-T "Strain" pattern (LVHand RVH)..252

Figure 6.29: Comparison of normal QRSto changes with RVH and LVH 253

Figure 6.30: Wolff-Parkinson-White Syndrome...257

Figure 6.31: Distribution of coronary arteries 260

Figure 6.32: ECG changes with infarction...261

Figure 6.33: Patterns of ischemia 262

Figure 6.34: Patterns of injury 263

Figure 6.35: Areas of the heart 264

Figure 6.36: Right ventricular and posterior leads 270

Table 6.1: Right Side and Posterior Leads 270

Chapter 7

Box 7.1: Cardiovascular Effects of Tobacco: Nicotine and Carbon Monoxide 288

Box 7.2: Causes of Resistant Hypertension 296

Table 7.1: Lipid levels 297

Table 7.2: LDL-C treatment goals in different patient populations 299

Table 7.3: Effect of lipid lowering drugs on LDL-C levels 301

Table 7.4: Effect of lipid lowering drugs on HDL-C levels and triglycerides..........................302

Box 7.3: Key Points Regarding Administration of Lipid Lowering Drugs 306

Box 7.4: Body Mass Index 309

Box 7.5: American Heart Association Recommendations for Healthy Eating and Lifestyle
Choices...309

Chapter 8

Table 8.1: Continuum of Coronary Artery Disease 325

Figure 8.1: Comparison of stable and vulnerable plaque...327

Figure 8.2: Early hyper acute T waves best seen in leads V_2, V_3, and V_4 336

Figure 8.3: Post hyper acute T waves in leads V_2, V_3, and V_4 337

Figure 8.4: Thrombus formation caused by plaque rupture resulting in complete
occlusion of coronary artery 338

Table 8.2: Cardiac Biomarker Summary 338

xix

Cardiovascular Nursing Practice: A Comprehensive Resource Manual and Study Guide for Clinical Nurses

Figure 8.5: Acute J point and ST segment elevation in the inferior leads with reciprocal depression in the high lateral leads, particularly lead aVL. ST segment depression in leads V_1-V_3 represent reciprocal changes related to co-existing posterior wall injury 339

Figure 8.6: Acute J point and ST segment elevation in the septal, anterior, and lateral leads. Reciprocal ST segment depression in the inferior leads from the high lateral wall injury 341

Figure 8.7: Subtle ST segment elevation in leads I and aVL representing high lateral wall injury. Reciprocal ST segment depression in the inferior leads 342

Figure 8.8: ST segment elevation in V_4R, V_5R, and V_6R confirming a right ventricular infarct in the presence of an inferior and posterior wall MI 343

Figure 8.9: ST elevation in leads 1, aVL, and V_1-V_5 in the presence of a RBBB 345

Figure 8.10: Inferior posterior MI in presence of LBBB 346

Figure 8.11: Diffuse ST elevation of classic pericarditis 347

Figure 8.12: Terminal T wave inversion in leads V_2 and V_3 and symmetrical T wave inversion in lead V_4 showing the evolution of an ST segment elevation MI after an interventional procedure 349

Figure 8.13: Pseudo normalization of a T wave after a ST segment elevation MI, representing reocclusion of a vessel 354

Figure 8.14: Deep symmetrical T wave inversion of a non STEMI confirmed by positive cardiac biomarkers 355

Box 8.1: Safe Activities (3 MET) During the Immediate Post Dischage Period.....................363

Box 8.2: Weight Lifting Restriction Guidelines..363

Chapter 9

Table 9.1: Stages of Heart Failure 376

Figure 9.1: Normal left ventricle (A), ventricle with systolic dysfunction and eccentric hypertrophy (B) 377

Figure 9.2: Relationship of pathophysiology of left ventricular systolic failure to clinical presentation 378

Figure 9.3: Normal left ventricle (A), ventricle with diastolic dysfunction and concentric hypertrophy (B) 378

Figure 9.4: Concentric hypertrophy (A), Eccentric hypertrophy (B).....................................379

Table 9.2: Summary Comparison of Systolic and Diastolic Dysfunction 379

Table 9.3: Comparison of Signs and Symptoms of Right- and Left-sided Heart Failure 380

Figure 9.5: Sympathetic nervous system receptors and response 381

Figure 9.6: Renin Angiotensin Aldosterone System (RAAS) 382

Figure 9.7: The vicious cycle of heart failure caused by uninterrupted neurohormonal response 383

Table 9.4: Summary of Results of Neurohormonal Stimulation in Heart Failure 384

Table 9.5: The New York Heart Association Functional Classifications 385

Table 9.6: ACE Inhibitor Dosing in Heart Failure 388

Table 9.7: Angiotensin II Receptor Blockers Dosing in Heart Failure 389

Table 9.8: Beta Blocker Dosing in Heart Failure..390

Table 9.9: Summary of Heart Failure Medications by Class 393

Cardiovascular Nursing Practice: A Comprehensive Resource Manual and Study Guide for Clinical Nurses

Table 9.10: Specific Medications By Class 393

Figure 9.8: Placement of the left ventricular lead in resynchronization therapy 395

Figure 9.9: Paced complex with standard right ventricular pacing (top) compared to biventricular pacing (bottom)...395

Table 9.11: Clinical Presentation in Decompensated Heart Failure................................398

Table 9.12: Clinical Signs of Fluid Overload and Hypoperfusion.................................398

Table 9.13: Patient Education Checklist...404

Chapter 10

Figure 10.1: Comparison of the normal left ventricle (A) with the abnormal left ventricle of DCM (B), RCM (C), and HCM (D) 415

Table 10.1: American Heart Association/American College of Cardiology Staging of Heart Failure 415

Table 10.2: Causes of Dilate Cardiomyopathy...416

Figure 10.2: Physiologic changes in dilated cardiomyopathy 417

Figure 10.3: Drawing representing the alternating pulse amplitude with pulsus alternans 418

Figure 10.4: Drawing indicating the location of an S3 in relation to a normal S1 and S2 418

Figure 10.5: Drawing demonstrating the holosystolic plateau murmur of mitral regurgitation......419

Table 10.3: Causes of Restrictive Cardiomyopathy 425

Figure 10.6: Drawing indicating the location of an S4 in relation to a normal S1 and S2 426

Table 10.4: Clinical Features of Constrictive Pericarditis and Restrictive Cardiomyopathy......427

Figure 10.7: Drawing of the difference between normal myocardial cells and the myocardial disarray with HCM 430

Figure 10.8: Asymmetrical HCM...431

Figure 10.9: Asymmetrical septal hypertrophy involving the upper portion of the septal wall......431

Figure 10.10: Hypertrophic obstructive cardiomyopathy during ventricular diastole (A) and ventricular systole (B) 432

Figure 10.11: Drawing representing the early collapse and the secondary rise of impulse that is characteristic of Pulsus Bisferiens in the patient with HOCM 434

Figure 10.12: Drawing demonstrating the subvalvular left ventricular outflow obstruction systolic murmur of HOCM 435

Table 10.5: Maneuvers Decreasing Venous Return to the Heart 435

Figure 10.13: Surgical myectomy...439

Figure 10.14: Alcohol septal ablation 440

Figure 10.15: Right ventricular outflow tract tachycardia in a patient diagnosed with arrhythmogenic cardiomyopathy 444

Figure 10.16: Idiopathic right ventricular outflow tract tachycardia in a structurally normal heart 445

Chapter 11

Figure 11.1: The cardiac cycle (A,B,C,D) 452

Figure 11.2: Normal aortic valve closed (left) and open (right) 453

Figure 11.3: Aortic recoil 453

Figure 11.4: Perfusion to the coronary arteries 454

Figure 11.5: Drawing representing the systolic ejection murmur of aortic stenosis 457

xxi

Cardiovascular Nursing Practice: A Comprehensive Resource Manual and Study Guide for Clinical Nurses

Figure 11.6: Drawing indicating the location of an S4 in relation to a normal S1 and S2 457

Figure 11.7: Drawing indicating the location of an S3 in relation to a normal S1 and S2 457

Table 11.1: ACC/AHA Recommendations for Aortic Valve Replacement in Aortic Stenosis 462

Figure 11.8: Bileaflet mechanical valve 463

Figure 11.9: Stented heterograft 464

Figure 11.10: Drawing representing the diastolic decrescendo murmur of AR.........................470

Table 11.2: ACC/AHA Recommendations for Aortic Valve Replacement/Repair in Aortic
　　　　　Regurgitation 475

Figure 11.11: Normal mitral valve 479

Figure 11.12: Drawing representing the abnormal leaflet closure in mitral valve prolapse......479

Figure 11.13: Drawing demonstrating the holosystolic plateau murmur of MR......................481

Table 11.3: ACC/AHA Recommendations for Mitral Valve Repair/Replacement in Mitral
　　　　　Regurgitation 485

Figure 11.14: Drawing demonstrating the diastolic crescendo murmur of MS with an
　　　　　opening snap (OS) 490

Table 11.4: ACC/AHA Recommendations for Anticoagulation in Patients with Mitral Stenosis 493

Table 11.5: ACC/AHA Recommendations for Percutaneous Mitral Balloon Valvotomy 495

Table 11.6: ACC/AHA Recommendations for Mitral Valve Surgery in Mitral Stenosis 497

Chapter 12

Figure 12.1: Layers of the heart 505

Table 12.1: Etiologies of Pericarditis 507

Figure 12.2A: Concave ST seen in pericarditis. B. Convex ST seen in acute myocardial
　　　　　infarction 509

Figure 12.3: ECG of patient presenting with acute chest pain with normal cardiac
　　　　　catheterization 509

Table 12.2: Clinical Features of Constrictive Pericarditis and Restrictive Cardiomyopathy......520

Table 12.3: Duke Criteria for Diagnosis of Infective Endocarditis 530

Table 12.4: Proposed Modifications to the Duke Criteria for Diagnosing
　　　　　Infective Endocarditis 531

Chapter 13

Figure 13.1: Arm and ankle blood pressure cuffs used to obtain ABI measurement 545

Box 13.1: Six Ps of Acute Limb Ischemia..550

Figure 13.2: Lower extremity arterial anatomy 553

Table 13.1: Classification of Lesions 553

Figure 13.3: Aortobifemoral bypass 554

Figure 13.4: Femoral-popliteal bypass 555

Figure 13.5: Location of renal arteries off abdominal aorta 558

Figure 13.6: Abdominal aortic aneurysm and graft repair 562

Table 13.2: Classification of Abdominal Aortic Aneurysms 563

Figure 13.7: Stent graft used in endovascular repair of abdominal aortic aneurysm. 565

Figure 13.8: Aortic dissection 569

Figure 13.9: Type A and Type B aortic dissections 570

Figure 13.10: Central nervous system anatomy 574

Cardiovascular Nursing Practice: A Comprehensive Resource Manual and Study Guide for Clinical Nurses

Figure 13.11: Lobes of cerebral hemispheres 575

Figure 13.12: Cerebral circulation 575

Figure 13.13: Circle of Willis 576

Figure 13.14: Areas of injury in an ischemic stroke 578

Table 13.3: Fibrinolytic Therapy 579

Table 13.4: Changes with Right and Left Brain Strokes 581

Figure 13.15: Carotid endarterectomy 582

Chapter 14

Figure 14.1: Preload 591

Figure 14.2: LV afterload 592

Figure 14.3: Contractility 593

Figure 14.4: Sympathetic nervous system 596

Figure 14.5: Renin-Angiotensin-Aldosterone System (RAAS) 597

Table 14.1: ACE Inhibitors 600

Table 14.2: Angiotensin II Receptor Blockers (ARB) 601

Table 14.3: Indications for Beta Blocker Therapy 603

Table 14.4: Beta Blockers 605

Table 14.5: Indications for Calcium Channel Blockers 608

Table 14.6: Calcium Channel Blockers 609

Table 14.7: Diuretics 611

Figure 14.6: Sites of sympathomimetic drugs 612

Figure 14.7: Plaque rupture in coronary artery 624

Figure 14.8: Pathways for platelet activation 625

Figure 14.9: Extrinsic pathway/sites of action. Heparin and Warfarin. 626

Table 14.8: Fibrinolytics 638

Table 14.9: Classification of Antiarrhythmic Drugs 641

Figure 14.10: Site of action: antiarrhythmic drugs...................................642

Figure 14.11: Major effects of Class I and Class III agents 642

Figure 14.12: Heart rate and rhythm control drugs 643

Table 14.10: Drugs Used for Heart Rate and Rhythm Control 644

Table 14.11: Anti-Lipid Drugs 654

Chapter 15

Figure 15.1: Femoral access sites..664

Figure 15.2: Intracardiac catheter placement 664

Figure 15.3: Angiographic views of coronary arteries...............................665

Figure 15.4: Left ventriculogram 665

Table 15.1: Indications for Percutaneous Coronary Intervention..................669

Figure 15.5: Balloon positioned across plaque 672

Figure 15.6: Cutting balloon...672

Figure 15.7: Balloon-mounted stent deployment in a coronary artery 672

Figure 15.8: Directional atherectomy device 674

Figure 15.9: Rotational atherectomy device...674

xxiii

Figure 15.10: Transluminal extraction catheter 675

Figure 15.11: IVUS image of a coronary artery with plaque..........................675

Figure 15.12: Comparison of skin and femoral artery puncture sites 681

Chapter 16

Table 16.1: Preoperative Discontinuation Time Frames for Drugs Impacting Coagulation 692

Figure 16.1: Cardiopulmonary bypass or heart/lung machine 695

Figure 16.2: Oxygenator..........................696

Figure 16.3: Cardiopulmonary bypass circuit 697

Figure 16.4: A) Bicaval cannulation; B) Cannulation via single cannula 698

Figure 16.5: Arterial cannulation sites 699

Table 16.2: Summary of Cardioplegia Administration..........................700

Figure 16.6: Saphenous vein graft and internal mammary artery graft 711

Table 16.3: Intra-operative Factors Impacting Postoperative Pulmonary Function..........................717

Table 16.4: Postoperative Strategies for Improving Pulmonary Function 718

Table 16.5: Benefits of Early Extubation in Appropriate Patients 718

Table 16.6: Exclusion Criteria for Early Extubation 719

Table 16.7: Weaning and Extubation Criteria..........................720

Table 16.8: Signs of Weaning Failure..........................720

Chapter 17

Figure 17.1: Anterolateral position for placing paddles or hands-free adhesive pads for defibrillation 745

Figure 17.2: Cardioversion 747

Table 17.1: Energy Levels for Cardioversion..........................747

Table 17.2: NBG Code for Pacing Nomenclature 752

Figure 17.3: Pacing systems 753

Figure 17.4: Ventricular pacing using transvenous wire 754

Figure 17.5: Epicardial pacing 755

Figure 17.6: Transcutaneous pacing 756

Figure 17.7: Normal VVI pacemaker function..........................757

Figure 17.8: AV interval 763

Figure 17.9: Atrial escape interval 763

Figure 17.10: Total atrial refractory period (TARP)..........................764

Figure 17.11: Post ventricular atrial refractory period (PVARP)..........................764

Figure 17.12: Ventricular blinking period (VBP)..........................764

Figure 17.13: Maximum tracking interval (MTI)..........................765

Figure 17.14: Wenkebach upper rate response 771

Figure 17.15: Block upper rate response 771

Figure 17.16: Mechanism of PMT 772

Figure 17.17: Normal ventricular function..........................774

Figure 17.18: Electrical and mechanical abnormalities 775

Figure 17.19: Cardiac resynchronization therapy (CRT) 775

Figure 17.20: ICD generator and lead 781

Cardiovascular Nursing Practice: A Comprehensive Resource Manual and Study Guide for Clinical Nurses

Figure 17.21: Tach zones 782

Figure 17.22: Catheter placement..788

Figure 17.23: Intracardiac recordings...789

Figure 17.24: AV nodal re-entry tachycardia (AVNRT)...................................790

Figure 17.25: Circus movement tachycardia (CMT) 791

Chapter 18

Figure 18.1: Infiltrates on chest x-ray 818

Figure 18.2: Closed (simple) pneumothorax 824

Figure 18.3: Tension pneumothorax 825

Figure 18.4: Open pneumothorax 825

Table 18.1: Types of Hypotonic Hyponatremia 829

Table 18.2: Causes of Hypocalcemia 838

Table 18.3: Signs and Symptoms of Hypocalcemia 838

Box 18.1: Signs and Symptoms of Hypercalcemia 840

Table 18.4: Signs and Symptoms of Hypomagnesaemia 842

Figure 18.5: Overview of kidney anatomy 845

Figure 18.6: Major components of nephron 846

Figure 18.7: Process of filtration, secretion, and reabsorption in the formation of urine 846

Table 18.5: Diagnostic Parameters for Assessment of Renal Function 848

Table 18.6: Stages of Acute Kidney Injury 850

Figure 18.8: Arteriovenous fistula 858

Table 18.7: Summary of the Differences in CEBT Strategies 860

Table 18.8: Definitions and Criteria Related to Sepsis and Septic Shock 862

CHAPTER 1:
CARDIOVASCULAR ANATOMY AND PHYSIOLOGY

INTRODUCTION

Cardiac anatomy and physiology form a critical foundation for understanding cardiovascular nursing. All clinical application builds on this foundation. Even in the field of medicine, *"in this technology driven era, a new appreciation of cardiac anatomy has emerged as the cornerstone for clinical cardiology"* (Fuster et al., 2001, p. 45).

BASIC CARDIAC ANATOMY

The heart is a hollow, muscular, four-chambered organ. It is positioned in the mediastinum (middle of the thoracic cavity) between the lungs, above the diaphragm and in front of the esophagus. The heart is attached to the thorax by the great vessels. The great vessels include the aorta, pulmonary artery, inferior vena cava, and superior vena cava. The adult heart is approximately 5 inches by 3½ inches by 2½ inches or roughly the size of a person's fist. The tip of the left ventricle forms the apex (bottom) of the heart. The apex is located at about the fifth intercostal space, at the left midclavicular line. The base, or top, of the heart is located at approximately the second intercostal space (Figure 1.1).

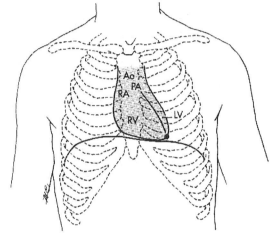

Figure 1.1: Location of the heart in the chest cavity. (Ao: Aorta; PA: Pulmonary artery; RA: Right atrium; RV: Right ventricle; LV: Left ventricle.
From Pass CCRN (2nd ed.), by R.D. Dennison, 2000, St. Louis: Mosby. Reprinted with permission from Elsevier.

Cardiac Chambers

The right and left atria (upper chambers) are separated by a mass of connective tissue called the interatrial septum. The right and left atria are low-pressure, thin-walled chambers that receive blood and act as reservoirs. The right atrium receives deoxygenated blood from the venous system via the inferior and superior venae cavae, as well as from the coronary sinus (the primary coronary vein). The left atrium receives oxygenated blood from the pulmonary veins after the blood has traveled through the lungs (Figure 1.2). Both the right and left atria have an ear like structure attached to the atrium called the atrial appendage. Patients with atrial fibrillation, mitral valve disease and other disorders are at a high risk for the development of thrombus in the atrial appendage due to the relative static nature of the blood in the atrial appendage. The right and left ventricles (lower chambers) are the pumping chambers of the heart and receive blood from the atria. The ventricles are separated by the interventricular septum. The right ventricle is a thin-

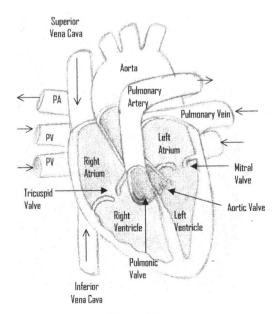

Figure 1.2

walled, low-pressure pump that receives deoxygenated blood from the right atrium. This ventricle pumps blood into the pulmonary artery, which carries the blood to the lungs to exchange carbon dioxide for oxygen. The left ventricle is a thick-walled, high-pressure pump that receives oxygenated blood from the left atrium and pumps blood into the aorta for distribution throughout the circulatory system.

Layers of the Heart

The three layers of the heart are the endocardium, myocardium, and epicardium. The pericardium is an additional layer that surrounds the heart (Figure 1.3).

Endocardium

The endocardium is a serous membrane consisting of connective tissue, elastic fibers, and a thin layer of epithelial cells that form a smooth surface for the movement of blood and prevention of clot formation.

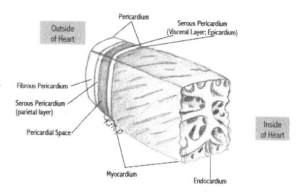

Figure 1.3: Layers of the heart.

The endocardium is not only the inner surface of the heart chambers and valves, but also covers the walls of the vessels of the entire vascular system, creating a closed circulatory system. Inflammation of the endocardium or heart valves is called endocarditis.

Myocardium

The myocardium is the thick middle layer of the heart. The largest layer of the heart, the myocardium contains cardiac muscle fibers that have the ability to contract and to conduct electrical stimuli. The myocardium of the ventricles is thicker than the myocardium of the atria. The left ventricle has the thickest myocardium due to the high pressure in the aorta that the ventricle must pump against in order to eject its contents. As patients develop myocardial hypertrophy (increased cell size), this layer of the heart becomes larger. Damage to the myocardial layer of the heart, such as that which occurs with myocardial infarction, results in a decreased ability for the heart to contract, resulting in an impaired ability to eject blood from the ventricle (systolic dysfunction).

Epicardium

The epicardium is the smooth outer layer of the heart that contains the network of coronary arteries and veins, the autonomic nerves, the lymphatic system, and fat tissue. Coronary blood vessels that supply the myocardium and endocardium with oxygen-rich blood must first cross the epicardium before entering the myocardium, and, finally, the endocardium. Advanced age and obesity increase the amount of fat tissue in the epicardial layer, resulting in an increase in the amount of tissue that must be supplied with oxygen-rich blood before supplying the myocardium and endocardium (Fuster et al., 2004). The epicardium is also called the visceral layer of the pericardium. An increasing amount of adipose tissue in the epicardium can increase a person's risk of myocardial rupture during or after an acute myocardial infarction (MI).

Pericardium

The thin sac surrounding the heart is called the pericardium. This fibrous sac protects the heart from infection and traumatic injury. The pericardium has little elastic tissue and cannot expand easily. Almost the entire ascending aorta (beyond the origin of the coronary arteries), the main pulmonary artery, all four pulmonary veins, and portions of the inferior and superior venae cavae are contained within the pericardial sac

Cardiovascular Anatomy and Physiology

(Fuster et al., 2004). The pericardium has several layers (Figure 1-3). The external cover of the pericardium is called the fibrous pericardium and is continuous with the external walls of the great vessels. The parietal pericardium is the inner lining of the fibrous pericardium. The visceral pericardium is another name for the epicardium. This inner lining of the pericardium forms the outer lining of the heart and great vessels. The space between the parietal and visceral layers of the pericardium contains a small amount of lubricating fluid, approximately 10 to 30 ml (Bond, 2005). This fluid prevents friction between the epicardium and the fibrous pericardium during each cardiac contraction. Pericardial disease can interfere with the ability of the ventricles to fill during diastole. Pericarditis is inflammation of the pericardium. If the aorta ruptures or dissects, the pericardium can rapidly fill with blood. Rapid filling of the pericardial sac can produce fatal results, including cardiac tamponade and death.

Cardiac Valves

The four cardiac valves located within the heart are designated as either atrioventricular (AV) valves or semilunar valves (Figure 1.4). The valves located between the atria and ventricles are AV valves. The tricuspid valve is located between the right atrium and right ventricle, and the mitral valve is located between the left atrium and left ventricle. The two semilunar valves are located between the ventricles and the great vessels. The pulmonic valve is located between the right ventricle and the pulmonary artery, and the aortic valve is located between the left ventricle and the aorta.

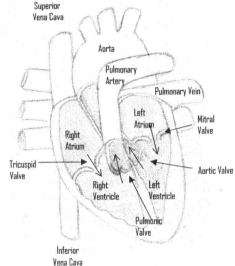

Figure 1.4: Cardiac valves.

Atrioventricular Valves

The AV valves are anatomically different from the semilunar valves. Papillary muscles project from the inner surface of the ventricle and attach to delicate strands of fibrous material called chordae tendineae. The chordae tendineae attach to the valve leaflets (see Figure 1.5). The leaflets form the valve cusps (three cusps for the tricuspid, two for the mitral). The uppermost portions of the valve cusps are joined together by a fibrous ring at the top of the valve, called the annulus. The AV valves open passively during diastole, forming a funnel-like shape that allows blood to flow from the atria to the ventricles. At the end of diastole, ventricular pressure increases and forces the valve leaflets to come together and close the valve opening between the atrium and the ventricle.

As the ventricle contracts to eject blood, the papillary muscles contract to prevent the valve leaflets from prolapsing into the atrium. The closure of the leaflets prevents the backward flow of blood from the ventricle to the atrium. At the end of systole, when the ventricle relaxes, the AV valves open again and the cycle is repeated.

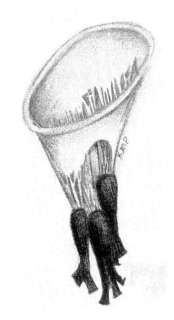

Figure 1.5: AV valve showing the papillary muscles and chordae tendineae.

During an acute MI of the left ventricle, a papillary muscle of the mitral valve can become weakened and potentially rupture. If a papillary muscle ruptures, the mitral valve can no longer maintain unidirectional blood flow. As a result, blood backs up into the left atrium during ventricular contraction, causing acute left-sided heart failure.

Chapter 1

Semilunar Valves

Each semilunar valve consists of an annulus and three cusps (Figure 1.6). The pulmonic and aortic valves have the same structure; however, the aortic valve leaflets are heavier and thicker due to the increased pressure system in the left side of the heart. The pulmonic valve is located between the right ventricle and the pulmonary artery, and the aortic valve is located between the left ventricle and the aorta. These valves function by pressure changes in the heart and the great vessels. During diastole, the semilunar valves are closed as the ventricles fill with blood from the atria. As systole begins, the ventricles begin to contract, and the AV valves close. Once the pressure in the ventricles is greater than the pressure on the other side of the semilunar valves, the valves are forced open, ejecting blood out of the ventricles into the great vessels. When ventricular ejection is complete, diastole begins, and the pressure in the ventricles falls below the pressure in the great vessels, causing the semilunar valves to close tightly. Tight closure prevents the backward flow of blood from the great vessels to the ventricles. The cycle then begins again.

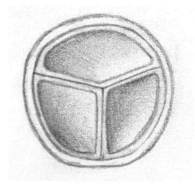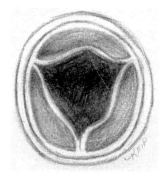

Figure 1.6: Closed aortic valve (left); Open aortic valve (right).

When auscultating the heart, the first heart sound (S1), referred to as "lub," is associated with closure of the AV valves. The second heart sound (S2), referred to as "dub," is associated with closure of the semilunar valves. These two sounds together form the "lub-dub" of cardiac auscultation. S1 ("lub") represents the beginning of ventricular systole or contraction, and S2 ("dub") represents the beginning of ventricular diastole, or relaxation.

When cardiac valves function correctly, they permit forward flow of blood when the valve is open and prevent backward flow of blood when the valve is closed. During ventricular systole, the tricuspid and mitral valves close to prevent backward flow of blood from the ventricles into the atria. During ventricular systole, all blood forced from the ventricles during ejection is propelled forward, through open pulmonic and aortic valves, into the pulmonary and systemic vascular beds. During ventricular diastole, the tricuspid and mitral valves open, allowing filling of the ventricles from the atria. When the pulmonic and aortic valves close properly during ventricular diastole, they prevent the backward flow of blood from the pulmonary and systemic vascular beds into the ventricles.

CIRCULATORY SYSTEM

The heart and blood vessels work together for one primary purpose: the delivery of oxygen and other nutrients to the cellular level. The capillaries are the location where oxygen and nutrients are exchanged.

Arterial System

Oxygenated blood leaves the left ventricle and travels to the tissue level via the systemic arterial system. Arteries are made up of elastic tissue that allows them to respond to the higher pressures associated with the force of left ventricular contraction. Large arteries also contain smooth muscle. All arteries have three layers of tissue that surround the open lumen (Figure 1.7).

Cardiovascular Anatomy and Physiology

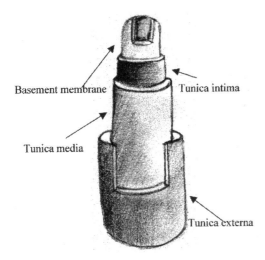

Figure 1.7 Layers of the arterial wall.

The inner layer, called the intima, has a thin lining of endothelium that contains epithelial cells. The intima decreases resistance to flow and minimizes the chance of platelet aggregation. The media, the middle layer, is comprised of smooth muscle and elastic connective tissue. The media is responsible for changes in the diameter of the vessel, as needed, to assist with blood pressure control. The fibrous outer layer, called the adventitia, is designed to protect the vessel and provide connection to other internal structures. Arteries have the ability to expand or contract in response to the body's cardiac output needs.

Arterioles

The large arteries carry blood from the aorta to the rest of the body. The arteries divide and become smaller as they move away from the aorta. The smallest arteries branch into arterioles. Arterioles connect to the capillary bed. At the arteriole level of the capillary is smooth muscle that is referred to as the precapillary sphincter. The arterioles and the precapillary sphincter regulate blood flow to the capillaries. This regulation of blood flow is primarily determined by the oxygen needs of the tissue through a process called autoregulation. When oxygen needs increase, the arterioles dilate. This dilatation decreases resistance to flow and results in increased flow to the capillaries (Darovic, 2002).

Capillary System

When oxygenated blood reaches the capillary level, oxygen and other nutrients are exchanged. Because capillary walls are only one cell thick, gases and nutrients pass through the walls easily. Miles of capillaries are located near almost all body cells. The capillaries contain no smooth muscle (Bridges, 2005b). Therefore, capillary tone depends on the tone of the vessel located just before and after the capillary. Four pressures influence the movement of fluids across capillary membranes: capillary hydrostatic pressure, interstitial hydrostatic pressure, capillary oncotic pressure, and interstitial colloidal oncotic pressure (Opie, 2004). Once oxygen and nutrients are exchanged for waste products, deoxygenated blood is returned to the right atrium from the capillaries via the venous system.

Venous System

The venous system is a low-pressure system compared to the arterial system. Because veins are not subject to the high pressures of the arterial system, their walls are much thinner than those of arteries. Thinner walls allow for much more distensibility. At any given time, the venous system generally holds 65% to 70% of the body's total blood volume (Bridges, 2005b), and the venous system can regulate the amount of blood returning to the heart. Vasoconstriction of veins increases blood flow to the heart by decreasing the amount of blood held in the vascular bed. Vasodilatation decreases blood flow to the heart by increasing the vascular bed to hold more volume.

The venous system is strongly influenced by gravity and relies on one-way valves (Figure 1.8) that help prevent backward flow of blood through the low-pressure venous system. These venous valves, absent in a small percentage of people, can be damaged by age or by catheter insertion (Fuster et al., 2004). Venous return is also augmented by contraction of skeletal muscles, which compress veins and help to propel blood forward. Weakened vein valves cause varicose (dilated) veins. Age, prolonged standing, and pregnancy contribute to varicose veins. In right-sided heart failure, venous valves are important in maintaining the unidirectional flow of blood back to the right side of the heart.

Endothelium

The endothelium is a single cell layer lining the entire vascular bed. It is a highly dynamic, autocrine and paracrine organ that regulates vascular tone and the interaction of the vessel wall with circulating substances and blood cells. The endothelium produces both vasodilators and vasoconstrictors. The major vasodilator, nitric oxide, provides vascular protective actions. The endothelium exerts influence over

- coagulation
- arterial tone
- vascular growth.

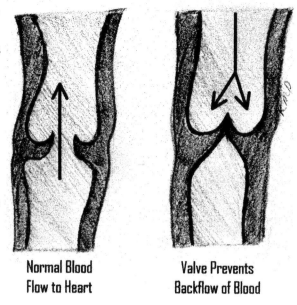

Figure 1.8: One-way vein valves.

The endothelium releases both vasoconstrictive (endothelin) and vasodilatory substances (nitric oxide). Endothelial dysfunction plays a major role in most pathological conditions, including hypertension, diabetes, coronary artery disease and heart failure.

Normal Circulatory Patterns

The thoracic aorta arises from the aortic valve, which is divided into three segments: ascending aorta, aortic arch, and descending thoracic aorta. The origin of the coronary arteries is located in the ascending aorta immediately above the aortic valve. The location of the origin of the coronary arteries allows them to receive blood that is rich in oxygen. The aortic arch has three branches: brachiocephalic artery, left common carotid artery, and left subclavian artery (Figure 1.9). These branches are responsible for blood flow from the heart to the upper torso, neck, head, brain, and arms. The thoracic aorta, which is located below the aortic arch, branches off to supply blood to the torso, including the thoracic cavity and the lungs.

The abdominal aorta supplies blood to the abdominal organs and the kidneys. At approximately the fourth lumbar vertebra, the aorta divides into the internal iliac arteries. The lower trunk, including the reproductive organs and the legs, receive their blood supply from the internal iliac arteries.

The venous system mimics the arterial system in returning blood to the heart. Prior to entering the heart, the entire venous system enters into the superi-

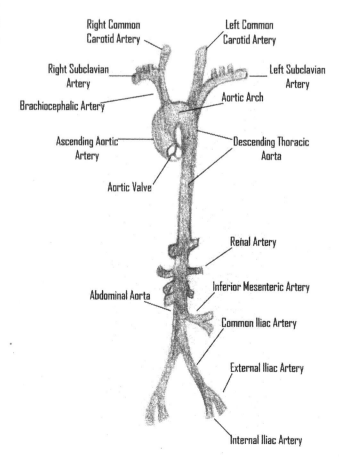

Figure 1.9: Arterial trunk of normal circulation.

or vena cava or the inferior vena cava. The superior vena cava receives venous blood returning from the head, neck, upper extremities, and thorax. The inferior vena cava receives blood from below the level of the diaphragm, including the abdomen, pelvis, and lower extremities. The superior and inferior venae cavae empty the returning deoxygenated blood into the right atrium. The coronary veins also drain into the coronary sinus, which then empties directly into the right atrium.

Circulation Through the Heart

Once deoxygenated blood is received by the right atrium, it moves to the right ventricle through the tricuspid valve during ventricular diastole (Figure 1.10). After the right ventricle fills, the tricuspid valve closes, and the ventricle contracts and ejects the blood through the open pulmonic valve into the pulmonary artery. The pulmonary artery divides into the right and left pulmonary arteries and carries blood to the pulmonary capillaries, where gas exchange occurs. Blood leaving the right ventricle is low in oxygen and high in carbon dioxide. When gas exchange occurs, oxygen enters the blood, and carbon dioxide leaves the blood and is exhaled. The pulmonary veins return oxygenated blood to the left side of the heart via the left atrium. The blood in the left atrium moves through the open mitral valve into the left ventricle during ventricular diastole. At the end of diastole, the mitral valve closes, and the left ventricle contracts, forcing the aortic valve open and ejecting the oxygenated blood into the aorta for participation in systemic circulation.

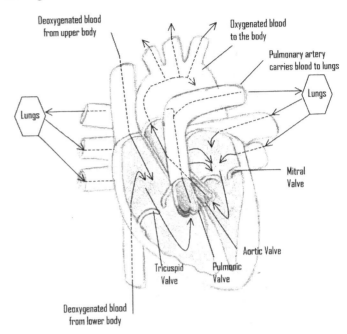

Figure 1.10: Blood flow through the heart.

CARDIAC CYCLE

Systole is contraction of the heart muscle, resulting in ejection of blood from the chamber. Diastole is relaxation of the heart muscle, allowing for filling of the chamber. Each of the atria and ventricles undergo systole and diastole. In a resting adult, each cardiac cycle lasts approximately 0.8 second (Opie, 2004). The efficiency of the cardiac cycle depends on the health of the cardiac muscle, valves, and conduction system. The heart's conduction system provides the timing of events for atrial and ventricular systole.

Ventricular Diastole

Ventricular diastole begins when ventricular contraction is complete. Once ventricular contraction is complete, the pressure in the pulmonary vascular bed and the aorta exceeds the pressure in the right and left ventricles, this causes the semilunar valves (pulmonic and aortic) to close. Simultaneously, the pressure in the atria which continued to receive blood from the venous system (right atrium) and the pulmonary artery (left atrium) during ventricular systole, exceeds the pressure in the nearly empty ventricles and the AV valves (tricuspid and mitral) open. Once the tricuspid and mitral valves open, a rapid, passive filling of the ventricles occurs as blood moves from the atria through the open valves into the ventricles. Approximately 75% of ventricular filling occurs during this early passive filling phase (Figure 1.11). This phase of the cardiac cycle is also known as cardiac diastole as both the atrium and the ventricles are at rest. The remainder of ventricular filling occurs late in ventricular diastole with atrial contraction. This contraction of the atria is known as atrial systole.

Atrial systole (Figure 1.12) is commonly referred to as atrial kick and contributes as much as 25% of the ventricular volume (Bond, 2005). In atrial fibrillation, the atrial contribution to left ventricular filling is lost because the atria do not contract. This loss of atrial kick can result in enough decrease in stroke volume to cause a decrease in cardiac output and, ultimately, symptoms of decreased perfusion.

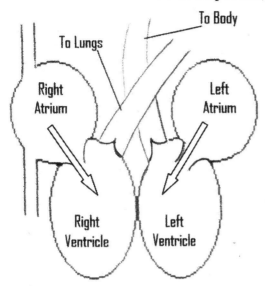

Figure 1.11: Early ventricular diastole. Passive ventricular filling phase. Cardiac diastole.

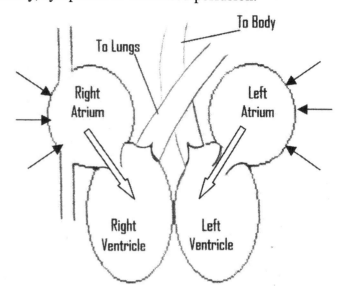

Figure 1.12: Atrial systole. Late ventricular diastole. Active ventricular filling. (Black arrows indicate atrial contraction.)

Ventricular Systole

After atrial contraction, the pressure in the atria and ventricles equalizes, the AV valves partially close, and ventricular systole begins. Ventricular systole has two phases. The first phase is isovolumic or isovolumetric contraction, so named because the volume of blood in the ventricles does not change during this phase. During isovolumic contraction, the ventricular walls tense and press toward the center of the ventricular cavity. This tensing of the walls increases the pressure in the ventricles. When the pressure in the ventricles exceeds that in the atria, the AV valves close quickly, preventing backward flow of blood into the atria. At this point in the cardiac cycle, all valves are closed (Figure 1.13).

In order for ejection of the ventricular contents to occur, the myocardial walls of the ventricles must develop enough pressure to force the semilunar (aortic and pulmonic) valves open. Once the pressure in the ventricles exceeds the pressure in the aorta and pulmonary artery, the aortic and pulmonic valves open. The second phase of systole is ejection (Figure 1.14), during which blood is ejected into the systemic and pulmonary circulation. At peak systole, pulmonary artery systolic pressure equalizes with right ventricular systolic pressure; and aortic systolic pressure equalizes with left ventricular systolic pressure. The semilunar valves close at the end of systole, when the pressure in the arteries exceeds the pressure in the ventricles. Normally, ventricular diastole (ventricular filling) is two times longer than ventricular systole (ventricular emptying). As heart rate increases, ventricular diastolic time shortens while ventricular systolic time essentially stays the same. Therefore, an increased heart rate decreases the time available to fill the ventricles and the coronary arteries.

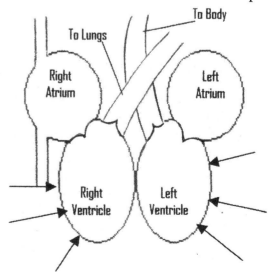

Figure 1.13: Isovolumic contraction – ventricular systole. (Black arrows indicate ventricular contraction.)

Cardiovascular Anatomy and Physiology

CORONARY CIRCULATION

The coronary arteries begin in the epicardial layer of the heart. These arteries then travel through the myocardium and ultimately to the endocardium to provide oxygen-rich blood to the entire cardiac musculature. Since the endocardium is the last layer of the heart to receive oxygenated blood it is usually the first layer of the heart to be damaged when oxygen supply is decreased. During systole, as the heart contracts, blood flow through the coronary arteries is markedly reduced due to compression on the vessels by contracting muscle. Therefore, coronary artery perfusion occurs primarily during diastole, when the ventricles are relaxed. Aortic recoil and the origin of the coronary arteries play a key role in coronary artery perfusion. There are two main coronary arteries, the left main coronary artery and the right coronary artery. These two arteries divide into several branches and will be discussed later in the chapter.

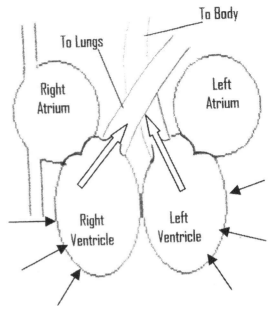

Figure 1.14: Ventricular systole. (Black arrows indicate ventricular contraction.)

Aortic Recoil and Coronary Artery Perfusion (Figure 1.15)

Ejection of blood from the left ventricle through the aortic valve to the aorta causes the normal compliant aorta to distend as it accepts the volume from the ventricle. At the end of ventricular ejection, the pressure in the aorta becomes greater than the pressure in the left ventricle. Once this pressure gradient occurs the walls of the distended aorta naturally recoil, displacing blood forward and backward. The forward displacement of blood provides cardiac output to the systemic system. The backward displacement of blood towards the aortic valve forces the normal aortic valve to rapidly close and prevent backflow of blood into the left ventricle. The blood that is displaced backwards collects at the cusps of the aortic valve where the origins to the right and left coronary artery are located (Fig. 1.16). The area where the blood enters the coronary artery is known as the sinus of valsalva. There is a right aortic sinus where the origin of the right coronary is located, a left aortic sinus where the origin of the left coronary is located and a third sinus is known as the non-coronary or posterior sinus where no coronary arteries are located. This system provides highly oxygenated blood to fill the coronary arteries.

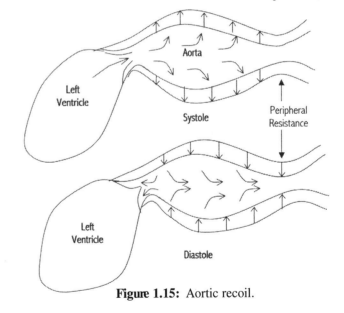

Figure 1.15: Aortic recoil.

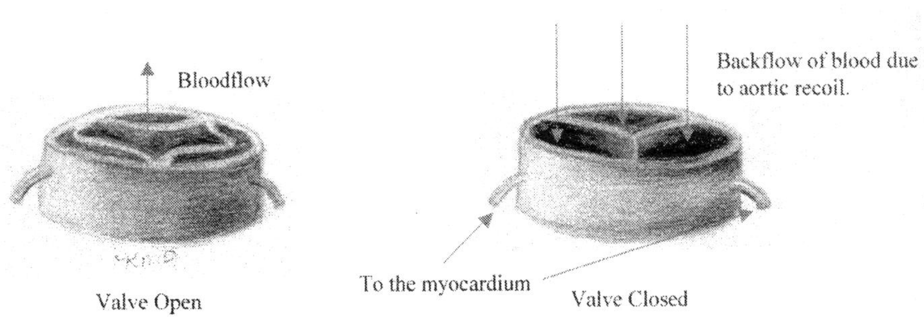

Figure 1.16: Perfusion of the coronary arteries.

Left Coronary Artery System

The left main coronary artery, which supplies oxygenated blood to the largest portion of the myocardium, travels a short distance before dividing into the left anterior descending artery (LAD) and left circumflex artery (LCX) (Figure 1.17).

Left Anterior Descending Artery

The LAD supplies oxygenated blood to the anterior wall of the left ventricle, with some perfusion of the right ventricle as well. The septal perforating branches of the LAD supply the septum and the bundle branches, while the diagonal branches supply the anterior left ventricular free wall.

Left Circumflex Artery

The LCX supplies oxygenated blood to the lateral wall and the posterolateral wall of the left ventricle as well as the left atrium. The LCX may also supply the inferior wall of the left ventricle in some people. The sinoatrial (SA) node receives blood from the LCX in 45% of the population (Bond, 2005; Fuster et al. 2004), and the AV node receives its blood from the LCX in 10% of the population (Bond, 2005).

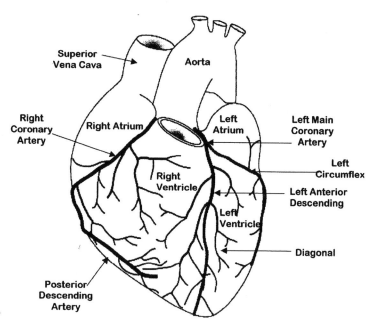

Figure 1.17 The coronary arteries.

Ramus Intermediate Artery

Some patients have a third branch of the left main coronary artery that is located between the left anterior descending artery and the circumflex artery. This artery is called the ramus intermediate artery. This artery may provide circulation to the posterolateral wall of the left ventricle.

Right Coronary Artery System

The right coronary artery (RCA) comes from the right side of the aorta. The RCA supplies oxygenated blood to the right atrium and right ventricle, as well as the inferior and posterior walls of the left ventricle, in most people. A branch of the RCA supplies the SA node in 55% the population (Bond, 2005; Fuster et al., 2004), and the AV nodal branch of the RCA supplies the AV node in about 90% of the population (Bond, 2005). The posterior branch of the left bundle branch system receives oxygenated blood from the RCA in addition to the LAD.

Dominance

The term right or left dominance refers to the vessel (LCX or RCA) from which the posterior descending artery (PDA) arises. In 70% of the population, the PDA arises from the RCA (Fuster et al., 2004). In the remainder of the population, the PDA arises from the LCX. The PDA supplies oxygenated blood to the posterior portions of the right and left ventricles, as well as to the posterior one third of the septum.

Collateral Circulation

Collateral circulation provides communication between the major coronary arteries and their branches. When stenosis of one artery produces a pressure gradient, the collateral vessels can dilate with time and provide a natural bypass for blood flow beyond the stenosis or narrowing. The coronary arterioles lie

Cardiovascular Anatomy and Physiology

Table 1.1 Coronary Artery Supply	
Coronary Artery	**Circulation Supplied To**
Left Anterior Descending Artery	Anterior Left Ventricle Anterior two-thirds of Septum His Bundle and Bundle Branches
Left Circumflex Artery	Left Atrium SA Node (45% of population) AV Node (10% of population) Lateral Left Ventricle Posterior Left Ventricle (10% of population) Posterior Septum (20% of population) Posterolateral Left Ventricle
Right Coronary Artery	Right Atrium SA Node (55% of population) AV Node (90% of population) Inferior Left Ventricle Posterior Septum (80% of population) Right Ventricle Posterior Left Ventricle (90% of population) Left Posterior Bundle Branch

within the myocardium and supply the capillaries. The capillary system is also referred to as the microcirculation. Abnormalities in microcirculation can cause cardiac symptoms in the presence of normal epicardial coronary arteries.

The location of occlusion of a coronary artery provides important information about the structures of the myocardium affected by the occlusion. For example, a total occlusion of the LAD artery produces a left ventricular anterior wall MI with potential for right and left bundle branch blocks, as well as left ventricular failure. Occlusion of the RCA commonly produces AV heart blocks because the RCA supplies the AV node in approximately 90% of the population.

Cardiac Veins

The cardiac veins drain into the coronary sinus, which empties into the right atrium. In nearly all people, the coronary veins run parallel to the coronary arteries.

CARDIAC ACTION POTENTIAL

An action potential (AP) is a time dependent change in electrical voltage across a cardiac cell membrane during depolarization and repolarization of the cell (Wit & Rosen, 1981a). These voltage changes are due to the movement of ions (primarily Na^+, Ca^{++}, and K^+) across the semi-permeable membrane of a cardiac cell. When one cell develops an action potential (i.e. depolarizes) it triggers adjacent cells to develop their own action potential, causing the electrical activity to travel through the heart. It is the job of the cardiac conduction system to spread this electrical activity in an orderly fashion from atria to ventricles. The action potential can be considered to be the electrocardiogram (ECG) of a single cardiac cell as it depolarizes and repolarizes. When all the action potentials of all the cardiac cells are recorded from surface electrodes on the body, the result is what we know as the ECG.

There are two major types of action potentials in the heart: 1) The "slow response" action potential, characteristic of pacemaker cells in the sinus node and the AV node, which is primarily dependent on calcium ions, 2) the "fast response" type that is dependent on sodium ions and occurs in Purkinje fibers and the working cells of the atria and ventricles. Figure 1.18 illustrates both types of action potentials. The following description of the phases of the action potential applies to Purkinje cells and atrial and ventricular muscle cells. The action potential of sinus node and AV node cells is described later.

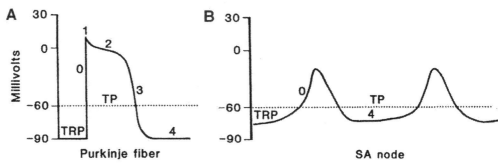

Figure 1.18: A. Action potential of a Purkinje fiber. Atrial and ventricular muscle cell APs are similar. B. Action potential of a sinus node cell. AV node AP is similar.

Transmembrane Resting Potential (TRP)

At rest (during diastole) the cell has a positive charge on the outside of its membrane and a negative charge inside due to:

- The presence of non-diffusible negatively charged ions inside the cell that trap negative charges within the cell.

- Higher concentration of Na⁺ outside the cell (i.e. 140 mEq/L outside compared to 14 mEq/L inside) and a higher concentration of K⁺ inside the cell (i.e. 140 mEq/L inside compared to 4 mEq/L outside, Guyton & Hall, 2000). At rest, the membrane is permeable to K⁺ but relatively impermeable to Na⁺ and other ions. This causes K⁺ to leak out of the cell along its concentration gradient, carrying positive charges to the outside of the cell.

- The combination of these two mechanisms causes the inside of the cell to be approximately -80 to -90 mV negative, with respect to the outside of the cell at rest.

- K⁺ is the most important ion in determining the TRP. Both hypokalemia and hyperkalemia can cause arrhythmias by changing the TRP.

TRP is partly maintained by the Na-K pump, which actively transports Na⁺ and K⁺ ions against their concentration gradients (i.e. removes Na⁺ from the inside and returns K⁺ that has leaked out back to the inside of the cell). This pump moves 3 Na⁺ ions out for every 2 K⁺ ions in, thus helping maintain normal intracellular negativity.

- The Na-K pump is dependent on ATP (adenosine triphosphate) to supply the energy necessary to transport ions against their concentration gradients. An adequate supply of ATP is dependent on an adequate supply of O_2 to the heart.
    - Ischemia and hypoxia contribute to arrhythmias because they cause a decrease in TRP (i.e. from -90 mV to -70 mV) by decreasing the amount of O_2 available to maintain the Na-K pump activity.
    - Digitalis and other drugs that interfere with the operation of the Na-K pump also decrease TRP and can cause arrhythmias.

Threshold Potential (TP)

The threshold potential is the level to which the membrane potential must be lowered in order for an action potential to develop. Threshold in atrial and ventricular muscle cells is about -60 to -70 mV.

Cardiovascular Anatomy and Physiology

Phases of the Action Potential (Figure 1.19)

Phase 0 – rapid membrane depolarization (upstroke of AP)

◆ Rapid influx of Na^+ into the cell due to opening of specialized "fast Na^+ channels" in the membrane when the cell is stimulated.

 ❖ The number of Na^+ channels available depends on the level of TRP at the time of stimulation (Wit & Rosen, 1981b).

 ❖ At normal TRP (-80 to -90 mV), most channels are available and Phase 0 rises rapidly; at reduced TRP (-60 mV), only half are available and Phase 0 rises more slowly; at TRP of –50 mV, most channels are inactivated and depolarization is dependent on Ca^{++} channels.

 ☆ When the membrane depolarizes to about -60 mV, the "slow Ca^{++} channels" open and both Na^+ ions and Ca^{++} ions enter the cell and contribute to depolarization.

 ☆ The rate of rise of Phase 0 reflects conduction time from cell to cell and is dependent on the level of the membrane at the time of stimulation.

 ✳ The more negative the TRP, the more rapid the rise of Phase 0, and the faster the conduction time through the heart.

 ✳ When TRP is reduced (i.e. at -60 mV), conduction velocity is slowed. This is why ischemia, which reduces TRP by decreasing the amount of O_2 available to maintain the Na-K pump, creates areas of slow conduction in the heart and can contribute to arrhythmias.

◆ Phase 0 of ventricular cells corresponds to the QRS complex on the ECG.

Phase 1 – early rapid repolarization due to decreased permeability of the membrane to Na^+.

Phase 2 – plateau phase, where membrane potential is maintained near 0 mV.

◆ A balanced influx of positive ions (Na^+ and Ca^{++}) and negative ions (Cl-) is the proposed explanation for maintaining this membrane potential.

◆ Ca^{++} channels remain open longer than Na^+ channels, so Ca^{++} continues to enter the cell, carrying positive charges with it and contributing to the plateau phase.

◆ Ca^{++} enters the cell to trigger mechanical contraction.

◆ Phase 2 of the action potential corresponds to the ST segment on the ECG.

Phase 3 – repolarization

◆ K^+ channels open and K^+ flows rapidly out of the cell, carrying positive charges to the outside and returning the membrane potential to its resting state.

◆ Phase 3 corresponds to the T wave on the ECG.

Phase 4 – resting state (TRP)

◆ Contracting muscle cells in atria and ventricles and Purkinje fibers have a stable TRP and depend on an outside stimulus (i.e. a propagated AP from the sinus node or a pacemaker stimulus) for depolarization.

 ❖ TRP is –85 to –90 mV; Phase 0 has a rapid upstroke, and conduction velocity is fast. Figure 1.18A illustrates a Purkinje cell AP.

◆ Phase 4 corresponds to the T-P segment between beats on the ECG.

◆ Cells in the SA and AV nodes have an unstable Phase 4 where TRP gradually decreases until threshold is reached and an AP is generated.

 ❖ TRP in these cells is –60 to –70 mV; Phase 0 has a slow upstroke, and conduction velocity is slow. Figure 1.18B illustrates a SA node AP.

- ❖ AP development is thought to be due to slow Ca^{++} channels, since most of the Na$^+$ channels are inactivated at this low resting potential.
- ❖ The sinus node is the normal pacemaker of the heart because the TRP in SA node cells has the fastest spontaneous rise to threshold.
- ❖ Other cells in the conduction system (e.g. AV node cells and some ventricular cells) also have a TRP that can spontaneously depolarize to threshold and create an AP, but at much slower rates than SA node cells. These cells are normally "overdrive suppressed" by the faster SA node cells, and they only become pacemaker cells when the SA node fails to function as a pacemaker (i.e. junctional or ventricular escape beats).

Refractory Period

The refractory period is a period of time following depolarization during which a cell cannot respond to a stimulus by propagating another AP. Figure 1.19 illustrates the refractory periods of a cardiac cell.

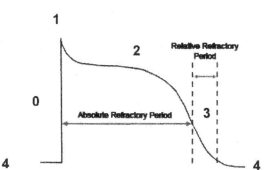

Figure 1.19: Phases of the action potential (0, 1, 2, 3, 4) and absolute and relative refractory period.

- ◆ Absolute refractory period (ARP) or effective refractory period (ERP) – period of time after stimulation during which a cell cannot respond to another stimulus, regardless of stimulus strength.
- ◆ Relative refractory period (RRP) – period of time following the ARP during which a cell can respond to a strong stimulus but the response is abnormal (conduction velocity is slow).

CONTRACTILE PROPERTIES OF CARDIAC MUSCLE

The heart is composed of two major types of cells: contracting cells and conducting cells. The atrial and ventricular walls are composed of contractile muscle cells called myocytes that are capable of shortening to eject blood from the chamber. The conducting cells are responsible for initiating and conducting the electrical impulse through the heart. The adult heart has approximately 19 billion cardiac cells (Bond, 2005). Millions of cardiac cells are lost with each year of life (Opie, 2004).

Cardiac muscle cells differ from skeletal muscle cells in that they are shorter, broader, and more interconnected. Each cell is structurally distinct, but there are many end-to-end and side-to-side connections that allow the electrical impulse to activate all contracting cells within a chamber in a sequential manner that causes the cells to function as an integrated unit. These connections allow both atria to contract together and both ventricles to contract together. Because of this unique system, the heart uses very little neural tissue (Morton et al., 2005).

Cardiac muscle cells are more metabolically active, require more energy, and experience more prolonged contractions than skeletal muscle cells. The prolonged contraction prevents impulses from coming rapidly enough to produce a sustained contraction, thereby preventing cardiac muscle from running low on adenosine triphosphate (ATP) and becoming fatigued (Opie, 2004).

Myofibrils

Myofibrils are the contractile elements of a cardiac cell. They run the entire length of the cell and are composed of a series of sarcomeres (Figure 1.20). Sarcomeres are the structural and functional units of contraction and consist of overlapping thick (myosin) and thin (actin) protein filaments. Myosin filaments have projections or "heads" on them that have the potential to attach to binding sites on actin filaments.

Cardiovascular Anatomy and Physiology

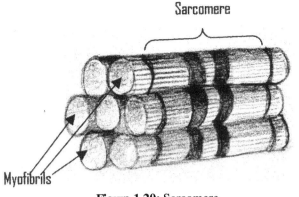

Figure 1.20: Sarcomere.

At rest, during diastole, there are no connections between myosin and actin filaments. During depolarization, calcium ions move into the myocardial cell and bind to troponin located on actin filaments. Calcium bound troponin allows the myosin head to bind to actin, creating a cross-bridge. There is a rapid and successive uncoupling and reattachment of myosin cross-bridges to new actin binding sites, which pulls the actin filaments in toward the center of the sarcomere, resulting in shortening of the sarcomere. When all sarcomeres in the myofibrils shorten, the entire fiber shortens; when all fibers shorten, the muscle contracts. In order for contraction to occur, there must be an adequate amount of Ca^{++} and an adequate supply of energy in the form of ATP. The amount of ATP that is available is dependent on an adequate O_2 supply to the myocardium. This is why ischemia and hypoxia, two causes of reduced myocardial O_2 supply, result in decreased contractility.

Contraction stops when the influx of calcium ions stops and calcium is returned to its storage sites on the sarcoplasmic reticulum and the T tubules (discussed below). Without calcium, the actin and myosin filaments separate and slip past each other in the reverse direction, lengthening the sarcomere to its relaxed state (Guyton & Hall, 2000).

Sarcoplasmic Reticulum

Cardiac muscle fibers have invaginations of the cell membrane called transverse (T) tubules that penetrate all the way from one side to the other side (of the fiber) and function to spread the action potential all the way through the fiber. These T tubules communicate with another system of longitudinal (L) tubules inside the fiber that runs parallel to the fiber and ends in chambers called *cisternae* (Figure 1.21). The L tubules and the cisternae make up the sarcoplasmic reticulum (SR), which contains large amounts of Ca^{++} ions that are released when the AP spreads to the interior of the cell through the T tubules (Guyton & Hall, 2000).

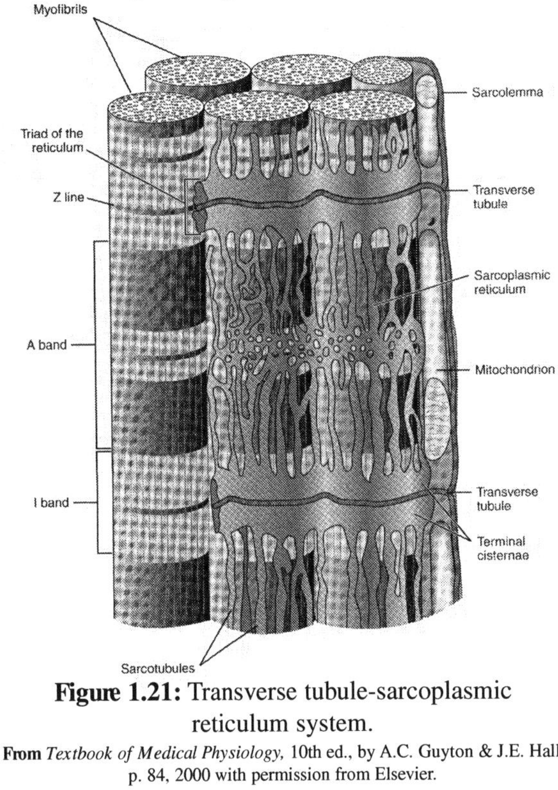

Excitation-Contraction Coupling

Normal cardiac muscle cells contract in response to depolarization; this is termed excitation-contraction coupling. When an AP propagates along a cardiac muscle cell membrane, it travels to the interior of the cell through the T tubules, spreading along the sarcoplasmic reticulum where Ca^{++} ions are stored and triggering the release of Ca^{++} ions from the SR (Morton et al., 2005; Guyton & Hall, 2000). The combination of the released Ca^{++} ions and the influx of calcium during depolarization provides the calcium ions necessary to facilitate actin-myosin interaction, thus causing the muscle to contract.

Figure 1.21: Transverse tubule-sarcoplasmic reticulum system.
From *Textbook of Medical Physiology,* 10th ed., by A.C. Guyton & J.E. Hall, p. 84, 2000 with permission from Elsevier.

Depolarization does not guarantee contraction. If a cardiac muscle cell has been damaged, normal contraction might not occur even when the cell is stimulated. Clinically, this results in electrical activity (i.e. a cardiac rhythm), but no mechanical contraction (i.e. no pulse), and is called electromechanical dissociation or pulseless electrical activity (PEA).

CARDIAC CONDUCTION SYSTEM

Contraction of the chambers of the heart in a coordinated fashion is necessary for normal function of the heart. The cardiac conduction system (Figure 1.22) is responsible for initiating the electrical impulse and transmitting it in a systematic way through the heart.

SA Node

Stimulation of cardiac muscle cells is initiated in a small group of pacemaker cells located in the center of the SA node. The SA node is the natural pacemaker of the heart and sets a heart rate of 60 to 100 beats per minute. External nervous system stimulation is not necessary for SA node activity, but can impact SA node activity. The SA node is located close to the junction between the superior vena cava and the right atrium (Opie, 2004). The SA node is supplied by the RCA in 55% of the population, and by the LCX in the remaining 45% of the population. From the SA node, the depolarization travels through the right atrial tissue via internodal pathways and through the left atrial tissue via Bachmann's Bundle. From the internodal pathways the impulse travels to the AV node.

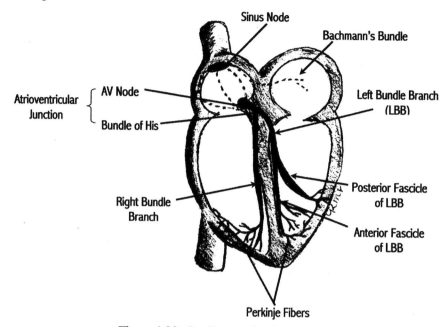

Figure 1.22: Cardiac conduction system.

AV Node

The AV node slows conduction from the atria to the ventricles. Conduction is slowed to assure that the ventricles are relaxed at the time of atrial contraction, allowing them to fill completely before contracting. The AV node is located in the posterior wall of the low right atrium behind the tricuspid valve and next to the os of the coronary sinus (Guyton & Hall, 2000; Opie, 2004).

His Bundle

From the AV node, the electrical impulse travels along the His Bundle, which divides into the bundle branches.

AV Junction

The AV node and the His Bundle are surrounded by tissue that is infiltrated with cells that have automaticity (pacemaker cells). This is referred to as the AV Junction. The AV junction has the ability to initiate a heart rate of 40-60 beats per minute if the sinus node fails as the normal pacemaker.

Bundle Branches

The right bundle branch carries the impulse to the right ventricle. The left bundle branch divides into the left posterior fascicle, which carries the impulse to the posterior and inferior left ventricles, and to the left anterior fascicle, which carries the impulse to the anterior and superior left ventricle. Blocks of the posterior fascicle of the left bundle branch are rare, as the posterior fascicle has a dual blood supply and receives oxygenated blood from the LAD and the RCA. The tissue of the posterior fascicle itself is also very thick and dense compared to the thin band of tissue that makes up the anterior fascicle of the left bundle branch and the right bundle branch making the posterior fascicle less susceptible to injury or ischemia.

Purkinje Fibers

From the bundle branches, the impulse travels to the Purkinje fibers, where the depolarization is carried through the subendocardial layers of the heart. Some Purkinje cells can function as pacemaker cells and initiate a heart rate of 20 to 40 beats per minute if no impulse is received through the normal conduction system.

HEMODYNAMIC PRINCIPLES

Cardiac Output

Perfusion of the body with oxygenated blood is dependent on cardiac output. Cardiac output (CO) is the amount of blood ejected by the left ventricle every minute. Heart rate (HR) and stroke volume (SV) are the primary determinants of cardiac output (see Figure 1.23).

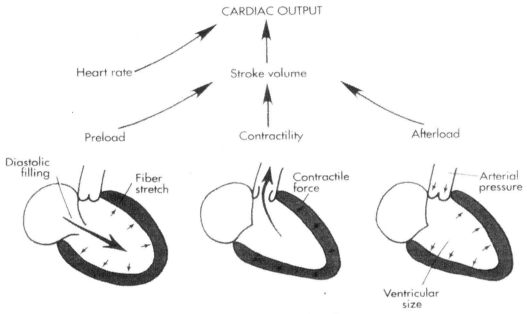

Figure 1.23: Components of cardiac output.
From *Pass CCRN* (2nd ed.), by R.D. Dennison, 2000, St. Louis: Mosby. Reprinted with permission.

Stroke volume is the volume of blood ejected by the left ventricle with each beat. Each ventricle holds about 150 ml when full and ejects about 50% to 60% of its volume with each beat (Dennison, 2000). The percentage of volume ejected with each beat is termed the ejection fraction (EF). Stroke volume has three components: preload, afterload, and contractility.

Changes in heart rate, preload, afterload, or contractility change cardiac output (Table 1.2). Additionally, increasing any one of these factors increases myocardial oxygen demand.

Table 1.2 Key Definitions Relating to Cardiac Output (1 of 2)	
Cardiac Output	Volume of blood ejected by ventricle every minute. Cardiac Output = Heart Rate x Stroke Volume.

Chapter 1

Table 1.2
Key Definitions Relating to Cardiac Output (2 of 2)

Stroke Volume	Volume of blood ejected by ventricle each beat. Components of SV: Preload, Afterload, Contractility.
Ejection Fraction	Percentage of volume in ventricle ejected with each beat.
Preload	Stretch on the ventricular myocardial fibers at the end of ventricular diastole. The result of the volume in the ventricle at the end of diastole.
Afterload	Pressure the ventricle must overcome to eject its contents.
Contractility	Ability of the ventricle to pump independent of preload or afterload.

Determinants of Cardiac Output

Heart Rate. The heart rate is defined as the number of times the heart beats every minute. Normal heart rate in an adult ranges from 60 to 100 beats per minute. During exercise, the heart rate naturally increases to meet the increased metabolic needs of the body. Heart rate also decreases as the body's needs decrease, such as during sleep. However, extremely slow heart rates (less than 40 beats per minute) and extremely high heart rates (greater than 150 beats per minute) experienced over a prolonged period, can negatively affect cardiac output. High heart rates do not allow adequate time for ventricular filling (shortens diastole), and low heart rates do not provide an adequate number of ejections per minute (CO= HR x SV).

Preload. Preload (Figure 1.23), one of the determinants of stroke volume, is defined as the stretch on the ventricular myocardial fibers at the end of ventricular diastole. The volume of blood filling the ventricles causes the myocardium to stretch. According to Starling's law, the larger the volume of blood in the ventricle at the end of diastole (within physiologic limits), the greater the energy of the subsequent contraction (Opie, 2004). Therefore, as the filling of the ventricle increases, the strength of the subsequent contraction also increases, resulting in a greater stroke volume. Venous return to the heart determines the amount of blood entering the ventricles that stretches the myocardial fibers. The amount of venous blood returned to the right atrium ultimately enters the right and left ventricles. It is this volume of blood that produces the stretch in the ventricles during diastole. If venous return decreases, as with hypovolemia, preload decreases. When preload decreases, stroke volume decreases.

Afterload. Afterload (Figure 1.23) is the workload of the ventricle, or the pressure the ventricle must overcome to eject its contents. Afterload is affected by both anatomical structures and physiological changes that may impede the ejection of ventricular contents. These structures and changes include aortic or pulmonic valve function, arterial or pulmonary arterial pressures (vascular resistance), compliance of vascular walls, and diastolic pressure in the great arteries.

If the ventricular contents are to be ejected, the pressure in the ventricles must become great enough to force the aortic and pulmonic valves open. A stenotic valve is much more difficult to open due to the abnormalities in the valve. Therefore, aortic or pulmonic stenosis increases afterload. The overall resistance the left ventricle must pump against, known as systemic vascular resistance, is determined primarily by the systemic arterioles (Opie, 2004). Arterioles are small arteries with thick muscular walls. When the arterioles dilate, systemic vascular resistance decreases; when they constrict, systemic vascular resistance increases.

Arterioles respond to systemic changes and can vasoconstrict or vasodilate depending on the hemodynamic needs of the body. Noncompliant vascular walls, which exist in hypertension, do not relax easily and increase afterload. The vascular resistance the right ventricle must pump against is the pulmonary vascular resistance, which is determined by the pulmonary artery pressures.

Blood pressure is not equal to systemic vascular resistance. Cardiac output times the systemic vascular resistance determines blood pressure. Blood pressure, however, is a noninvasive method of evaluating systemic vascular resistance. Generally, as diastolic pressure rises, so does systemic vascular resistance.

Contractility. The third and final component of the stroke volume equation is contractility (Figure 1.23). Contractility is the ability of the ventricle to contract independent of preload or afterload. Contractility is referred to as the inotropic state of the myocardium and is a major component of systole. During ventricular contraction, the sarcomere (repeating unit of the myofibril), or cardiac muscle, shortens (Bond, 2005). The extent of myofibril shortening determines the velocity of the ejection of the myocardial contents. Damage to the myocardial muscle cells, as occurs in MI, decreases the ability of the myofibrils to shorten and impairs the ability of the ventricle to contract. Overstretch of the myofibrils also results in myofibrils that can no longer shorten effectively.

Additional Factors Contributing to Cardiac Output

Ventricular Synergy. The shape of the left ventricle is designed to provide a contraction that is generally an inward movement. This inward movement occurs simultaneously among all walls of the ventricle. This normal inward contraction of the ventricle is referred to as normal muscular synergy (Darovic, 2002). This normally coordinated contraction may become uncoordinated due to a variety of conditions. The ventricle may become damaged due to ischemic heart disease or aneurysms. Abnormalities in conduction, such as bundle branch blocks and ventricular ectopy, can also alter normal contraction patterns. Finally, changes in ventricular size caused by dilatation or fibrosis can also alter normal muscular synergy. Dysynergy can result in an increase in the energy needed for contraction and a decrease in cardiac output.

Ventricular Synchrony. The right and left ventricles are designed to contract simultaneously. Simultaneous contraction is referred to as ventricular synchrony. Ventricular dysynchrony occurs when the right and left ventricles do not contract at the same time. This dysynchrony is commonly demonstrated by a bundle branch block pattern on an electrocardiogram. If the right and left ventricles do not contract synchronously, cardiac output and performance are compromised.

Impact of Ventricular Septum. The interventricular septum functions as part of the left ventricle and contributes to left ventricular ejection by moving towards the left ventricular free wall during systole. Anything that alters septal motion (e.g. septal infarction, right ventricular volume or pressure overload) or prevents it from contracting with the left ventricle (e.g. left bundle branch block, septal infarction) can result in reduction of stroke volume and cardiac output.

THE CARDIOPULMONARY CIRCUIT AND DELIVERY OF OXYGEN

The heart and lungs work together to form the cardiopulmonary circuit (Figure 1.24). The purpose of the cardiopulmonary circuit is to deliver oxygen to all the tissues of the body. The amount of oxygen delivered to the tissues is determined by three factors:

◆ cardiac output
◆ hemoglobin level
◆ oxygen saturation.

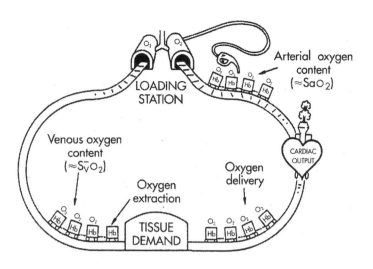

Figure 1.24: Schematic of the cardiopulmonary circuit.
From *Pass CCRN* (2nd ed.), by R.D. Dennison, 2000, St. Louis: Mosby. Reprinted with permission.

Under normal conditions, approximately 1,000 ml of oxygen, attached to hemoglobin, is delivered to the tissues each minute via the arterial system, and the tissues of the body extract 25% of the oxygen delivered to them (Dennison, 2000), leaving a 75% reserve. If the cardiopulmonary circuit fails to deliver enough oxygen to meet the needs of the tissues, the amount left in the reserve diminishes. The oxygen reserve is measured by assessing the percent of oxygen saturation of venous blood (SVO_2).

When oxygenated blood reaches the capillary level, oxygen and other nutrients are exchanged for waste products. Once this exchange occurs, deoxygenated blood is returned to the right atrium from the capillaries via the venous system (Figure 1.25).

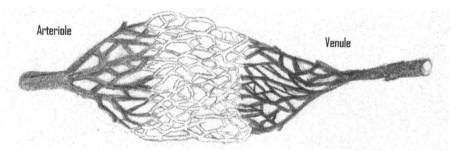

Figure 1.25: Capillary network.

Myocardial Oxygenation

The balance of myocardial oxygen supply and demand is key in providing cardiac muscle with the proper amount of oxygen to maintain optimum function. The ability of the myocardium to contract effectively is directly related to the amount of oxygen that is supplied to the heart. The myocardium is unique because the left ventricle extracts approximately 75% of the oxygen that is delivered, as opposed to the normal 25% that is extracted by other tissues. Two-thirds of myocardial oxygen extraction occurs during isovolumic contraction (Darovic, 2002). Because there is little oxygen reserve to be utilized during periods of increased need, the myocardium becomes very dependent on flow from the coronary arteries. The body inherently changes the diameter of the coronary arteries to change the delivery of oxygen. As myocardial oxygen demand increases, the coronary arteries dilate, if they are able, to deliver more oxygen-rich blood to the myocardium. As myocardial oxygen demand increases, so must the myocardial oxygen supply. Myocardial oxygen demand increases with an increase in any of the four components of cardiac output (heart rate, preload, afterload, or contractility). If myocardial oxygen supply cannot be increased during periods of increased demand, then ischemia occurs.

In patients with coronary artery disease, narrowed blood vessels are often unable to dilate enough to provide the necessary oxygen supply and, therefore, angina occurs during periods of increased metabolic demand. The inability to adequately dilate is why stable angina generally occurs with activity and subsides when activity is stopped.

Cardiovascular Anatomy and Physiology

Myocardial oxygen supply depends on cardiac output, hemoglobin level, and oxygen saturation. Hemoglobin is the primary transporter of oxygen. Low hemoglobin levels can exacerbate ischemia in patients with coronary artery disease. If hemoglobin levels become critically low, ischemia can occur, even in patients without coronary artery disease. Oxygen saturation levels also affect the delivery of oxygen to myocardial tissue. Oxygen saturation levels can drop during periods of critical illness. Low oxygen saturation levels are commonly caused by pulmonary conditions, in which the diffusion of oxygen across the alveolar membrane and into the pulmonary capillaries is impaired.

NEUROLOGICAL CONTROL OF THE HEART AND BLOOD PRESSURE

Both branches of the autonomic nervous system, the sympathetic nervous system (SNS) and the parasympathetic nervous system (PNS), innervate the heart. The sympathetic nervous system allows the body to function under stress, and the parasympathetic nervous system helps the body conserve and restore resources. Both branches of the autonomic nervous system contribute to regulation of the major components of cardiac output. Because blood pressure is the product of cardiac output and systemic vascular resistance, it is also impacted by the autonomic nervous system.

Sympathetic Nervous System (Adrenergic Response)

The SNS has two key neurotransmitters, or messengers: epinephrine (or adrenalin) and norepinephrine (also called noradrenalin). These neurotransmitters, also called catecholamines, are excitatory messengers that are released in response to excitation or stress. The stress can be as simple as waking up or as severe as extreme fright.

The major effects of norepinephrine include increased heart rate, increased systolic and diastolic blood pressures, and decreased blood flow to the extremities (Opie, 2004). The major effects of epinephrine release are increased heart rate (*chronotropic* response), increased conduction from the SA node to the AV node (*dromotropic* response), increased stroke volume, increased contractility (*inotropic* response), increased systolic blood pressure with decreased diastolic blood pressure (resulting in an increase in pulse pressure), and increased blood flow to the extremities (Opie, 2004).

Sympathetic nerve fibers supply the SA node, the AV node, and the myocardium of the atria and ventricles. Once the neurotransmitters are activated by the SNS, the exact impact depends on the specific receptors stimulated.

Beta$_1$-adrenergic receptors are located in the heart and, when stimulated, cause an increase in heart rate, conductivity, and contractility. Beta$_2$-adrenergic receptors are located in the lungs and periphery and, when stimulated, cause bronchial and peripheral vasodilatation. Alpha$_1$-adrenergic receptors are located in the vessels of vascular smooth muscle and affect the tone of the small arterioles responsible for determining systemic vascular resistance. Alpha$_1$ and Beta$_2$ stimulation oppose each other in the periphery and their impact on systemic vascular resistance. The net result of SNS stimulation on alpha- and beta-receptors depends on the degree to which each receptor is stimulated. In general, alpha-receptors are more sensitive to norepinephrine, and beta receptors are more sensitive to epinephrine (Clinical Pharmacology Database, 2004). The renal, mesenteric, and coronary blood vessels also contain dopaminergic receptors. Stimulation of dopaminergic receptors results in vasodilatation. Table 1.3 describes SNS receptors and their response to stimulation.

21

Table 1.3
Adrenergic Receptor Location and Response

Receptor	Location of Receptor	Response to Stimulation
Alpha$_1$	Vascular smooth muscles	Vasoconstriction
Beta$_1$	Heart – SA node, AV node and myocardium	Increased Heart Rate (Chronotropic) Increased Conduction (Dromotropic) Increased Contractility (Inotropic)
Beta$_2$	Vascular and bronchial smooth muscles	Bronchodilatation Vasodilatation
Dopaminergic	Vascular smooth muscle – renal, coronary and mesenteric	Vasodilatation

Parasympathetic Nervous System (Vagal Response)

The PNS innervates the SA node, AV node, AV junction, and myocardium of the atria (Dennison, 2000). There is minimal parasympathetic innervation of the ventricles. When the PNS is stimulated, the response is called a cholinergic, or vagal response. Acetylcholine is the neurotransmitter that is released when parasympathetic nerve fibers are stimulated. Acetylcholine binds to the parasympathetic receptors. Cholinergic receptors are classified into two types: nicotinic and muscarinic. Parasympathetic receptors located in the heart and smooth muscles are called muscarinic receptors.

Stimulation of the PNS decreases heart rate (decreased chronotropic response) and slows conduction (decreased dromotropic response). PNS stimulation has very little effect on the force of ventricular contraction because of the minimal innervation of the PNS in the ventricles. When the PNS is stimulated, acetylcholine is released, which results in a cholinergic, or vagal, response. Acetylcholine directly inhibits the SA node, thus decreasing heart rate. Stimulation of the PNS also causes vasodilatation due to nitric oxide release from the endothelium (Opie, 2004). Venous vasodilatation decreases preload, and arterial vasodilatation decreases afterload.

Vagal tone is more pronounced during sleeping hours. When blood pressure is elevated, the feedback from the baroreceptors (discussed below) causes parasympathetic stimulation, which results in slower heart rate, decreased force of contraction, and vasodilatation. The slower heart rate, decreased force of contraction, and vasodilatation result in lower cardiac output and blood pressure. The activation of the PNS during an acute hypertensive crisis explains the reflex bradycardia commonly seen in this clinical situation. Conversely, low blood pressure causes reflex tachycardia.

Baroreceptors

Baroreceptors are specialized nerve tissues located in the aortic arch and carotid sinus (the origin of the internal carotid artery) (Figure 1.26). Baroreceptors function as sensors in the nervous system and are sensitive to wall tension within the arterial vessels. An increase or decrease in wall tension and pressure sends signals to the vasomotor center in the brain stem (Opie, 2004). The medulla is the vasomotor center of the brain and interprets all the information it receives from the baroreceptors via the afferent pathways. The medulla transmits information back to the heart and blood vessels via the motor nerves called efferent pathways (Opie, 2004). Impulses from this center control the diameter of blood vessels.

When blood pressure is increased, baroreceptors recognize the increased wall tension and send a message to inhibit the SNS and stimulate the PNS. Heart rate slows and veins and arteries dilate throughout the system. These changes result in decreased blood pressure. When blood pressure decreases, wall tension decreases. The opposite effects, increased heart rate and vasoconstriction, occur with stimulation of the SNS. Rapid adjustments in BP are controlled by baroreceptor reflexes. Reflexes are sluggish in orthostatic hypotension.

Two baroreceptor reflexes control release of adrenergic (SNS) or cholinergic (PNS) neurotransmitters.

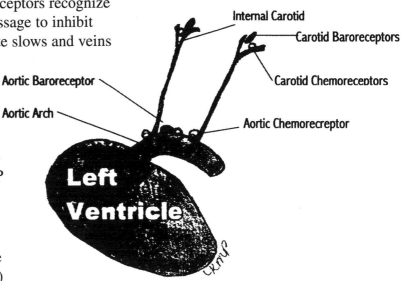

Figure 1.26

Aortic Reflex

Increase in arterial BP
→ Stimulation of baroreceptors located in the aortic arch
→ Parasympathetic (Vagal) stimulation from the medulla
→ HR and CO decrease
→ BP decreases

Bainbridge Reflex

Increase in venous BP
→ Stimulates baroreceptors located in the aortic arch
→ Increased sympathetic stimulation
→ Heart rate increases to handle increased venous return

When the vagal maneuver of carotid massage is performed, baroreceptors in the carotid arteries are manually stimulated to decrease rate of SA node and slow conduction through the AV node, resulting in decreased heart rate and potentially causing AV block.

Chemoreceptors

The carotid arteries also contain chemoreceptors, which respond to changes in blood chemistry, including arterial oxygen content, arterial carbon dioxide levels, and arterial pH. As blood pressure lowers to a critical point, the delivery of oxygen also decreases to a critical point. As oxygen delivery decreases, carbon dioxide levels increase. When stimulated by an elevated arterial carbon dioxide level, chemoreceptors send a message to the vasomotor center to stimulate cardiac activity via the SNS. Heart rate increases and vasoconstriction occurs, causing an increase in blood pressure with a resultant increase in oxygenation.

Role of the Renin-Angiotensin-Aldosterone System (Figure 1.27)

Renin is released from the kidneys in response to low circulating volume, low cardiac output, or poor kidney perfusion. Activation of the SNS and increased catecholamines stimulate renin release. Once renin is released into the circulation, it joins with angiotensinogen to form angiotensin I. Angiotensin I is

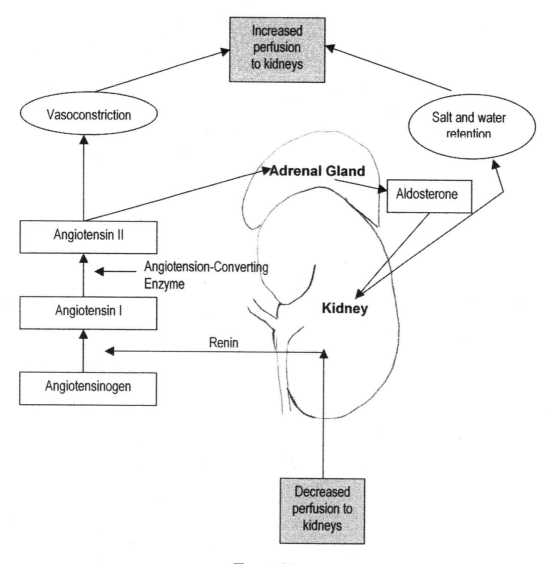

Figure 1.27

converted to angiotensin II in the presence of angiotensin-converting enzyme. Angiotensin-converting enzyme is found in the capillary bed of the lungs and other tissues. The important end result of the renin-angiotensin-aldosterone system (RAAS) is caused by the effects of circulating angiotensin II.

Angiotensin II has three primary effects:

1. arterial vasoconstriction
2. stimulation of thirst
3. stimulation of the adrenal cortex to secrete aldosterone (aldosterone increases sodium and water reabsorption).

As the blood vessels constrict and water is reabsorbed and retained, blood pressure increases and perfusion to the body, including the kidneys, improves. This increased perfusion then decreases the production of renin by the kidneys.

The end result of stimulation of the RAAS includes arterial vasoconstriction and aldosterone secretion. Arterial vasoconstriction increases afterload, and aldosterone secretion increases preload. These effects are clinically important in patients with heart failure who have chronic stimulation of the RAAS.

REGULATION OF FLUID BALANCE

The regulation of fluid balance occurs through three mechanisms:

◆ Fluid intake
◆ Hormonal control
    ❖ Vasopressin (antidiuretic hormone-ADH)
    ❖ Aldosterone
◆ Fluid output.

Fluid Intake

Fluid intake is regulated by the thirst mechanism. Osmoreceptors in the hypothalmus are stimulated by an increase in osmotic pressure of body fluids and cause thirst. Osmoreceptors are also stimulated by a decrease in extracellular fluid volume. A decrease in salivary secretions from certain medications (e.g. anticholinergics) also stimulates thirst.

Hormonal Control

Hormonal control is regulated by vasopressin (ADH) and aldosterone. Vasopressin, which is produced in the hypothalamus and stored in the posterior pituitary, functions as the water conservation hormone. Vasopressin regulates the osmotic pressure of extracellular fluid by regulating the amount of water reabsorbed in the renal tubules. Vasopressin release is stimulated by an increase in osmotic pressure. Increased vasopressin causes water reabsorption in the renal tubules, which dilutes the blood in an attempt to return osmotic pressure to normal. Excreted urine volume is decreased and the concentration of urine is increased as more fluid is returned to the circulation.

Aldosterone is secreted from the adrenal cortex. It regulates extracellular fluid volume by increasing reabsorption of sodium and chloride in the renal tubules. With an increased reabsorption of sodium, water retention follows. Aldosterone promotes excretion of potassium and hydrogen.

Aldosterone production is increased in healthy persons in the following circumstances:

◆ Low fluid volume
◆ Low blood sodium
◆ High blood potassium.

Cushing's Syndrome causes an overproduction of aldosterone; aldosterone is under produced with adrenalectomy, AIDS, and metastatic cancer.

Fluid Output

A change in extracellular fluid results in altered intravascular volume and venous return to the heart. Alterations in cardiac output result in changes in arterial pressure. The kidneys sense these changes in arterial pressure and respond by altering fluid excretion. Fluid is also lost through the gastrointestinal tract, skin, and lungs.

Distribution of Body Fluid (Figure 1.28)

Intracellular fluid volume accounts for 40% of adult body weight.

Extracellular fluid volume accounts for about 20% of adult body weight.

Extracellular fluid consists of intravascular volume (fluid within the blood vessels) and fluid in the interstitial space (between vessels and cells).

Fluid is not static and is capable of moving between the intravascular space and interstitial space, as well as moving between extracellular and intracellular space.

Movement of Fluid and Electrolytes

The movement of fluids and electrolytes is influenced by the following physiological concepts:

- Capillary Permeability
- Diffusion
- Osmosis
- Active Transport
- Hydrostatic Pressure
- Filtration
- Colloidal Osmotic Pressure.

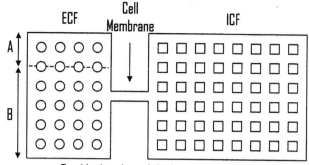

Figure 1.28: Distribution of body fluid.

Capillary Permeability

All capillary walls do not have the same permeability; for example, proteins can cross membranes in the liver but not in the kidneys.

Diffusion

Diffusion is the movement of solute in a solution or across a permeable membrane. The solute can be a gas or a substance.

The solute moves from an area of higher concentration to an area of lower concentration (Figure 1.29). Diffusion can be simple as in the diffusion of oxygen across the alveolar capillary membrane, or it can be facilitated as in the diffusion of glucose into the cell facilitated by insulin.

Osmosis

Osmosis is the movement of a pure solvent (water) from an area less concentrated to an area more concentrated (Figure 1.30). Osmosis is a passive process. The solvent moves but not the solute because of a semi-permeability of a membrane. Osmosis stops when there is equilibrium.

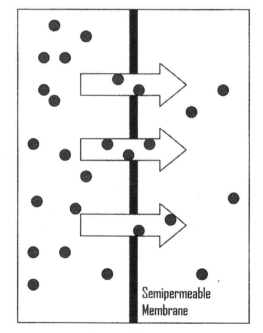

Figure 1.29: Diffusion.

Active Transport

Active transport is used when electrolytes have to move from an area of lesser concentration to an area of greater concentration against a concentration gradient. This is the mechanism involved in the sodium potassium pump discussed earlier in this chapter.

Hydrostatic Pressure (Pushing Pressure)

Hydrostatic pressure is the force of fluid pressing against vessel walls. It is determined by weight of blood and the blood pressure. Hydrostatic pressure at the arterial end of capillaries is twice as great as at the venous end.

Cardiovascular Anatomy and Physiology

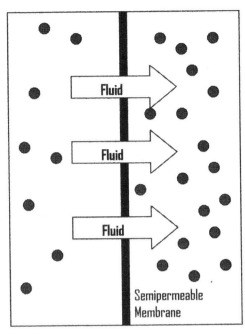

Figure 1.30: Osmosis.

Filtration

During filtration both solute and solvent move together in response to hydrostatic pressure. During tissue perfusion water and nutrients are exchanged as a result of differences in hydrostatic pressure between the capillaries and tissues. Filtration is also used to remove solute and solvent during renal replacement therapies.

Osmolality

Osmolality is the number of osmotically active particles per kilogram of water. It is measured in milliosmoles per kilogram of water. Extracellular osmolality is determined predominantly by the concentration of sodium. Sodium is the most prevalent extracellular cation and provides 90-95% of the osmotic pressure. Intracellular and extracellular fluids have approximately the same osmolality.

Normal serum osmolality = 280-294 mOsm/kg.

Specific Gravity

Specific gravity is the weight of a solution compared to an equal amount of distilled water (can be used to estimate osmolality). Urine osmolality, however, is a more specific measurement of renal function than specific gravity. The kidneys respond to changes in osmolality rather than specific gravity.

Osmotic Pressure (Pulling Pressure)

Osmotic pressure (oncotic pressure) is the pull determined by the number of plasma colloids (or solute) on the concentrated side. Osmotic pressure is determined by osmolality. Osmotic pressure affects osmosis. For example: Intravascular fluid has more protein than interstitial fluid; therefore, it has a higher oncotic pressure. Intravascular oncotic (pulling) pressure is greater at the venous end than intravascular hydrostatic pressure; therefore, the net result is that fluids are pulled into the intravascular space.

Extracellular Fluid Volume Deficit

When extracellular fluid volume is low:

- Remaining fluid is more concentrated (hypertonic).
- Cellular dehydration occurs as fluid leaves the cells.
- Elderly are at risk due to:
    - Decrease in total body water
    - Reduced sense of thirst
    - Reduced ability of kidneys to concentrate urine.
- Hematocrit increases due to hemoconcentration.
- Sodium levels increase due to decrease in fluid volume (hyperosmolar hypernatremia).
- Urine specific gravity increases.

Chapter 1

Extracellular Fluid Volume Overload

◆ Normal compensatory changes that occur when extracellular fluid volume is high:

→ Excess ECF

→ Water moves into cells

→ Osmoreceptors respond

→ Decreased release of vasopressin (ADH)

→ Increased urine output

◆ Does not occur as a primary problem unless compensatory mechanisms fail:

❖ Kidney disease

❖ Decreased cardiac output

❖ Excessive ADH

★ Fear

★ Pain

★ Acute infection

★ Analgesics

★ Trauma

★ Acute stress.

◆ Extracellular fluid volume excess results in:

❖ Decreased oncotic pressure

❖ Fluid moves into cells

★ Cellular swelling.

Fluid Shifting

During fluid shifting, large quantities of fluid shift from intravascular to extravascular space. Fluid shifting can be caused by:

◆ Increased capillary permeability, allowing plasma protein to leak into interstitial spaces

◆ Decreased intravascular oncotic pressure

◆ Lymphatic blockage.

Phases of Fluid Shifting

Phase I: Fluid shifts out of vascular space and symptoms resemble fluid volume deficit because circulating volume is decreased.

Phase II: Fluid is reabsorbed and moves back into vascular space. The process occurs gradually and does not cause signs of fluid overload.

Cardiovascular Anatomy and Physiology

Linking Knowledge to Practice

✔ *The body tolerates bradycardia better than tachycardia.*

✔ *Anything that increases heart rate will decrease diastolic filling time. Decreased diastolic filling time resulting in a smaller ventricular volume available for ejection from the ventricle (decrease preload) as well as, a decreased time for perfusion of the coronary arteries.*

✔ *Preload, afterload, contractility and heart rate (components of cardiac output) work in harmony with each other to maintain cardiac output. For example, if preload decreases, heart rate and afterload will increase to compensate for the decreased volume.*

✔ *The components of cardiac output are the same components that determine myocardial oxygen demand (MVO_2). Therefore, any impact on the components of cardiac output will have an impact on MVO_2. Most importantly, increases in afterload or contractility significantly impact myocardial oxygen needs.*

✔ *The electrical conduction system runs close to the mitral and aortic valves. Patients undergoing mitral or aortic valve surgery may develop a temporary or permanent block in the AV conduction system.*

✔ *Stimulation of the ventricle during the relative refractory period can result in ventricular tachycardia or fibrillation.*

✔ *The thin wall of the right ventricle makes it susceptible to dysfunction in response to small changes in pulmonary vascular resistance.*

✔ *Excess volume in the left ventricle at the end of diastole leads to stretching of the ventricle. Stretching of the left ventricle will also result in stretching of mitral valve annulus resulting in mitral regurgitation.*

✔ *Coronary circulation begins with the epicardium and reaches the endocardium last; therefore, myocardial ischemia and infarction begin with the endocardial layer of the heart.*

✔ *A thickened myocardial wall (hypertrophy) results in decreased flow of oxygen-rich blood to the deep myocardium and endocardial layer. Angina can occur even without narrowing of coronary arteries.*

✔ *The amount of extracellular calcium ions affects the availability of calcium to enter the cardiac cells via the T channels. Low extracellular calcium ions can therefore affect the force of myocardial contraction. Calcium T channels are not affected by the administration of calcium channel blockers.*

✔ *In heart failure leading to pulmonary edema, the hydrostatic pressure in the lungs becomes increased. This increase in hydrostatic pressure exceeds the oncotic pressure in the capillaries, and fluid is pushed out into the interstitial spaces of the lung.*

✔ *High dose potassium solutions (cardioplegia solutions) used during cardiopulmonary bypass arrest the heart because high concentrations of extracellular potassium inhibit the sodium channel.*

✔ *Many medications impact the RAAS including beta blockers, ACE Inhibitors, angiotensin receptor blockers, and aldosterone antagonists.*

Chapter 1

TEST YOUR KNOWLEDGE

1. The thick middle layer of the heart is called the
   a. endocardium.
   b. myocardium.
   c. epicardium.
   d. pericardium.

2. The two atrioventricular valves are the
   a. tricuspid and pulmonic valves.
   b. aortic and pulmonic valves.
   c. tricuspid and mitral valves.
   d. aortic and mitral valves.

3. The layer of the arterial wall that is responsible for changes in the diameter of the artery is the
   a. media.
   b. intima.
   c. externa.
   d. adventitia.

4. The aortic and pulmonic valves are open during this part of the cardiac cycle:
   a. Atrial systole.
   b. Ventricular diastole.
   c. Ventricular systole.
   d. Isovolumic contraction.

5. The anterior left ventricle receives oxygenated blood via the
   a. left circumflex coronary artery.
   b. right coronary artery.
   c. posterior descending coronary artery.
   d. left anterior descending coronary artery.

6. Patients with occlusion of the right coronary artery are at high risk for the development of Mobitz Type I heart blocks because this part of the conduction system is supplied by the right coronary artery in the approximately 90% of the population.
   a. SA node
   b. AV node
   c. Bundle branches
   d. Purkinje fibers

Cardiovascular Anatomy and Physiology

7. During Phase 0 of the action potential, there is a rapid influx of which ion into the cell?
    a. K^+
    b. Ca^{++}
    c. Na^{++}
    d. Mg^+

8. If an electrical stimulus is applied to a cell during the absolutely refractory period, the cell
    a. will respond normally.
    b. will not respond.
    c. will only respond to a stronger than normal stimulus.
    d. will respond with a delayed response.

9. The three pacemakers of the heart are the SA Node, the AV Junction and the
    a. Bundle Branches.
    b. AV Node.
    c. Perkinje Fibers.
    d. His Bundle.

10. Stoke volume is defined as
    a. the volume of blood ejected by the ventricle each beat.
    b. the volume of blood ejected by the ventricle each minute.
    c. the percent of blood ejected from the ventricle each beat.
    d. the volume of blood in the ventricle available for ejection each beat.

11. The components of cardiac output include
    a. heart rate.
    b. preload.
    c. afterload.
    d. contractility.
    e. b, c, and d.
    f. all of the above.

12. The amount of oxygen delivered to the tissues is determined by what factors?
    a. Cardiac output
    b. Hemoglobin level
    c. Oxygen saturation
    d. All of the above.

Chapter 1

13. The ventricles of the heart are innervated by the
    a. parasympathetic nervous system.
    b. sympathetic nervous system.
    c. none of the above.
    d. All of the above.

14. Stimulation of the parasympathetic nervous system would result in
    a. decreased heart rate and decreased conductivity.
    b. increased heart rate and increased conductivity.
    c. decreased heart rate and increased conductivity.
    d. increased heart rate and decreased conductivity.

15. Activation of the Renin-Angiotensin-Aldosterone System results in
    a. arterial vasoconstriction, decreased retention of sodium and water.
    b. arterial vasodilation, decreased retention of sodium and water.
    c. arterial vasoconstriction, increased sodium and water reabsorption.
    d. arterial vasodilation, increased sodium and water reabsorption.

ANSWERS

1. B
2. C
3. A
4. C
5. D
6. B
7. C
8. B
9. C
10. A
11. F
12. D
13. B
14. A
15. C

Cardiovascular Anatomy and Physiology

REFERENCES

Alcomo, I.E. (1996). *Anatomy and physiology the easy way*. Hauppauge, NY: Barrons.

Bond, E.F. (2005). Cardiac anatomy and physiology. In S.L.Woods, E.S. Froelicher, S.U. Motzer, & E.J. Bridges (Eds.), *Cardiac nursing* (5th ed., pp. 3-48). Philadelphia: Lippincott, Williams and Wilkins.

Bridges, E.J. (2005). Systemic circulation. In S.L.Woods, E.S. Froelicher, S.U. Motzer, & E.J. Bridges (Eds.), *Cardiac nursing* (5th ed., pp. 49-70). Philadelphia: Lippincott, Williams and Wilkins.

Bridges, E.J. (2005). Regulation of cardiac output and blood pressure. In S.L.Woods, E.S. Froelicher, S.U. Motzer, & E.J. Bridges (Eds.), *Cardiac nursing* (5th ed., pp. 81-108). Philadelphia: Lippincott, Williams and Wilkins.

Darovic, G.O. (2002). *Hemodynamic monitoring: Invasive and noninvasive clinical application*. (3rd ed.). Philadelphia: Saunders.

Fischbach, F. (2004). *A manual of lab and diagnostic test* (7th ed.). Philadelphia: Lippincott, Williams and Wilkins.

Guyton, A.C. & Hall, J.E. (2000). *Textbook of medical physiology*. Philadelphia: Saunders.

Kumar, V., Abbas, A.K., & Fausto, N. (2005) *Pathologic basis of disease* (7th ed.). Philadelphia: Elsevier Saunders.

Marini, J.J. & Wheeler, A.P. (2006). *Critical care medicine the essentials* (3rd ed.). Philadelphia: Lippincott, Williams and Wilkins.

McCance, K.L. & Huether, S.E. (2006). *Pathophysiology: the biologic basis for disease in adults and children* (5th ed.). St. Louis: Elsevier.

Opie, L.H. (2004). *Heart physiology from cell to circulation* (4th ed.). Philadelphia: Lippincott, Williams and Wilkins.

Porth, C.M. (Ed.). (2004). *Essentials of pathophysiology: Concepts of altered health states*. Philadelphia: Lippincott, Williams and Wilkins.

Speakman, E. & Weldy, N.J. (2002). *Body fluids and electrolytes* (8th ed.). St. Louis, MO: Mosby.

Thibodeau, G.A. & Patton, K.T. (2003). *Anatomy and physiology* (5th ed.). St. Louis, MO: Mosby.

Wit, A.L. & Rosen, M.R. (1981a). Cellular electrophysiology of cardiac arrhythmias: Part I: Arrhythmias caused by abnormal impulse generation. *Modern Concepts in Cardiovascular Disease, 50*, 1-6.

Wit, A.L. & Rosen, M.R. (1981b). Cellular electrophysiology of cardiac arrhythmias: Part II: Arrhythmias caused by abnormal impulse conduction. *Modern Concepts in Cardiovascular Disease, 50*(2), 7-12.

CHAPTER 2:
CARDIOVASCULAR ASSESSMENT

INTRODUCTION

A well-organized and comprehensive assessment will provide the nurse with valuable information about the patient. Nurses at the bedside are the eyes and ears of the health care team twenty-four hours a day, seven days a week. An astute nurse with good assessment skills can recognize subtle changes in the patient's status, respond quickly to those changes, and notify the appropriate member of the health care team as needed. The assessment also provides the basis for the development of a nursing plan of care aimed at meeting mutually agreed upon goals with the patient.

HEALTH HISTORY

The health history provides information that drives the physical assessment as well as the diagnostic studies and treatment of the patient. The health history should encompass the physiological and the psychosocial aspects of the patient. During the process of collecting the health history, the nurse has the opportunity to develop a relationship with the patient that will lay the groundwork for future patient nurse encounters. In the acutely ill cardiac patient, the interview process may be brief, as acute interventions may be required; however, the health history is an important part of the assessment and should not be eliminated, as it may provide key information that may influence the treatment strategies.

History of Present Illness

- ◆ Chief Complaint/Present Illness
  - ❖ Determine why the patient is seeking help from the medical profession.
  - ❖ Ask the patient to use his or her own words to describe why he or she is seeking assistance.
  - ❖ Presenting Symptoms
    - ☆ Ask the patient to describe the symptoms associated with the illness.
    - ☆ Initiate a discussion of symptoms that should include a systemized approach to evaluating the symptoms. Utilization of the letters NOPQRST helps remind the interviewer of the appropriate questions to ask.
      - ✳ N = Normal: What is the patient's baseline? How does he or she normally feel? Is this an exacerbation of an already occurring illness or is it new?
      - ✳ O = Onset: When did the discomfort or symptom begin?
        - – Sudden or gradual?
        - – Time of day?
        - – Hour of day?
      - ✳ P = Precipitating, provoking or palliative factors?
        - – Precipitating (triggers): Stress, food, activity, position changes, movement, or deep breath?
        - – Provoking factors: Does anything make it worse, such as movement, deep breaths or palpation?
        - – Palliative: Does anything make it better?

- ✱ Q = Quality or quantity.
  - Describe the discomfort or symptom.
  - Ask the patient to describe the discomfort or symptom in his or her own words. Listen carefully. What one describes as pain may be pressure to another.
  - Assess for descriptors such as pain, pressure, or heaviness.
    - Is the discomfort continuous, intermittent, or stabbing?
    - Is the discomfort worse than normal?
    - Is the discomfort more or less than earlier?
- ✱ R = Radiation and region.
  - Where is the discomfort or symptom?
    - Have the patient point to the primary area of pain.
  - Does the discomfort radiate (travel) to another area?
- ✱ S = Severity and other symptoms.
  - Have the patient rate the severity utilizing an easily recognized pain scale.
  - Numeric: quantifies the pain using numbers. A generally accepted scale is the numeric scale of 0-10 (Figure 2.1).

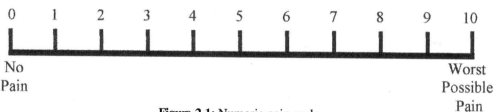

Figure 2.1: Numeric pain scale.

  - Visual: quantifies pain using pictures, such as the Wong-Baker Faces Pain Rating Scale.
  - Verbal: utilizes words such as low, mild, moderate, severe and excruciating.
  - What is the result of the discomfort or symptom?
  - Does it interfere with sleep?
  - Does it interfere with work?
  - Can it be ignored for any period of time?
  - Is it getting worse or better?
  - How severe was it at its worst?
  - Are there any other associated symptoms such as fatigue, shortness of breath, nausea, fever, etc.?
- ✱ T = Time and treatment.
  - Is the symptom or discomfort continuous or intermittent?
  - How long does it last?
  - Has the patient been treated in the past for this same concern? If so, what was the treatment and how effective was the treatment?

Assessment of Specific Chief Complaints Associated With the Cardiovascular Patient

- ◆ Chest Pain or Pressure
  - ❖ Is most common symptom in cardiovascular presentation.
  - ❖ Utilize the NOPQRST method of assessment.

Cardiovascular Assessment

❖ Normal
  ☆ May normally have angina that is now occurring more frequently or with greater severity.
  ☆ May describe "twinges" of discomfort previously, but severity or frequency has increased.
  ☆ May describe no discomfort prior to this incident.
❖ Onset
  ☆ Did the discomfort start suddenly or gradually? Most angina starts at a low intensity and builds gradually.
  ☆ What time of day did the discomfort start? Some myocardial infarctions occur in the morning after the patient rises and begins the activity for the day.
  ☆ Did the discomfort begin the day of presentation or has it been occurring for a period of time? There is often a history of discomfort that has been occurring that may have been different in severity or intermittent. This is important to determine.
  ☆ Myocardial infarctions may also occur with activity or after a heavy meal when myocardial oxygen demand is increased.
❖ Precipitation, provoking or palliation
  ☆ Chest pain caused by coronary artery disease is often precipitated by exertion of some type (emotional or physical).
  ☆ The increased demands placed on the system while trying to digest a large meal can result in angina.
  ☆ Exposure to cold may result in enough vasoconstriction to result in angina.
  ☆ Question the patient about any associated factors such as:
    ✳ Does the discomfort change with movement, a deep breath or position change? Anginal pain does not usually change with movement or position changes. Be cautious to rule out pericarditis in the patient with a history that is suspicious for pericarditis or pleuritic pain.
    ✳ Does the discomfort increase with palpation? Anginal pain should not change with palpation.
  ☆ Question the patient about anything that has been tried to relieve the discomfort and what the results of those efforts were.
    ✳ If sublingual nitroglycerin was taken, did the pain improve? How many nitroglycerin tablets were taken? If there was no relief from the discomfort determine if the nitroglycerin tablets were still effective. Nitroglycerin tablets have special storage requirements to help maintain potency:
      – Keep the medicine in the original glass, screw-cap bottle. For patients who wish to carry a small number of tablets with them for emergency use, a specially designed container is available. However, only containers specifically labeled as suitable for use with nitroglycerin sublingual tablets should be used.
      – Remove the cotton plug that comes in the bottle and do not put it back.
      – Put the cap on the bottle quickly and tightly after each use.
      – To select a tablet for use, pour several into the bottle cap, take one, and pour the others back into the bottle. Try not to hold them in the palm of your hand because they may pick up moisture and crumble.
      – Do not keep other medicines in the same bottle with the nitroglycerin since they will weaken the nitroglycerin effect.
      – Keep the medicine handy at all times, but try not to carry the bottle close to the body. Medicine may lose strength because of body warmth. Instead, carry the tightly closed bottle in your purse, the pocket of a jacket or other loose-fitting clothing whenever possible.

Chapter 2

- Store the bottle of nitroglycerin tablets in a cool, dry place. Store at average room temperature away from direct heat or direct sunlight is best. Do not store in the refrigerator or in a bathroom medicine cabinet because the moisture usually present in these areas may cause the tablets to crumble if the container is not tightly closed. Do not keep the tablets in an automobile glove compartment. (From http://www.nlm.nih.gov/medlineplus/druginfo/uspdi/202412.html).

★ Determine if stopping activity and resting resulted in a decrease in the discomfort. Relief of chest pain with cessation of activity is a good predictor of anginal discomfort.

- Angina is usually relieved by nitroglycerin or rest.

❖ Quality and quantity.

★ Anginal or ischemic discomfort has been described in many ways, including heaviness, pressure, tightness, or squeezing.

★ Stabbing, intermittent, knife-like descriptions are not likely to be due to a cardiac ischemia.

★ Remember to ask the patient to describe the discomfort. Discomfort caused by pericarditis is usually a stabbing type pain that may come and go. Cardiac patients may deny pain, as their discomfort is pressure or heaviness, not pain.

❖ Radiation and region.

★ The substernal region is the usual location for discomfort with a cardiac cause.

★ The anginal or ischemic discomfort is likely to radiate to the jaw, either arm, or the back.

★ The discomfort does not have to be substernal. Isolated discomfort in the jaw, the arm or back may still have a cardiac origin.

★ The region of discomfort for cardiac ischemia is usually larger than a fingertip and often times the size of a hand or closed fist.

❖ Severity and other symptoms.

★ Keep in mind that severity is a subjective evaluation of the discomfort.

★ Ischemic discomfort can range from mild to severe.

★ If the patient has described the discomfort as heaviness or pressure, ask him or her to rate the heaviness or pressure on a scale of 0-10. If he or she is asked to rate his or her level of pain and perceives no pain, but rather pressure or heaviness, the assessment may not be accurate.

★ Asking the patient to rate the discomfort is helpful in understanding his or her perception of the discomfort.

★ Assess for other symptoms, such as nausea, vomiting, dyspnea or diaphoresis that may be associated with the discomfort.

❖ Time and treatment.

★ The length of time since the onset of symptoms is an important factor in the treatment of myocardial infarctions.

★ Patients may report symptoms that last from 30 seconds to hours.

★ Anginal or ischemic pain is usually not intermittent (lasting less than 30 seconds at a time). The discomfort may wax and wane over a period of days or weeks, but is not usually intermittent over the course of a short period of time.

★ Determine if the patient has been treated for the same symptoms in the past. If they have been treated for these symptoms in the past what was the treatment and was the treatment helpful or not.

Cardiovascular Assessment

◆ Dyspnea
  ❖ Can indicate either a pulmonary or cardiac problem.
  ❖ Determine if the symptom occurs with activity or at rest.
  ❖ If with activity, determine the level of activity. The elderly tend to adjust their activity to lower levels as they age, assuming difficulty breathing is due to overwork and aging, not a pathological problem.
  ❖ Decreased activity tolerance demonstrated by dyspnea on exertion might be angina caused by a lack of cardiac supply to meet the increase in demand with activity.
  ❖ Determine onset of the symptom – sudden or gradual.
  ❖ Orthopnea: difficulty breathing when lying flat.
  ❖ Paroxysmal nocturnal dyspnea: breathing difficulties that begin 1-2 hours into sleep. Relieved by sitting up.
  ❖ Assess how many pillows the patient sleeps on at night. An increased number of pillows is the same as sleeping with the head of the bed elevated.

◆ Cough and hemoptysis
  ❖ Can be caused by heart failure or pulmonary embolus.
  ❖ May be an early sign of left-sided heart failure.
  ❖ Evaluate for wet or dry cough.
  ❖ Evaluate for frequency (chronic or new onset).
  ❖ Determine if it occurs only with activity.
  ❖ Evaluate for sputum production.
  ❖ If there is sputum, identify color, consistency and amount.
  ❖ If hemoptysis is present, assess to determine if the sputum is blood streaked, frothy or frank blood.
  ❖ Hemoptysis may be present in a variety of situations, including mitral stenosis, pulmonary embolus, pulmonary hypertension and tuberculosis.

◆ Palpitations
  ❖ Awareness of heart beat.
  ❖ May occur with fast or normal heart rate.
  ❖ May be irregular or regular.
  ❖ New onset atrial fibrillation with rapid ventricular rate may result in palpitations.
  ❖ Patients with hyperdynamic stroke volumes (aortic or mitral regurgitation, pregnancy) often feel their heart beating.
  ❖ May also be caused by premature atrial or ventricular beats.

◆ Syncope
  ❖ Differentiate between dizziness, fainting and syncope. If the patient reports dizziness described as the room spinning or whirling this usually indicates a vestibular disorder. If the patient describes symptoms of fading off or blacking out this is usually caused by an insufficient blood supply to the brain that results when the blood pressure or heart rate are low.
  ❖ Determine any associated activities, such as with exercise or when rising from a sitting position.
  ❖ Usually occurs when systolic blood pressure becomes less than 70 mmHg.

Chapter 2

Past Medical History

- Provides information about past events including chronic illnesses, surgeries and procedures.
- Review all systems
  - Neurological:
    - Cerebral vascular accident (stroke).
    - Transient ischemic attacks (TIA).
  - Pulmonary:
    - Primary lung disease (COPD, asthma, bronchitis).
  - Cardiovascular
    - Coronary Artery Disease:
      - Myocardial infarction
      - Angina
      - Percutaneous balloon angioplasty with or without intracoronary stent placement
      - Cardiac surgery.
    - Rheumatic heart disease.
    - Endocarditis.
    - Heart Failure:
      - Biventricular Pacemaker
      - Weight history
      - Ejection Fraction – if known.
    - Valve disease:
      - Murmur or known valve disease
      - Valve replacement / repair surgery.
    - Cardiac arrhythmias:
      - Pacemaker
      - Implantable cardioverter defibrillator
      - Cardiac Ablation
      - Cardiac Maze Procedure.
    - Peripheral vascular disease:
      - Claudication
      - Angioplasty with stent placement
      - Surgery.
    - Hyperlipidemia, dyslipidemia.
- Gastrointestinal
  - Appetite.
  - Ulcers.
  - GI Bleeding.
  - Chronic disorders.

Cardiovascular Assessment

- ◆ Genitourinary
  - ❖ Kidney disease.
  - ❖ Renal insufficiency.
  - ❖ Urination difficulties.
  - ❖ Menstruation/menopause.
- ◆ Endocrine
  - ❖ Diabetes mellitus:
    - ★ Type I.
    - ★ Type II.
  - ❖ Thyroid disease.
- ◆ Connective tissue disorders .
- ◆ Bleeding disorders.
- ◆ Anemia.
- ◆ Traumatic Injuries/Surgeries.
- ◆ Other hospitalizations not covered.
- ◆ Current Medications:
  - ❖ Include over the counter medications.
  - ❖ Include compliance with medication regime.
  - ❖ Determine patient's understanding of medications.
- ◆ Current vitamin or herbal supplements.
- ◆ Recreational drug use.
- ◆ Alcohol use.
- ◆ Allergies to medication and other substances and associated reactions.
- ◆ Immunizations: flu and pneumonia.

Risk Factor Profile
(See Chapter 7 for full discussion)

- ◆ Smoking
  - ❖ Packs per day and years of smoking.
- ◆ Cholesterol Level.
- ◆ Activity.
- ◆ Weight.
- ◆ Dietary patterns.
- ◆ Stress.

Family History for Cardiovascular Disease
(Include onset of disease process in family members)

- ◆ Include parents, siblings and children.
- ◆ Coronary artery disease.
- ◆ Cerebral vascular disease.
- ◆ Peripheral vascular disease.
- ◆ Diabetes mellitus.
- ◆ Hypertension.

41

Chapter 2

Social History

- Smoking.
- Alcohol use.
- Recreational drug use.
- Occupation.
- Stress level.
- Exercise habits.
- Dietary habits.
- Sleep patterns.
- Financial concerns.
- Barriers to learning.
- Education level.
- Learning preference.
- Cultural factors.
- Home situation.
    - Who does patient live with?
    - Is patient in a safe environment?
    - Is patient able to care for self?
    - Is patient capable of following medication regime?
    - If assistance is required, who is available to assist?
    - Are there any transportation needs?
    - Who provides meals? Is assistance needed?
    - What assistive devices are at home and what are needed?
        - Home oxygen.
        - Glucometer.
        - Scale.
        - Walker.

PHYSICAL ASSESSMENT

Utilizing a systematic approach to the cardiovascular physical assessment helps assure a complete assessment. As with any patient contact, the assessment should be completed with respect and recognition for patient privacy. The examiner should assure the patient and make him or her aware of what is to occur as the assessment progresses. The room should be quiet, and it is best if the examiner stands on the right side of the patient, as this is the best position for assessing heart sounds and jugular venous distention. The physical assessment starts with an overall visual assessment of the patient that usually occurs as the examiner is making an initial introduction to the patient. The examiner determines if the patient appears physically ill, appears his or her stated age, assesses overall alertness, respiratory pattern, body habitus and position, signs of pain and any other obvious signs of illness or distress. This chapter focuses on the cardiovascular assessment. While not all systems are covered in this text, an evaluation of all systems is necessary in a routine assessment, especially those systems associated with the past medical history or chief complaint.

Cardiovascular Assessment

Neurological Assessment

◆ Assessment of mental status may provide information regarding perfusion to the brain.

❖ When a patient demonstrates new signs of neurological deficit, the astute practitioner should assess for adequate perfusion of the brain. A decrease in cardiac output can result in a decreased perfusion to the brain.

◆ Assess for orientation and alertness.

Assessment of the Skin and Mucus Membranes

◆ Color

❖ Skin that is pink indicates adequate perfusion.

❖ Skin that is red, such as the pink to red cheeks of the patient with mitral regurgitation (mitral facieses), may indicate hyperperfusion.

◆ Skin turgor: Tenting is an indication of dehydration. Skin turgor is best assessed on the back of the hand or the forearm.

◆ Skin: Assessment of the skin temperature in conjunction with assessment of the lungs can provide a basic assessment of overall cardiac output. These two parameters together are described in Table 2-1.

Table 2.1 Assessment for Cardiac Perfusion and Pulmonary Congestion	
Warm and Dry No Congestion Normal Perfusion	**Warm and Wet** Congestion Normal Perfusion
Cold and Dry No Congestion Low Perfusion	**Cold and Wet** Congestion Low Perfusion

Nail Beds

◆ Capillary Refill

❖ Pressure is applied to the nail bed until it turns white (blanches).

❖ Once blanching occurs, pressure is released.

❖ Assess for the time it takes for color to return to the nail bed.

❖ Greater than 2 seconds is abnormal and can indicate:

★ Dehydration.

★ Shock.

★ Peripheral vascular disease.

★ Hypothermia.

◆ Clubbing of Fingers

❖ The loss of the normal angle between the nail bed and the skin.

❖ Variety of causes, but usually indicates chronic hypoxia.

❖ Develops over time.

❖ Can indicate pulmonary pathology including pulmonary fibrosis, cystic fibrosis, and interstitial lung disease.

❖ Can indicate cardiac pathology, including cyanotic congenital heart diseases, right-to-left shunting, and bacterial endocarditis.

Chapter 2

- ◆ Splinter hemorrhages
  - ❖ Thin red streaks under the nail beds that run from the base to the tip of the nail.
  - ❖ May indicate infective endocarditis.
- ◆ Osler's Nodes
  - ❖ Small dark pink to reddish-purple raised nodules.
  - ❖ May or may not have a whitish center.
  - ❖ Tender.
  - ❖ Usually found on the pads of the fingers, but may be found on the palms of the hands and the soles of the feet.
  - ❖ May be indicative of infective endocarditis.
- ◆ Janeway Lesions
  - ❖ Small, pink to red macular (flat discoloration) lesion.
  - ❖ Circular or oval in shape.
  - ❖ Non-tender.
  - ❖ Usually found on the palms of the hands and the soles of the feet.
  - ❖ May be indicative of infective endocarditis.

Cyanosis Assessment

- ◆ Central cyanosis
  - ❖ Occurs when more than 5 grams/dL of hemoglobin is deoxygenated.
  - ❖ Results in a bluish or steel-gray discoloration of the skin and mucous membranes. The bluish or steel-gray discoloration of the lips can be from central or peripheral cyanosis, therefore the oral mucosa or the tongue may be better tools for assessment of central cyanosis.
  - ❖ Central cyanosis is usually not seen until oxygen saturation drops to between 73% to 78%.
  - ❖ The absence of cyanosis does not exclude hypoxemia.
- ◆ Peripheral cyanosis
  - ❖ Caused by peripheral vasoconstriction and decreased local blood flow.
  - ❖ May occur with or without central cyanosis (i.e., with or without hypoxemia).
  - ❖ Peripheral cyanosis is usually observed in the nailbeds of the hands or feet, the earlobes or nose.
  - ❖ Peripheral cyanosis should improve with warming.

Vital Signs

- ◆ Temperature
  - ❖ High grade.
  - ❖ Low grade – not usually greater than 38.5° Celsius (101.5° Fahrenheit).
- ◆ Pulse – Heart Rate
  - ❖ Assess rate.
  - ❖ Assess for regularity.
  - ❖ Assess to assure apical and radial pulse rate the same (assures all beats are perfused).
  - ❖ For further discussion about peripheral pulses see extremity assessment.
- ◆ Respirations
  - ❖ Determine rate.
  - ❖ Assess respiratory effort.
    - ☆ Increased work of breathing, with use of accessory muscles, increases myocardial oxygen demand.

Cardiovascular Assessment

◆ Blood Pressure
  ❖ Blood pressure = Cardiac Output x Systemic Vascular Resistance.
  ❖ Systolic: maximum pressure in the arteries when blood is expelled from the left ventricle.
  ❖ Diastolic: represents the pressure in the arteries when the heart is at rest.
  ❖ Pulse Pressure: difference between systolic and diastolic pressure.
    ☆ Pulse pressure can provide good assessment information to the bedside practitioner.
      ✶ Trending of pulse pressure can provide information on cardiac output and volume status during acute illnesses.
      ✶ Assessment of pulse pressure in the patient without an acute illness can also assist in looking for signs of chronic compensation.
    ☆ Narrowed pulse pressure
      ✶ Situations that cause a decrease in cardiac output result in vasoconstriction and a narrowing of the pulse pressure. When cardiac output is compromised the heart rate usually begins to increase as arteries begin to vasoconstriction. This vasoconstriction will be noted by a rise in diastolic blood pressure and a narrowing of the pulse pressure.
      ✶ Pulse pressure may be chronically narrowed by chronic illness or may narrow with acute situations.
      ✶ Trending of pulse pressure over minute to hours may be helpful in assessing slow changes such as a slow loss of blood.
      ✶ Except in situations resulting in a vasodilatory shock, a patient with no blood pressure or very low blood pressure is experiencing vasoconstriction and therefore an increase in cardiac afterload.
      ✶ Situations that may cause the pulse pressure to narrow:
        – Vasoconstriction.
        – Dehydration.
        – Bleeding.
        – Cardiac Tamponade.
        – Mechanical obstruction to forward flow: aortic stenosis, mitral stenosis.
        – Backward flow of blood: acute aortic or acute mitral regurgitation.
    ☆ Widened pulse pressure
      ✶ As cardiac output increases the walls of the arterial vessels relax and pulse pressure widens.
      ✶ Situations that cause the pulse pressure to widen:
        – Vasodilation.
        – Fluid overload situations.
        – Aging / athersclerosis.
          • As the aorta becomes stiffer with age the systolic blood pressure rises, which is seen in isolated systolic hypertension.
        – Disease processes causing increased cardiac output:
          • Chronic aortic regurgitation.
  ❖ Assess blood pressure in both arms during initial assessment to detect differences.
  ❖ Utilize proper technique.
    ☆ Assure proper cuff size and location.
      ✶ Ideal width 40% of the circumference of the arm.

45

Chapter 2

* Cuff too small: falsely elevated blood pressure measurement.

* Cuff too large: falsely decreased blood pressure measurement.

☆ Support arm at heart level.

☆ Palpate brachial or radial artery while inflating the cuff.

☆ Once brachial pulse is obliterated, inflate the cuff 20-30 mm Hg more before deflating the cuff.

* Prevents over inflation of cuff, causing undue patient discomfort.

* Assures missing any auscultatory gap. This gap is noted as a period of abnormal silence that usually occurs shortly after the first appearance of Korotkoff sounds. This gap is often associated with atherosclerosis and noted in patients with hypertension.

☆ Variation of up to 10-15mm Hg between arms is a normal variant. Greater than 15 mm Hg indicates lower flow to arm with lower reading.

❖ BP in lower extremities is higher than blood pressure in the arms – as much as 10 mm Hg difference is normal.

❖ Orthostatic blood pressure should be assessed on the patients at risk, especially those with complaints of dizziness or syncope.

☆ Assesses homeostatic control of the blood pressure and heart rate in making the required adjustments for position changes.

☆ Orthostatic hypotension is a systolic fall of at least 20 mm Hg or a diastolic fall of at least 10 mm Hg within three minutes of standing.

☆ Procedure for assessing orthostatic blood pressure:

* All requirements for normal blood pressure assessment should be followed including cuff size, arm position etc.

* Measure lying blood pressure after the patient has been supine for a minimum of 5 minutes.

* Stand the patient. Measure the blood pressure after the patient has been standing for one minute.

* If the patient can continue to stand, measure the blood pressure at 3 minutes and again at five minutes.

* Note any symptoms the patient experiences.

* If the patient is unable to stand for 3 minutes measure the blood pressure at 1 and 2 minutes if able.

* Record the blood pressure, any symptoms and the time intervals of the standing pressures.

☆ Orthostatic hypotension results from many things including:

* Volume depletion.

* Autonomic insufficiency.

* Vasomotor abnormality.

Jugular Vein Evaluation

◆ Reflects volume and pressure in the right atrium.

◆ Total blood volume, distribution of blood volume, and right atrial contraction influence right atrial and central venous pressure (CVP).

◆ Venous return to the heart is non-pulsatile.

◆ Changes in flow and pressure caused by right atrial filling and pressure produces backward pulsations that are reflected in the central venous system and ultimately the jugular veins.

◆ To determine Jugular Venous **Distention** (JVD) (Figure 2.2).

Cardiovascular Assessment

- ❖ Elevate the head of the bed approximately 30-45 degrees.
  - ★ With the head of the bed elevated to 30-45 degrees the external jugular vein pulsation is normally seen to 1-3 cm above the angle of Louis (sternal angle), which is located where the manubrium and the body of the sternum meet at approximately the second rib.
  - ★ This angle also allows for differentiation of the internal jugular vein from the carotid artery. Pulsations from the internal jugular vein are different than the easily recognizable arterial pulsation in the carotid artery.
- ❖ Raise the level of the bed to a position that is comfortable and will provide good visualization of the neck veins.
- ❖ Stand on the right side of the patient with the patient's head turned slightly to the left.
- ❖ Expose the neck and the upper shoulders to allow for clear evaluation of the neck veins.
- ❖ An adequate light source with a strong beam of light should be used to allow for visualization of the highest point of venous pulsations. The light should be directed tangentially (allowing the light to silhouette or shadow the pulsations) at approximately a 45 degree angle from the right shoulder across the right side of the neck to the patient's midline.
- ❖ Slight elevation of the patient's chin may help in the visualization of the neck veins.
- ❖ If unable to differentiate venous pulse from arterial pulse placing the right thumb or index finger across the base of the neck with light pressure should obliterate the venous pulse and cause the veins to fill and distend.
- ❖ JVD should be assessed during expiration as JVD decreases during inspiration.
- ❖ Measure the distance (in centimeters) from the angle of Louis (horizontal line) to the top of the column of blood (vertical line) in the distended neck vein.
- ❖ Normal JVD at a 30-45 degree angle is 1-3 cm above the sternal angle.

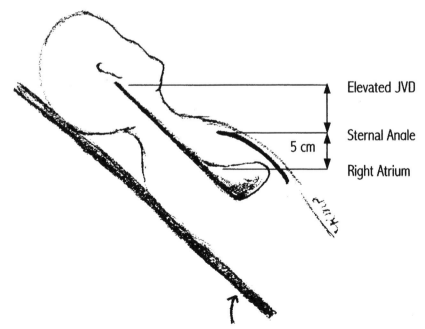

Figure 2.2: Assessment of JVD.

Chapter 2

◆ To determine Jugular Venous **Pressure** (JVP)
  ❖ JVP is an estimate of central venous pressure (CVP) or right atrial pressure (RA pressure).
  ❖ The angle of Louis is 5 cm above the midpoint of the right atrium (which is considered to be 0 cm).
  ❖ Adding this 5 cm to the measured JV**D** will provide an estimated JV**P** or CVP.
  ❖ For example: JVD of 3 cm + 5 cm = estimated JVP or CVP of 8 cm.
  ❖ Estimated CVP > 8 cm indicates elevated right atrial pressures.
    ☆ Increased preload / hypervolemia.
    ☆ Right ventricular failure.
    ☆ Tricuspid valve regurgitation.
    ☆ Pulmonary hypertension.
    ☆ Pericardial effusion/ cardiac tamponade.
    ☆ Superior vena caval obstruction (tumor).
  ❖ Conversely, flat neck veins in a supine position suggest hypovolemia.

Hepatojugular Reflux (HJR)
(Abdominojugular Reflux)

◆ Additional assessment for increased volume or pressure.
◆ An evaluation of neck vein distention occurs while assessing HJR so patient position is the same as with JVD assessment.
◆ Apply firm pressure over the liver (right upper quadrant of the abdomen) for approximately 30 seconds.
◆ A more pronounced rise in JVD indicates a positive test.
◆ Positive HJR indicates:
  ❖ Increased preload/hypervolemia.
  ❖ Right ventricular failure.

Cardiac (Precordial) Examination
◆ Palpation
  ❖ Identify the point of maximal impulse (PMI) – apical impulse.
    ☆ Identifies the apex of the heart.
    ☆ Left ventricle contracts and rotates forward during ventricular systole, causing the left ventricular wall to come in contact with the chest wall.
    ☆ Left ventricular apex is normally located at the 5th intercostal space, midclavicular line.
    ☆ Assess for PMI: stand on the patient's right side and place right palm on patient's chest, with heel of palm resting on the sternum, and fingertips below the nipple. *Note:* In female patients, the examiners hand must be placed beneath the patient's breast with the lateral wall of the index finger next to the inferior surface of the left breast. Special care should be taken to explain the examination to the patient prior to proceeding.
    ☆ The normal apical impulse can be covered by one finger.
    ☆ Note location of impulse.
      ✳ Enlarged left ventricle, as seen with left ventricular hypertrophy, aortic insufficiency, mitral regurgitation, etc. shifts the PMI down and to the left.
      ✳ Enlarged right ventricle as seen with right ventricular hypertrophy, pulmonary hypertension etc. shifts the PMI towards the mediastinum.

48

Cardiovascular Assessment

   ★ Not always able to palpate, especially with obesity and COPD.
       ✳ Placing patient in the left lateral decubitus position may enhance PMI.
   ★ Note intensity of impulse.
       ✳ PMI is normally a light pulsation.
       ✳ Increases with failure.
       ✳ Increases with chronic disease processes that result in hyperdynamic cardiac output, such as mitral regurgitation, aortic insufficiency, or ventricular hypertrophy.
       ✳ May increase with fever, anemia, hyperthyroidism and anxiety.
   ★ Thrill
       ✳ Palpable version of a murmur.
       ✳ Vibration that represents turbulence of blood.
       ✳ Usually felt with a grade 4/6 or greater murmur.
       ✳ May be present without an audible murmur, and a murmur may be present without a palpable thrill.
       ✳ Presence of a thrill without a murmur may indicate that a condition that can cause a murmur is present.

Heart Sounds – Auscultation

◆ Examination
   ❖ Best accomplished in a quiet room.
   ❖ Eliminate as many extraneous sounds as possible.
◆ Stethoscope
   ❖ Bell:
      ★ To assess low pitched sounds.
      ★ Utilize very light to no pressure.
      ★ Should listen at least 5 seconds at a site to appreciate low pitched sounds.
   ❖ Diaphragm:
      ★ To assess high pitched sounds.
      ★ Utilize firm pressure.
◆ Sounds are produced by vibrations from the heart walls, valves and turbulent blood flow.

The Cardiac Cycle

◆ Understanding the cardiac cycle and the opening and closing of the cardiac valves in relation to systole and diastole is key to understanding heart sounds.
◆ Atrial and Ventricular Diastole (A of Figure 2.3): passive ventricular filling from atrium.
   ❖ At the beginning of ventricular diastole as ventricular pressure falls below atrial pressure, the tricuspid and mitral valves open.
   ❖ Blood flows through the open tricuspid and mitral valves and begins to fill the ventricles.
   ❖ Also referred to as early diastolic filling time or early diastole.
   ❖ Pulmonic and aortic valves are closed.
◆ Atrial Systole (B of Figure 2.3): active ventricular filling with atrial contraction
   ❖ Atria contract to eject the remainder of their contents into the ventricles.
   ❖ Contraction know as "atrial kick."

49

- ❖ Also referred to as late diastolic filling time.
- ❖ Pulmonary and aortic valves remain closed, while tricuspid and mitral valves are open.
- ◆ Early Ventricular Systole (C of Figure 2.3): isovolumic contraction.
  - ❖ Walls of the ventricles begin to contract and the pressure in the ventricles becomes greater than the pressure in the atria, causing the tricuspid and mitral valves to close.
  - ❖ Contraction of the walls of the ventricles increases pressure in the ventricles.
  - ❖ All valves are closed for a brief moment.
  - ❖ Once pressure in ventricles becomes greater than the pressure on the other side of the pulmonic and aortic valves, the valves are forced open.
- ◆ Ventricular Systole (D of Figure 2.3): ejection.
  - ❖ Blood is ejected from the ventricles through the open pulmonic and aortic valves
- ◆ Ventricular Diastole
  - ❖ After ejection occurs the pressure in the ventricles becomes less than the pressure in the pulmonary and peripheral vascular systems and the pulmonic and aortic valves close.
  - ❖ As the ventricles relax, ventricular pressure falls below atrial pressure, causing the tricuspid and mitral valves to open. The cycle begins again.

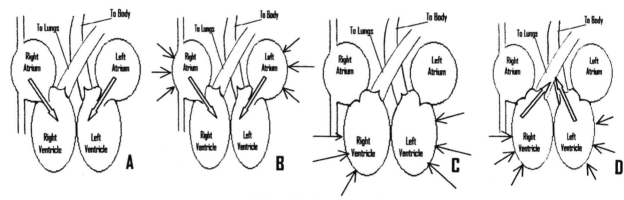

Figure 2.3: Cardiac cycle.

Auscultatory Areas (Figure 2.4)

- ◆ Locations where specific sounds are best heard.
  - ❖ Auscultation at all sites is necessary, as not all sounds are audible throughout the precordium.
  - ❖ Different sites offer different advantages.
  - ❖ Correlate with valves of the heart.
  - ❖ Auscultatory sites.
    - ★ Aortic Area
      - ∗ 2nd intercostal space right of the sternal border.
      - ∗ Sounds associated with aortic valve and aorta.
    - ★ Pulmonic Area
      - ∗ 2nd intercostal space left of the sternal border.
      - ∗ Sounds associated with pulmonic valve and pulmonary artery.

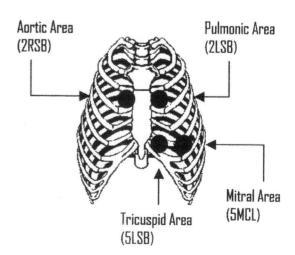

Figure 2.4: Auscultatory sites.

Cardiovascular Assessment

☆ Tricuspid Area

　　✱ 5th intercostal space left of the sternal border.

　　✱ Sounds associated with tricuspid valve and right ventricle.

☆ Mitral Area

　　✱ 5th intercostal space left midclavicular line.

　　✱ Sounds associated with mitral valve and left ventricle.

☆ Erb's Point

　　✱ 3rd intercostal space left of the sternal border.

　　✱ Not associated with a valve.

　　✱ Can often hear sound associated with aortic or pulmonic valve areas.

Characteristics of Heart Sounds

◆ Location

　❖ Anatomical area where sound is best heard.

◆ Intensity

　❖ Loudness or softness during auscultation.

　❖ Subjective data.

　❖ Can be affected by body habitus.

　❖ Can be affected by pathology, such as pericardial fluid.

　❖ Can be affected by velocity of blood flow.

◆ Duration

　❖ Length of time the sound is heard.

◆ Pitch

　❖ Refers to the frequency of the sound.

　❖ Sounds are usually low, medium or high pitched.

◆ Quality

　❖ Description of the sound.

　❖ Sharp, dull, harsh, blowing, musical, booming.

◆ Timing

　❖ Relates the timing of the sound to the cardiac cycle.

General Heart Sound Principles

◆ Right-sided heart sounds are heard better during inspiration.

◆ Left-sided heart sounds are heard better during expiration.

◆ Events on the left side of the heart occur before events on the right side of the heart.

First and Second Heart Sounds – S1 and S2

First Heart Sound – S1 "Lub Dub"

◆ Closure of the mitral and tricuspid valves.

◆ Beginning of ventricular systole and atrial diastole.

◆ Palpate the carotid pulse to assist with identification of S1. S1 occurs just before the carotid impulse.

◆ Location: heard best at mitral area – at the heart's apex.

- Intensity: directly related to force of contraction.
  - Louder with tachycardia or mitral stenosis.
- Duration: short.
- Quality: dull.
- Pitch: high.
- Split S1.
  - Mitral valve closes before tricuspid valve, but closure is usually heard as one sound. Referred as a normal split S1 if both sounds are heard.
  - Best heard over tricuspid area.
  - Abnormal split S1 (widened) occurs when activation of right sided events are delayed such as with late closure of tricuspid valve, right bundle branch block, or left ventricular pacing.
  - Split S1 usually becomes more prominent on inspiration.

Second Heart Sound – S2 "Lub Dub" (Figure 2.5)

- Closure of aortic and pulmonic valves.
- End of ventricular systole; beginning of ventricular diastole.
- Location: pulmonic area (or Erb's point).
- Intensity: directly related to closing pressure in the aorta and pulmonary artery.
- Duration: shorter than S1.
- Quality: booming.
- Pitch: high.
- Physiologic splitting of S2

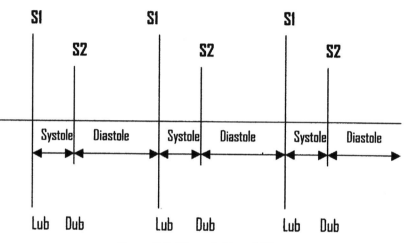

Figure 2.5: Normal S1 and S2.

  - Present during inspiration and not easily audible during expiration.
  - Inspiration causes increased venous return to heart, prolonging right ventricular systole and delaying closure of pulmonic valve.
  - Aortic valve closes before pulmonic valve.
  - Best heard at pulmonic area or Erb's point (4th intercostal space, left sternal border).
  - Referred as a physiological split S2.
  - Abnormal split S2 (audible during both inspiration and expiration).
    - Severe pulmonic stenosis, pulmonary hypertension, systemic hypertension.

Third and Fourth Heart Sounds – S3 and S4

- Ventricular diastolic filling sounds.
- Low frequency sounds.
- Produced by ventricular filling rather than valve closure.
- Normal in children and young adults.

Cardiovascular Assessment

Third Heart Sound – S3 "Lub DubDa" (Figure 2.6)
- Ventricular Gallop.
- Occurs during early ventricular diastole (Figure 2.8).
- Caused by increased atrial or ventricular pressure or resistance to filling. Most frequently associated with systolic dysfunction.
- Results from increased blood volume or increased resistance.
- Associated with right or left ventricular failure, ischemia, aortic regurgitation, mitral regurgitation or systolic dysfunction.
- May be normal in young children or during pregnancy.
- Left- or right-sided S3, depending on the ventricle affected.
- Best heard with patient in left lateral decubitus position.
- Location
  - Left-sided S3 – mitral area.
  - Right-sided S3 – tricuspid area.
- Intensity
  - Left-sided heard best during expiration.
  - Right-sided heard best during inspiration.
- Duration: short.
- Quality: dull, thud like.
- Pitch: low.
- May be normal in children, young adults (up to 35-40) and in the 3rd trimester of pregnancy.

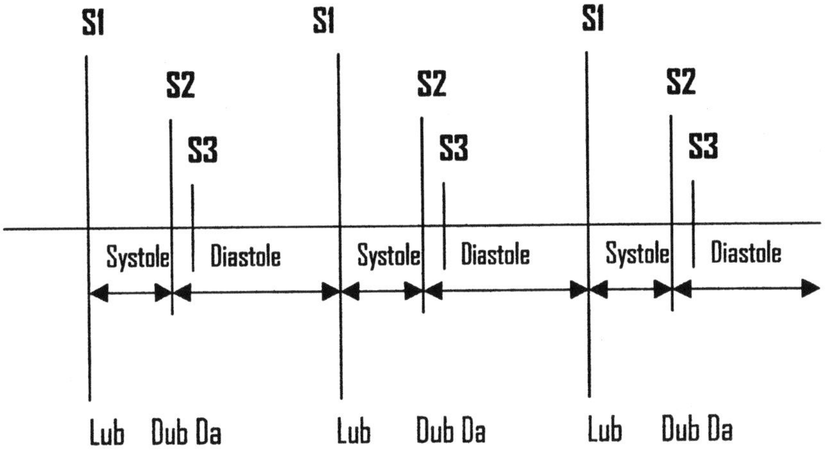

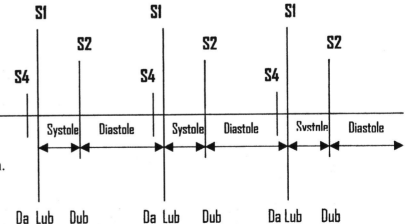

Figure 2.6: S1, S2 and S3.

Fourth Heart Sound – S4 "DaLub Dub" (Figure 2.7)
- Atrial gallop.
- Occurs during late ventricular diastole (Figure 2.8).
- Caused by atrial contraction and the propulsion of blood into a noncompliant (stiff) ventricle.
- Associated with systemic hypertension, restrictive cardiomyopathy, ischemia, aortic stenosis.
- May be normal in athletes.
- Left- or right-sided, depending on ventricle affected.
- Best heard with patient in left lateral decubitus position.
- Location
  - Left-sided S4 – mitral area.
  - Right-sided S4 – tricuspid area.
- Intensity
  - Left-sided louder on expiration.
  - Right-sided louder on inspiration.
- Duration: short.
- Quality: thudlike.
- Pitch: low.

Figure 2.7: S4, S1, and S2.

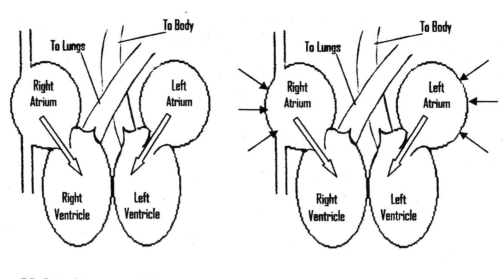

Figure 2.8: Early ventricular systole and Late ventricular diastole.

Summation Gallop (Figure 2.9)
- Some patients may have an S3 and S4, which result in what is referred to as a quadruple rhythm.
- If the heart rate is elevated (>100 beats per minute), the S3 and S4 merge as diastolic filling time decreases, resulting in a summation gallop.
- Results in single 3rd heart sound.
- Best heard with patient in left lateral decubitus position.
- Location
  - Left-sided S4 – mitral area.
  - Right-sided S4 – tricuspid area.
- Intensity: louder than an S3 or S4.
- Pitch: low.

Murmur Fundamentals
- Caused by turbulence of blood (Figure 2.10).
- Murmur: If turbulence is intracardiac.
- Bruit: If turbulence is extra cardiac.
- Stenotic Murmurs
  - Valve does not open appropriately.
  - Heard during the part of the cardiac cycle when the valve is open.
  - Heard when there is difficulty with forward flow through an open valve.

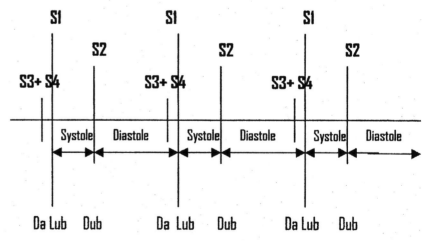

Figure 2.9: Summation gallop.

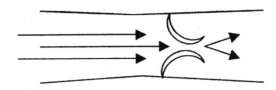
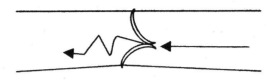

Forward flow through a stenotic valve.   Backward flow through an incompetent valve.

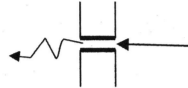

Flow through a septal defect or an AV fistula.   Flow into a dilated chamber or a portion of a vessel.

Figure 2.10: Drawing demonstrating turbulence of flow.

- ◆ Regurgitant Murmurs
    - ❖ Valve does not close appropriately.
    - ❖ Heard during the part of the cardiac cycle when the valve is to be closed.
    - ❖ Heard when there is backward flow through a valve that is not closing properly.
- ◆ Murmur Timing
    - ❖ Systolic:
        - ★ Holosystolic
        - ★ Ejection (midsystolic)
        - ★ Late.
    - ❖ Diastolic:
        - ★ Early
        - ★ Mid-diastolic
        - ★ Late.
- ◆ Murmur Location
    - ❖ Place murmur is heard the loudest.
- ◆ Radiation
    - ❖ Direction in which murmur radiates.
- ◆ Murmur Configuration
    - ❖ Crescendo: gets louder.
    - ❖ Decrescendo: gets softer.
    - ❖ Crescendo-decrescendo: gets louder then softer.
    - ❖ Plateau: even intensity throughout.

- Murmur Quality Descriptors
  - Soft.
  - Harsh.
  - Blowing.
  - Musical.
  - Rumbling.
  - Rough.
- Murmur Grading: Grade 1-6 Scale
  - Grade 1/6: faint, may be heard intermittently.
  - Grade 2/6: faint, usually heard as soon as stethoscope is placed on the chest.
  - Grade 3/6: easily heard, described as moderately loud.
  - Grade 4/6: loud, thrill (palpable vibration) present.
  - Grade 5/6: loud enough to be heard with only the edge of the stethoscope on the chest wall; almost always with a thrill; usually radiates.
  - Grade 6/6: loud enough to be heard with stethoscope close to but not touching chest wall; thrill present; radiates.

Systolic Murmurs

- Murmurs heard during ventricular systole.
- Most common systolic murmurs represent mitral regurgitation or aortic stenosis.
- Not all systolic murmurs represent pathological conditions. Some systolic murmurs referred to as "Innocent Systolic Murmurs" occur with when there is turbulence of blood through a normal valve.
- Located between S1 and S2.
- Tricuspid and mitral valves closed during ventricular systole.
  - Valves do not close completely.
  - Tricuspid regurgitation.
  - Mitral regurgitation.
- Pulmonic and aortic valves open during ventricular systole.
  - Valves do not open properly.
  - Pulmonic stenosis.
  - Aortic stenosis.

Aortic Stenosis Murmur (Figure 2.11)

- Systolic ejection murmur.
- Timing: mid systolic. This is an ejection murmur. Ejection occurs after isovolumic contraction, which is the earliest part of systole.
- Location: best heard over aortic area.
- Radiation: toward right side of neck.

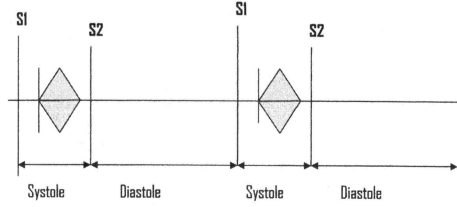

Figure 2.11: Murmur configuration for aortic or pulmonic stenosis.

- ◆ Configuration: crescendo-decrescendo.
- ◆ Pitch: medium to high.
- ◆ Quality: harsh.

Pulmonic Stenosis Murmur (Figure 2.11)
- ◆ Systolic ejection murmur.
- ◆ Timing: mid systolic. This is an ejection murmur. Ejection occurs after isovolumic contraction, which is the earliest part of systole.
- ◆ Location: best heard over pulmonic area.
- ◆ Radiation: left neck or left shoulder.
- ◆ Configuration: crescendo-decrescendo.
- ◆ Pitch: medium.
- ◆ Quality: harsh.

Tricuspid Regurgitation Murmur (Figure 2.12)
- ◆ Timing: holosystolic.
- ◆ Location: best heard over tricuspid area.
- ◆ Radiation: to the right of the sternum.
- ◆ Configuration: plateau.
- ◆ Pitch: high.
- ◆ Quality: scratchy or blowing.

Mitral Regurgitation Murmur (Figure 2.12)
- ◆ Timing: holosystolic.
- ◆ Location: best heard over mitral area.
- ◆ Radiation: to the left axilla.
- ◆ Configuration: plateau.
- ◆ Pitch: high.
- ◆ Quality: blowing, harsh or musical.

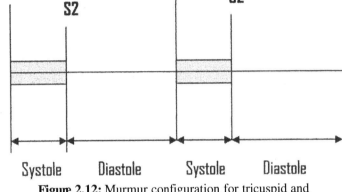

Figure 2.12: Murmur configuration for tricuspid and mitral regurgitation.

Diastolic Murmurs

- ◆ Murmurs heard during ventricular diastole.
- ◆ Diastolic murmurs are different from systolic murmurs as they do represent a pathological condition associated with the murmur. There are no "innocent" diastolic murmurs.
- ◆ Diastolic murmurs are more serious than systolic murmurs.
- ◆ Diastolic murmurs are never normal.
- ◆ Pulmonic and aortic valves closed during ventricular diastole.
    - ❖ Valves do not close properly.
    - ❖ Pulmonic regurgitation.
    - ❖ Aortic regurgitation.
- ◆ Tricuspid and mitral valves open during ventricular diastole.
    - ❖ Valves do not open properly.
    - ❖ Tricuspid stenosis.
    - ❖ Mitral stenosis.

Chapter 2

Pulmonic Regurgitation (Figure 2.13)
- Timing: early diastole.
- Location: best heard over pulmonic area.
- Radiation: towards apex.
- Configuration: decrescendo.
- Pitch: high.
- Quality: blowing.

Aortic Regurgitation (Figure 2.13)
- Timing: early diastole.
- Location: best heard over aortic area.
- Radiation: towards apex.
- Configuration: decrescendo.
- Pitch: high.
- Quality: blowing.

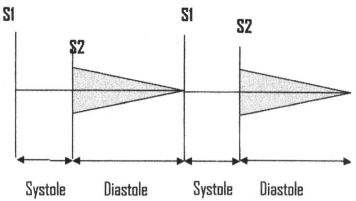
Figure 2.13: Murmur configuration for aortic or pulmonic regurgitation.

Tricuspid Stenosis (Figure 2.14)
- Timing: mid to late diastole.
- Location: best heard over tricuspid area.
- Radiation: none.
- Configuration: Begins with an opening snap. Cresendo-decrescendo with late crescendo (from atrial kick if in normal sinus rhythm).
- Pitch: low.
- Quality: rumbling.
- Increases during inspiration.

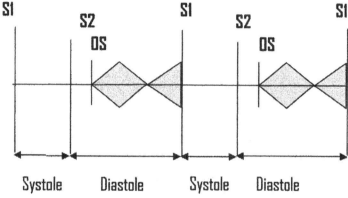
Figure 2.14: Murmur configuration for tricuspid stenosis.

Mitral Stenosis (Figure 2.15)
- Timing: mid to late diastole.
- Begins with an opening snap (OS).
- Location: best heard over mitral area.
- Radiation: none.
- Configuration: Begins with an opening snap with a late crescendo (from atrial kick if in normal sinus rhythm).
- Pitch: low.
- Quality: rumbling.

Other Cardiac Sounds
Pericardial Friction Rub
- Timing: systolic and early and late diastolic.
- Location: best heard over tricuspid or xyphoid areas.
- Radiation: may be heard across precordium.
- Pitch: high.
- Quality: grating, scratching.

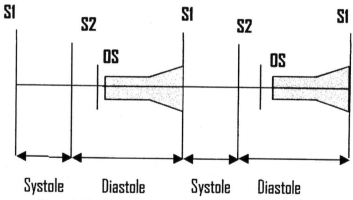
Figure 2.15: Murmur configuration for mitral stenosis.

♦ Increases with inspiration.

♦ May only last a few hours.

♦ Commonly heard after cardiac surgery and with large myocardial infarctions.

Ventricular Septal Defect or Rupture

♦ Timing: continuous.

♦ Location: 3rd or 4th intercostal space left of the sternum.

♦ Radiation: widely throughout the precordium.

♦ Configuration: plateau.

♦ Pitch: high.

♦ Quality: harsh.

Papillary Muscle Rupture

♦ Sudden onset.

♦ Same as murmur of mitral regurgitation.

Examination of Extremities

General Examination

♦ Note extremity color and temperature; look for symmetry.

♦ Note alteration in extremity skin condition: petechiae, jaundice, rashes, ulcerations.

Edema

♦ Note location of edema.

♦ Edema may be in dependent locations, such as the sacrum in the recumbent patient.

♦ Dependent edema is a sign of right ventricular failure.

♦ Can have multiple causes.

❖ Cardiac.

❖ Right ventricular failure.

❖ Constrictive pericarditis.

❖ Restrictive cardiomyopathy.

❖ Tricuspid valve disease.

♦ Pulmonary

❖ COPD.

❖ Pulmonary hypertension.

♦ Renal

❖ Renal failure.

❖ Nephrotic syndrome.

♦ Venous

❖ Deep vein thrombosis.

❖ Venous insufficiency.

♦ Miscellaneous

❖ Angioedema from an allergic reaction (usually facial).

❖ Burns.

❖ Liver Failure.

❖ Lymphedema.

Chapter 2

- ❖ Malnutrition.
- ❖ Myxedema.
- ❖ Increased capillary permeability.
- ❖ Proteinuria.
- ◆ Evaluated on a 4-point scale.
- ◆ 0 = None present.
- ◆ 1+ = 0 to ¼ inch   Trace.
- ◆ 2+ = ¼ to ½ inch   Mild.
- ◆ 3+ = ½ to 1 inch   Moderate.
- ◆ 4+ = > than 1 inch   Severe.
- ◆ Described as pitting or non-pitting.
- ◆ Anasarca: generalized edema.

Pulses

- ◆ Multiple locations
  - ❖ Carotid, radial, brachial, femoral, popliteal, posterior tibial, dorsalis pedis.
- ◆ Evaluate for
  - ❖ Presence.
  - ❖ Laterality.
  - ❖ Strength:
    - ★ 4 point scale (0-3).
    - ★ 0 = absent.
    - ★ 1+ = Palpable but thready and weak, easily obliterated.
    - ★ 2+ = Normal, easily identified, not easily obliterated.
    - ★ 3+ = Full, bounding, cannot obliterate.
  - ❖ Symmetry.
  - ❖ Alteration in pulse contour
    - ★ Pulsus Magnus:
      - ✳ Strong and bounding.
      - ✳ Rapid upstroke and downstroke.
      - ✳ Considered to be brisk.
      - ✳ Readily palpable.
      - ✳ Observed in patients with: hypertension, aortic regurgitation, thyrotoxicosis, patent ductus arteriosus, AV fistula.
    - ★ Pulsus Parvus:
      - ✳ Small pulse.
      - ✳ Weak.
      - ✳ Often referred to as "thready."
      - ✳ Observed in patients with: aortic or mitral stenosis, constrictive pericarditis, cardiac tamponade.
    - ★ Pulsus Alternans (Figure 2.16):
      - ✳ Large amplitude pulse, followed by a low amplitude pulse during a regular rhythm.
      - ✳ Observed in patients with left ventricular failure.

Cardiovascular Assessment

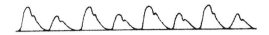

Figure 2.16: Configuration of pulsus alternans.

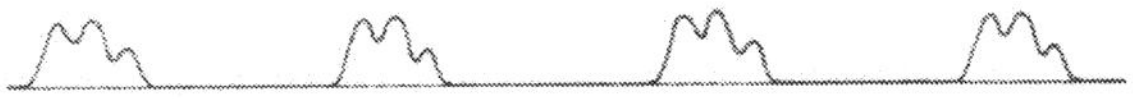

Figure 2.17: Configuration of bisferiens pulse.

- ☆ Pulsus Bisferiens (double peaked) (Figure 2.17):
    - ✱ Double peaked systolic impulse.
    - ✱ Observed in patients with hypertrophic cardiomyopathy, constrictive cardiomyopathy, aortic stenosis.
- ☆ Water-Hammer Pulse:
    - ✱ Rapidly rising and collapsing.
    - ✱ Common in patients with aortic regurgitation.

Arterial vs. Venous Disease

- ◆ See Table 2.2 for differentiation.

Table 2.2
Clinical Differentiation of Venous and Arterial Disease

	Arterial	Venous
Color	Ruddy when dependent Pale when elevated	Cyanotic when dependent
Temperature	Cool	Normal
Pulses	Diminished to absent	Present
Pain	Acute Occlusion: Severe to excruciating Chronic Occlusion: Intermittent claudication	Aching
Edema	Absent	Present
Skin Variations	Thin and shiny Loss of hair Thick toenails	Brown pigmentation at the ankles
Ulcerations	Toes At the site of an traumatic injury	Side of ankles

Signs of Acute Limb Ischemia – The 6 P's

- ◆ Pain
    - ❖ Not impacted by dependency.
    - ❖ May be decreased if collaterals are present.
- ◆ Paralysis.
- ◆ Parathesias.
- ◆ Pulselessness (pulses may be present if there is microembolization).
- ◆ Pallor (pallor early – followed by cyanosis if left untreated).
- ◆ Polar (cold) – unilateral.

Chapter 2

Other Assessment Considerations

There are special considerations in the physical assessment of the elderly, based on expected changes with the aging process. Some of these anticipated changes include: 1) increased systolic blood pressure, 2) risk of orthostatic hypotension, 3) decline in short term memory, 4) altered gait, 5) increased sensitivity to medications, 6) thinning of skin, 7) decreased appetite, and 8) decreased renal function.

Assessment is the primary starting point for developing a comprehensive plan of care. A diligent and complete assessment is the key to discovery.

Linking Knowledge to Practice

✔ *When questioning the patient about cardiac pain, remember to use descriptors other than "pain." Often the discomfort is pressure or heaviness, and the patient will deny pain.*

✔ *Cardiac pain does not usually change with movement or a deep breath.*

✔ *If the patient does not experience relief of chest pain from the nitroglycerin tablet taken at home, but does experience relief of chest pain with a nitroglycerin tablet provided by the paramedic or hospital, assess the age of the nitroglycerin that patient had at home. It may be necessary to provide the patient with education regarding nitroglycerin storage and replacement.*

✔ *Skin temperature and neurological status are two quick ways to assess perfusion.*

✔ *Blood pressure is another simple way to assess perfusion and fluid status. A narrowed pulse pressure is a sign of volume depletion and decreased perfusion, while a widened pulse pressure can indicate normal volume status with normal or increased perfusion.*

✔ *Careful auscultation of heart sounds may provide early clues to valvular heart disease.*

✔ *The systolic murmurs of mitral regurgitation and aortic stenosis are the most frequently heard murmurs.*

TEST YOUR KNOWLEDGE

1. When assessing chest pain which of the following is not a common characteristic of discomfort caused by angina?

    a. Discomfort that is precipitated by exertion.

    b. Discomfort that is described as pressure or tightness.

    c. Discomfort is intermittent and comes and goes (lasting about 30 seconds).

    d. Discomfort that is relieved with rest or nitroglycerin.

2. A patient presents in acute distress with audible crackles 1/2 the way up bilaterally, extremities are cool to the touch, and elevated JVD is present. With this information you would assess his cardiac perfusion and pulmonary congestion status to be which of the following?

    a. No congestion, normal perfusion

    b. Congestion, normal perfusion

    c. Congestion, low perfusion

    d. No congestion, low perfusion

Cardiovascular Assessment

3. Which of the following would lead you to determine the patient has central cyanosis?

    a. A bluish discoloration of the skin and mucous membranes, especially the oral mucosa.

    b. A bluish discoloration of the nailbeds, earlobes, lips or nose.

    c. A bluish discoloration that improves as the patient is warmed.

    d. A bluish discoloration of the lips with normal coloration of the tongue and oral mucosa.

4. After return from a cardiac catheterization you monitor patient vital signs along with groin assessments as per protocol. Your vital signs are as follows:

    10:00am   140/60   Heart Rate 64
    10:15am   140/64   Heart Rate 68
    10:30am   138/68   Heart Rate 70
    10:45am   140/72   Heart Rate 72
    11:00am   140/78   Heart Rate 78
    11:30am   138/84   Heart Rate 82
    12:00 n   138/88   Heart Rate 90

    Your evaluation of the vital signs would lead you to assess for all of the following except:

    a. Groin hematoma

    b. Development of sepsis

    c. Retroperitoneal bleeding

    d. Dehydration

5. Which of the following blood pressure parameters meet criteria for a orthostatic hypotension?

    a. Lying blood pressure of 134/78 with standing blood pressure of 144/78.

    b. Lying blood pressure of 134/78 with standing blood pressure of 134/70.

    c. Lying blood pressure of 134/78 with a standing blood pressure of 124/70.

    d. Lying blood pressure of 134/78 with a standing blood pressure of 114/78.

6. To correctly estimate jugular venous distention, the patient should be placed on his/her back with the head of the bed elevated

    a. 15-35 degrees.

    b. 30-45 degrees.

    c. 45-60 degrees.

    d. None of the above.

7. The cardiologist has documented that your patient's JVD is 5 cm. What is your patient's estimated CVP?

    a. 5

    b. 8

    c. 10

    d. 15

Chapter 2

8. When listening to heart sounds, S1 signifies
   a. beginning of ventricular systole.
   b. beginning of ventricular diastole.
   c. propulsion of blood into a non compliant ventricle.
   d. blood entering an already full ventricle.

9. When listening to heart sounds, S1 signifies
   a. closure of aortic and pulmonic valves.
   b. opening of aortic and pulmonic valves.
   c. opening of mitral and tricuspid valves.
   d. closure of mitral and tricuspid valves.

10. You are caring for a patient in congestive heart failure. An early ventricular diastolic filling sound you would expect to hear would be
    a. Split S1.
    b. Split S2.
    c. S3.
    d. S4.

11. When listening to your patient's heart sounds, you hear a murmur. Upon further assessment you note that the murmur is best heard between S1 and S2. You would identify this murmur as
    a. systolic murmur.
    b. diastolic murmur.
    c. both a and b.
    d. None of the above.

12. As you continue to assess the above noted murmur, you recognize that this murmur could possibly be which of the following?
    a. Aortic regurgitation, pulmonic stenosis, mitral regurgitation, tricuspid stenosis
    b. Aortic regurgitation, pulmonic regurgitation, mitral stenosis, tricuspid stenosis
    c. Aortic stenosis, pulmonic regurgitation, mitral stenosis, tricuspid regurgitation
    d. Aortic stenosis, pulmonic stenosis, mitral regurgitation, tricuspid regurgitation

13. As you continue to assess the above patient's murmur, you note that the murmur is best heard at the 2nd intercostal space right of the sternal border. You identify the murmur as
    a. pulmonic regurgitation.
    b. pulmonic stenosis.
    c. aortic stenosis.
    d. aortic regurgitation.

Cardiovascular Assessment

14. Signs of venous peripheral vascular disease in the legs include:
    a. Brown pigmentation at the ankles, warm legs, open area over the left lateral malleolus
    b. Shiny skin with no hair, pale extremities, pain with ambulation
    c. Normal color, severe pain, open sore at the end of the great toe on the right foot
    d. 2+ Edema, absent pulses, thick toenails, feet become cyanotic when dependent

15. The six P's of acute limb ischemia include all of the following except
    a. pain.
    b. purple.
    c. pulselessness.
    d. polar.

ANSWERS

1.	C	9.	D
2.	C	10.	C
3.	A	11.	A
4.	B	12.	D
5.	D	13.	C
6.	B	14.	A
7.	C	15.	B
8.	A		

REFERENCES

Alspach, J.G. (2006). *Core curriculum for critical care nursing* (6th Ed.). St. Louis: Saunders.

Bloomquist, J. & Love, M.M. (2000). Cardiovascular assessment and diagnostic procedures. In L.D. Urden & K.M. Stacy, (Eds.) *Priorities in critical care nursing* (pp. 99-145). St Louis: Mosby.

The Consensus Committee of the American Autonomic Society and the American Academy of Neurology. Consensus statement on the definition of orthostatic hypotension, pure autonomic failure, and multiple system atrophy. *Neurology 1996;46*:1470.

Darovic, G.O. (2002). *Hemodynamic monitoring: Invasive and noninvasive clinical application* (3rd ed.). Philadelphia: Saunders.

Kumar, V., Abbas. A.K., & Fausto, N. (2005). *Pathologic basis of disease* (7th ed.). Philadelphia: Elsevier Saunders.

Lewis, S.M., Heitkemper, M.M., & Dirksen, S.T. (2004). *Medical surgical nursing: assessment and management of clinical problems* (6th ed.). St. Louis: Mosby.

Chapter 2

Massie, B.M. & Amiodon, T.M. (2004). Heart. In L.M. Tierney, Jr., S.J. McPhee, & M.A. Papadakis, *Current medical diagnosis and treatment* (43rd ed., pp. 315-400). New York: McGraw-Hill.

Moore, K.L. & Dalley, A.F. (1999). *Clinically oriented anatomy* (4th ed.). Philadelphia: Lippincott, Williams and Wilkins.

Morton, P.G., Tucker, T., & Rueden, K.V. (2005). Patient assessment: cardiovascular system. In P.G. Morton, D. Fontaine, C.M. Hudak, & B.M. Gallo, (Eds.), *Critical care nursing: a holistic approach* (8th ed.) (pp. 211-291). Philadelphia: Lippincott, Williams and Wilkins.

CHAPTER 3:
OXYGENATION AND PULMONARY PHYSIOLOGY

OVERVIEW

Control of Breathing

The central nervous system (brain and spinal cord) is key to proper pulmonary function because the respiratory muscles do not contract spontaneously like cardiac muscles. The medulla is the respiratory center of the brain. The respiratory center is located in the reticular formation of the medulla beneath the floor of the 4th ventricle.

Breathing is automatically generated by neurons located in the respiratory control center of the brainstem. This center is responsible for automatic inspiration and expiration, and is able to alter these functions to meet increased metabolic need during exercise and to suppress them during speech or breath holding.

The respiratory control center in the brainstem affects the control of breathing via a final common pathway including:

◆ Spinal cord.

◆ Nervous system innervation of the muscles of respiration (such as phrenic nerve).

◆ Respiratory muscles.

The spontaneous generation of the inspiratory and expiratory cycle can be altered by several factors:

◆ Reflexes in the lungs and airways.

◆ Reflexes in the cardiovascular system.

◆ Receptors in contact with cerebral spinal fluid.

◆ Commands from higher centers in the brain: pons, hypothalamus, centers of speech, other areas of the cortex.

Effective pulmonary function also requires an intact chest wall and functioning muscles of the respiratory system.

Muscles of Inspiration and Expiration

The most important muscle of inspiration is the diaphragm. The diaphragm is a thin, dome-shaped sheet of muscle attached to the lower ribs and spine. Two phrenic nerves that originate from cervical segments 3-5 innervate the diaphragm. If one phrenic nerve is damaged, half of the diaphragm will be paralyzed.

The external intercostal muscles are supplied by the intercostal nerves that branch off the spinal cord at the same level. The external intercostal muscles assist the diaphragm with inspiration.

Expiration is passive during quiet breathing, but is very active during exercise. The abdominal wall muscles are the most important muscles of active expiration. During contraction of these muscles, the diaphragm is pushed up in response to an increase in intra-abdominal pressure. The internal intercostal muscles also assist with active expiration.

Inspiratory muscles

◆ Diaphragm (primary muscle of inspiration)
   ❖ Innervated by phrenic nerves (leave spinal cord at cervical spaces 3 through 5).

Chapter 3

◆ External intercostals.

◆ Accessory muscles of inspiration.

Expiratory Muscles

◆ Abdominal muscles.

◆ Internal intercostals.

◆ *Note:* Expiration is normally passive and requires no muscles. Active expiration, however, occurs normally while speaking, singing or exercising.

Normal negative intrathoracic pressure refers to the pressure of –3 to –5 cm H_2O (below atmospheric pressure) in the intrapleural space, even when no respiratory muscles are contracting. The intrapleural space is the fluid-filled space between the visceral and parietal pleural. There is 15-25 ml of serous fluid in the intrapleural space in the average adult.

Process of Inspiration

Inspiration is accomplished by causing alveolar pressure to fall below atmospheric pressure. This is called negative pressure breathing because atmospheric pressure is considered 0 cm H_2O. Normal negative pressure breathing is caused by the contraction of the inspiratory respiratory muscles, which drops the diaphragm, increases thoracic volume, and lowers intrathoracic pressure. The lowering of the intrathoracic pressure influences the alveolar pressure. A decrease in intrathoracic pressure creates a pressure gradient, referred to as the transpulmonary or distending pressure. This distending pressure causes the alveoli to expand, thus lowering alveolar pressure to allow for inspiration.

Positive pressure breathing occurs when pressure at the nose or mouth is raised above alveolar pressure. Positive pressure breathing is used during mechanical ventilation.

Linking Knowledge to Practice

✔ *Patients with difficulty breathing prefer to be sitting in a fully upright position because this position helps in dropping the diaphragm and displacing the abdominal contents.*

Anatomy of the Pulmonary System

◆ Thorax

❖ Thoracic cage: 12 vertebrae, each with a pair of ribs.

❖ Posteriorly, each rib is attached to a vertebrae.

❖ Anteriorly, the first seven ribs are attached to the sternum.

❖ Ribs 8-10 are attached by cartilage to the rib above.

❖ Ribs 11 and 12 are called floating ribs.

◆ Muscles of ventilation

◆ Lungs – only attached to the body at the mediastinum by the pulmonary ligament

❖ Right lung has 3 lobes.

❖ Left lung has 2 lobes (space limitation due to heart).

❖ Lobes are further divided into bronchopulmonary segments.

❖ Lobules are the smallest, gross anatomic unit of the lung. Lobules contain the gas exchange components of terminal bronchioles, alveolar ducts, and alveolar sacs.

❖ The lymphatic system surrounds the lobules to drain off excess fluid and to remove any inhaled particles.

Oxygenation and Pulmonary Physiology

- Pleural Space
  - Parietal pleura lines the chest wall and contains many nerve fibers.
  - Visceral pleura lies over the lung parenchyma and does not contain nerve fibers.
  - Small amount of serous fluid between the parietal and visceral pleura allows the pleurae to slide over each other during inspiration and expiration.
  - Pressure within pleural space is called intrapleural pressure.
  - Intrapleural pressure is less than the pressure in the lungs, and this negative pressure keeps the lungs inflated (loss in negative pressure results in pneumothorax).
  - Abnormal fluid accumulation in the pleural space is called pleural effusion.
- Mediastinum
  - Space between the two lungs containing the heart, great vessels, thymus gland, esophagus, lymph nodes, and nerve fibers.

Conducting Airways

No gas exchange occurs in the conducting airways (Figure 3.1). This space is known as anatomical dead space. The majority of the airway is lined with ciliated cells and mucous secreting cells. These mechanisms serve to protect the lungs.

- Nose.
- Pharynx: located posterior to mouth and nasal cavities.
- Larynx: structure consists of muscles, ligaments, and incomplete rings of cartilage.
  - Vocal cords are the location of the narrowest part of conducting airway. The opening between vocal cords is called the rima glottis.
  - Epiglottis.
    - The epiglottis is located posterior to the root of the tongue. It is a piece of cartilage that is able to move up and down. During inhalation it moves upward to allow air to flow into the trachea. During swallowing it moves down to cover the larynx and allow food to enter the esophagus.
    - During straining with defecation, air is held in the lungs due to closure of the epiglottis. Contraction of the intra-abdominal muscles causes an increase in intrathoracic pressure. This is called the Valsava maneuver.
  - Cricoid cartilage: only complete rigid ring.
- Trachea (beginning of tracheobronchial tree which branches multiple times before reaching the alveoli). The trachea is a fibromuscular tube that contains incomplete cartilage rings. These rings stabilize the airway and prevent collapse during coughing. The trachea also contains mucosal cells and cilia to trap foreign material and propel up the airway. Cartilage disappears in the distal airways.
- Right and left bronchi.

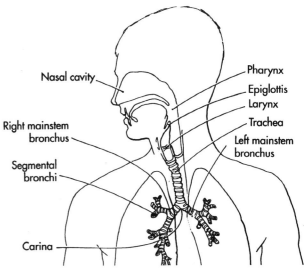

Figure 3.1: Conducting airways of the respiratory system.
From *Pass CCRN* (2nd ed.), R.D. Dennison, 2000. St. Louis: Mosby. Reprinted with permission from Elsevier.

- Non-respiratory terminal bronchioles. Progressive loss of cilia. Bronchioles and alveolar sacs contain no cartilage and therefore are capable of collapse and bronchospasm. Smooth muscle is located throughout the airways, even to the level of the alveolar ducts.

Gas Exchange Airways (Respiratory Zone of the Lung)

- Respiratory bronchioles (transition between conducting airways and gas exchange airways. Alveoli begin to appear here.) Each portion of the lung supplied by a terminal respiratory bronchiole is called the acinus.
- Alveolar ducts.
- Alveolar sacs (alveoli are structurally interdependent – this helps prevent the collapse of individual alveoli).

The alveolar structures are made up of two types of alveolar cells: Type I and II. Type I alveolar cells are flat, squamous epithelial cells and comprise approximately 90% of the alveolar surface area. These cells are designed for gas exchange and are sensitive to injury. They help prevent fluid entry into the alveoli.

Type II alveolar cells secrete key components for pulmonary surfactant synthesis and are also capable for generating into Type I cells in response to injury (Levitzky, 2003).

Surfactant is a phospholipid responsible for decreasing surface tension in the alveoli in response to decreased volume. This decrease in surface tension accomplishes two goals: 1) keeps smaller airways open during expiration; 2) improves the ease of opening alveoli during inspiration. A decrease in surfactant results in an increase in surface tension and increased pressure required to open the alveoli.

In addition to Types I and II alveolar cells, there are alveolar macrophages that engage in the phagocytosis of foreign materials.

Lung Volumes (Table 3.1)

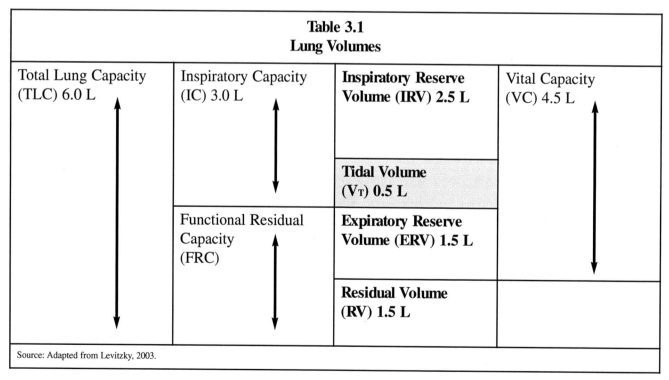

Table 3.1 Lung Volumes

Total Lung Capacity (TLC) 6.0 L	Inspiratory Capacity (IC) 3.0 L	Inspiratory Reserve Volume (IRV) 2.5 L	Vital Capacity (VC) 4.5 L
		Tidal Volume (V_T) 0.5 L	
	Functional Residual Capacity (FRC)	Expiratory Reserve Volume (ERV) 1.5 L	
		Residual Volume (RV) 1.5 L	

Source: Adapted from Levitzky, 2003.

Tidal Volume (V_T): Volume of air entering or leaving the nose or mouth per breath.

Normal is 500 ml for 70 kg adult.

Tidal volume increases with exercise.

Inspiratory Reserve Volume (IRV): Volume of air inhaled into the lungs during maximal forced inspiration, beginning at the end of normal tidal inspiration.

Expiratory Reserve Volume (ERV): Volume of air expelled during maximal forced expiration, beginning at the end of normal tidal expiration.

Residual Volume (RV): Volume of air left in lungs after maximal forced expiration.

Prevents lungs from collapsing in healthy persons.

Increases in emphysema.

Functional Residual Capacity (FRC): Volume of air in lungs at end of normal tidal expiration.

Inspiratory Capacity (IC): Volume of air inhaled into the lungs during a maximal inspiratory effort that begins at the end of normal tidal expiration.

Total Lung Capacity (TLC): The volume of air in the lungs after maximal inspiratory effort.

Vital Capacity (VC): Volume of air expelled from the lungs during maximal forced expiration after maximal forced inspiration.

VT, IRV, ERV, IC, and VC can all be measured with a spirometer. The RV, FRC, and TLC cannot be measured with spirometry because the patient cannot exhale all the air in the lungs; other techniques such as nitrogen-washout, helium-dilution, or body plethysmography must be used.

PULMONARY PHYSIOLOGY

Outline

- Ventilation (occurs simultaneously with perfusion).
- Perfusion of Blood to Pulmonary Capillaries.
- Diffusion of Oxygen Across the Alveolar Capillary Membrane.
- Transport of Gases in Blood.
- Oxygen Delivery to the Tissues.
- Cellular Respiration.

Ventilation

Ventilation is the movement of air between the atmosphere and alveoli and the distribution of air within the lungs to maintain appropriate concentrations of oxygen and carbon dioxide in the blood. The process of ventilation occurs through inspiration and expiration. Effective ventilation is influenced by the work of breathing. The work of breathing is impacted by <u>compliance</u> (elastic work of breathing), and <u>airway resistance</u> (resistive work of breathing).

Compliance (also called elastic work of breathing)

- Compliance is the ease with which the lung can be stretched. It is impacted by compliance of the lung and compliance of the chest wall. Compliance is the opposite of elastic recoil.
- Dynamic compliance is the compliance assessed during the course of a breath.
- Compliance affects the relationship between volume and pressure. A noncompliant lung produces higher pressures in response to normal volumes. Normal lung tissue is more compliant at lower volumes and becomes less compliant with higher volumes.

Chapter 3

◆ Lung tissue is made of elastin and collagen fibers. Collagen fibers resist stretching and elastin fibers aid in stretching.

◆ Pulmonary surfactant reduces the surface tension of the fluid lining of the alveoli and reduces elastic recoil of the lung, therefore increasing compliance. This decreases the work of inspiration. Surfactant is a lipoprotein that is secreted by Type II alveolar cells.

◆ Restrictive diseases restrict lung expansion due to decreased lung compliance. Atelectasis decreases lung compliance and increases elastic recoil. In pulmonary fibrosis and interstitial lung disease, elastin fibers are replaced with scar tissue; causing a decrease in compliance. Obesity and musculoskeletal disorders can also decrease chest wall compliance.

◆ People with decreased lung compliance must do more work of breathing to achieve effective inspiration.

Linking Knowledge to Practice

Nursing interventions to increase compliance:
✔ *Deep breath and hold.*
✔ *Incentive spirometry (10 breaths per hour).*

Airway Resistance (also called resistive work of breathing)

◆ In normal circumstances, airway resistance is low and only small changes in pressure are needed to move large amounts of air into the lungs.

◆ Small changes in airway diameter can have significant impact on airway resistance.

◆ Airway resistance is complicated because of the branching and progressive narrowing of the airway system. The large number of small airways offsets the increased resistance created by the small diameter of the airways. The overall resistance of the small airways is low during normal breathing, The greatest resistance normally occurs in the bronchi.

◆ In normal lungs, airway resistance is higher with low lung volumes (forced expiratory effort) and lower with high lung volume (deep inspiratory effort).

◆ Assessment of expiratory airway resistance can be done by assessing forced expiratory volume in the first second (FEV_1). Eighty percent of forced vital capacity (FVC) should occur within the first second of forced expiratory effort. A patient with airway obstruction caused by asthma exhales far less than 80% of the FVC within 1 second. Patients with airway obstruction also have a decreased peak expiratory flow (PEF).

◆ Obstructive diseases interfere with airflow and increase resistance.
 ❖ Asthma.
 ❖ Emphysema.
 ❖ Bronchitis.
 ❖ Foreign body causes a fixed obstruction.
 ❖ Sleep apnea can be an obstructive disorder.

◆ Bronchial smooth muscle is under control of the autonomic nervous system. Stimulation of the parasympathetic system causes constriction of smooth muscle and an increase in mucous secretion.

◆ Stimulation of the sympathetic nervous system causes dilation of the bronchial smooth muscle and a reduction of mucous secretion.

Oxygenation and Pulmonary Physiology

◆ The dilation of bronchial smooth muscle is achieved through stimulation of the beta 2 receptors located in the airways. Nitric oxide also dilates bronchial smooth muscle. Bronchial smooth muscle is normally under more dominant parasympathetic tone than sympathetic tone.

◆ Inhalation of irritants such as smoke and dust cause reflex constriction of the airways. Histamine, leukotrienes, alpha agonists, thromboxane A2, and serotonin can also cause reflex constriction.

Linking Knowledge to Practice

Nursing interventions to decrease resistance:

✔ *Decrease endotracheal tube resistance.*

❖ *> 8 mm*

❖ *Short tubes*

✔ *Bronchodilators.*

✔ *Suctioning.*

Minute Ventilation

Minute Ventilation

Minute ventilation (V_E) is the volume of air entering the nose or mouth each minute.

Minute ventilation = rate x tidal volume (V_T).

Normal minute ventilation is approximately 12 x 500 ml = 6000 ml.

Minute ventilation is not equal to the volume of air entering and leaving the alveoli per minute (alveolar ventilation [V_A]). This is due to anatomical dead space. Anatomical dead space is the last part of each inspiration (and expiration) remaining in the conducting airways, and does not participate in gas exchange. Approximately 30% of V_T does not participate in gas exchange. Minute ventilation is composed of both alveolar ventilation and dead space ventilation.

Alveolar Ventilation

Alveolar Ventilation

Alveolar ventilation (V_A) = V_T – anatomical dead space.

Alveolar minute ventilation is approximately 350 ml per breath.

Alveolar ventilation is decreased with an increase in dead space.

Bronchial constriction decreases anatomical dead space and bronchial vasodilation increases anatomical dead space.

Chapter 3

Assessment of Ventilation

◆ Efficiency and effectiveness of alveolar ventilation is measured by $PaCO_2$.
  ❖ $PaCO_2$ is the arterial CO_2 pressure.
  ❖ $PaCO_2$ = VCO_2 (CO_2 production) / V_A (alveolar ventilation).
  ❖ $PaCO_2$ is directly related to CO_2 production and indirectly related to alveolar ventilation.
  ❖ **$PaCO_2$ > 45 mm Hg indicates alveolar hypoventilation.**
    ★ The only physiologic reason for elevated $PaCO_2$ is inadequate alveolar ventilation.
  ❖ $PaCO_2$ < 35 mm Hg indicates alveolar hyperventilation.
◆ CO_2 is the byproduct of aerobic metabolism.
◆ The brain adjusts alveolar ventilation to keep arterial PCO_2 at approximately 40 mm Hg.
  ❖ Central chemoreceptors located near medulla respond to pH of surrounding fluid: decreased pH = increased ventilation
  ❖ Peripheral chemoreceptors located in carotid and aortic bodies sensitive to hypoxemia: low PaO_2 = increased ventilation.
  ❖ Many other receptors located in the pulmonary system that impact ventilation.
◆ Hypoventilation can occur with a normal respiratory rate if tidal volume is inadequate.
  ❖ Example: Shallow breathing due to postoperative abdominal pain.
  ❖ When a patient has a decrease in tidal volume, the patient's dead space does not change, this results in a decrease in alveolar ventilation.

Linking Knowledge to Practice

✔ *Untreated alveolar hypoventilation leads to hypoxemia. In acute respiratory failure, a blood gas is necessary to assess the $PaCO_2$ to determine if inadequate ventilation contributed to the hypoxemia.*

Treatment of Ventilation Problems

Minute ventilation can be altered by changing rate or tidal volume. Treatment for inadequate ventilation includes improving rate or tidal volume by:

◆ Reversing sedation if applicable.
◆ Ventilation with ambu bag.
◆ Intubation and mechanical ventilation.

Linking Knowledge to Practice

✔ *Patients with chronic obstructive lung disease may retain CO_2. Although their CO_2 levels are high, they have compensated and have a normal pH. In these patients, a low pH rather than a high PCO_2 is used as an assessment of respiratory failure. Also, when treating these patients, ventilation is adjusted to return the pH to normal rather than returning the CO_2 to normal.*

Perfusion

Perfusion is the movement of blood through the pulmonary capillaries and occurs simultaneously with ventilation. Blood is supplied to the lung by the pulmonary artery. The main pulmonary artery branches like the airway system. Pulmonary arteries follow the bronchi down the center of the lobules as far as the terminal bronchioles. Beyond that point, the pulmonary capillary bed lies in the alveolar walls. After gas exchange, oxygenated blood is collected by the pulmonary venous system and returned to the left atrium.

Oxygenation and Pulmonary Physiology

The entire output of the right ventricle is ejected into the pulmonary artery. Pulmonary blood flow contains mixed venous blood that was returned to the right atrium through the inferior and superior vena cavae, and from the heart muscle itself through the coronary sinus. It is mixed venous blood that participates in gas exchange with alveolar air at the capillary level.

Pulmonary capillaries are slightly smaller than the average erythrocyte, so the erythrocyte must change shape to pass through the pulmonary capillary. Gas exchange actually starts in smaller pulmonary arterial vessels that are not true capillaries. These are called functional pulmonary capillaries. At rest each red blood cell spends only about 0.75 seconds in the pulmonary capillary (Levitzky, 2003). During exercise, the time for gas exchange is much less.

There are approximately 280 billion capillaries that supply 300 million alveoli. Alveoli are completely enveloped in pulmonary capillaries (Figure 3.2). The estimated potential surface area for gas exchange is 50-100 m² (Levitzky, 2003).

The pressure around the pulmonary capillaries is called the alveolar pressure. As the lung expands, these capillaries are pulled open by the elastic lung parenchyma that surrounds them.

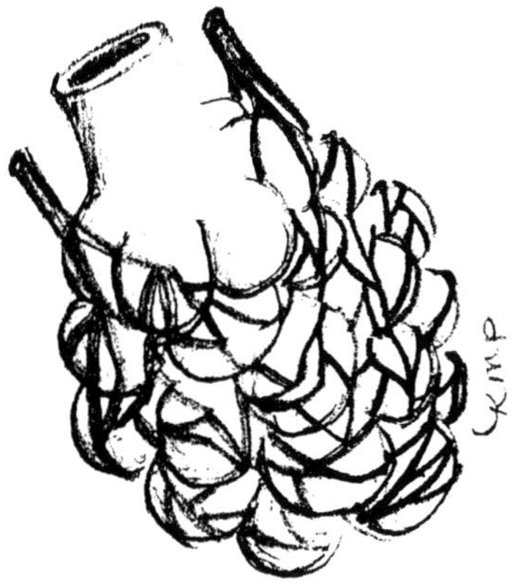

Zones of Perfusion

Ventilation and perfusion patterns vary in the upright lung due to gravity. The ratio of ventilation to perfusion is higher in the upper areas of the lungs, compared to the gravity dependent areas of the lung. This is because there is much less blood flow to the upper areas of the lung.

Figure 3.2: Alveoli surrounded by pulmonary capillaries.

The ratio of ventilation to perfusion is lower in the lower lobes (gravity dependent regions) of the lung. Gravity dependent areas of the lung receive more perfusion per alveolar unit. Blood also travels through the gravity dependent regions at a faster rate. There is actually more overall gas exchange in the lower lobes of the lung due to the increased amount of perfusion.

The lungs are divided into 3 zones (Figure 3.3).

◆ Zone 1: Least gravity dependent area. There may be no blood flow because alveolar pressure is greater than the pressure in both pulmonary arterioles and pulmonary venules.

◆ Zone 2: Pulmonary arteriole pressure is greater than alveolar pressure; however, alveolar pressure is greater than pulmonary venule pressure. This allows for intermittent blood flow during the cardiac cycle.

◆ Zone 3: This zone is always perfused because pressure in both the pulmonary arterioles and the pulmonary venules exceeds the alveolar pressure. There is constant flow during the cardiac cycle.
   Note: These zones are not static. Any part of the lung can take on characteristics of any zone based on hemodynamic and ventilatory changes (Darovic, 2002).

Note: The lungs also receive some arterial blood flow from the left ventricle. This is bronchial blood flow, which supplies systemic oxygenated blood to parts of the lung. Bronchial blood flow pressure is the same as pressure in other systemic arteries. Bronchial venous blood enters the pulmonary veins and returns to the left atrium without participating in gas exchange. This contributes to the normal anatomic right to left shunt. Part of tracheal bronchial tree (the respiratory bronchioles, alveolar ducts, alveolar sacs, and alveoli) receives oxygen by diffusion of the alveolar air.

Pulmonary Vascular Resistance Overview

Pulmonary vessels are thin walled and have less vascular smooth muscle than vessels in the systemic circulation. Normal pulmonary vascular resistance (PVR) is about 1/10 of systemic vascular resistance. Pulmonary vascular resistance is evenly distributed between the pulmonary arteries, the pulmonary capillaries, and the pulmonary veins. This is compared to systemic circulation whereby approximately 70% of the resistance comes from the arterioles (Levizky, 2003).

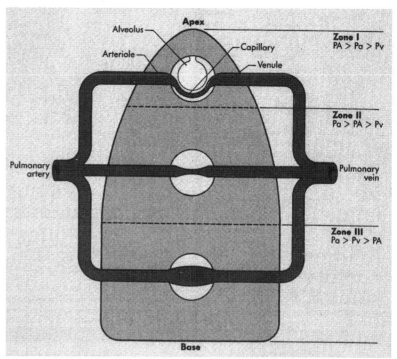

Figure 3.3: Zones of distribution of perfusion.
From *Pass CCRN* (2nd ed.), R.D. Dennison, 2000. St. Louis: Mosby. Reprinted with permission from Elsevier.

Pulmonary Artery Pressures

Mean pulmonary artery pressure is ≈ 15 mm Hg.

Pulmonary artery systolic is ≈ 25 mm Hg.

Pulmonary artery diastolic is ≈ 8-10 mm Hg.

The total pressure drop from the pulmonary artery to the left atrium is approximately 10 mm Hg.

Physiological Alterations in Pulmonary Vascular Resistance

◆ Extravascular effects (gravity, body position, lung volume, alveolar and intrapleural pressure, and right ventricular output) have more influence on PVR than the tone of the vascular smooth muscle. The resistance of both alveolar vessels (capillaries between the alveoli) and extra-alveolar vessels contribute to the total PVR.

◆ During positive pressure mechanical ventilation, both the alveolar and extra-alveolar vessels are compressed during lung inflation. With the addition of PEEP (positive end expiratory pressure), these vessels remain compressed during expiration as well. PVR is thus increased.

◆ An increase in cardiac output from the right ventricle (as during exercise) causes a slight increase in pulmonary artery pressure (PAP) and also causes a decrease in PVR. The reasons for this decrease in PVR in response to an increased blood flow include recruitment and distention.

Oxygenation and Pulmonary Physiology

❖ During periods of normal cardiac output, not all pulmonary capillaries are perfused. When pulmonary artery pressure rises, some capillaries not previously opened will open. This opening of capillaries is called capillary recruitment. Capillary recruitment allows more pathways for blood flow, and overall resistance to flow is lowered. A decrease in cardiac output can cause a derecruitment of pulmonary capillaries.

❖ In response to higher pulmonary artery pressure, capillaries distend and change shape to a more circular shape, thus decreasing PVR.

◆ Lung volumes also affect pulmonary vascular resistance. At high lung volumes, pulmonary alveolar vessels are pulled open and pulmonary vascular resistance is low. When lung volume is low, there is a high resistance. However, pulmonary capillary resistance can rise if alveolar pressure rises.

◆ Causes of Increased PVR

   ❖ Epinephrine and norepinephrine.

   ❖ Histamine / influx of inflammatory mediators.

   ❖ Thromboxane / platelet activation and aggregation.

   ❖ Alveolar hypoxia (local vasoconstriction).

   ❖ Hyercapnea / acidosis.

   ❖ Hypothermia.

   ❖ Pulmonary endothelial dysfunction.

◆ Hypoxic Pulmonary Vasoconstriction

   ❖ Localized hypoxic pulmonary vasoconstriction serves a physiologic purpose by diverting mixed venous blood away from localized, poorly ventilated alveoli caused by conditions such as atelectasis or airway obstruction. The diverted mixed venous blood is sent to well-ventilated alveoli to participate in gas exchange. Increased levels of alveolar PCO_2 also causes pulmonary vasoconstriction.

   ❖ The mechanism of hypoxic pulmonary vasoconstriction is not fully understood. Hypoxia may cause a release of vasoconstrictor substances from the pulmonary parenchyma or nearby mast cells. It may also decrease the release of nitric oxide, a vasodilator. Hypoxia can act directly on vascular smooth muscle by allowing more calcium to enter the cells, and therefore cause direct vasoconstriction.

   ❖ Hypoxic pulmonary vasoconstriction also occurs in response to more global hypoxia as a result of hypoventilation. This general constrictive response increases pulmonary artery pressure and helps recruit additional pulmonary capillaries, which aids in better ventilation and perfusion matching.

   ❖ Hypoxic pulmonary vasoconstriction has limitations because of the relatively small amount of vascular smooth muscle found in the pulmonary arteries. In addition, pre-existing high pulmonary artery pressures and alkalosis can interfere with the ability of the vessels to constrict in response to hypoxia.

   ❖ Entire lung hypoxic vasoconstriction greatly increases the workload of the right ventricle, and increased pulmonary artery pressure may lead to pulmonary edema.

◆ Pulmonary Vasodilators

   ❖ IV

      ★ Nitroglycerin.

      ★ Sodium nitroprusside (Nipride).

      ★ Prostaglandins (PGE1, PGI2).

      ★ PDE1 (phosphodiesterase enzyme 1) inhibitor.

❖ Inhaled
  ★ Any of the above IV medications.
  ★ Nitric oxide.
  ★ Prostacyclin (PGI2, Epoprostenol, Flolan), or derivative Iloprost.

Alveolar Dead Space

Alveolar dead space refers to ventilated alveoli that receive no perfusion. A pulmonary embolus results in alveolar dead space. When alveolar pressure exceeds pulmonary arterial pressure, there is also no perfusion to those alveoli. In healthy people, pulmonary artery pressure is greater than alveolar pressure, even in the uppermost regions of the lung, so there is no alveolar dead space. Patients on mechanical ventilation with positive end expiratory pressure (PEEP) may have increased amounts of alveolar dead space because alveolar pressures are always high.

Arterial Blood Supply to the Lungs

The bronchial artery system supplies arterial blood to the level of the terminal bronchiole. The alveoli receive its blood supply from the pulmonary circulation.

Diffusion of Oxygen Across Alveolar Capillary Membrane (Gas Exchange)

The primary purpose of the pulmonary system is gas exchange. Gas exchange occurs at the alveolar capillary unit. Effective ventilation and perfusion must take place simultaneously for the diffusion of gases to occur.

Oxygen enters the alveoli through the conducting airways by bulk flow, which occurs when gases move in response to differences in total pressure (Figure 3.4). Diffusion is the net movement of molecules from an area where a gas exerts a higher partial pressure to an area where the gas exerts a lower partial pressure. Each gas moves according to its individual partial pressure.

Normal alveolar gas pressures: $PAO_2 = 100$ mm Hg
$PACO_2 = 40$ mm Hg

Normal mixed venous blood gas pressures:
$PvO_2 = 40$ mm Hg
$PvCO_2 = 45$ mm Hg

Gas exchange occurs at the alveolar capillary membrane (Figure 3.5). A thin layer of squamous epithelial cells covers the alveolar surface. In addition there is a layer of cells that also produces a fluid lining. A thin layer of squamous epithelial cells also forms pulmonary capillaries. Gas exchange must occur across 1) the alveolar epithelium; 2) the alveolar fluid lining; 3) the capillary epithelium; and 4) the interstitial space that exists between the two.

Both oxygen and CO_2 diffuse across the alveolar capillary membrane. However, CO_2 is more diffusible than oxygen, and barriers to diffusion impact the diffusion of oxygen more than the diffusion of CO_2. Therefore, in discussing diffusion, the focus is on the diffusion of oxygen across the alveolar capillary membrane.

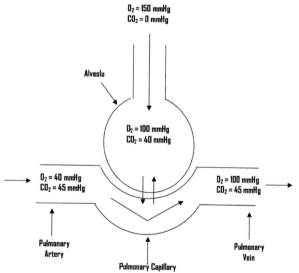

Figure 3.4: Diffusion of oxygen across the alveoli capillary membrane.

Oxygenation and Pulmonary Physiology

Determinants of Diffusion

The following factors impact how well oxygen is able to diffuse from the alveoli through the alveolar capillary membrane and into the blood.

- Surface area available
    - Decreased in:
        - Pulmonary resection.
        - Emphysema.
        - Tumors.
        - Any ventilation to perfusion mismatching.
    - Increase in exercise
- Thickness of alveolar capillary membrane
    - Increased with interstitial or alveolar edema.
    - Increased with interstitial or alveolar fibrosis.
- Driving pressure (partial pressure difference of gas across the barrier)
    - Negatively affected by low inspired fraction of O_2 (smoke inhalation), or by low barometric pressure (high altitudes).

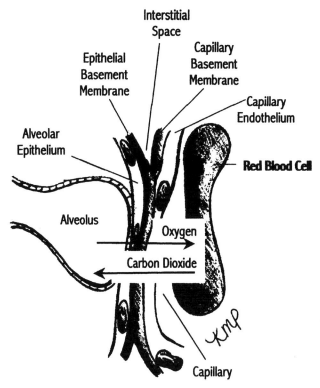

Figure 3.5: Gas exchange at the alveolar capillary membrane.

Poor diffusion of oxygen results in poorly oxygenated blood returning to the left side of the heart and entering the systemic circulation. A diffusion abnormality is often referred to as an oxygenation problem because the result is low PaO_2 and low oxygen saturation.

Assessment of Diffusion (Oxygenation)

Blood Gasses

- The oxygen saturation and the PaO_2 on a blood gas are used to assess the adequacy of oxygen diffusion from the alveoli into the blood.

A (alveolar) –a (arterial) Gradient ($PAO_2 - PaO_2$)

- The A-a gradient is the alveolar to arterial oxygen pressure difference.
- Difference between alveolar and arterial oxygen should be small.
    - Normal A-a Gradient = 5-15 mm Hg.
        - PAO_2 = 100 mm Hg.
        - PaO_2 = 80 to 100 mm Hg.
- The A-a gradient provides an index of gas transfer (diffusion).
    - A large A-a gradient (a significant amount of alveolar oxygen not diffusing into the blood) generally indicates that the lung is the site of dysfunction, and there is a diffusion problem.
- Causes of increased alveolar/arterial PO_2 gradient:
    - Simple diffusion impairment, such as in pulmonary edema where interstitial fluid creates a barrier to diffusion.
    - Diffusion impairment caused by significant ventilation and perfusion mismatching, i.e. intrapulmonary shunt (discussed later in chapter).

Chapter 3

Reference Equation for Alveolar O_2 (PAO_2)

Alveolar Gas Equation (calculated – not directly measured):

$$PAO_2 = FIO_2 (PB - 47) - PaCO_2/0.8$$

- PAO_2 = partial pressure of alveolar oxygen.
- FIO_2 = fraction of inhaled oxygen.
- PB = barometric pressure (sum of all the gas pressures).
- P_{H_2O} = 47 mm Hg = water vapor pressure.
- $PaCO_2$ = partial pressure of arterial carbon dioxide.
- 0.8 = respiratory quotient.

PaO_2/ FIO_2 Ratio

The PaO_2/FIO_2 ratio is determined by dividing the PaO_2 by the FIO_2 (in decimal form).

- Normal > 350.
- Acute lung injury < 300.
- ARDS < 200.

Linking Knowledge to Practice

- ✔ *Healthy patient with a PaO_2 of 95 mm Hg on room air:*
  - ❖ *PaO_2/FIO_2 ratio is 95/.21 = **452**.*
- ✔ *Patient presenting in respiratory distress has an initial PaO_2 of 60 mm Hg on room air.*
  - ❖ *PaO_2/FIO_2 ratio is: 60/.21 = **286**.*
- ✔ *Above patient is placed on a 100% non-rebreather mask with the repeat blood gases showing a PaO_2 of 80 mm Hg.*
  - ❖ *PaO_2 ratio is 80/1.0 = **80**.*
  - ❖ *This indicates the patient is deteriorating, despite a PaO_2 of 80 mm Hg.*

- ✔ *The PaO_2/FIO_2 ratio can be used to trend improvement or worsening of a patient's oxygenation status.*

More on PaO_2 Assessment

- PAO_2 (alveolar oxygen) affects PaO_2 (arterial oxygen).
  - ❖ An increase in FIO_2 increases PAO_2, and therefore increases PaO_2 in the absence of a diffusion abnormality.
  - ❖ An increase in $PaCO_2$ decreases PAO_2, and therefore decreases PaO_2.
- PaO_2 of 80-100 is normal if the patient is breathing room air (FIO_2 0.21).
- Always relate PaO_2 to FIO_2.
  - ❖ One way to do this is by using the PaO_2 / FIO_2 as described above.
  - ❖ Another way is to determine the expected PaO_2 for the given FIO_2.
    - ★ Expected PaO_2 = (FIO_2 % x 6) – $PaCO_2$.

80

Treatment of Diffusion Problems

Oxygen therapy (increased FIO_2), and positive end expiratory pressure (PEEP) or continuous positive airway pressure (CPAP), are used to promote the diffusion of oxygen across the membrane.

Linking Knowledge to Practice

✔ *Hypoxemia due solely to a diffusion abnormality is typically improved by breathing 100% oxygen.*

Ventilation / Perfusion Ratio (V/Q)

Abnormalities in the matching of ventilation and perfusion impact the diffusion of oxygen, and therefore oxygenation.

- Ventilation (V): Alveolar minute ventilation = 4 to 6L.
- Perfusion (Q): Normal cardiac output = 5L/min.
- Normal V/Q ratio 0.8 to 1.2
- Ventilation and perfusion must be matched at the alveolar capillary level for optimal gas exchange.

Increased V/Q Ratio

- Alveolar dead space – ventilation is greater than perfusion
    - Occurs when air enters non perfused alveoli (Figure 3.6).
    - V/Q ratio > 0.8 (increased V/Q ratio).
    - Alveolar PO_2 rises.
    - Alveolar PCO_2 falls.
    - Situations that increase alveolar dead space
        - Pulmonary embolism.
        - Decreased right ventricular cardiac output.
        - High alveolar pressure (positive pressure ventilation with PEEP).

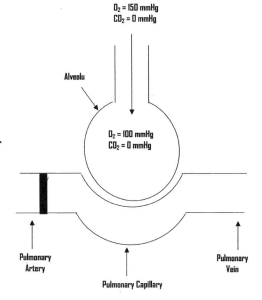

Figure 3.6: Increased V/Q ratio.

Decreased V/Q Ratio

- Intrapulmonary shunt - mixed venous blood perfuses totally collapsed or unventilated alveoli (Figure 3.7).
    - No gas exchange occurs and poorly oxygenated blood returns to the left side of the heart.
    - Increasing the FIO_2 improves oxygenation to minimal extent when there is significant intrapulmonary shunting.
- V/Q ratio < 0.8 (decreased V/Q ratio).
- Alveolar PO_2 falls.
- Alveolar PCO_2 rises.

An alveolar unit that is neither ventilated nor perfused is called a silent unit.

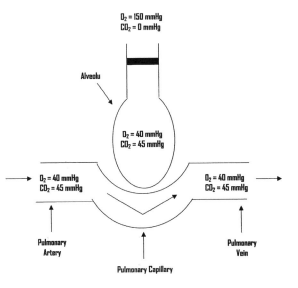

Figure 3.7: Decreased V/Q ratio.

Chapter 3

Causes of non-uniform ventilation:

◆ Uneven resistance to airflow.

  ☆ Collapsed airways (emphysema).

  ☆ Bronchoconstriction (asthma).

  ☆ Inflammation (bronchitis).

◆ Non-uniform compliance throughout the lung.

  ☆ Fibrosis

  ☆ Pulmonary edema

  ☆ Pneumonia

  ☆ Atelectasis

  ☆ Pneumothorax

  ☆ Tumors

  ☆ Emphysema

  ☆ Decreased surfactant.

Causes of non-uniform perfusion:

◆ Emboli.

◆ Compression of pulmonary capillaries by high alveolar pressures.

◆ Tumors.

◆ Pneumothorax.

◆ Collapse of alveoli.

◆ Pulmonary vascular hypotension.

Transport of Gases in the Blood

Oxygen and carbon dioxide move together through the circulatory system; oxygen is moved from the alveolus to the tissues for utilization, and carbon dioxide is moved from the tissues back to the alveolus for exhalation.

After the diffusion of oxygen across the alveolar capillary membrane, some oxygen remains physically dissolved in plasma, but the majority enters the erythrocyte and chemically binds with hemoglobin (Hb). The binding between oxygen and hemoglobin is reversible at the tissue level. Much more oxygen is combined with hemoglobin than physically dissolved in blood.

◆ Hemoglobin: 97% of oxygen is combined with hemoglobin

  ❖ Represented by the SaO_2.

  ❖ Percentage of hemoglobin saturation = O_2 bound to Hb, divided by the O_2 capacity of hemoglobin x 100%.

◆ Plasma: 3% of oxygen is dissolved in plasma.

  ❖ Represented by the PaO_2 (partial pressure of oxygen in plasma).

The amount of oxygen dissolved in plasma is not sufficient to meet the oxygen demands of the tissues; however, it is the primary factor in determining the amount of O_2 that binds to hemoglobin.

Each gram of hemoglobin, when fully saturated with oxygen, can combine with approximately 1.39 ml of oxygen. The oxygen carrying capacity is determined by the amount of hemoglobin in the blood. The percent of Hb saturation does not reflect the total amount or volume of oxygen.

Variations in the hemoglobin structure can have significant physiological effects. Alterations in hemoglobin can impact the affinity hemoglobin has for oxygen and other substances, and can change the physical properties of hemoglobin. One abnormal variant of hemoglobin is hemoglobin S, which is present in sickle cell disease. When hemoglobin S is not combined with oxygen, it crystallizes in the cytosol of the red blood cell. This crystallization of the hemoglobin causes it to be less soluble within the red blood cell and changes the shape of the cell to a sickle shape. These sickle cells are more fragile than normal cells and also stick together more easily, increasing blood viscosity and risk of thrombosis.

Oxyhemoglobin Dissociation Curve

- The partial pressure of the oxygen (PaO$_2$) in the plasma determines the amount of oxygen that binds with hemoglobin. When the PaO$_2$ is high, hemoglobin is highly saturated with oxygen, and when the PaO$_2$ is low, oxygen is released from hemoglobin. This relationship is displayed in the oxyhemoglobin curve (Figure 3.8).
- The oxyhemoglobin curve shows the relationship between PaO$_2$ and SaO$_2$. The curve is said to be S-shaped.
    - The upper part of the curve shows that a PaO$_2$ above 60 mm Hg results in minimal changes in oxygen saturation. This flat part of the curve protects the body by allowing the hemoglobin to remain highly saturated when the PaO$_2$ ranges from 60 to 100 mm Hg.
        - The significance is that between a PaO$_2$ of 70 mm Hg and a PaO$_2$ of 100 mm Hg, there is only a small change in the oxygen content of the blood.
        - Hemoglobin is about 97% saturated at a PaO$_2$ of 100 mm Hg, so raising the alveolar PaO$_2$ above 100 can add little more oxygen to the hemoglobin. Hemoglobin becomes fully saturated with the PaO$_2$ of about 250 mm Hg.
    - The lower part of the curve shows that a PaO$_2$ below 60 results in a significant decrease in oxygen saturation. This allows the tissues to extract large amounts of oxygen with only small changes in PaO$_2$.
- On a normal oxyhemoglobin curve, a PaO$_2$ of 60 mm Hg = SaO$_2$ of 90%.
- As the blood passes into the systemic capillaries, it is exposed to lower PaO$_2$ levels, and oxygen is released from the hemoglobin into the plasma. This dissociation of oxygen into the plasma allows for O$_2$ to diffuse into the tissues for use at the cellular level. The PaO$_2$ in the capillaries varies from tissue to tissue. The PaO$_2$ in the myocardium is very low. The oxyhemoglobin curve is steep so a small drop in PaO$_2$ can lead to a substantial dissociation of oxygen from hemoglobin. This unloads more oxygen for use by the tissues.
- Four main factors alter the normal association between oxygen and hemoglobin. They are alterations in: pH, PCO$_2$, temperature of the blood, and concentration of 2, 3, DPG in the erythrocytes.

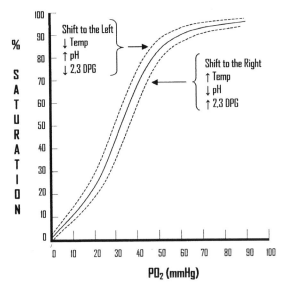

Figure 3.8: Oxyhemoglobin dissociation curve.

Chapter 3

Shifts in Oxyhemoglobin Curve

◆ The normal oxyhemoglobin curve occurs at 37 degrees, pH 7.4, and PCO_2 of 40 mm Hg. The impact of changes in pH, $PaCO_2$, and temperature on the oxyhemoglobin curve are seen in Figure 3.8.

◆ Shifts in the oxyhemoglobin curve are more pronounced when PaO_2 levels are low rather than high. Therefore, shifts have a more profound effect with unloading of oxygen at the tissue level than with the uptake of oxygen in the lungs.

◆ Shift to the Left.

❖ Hemoglobin has a higher affinity for oxygen. It is easier for hemoglobin to pick up oxygen at the lung level, and more difficult to drop it off at the tissue level.

❖ Hemoglobin is more saturated for a given PaO_2.

❖ Less oxygen is unloaded at the tissue level for a given PaO_2. This results in decreased tissue perfusion despite a higher SaO_2.

❖ Causes of shift to left.

    ☆ Decreased temperature (hypothermia)

    ☆ Decreased 2,3 – DPG

    ☆ Hypocapnia

    ☆ Alkalemia.

◆ Shift to the Right

❖ Hemoglobin has less affinity for oxygen. It is more difficult for hemoglobin to pick up oxygen at the lung level, but easier to drop off at the tissue level.

❖ Hemoglobin is less saturated for a given PaO_2, and more oxygen is unloaded for a given PaO_2.

❖ Causes of shift to right.

    ☆ Increased temperature (hyperthermia).

    ☆ Increased hydrogen ions (hypercapnia, acidemia).

    ☆ Increased 2,3 – DPG.

        ✳ 2,3-Diphosphoglycerate is a substance produced by erythrocytes during their normal glycolysis, which binds to hemoglobin and decreases the affinity of hemoglobin for oxygen.

        ✳ Conditions with increased 2,3-Diphosphoglycerate include chronic hypoxemia, anemia, and hyperthyroidism.

        ✳ Condition with decreased 2,3-Diphosphoglycerate include massive transfusion of stored blood (banked blood stored for as little as one week has low levels of 2,3 –DPG), hypophosphatemia, and hypothyroidism.

Rise

In

2, 3-DP**G**

H+

Temperature

Figure 3.9: Shift to the right mnemonic.

Helpful Hint: A way to remember the causes for a shift to the right are found in Figure 3.9.
Rise **I**n 2, 3-DP**G**, **H**ydrogen ions, and **T**emperature is used to spell "right."

Oxygenation and Pulmonary Physiology

Other factors affecting oxygen transport

Carbon monoxide. Carbon monoxide has a high affinity for hemoglobin and limits the ability of oxygen to bind with hemoglobin. It also shifts the oxyhemoglobin curve to the left and prevents the unloading of oxygen at the tissues. Carbon monoxide is very dangerous because low levels of carbon monoxide can result in dangerously high levels of carboxyhemoglobin. Carbon monoxide is colorless, odorless, and tasteless. Smoking and or living in urban areas can cause small amounts of carboxyhemoglobin to be present in the blood.

Methemoglobin. Methemoglobin is hemoglobin with iron in the ferric state. Iron atoms in the ferric state will not bind with oxygen. Methemoglobin can be caused by nitrite poisoning or toxic reactions to oxidant drugs.

Artifical Blood. Fluorocarbons are used to transport oxygen in artificial blood products. They have less oxygen carrying capacity than hemoglobin, but a higher oxygen carrying capacity than plasma.

Definitions

<u>Hypoxemia</u> – defined as insufficient oxygenation of the blood.
- Mild hypoxemia: $PaO_2 < 80$ mm Hg or SaO_2 95%.
- Moderate hypoxemia: $PaO_2 < 60$ or mm Hg or SaO_2 90%.
- Severe hypoxemia: $PaO_2 < 40$ mm Hg or SaO_2 75%.

<u>Hypoxia</u> – insufficient oxygenation of tissues. It is determined by a combination of cardiac index, Hgb, SaO_2, patency of the vessels, and cellular demand. Hypoxia is not directly measured. End organ function is used to evaluate tissue hypoxia.

<u>Cyanosis</u> – a bluish purple discoloration of the skin, nail beds, and mucous membranes. Occurs when more than 5 g Hb/100 ml of arterial blood is in the deoxygenated state.

The absence of cyanosis does not exclude hypoxemia. An anemic patient with hypoxemia may not have enough hemoglobin to express signs of cyanosis. In contrast, patients with polycythemia may look cyanotic without being hypoxemic.

Oxygen Delivery to Tissues

Oxygen delivery is the volume of oxygen delivered to tissues each minute and is expressed as DO_2.

Delivery of Oxygen

DO_2 (ml/min) = cardiac output (CO) (L/min) x arterial oxygen content (CaO_2) (ml/dl) x 10.

CaO_2 is the amount of oxygen bound to hemoglobin + the amount of oxygen dissolved in plasma. It is measured in ml/dl. Multiplying by a factor of 10 in the above equation adjusts the two factors to the same scale, so the product will be in ml (Darovic, 2002).

Chapter 3

Arterial Oxygen Content

$CaO_2 = Hb \times 1.36$ (oxygen carrying capacity) $\times SaO_2$ (decimal) $+ PaO_2 \times (0.003$ /solubility constant).

Percent saturation is not interchangeable with oxygen content. Anemia does not alter saturation but does alter arterial oxygen content.

Linking Knowledge to Practice

✔ *The major determinants of arterial oxygen content are hemoglobin and saturation. Increasing PaO_2 is not the main strategy to increase oxygen-carrying capacity unless hemoglobin and saturation cannot be further improved, such as in carbon monoxide poisoning.*

❖ *Normal CaO_2 is approximately 20 ml/dL.*

❖ *Normal DO_2 = 900- 1100 ml/min (1000).*

❖ *Normal DO_2I = 550 – 650 ml/min.*

✔ *Oxygen delivery to patient can be improved by increasing cardiac output, Hb or SaO_2. Low cardiac output significantly reduces delivery of oxygen to the tissues, even in the presence of adequate hemoglobin and oxygen saturation.*

Oxygen Consumption

Oxygen consumption is the volume of oxygen consumed by the tissues each minute and is measured as VO_2.

VO_2 is determined by comparing the oxygen content in arterial blood (CaO_2) to the oxygen content in mixed venous blood (CvO_2). Normal CaO_2 is approximately 20 ml/dL and normal CvO_2 is approximately 15 ml/dL. This comparison demonstrates that tissues consume approximately 25% of what is delivered.

◆ Normal VO_2 is 200 – 300 ml/min (250 ml/min)

Oxygen Consumption

VO_2 (ml/min) = CO x Hb x 1.36 x 10 x ($SaO_2 - SvO_2$)

The actual percentage of oxygenation utilization is different in different tissues. The heart, for example, utilizes the majority of the oxygen it receives.

Oxygen Reserve in Venous Blood

Oxygen reserve is measured by mixed venous (blood mixed from inferior and superior vena cavae and coronary sinus) oxygen saturation. Mixed venous blood has a PO_2 of 40 mm Hg, with a corresponding saturation of approximately 75%.

Oxygenation and Pulmonary Physiology

Mixed venous oxygen saturation is SVO_2.

◆ Normal SVO_2 is 60-80%, or approximately 75%.

Delivery/Consumption/Reserve Review

◆ Tissues are delivered approximately 1000 ml/min (DO_2).

◆ Tissues use approximately 250 ml/min (VO_2).

◆ This leaves a 75% reserve in venous blood (SVO_2).

The tissues utilize approximately 25% of the delivered oxygen. This is called the oxygen extraction ratio (O_2ER).

Relationship Between Oxygen Consumption and Oxygen Delivery

◆ Oxygen delivery and oxygen consumption are independent of each other in normal circumstances. This means that tissues extract the amount of oxygen needed independent of delivery because delivery exceeds need. In this independent state, there is always an acceptable reserve.

◆ Because the normal reserve is approximately 75%, there is some room in the independent state for delivery to fall or for consumption to increase.

Linking Knowledge to Practice

✔ *When oxygen delivery and oxygen consumption are independent, the tissues continue to extract the amount of required oxygen when a small drop in hemoglobin decreases oxygen delivery. Delivery is decreased and consumption stays the same, so the venous reserve is decreased. The oxygen reserve is impacted but tissue oxygen is preserved.*

✔ *When delivery and consumption are in the independent state and there is a fall in delivery, the reserve also falls because consumption stays the same. In this situation an increase in delivery (cardiac support, blood administration, improved oxygenation) results in an increase in reserve. Table 3.2 demonstrates these relationships.*

Table 3.2
Relationship Between Delivery and Reserve

DO_2	VO_2 (extraction is independent of delivery)	SVO_2 (SVO_2 improves when delivery is increased)
1000 cc	250 cc (25%)	75%
750 cc	250 cc (33%)	67%
500 cc	250 cc (50%)	50%

◆ At a critical level of DO_2 (approximately 420 ml/mm^2) (FCCS, 2006), the tissues no longer extract and consume oxygen independent of delivery. This is called a dependent state because the tissues alter their consumption based on low levels of delivery. Anaerobic metabolism occurs here because there is an oxygen deficit. Anaerobic metabolism leads to the production of lactic acid. Delivery of oxygen should be kept > 500 ml per minute at all times to assure that consumption is independent of delivery.

Chapter 3

Linking Knowledge to Practice

✔ *SVO₂ does not increase with increased delivery while in this dependent state. The development of lactic acidosis is a grave sign. Therefore, it is important to recognize and treat a decrease in oxygen delivery while oxygen consumption is still in the independent state.*

<u>Increased VO₂</u> – in addition to a decrease in oxygen delivery, critically ill patients can have an increase in oxygen consumption that places tissue oxygenation at risk. The following can increase oxygen consumption in the critically ill patient:

◆ Fever
◆ Shivering
◆ Suctioning
◆ Sepsis
◆ Non-family visitor
◆ Position change
◆ Sling scale weight
◆ Bath
◆ Chest x-ray
◆ Multi-organ failure
◆ Other conditions that increase physiological or psychological stress.

SVO₂ Monitoring

SVO₂ is a global indicator of the balance between oxygen supply and demand. SVO₂ is influenced by both oxygen delivery and oxygen extraction. SVO₂ reflects mixing of venous blood from superior vena cava, inferior vena cava and coronary sinus. SVO₂ is measured using a pulmonary artery fiberoptic catheter. Normal SVO₂ value is approximately 70-75%.

◆ Causes of low SVO₂ (< 60%) include:
  ❖ Decreased delivery.
  ❖ Increased consumption.
◆ Causes of high SVO₂ (> 80%) include:
  ❖ Increased delivery.
  ❖ Decreased demand.
  ❖ Sepsis (tissues cannot extract).
  ❖ Wedged catheter.
◆ A clinically significant change in SVO₂ is + or – 5-10% over 3 to 5 minutes.
◆ SVO₂ < 40% represents limits of compensation where extraction and consumption become dependent on delivery, and lactic acidosis occurs. In this state, oxygen demand is greater than oxygen delivery and reserve can be depleted, leading to oxygen debt.

Oxygenation and Pulmonary Physiology

ScVO₂

$ScVO_2$ reflects oxygen saturation of blood returning to right atrium via the superior vena cava. This measurement can be obtained without a pulmonary artery catheter, using a modified central venous catheter with fiberoptic technology.

◆ Normal value is > 70%.

◆ $ScVO_2$ trends higher than SVO_2 but trends with SVO_2.

Cellular Respiration

Cellular respiration refers to the utilization of oxygen by the cell. Oxygen is used by the mitochondria in the production of cellular energy. Prolonged oxygen deficit can result in lethal cell injury. Cellular respiration is not directly measured, but is estimated based on the amount of oxygen consumed and the amount carbon dioxide produced.

Anaerobic metabolism produces a spiraling downhill cycle:

◆ Decrease adenosine triphosphate (ATP) → Failure of Na+ and K+ pump.

◆ Increased Lactic Acid → Metabolic acidosis → Cellular Dysfunction → Organ Failure.

Cellular respiration is affected by delivery of oxygen to the tissues. It is also affected by the following, even in the presence of normal delivery of oxygen:

1) Metabolic demands of the tissue exceed even normal supply.

2) Tissue edema or fibrosis can interfere with the ability of oxygen to diffuse into the tissues.

3) Inability of the cell to use oxygen to produce energy (produces an elevation in SVO_2).

OXYGEN THERAPY AND MECHANICAL VENTILATION

Oxygen Delivery Systems

Oxygen is used to increase the delivery of FIO_2 beyond 0.21 in response to a low oxygen saturation level.

◆ Cannula: < 40 - 50% FIO_2

  ❖ Low flow delivery system.

◆ Simple mask: 40-60% FIO_2

  ❖ If mist disappears during inspiration, there is an entrainment of air. Flow is not adequate to meet inspiratory demand and should be increased.

◆ Venturi mask: Up to 40% FIO_2

  ❖ Air is entrained to deliver a specific FIO_2.

◆ Non-rebreathing mask: 80-100% FIO_2

  ❖ Bag is filled with 100% oxygen and is fully or partially inflated.

◆ Bag valve mask

  ❖ High flow > 15L/min

  ❖ Very little air entrainment with a firm fit.

Low Flow Oxygen Delivery

◆ Doesn't provide total inspired gas.

◆ Patient breathes varying amounts of room air.

◆ FIO_2 depends on rate and depth of ventilation and fit of device.

Chapter 3

- ◆ Doesn't have to mean low FIO_2.
- ◆ Nasal cannula is a low-flow oxygen delivery system.
- ◆ Simple face mask is a moderate flow delivery system.
- ◆ <u>Guidelines for estimating FIO_2 with low flow oxygen devices</u>
  - ❖ Approximately 4% increase in FIO_2 for each 1L nasal cannula.
  - ❖ Non-breather mask is the closest device to 100% FIO_2 without the use of mechanical ventilation.

High Flow Oxygen Delivery

- ◆ Provides entire inspired gas by high flow of gas.
- ◆ Provides a predictable FIO_2.
- ◆ Doesn't mean a high FIO_2.
- ◆ 100% non-rebreather masks, venturi masks and mechanical ventilators are examples of higher flow oxygen delivery systems.

Complications of Oxygen Therapy

Special Considerations in Patients with Hypoxic Drive

Patients who are chronic CO_2 retainers use a hypoxic drive rather than CO_2 level to trigger their drive to breathe. Caution is used in these patients when administering oxygen therapy. The hypoxic drive typically occurs with an oxygen saturation of approximately 90-92%. Utilizing oxygen therapy to raise the oxygen saturation above this level may eliminate the hypoxic drive. It is important to note that oxygen saturation, not the amount or delivery of oxygen, determines the hypoxic drive.

Oxygen Toxicity

Oxygen toxicity results in alveolar capillary membrane damage, alveolar collapse, and, ultimately, fibrosis and non-compliant lung tissue. The onset is related to both the concentration and duration of FIO_2. Oxygen toxicity has been associated with 100% FIO_2 for > 24 hours or with > 50% FIO_2 for longer than 3 weeks. Symptoms of oxygen toxicity include:

- ◆ Dyspnea.
- ◆ Decreased lung compliance.
- ◆ Retrosternal pain.
- ◆ Parasthesia in the extremities.

Guidelines to reduce the risk of oxygen toxicity include:

- ◆ 100% for no more than 24 hours.
- ◆ 60% for no more than 2-3 days.
- ◆ 40% or less for more than 2-3 days.

Other Complications of Oxygen Therapy

- ◆ Absorption atelectasis: With high FIO_2, nitrogen is washed out of airways, leaving only O_2, CO_2 and water vapors. When oxygen diffuses into the capillary, the alveoli can collapse.
- ◆ Decreased hypoxic drive (potential in chronic CO_2 retainers): hyopoxic drive is usually stimulated at a SaO_2 of about 90-92%.

Oxygenation and Pulmonary Physiology

Mechanical Ventilation

Mechanical ventilation is the delivery of positive pressure ventilation. This is different from the normal negative pressure ventilation that occurs with spontaneous breathing. In response to the initiation of positive pressure ventilation, some patients develop hypotension due to the change in intrathoracic pressure. Patients may also be hypotensive due to the sedation used during intubation. A pneumothorax should always be considered when profound hypotension occurs. A chest tube is required when a patient with a pneumothorax is on positive pressure ventilation. A pneumothorax results in a sudden increase in peak inspiratory pressure (discussed below).

Indications for Mechanical Ventilation

◆ Respiratory failure.
  ❖ Hypercapnic.
  ❖ Hypoxemic.
◆ Excessive work of breathing.
  ❖ Tachypnea
  ❖ Accessory muscle use
  ❖ Tachycardia
  ❖ Diaphoresis
◆ Protection of airway.

Goals for Mechanical Ventilation

◆ Achieve adequate ventilation.

◆ Achieve adequate oxygenation.

◆ Provide decreased work of breathing, patient comfort and synchrony with the ventilator.

◆ Protect the lungs from further injury.

Linking Knowledge to Practice

✔ *Increased work of breathing steals significant cardiac output away from other organs. Increased work of breathing should always be aggressively treated, even if initial oxygen saturation is adequate. Tachypnea is an important sign of impending risk to the patient.*

Noninvasive Positive Pressure Ventilation (NPPV)

Noninvasive positive pressure ventilation is mechanical ventilation without endotracheal intubation. A nasal or face mask is utilized. It can be used in hypercapnic or hypoxemic respiratory failure. It is most successful when used with a patient who is alert, oriented, and cooperative. The contraindications include:

◆ Decreased level of consciousness.

◆ Gastrointestinal bleeding.

◆ Hemodynamic instability.

◆ Progressive decline in respiratory status
(FCCS, 2006).

91

Chapter 3

Continuous Positive Airway Pressure (CPAP)

CPAP maintains positive airway pressure at the end of expiration, rather than allowing pressure to return to zero (Figure 3.10). There are no machine delivered breaths. The patient controls rate and V_T. Continuous positive airway pressure accomplishes what PEEP accomplishes as an adjunct to other modes of mechanical ventilation.

Biphasic Positive Airway Pressure (BiPAP)

Combines CPAP with pressure support during inspiration.

Types of Breaths Used in Mechanical Ventilation

It is important to understand the types of breaths that can be delivered by mechanical ventilators in order to understand the modes of mechanical ventilation.

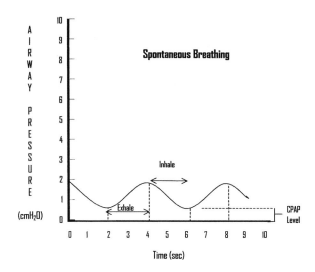

Figure 3.10: Continuous positive airway pressure.

- Volume cycled breath: Breath is delivered at a preset tidal volume. Exhalation begins after the set volume has been delivered. Volume cycled breathing is used in volume control ventilation.

- Time cycled breath: A pressure control breath is delivered at a constant pressure (i.e. 20 cm H_2O) for a preset time (i.e. 2 seconds). Time cycled breathing is used in pressure control ventilation.

- Flow cycled breath: A flow cycled breath is a pressure support breath. It allows a constant pressure during inspiration. There is no set time in a flow cycled breath. Once a set amount of the peak flow has been delivered, exhalation begins. Flow cycled breaths are used in pressure support ventilation.

Modes of Ventilation

Assist Control (AC) Mode. In assist control ventilation, a minimal respiratory rate is set. The ventilator assures that the patient receives a set number of breaths delivered at the preset parameters based on either volume cycled or time cycled breaths. The patient is allowed to initiate breaths above the preset respiratory rate. When the patient triggers a spontaneous breath, the ventilator assures the delivery of the breath at the same settings as the ventilator initiated breaths. The AC mode differs from controlled mandatory ventilation (CMV) where no spontaneous breaths are allowed. Current ventilators have no direct setting for CMV; however, this mode is essentially achieved in the AC mode in patients who are heavily sedated or paralyzed, or who have no spontaneous respiratory activity.

- Allows the patient to assist with initiation of breaths, yet maintains control of patient breaths once initiated (Figure 3.11).

- Is effective in decreasing the work of breathing when used with appropriate sedation via a sedation protocol.

- Can use volume targeted (volume cycled breaths) or pressure targeted (time cycled) breaths.

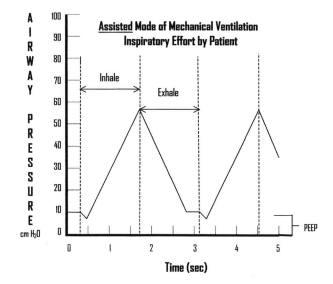

Figure 3.11: Assist control ventilation.

Oxygenation and Pulmonary Physiology

- Volume targeted with volume cycled breaths delivers a preset tidal volume.
  - ❖ Delivers constant tidal volume regardless of peak airway and alveolar pressure
- Pressure targeted with time cycled breaths delivers a preset pressure for set amount of time (called pressure controlled).
  - ❖ Delivers constant peak airway pressure and alveolar pressure, regardless of tidal volume delivered.
  - ❖ Primary advantage is that a decreased level of tidal volume is automatically delivered when there is any impedance to ventilation.

Example: AC using volume cycled breaths is set at a respiratory rate of 12 per minute and a tidal volume of 600. The patient is breathing spontaneously 8 times a minute above the preset rate of 12, for a total respiratory rate of 20 breaths per minute. Each of the 20 breaths is delivered at a tidal volume of 600 ml.

Synchronized Intermittent Mandatory Ventilation (SIMV). Like AC ventilation, SIMV delivers a set number of ventilator breaths at preset parameters and also allows the patient to initiate breaths above the preset rate. However, patient initiated breaths in SIMV are patient dependent and not guaranteed to achieve ventilator set parameters.

- SIMV can be used for volume targeted (volume cycled breaths) or pressure targeted (time cycled breaths) ventilation.
- Pressure support is often used during spontaneous breaths.
- The primary disadvantage of SIMV is the increased work of breathing in the patient with respiratory distress.

Example: SIMV using volume cycled breaths is set at a respiratory rate of 8 per minute and a tidal volume of 600. The patient is breathing spontaneously 8 times a minute above the preset rate of 8, for a total respiratory rate of 16 breaths per minute. Only the 8 preset ventilator breaths are delivered at a tidal volume of 600 ml. The tidal volume on the 8 additional patient initiated breaths is completely determined by the patient. For this reason, SIMV is not a mode of choice for a patient with respiratory distress.

Pressure Support Ventilation. Pressure support ventilation combines mechanical ventilation with spontaneous breathing. This mode of ventilation allows for spontaneous breathing through all phases of the respiratory cycle. Pressure support during inspiration can be combined with continuous positive airway pressure (CPAP), which maintains a positive pressure at the end of expiration.

Airway Pressure Release Ventilation (APRV). APRV is a mode of ventilation aimed at opening alveoli and is called an open lung strategy. This mode combines mechanical ventilation with spontaneous breathing. A high level of CPAP is used during spontaneous breathing with a release level (the release level allows CO_2 to be cleared). Spontaneous breathing is required throughout airway pressure release ventilation. The patient breathes small tidal volumes in this mode.

- Two pressure levels are used.
  - ❖ P High (the high pressure is typically set at 20-30 cm H_2O).
  - ❖ P Low (the low pressure is typically set at 0 cm H_2O). P low is also known as the release pressure.
- One inspiratory time is used: T High (this is the amount of time the patient will breathe at the high pressure, typically 4 to 6 seconds).
- One expiratory time is used: T Low (this is the amount of time allowed for the release or low pressure. It is typically a very short time, such as 0.8 seconds).
- Advantages:
  - ❖ Prevents lung overdistention.
  - ❖ Lower mean and peak airway pressures prevent barotrauma.

Chapter 3

- ❖ Spontaneous breathing during all cycles decreases use of sedatives and paralytics.
- ❖ Less cardiac compromise.
- ◆ Barriers to Use:
  - ❖ Potential derecruitment of alveoli during release phase.
  - ❖ Minute ventilation needs to be monitored.
  - ❖ Learning curve required.

High Frequency Oscillatory Ventilation. This mode of ventilation is another mode aimed at recruiting (opening) alveoli, and is also referred to as an open lung strategy.

- ◆ Oscillates gas (not jet ventilation) and maintains a constant mean airway pressure.
- ◆ Recruits alveoli and also prevents derecruitment.
- ◆ Gas is both delivered and removed; 1/3 time delivery in and 2/3 time delivery out.
- ◆ Tidal volume is small between 1-3 ml/kg.
- ◆ Initial setting usually at 5 to 6 HZ (60 oscillations/HZ).
- ◆ Visible chest movement occurs in response to oscillation.
- ◆ Jugular venous distention occurs as a result of the effects (tamponade-like effect) of continuous oscillation.
- ◆ Minimizes barotrauma and oxygen toxicity.

Adjuncts of Mechanical Ventilation

- ◆ PEEP – Positive End Expiratory Pressure – maintains positive pressure at the end of exhalation and does not allow pressure to return to zero. Provides results similar to continuous positive airway pressure (CPAP).
  - ❖ PEEP is used to improve oxygenation by increasing mean airway pressures and increasing the driving pressure of oxygen across the alveolar capillary membrane. PEEP is also associated with potential complications:
    - ☆ Barotrauma – from increased pressure at the end of expiration. This risk is increased with high levels of PEEP and in patients with emphysema.
    - ☆ Decreased cardiac output – from decreased venous return to the heart as a result of increase in intrathoracic pressure. PEEP should not be initiated in hypovolemic states.
    - ☆ Regional hypoperfusion – from compression of capillaries surrounding over-distended alveoli.
- ◆ Pressure Support Ventilation (PSV) – provides positive pressure for spontaneous breaths during SIMV.

Oxygenation and Pulmonary Physiology

Initial Ventilator Settings in Acute Respiratory Failure

(*Note:* Most common initial mode of ventilation used in critical care for respiratory failure is AC with volume cycled breaths.)

Tidal volume: (V_T): Usually set at 8-10 ml/kg of ideal body weight. The lower end of the range is typically used. For patients with acute lung injury, lower tidal volumes of 5-8 ml/kg of ideal body weight are used to prevent additional lung injury.

Respiratory Rate: Usually set at 12-16 breaths per minute.

Fraction of Inspired Oxygen (FIO_2): Started at 1.0 or 100%. Wean as quickly as possible to 0.4 or 40%, while maintaining an oxygen saturation of 92-94%.

PEEP: Usually started at 5 cm of H_2O. PEEP is titrated up as needed to achieve adequate oxygenation. > 15 cm H_2O of PEEP is rarely used.

Other ventilator settings:

◆ Peak Flow (gas flow): Speed and method of V_T delivery, velocity of air flow in liters per minute.

◆ Sensitivity: Determines patient's effort to initiate an assisted breath.

◆ I:E ratio (inspiratory to expiratory ratio): Typically set at 1:2 (can be altered to facilitate gas exchange).

Measured Parameters During Mechanical Ventilation

Peak Inspiratory Pressure (PIP) (Figure 3.12)

◆ Pressure needed to get air through airways and distend the lung.

◆ Accounts for both airway resistance (tubing and patient airways) and lung and chest wall compliance.

◆ Used to set high and low alarm limits.
   ❖ High pressure limit is maximum pressure the ventilator can generate to deliver the preset tidal volume, usually 10-20 cm H_2O above the Peak Inspiratory Pressure.

◆ Peak Inspiratory Pressure is different from peak flow that is set on the ventilator.

Linking Knowledge to Practice

✔ *A high peak inspiratory pressure can result from a problem with airway resistance caused by excessive secretions or bronchospasm, or can be caused by a decrease in lung compliance, such as in pulmonary fibrosis. Decreased lung compliance can also occur in acute conditions, such as pulmonary edema.*

Inspiratory Plateau Pressure (IPP) (Figure 3.12)

◆ The inspiratory plateau pressure is measured by holding inspiration after delivered tidal volume is complete. This measurement takes airway resistance out of the equation.

◆ The plateau pressure is reflective of the pressure in the alveoli at the end of inspiration. This is the pressure needed to keep alveoli distended (independent of resistance).

◆ The plateau pressure therefore reflects lung and chest wall compliance.

◆ Decreasing V_T is a strategy to lower plateau pressure. A lower V_T may cause an increase in $PaCO_2$. Permissive hypercapnea (acceptance of increased $PaCO_2$) may be indicated in order to reduce the plateau (and peak) airway pressure and protect the lung. Permissive hypercapnea is contraindicated with increased intracranial pressure.

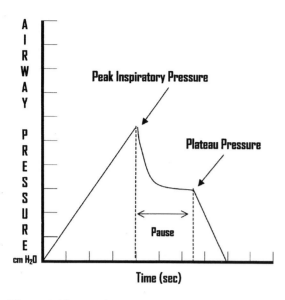

Figure 3.12: Peak inspiratory and plateau pressures.

Linking Knowledge to Practice

✔ *An increase in airway resistance from excessive secretions or bronchospasm does not impact plateau pressures (only peak inspiratory pressures). However, decreased alveolar compliance from ARDS impacts both peak inspiratory pressure and plateau pressure.*

✔ *When peak pressure is increased but plateau pressure is unchanged, the problem is related to an increase in airway resistance (e.g. tracheal tube obstruction, airway obstruction from secretions, or acute bronchospasm). Key interventions include suctioning and the administration of bronchodilators.*

✔ *When there is an increase in both peak and plateau pressures, consider conditions that decrease compliance of the lung tissue or chest wall (e.g. pneumothorax, lobar atelectasis, pulmonary edema, worsening pneumonia, ARDS).*

Interventions to Decrease Airway Resistance
- Bronchodilators such as albuterol (Ventolin; Proventil) or ipratropium bromide (Atrovent).
- Steroids for bronchospasm.
- Repositioning and suctioning to mobilize and aspirate secretions.

Interventions to Improve Lung Compliance
- Prevent abdominal distention.
- Thoracentesis or chest tube for pleural effusion.
- Diuretics for pulmonary edema.
- Antibiotics for pneumonia
  (Bojar, 2005).

Mean Airway Pressure.
The mean airway pressure is the constant opening pressure in the airway. It is a reflection of the mean pressure throughout the respiratory cycle. An adequate mean airway pressure is needed for optimal oxygenation. Lung recruitment efforts involve a sustained increase in airway pressure.

The use of PEEP increases mean airway pressure in mechanically ventilated patients. The use of pressure support and CPAP during non-invasive mechanical ventilation also increases mean airway pressure. In addition, an increase in inspiratory time increases mean airway pressure.

I:E Ratio.
The inspiratory/expiratory ratio is monitored during mechanical ventilation. The normal ratio is 1:2. Patients with COPD require longer expiratory times (1:3, 1:4 or perhaps longer).

The I:E ratio can be adjusted during mechanical ventilation to optimize oxygenation. Increasing inspiratory time increases mean airway pressure. Increasing V_T and decreasing peak flow rate (gas takes longer to enter alveoli) increases inspiratory time. When inspiratory time increases, expiratory time decreases, and there is the risk for auto PEEP.

Oxygenation and Pulmonary Physiology

When expiration time is too short, patients can develop auto PEEP. The lung volume at end expiration should reflect functional residual capacity (FRC). Auto PEEP causes the lung volume at end of expiration to be greater than functional residual capacity (FRC). The arrow in Figure 3.13 shows the failure of the waveform to return to baseline during expiration. This represents auto PEEP.

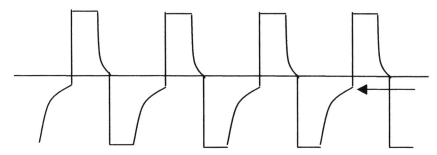

Figure 3.13: Auto PEEP.

A high respiratory rate shortens the time available for expiration and can result in auto PEEP. In addition, a high V_T increases inspiratory time, therefore shortening expiratory time and placing the patient at risk for auto PEEP. Decreasing V_T is an effective intervention to decrease inspiratory time, and therefore increase expiratory time. Auto PEEP increases all airway pressures and decreases venous return to the heart.

Interventions to Increase Expiratory Time:
- Decrease tidal volume.
- Increase Peak Gas Flow.
- Decrease respiratory rate.

Lung Protective Strategies

The goal of lung protective strategies is to avoid ventilator induced lung injury. Types of lung injury are:
- Barotrauma (caused by excessive pressure).
- Volutrauma (caused by excessive volume).
- Ateletrauma (caused by low volume resulting in repetitive opening and closing of distal lung units).
- Biotrauma (caused by biochemical mediators released in response to mechanical ventilation, as opposed to a mechanical complication)
  (Slutsky, 1999)

Current lung protective strategies include:
- Low tidal volume (6 ml/kg) with permissive hypercapnea.
- Maintain plateau pressure < 30 cm H_2O.

Hemodynamic Effects of Mechanical Ventilation

- Decreased venous return (decreased right ventricular preload).
- Pulmonary capillary compression and increased right ventricular afterload.
- Decreased right ventricular stroke volume.
- Decreased left ventricular afterload.
- State of baseline left ventricular function impacts hemodynamic effects.

Chapter 3

Linking Knowledge to Practice

When a patient develops hypotension during mechanical ventilation, assessment should be made for one of the following related factors:

✔ *Conversion to positive pressure ventilation.*
 ❖ *Assure adequate circulating fluid volume.*
✔ *Tension Pneumothorax.*
 ❖ *Chest tube required.*
✔ *Development of auto PEEP.*
 ❖ *Increase expiration time.*

Sedation During Mechanical Ventilation

Patients on mechanical ventilation should be adequately sedated in addition to receiving adequate analgesia. Under sedation is a common clinical error. However, over sedation also leads to increased clinical complications. Sedation protocols are effective tools for achieving optimal patient sedation. Long acting agents provide more consistent levels of sedation and can be used when near term extubation is not planned. Lorazepam, a benzodiazepine, for example, has a longer elimination half-life and would not be appropriate in patients only requiring short term intubation. Analgesics, in addition to sedative and anxiolytic agents, should be used for patient comfort. All patients receiving sedation while on mechanical ventilation should undergo a daily awakening trial (sedation vacation). After the awakening trial, the patient needs to be reassessed for the continued need for sedation and for the appropriate level of sedation. The most important goals for analgesia and sedation during mechanical ventilation are patient comfort and ventilator synchrony.

Benefits of Sedatives During Mechanical Ventilation

* Reduce anxiety.
* Amnesia, particularly during use of neuromuscular blocking agents.
* Prevent recall of unpleasant experience.
* Decrease level of stress hormones.
* Reduce tissue oxygen consumption.
* Improve ventilator synchrony.

Neuromuscular Blocking Agents (Paralytics)

Most patients on mechanical ventilation do not require neuromuscular blockade (paralysis). Low tidal volume ventilation is usually tolerated well with adequate sedation. Administration of neuromuscular blockade should be preceded by adequate sedation, and sedation must be continued throughout neuromuscular blockade. Neuromuscular blocking agents should always be given in the lowest possible dose for the shortest amount of time.

Possible indications for neuromuscular blockade in the patient receiving mechanical ventilation include:

◆ Endotracheal intubation. There is the potential risk of loss of airway when paralytics are used to facilitate intubation.

◆ Facilitation of tolerance to mechanical ventilation. This may be indicated, especially with high levels of PEEP, airway pressure release ventilation, or inverse I:E ratio ventilation.

◆ Reduction in oxygen consumption. Adequate sedation, however, is also effective in decreasing oxygen consumption.

98

Oxygenation and Pulmonary Physiology

There are 2 groups of neuromuscular blocking agents: depolarizing and non-depolarizing.

Depolarizing agents

Depolarization occurs by acetylcholine binding to muscle receptors and producing a sodium – potassium discharge. Repolarization is able to occur because acetylcholine is inactivated by acetylcholinesterase. Depolarizing agents work by mimicking the effect of acetylcholine on the neuromuscular junction at the motor end plate and producing a depolarization. Depolarization results in the fasciculation of skeletal muscle, followed by paralysis. Depolarizing agents are resistant to acetylcholinesterase. However, a second plasma enzyme, pseudocholinesterase is able to metabolize both acetylcholine and acetylcholine-like agents (Clinical Pharmacology Database, 2007; Marini & Wheeler, 2006)

Succinylcholine, a depolarizing agent, has a very rapid onset of action (within seconds) and a short duration of action (less than 10 minutes). If given in repeat doses, it produces a vagal response. The depolarization process produces a muscle contraction and release of potassium. Significant hyperkalemia can develop in high-risk patients. Vomiting, increased intraocular pressure, and post paralysis muscle pain are other potential side effects (Marini & Wheeler, 2006).

Non-depolarizing agents

Non-depolarizing agents work instead by occupying the binding sites for acetylcholine at the post-junctional membrane. This prevents the action of acetylcholine. There is no depolarizing effect. These agents are not resistant to the antagonistic effects of acetylcholinesterase. Many of these medications have a chemical structure that resembles corticosteroids (Clinical Pharmacology Database, 2007; Marini & Wheeler, 2006). Non-depolarizing agents are commonly classified by their duration of action ranging from short duration (20 minutes) to long duration (greater than one hour). Vecuronium and atracurium are the agents most used in the critical care setting (Ellstrom, 2006).

Table 3.3 lists commonly used neuromuscular blocking agents.

Table 3.3 Classification of Neuromuscular Blocking Agents	
Depolarizing	**Non-depolarizing**
Succinylcholine	Mivacurium – Short duration
	Vecuronium – Intermediate duration Atracurium – Intermediate duration
	Doxacurium – Long duration Pipecuronium – Long duration Pancuronium – Long duration
(Marini & Wheeler, 2006).	

Many different drugs can enhance or antagonize neuromuscular blocking effects. In the cardiac patients it is important to know that beta blockers and calcium channel blockers, certain antiarrhythmics, acidosis, hyponatremia, hypocalcemia, and hypothermia enhance neuromuscular blocking effects (Marini & Wheeler, 2006).

Linking Knowledge to Practice

✔ *Paralytic agents interfere with the ability to assess for many complications, including ischemia, stroke, hypoglycemia, and seizures. The lack of ability to assess for seizure activity becomes increasingly important when paralytics are used to treat shivering during hypothermia therapy post-cardiac arrest. These patients in particular are at high risk for seizure activity from hypoxic neurological injury.*

Complications of neuromuscular blockade

There are many potential side effects of long term use, including the development of deep vein thrombosis, muscle atrophy, and nerve compression syndromes. Acute quadriplegic myopathy syndrome, or critical illness polyneuropathy, is a serious complication of neuromuscular blockade in which patients are left with residual weakness after long term use of neuromuscular blockade (Marini & Wheeler, 2006).

Assessment with neuromuscular blocking agents

Peripheral nerve stimulators (Figure 3.14) are used to objectively assess patients on neuromuscular blockade. The most commonly used nerve-muscle combinations are the facial nerve and orbicularis oculi, and the ulnar nerve and adductor pollicus.

The nerve is stimulated with 4 electrical stimuli, and the response is observed in terms of the number of twitches. There is the potential for four possible twitches. Blockade of 90-95% of the receptors results in a one-twitch response. The goal is to have one or two twitches in response to nerve stimulation. Complete obliteration of the twitches implies paralytic overdose. However, there may be occasions when patients require excessive peripheral blockade in order to achieve diaphragmatic paralysis and ventilator synchrony (Marini & Wheeler, 2006).

Another technique to prevent excessive neuromuscular blockade is to allow the patient to move before giving any additional doses of neuromuscular blockade. This technique may reveal that paralysis is no longer needed or sedation is inadequate. This may also allow for the assessment of any symptoms that have been masked.

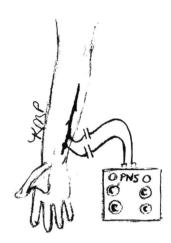

Figure 3.14: Peripheral nerve stimulator.

Patient Care and Monitoring During Mechanical Ventilation

Pulse Oximetry

SpO_2 (pulse oximetry) monitoring is routinely used to assess the patient's oxygenation status. Blood gases to evaluate pH and $PaCO_2$ are used to assess the patient's ventilaton status. Pulse oximetry is used to estimate oxyhemoglobin. The SpO_2 generally correlates with the SaO_2 + or - 2%. The goal in most patients is to keep the oxygen saturation equal to or greater than 92-94%. In African Americans the SpO_2 should be a little higher (FCCS, 2006). Accurate pulse oximetry requires the presence of a pleth wave detecting an accurate pulse. Patients receiving administration of high fat content such as with propofol or TPN can have a falsely high SpO_2. In addition, several factors can interfere with the accuracy of pulse oximetry.

- Hemoglobin < 5 g/dL or hematocrit <15%.
- Abnormal hemoglobin, such as carboxyhemoglobin or methemoglobin.
- SpO_2 below 70%.
- State of low blood flow, such as with hypotension or vasoconstriction.
- IV dyes, fingernail polish, and some skin pigmentations
  (FCCS, 2006 and Ellstrom, 2006).

End Tidal CO2 Monitoring

Patient End Tidal CO_2 ($PetCO_2$) is a noninvasive assessment of $PaCO_2$. Expired CO_2 can be measured, directly at the patient and ventilator interface. Airway adapter should be placed as close to the patients airway as possible. End exhalation is assumed to represent alveolar gas, and under normal circumstances, parallels $PaCO_2$. The normal gradient between $PaCO_2$ and $PetCO_2$ is 1-5 mm Hg. Several factors can interfere with the correlation, including body temperature, pulmonary disease and cardiac status. For example in pulmonary embolus, shock, or other critical conditions there is an increase in PaCO$_2$, and the gradient between PaCO$_2$ and PetCO$_2$ widens. PetCO$_2$ monitoring has limited applications for assessing changes in alveolar ventilation. It can be used to detect changes over time and should be considered in patients who are undergoing deep sedation.

Additional Considerations During Mechanical Ventilation

Excessive intake of carbohydrates and fats can increase CO$_2$ production. Tube feedings designed for patients with pulmonary disease and those on mechanical ventilation are available.

Systemic hydration and humidification of ventilator circuit are necessary to prevent drying and thickening of secretions.

Prevention of Ventilator Acquired Pneumonia
- Hand hygiene.
- Oral care, including brushing of teeth, gums, and tongue.
- HOB elevated 30 to 40 degrees.
- Suction only when necessary (not routine).
- Routine installation of NS not recommended.
- Cover yankauer catheters when not in use.
- Ventilator circuit changes only when soiled, or weekly.
- Adequate endotracheal tube cuff pressure:
  - Maintain at < 20 mm Hg or < 25 cm H$_2$O to not exceed capillary filling pressure of trachea.
  - Low pressure high volume cuffs typically used.
  - Inflate to assure no or minimal leak during inspiration.
  - Need for increasing air may be due to tracheal dilation or leak in cuff or pilot balloon valve (tube must be replaced if leak present).
  - Cuff pressures measured routinely every 8-12 hours and with any change in tube position (Ellstrom, 2006).
- Subglottic suctioning prior to repositioning or deflating cuff (Figure 3.15).
- Hold tube feedings if residuals > 150 cc.
- Discontinue NG tubes as soon as possible.
- Extubate as soon as possible.
- Avoid nasal intubation.
- Stress ulcer prophylaxis with sucralfate rather than H$_2$ blockers or proton pump inhibitors is thought to have the potential advantage of not promoting bacterial colonization of the gastrointestinal tract because it does not raise gastric pH.
- Avoid overuse of antibiotics.

Tracheostomy

Indications for tracheostomy include to:
- Bypass an upper airway obstruction.
- Decrease dead space ventilation.
- Facilitate in removal of secretions.

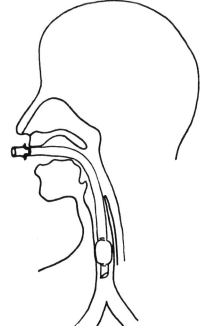

Figure 3.15: Endotracheal tube location.
From *Pass CCRN* (2nd ed.), R.D. Dennison, 2000. St. Louis: Mosby. Reprinted with permission from Elsevier.

Chapter 3

- Prevent/limit aspiration (cuffed tubes are usually used when patient is receiving mechanical ventilation).
- Provide patient comfort for prolonged mechanical ventilation

(Ellstrom, 2006).

A tracheostomy should be considered for patients requiring mechanical ventilation longer than 2 weeks. The most common method of tracheostomy placement is with a percutaneous dilational technique using bronchoscopic guidance (Bojar, 2005). Benefits to tracheostomy placement for ventilator dependent patients include:

- Decreased laryngeal damage, swallowing dysfunction, and glottic trauma.
- Decreased in airway resistance.
- Improved ability to suction lower airways.
- Decreased risk of sinusitis.
- Improved patient comfort and mobility

(Bojar, 2005).

Care of a tracheostomy includes:

- Keep tube secure. Risk for dislodgement is high for first 3 to 5 days after insertion.
- Keep the stoma clean and dry and assess for skin breakdown under and around the neck plate. Treat new tracheostomy as a surgical wound.
- Exchange (if disposable) or clean the inner cannula. Be prepared for complications by having the following readily available: ambu bag and mask, suction equipment, tube obturator, and intubation supplies.

(Ellstrom, 2006).

Ventilator Weaning

Most patients are weaned by using a spontaneous breathing trial on T-piece with CPAP. T-piece spontaneous breathing trials are done for only short periods of time. Inspiratory pressure support may also be added during the weaning process to overcome the resistance of the endotracheal tube and the ventilator circuit.

Other methods of weaning include decreasing the rate of SIMV and adding pressure support to spontaneous breaths. Pressure support for spontaneous breaths is then progressively lowered.

Weaning Criteria

- Resolution of acute process.
- Hemodynamic stability.
- Adequate nutritional status.
- Adequate level of consciousness, ability to cooperate, and psychological preparedness

Minimal Weaning Parameters

- Spontaneous respiratory rate < 30 breaths per minute.
- Spontaneous tidal volume: > 5ml/kg.
- Vital capacity: > 10 ml/kg, ideally 15ml/kg.
- Minute ventilation: < 10L.
- Negative inspiratory pressure: more negative than -25 to -30 cm H_2O.
- FIO_2: < 0.50.
- PaO_2 / FIO_2 ratio > 200.

A sensitive indicator for weaning readiness is the rapid, shallow breathing index: the respiratory rate divided by average V_T in liters during 1 minute of spontaneous breathing. An index of < 100 breaths/min/L is associated with successful weaning (Raoof & Khan, 1998).

Oxygenation and Pulmonary Physiology

Examples:

Patient has a spontaneous respiratory rate of 16 with an average tidal of volume of 500 ml per breath. The rapid shallow breathing index is: 16/0.5L = 32.

Patient has a spontaneous respiratory rate of 32 with an average tidal volume of 300 ml per breath. The rapid shallow breathing index is: 32/0.3L = 107.

Weaning with a tracheostomy involves cuff deflation with periods of capping the tube opening to allow for breathing through the upper airway.

Post Extubation Issues

◆ Laryngotracheal edema may occur post-extubation in patients who have been intubated for several days. This may result in upper airway obstruction. Treatment includes epinephrine and steroids.

◆ Patients who have been intubated for a long period of time should be assessed for adequate swallowing ability in order to avoid aspiration.

◆ Patients may have vocal cord damage as a result of prolonged intubation.

◆ Moving from positive pressure breathing back to spontaneous negative pressure breathing changes the intrapleural pressure from positive to negative and increases left ventricular afterload. Patients with severe left ventricular dysfunction may not tolerate this increase in afterload.

◆ Sealing of tracheostomy incision occurs within 72 hours of extubation. Until this time patients are unable to produce adequate coughing pressure (Ellstrom, 2006).

ACID–BASE BALANCE

Definitions

◆ Acid: Substance that can give up a H^+ ion.

◆ Acidemia: Blood pH below 7.35.

◆ Acidosis: Condition that causes acidemia.

◆ Base: Substance that can accept an H^+ ion.

◆ Alkalemia: Blood pH above 7.45.

◆ Alkalosis: Condition that causes the alkalemia.

Blood pH

◆ Indirect measurement of hydrogen ion activity or hydrogen ion concentration.

◆ Reflection of balance between carbonic acid and bicarbonate (base).

◆ Inversely proportional to hydrogen ion concentration (acids donate H^+ ions).

  ❖ ▲H^+ concentration = ▼pH, more acid.

  ❖ ▼H^+ concentration = ▲pH, less acid.

  ❖ pH < 6.9 or > 7.8 is incompatible with life.

Production and Removal of Acids in the Body

Cellular metabolism produces most acids in the body. These acids are waste products of ingested foods. Carbon dioxide is produced as the end product of the oxidation of glucose and fatty acids during aerobic metabolism. The hydration of carbon dioxide results in the formation of carbonic acid (H_2CO_3) (volatile acid), which can dissociate into a hydrogen ion and a bicarbonate ion. Large amounts of CO_2 are removed from the body during ventilation.

103

Chapter 3

About 5-10% of CO_2 carried in the blood is physically dissolved in solution. (Carbon dioxide is about 20 times more soluble in plasma than oxygen.) About 5-10% of carbon dioxide travels in the form of carbamino compounds (e.g. carbaminohemoglobin where the carbon dioxide is bound to the amino acids of hemoglobin). Deoxyhemoglobin can bind more carbon dioxide than oxyhemoglobin. When hemoglobin in pulmonary capillaries binds with oxygen, it releases carbon dioxide. About 80-90% of carbon dioxide in the blood is carried as bicarbonate ions. Red blood cells play an important role in facilitating the chemical reaction that produces bicarbonate ions.

$$\text{(Lungs) } CO_2 + H_2O \leftrightarrow H_2CO_3 \leftrightarrow HCO_3^- + H^+ \text{ (Kidneys).}$$

Other acids (non-volatile acids) produced in much smaller quantity during metabolism include sulfuric acid, phosphoric acid, hydrochloric acid, and lactic acid. The removal of these acids is accomplished mainly by the kidneys.

Buffers

◆ Bicarbonate (HCO_3^-).
  ❖ Generated by kidney.
  ❖ Aids in elimination of H^+.
  ❖ Most important buffer system in the body.
◆ Phosphate
  ❖ Aids in excretion of H^+ ions by the kidneys.
◆ Proteins

Role of Respiratory System

◆ Respiratory system can only compensate for metabolic disorders. Responds within minutes.
◆ Regulates the excretion or retention of carbonic acid.
  ❖ If pH is down (metabolic acidosis): increase rate and depth of respiration to blow off CO_2 (increases alveolar ventilation).
  ❖ If pH is up (metabolic alkalosis): decrease rate and depth of respiration to retain CO_2 (decreases alveolar ventilation).

Role of Renal System

◆ Renal system can compensate for respiratory disorders and for metabolic disorders not involving the kidneys. Responds within 48 hours, but complete compensation may take several days.
◆ Regulates excretion or retention of HCO_3^- and the excretion of H^+ and non-volatile acids.
  ❖ If pH is down (acidosis): Kidney retains HCO_3^- and excretes fixed acids.
  ❖ If pH is up (alkalosis): Kidney decreases HCO_3^- reabsorption and decreases hydrogen ion secretion. *Note:* There is an inverse relationship between renal K+ secretion and renal H^+ secretion. Therefore, alterations in acid base balance cause an alteration in K+ balance.
◆ Normally the kidneys secrete about 70 mEq of H^+ and reabsorb about 70 mEq of HCO_3^- daily. This process can increase greatly during acidosis, acidifying the urine to a pH as low as 4.0 to 5.0.

Oxygenation and Pulmonary Physiology

ABG Analysis

- Evaluate ventilation: $PaCO_2$.
- Evaluate acid-base status: pH.
- Evaluate source of abnormal pH: respiratory or metabolic.
- Evaluate oxygenation: PaO_2, SaO_2.

Normal Parameters

- pH
  - Normal 7.35-7.45.
  - < 7.35 Acidosis.
  - > 7.45 Alkalosis.
- $PaCO_2$
  - Normal 35-45 mm Hg.
  - < 35 mm Hg respiratory alkalosis or respiratory compensation for metabolic acidosis.
  - > 45 mm Hg respiratory acidosis or respiratory compensation for metabolic alkalosis.
- HCO_3^-
  - Normal 22-26 mEq/L.
  - < 22 metabolic acidosis or metabolic compensation for respiratory alkalosis.
  - > 26 metabolic alkalosis or metabolic compensation for respiratory acidosis.
- Base Excess (BE): The base excess or base deficit is the number of mEq of acid or base needed to titrate one liter of blood to a pH of 7.4 at a temperature of 37 degrees Celsius and with a constant PCO_2 of 40 mm Hg.
  - Normal + 2 to –2 mEq/L.
  - > +2 = metabolic alkalosis or metabolic compensation for respiratory acidosis.
  - < -2 (base deficit) = metabolic acidosis or metabolic compensation for respiratory alkalosis.
    - ☆ *Note:* Base deficit can be used to estimate how much sodium bicarbonate (in mEq) to give a patient. This is determined by multiplying the base deficit by the patient's estimated extracellular fluid space. Extracellular fluid space is estimated at 0.3 times the lean body mass in kilograms.
- PaO_2
  - Normal 80-100 mm Hg (for FIO_2 0.21).
  - > 100 hyperoxemia.
  - < 80 mild hypoxemia.
  - < 60 moderate hypoxemia.
  - < 40 severe hypoxemia.
- SaO_2
  - Normal 95% or >.
  - < 95% mild desaturation of hemoglobin.
  - < 90% moderate desaturation of hemoglobin.
  - < 75% severe desaturation of hemoglobin.

Chapter 3

Compensation

An acidosis or alkalosis for which there has been compensation causes the pH to return to the normal range while leaning toward the initial disorder. The body never overcompensates. A non-leaning pH with two abnormal indicators suggests a mixed disorder (one alkalotic and one acidotic process). An example is primary respiratory alkalosis and primary metabolic acidosis.

Anion Gap

The anion gap is used to help determine the cause of the patient's metabolic acidosis. The anion gap is determined by summing the plasma chloride and bicarbonate levels, then subtracting from the patient's sodium level.

- Anion Gap = $Na+ - [Cl- + HCO_3-]$.
- A normal anion gap is 12 + or – 4 mEq/L. An increased anion gap typically indicates an increased concentration of anions other than Cl- and HCO_3-. Causes of increased concentrations of these other anions include lactic acidosis, ketoacidosis, ingestion of anions such as salicylate, or renal retention of anions such as sulfate, phosphate, and urate.

Causes of Respiratory Acidosis (any cause of alveolar hypoventilation)

- Depression of respiratory control centers.
- Neuromuscular disorders.
- Chest wall restriction.
- Lung restriction.
- Airway obstruction.
- Pulmonary parenchymal disease/injury.

Causes of Respiratory Alkalosis (any cause of alveolar hyperventilation)

- Central nervous system disorders.
- Drugs.
- Hormones.
- Bacteremia.
- Over mechanical ventilation.
- High Altitude.
- Acute Asthma.
- Pulmonary Embolism.

Causes of Metabolic (Non-Respiratory) Acidosis

- Ingested toxic substances.
- Loss of bicarbonate ions.
- Lactic acidosis.
- Ketoacidosis.
- Renal failure.

Oxygenation and Pulmonary Physiology

Causes of Metabolic Alkalosis

◆ Loss of hydrogen ions.
  ❖ Vomiting.
  ❖ Diuretics.
  ❖ Steroids.
◆ Excess bicarbonate.

LET'S PRACTICE – ABG ANALYSIS ON ROOM AIR *(answers at end of chapter)*

1. pH   7.30
    $PaCO_2$ 54
    HCO_3^- 26
    PaO_2 64

2. pH   7.48
    $PaCO_2$ 30
    HCO_3^- 24
    PaO_2 96

3. pH   7.30
    $PaCO_2$ 40
    HCO_3^- 18
    PaO_2 85

4. pH   7.50
    $PaCO_2$ 40
    HCO_3^- 33
    PaO_2 92

5. pH   7.35
    $PaCO_2$ 54
    HCO_3^- 30
    PaO_2 55

6. pH   7.21
    $PaCO_2$ 60
    HCO_3^- 20
    PaO_2 48

Chapter 3

7. pH   7.54
   $PaCO_2$ 25
   HCO_3^- 30
   PaO_2 95

TEST YOUR KNOWLEDGE

1. A shift in the oxyhemoglobin curve to the left means

    a. hemoglobin releases oxygen more easily.

    b. hemoglobin binds with oxygen more tightly.

    c. tissues have improved oxygenation due to increased SaO_2.

    d. the SaO_2 for a PaO_2 of 60 mm Hg is expected to < 90%.

2. A patient has a low PaO_2 and normal $PaCO_2$ on blood gas. The low PaO_2 is corrected with oxygen therapy. This pulmonary problem is best described as

    a. a ventilation problem.

    b. a significant shunt.

    c. chronic COPD.

    d. a diffusion problem.

3. Blood gases after intubation and on a mechanical ventilator with an FIO_2 of 100% are: pH 7.21 $PaCO_2$ 42 mm Hg, PaO_2 51 mm Hg, and SaO_2 of 85%. Based on the above, you know:

    a. These gases represent a respiratory acidosis.

    b. PEEP can be added or increased to improve oxygenation.

    c. The patient has a significant intrapulmonary shunt.

    d. An increase in TV will be ordered.

    e. b and c only.

    f. All of the above.

4. Effectiveness of ventilation is evaluated by

    a. $PaCO_2$.

    b. SaO_2.

    c. pulmonary function studies.

    d. arterial pH.

Oxygenation and Pulmonary Physiology

5. Which of the following is not an indication for a tracheostomy:

    a. To decrease dead space.

    b. To prevent aspiration.

    c. To deliver a higher percentage FIO_2.

    d. To deliver mechanical ventilation over an extended period of time.

6. Your patient is on a mechanical ventilator: SIMV with a rate of 8, TV 700, FIO_2 0.40 and 5 cm of PEEP. His blood gases reveal pH 7.30, PCO_2 of 50 PaO_2 of 79, and a saturation of 95%. Most likely, ventilator change will include:

    a. Increased PEEP to 7.5.

    b. Increased FIO_2 to 0.45.

    c. Increased TV to 800.

    d. Changed to AC mode rate of 12 and provide sedation.

7. One of the goals in treating ARDS is to reduce oxygen consumption. This can be achieved by all of the following, except

    a. suctioning routinely every two hours.

    b. assuring adequate sedation.

    c. decreasing core body temperature.

    d. alternating nursing interventions with periods of rest.

8. You are working in the emergency department and draw blood gases on a patient not yet diagnosed. The blood gases on 4L nasal cannula are: pH 7.24, $PaCO_2$ 55, PaO_2 50, HCO_3^- 18. Your interpretation of these blood gases is

    a. respiratory acidosis.

    b. metabolic acidosis with mild hypoxemia.

    c. mixed respiratory and metabolic acidosis with significant hypoxemia.

    d. respiratory acidosis attempting to try to compensate.

9. A patient with pulmonary edema has impaired diffusion due to

    a. increased thickness of the alveolar capillary membrane.

    b. retaining PCO_2.

    c. an elevated body temperature associated with pulmonary edema.

    d. low barometric pressure.

Chapter 3

10. When monitoring a patient's SaO_2, you know the following:

    a. Keeping the SaO_2 > 90% is important.

    b. SaO_2 is not a sensitive indictor of ventilation.

    c. SaO_2 drops in a patient with a diffusion problem, intrapulmonary shunt, or untreated hypoventilation.

    d. All of the above.

11. When caring for a patient with COPD who chronically retains $PaCO_2$, you know the following to be true about delivering oxygen therapy:

    a. The patient should never be given more than 2L via nasal cannula.

    b. It is important to avoid oxygen saturations > 92% to protect the patient's hypoxic drive to breathe.

    c. It is safe to place the patient on a 100% non-rebreather as long as you check a pulse oximeter reading every 4 hours.

    d. Delivering oxygen decreases the PCO_2 which is the patient's drive to breathe.

12. A rise in hydrogen ions (acidosis) causes the oxyhemoglobin curve to shift

    a. right.

    b. left.

    c. no effect.

    d. right or left depending on the patient SaO_2.

13. The best indicator of global oxygenation is

    a. CO_2.

    b. SaO_2.

    c. SVO_2.

    d. DO_2.

14. Your patient has a cardiac index of 1.9, a Hb of 9.8 and an SaO_2 of 88%. What interventions would improve your patient's delivery of oxygen?

    a. Increase the cardiac index to 2.4.

    b. Increase the hemoglobin to 12.0.

    c. Increase the SaO_2 to 95%.

    d. All of the above.

Oxygenation and Pulmonary Physiology

15. Oxygen consumption (VO_2) in a healthy person is approximately what percent of oxygen delivery?
    a. 15%
    b. 25%
    c. 50%
    d. 75%

16. Which of the following statements is true?
    a. When oxygen reserve falls below 75%, anaerobic metabolism occurs.
    b. When you increase delivery of oxygen to tissues, they automatically consume more oxygen, keeping the reserve at a constant.
    c. A high SVO_2 always indicates excellent oxygenation.
    d. Oxygen consumption should be independent of oxygen delivery in a healthy person.

17. Your patient is on 60% FIO_2 and has a PaO_2 of 70 mm Hg. With this information, what do you know to be true?
    a. Your patient's oxyhemoglobin curve has shifted to the right and his SaO_2 will be lower than expected.
    b. Your patient has a clinically significant intrapulmonary shunt such as that caused by ARDS.
    c. Your patient's expected PaO_2 is only 90 mm Hg, so he has only a minor intrapulmonary shunt.
    d. Your patient's oxyhemoglobin curve has shifted to the left and his SaO_2 will be higher than expected.

18. If a patient has a normal PAO_2 (alveolar oxygen pressure) and a low PaO_2, this indicates a larger than normal A-a gradient and therefore a diffusion problem caused by some type of pathology at the location of the lungs.
    a. True.
    b. False.

19. If a patient has a low PAO_2 and a low PaO_2 resulting in hypoxemia but a normal A-a gradient, this suggests there is a ventilation problem.
    a. True.
    b. False.

20. Optimal PEEP is best defined as
    a. 5-10 cm in an intubated and ventilated patient.
    b. the amount of PEEP calculated based on the patient BSA.
    c. the amount of PEEP needed to achieve optimal oxygenation without causing a decrease in cardiac output or other complications.
    d. the amount of PEEP needed to allow your tidal volume and rate to be set at the lowest levels.

Chapter 3

21. All of following can cause a high inspiratory plateau pressure:

   a. ARDS

   b. Bronchospasm

   c. Increased upper airway secretions

   d. All of the above.

22. The preferred method of ventilation to decrease the work of breathing in a patient with respiratory failure is

   a. SIMV.

   b. assist control with adequate sedation.

   c. noninvasive ventilation with BiPAP.

   d. SIMV with pressure support.

23. Interventions to decrease peak inspiratory pressure in the presence of a normal plateau pressure may include

   a. suctioning.

   b. utilizing an endotracheal tube size 8 or >.

   c. albuterol or other bronchodilator.

   d. All of the above.

24. In a patient who develops auto PEEP, appropriate interventions to increase expiratory time may include

   a. increase respiratory rate.

   b. decrease tidal volume.

   c. increase tidal volume.

   d. decrease peak gas flow.

25. Possible causes of hypotension during mechanical ventilation include all of the following, except:

   a. development of auto PEEP.

   b. initial adjustment to positive pressure ventilation.

   c. increased venous return due to an increased level of PEEP.

   d. tension pneumothorox.

PRACTICE ABG ANSWERS

1. Respiratory acidosis with mild hypoxemia.
2. Respiratory alkalosis.
3. Metabolic acidosis.
4. Metabolic alkalosis.
5. Compensated respiratory acidosis with moderate hypoxemia.
6. Respiratory and metabolic acidosis with moderate hypoxemia.
7. Mixed respiratory and metabolic alkalosis.

ANSWERS

1.	B	14.	D
2.	D	15.	B
3.	E	16.	D
4.	A	17.	B
5.	C	18.	A
6.	D	19.	A
7.	A	20.	C
8.	C	21.	A
9.	A	22.	B
10.	D	23.	D
11.	B	24.	B
12.	A	25.	C
13.	C		

REFERENCES

Alcomo, I.E. (1996). *Anatomy and physiology the easy way.* Hauppauge, NY: Barrons.

Clinical Pharmacology Database. (2007). Gold Standard Inc. http://www.clinicalpharmacology.com

Burns, S.M. (2005). Mechanical ventilation of patients with acute respiratory distress syndrome and patients requiring weaning: The evidence guiding practice. *Critical Care Nurse, 25*(4), 14-23.

Dennison, R.D. (2000). *Pass CCRN* (2nd ed.). St. Louis: Mosby.

Ellstrom, K. (2006). The pulmonary system. In J.G. Alspach (Ed.), *Core curriculum for critical care nursing* (pp. 45-170). St. Louis: Saunders.

Kumar, V., Abbas, A.K., & Fausto, N. (2005). *Pathologic basis of disease* (7th ed.). Philadelphia: Elsevier Saunders.

Levitzky, M.G. (2003). *Pulmonary physiology* (6th ed.). New York: McGraw-Hill.

Lewis, S.M., Heitkemper, M.M., & Dirksen, S.T. (2004). *Medical surgical nursing: Assessment and management of clinical problems* (6th ed.). St. Louis: Mosby.

Marini, J.J. & Wheeler, A.P. (2006). *Critical care medicine the essentials* (3rd ed.). Philadelphia: Lippincott, Williams and Wilkins.

Melander, S.D. (2004). *Case studies in critical care nursing: A guide for application and review.* Philadelphia: W.B. Saunders Company.

Moore, K.L. & Dalley, A.F. (1999). *Clinically oriented anatomy* (4th ed.). Philadelphia: Lippincott, Williams and Wilkins.

Morton, P.G., Fontaine, D., Hudak, C.M., & Gallo, B.M. (Eds.). (2005). *Critical care nursing* (8th ed.). Philadelphia: Lippincott, Williams and Wilkins.

Porth, C.M. (Ed.). (2004). *Essentials of pathophysiology: Concepts of altered health states.* Philadelphia: Lippincott, Williams and Wilkins.

Raoof, S. & Faroque, K.A. (1998). *Mechanical ventilation manual.* Philadelphia, PA: American College of Physicians.

Schell, H.M. & Puntillo, K.A. (2001). *Critical care nursing secrets.* Philadelphia: Hanley and Belfus, Inc.

Slutsky, A.S. (1999, July). Lung Injury Caused by Mechanical Ventilation. *Chest, 116*, 9-15.

St. John, R.E. (2003, Aug). End Tidal Carbon Dioxide Monitoring. *Critical Care Nurse, 23*(4), 83-88.

Thelan, L.A., Davie, J.K., Urden, L.D. & Lough, M.E. (1994). *Critical care nursing: Diagnosis and management* (2nd ed.). St. Louis: Mosby.

Thibodeau, G.A. & Patton, K.T. (2003). *Anatomy and physiology* (5th ed.). St. Louis: Mosby.

Urden, L.D. & Stacy, K.M. (2000). *Priorities in critical care nursing* (3rd ed.). St. Louis: Mosby, Inc.

West, J.B. (2001). *Pulmonary physiology and pathophysiology: An integrated, case-based approach.* Philadelphia: Lippincott, Williams and Wilkins.

CHAPTER 4:
HEMODYNAMICS / SHOCK STATES / INTRA-AORTIC BALLOON PUMP THERAPY

HEMODYNAMIC CONCEPTS

Cardiac Output

Cardiac output is the volume of blood ejected by the ventricles each minute, normally 4-8 L/min. Cardiac output is used to assess the adequacy of blood flow. The cardiac index is a more patient specific indicator because it adjusts cardiac output to body surface area. The normal cardiac index is 2.5-4 L/min/m². The formula for cardiac output is stroke volume times heart rate: CO = SV x HR. When evaluating cardiac output there are 4 factors to consider (Figure 4.1):

- The 3 determinants of stroke volume:
  - Preload
  - Afterload
  - Contractility.
- Heart Rate

Note: The same 4 components also determine myocardial oxygen demand.

Determinants of Cardiac Output

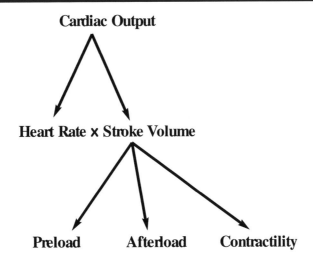

Figure 4.1: Cardiac output.

Chapter 4

Stroke Volume

Stroke volume is the amount of blood ejected from the ventricle with each beat. The normal stroke volume is 60-100 ml per beat. Normal stroke volume index is 35-60 ml/beat/m². Stroke volume provides a more specific assessment of left ventricular function than cardiac output because tachycardia has the potential to increase cardiac output to normal or near normal levels in the presence of low stroke volume.

Low stroke volume can be due to low preload, decreased contractility, or high afterload. Valvular dysfunction, such as mitral regurgitation, can also cause a decreased stroke volume. High stroke volume can be caused by low afterload or increased contractility.

Preload

Preload is the stretch on the myocardial muscle fibers at the end of diastole and is determined by the volume of blood filling the ventricle at the end of diastole. As shown in Figure 4.2, the greater the volume and therefore the stretch (muscle fiber length), the greater the force of contraction and stroke volume. This occurs to a point where increased volume and stretch no longer produce an increase in stroke volume. Excessive preload results in congestion, increased resistance to coronary blood flow, and increased myocardial oxygen consumption.

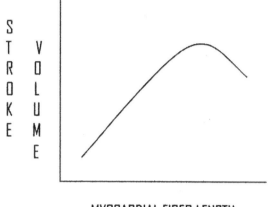

Figure 4.2: Preload.

Right Ventricular Preload

- Measured by right atrial pressure (RAP) or central venous pressure (CVP).
  - Normal: 2-6 mm Hg.
- Volumetric catheters allow for the measurement of right ventricular end diastolic volume (RVEDV).
  - Normal: 100-160 ml.

Left Ventricular Preload

- Measured by the mean pulmonary artery occlusive pressure (PAOP).
- Measures left atrial pressure by occluding blood flow distal to the catheter tip and creating a static column of blood that reflects pressure back from the left atrium (Figure 4.3).
- Normal: 5-12 mm Hg.
- PAOP pressures are not an accurate reflection of left ventricular filling volume in the presence of mitral valve disease or decreased LV compliance.

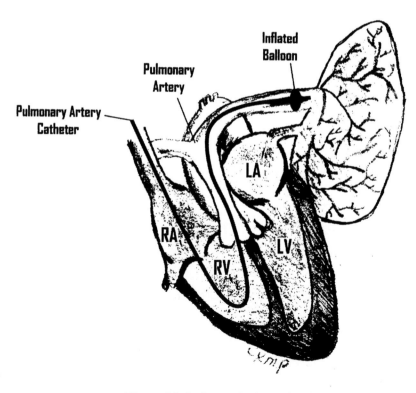

Figure 4.3: Left ventricular preload.

- The pulmonary artery diastolic pressure (PAd) can be used in place of the PAOP to assess left ventricular filling pressure if no pulmonary hypertension is present. The mean left atrial pressure can also be used if a left atrial catheter is in place.

Noninvasive Assessment
- Noninvasive assessment parameters for increased preload include:
  - Right ventricular: jugular venous distention, hepatojugular reflux, and pitting peripheral edema.
  - Left ventricular: shortness of breath, inspiratory crackles, decreased oxygen saturation, and chest radiograph findings consistent with congestion.
  - Daily weights used to assess total body fluid status and can be incorporated into the noninvasive assessment for increased right and left ventricular preload.
  - Echocardiography can also be used in the assessment of filling volumes.
- Noninvasive assessment parameters for decreased preload include:
  - Decreased blood pressure.
  - Decrease urine output.
  - Flat neck veins.

Preload and Ventricular Compliance
It is important to understand that when assessing preload using a pulmonary artery catheter, pressure is used to reflect end diastolic volume. In a normal ventricle, there is an expected relationship between volume and pressure (Figure 4.4). There are several situations however where pressure will not accurately reflect end diastolic volume.

An increase in pressure does not always equal an increase in volume. A stiff or noncompliant ventricle can produce a higher pressure with a normal volume status. Conversely, a large dilated ventricle (more compliant) will not produce a high pressure, even when the volume in the ventricle is higher than normal. Therefore, a change in pressure accurately reflects a change in volume only in the presence of a normally compliant ventricle.

Increased compliance is seen in dilated cardiomyopathy and mild to moderate aortic regurgitation. A decrease in ventricular compliance is seen with diastolic dysfunction, ischemia, hypertrophic cardiomyopathy, and restrictive pericarditis. Elevated preload and increases in intra-thoracic and intra-pericardial pressures will also decrease the compliance of the ventricle.

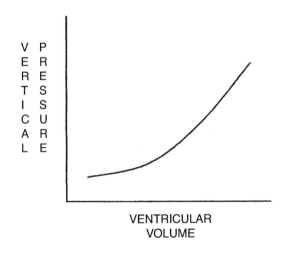

Figure 4.4: Relationship between volume and pressure in normal compliant ventricle.

Linking Knowledge to Practice

✔ *An increase in PAOP or PAd pressure may indicate myocardial ischemia, causing acute diastolic dysfunction and reduced ventricular compliance. Additional assessment parameters, including pain assessment, 12-lead ECG and ST-segment monitoring are indicated in patients who have a sudden increase in PAOP or PAd pressures without other clear evidence of fluid overload.*

Chapter 4

Linking Knowledge to Practice

✔ *Due to the variability of ventricular compliance in patients with cardiac disease, there is no specific number representing optimal preload. Optimal preload is best defined as the preload that provides optimal stroke volume while at the same does not produce congestion or ischemia.*

Factors Influencing Preload

There are several factors that influence preload. These include:

◆ Volume status and amount of blood in the vascular space.

◆ Venous tone and body position.

◆ Intra-thoracic pressure and intra-pericardial pressure.

◆ Atrial kick.

◆ Diastolic relaxation (compliance) and filling time.

◆ Tachyarrhythmias.

◆ Left ventricular function (contractility).

◆ Body temperature.

Causes of Decreased Preload

◆ Decrease in circulating volume:
  ❖ Hemorrhage.
  ❖ Dehydration.
  ❖ Burns.
  ❖ Excessive diuresis.
  ❖ Third space shifting.

◆ Changes in size of vascular space (excessive vasodilation producing relative hypovolemia)
  ❖ Sepsis.
  ❖ Anaphylaxis.
  ❖ Venous vasodilators.

Causes of Increased Preload

◆ Increase in circulating volume
  ❖ Over hydration.
  ❖ Heart failure (backward failure results in pulmonary and systemic venous congestion).
  ❖ Renal disease.

Correcting Preload

◆ To increase preload:
  ❖ Volume
    ★ Isotonic crystalloids.
    ★ Colloids (Hetastarch or Albumin).
    ★ Blood or blood products when clinically indicated.
  ❖ Decrease vasodilators.
  ❖ Rhythm control (decrease heart rate and restore atrial kick).
  ❖ Change position (elevate feet).

- ❖ Treat hyperthermia.
- ◆ To decrease preload
  - ❖ Diuretics.
  - ❖ Venous Vasodilators.
    - ★ NTG
    - ★ Morphine Sulfate
    - ★ Nesiritide.
  - ❖ Increase contractility to improve forward flow.
  - ❖ ACE inhibitors, angiotensin II receptor blockers, and aldosterone antagonists can also be used to manage preload.

Linking Knowledge to Practice

✔ *Reducing preload reduces myocardial oxygen consumption. Preload reduction is the mechanism of action in low dose intravenous nitroglycerin used to treat ischemic chest pain. However, if preload is reduced to a level that is too low, cardiac output and blood pressure will fall.*

Afterload

Afterload is the force the ventricle needs to overcome to eject blood volume. Afterload is therefore measured during systole. Afterload is inversely related to stroke volume (Figure 4.5). An increase in afterload results in a decrease in stroke volume and increases myocardial oxygen consumption. Blood pressure is related to afterload, but it is not synonymous with afterload. Both cardiac output and systemic vascular resistance (SVR) determine blood pressure.

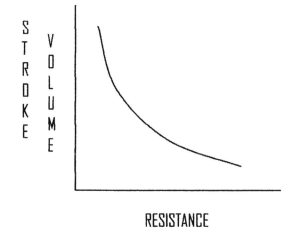

Figure 4.5: Afterload.

Components of afterload include:
- ◆ Vascular resistance (most important component).
- ◆ Valve compliance.
- ◆ Blood viscosity.
- ◆ Aortic compliance.
- ◆ Arterial wall compliance.

More About Vascular Resistance

The diameter of the blood vessels is the primary factor in determining vascular resistance. There can be systemic as well as regional vasoconstriction, causing changes in vascular resistance. When resistance increases, the mean arterial blood pressure must increase to assure adequate flow through the vessels.

Measurement of Vascular Resistance

Vascular resistance is calculated rather than directly measured.

Vascular Resistance = pressure gradient across the circulation x cardiac output.

Metric units, dynes/sec/cm;[5] are the measurement units most commonly used in clinical practice. To obtain metric units, the above formula is multiplied by 80, which is a conversion factor for converting the measurement to dynes/sec/cm.[5]

Chapter 4

SVR

SVR represents the average resistance to flow throughout systemic circulation and does not reflect regional changes in vascular resistance.

Formula for SVR

SVR = MAP - CVP / CO x 80.

PVR

PVR represents the average resistance to flow throughout the pulmonary circulation.

Formula for PVR

PVR = Mean PAP - PAOP / CO x 80

RV Afterload
◆ Right ventricular afterload is reflected by pulmonary vascular resistance (PVR).
◆ Normal: < 200 dynes/sec/cm.$^{-5}$

LV Afterload
◆ Left ventricular afterload is reflected by SVR.
◆ Normal: 800-1200 dynes/sec/cm.$^{-5}$
◆ Diastolic blood pressure is the closest non-invasive measurement

Note: PVR and SVR are used to estimate right and left ventricular afterload. They are only an estimate because they do not account for the other factors determining afterload such as valve resistance or blood viscosity.

Noninvasive Assessment
◆ Hypoxemia and acidemia result in an increase in PVR.
◆ Diastolic blood pressure is the closest non-invasive assessment of SVR.
◆ Pulse pressure is also used to assess SVR. An acute decrease in pulse pressure (narrow pulse pressure) represents an increase in SVR.

Factors Influencing Left Ventricular Afterload
◆ Sympathetic nervous system stimulation and arterial tone.
◆ Aortic pressure and compliance.
◆ Ventricular outflow tract obstructions: aortic stenosis, hypertrophic obstructive cardiomyopathy.
◆ Increased blood viscosity.
◆ Intra-thoracic pressure.

Causes of Decreased Left Ventricular Afterload
◆ Vasodilation
    ❖ Sepsis.
    ❖ Anaphylaxis.
    ❖ Vasodilators.

Hemodynamics/Shock States/Intra-Aortic Balloon Pump Therapy

❖ Hyperthermia.

❖ End stage cirrhosis.

◆ Increased intra-thoracic pressure (PEEP).

◆ Severe anemia (decrease in blood viscosity).

Note: An increase in cardiac output will cause a decrease in PVR and SVR.

Causes of Increased Left Ventricular Afterload

◆ Vasoconstriction

❖ Hypertension.

❖ Vasopressors.

❖ Late sepsis.

❖ Hypothermia.

❖ Compensation for hypovolemia or low cardiac output.

❖ Excessive sympathetic nervous system response.

Causes of Increased Right Ventricular Afterload

◆ Large pulmonary embolism.

◆ Pulmonary edema.

◆ Hypercapnea.

◆ Hypoxemia.

◆ Primary pulmonary hypertension.

Correcting Afterload

◆ To increase Afterload:

❖ Vasopressors

☆ Sympathomimetics.

✶ Epinephrine.

✶ Norepinephrine.

✶ Dopamine.

✶ Phenylephrine.

☆ Vasopressin (used when patient not responsive to sympathomimetics).

Note: A 5- to 10-minute response time between dose adjustments should be used when titrating vasopressors (PACEP, 2006). A normal patient response to a vasopressor is a rapid rise in blood pressure.

Note: Many patients with vasodilation and decreased SVR also have decreased preload and need volume administration.

◆ To decrease Afterload:

❖ Arterial Vasodilators

☆ Direct arterial vasodilators/smooth muscle relaxants.

✶ Sodium Nitroprusside.

✶ Hydralazine.

☆ ACE inhibitors.

☆ Calcium channel blockers.

☆ Nesiritide.

❖ IABP

❖ Special considerations in reducing right ventricular afterload include the use of oxygen and pulmonary vasodilators.

Chapter 4

Linking Knowledge to Practice

✔ *Vasopressors are given to achieve an adequate mean arterial pressure to perfuse the organs. However, vasopressors may not always improve tissue oxygenation, despite an increase in blood pressure. Severe vasoconstriction can impair tissue perfusion. End organ tissue perfusion should be a key assessment parameter during the use of vasopressors.*

✔ *In addition, vasopressors and increased afterload in patients with left ventricular dysfunction can result in decreased cardiac output and increased myocardial oxygen consumption, therefore worsening the clinical picture.*

Contractility

Contractility is the velocity and extent of myocardial fiber shortening independent of preload and afterload. The state of contractility is called the inotropic state. An increase in contractility increases myocardial work and myocardial oxygen consumption.

Although the true contractile ability of the myocardium is assessed independent of preload and afterload, the overall effectiveness of contractility is related to the degree of myocardial fiber stretch (preload) and wall tension (afterload).

◆ During contraction, the ventricle moves globally in an inward movement. This is called synergy of contraction. Dyssynergy, uncoordinated ventricular contraction, results in impaired pump function.

Contractility can be non-invasively evaluated with echocardiography or nuclear imaging. Contractility can be estimated invasively with a pulmonary artery catheter, using a calculated left ventricular stroke work index (LVSWI) and a right ventricular stroke work index (RVSWI).

◆ LVSWI normal value: 50-62 gm-m/m²/beat.
◆ RVSWI normal value: 5-10 gm-m/m²/beat (Martin, 2006).

Factors Influencing Contractility
◆ Sympathetic nervous system and the adrenals (which release catecholamines).
◆ Ventricular muscle mass.
◆ Alterations in metabolic state.
◆ Medications: inotropes.
◆ Dyssynergy
  ❖ Regional wall motion abnormalities.
  ❖ Ventricular ectopic beats or conduction abnormalities.
  ❖ Significant ventricular fibrosis and dilation.

Causes of Decreased Contractility
◆ Excessive preload or afterload.
◆ Drugs – negative inotropes.
◆ Myocardial damage.
◆ Ischemia.
◆ Cardiomyopathy.
◆ Changes in ionic environment: hypoxia, acidosis or electrolyte imbalance.
  ❖ Acidosis alters available calcium for actin-myosin interaction.
  ❖ Hypoxia deceases the amount of intracellular ATP.

Hemodynamics/Shock States/Intra-Aortic Balloon Pump Therapy

Causes of Increased Contractility
- Positive inotropes.
- Hyperthyroidism.
- Adrenal Medulla tumor.

Improving Contractility
- To increase contractility:
  - Inotropes
    - Sympathomimetics
      - Dobutamine.
      - Epinephrine (dose dependent).
      - Dopamine (dose dependent).
    - Phosphodiesterase (PDE) inhibitors (e.g. milrinone).
    - Digoxin (not used to increase contractility in acute situations).
- To decrease contractility. (*Note:* Medications given to decrease contractility are given with the therapeutic purpose of decreasing myocardial oxygen demand or to reduce outflow tract obstruction in hypertrophic cardiomyopathy.)
  - Beta blockers.
  - Calcium channel blockers.

Linking Knowledge to Practice

✔ *Low cardiac output does not necessarily mean diminished contractility. Preload and afterload abnormalities may cause low cardiac output in a patient with normal contractility. Correct preload and afterload problems first because medications to increase contractility cause a significant increase in myocardial oxygen demand.*

Heart Rate

An increase in heart rate increases cardiac output and compensates for a low stroke volume until a physiological limit is reached where filling time decreases, resulting in decreased stroke volume and cardiac output. Tachycardia also decreases coronary artery perfusion time and increases myocardial oxygen consumption.

Left Ventricular Function Curves

Figure 4.6 shows the left ventricular function curve relating left ventricular preload (PAOP) to cardiac index. The shape of the curve shows that an increase in preload increases cardiac index to a point where there is a physiological limitation. The top curve shows normal left ventricular function, and the bottom curve shows depressed left ventricular function.

Figure 4.7 demonstrates the impact of altering preload on left ventricular function. Altering preload changes the location on the patient's existing left ventricular function curve in the following way:

- Administering fluid increases preload and moves a patient from A to B along the curve.

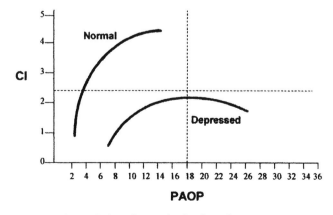

Figure 4.6: Left ventricular function curve.

- ◆ Diuretics or venous dilators (i.e. preload reduction) move the patient from B to A.

Figure 4.8 demonstrates that improving the contractile performance of the ventricle moves the patient to a higher left ventricular function curve (i.e. from A to B).

Figure 4.9 demonstrates the impact of afterload reduction on left ventricular function. When afterload is reduced, forward flow is improved and, as a result, preload is also reduced. Therefore, a reduction in afterload improves ventricular function by moving the curve up and to the left.

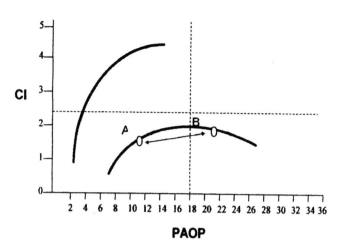

Figure 4.7: Impact of altering preload on left ventricular function.

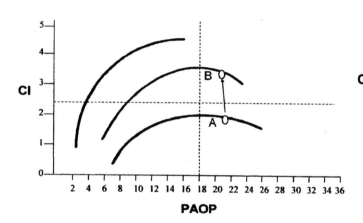

Figure 4.8: Improved contractile performance.

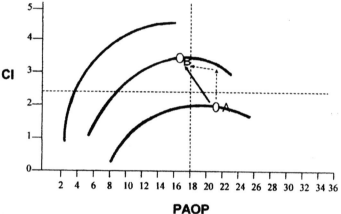

Figure 4.9: Impact of afterload reduction on left ventricular function.

Oxygen Delivery To Tissues

Oxygen delivery is the volume of oxygen delivered to tissues each minute, and is expressed as DO_2.

Formula for Delivery of Oxygen

DO_2 (ml/min) = cardiac output (CO) (L/min) x arterial oxygen content (CaO_2) (ml/dL) x10

CaO_2 is the amount of oxygen bound to hemoglobin + the amount of oxygen dissolved in plasma. It is measured in ml/dL. Multiplying by a factor of 10 in the above equation, the two factors are adjusted to the same scale, so the product is in ml (Darovic, 2002).

Hemodynamics/Shock States/Intra-Aortic Balloon Pump Therapy

Formula for Arterial Oxygen Content

CaO_2 = Hgb x 1.36 (oxygen carrying capacity) x SaO_2 (decimal) + PaO_2 x 0.003 (solubility constant)

Percent saturation is not interchangeable with oxygen content. Anemia does not alter saturation but does alter arterial oxygen content.

- ◆ Normal CaO_2 is approximately 20 ml/dL.

Linking Knowledge to Practice

- ✔ *The major determinants of arterial oxygen content are hemoglobin and saturation. An increase in PaO_2 is not the main strategy to increase oxygen carrying capacity unless hemoglobin and saturation cannot be further improved, such as in carbon monoxide poisoning.*
  - ❖ Normal DO2 = 900-1100 ml/min (1000).
  - ❖ Normal DO2I = 550-650 ml/min.
- ✔ *Oxygen delivery can be improved by increasing cardiac output, hemoglobin or SaO_2. Cardiac output is the major determinant of oxygen delivery so that low cardiac output significantly reduces delivery of oxygen to the tissue, even in the presence of adequate hemoglobin and oxygen saturation.*

Oxygen Consumption

Oxygen consumption is the volume of oxygen consumed by the tissues each minute and is measured as VO_2. VO_2 is determined by comparing the oxygen content in arterial blood (CaO_2) to the oxygen content in mixed venous blood (CvO_2). Normal CaO_2 (oxygen content in arterial blood) is approximately 20 ml/dL and normal CvO_2 is approximately 15 ml/dL. This comparison demonstrates that the tissues consume approximately 25% of what is delivered.

Normal VO_2 is 200-300 ml/min (250 ml/min).

Formula for Oxygen Consumption

VO_2 (ml/min) = CO x Hgb x 1.36 x 10 x (SaO_2 - SvO_2).

Oxygen Reserve in Venous Blood

Oxygen reserve is measured by mixed venous (blood mixed from inferior and superior vena cavae and coronary sinus) oxygen saturation ($SmvO_2$). Mixed venous blood has a PO_2 of 40 mm Hg with a corresponding saturation of approximately 75%.

Normal $SmvO_2$ is 60-80%, or approximately 75%.

Chapter 4

Delivery/Consumption/Reserve Review

◆ Tissues are delivered approximately 1000 ml/min (DO_2).

◆ Tissues use approximately 250 ml/min (VO_2).

◆ This leaves an approximate 75% reserve in venous blood ($S_{MV}O_2$).

The tissues utilize approximately 25% of the delivered oxygen. This is called the oxygen extraction ratio (O_2ER).

Relationship Between Oxygen Consumption and Oxygen Delivery

◆ Oxygen delivery and oxygen consumption are independent of each other in normal circumstances. This means tissues will extract the amount of oxygen needed independent of delivery because delivery exceeds need. In this independent state there is always an acceptable reserve.

◆ Because the normal reserve is approximately 75%, there is some room in the independent state for delivery to fall or for consumption to increase.

Linking Knowledge to Practice

✔ *For example: When oxygen delivery and oxygen consumption are independent, the tissues continue to extract the amount of required oxygen when a small drop in hemoglobin decreases oxygen delivery. Delivery is decreased and consumption stays the same, so the venous reserve is decreased. The oxygen reserve is impacted, but tissue oxygen is preserved.*

✔ *When delivery and consumption are in the independent state and there is a fall in delivery, the reserve also falls because consumption stays the same. In this situation an increase in delivery (cardiac support, blood, improved oxygen) results in an increase in reserve. (See Table 4.1.)*

Table 4.1 Relationship Between Delivery and Reserve		
DO_2	VO_2 (extraction is independent of delivery)	$SMVO_2$ ($SMVO_2$ improves when delivery increases)
1000 ml	250 cc (25%)	75%
750 ml	250 cc (33%)	67%
500 ml	250 cc (50%)	50%

At a critical level of DO_2 (approximately 420 ml/mm²) (FCCS, 2006), the tissues no longer extract and consume oxygen independent of delivery. This is called a dependent state because the tissues alter their consumption based on low levels of delivery. Anaerobic metabolism occurs here because there is an oxygen deficit. Anaerobic metabolism leads to the production of lactic acid. Delivery of oxygen should be kept > 500 ml per minute at all times to assure that consumption is independent of delivery.

Linking Knowledge to Practice

✔ *$S_{MV}O_2$ does not increase with increased delivery while in this dependent state. The development of lactic acidosis is a grave sign. Therefore, it is important to recognize and treat a decrease in oxygen delivery, while oxygen consumption is still in the independent state.*

Hemodynamics/Shock States/Intra-Aortic Balloon Pump Therapy

Increased VO₂

In addition to a decrease in oxygen delivery, critically ill patients can have an increase in oxygen consumption that places tissue oxygenation at risk.

- Fever.
- Shivering.
- Suctioning.
- Sepsis.
- Non family visitor.
- Position change.
- Sling scale weight.
- Bath.
- CXR.
- Multi-organ failure.

S$_{MV}$O₂

S$_{MV}$O₂ is a global indicator between oxygen supply and demand. S$_{MV}$O₂ is influenced by both oxygen delivery and oxygen extraction. S$_{MV}$O₂ reflects mixing of venous blood from superior vena cava, inferior vena cava and coronary sinus. S$_{MV}$O₂ is measured using a pulmonary artery fiberoptic catheter.

INVASIVE HEMODYNAMIC MONITORING

Pulmonary Artery Catheter

The basic PA catheter is a multilumen catheter that is 110 cm long with a proximal port, a distal port, an inflatable balloon, and a thermistor that measures blood temperature (Figure 4.10). When in correct position in the body (Figure 4.11), the proximal port opens into the RA and is used to measure RA pressure and inject fluid for obtaining cardiac output measurements. The distal port is in a branch of the pulmonary artery and is used to measure PA pressure. The balloon at the end of the catheter can be inflated to obtain pulmonary artery occlusive pressure (PAOP), also called pulmonary artery wedge pressure (PAWP), as explained below. Some models of the PA catheter have an infusion port that opens into the RA just distal to the injection port, through which fluids can be infused. Other models contain fiberoptics that can be used to measure mixed venous oxygen saturation (S$_{MV}$O₂).

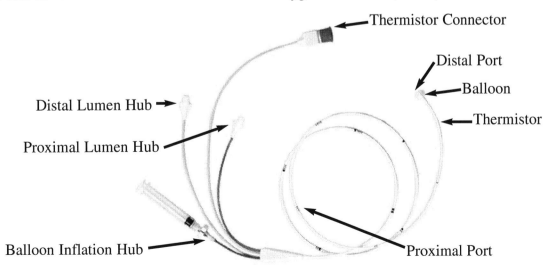

Figure 4.10: Basic PA catheter.
(Courtesy of Edwards Critical Care)

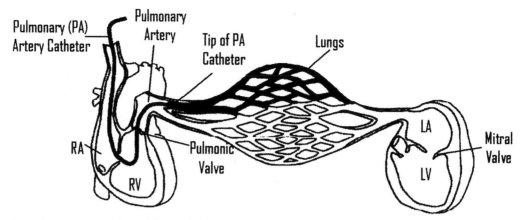

Figure 4.11: PA catheter in proper position with proximal port in right atrium and distal port in a branch of the pulmonary artery.

The pulmonary artery catheter is typically inserted via the jugular or subclavian vein. The femoral vein may also be used, although this limits patient mobility and there is increased concern for infection.

The balloon is inflated during insertion to allow blood flow to direct the catheter to the desired location, and to protect the endocardial structures and the pulmonary vessels from the hard tip of the catheter. The distal tip of the catheter is not covered during balloon inflation; therefore, intracardiac pressures and pressure in the pulmonary artery can be recorded, and the waveforms displayed during insertion. The first pressure to be measured during insertion is the right atrial pressure, then right ventricular pressure, followed by the pulmonary artery pressure. After insertion, the proper placement of the pulmonary artery catheter should be confirmed by chest x-ray.

Pressure Monitoring System

Pulmonary artery pressure monitoring requires a fluid system and an electrical system in order to display pressures and waveforms on a bedside monitor (Figure 4.12).

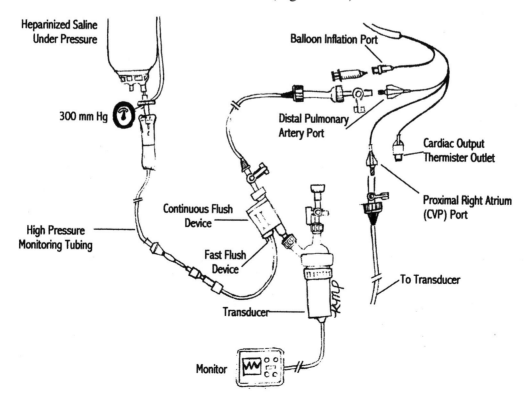

Figure 4.12: Pulmonary artery pressure monitoring system.

Hemodynamics/Shock States/Intra-Aortic Balloon Pump Therapy

Fluid System

◆ Fluid source: IV bag of D₅W or NS spiked with regular IV tubing to create a continuous fluid filled line from the IV bag to the transducer.

◆ Pressure bag around fluid source: IV bag must be pressurized at 300 mm Hg to overcome the resistance of the flush device in the transducer and to deliver 3-5 ml/hr through the catheter to keep the line patent.

◆ High-pressure tubing: Rigid tubing from the transducer to the catheter is necessary to accurately transmit the pressure signal to the transducer.

◆ Flush device: Located on the transducer. Contains a one-way valve that allows 3-5 ml/hr of fluid to pass through unless the resistance is released by pulling the tail or pushing the lever on the device; this allows the line to run wide open.

◆ Pulmonary artery catheter: Designed to pick up pressure waves.

Electrical System

◆ Transducer: contains fine wires that move back and forth with pressure changes and convert the pressure (mechanical signal) to an electrical signal that is sent to the monitor. Must be filled with fluid and be bubble free to accurately transmit pressure. The transducer is the link between the fluid filled tubing and the electronic system.

◆ Connecting cable: connects the transducer to the bedside monitor and transmits the electrical signal to the monitor.

◆ Monitor: converts and amplifies the electrical signal to an analog waveform, then displays it on the screen along with a digital output.

Pressures within the cardiovascular system must be transmitted through the fluid in the catheter and tubing to the transducer. Therefore, recorded pressures lag slightly behind the physiological pressure changes. The pressure tubing must be kept as short as possible to minimize this lag time.

Once in place, several direct measurements and additional calculated measurements can be obtained.

Direct Measurements

◆ Right atrial (RA) pressure (measures CVP).

◆ Pulmonary artery pressure (PA).

◆ Pulmonary artery occlusive pressure (PAOP, also called wedge pressure).

◆ Cardiac output (intermittent or continuous).

◆ Venous oxygen saturation (SVO₂).

Indirect/Calculated Measurements

◆ Stroke volume (SV) and stroke volume index (SVI).

◆ Systemic vascular resistance (SVR).

◆ Pulmonary vascular resistance (PVR).

◆ Left ventricular stroke work index (LVSWI).

◆ Right ventricular stroke work index (RVSWI).

◆ Cardiac Index (CI).

Some catheters can calculate RV volumes and ejection fraction (EF).

Principles for Accurate Monitoring

◆ All air must be eliminated from the tubing, stopcock, and transducer. Air transmits impulses differently from fluid and causes inaccuracies in the system.

- All connections should be tightened. All vented caps should be replaced with dead end caps. All stopcocks should be closed to air.
- Avoid adding extra stopcocks or extension tubing.
- Air should be removed from the fluid source before priming.
- The fluid source is maintained under 300 mm Hg pressure to allow continuous infusion through the flush device, tubing, and catheter. Keep solution bag adequately filled.
- A brief fast flush should be done through open stopcocks after zeroing or blood sampling.
- Tiny air bubbles can escape the fluid solution, so periodic assessment, "flicking" of tubing and stopcocks, and flushing the tubing helps eliminate these bubbles.
- The phlebostatic axis should be marked on the patient's chest with non-washable marker.
  - Approximates the level of the left atrium and the tip of the PA catheter.
  - Located at 4th intercostal space, mid-anterior-posterior chest (Figure 4.13).
- The air reference stopcock is zeroed at the level of the phlebostatic axis. Zeroing (opening the transducer to air) establishes atmospheric pressure as zero.
- Zero the system on initial setup and if any part of the electrical system (transducer, cables) becomes disconnected.
- All readings must be at the level of the phlebostatic axis.
  - For each 1 cm that the transducer is above or below the phlebostatic axis, 0.74 mm Hg hydrostatic pressure is added or subtracted.
  - For example: If the transducer is 10 cm below the phlebostatic axis, the measured pressure will be overestimated by 7.4 mm Hg.
  - The impact of hydrostatic pressure is especially important in the assessment of RA and PAOP pressures.

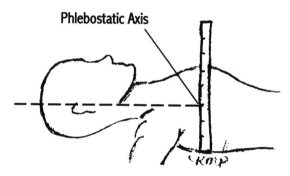

Figure 4.13: Marking of phlebostatic axis.

- Re-level with any change in patient position or change in transducer/stopcock position.
- Measurements can be obtained with backrest elevation from 0 to 45-60 degrees.
- Waveforms should be read at end-expiration.
- Use a graphic analog tracing to obtain RA, PA, and PAOP readings.
- Correlate RA and PAOP readings to the ECG tracing to assist with *a* wave and *v*-wave identification. This is discussed later in this chapter.
- Perform a square wave test (also called fast flush test or dynamic response test) to determine the system accuracy. This procedure is described below (AACN, 2004; Bridges, 2006; Bridges, 2005c; Darovic, 2002; Wiegand & Carlson, 2005; McGhee & Bridges, 2002).

Procedure for Square Wave Testing (also called Dynamic Response Testing)
- Use fast flush for square wave testing. The square wave test assesses the natural frequency response and damping characteristic of the system.
- A square wave is produced by a fast flush that is obtained by rapid push and then release of the fast flush device. The fast flush test should be repeated 2-3 times, and the response recorded on a graphic recorder for evaluation.

- There are three steps involved in the square wave test:
  - Determination of the natural frequency.
  - Indirect determination of the damping co-efficient (by determining the amplitude ratio of two consecutive fast flush oscillation).
  - Evaluation of the overall dynamic response as optimal, adequate, underdamped, overdamped, or unacceptable.
- The natural frequency is the speed at which the system vibrates when excited by a signal. The higher the natural frequency, the better the dynamic response of the system.
  - The number of blocks (small boxes on the ECG graph paper) between the bounces assesses the frequency of the system. Ideally there should be space of < 1 block between bounces, indicating that the frequency response is optimal, and the system should function properly with any degree of damping.
  - If there are between 1.5 and 2.0 blocks, it is important to assess damping and assure that the height of the 2nd bounce is ≤ ⅓ of the first bounce.
  - If there are > 2.0 to 2.5 boxes between the bounces, the system is inaccurate due to poor frequency response, regardless of the damping assessment (height of the 2nd wave). Proper damping in this situation will not compensate for poor frequency response.
- Damping represents how quickly there is the loss of vibrating energy of the physiological signal. All hemodynamic systems have damping. Without damping, the vibrations would continue indefinitely and an accurate waveform could not be recorded.
  - The square wave should return quickly to baseline.
  - There should be 1 to 2 bounces after the square wave before returning to the PA waveform.
  - The second bounce should be ≤ ⅓ the height of the first bounce. The height of the waves assesses damping.

(Darovic, 2002; McGhee & Bridges, 2002).

A normal square wave test for frequency is demonstrated in Figure 4.14.

Poor Frequency and Underdamped System (Figure 4.15)
- Greater than 2 blocks between bounces (poor frequency).
- Second bounce close to height of 1st bounce. or ringing occurs after release of fast flush (underdamped).
- System is inaccurate with falsely high (overestimated) systolic pressures and falsely low (underestimated) diastolic pressures due to artifact.
- Pressure monitoring systems often have low natural frequency and a tendency to be underdamped.
- Underdamping is also associated with certain patient conditions, including hypertension and hyperdynamic states. The dynamic response test is used to differentiate system problems from patient problems

(Darovic, 2002; McGhee & Bridges, 2002).

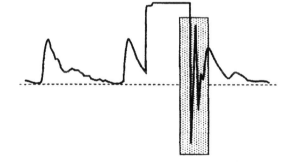

Figure 4.14: Normal square wave test.
From *Pass CCRN* (2nd ed.), by R.D. Dennison, 2000, St. Louis: Mosby. Reprinted with permission from Elsevier.

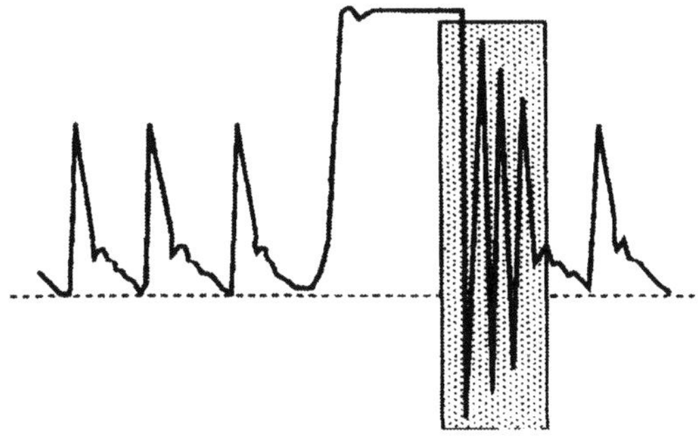

Figure 4.15: Poor frequency and underdamped system.
From *Pass CCRN* (2nd ed.), by R.D. Dennison, 2000, St. Louis: Mosby. Reprinted with permission from Elsevier.

Overdamped System (Figure 4.16)

- Absence of bounces (oscillations) or sluggish response.
- Gradual descent to baseline.
- The pressure waveform looks unnaturally smooth.
- System is inaccurate with falsely low (underestimated) systolic pressures and falsely high (overestimated) diastolic pressures (Darovic, 2002; McGhee & Bridges, 2002).
- Overdamped waveforms can also occur as a result of some clinical conditions, such as those with low cardiac output states. The dynamic response test is used to differentiate system problems from patient problems.

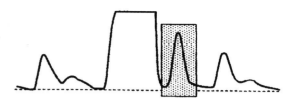

Figure 4.16: Overdamped system.
From *Pass CCRN* (2nd ed.), by R.D. Dennison, 2000, St. Louis: Mosby. Reprinted with permission from Elsevier.

Patient characteristics can cause overdamping and underdamping. The dynamic response or square wave test is used to differentiate if there is a patient or system problem.

Interventions for Square Wave or Dynamic Response Testing Failure:
- Assure all small air bubbles are removed from the system.
- Assure wide bore high pressure tubing is used that is no longer than 48 inches.
- Assure that all connections are tight.
- Avoid any extra stopcocks.
- Assess for any obstruction in the system.

Linking Knowledge to Practice

✔ *Over and underdamping of the pressure monitoring system have a greater impact on systolic and diastolic pressures than on mean pressures.*

Waveform Analysis

Changes in hemodynamic pressures are related to mechanical events in the heart. Blood flow through the heart or changes in myocardial tension can cause changes in hemodynamic pressure readings. Mechanical events of the heart are always preceded by electrical events, so hemodynamic pressure readings should be correlated with the cardiac rhythm.

RA Waveform (Figure 4.17)
- *a* wave = atrial contraction
  - Occurs after the P wave (or right after the PR interval).
- *c* wave = closure of tricuspid valve
  - Often not visible.
  - Occurs at end of QRS complex.
- *v* wave = atrial filling
  - Blood entering atrium from superior and inferior vena cavae.
  - Occurs near the end of the T wave.
- x descent = downstroke following the *a* wave
- y descent = downstroke following the *v* wave
  - Represents the opening of the tricuspid valve and passive atrial emptying.
- RA pressure is the clinical indicator of RV preload.
- Document the mean of the *a* wave for RA pressure.

Hemodynamics/Shock States/Intra-Aortic Balloon Pump Therapy

❖ The mean of the *a* wave approximates end diastolic pressures because it gives a value close to the end of the QRS complex, which approximates the end of diastole.

◆ Normal value: 2-6 mm Hg.

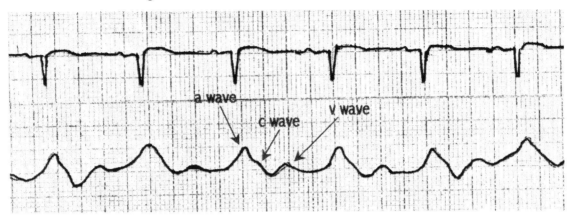

Figure 4.17: RA waveform.

RV Waveform (Figure 4.18)

◆ Measured only during insertion or removal of catheter.
◆ PVCs or RBBB may occur as catheter is floated through the right ventricle.
◆ Waveform has sharp rapid upstroke and rapid downstroke.
◆ Normal value: 15-30 / 2-7 mm Hg.
◆ If an RV waveform is observed during monitoring, the catheter must be re-positioned.
   ❖ Advance into the PA via balloon inflation.
   ❖ Pull the catheter back into the RA.

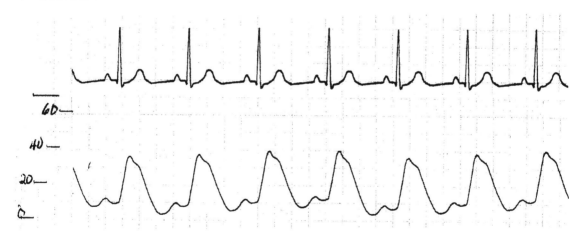

Figure 4.18: RV waveform.

PA Waveform

◆ Systolic pressure almost same as RV systolic pressure.
   ❖ Peak systolic pressure is within the T wave.
◆ Rapid upstroke and downslope related to systolic ejection into pulmonary artery.
◆ Diastolic pressure rises compared to RV diastolic pressure (Figure 4.19).
   ❖ LV end diastolic pressure occurs at the end of QRS complex.
   ❖ Diastolic pulmonary artery pressure is an indirect reflection of left ventricular end diastolic pressure (preload) in the absence of pulmonary disease, pulmonary hypertension or mitral stenosis. (*Note:* Even temporary hypoxia negates the ability to use the PAd as an assessment of left ventricular function because hypoxia causes pulmonary vasoconstriction.)

Chapter 4

- ❖ PAd is normally 1-4 mm Hg higher than mean PAOP.
- ◆ Dicrotic notch represents the closure of the pulmonic valve
- ◆ Normal value: 15-30 / 6-15 mm Hg with a mean of 9-17 mm Hg.

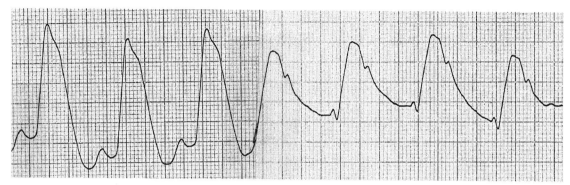

Figure 4.19: Diastolic pressure increase compared to RV diastolic pressure.

Pulmonary Artery Occlusive Pressure (PAOP)

- ◆ The PAOP is an intermittently assessed waveform obtained by inflating the balloon.
- ◆ Inflation of the balloon stops forward flow of blood past the catheter tip, resulting in a static column of blood between the tip of the catheter and the left atrium (Figure 4.20).
- ◆ Pressure in the left atrium is transmitted back to the catheter tip; therefore, PAOP is an indirect reflection of left atrial pressure.
- ◆ The mean PAOP is normally 1-4 mm Hg lower than the PA diastolic pressure (PAd). Figure 4.21 shows transition of PA pressure to PAOP pressure.
  - ❖ PAOP is never higher than the PAd, except in the presence of significant mitral regurgitation.

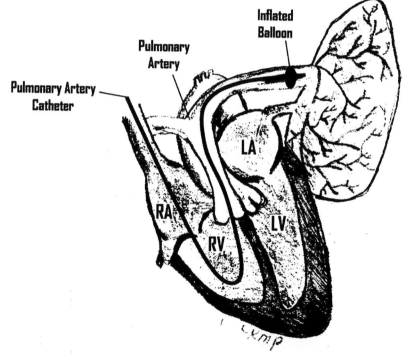

Figure 4.20: Pulmonary artery occlusive pressure (PAOP).

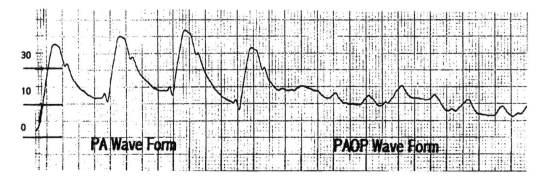

Figure 4.21: Transition of PA pressure to PAOP pressure.

PAOP Waveform (Figure 4.22)
- *a* wave = atrial contraction
  - Occurs usually in or at the end of the QRS complex rather than in the PR interval.
- *c* wave = closure of mitral valve
  - Not typically seen.
- *v* wave = atrial filling
  - Occurs after T wave in the TP interval.
- x descent = downstroke following the *a* wave
- y descent = downstroke following the *v* wave
  - Represents the opening of the mitral valve and passive atrial emptying
- Document the mean of the *a* wave for PAOP.
  - The mean of the *a* wave approximates end diastolic pressures because it gives a value close to the end of the QRS complex, which approximates the end of diastole.
- Normal value: 5-12 mm Hg.

Note: When correlating *a* waves and *v* waves with the ECG tracing it is important to understand the reasons why correlation varies between the RA pressure and the PAOP. PAOP waves are delayed slightly (approximately 0.10 seconds) when compared to RA waves. There are two reasons for this delay: 1) left atrial contraction follows right atrial contraction, and 2) there is a delay in transmitting the impulse from the left atrium to the PA catheter (Ahrens & Taylor, 1992).

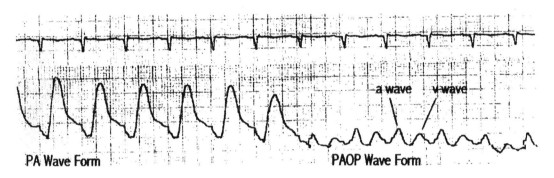

Figure 4.22: PAOP waveform.

Linking Knowledge to Practice

✔ It is important to manually locate the a *wave on RA and PAOP tracings through correlation with the cardiac rhythm strip. After the* a *wave is located, the mean of the* a *wave can be determined. The mean of the* a *wave is determined by averaging the top of the* a *wave and the bottom of the x descent. This can be seen in Figure 4.23.*

Limitations of PAOP
- PAOP does not always accurately reflect the volume in the ventricle at end diastole.
- PAOP is not an accurate assessment of LVEDV with mitral valve disease, pulmonary vein disease, abnormalities with ventricular compliance, high alveolar pressures, and tachycardia.
- PEEP > 10 cm H_2O may falsely elevate PAOP.

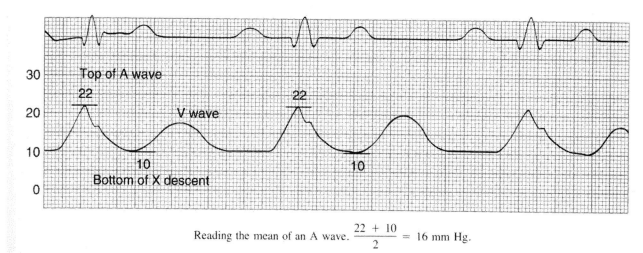

Reading the mean of an A wave. $\frac{22 + 10}{2} = 16$ mm Hg.

Figure 4.23: Example of correct measurement of an RA tracing.
From *Hemodynamic Waveform Analysis*, by T.S. Ahrens & L.A. Taylor, 1992, Philadelphia: Saunders. Reprinted with permission from Elsevier.

Safety Principles with PAOP Measurements
- Never inject > 1.5 cc of air into the balloon.
- Stop injection of air when waveform changes to PAOP waveform. A PAOP waveform that rises after inflation indicates over inflation of the balloon.
- Use minimal amount of inflation time; do not exceed 15 seconds.
- Allow air to passively escape from the balloon; never aspirate air.
- Never inject anything other than air into the balloon.
- Always display waveform from distal tip on monitor.
  - PA waveform should always be visible unless balloon is inflated.
  - The presence of a PAOP waveform in the absence of balloon inflation indicates catheter migration, and the catheter needs to be withdrawn slowly until the PA waveform reappears. In addition, if the PAOP waveform is produced with less than 1.25 cc of air, the catheter may be too distal and need to be pulled back.
- The introducer sheath should be securely sutured in place and catheter tip placement confirmed via chest x-ray.

A waves and V waves in CVP and PAOP Waveforms

A waves occur during atrial contraction. Large *a* waves (Figure 4.24) can occur with tricuspid or mitral stenosis, decreased ventricular compliance, with ventricular ectopic beats, and when there is any loss of AV synchrony. Large *a* waves are not an accurate reflection of filling pressures. Large *a* waves are called cannon waves when due to an arrhythmia.

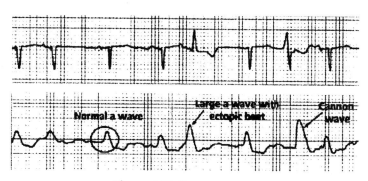

Figure 4.24: Large *a* waves.

A waves are absent in atrial fibrillation and in rhythms without atrial activity. Figure 4.25 shows a rhythm change from sinus to atrial fibrillation and the change in the RA pressure tracing. Note the presence of definite *a* waves during sinus rhythm and the lack of defined *a* waves during atrial fibrillation. When *a* waves are absent, the PAOP is read at the end of the QRS complex as illustrated. Note the close correlation between the mean of the *a* wave and the end of the QRS complex.

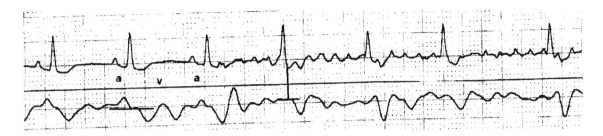

Figure 4.25: Rhythm change from sinus to atrial fibrillation and the change in the RA pressure tracing.

V waves occur during atrial filling. The peak of the *v* wave occurs after the T wave. Large *v* waves (Figure 4.26) can occur with tricuspid or mitral regurgitation, or with non-compliant atria. Read the CVP or PAOP the same way as always: locate the *a* waves and document the mean of the *a* wave for CVP and PAOP pressures.

Note: The sudden appearance of large *v* waves in a PAOP waveform suggests acute mitral valve regurgitation. Large *v* waves may cause the tracing to look more like a PA waveform, giving the impression that the catheter did not wedge.

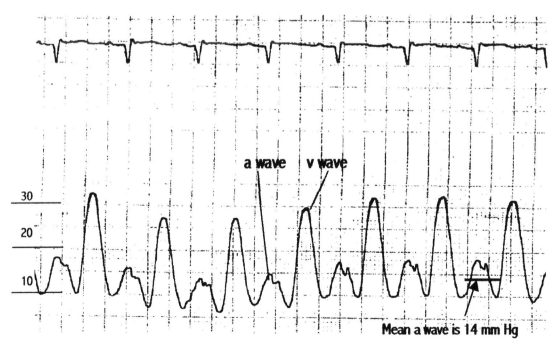

Figure 4.26: Large *v* waves.

Chapter 4

Impact of Respiratory Cycle on Hemodynamic Pressures and Waveform Assessment

Figure 4.27 demonstrates the impact of the respiratory cycle on hemodynamic pressure waveforms both during spontaneous breathing and mechanical ventilation.

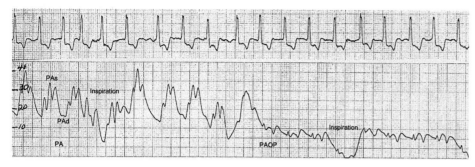
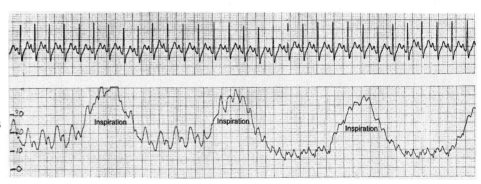

Figure 4.27: Impact of respiratory cycle on hemodynamic pressure waveforms. Both tracings show the conversion of a PA tracing to a PAOP tracing and the impact of the respiratory cycle on the waveforms. Top tracing is from a patient who is breathing spontaneously and the bottom trace is from a patient who is mechanically ventilated.

- ◆ Spontaneous Breathing
    - ❖ Waveforms drop during inspiration.
    - ❖ Waveforms rise during expiration.
- ◆ Positive Pressure Breathing (Mechanical Ventilation)
    - ❖ Waveforms rise during inspiration.
    - ❖ Waveforms drop during expiration.
- ◆ All hemodynamic pressure readings should be taken at the end of expiration where pleural pressure is closest to zero.
    - ❖ In spontaneous breathing, read the waveform just before it drops with inspiration. Figure 4.28 shows a PA to PAOP tracing in a spontaneously breathing patient. Pressures are read just before the inspiratory drop in the waveform.

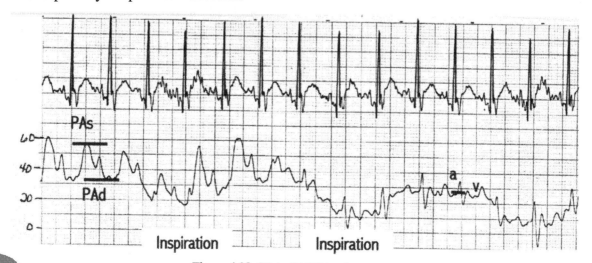

Figure 4.28: PA to PAOP tracing.

- ❖ In positive pressure mechanical ventilation, read the waveform just before it rises with the ventilator breath. Figure 4.29 show a PA pressure tracing in a ventilated patient. Pressure is read just before the inspiratory rise in the waveform (ventilator breath).

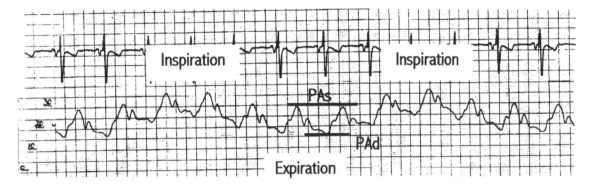

Figure 4.29: Correct reading of a PA pressure tracing on a ventilated patient.

Cardiac Output Measurement

Cardiac output (CO) can be measured at the bedside in a number of ways: thermodilution method using intermittent bolus injections of fluid, continuous measurement, using a specialized catheter that emits heat, or noninvasively, using transthoracic impedance measurement. This section covers thermodilution and continuous cardiac output measurement techniques.

Thermodilution Cardiac Output Measurement

This method of measuring CO involves the injection of a known amount of room temperature or iced D5W or NS into the RA through the proximal port of the PA catheter. The injectate fluid is warmed by the blood, and the temperature of the blood flowing past the thermistor at the distal end of the catheter is measured. The CO computer calculates CO based on the temperature change between the injectate and the blood flowing past the thermistor; the more blood (higher CO), the more the temperature change. The less blood (low CO), the less the temperature change.

- ◆ Injectate can be iced or at room temperature. Five or 10 ml can be used.
  - ❖ Five ml injectate has more potential for error (PACEP, 2006).
- ◆ A cardiac output constant is set in the computer to match the catheter type, injectate volume, and injectate temperature.
- ◆ Complete injection of the bolus should occur within 4 seconds. Injection should be smooth.
- ◆ At least 3 bolus measurements are obtained (to be averaged) with each assessment.
- ◆ The monitor displays the injection curve upon which its CO calculation is based. Each curve is evaluated to determine if it will be included in the measurements to be averaged. Irregular or notched curves are deleted. The goal is for the measurements of all included curves to be within 10% of each other.
- ◆ Triscuspid regurgitation or septal defects do not allow for accurate cardiac output assessment. Dysrhythmias can also interfere with an accurate measurement.

Continuous Cardiac Output

This method of CO measurement utilizes a catheter that emits frequent bursts of heat to warm the blood in the RA, and calculates CO based on the temperature difference between RA and blood flowing past the thermistor. CO is continuously displayed on the monitor.

- ◆ Cardiac output values are averaged over 3 to 6 minutes and updated every 30 to 60 seconds.
- ◆ Displayed values can be delayed by as much as 10 minutes with changes in CO (Bridges, 2005c).

Chapter 4

S$_{MV}$O$_2$ (Saturation of Mixed Venous Blood) Monitoring

The S$_{MV}$O$_2$ can be measured using a PA catheter that contains fiberoptic channels that emit light pulses from the tip of the catheter, and detect the amount light reflected from hemoglobin (Hgb). The amount of light reflected depends on the amount of oxygenated versus deoxygenated Hgb present. Reflected light is detected by an optical module that is connected to the catheter, and a microprocessor in the module calculates S$_{MV}$O$_2$ based on the amount of reflected light.

Cardiac output provides information about the ability of the cardiovascular system to deliver blood to the body, but it does not assess O$_2$ supply to the tissues or O$_2$ utilization by tissues. The S$_{MV}$O$_2$ is a global measure of O$_2$ delivery and consumption by the body, and is affected by changes in both delivery and consumption. The normal value is 60 to 80%.

Causes of low S$_{MV}$O$_2$ (< 60%) include:

◆ Decreased delivery.
◆ Increased consumption.

Causes of high S$_{MV}$O$_2$ (> 80%) include:

◆ Increased delivery.
◆ Decreased demand.
◆ Sepsis (tissues cannot extract).
◆ Wedged catheter.
◆ Arteriovenous fistula.

Note: A high S$_{MV}$O$_2$ can also represent a threat to tissue oxygenation. A clinically significant change is + or - 5 to 10% over 3 to 5 minutes.

S$_{MV}$O$_2$ < 40% represents limits of compensation where extraction and consumption become dependent on delivery and lactic acidosis occurs. In this state, oxygen demand is greater than oxygen delivery, and reserve can be depleted, leading to oxygen debt.

S$_{CV}$O$_2$ (Saturation of Central Venous Blood) Measurement

S$_{CV}$O$_2$ reflects oxygen saturation of blood returning to right atrium via the superior vena cava. This measurement can be obtained without a pulmonary artery catheter, using a modified triple lumen central venous catheter with oximetry capabilities. These catheters are frequently used in providing early goal directed therapy in sepsis.

◆ Normal value is 65 to 85%.
   ❖ Central venous blood in the SVC does not include blood returning to the heart from the lower extremities, abdominal organs, or the heart muscle itself; therefore the O$_2$ saturation in the SVC is slightly higher than true mixed venous blood.
◆ S$_{CV}$O$_2$ trends higher than S$_{MV}$O$_2$, but trends with S$_{MV}$O$_2$.

Linking Knowledge to Practice

✔ *The nurse must assure the accuracy of recorded hemodynamic values to use information obtained from a PA catheter to guide clinical decision-making. Several important components of nursing knowledge and skill can assure the recorded hemodynamic values are accurate. These practice components include: leveling of the transducer, correlation of waveforms with the ECG recording and respiratory patterns, and square wave testing.*

Hemodynamics/Shock States/Intra-Aortic Balloon Pump Therapy

Potential Complications of PA Catheter

Potential complications related to the insertion and maintenance of a pulmonary artery catheter are outlined in Table 4.2.

Table 4.2 Potential Complications of PA Catheter	
During Insertion	◆ Arterial puncture while attempting central venous access. ◆ Pneumothorax / hemothorax. 　• Avoid subclavian entry in COPD patients with hyperinflated lungs. ◆ Air embolism. ◆ Ventricular arrhythmias. ◆ Heart block. 　• Avoid insertion with LBBB or have pacing equipment available. ◆ Catheter knotting or kinking.
After Insertion	◆ PA rupture. ◆ PA infarction. ◆ Infection. ◆ Ventricular arrhythmias. ◆ Heparin induced thrombocytopenia (HIT) from heparin coated catheters. ◆ Venous thrombosis. ◆ Endocardial / valvular damage.

Prevention of PA Rupture / Infarction

◆ Avoid distal migration of catheter tip.
◆ Use PAd instead of PAOP if accurate.
◆ Inflate with only the amount of air needed for occlusion and for the least amount of time possible.
◆ Observe for spontaneous PAOP pressure, indicating need to pull back PA catheter tip.
◆ Pulling back indicated if able to wedge with < 1.25 cc of air.
◆ Pull back catheter tip before the initiation of cardiopulmonary bypass.

Treatment for Pulmonary Artery Catheter Rupture

◆ Deflate balloon/pull back catheter tip.
◆ Stop anticoagulants.
◆ Place patient in lateral position with affected side down.
◆ Selective bronchial intubation.
◆ PEEP.
◆ Surgical repair.

Chapter 4

Strategies to Prevent Infection

◆ Strict sterile technique during insertion.

◆ Dead end caps on all stopcocks.

◆ Sterile sleeve over catheter.

◆ Avoid glucose in IV solutions.

◆ Change solution and lines no more frequently than every 72 to 96 hours.

◆ Remove catheter as soon as clinically indicated.

Due to the complications associated with PA catheters and the lack of research to show improved outcomes, many patients post CABG have fluid status monitored by central venous pressure monitoring only.

Alternatives to PA Catheter Monitoring

Current questions remain regarding the safety and efficacy of pulmonary artery catheter use, thus use of the pulmonary artery catheter has declined for this reason. In addition, less invasive alternatives for hemodynamic monitoring are being utilized (McLean, 2004). Alternative methods to assess cardiac output include: esophageal Doppler, pulse contour analysis, and thoracic bioimpedance. In addition to being less invasive, these methods offer continuous beat-to-beat assessment.

◆ Transesophageal Doppler: This technique assesses hemodynamic function by measuring blood flow velocity in the descending aorta using a Doppler transducer on the tip of a flexible probe. Patients must be mechanically ventilated and sedated for this method of assessment.

◆ Pulse contour analysis (PiCCO): This technique requires central venous access and arterial access, but does not require catheter placement in the right heart. By evaluating the arterial pulse contour, continuous cardiac output is calculated. Additional parameters are also measured to aid in the assessment of preload, afterload, and contractility.

◆ Lithium derived continuous cardiac output (LiDCO): Similar to the PiCCO system, LiDCO utilizes an arterial line and either a central or peripheral venous line. The system is calibrated using a small dose of lithium chloride. The system utilizes the arterial blood pressure system to calculate continuous stroke volume, cardiac output and other hemodynamic measurements.

◆ Transthoracic electrical bioimpedance: This technology is based on assessing the change in impedance that occurs as blood is ejected into the aorta. Electrodes on the neck and chest are used to assess electrical impedance. Blood ejected into the aorta results in a decrease in impedance proportional to the volume of ejected blood. The magnitude of the decrease in impedance allows for a calculation of cardiac output via various algorithms. The calculation of blood flow is displayed in real time. A number of patient factors can interfere with the accuracy of this technique in measuring cardiac output. In addition, this technique does not provide an assessment of cardiac preload (McLean, 2004). There is insufficient evidence at this time to support the routine use of this technique.

Linking Knowledge to Practice

✔ *Key to the effectiveness of any type of continuous hemodynamic monitoring is the availability of protocols to allow the nurse to immediately act on the data. Assessment without intervention will not result in improved outcomes.*

Hemodynamics/Shock States/Intra-Aortic Balloon Pump Therapy

Table 4.3 Normal Hemodynamic Values	
Cardiac Output (CO)	4-8 L/min
Cardiac Index (CI)	2.5-4.0 L/min/m^2
Stroke Volume (SV)	60-100 ml/beat
Stroke Volume Index (SVI)	35-60 ml/beat/m^2
Right Atrial Pressure (RA)	2-6 mm Hg
Pulmonary Artery Pressure (PA) Systolic/Diastolic	15-30/6-15 mm Hg
Pulmonary Artery Pressure (PA) Mean	9-17 mm Hg
Pulmonary Artery Occlusion Pressure (PAOP)	5-12 mm Hg
Right Ventricular End Diastolic Volume (RVEDV)	100-160 ml
Systemic Vascular Resistance (SVR)	800-1200 dynes/sec/cm^{-5}
Pulmonary Vascular Resistance (PVR)	< 200 dynes/sec/cm^{-5}
Mean Arterial Pressure (MAP)	70-110 mm Hg

(Martin, 2006).

Arterial Line Monitoring

Indications

Arterial line monitoring is indicated for continuous blood pressure assessment during titration of vasoactive drugs. An arterial line is also indicated for multiple (> 4 per day) daily blood gas samples.

Blood Pressure Measurements

Systolic (SBP), diastolic (DBP), and mean pressures can be obtained from arterial blood pressure assessment. Mean arterial pressure (MAP) is the product of systemic vascular resistance and cardiac output. The MAP reflects the mean perfusion pressure throughout the cardiac cycle. It is the MAP that is sensed by the baroreceptors and is the foundation for autoregulation in the brain, heart, and kidneys. There are two formulas for calculating MAP. These formulas are only accurate when the heart rate is close to 60 bpm. Non-invasive blood pressure cuffs and invasive monitoring systems directly calculate the MAP.

◆ MAP = DBP + (SBP-DBP)/3.

◆ MAP = SBP + (DBP x 2)/3.

(McGhee & Bridges, 2002).

The mean arterial pressure is a more stable pressure and is less impacted by technical factors of invasive monitoring than the systolic or diastolic blood pressure. The MAP is a more accurate assessment of the patient's overall hemodynamic status.

Pulse pressure is the difference between systolic and diastolic blood pressure. A normal pulse pressure is approximately 40 mm Hg. An acute decrease in pulse pressure (narrow pulse pressure) is caused by a decrease in stroke volume or an increase in SVR. An increased or widened pulse pressure can be caused by several factors, resulting in an increased stroke volume: fever, exercise, anemia, hyperthyroidism, bradycardia, aortic regurgitation, and increased intracranial pressure.

Normal Arterial Waveform (Figure 4.30)

- Rapid upstroke (anacrotic limb) produced by left ventricular contraction.
- Rounded peak (systolic ejection) – reflects the displacement of ejected blood volume.
- Rapid downstroke.
- Dicrotic notch on downstroke – represents closure of aortic valve.
- Gradual decline (diastolic run off) until next upstroke.

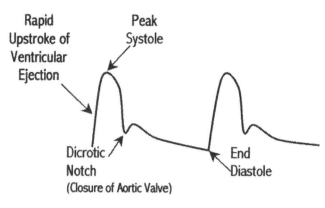

Figure 4.30: Normal arterial waveform.

The analog arterial waveform is affected by two factors: 1) the forward pressure pulse, and 2) the backward reflection of the pressure wave. Hypertension and vasoconstrictive states cause an increase in the backward reflection of the pressure wave and can cause an overestimation of systolic pressure. The waveform in these conditions may appear underdamped.

Technical Issues

- Arterial line pressures should be referenced to the phlebostic axis to eliminate any effects of hydrostatic pressure.
- Systolic blood pressure increases the further the monitoring site is from the central aorta, due to the effects of hydrostatic pressure. Radial and dorsalis pedis arteries may have systolic blood pressures 20 to 25 mm Hg higher than central aortic pressures (McGhee & Bridges, 2002).
- The dicrotic notch becomes less distinct the farther the monitoring site is away from the central aorta
- Arterial line and cuff pressures may differ because the arterial line measures pressure while the cuff measures flow, and the two do not necessarily correlate. However, the MAP will closely correlate between the two.
- A technically correct arterial line pressure is more accurate than a cuff pressure.

Linking Knowledge to Practice

✔ *Utilizing direct assessment of arterial blood pressure allows for a beat-to-beat assessment of changes in blood pressure. This allows the nurse to accurately assess for blood pressure responses to changes in therapy or in the patient condition.*
  - *Blood pressure response to changes in positive end expiratory pressure on the ventilator.*
  - *Blood pressure response to changes in cardiac rhythm.*
  - *Blood pressure response can be used to determine optimum pacing rate and/or AV delay with temporary pacemakers.*

Hemodynamics/Shock States/Intra-Aortic Balloon Pump Therapy

ALTERED HEMODYNAMIC STATES: VALVULAR HEART DISEASE

Mitral Stenosis

Obstruction of flow through the mitral valve results in a progressive rise in left atrial pressure and a decrease in left ventricular filling. Left ventricular filling is more dependent on atrial kick when there is mitral stenosis.

The increase in left atrial pressure is transmitted to the pulmonary circulation, resulting in what is called passive pulmonary hypertension. The PAd and PAOP rise in proportion to each other, but neither is a reflection of LV end diastolic pressure or volume. The increase in pulmonary pressures places the patient at risk for the development of pulmonary edema. Compensatory mechanisms occur to prevent pulmonary edema, including: 1) enlargement of left atrium to hold more blood; 2) increase in pulmonary lymph flow to remove more fluid; 3) decrease in alveolar capillary permeability; 4) hypertrophy of pulmonary arterioles, increasing their ability to constrict and reduce flow through the capillary bed. This constriction of the pulmonary arterioles leads to a more active pulmonary hypertension. This causes a widening of the gradient between the PAd and the PAOP.

Linking Knowledge to Practice

✔ *Patients with mitral stenosis can have a deterioration in their hemodynamic status due to poor ventricular filling and low stroke volume when they develop atrial fibrillation and lose atrial kick. Patients with mitral stenosis are also at risk for the development of pulmonary edema anytime there is an increase in venous return to the heart.*

Mitral Regurgitation

Hemodynamic changes are different for chronic versus acute mitral regurgitation. In chronic mitral regurgitation, the left atrium dilates to compensate for the increase in volume, and left atrial and pulmonary artery pressures can remain normal or only slightly elevated. The PAd rises in proportion to the PAOP. The degree of elevation in PAOP and PA pressures is dependent on the amount of regurgitation, the compliance or size of the left atrium, and the function of the left ventricle (described below).

Mitral regurgitation is the only condition in which the PAOP can be greater than the PAd pressure. The measured PAOP also has the potential to overestimate the left ventricular end diastolic filling pressure because of the large *v* waves. *V* waves become more diminished as the left atrium dilates and compensates. *V* waves are discussed earlier in this chapter.

The left ventricle receives extra volume during diastole (normal pulmonary venous return plus the regurgitant volume from systole). The left ventricle also enlarges to accommodate this increase in volume. During systole, not all left ventricular stroke volume ends up in the systemic circulation. Some of the stroke volume is regurgitated back into the left atrium, and systemic stroke volume is reduced. Left ventricular function is enhanced to increase stroke volume. This assures an adequate amount for systemic circulation and also helps eliminate the increase in end diastolic volume.

Acute mitral regurgitation results in hemodynamic compromise because the left atrium and left ventricle do not have time to compensate as they do in chronic mitral regurgitation. Acute mitral regurgitation can occur with endocarditis or papillary muscle ischemia/rupture, and causes sudden pulmonary edema and systemic hypoperfusion. SVR increases to compensate for perfusion failure and results in an impedance to forward flow and an increase in regurgitation.

145

Chapter 4

Aortic Stenosis

An increase in left ventricular systolic pressure is required to eject an adequate volume of blood through the stenotic valve. This increase in systolic pressure results in an increase in myocardial oxygen demand. In response to this increased need for left ventricular work, the left ventricle develops concentric hypertrophy (thickening of ventricular muscle wall, but no increase in cavity size). Concentric hypertrophy results in decreased ventricular compliance and impaired diastolic filling. Atrial kick becomes more important in maintaining adequate left ventricular end diastolic volume. Secondary left atrial enlargement develops in response to the hypertrophied left ventricle.

Linking Knowledge to Practice

✔ *Patients can have hypovolemia with normal left ventricular end diastolic filling pressures due to the noncompliant left ventricle. A decrease in stroke volume can occur with even small fluid losses and with any loss in atrial kick.*

Aortic Regurgitation

During compensated aortic regurgitation, the left ventricle enlarges (both wall thickness and chamber size) to accommodate the normal volume received from the left atrium, plus the regurgitant volume. The left ventricle becomes capable of ejecting up to two times the normal stroke volume. In addition, a decrease in SVR helps maintain forward flow. Patients with aortic regurgitation develop hyperdynamic circulation where aortic systolic pressure is high from the increased stroke volume, but aortic diastolic pressure is low from the decreased SVR and diastolic regurgitation.

If the volume of regurgitant flow exceeds the limits of compensation, then pathological ventricular dilatation occurs, resulting in decreased contractility and resultant heart failure. In response to a decrease in stroke volume, SVR increases, further impedes ejection, and worsens the amount of regurgitant flow. A vicious cycle exists of perfusion failure and worsening regurgitation. Pulmonary edema does not usually develop because the mitral valve closes early to protect the pulmonary circulation from the increase in end diastolic volume.

In acute, severe aortic regurgitation, the left ventricle is not able to compensate for the regurgitant flow. Forward flow is substantially decreased. In response, SVR increases and the regurgitant flow is increased; forward flow is decreased. Perfusion failure results quickly, and emergency surgical intervention is required to prevent circulatory collapse and death.

ALTERED HEMODYNAMIC STATES: TAMPONADE

Cardiac tamponade is a clinical syndrome that occurs when the accumulation of pericardial content causes compression of the heart and impedes normal cardiac function. As the compression of the heart increases, cardiac output decreases. It is not the volume of the pericardial content that determines the significance of the tamponade, but the amount of compression. The significance of the tamponade is most often directly proportional to the speed in which the pericardial contents are accumulated.

As the volume in the pericardial space increases for whatever reason, a larger space is required to hold the volume. Since the fibrous pericardium is not easily distensible, the only place for the pericardial space to expand is inward. As the pericardial space expands inward, the heart is compressed. The pericardial space is a continuous space that covers the entire surface of the heart. As volume increases, it is distributed over the entire surface area of the heart so all areas of the heart are equally compressed. As the intra-pericardial pressure increases, the intra-cardiac pressures all increase. Compression of the heart results in a reduction

Hemodynamics/Shock States/Intra-Aortic Balloon Pump Therapy

in filling. The ventricle is unable to expand during diastolic filling, resulting in a decreased stroke volume and cardiac output. Venous return to the heart is also altered, and right atrial collapse occurs. Blood accumulates in the venous system, and signs of right-sided failure occur.

Hemodynamic changes in tamponade include:

◆ Equalization of filling pressures. As the intra-pericardial pressure increases, the RA pressure, the PAd pressure and the PAOP (wedge) all "rise to equalize" and will usually move to within 5 mm Hg of each other.

◆ Note: After open heart surgery, more localized bleeding can also cause a tamponade effect. Clot formation next to the right or left atria may cause pressure increases consistent with either right or left heart failure, as opposed to pressure changes consistent with classic cardiac tamponade.

◆ An evaluation of the RA pressure waveform demonstrates a loss of the Y descent that occurs when the tricuspid valve opens and the atrium empties into the right ventricle. An increased intra-pericardial pressure prevents passive diastolic filling, thereby eliminating the Y descent on the RA pressure waveform. The RA waveform then only has one negative waveform (the X descent) that occurs just after atrial contraction and indicates atrial relaxation. Atrial pressures fall during systole due to decreased volumes, and the X descent is preserved (DeCastro and Schwartz, 2003).

ALTERED HEMODYNAMIC STATES: SHOCK STATES

Adequate oxygenation of the tissues is the result of the body's carefully orchestrated match between oxygen supply and oxygen demand. When delivery of oxygen to the tissues is no longer adequate to meet the metabolic needs, cellular hypoxia occurs and metabolic wastes (lactic acid) build up in the tissues. If the mismatch in supply and demand cannot be corrected, organ dysfunction and ultimately death occur. Shock states are those clinical conditions resulting in hypoperfusion and tissue hypoxia.

Pathophysiology of Shock

Adequate perfusion is dependent on the ability of oxygenated blood to reach the cells and organs. The major components of delivery of oxygen include: oxygen, hemoglobin and cardiac output. Cardiac output plays the most significant role in the delivery of oxygen to the tissues.

In most clinical situations as oxygen needs increase, hemodynamic adjustments are made by the body to meet the increased demand. With 75% of the delivered oxygen returning to the heart unused in normal circumstances, the oxygen reserve is usually adequate to provide for the increased needs of the body. Shock states occur when delivery of oxygen is insufficient to provide for the normal needs of the tissues or in times of increased physiological stress, and when the normal compensatory mechanisms are not adequate to meet the needs of the system. During shock states, oxygen demand exceeds oxygen delivery. The goals of treatment focus on increasing delivery while decreasing metabolic demand.

Stages of Shock

The severity of shock may be related to the calculated cardiac index. The bedside practitioner can also determine the severity of the shock state by the clinical signs of hypoperfusion demonstrated by the patient, which include: tachycardia, cool pale skin, hypotension, narrow pulse pressure, reduced urine output, and changes in mental status.

◆ Cardiac Index 2.2-2.5 = subclinical hypoperfusion: No clinical indications of hypoperfusion, but there is clinical suspicion that something is not normal.

Chapter 4

◆ Cardiac Index 2.0-2.2 = compensatory stage with sympathetic stimulation: The sympathetic nervous system activates to compensate for the decrease in perfusion. Tachypnea occurs as the pulmonary system attempts to increase the intake of oxygen with deeper and faster respirations.

The cardiovascular system in an attempt to increase cardiac output increases heart rate, increases contractility and SVR, which results in a narrowing pulse pressure (difference between systolic and diastolic pressure). Venous vasoconstriction increases preload. Skin temperature becomes cooler as vasoconstriction occurs.

The decreased perfusion to the kidney activates the renin-angiotensin-aldosterone system (RAAS), and water and sodium are preserved, increasing circulating volume and enhancing preload. The RAAS causes additional vasoconstriction.

The endocrine system responds to the decreased perfusion with release of anti-diuretic hormone, and further sodium and water reabsorption occurs as urine output decreases.

Bowel sounds decrease as blood is redirected to vital organs. The patient may become restless and confused as the perfusion to the brain deteriorates.

◆ Cardiac Index < 2.0 = shock with progressive hypoperfusion: Hypotension develops as the cardiac output and SVR are no longer able to maintain an adequate blood pressure. Tachycardia continues to increase as the sympathetic nervous system continues to try to increase cardiac output. Further vasoconstriction results in cold, clammy skin.

Anuria develops as the compensatory mechanisms continue to conserve water and sodium. Bowel sounds disappear, as perfusion of the gut is no longer possible because all resources are utilized for the vital organs.

Dysrhythmias develop as lactic acid builds in the system from anaerobic metabolism.

Neurological status continues to deteriorate as brain perfusion decreases, resulting in lethargy or even coma.

◆ Cardiac Index <1.8 = shock with refractory, profound hypoperfusion:
Lactic acid continues to develop from the persistent anaerobic metabolism and life-threatening dysrhythmias develop.

Hypotension becomes so severe that ,vasopressors become ineffective.

End organ failure occurs with the development of adult respiratory distress syndrome, hepatic failure with clotting abnormalities, and acute tubular necrosis. Mesenteric, myocardial and cerebral ischemia or infarctions are imminent.

Linking Knowledge to Practice

✔ *Careful evaluation of pulse pressure can aid in the early detection of compensatory mechanisms in response to low cardiac output. An increase in SVR initially narrows pulse pressure by increasing diastolic pressure while maintaining a normal systolic blood pressure. Assessment and response to a narrowing pulse pressure can allow for earlier intervention. Hypotension is a later sign of shock.*

Hemodynamics/Shock States/Intra-Aortic Balloon Pump Therapy

Classifications of Shock

Shock states are classified as hypovolemic, cardiogenic, obstructive, and distributive. (Table 4.4) Cardiogenic shock is often referred to as pump failure, while hypovolemic, distributive and obstructive shock are often referred to as circulatory failure.

Table 4.4 Classifications of Shock			
Hypovolemic (Hemorrhagic)	**Cardiogenic**	**Distributive** (Anaphylactic, Neurogenic, Septic)	**Obstructive**
Due to loss of circulating volume	Due to impaired ability of the myocardium to contract	Due to massive vasodilation (which results in relative hypovolemia)	Due to impaired ability of heart to adequately fill due to obstruction, such as in pulmonary embolus or cardiac tamponade.

Hypovolemic Shock

Hypovolemic shock is due to a loss in circulating volume. Hypovolemic shock is also referred to as hemorrhagic shock when the cause is blood loss.

Causes

The loss in circulating volume may be due to a variety of causes. Frank blood loss from traumatic injury results in a sudden decrease in intravascular volume. Circulating volume may also decrease as a result of fluid shifts. Burn patients, patients with acute severe pancreatitis, and patients after long cardiopulmonary pulmonary bypass times, experience a shift of fluid from the intravascular space to the interstitial spaces causing hypovolemia. Disease that results in loss of fluid, such as diabetes insipidus, diabetic ketoacidosis and hyperosmolar hypertonic nonketotic state, all result in an excessive diuresis, leaving a low circulating volume. Shock occurs when there is a loss of 15-20% of the circulating volume (Porth 2004).

Hemodynamic Alterations

The decreased circulating volume results in decreased venous return to the heart. With a lower venous return, the ventricle is underfilled during diastole. The decreased filling (ventricular preload) results in a decreased cardiac output. With a lower cardiac output, blood pressure drops and heart rate elevates in an attempt to compensate. The sympathetic nervous system also responds with an increase in SVR to elevate the blood pressure. The respiratory effort increases with faster and deeper respirations. If the volume is not restored, tissue perfusion decreases and cell and tissue death ultimately occur.

Chapter 4

A summary of characteristic hemodynamic alterations in hypovolemic shock is displayed in Table 4.5

Table 4.5 Hemodynamic Profile in Hypovolemic Shock	
Heart Rate	Increased
Preload (RAP, PAOP)	Decreased
Afterload (SVR)	Increased
Contractility	Neutral
Stroke Volume	Decreased
Cardiac Output	Decreased
Blood Pressure	Narrow pulse pressure, hypotension
SVO$_2$	Decreased

Clinical Findings

The clinical findings are directly related to the size of the volume loss. A loss of approximately 10% of the total volume is readily tolerated in the healthy person with no significant decrease in cardiac output (Porth, 2004). A volume loss of greater than 10% activates normal compensatory mechanisms, as the cardiac output begins to drop. Shock, as defined as a decrease in perfusion of tissues and organs, occurs when the loss is 15 to 20% of the total volume. Loss of 35 to 45% of the total blood volume causes inability to maintain a blood pressure (Porth, 2004). An estimation of the volume lost can be made by the clinical presentation of the patient. Table 4.6 reviews the clinical findings associated with blood loss.

When evaluating patients for early signs of volume depletion, the blood pressure and pulse can provide valuable information. As circulating volume decreases, the sympathetic system intervenes and increases heart rate to try to improve cardiac output. Simultaneously, blood pressure changes begin to occur. The pulse pressure (systolic pressure minus diastolic pressure) can provide good information as to fluid status. As volume is lost in the system, the diastolic blood pressure begins to rise while vasoconstriction occurs, with little effect on the systolic blood pressure. Systolic blood pressure drops when vasoconstriction is not able to maintain a normal systolic pressure. A narrowed pulse pressure can indicate lowered volume status with vasoconstriction. The pulse pressure and heart rate, when trended over time, can be helpful in identifying a slow volume loss and may help the clinician identify a potential issue before decompensation occurs.

Hemodynamics/Shock States/Intra-Aortic Balloon Pump Therapy

Table 4.6 Clinical Findings Associated with Progressive Loss of Blood	
Estimated Loss	**Clinical Presentation**
< 500cc	No signs or symptoms.
500-1,000 cc	Heart rate up to 20% above baseline. Systolic blood pressure 10% below baseline. Decreased urine output. Weakening pulse. Skin cool to touch. Cardiac output within normal limits with an elevated SVR. Mild acidosis.
1,000-2,000 cc	Heart rate 20 to 30% above baseline. Systolic blood pressure 10 to 20% below baseline. Respiratory rate 10% above baseline. Oxygen saturation may continue to remain normal if receiving supplemental oxygen. $SvO_2 < 60\%$. Urine output less than 30 cc/hour. Changes in level of consciousness. Skin cool and diaphoretic. Peripheral pulses weak and thready. Cardiac output decreased with elevated SVR. Progressive acidosis.
2,000-3,000 cc	Heart rate 20 to 30% above baseline. Systolic blood pressure 10 to 20% below baseline. Respiratory rate 10 to 20% above baseline. Oxygen saturation decreased. $SvO_2 < 55$ to 60%. Oliguria or anuria. Mental stupor. Extremities cold. Peripheral pulses poor. Peripheral cyanosis. Cardiac output decreased with elevated SVR. Severe acidosis.

(Adapted from Porth, 2004)

Treatment

The goal of treatment is to maximize the delivery of oxygen to the tissues. Delivery of oxygen is dependent on arterial oxygen content, hemoglobin and cardiac output. To effectively treat shock, the underlying cause must be treated.

Volume replacement is the first line of treatment. Preferably, two large bore intravenous catheters are placed to provide quick infusion of volume. For hypovolemic shock, isotonic crystalloid solutions are first line treatment. Isotonic solutions (0.9 NS or Lactated Ringers) are used because their osmolality is

Chapter 4

close to blood osmolality and they remain in the vascular space. Hypotonic solutions, such as 0.45% normal saline, have a lower osmolality and fluid leaves the vascular space and enters the cells.

Volume should be replaced at a rate of 3 cc of crystalloid for every 1 cc of volume lost. Typically a fluid challenge of 250 cc to 500 cc is attempted. Fluid is continued until there is a positive blood pressure response or the patient exhibits signs of fluid overload.

Colloids (Albumin human (5%), hetastarch, Dextran 40, Dextran 70, Dextran 75) can also be used during fluid resuscitation. Crystalloids are considered as effective as colloids in expanding volume and are used as first line therapy in fluid resuscitation. However, non-protein colloids (Hetastarch or a Dextran preparation) are considered when the patient has not responded to crystalloid resuscitation (4 liters of crystalloid over 2 hours) (Medscape, 2006). Non-protein colloids are generally preferred over albumin human, a protein colloid, based on cost. Both protein and non-protein colloids work by increasing the colloidal osmotic (oncotic) pressure and hold fluid in the vascular compartment. Less volume of colloid is used compared to crystalloid administration. Differences in colloid solutions are outlined in Table 4.7.

It is important to remember that neither crystalloids nor colloids increase oxygen carrying capacity. If hypovolemic shock is the result of blood loss, hemoglobin should be replaced using packed red blood cells to improve oxygen carrying capacity. Crystalloid fluid resuscitation is initiated prior to the administration of blood products to restore circulating volume.

Table 4.7 Colloids	
Albumin human	◆ Protein colloid. ◆ Sterile solution of human serum albumin. ◆ Solution containing 5% albumin human used in hypovolemia.
Hetastarch	◆ Non-protein colloid. ◆ Comparable with albumin human as volume expander. ◆ Little or no antigenic properties. ◆ May interfere with platelet function; large volume administration may transiently prolong bleeding times.
Dextran 70 / Dextran 75	◆ Non-protein colloid. ◆ Antigenic properties (uticaria, wheezing, mild hypotension). ◆ Need to observe for anaphylactoid reaction. ◆ May interfere with platelet function; large volume administration may transiently prolong bleeding times.
Dextran 40	◆ Non-protein colloid. ◆ Differs in molecular weight from Dextran 70 and Dextran 75. ◆ Appears to improve microcirculation. ◆ Has been used as prophylaxis to prevent venous thrombosis in patients undergoing surgery.

Hemodynamics/Shock States/Intra-Aortic Balloon Pump Therapy

Cardiogenic Shock

Causes

Cardiogenic shock is caused by a massive insult (usually myocardial infarction) to the left ventricle, resulting in profound left ventricular dysfunction. A large myocardial infarction with failed reperfusion and poor collateral circulation is a common cause of cardiogenic shock. However, any myocardial infarction in a patient with pre-existing left ventricular dysfunction can lead to cardiogenic shock. Early reperfusion therapy preserves myocardium and minimizes the risk for development of cardiogenic shock.

Cardiogenic shock can also occur as a complication of CABG in patients with poor left ventricular function or at the end stage of many types of heart disease. Cardiogenic shock can be triggered by a variety of cardiac and non-cardiac factors that depress myocardial function and result in a decrease in cardiac output. Cardiogenic shock can also result when patients require a higher than normal cardiac output, and the heart is unable to meet the increased demand. This may occur in anemia, hyperthyroidism or sepsis.

Cardiogenic shock as the result of an acute myocardial infarction and pump failure is used as the prototype for the rest of the discussion.

Hemodynamic Alterations

Decreased contractility from left ventricular failure results in a decreased stroke volume and decreased cardiac output. Heart rate increases in an attempt to increase cardiac output. However, patients with myocardial infarction are prone to arrhythmias that may further decrease cardiac output.

A compensatory response to a decrease in stroke volume is an increase in SVR in an effort to shunt the decreased stroke volume to vital organs and to preserve an adequate mean arterial pressure. This increase in SVR impedes ejection and forward flow of blood (decreases stroke volume) increases afterload, and increases myocardial oxygen demand and consumption.

Some patients with myocardial infarction have an abnormal vascular response, and the typical increase in SVR is not seen. This abnormal response is related to the activation of stretch receptors in the left ventricle, predominant in the inferior wall. Stimulation of these stretch receptors causes parasympathetic nervous system stimulation and results in bradycardia and vasodilation. This response is known as the Bezold-Jarisch reflex (Darovic, 2002).

As a result of left ventricular dysfunction, backward failure can occur, resulting in an elevation of left atrial and pulmonary pressures. This increase in pressures can lead to pulmonary edema and ultimate right ventricular failure. However, patients with chronic heart disease often require higher filling pressures (15 to 18 mm Hg or higher) for optimal stroke volume. Patients with acute right ventricular failure may require a right ventricular filling pressure as high as 15 mm Hg to provide adequate preload to the left ventricle (Darovic, 2002).

There are other factors that impact preload in cardiogenic shock. Diuretic therapy, diaphoresis, vomiting, and third spacing can complicate volume status. In addition, diastolic dysfunction from ischemia decreases the compliance of the ventricle and raises PAOP pressure higher than expected for a given end diastolic volume. Also, patients with co-existing right ventricular failure may have septal shifting into the left ventricle, resulting in decreased volume capacity of the left ventricle. This also may raise PAOP higher than expected for a given left ventricular diastolic volume. Interpretation of PAOP must be considered in light of the patient's clinical presentation.

Chapter 4

The characteristic hemodynamic profile of cardiogenic shock is described in Table 4.8.

Table 4.8 Hemodynamic Profile in Cardiogenic Shock	
Heart Rate	Increased
Preload (RAP, PAOP)	Increased *
Afterload (SVR)	Increased *
Contractility	Decreased
Stroke Volume	Decreased
Cardiac Output	Decreased
Blood Pressure	Narrow pulse pressure, hypotension
SVO₂	Decreased

* Hemodynamic parameters of preload and afterload can vary, based on the factors described above.

Clinical Findings
◆ Systolic BP < 90 mm Hg.
◆ Decreased sensorium.
◆ Cool, pale, moist skin.
◆ Peripheral cyanosis.
◆ Decreased urine output.
◆ Tachycardia.
◆ Weak, thready peripheral pulses.
◆ Tachypnea.
◆ Hypoxia.
◆ Muffled heart sounds due to decreased contractility.
◆ S3, S4 (may be difficult to hear).
◆ Distended neck veins if right-sided failure.
◆ Crackles or other adventitious lung sounds if pulmonary edema.

Linking Knowledge to Practice
✔ *Tachypnea and an increased work of breathing diverts an increased amount of cardiac output to the respiratory muscles and thus reduces the amount of blood flow to other vital organs. Any critically ill patient with an increased work of breathing needs to be intubated, sedated, and mechanically ventilated to decrease work of breathing and optimize cerebral, coronary and renal blood flow.*

Treatment
The treatment goal, as in all shock states, is to maximize the delivery of oxygen to the tissues. In cardiogenic shock there are the additional goals of increasing myocardial oxygen supply and decreasing myocardial oxygen demand. Because there is left ventricular pump failure in cardiogenic shock, the focus is on improving contractility with supportive measures (optimizing preload and afterload) to maximize stroke volume.

Hemodynamics/Shock States/Intra-Aortic Balloon Pump Therapy

Revascularization with emergency PCI should be considered in all patients where ischemia or infarct is the cause of the cardiogenic shock. Inotropic agents, such as dobutamine or milrinone, can be used to improve left ventricular contractility.

Preload reduction is needed when PAOP is > 20-22 mm Hg or when pulmonary edema develops. Diuretics and venous vasodilators are used to treat elevated preload. Preload may also need to be optimized with fluid therapy based on the circumstances described above.

Afterload reduction may be important to improving stroke volume. A failing left ventricle is not able to pump against high resistance. Caution must be used in reducing left ventricular afterload in the presence of hypotension. In addition, it is also important to consider the adverse impact of vasopressors in the presence of left ventricular failure. It is important to maintain an adequate mean arterial pressure to support perfusion, but at the same time reduce afterload to allow the ventricle to more easily eject its contents. Blood pressure is maintained if afterload reduction results in an improvement of stroke volume.

The mechanical support of an intra-aortic balloon pump is an effective method of reducing afterload in a patient with hypotension who cannot tolerate vasodilator therapy. In addition to reducing afterload, an intra-aortic balloon pump can improve myocardial perfusion in a patient with ischemia. Intra-aortic balloon pumping is discussed in detail later in this chapter. Left ventricular circulatory assist devices may also be considered.

Supportive measures in cardiogenic shock to improve delivery of oxygen include oxygenation, mechanical ventilation, and administration of packed red blood cells if hemoglobin is low.

The prevention and correction of metabolic acidosis is an outcome goal for all forms of shock.

Distributive Shock
Distributive shock includes anaphylactic shock, neurogenic shock, and septic shock. All 3 of these shock states result in severe peripheral vasodilation and expansion of vascular space with relative reduction in circulating volume. Acute adrenal insufficiency can also cause distributive shock.

All types of distributive shock have a similar hemodynamic profile.

Table 4.9 Hemodynamic Profile in Distributive Shock	
Heart Rate	Increased
Preload (RAP, PAOP)	Decreased
Afterload (SVR)	Decreased
Contractility	Neutral
Stroke Volume	Increased early, decreased late
Cardiac Output	Increased early, decreased late
Blood Pressure	Widened pulse pressure
SVO$_2$	Decreased (increased in late septic shock when tissues cannot extract oxygen).

Chapter 4

Anaphylactic Shock

Anaphylactic shock occurs when there is a severe antibody-antigen response, resulting in a release of multiple biochemical mediators from the mast cells. One of the released biochemical mediators is histamine, a potent vasodilator. The result is vasodilation, which causes a relative hypovolemia (i.e. no actual loss of volume, but existing volume is no longer adequate to fill up the dilated vascular space). Pooling of blood and an increase in capillary permeability also occur in anaphylactic shock.

Anaphylactic shock can result from a reaction to drugs, ionic contrast, foods, food additives, latex, blood products, insect venom, and other biological or environmental agents.

Clinical Finding Specific to Anaphylactic Shock
◆ Apprehension.
◆ Pruritus (itching), or warm burning sensation of skin.
◆ Generalized erythema or urticaria (hives).
◆ Angioedema (swelling of face and throat).
◆ Bronchoconstriction, increased mucous secretions.
◆ Cramping from contraction of gastrointestinal, uterine, and vascular smooth muscle.
◆ Coughing, choking, wheezing, shortness of breath.
◆ Chest tightness from coronary vasoconstriction.

Treatment Specific to Anaphylactic Shock
◆ Manage airway (high risk for airway obstruction).
◆ Remove offending agent or slow absorption (ice, flush skin, lavage).
◆ Modify or block effects of mediators.
◆ Epinephrine.
◆ Antihistamines.
◆ Diphenhydramine (H_1 blocker).
◆ Ranitidine (H_2 blocker).
◆ Corticosteroids (decrease capillary permeability, prevent delayed reaction).

Neurogenic Shock

Neurogenic shock is the least common form of shock and caused by a loss of autonomic control due to either a defect in the vasomotor center of the brainstem or an interruption in the outflow communicating pathways to the vessels. Spinal cord injury above the level of T_6 is the most common cause. Anesthesia, drugs, CNS problems, hypoxia, hypoglycemia, pain and emotional stress can also cause neurogenic shock.

The lack of sympathetic nervous system response results in a profound venous and arterial vasodilation leading to a reduction in both preload and afterload. Due to the lack of sympathetic nervous system response and predominant parasympathetic control, the heart rate is not able to increase to compensate for a decrease in cardiac output.

There is a loss of vasomotor control in the surface vessels that control heat loss and, consequently, the patient becomes hypothermic and the skin is warm and dry to touch. In patients with spinal cord injury, there is no ability to sweat below the level of injury.

Clinical Findings Specific to Neurogenic Shock
- Hypotension with bradycardia.
- Hypothermia.
- Warm, dry skin.

Treatment Specific to Neurogenic Shock

Intervening to preserve spinal cord function is key if spinal cord injury is the cause of neurogenic shock. Colloids are often used to limit the amount of fluid given to avoid any further spinal cord edema. Hypotonic solutions are also avoided to prevent any further spinal cord edema. Patients may have an atypical response to vasopressors due to the interruption in sympathetic nervous system communicating pathways. Vasopressin may be utilized if patient does not respond to sympathomimetics. Atropine is given for bradycardia.

Septic Shock

Septic shock is discussed in detail in Chapter 18 where the continuum from sepsis to septic shock is fully explained.

Obstructive Shock

Obstructive shock is a result of obstruction of ventricular filling or the obstruction of blood flow through the heart or great vessels, resulting in a decrease in cardiac output. Pulmonary embolus, cardiac tamponade, constrictive pericarditis, pneumothorax, hemothorax, and dissecting aneurysm can all cause obstructive shock. Pulmonary embolus and pneumothorax are discussed in Chapter 18; constrictive pericarditis and cardiac tamponade are discussed in Chapter 12; and dissecting aortic aneurysm is discussed in Chapter 13.

The focus of treatment of obstructive shock involves removing the obstruction to flow. This typically involves surgery or the administration of a fibrinolytic drug in the case of pulmonary embolus.

INTRA-AORTIC BALLOON PUMPING

The intra-aortic balloon pump (IABP) is a temporary cardiac assist device that utilizes counterpulsation therapy. This means the intra-aortic balloon is inflated during diastole and deflated during systole. The balloon is also a volume displacement device and displaces blood during inflation.

The intra-aortic balloon is placed in the descending thoracic aorta 1 to 2 cm below the left subclavian artery origin and above the renal and mesenteric arteries (Figure 4.31). The tip of the balloon should be between the 2nd and 3rd intercostal space on the chest x-ray. A chest x-ray should be done as soon as possible after placement if fluoroscopy was not used.

The balloon catheter is connected to pressure tubing maintained under 300 mm Hg pressure. The balloon catheter should not be used for drawing blood and when flushed, a long flush of 15 to 20 seconds should be used.

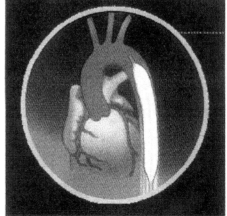

Figure 4.31: Intra-aortic balloon pump (IABP) placement.
(Courtesy of Datascope®)

Chapter 4

There are several hemodynamic effects of intra-aortic balloon pumping.

- Increased diastolic aortic pressure .
- Increased coronary blood flow with potential improvement in collateral circulation due to increased coronary perfusion pressure.
- Increased cardiac output, ejection fraction, and forward flow.
- Increased cerebral and renal blood flow.
- Increased systemic perfusion.
- Increased coronary and systemic oxygen supply.
- Increased hemodynamic pulse rate caused by balloon inflation.
- Decreased systolic aortic pressure.
- Decreased afterload.
  - ❖ Decreased MVO_2. MVO_2 decreases approximately 5% for every 10 mm Hg decrease in aortic valve opening pressure.
- Decreased LV wall tension – the isovolumetric phase of contraction is shortened.
- Decreased preload.
  - ❖ Decreased pulmonary congestion.
- Decreased compensatory chronotropic response

Indications for IABP

- Cardiogenic Shock.
- Extending MI .
- Unstable Angina.
- Intractable Ventricular Dysrhythmias.
- Support for high risk intervention.
- Bridging Device.
- Mechanical Defects.
- Post-operative myocardial dysfunction.

Contraindications

Absolute contraindications include aortic valve insufficiency and dissecting aortic aneurysm. Relative contraindications include: calcific aortic iliac disease, peripheral arterial disease, and severe obesity.

Inflation Overview (Figure 4.32)

Inflation of the intra-aortic balloon (IAB) during diastole increases aortic volume and pressure. The balloon is inflated immediately upon closure of the aortic valve.

Goals of Inflation

- Increase coronary perfusion pressure and coronary oxygen supply.
- Increase systemic perfusion pressure and peripheral oxygen supply.
- Increase baroreceptor response and decrease SNS stimulation.
  - ❖ Decrease SVR.
  - ❖ Decrease HR.

Hemodynamics/Shock States/Intra-Aortic Balloon Pump Therapy

Deflation Overview (Figure 4.32)

IAB deflation just prior to systole creates a potential space in the aorta. This reduces aortic volume and pressure. The balloon must be deflated before the full onset of systole.

Goals of Deflation
- Decrease afterload
  - Decrease MVO$_2$.
  - Decrease assisted peak systolic pressure.
  - Increase cardiac output and ejection fraction (increase forward flow).

Trigger

Triggering is a safety component of the IABP. The trigger is a reference point for balloon activation and deactivation and protects the patient against extreme errors in operator timing. The IABP is set to trigger off the R wave of the cardiac rhythm whenever this is a viable option. Different

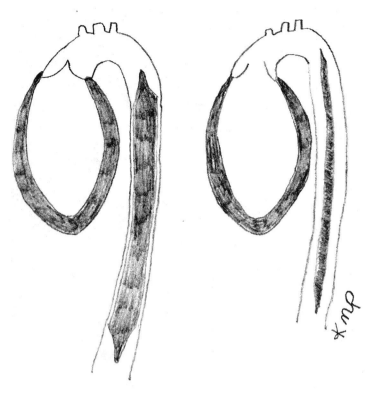

Figure 4.32: Intra-aortic balloon pump inflation and deflation. Balloon inflated during ventricular diastole (left) and balloon deflated during ventricular systole (right).

machines have different trigger modes for special rhythms, such as paced rhythms, rhythms with wide QRS complexes, and atrial fibrillation. The IABP is also capable of triggering off the arterial pressure waveform when there is an adequate upstroke. During CPR, the arterial pressure trigger is the preferred mode. However, if CPR cannot generate an adequate trigger, then there is an internal automatic trigger where a predetermined rate is used to deliver counterpulsation therapy. This mode does not synchronize counterpulsation with the patient's cardiac activity, so it can only be used if the patient is in cardiac arrest.

Linking Knowledge to Practice

✔ It is important to maintain balloon inflation whenever possible during CPR because the balloon cannot be reinflated once it has not been used for 30 minutes, due to the risk of cerebral emobilization.

Arterial Pressure Timing

Intra-aortic balloon action is mechanical, so the effectiveness of the balloon inflation and deflation is evaluated by a mechanical event.

The arterial waveform is used to assess timing. The IABP is placed in the 1:2 assist mode to evaluate timing. The screen is placed in the freeze mode, and the IABP is returned to preset assist mode, while timing is evaluated on the frozen screen.

Timing Assessment Points (Figure 4.33)
- PAEDP: Patient's end diastolic pressure: This point determines afterload and is a major determinate of MVO$_2$.
- PSP: Patient Systolic Pressure (unassisted). Pressure generated by the LV during mechanical contraction; 65-75% of stroke volume has been delivered. No IAB effect with this point.

- DN or Dicrotic notch: Signifies the beginning of diastole when the aortic valve closes. Remainder of stroke volume is delivered by this point.
- PDP or Peak Diastolic Augmented Pressure: Pressure generated in the aorta as a result of balloon inflation during diastole. During inflation aortic pressure increases. Also, each balloon inflation creates an additional mechanical pulse.
- BAEDP or Balloon-Assisted End Diastolic Pressure: Lowest aortic pressure produced by the deflation of the IAB during isovolumetric contraction. Results in reduced afterload and preload and, therefore, decreased MVO_2.

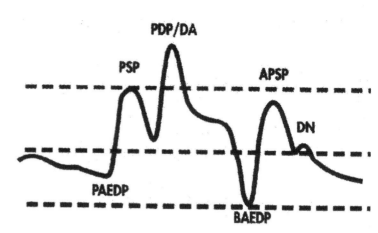

Figure 4.33: Timing assessment points.
(Courtesy of Datascope®)

- APSP or Assisted Patient Systole: The systole following IAB deflation. This pressure should be lower than PSP, reflecting a decrease in LV work as a result of the shortened isovolumetric contraction phase and lower resistance to systolic ejection.

Monitoring Issues with IABP Therapy

- Bedside monitors typically average the patient's systolic pressure and peak augmented diastolic pressure to determine a systolic reading.
- Noninvasive blood pressure monitors generally read the first event as the peak augmented diastolic pressure.
- It is therefore important to carefully document each individual pressure to accurately assess the optimal function of the IABP and the patient's clinical response.

IAB Inflation

Augmented Diastolic Pressure (Peak Diastolic Pressure)

The augmented or peak diastolic pressure is caused by increased pressure (volume) in the aorta during diastole. The augmented diastolic pressure should be greater than the patient's systolic pressure. The amount of augmentation is affected by the timing of balloon inflation. Maximal augmentation occurs when balloon inflation occurs 40 msec prior to the dicrotic notch.

The augmented diastolic pressure creates an additional perfusion event with an additional mechanical pulse. Perfusion is a result of both pressure and time. The coronary and peripheral circulations both receive additional perfusion; however, the coronary system receives greatest benefit due to proximity to balloon. The additional perfusion of the augmented diastolic pressure is generated with no additional myocardial oxygen consumption. The augmented diastolic pressure affects several regulatory and compensatory systems, as listed below.

- Baroreceptor Control
  - Baroreceptors are located in the aortic arch and carotid arteries.
  - Augmented diastolic pressure stimulates the baroreceptor response to decrease sympathetic nervous system stimulation and increase parasympathetic nervous system stimulation.
  - This results in vasodilation (decreased SVR) and decreased heart rate, which reduce myocardial oxygen consumption.

Hemodynamics/Shock States/Intra-Aortic Balloon Pump Therapy

◆ Metabolic Factors
   ❖ Increased capillary perfusion results in increased washout of metabolic waste and a decrease in metabolic acidosis.

Factors Impacting Augmentation
◆ Physical Factors
   ❖ Position: The closer the balloon is to the aortic valve, the higher the augmentation. However, there is a higher risk of cerebral embolism with a closer proximity to the aortic valve. General placement is 1 to 2 cm below the left subclavian artery opening.
   ❖ Volume: Balloon volume ranges from 30 to 50 cc. Volume may be increased to increase augmentation, as long as the aorta is not completely occluded.
   ❖ Diameter of balloon: The average balloon size is 15 to 18 mm, and average size of the aorta is 16 to 30 mm.
   ❖ Occlusiveness: The goal is to achieve 90% occlusiveness on inflation. This minimizes aortic wall trauma and damage to red blood cells and platelets.
   ❖ Drive Gas: Helium is the gas of choice. It has a low molecular weight and a fast transit time.
   ❖ Duration of Inflation: The faster the heart rate, the less time for inflation of the balloon.
   ❖ Efficiency of the System: Dehumidifying the gas is important because water droplets impair the efficiency of inflation and deflation.
   ❖ Timing: Early or late inflation times impair optimal augmentation.
◆ Biological Factors
   ❖ Arterial Pressure: Augmentation is impaired when mean arterial pressure (MAP) is < 40 mm Hg or > 100 mm Hg. When MAP is between 40 and 100 mm Hg, 10 to 25 mm Hg augmentation is expected.
   ❖ Aortic Pressure / Volume Relationship: There are 3 factors that determine the relationship between aortic pressure and volume.
      ✶ Windkessel Effect – lowest point of aortic flow correlates with aortic valve closure.
      ✶ Aortic Compliance.
      ✶ Stroke Volume.
      ✶ As aortic pressure and volume are reduced, diastolic augmentation is reduced.

High Augmentation
◆ Risks of increased augmentation (or PDP) are mechanical:
   ❖ Aortic valve regurgitation.
   ❖ Aortic wall damage/aortic dissection.
   ❖ Red blood cell destruction.
◆ In low cardiac output states, the benefits outweigh the risks.

High Augmentation Post Cardiac Surgery
◆ Benefits: maintenance of coronary graft patency.
◆ Risks: bleeding and disruption of suture sites.
◆ Strategies to decrease risks: use of vasodilators and lower placement.

Low Augmentation
◆ Weaning states: Augmentation decreases as the patient's hemodynamic condition improves.
◆ Low volume or output states: When stroke volume is < 25 cc, augmentation is low.
◆ Low augmentation causes reduced peripheral flow and stagnation of blood.

Chapter 4

Inflation Timing Principles

Timing is assessed using dicrotic notch to dicrotic notch. The IABP is placed in the 1:2 assist mode. Figure 4.34 demonstrates correct inflation timing. The timing points are described below:

1. Patient's end diastolic pressure.
2. Patient's systolic pressure (unassisted).
3. Dicrotic notch.
4. Peak diastolic augmented pressure.
5. Balloon assisted end diastolic pressure.
6. Assisted patient systole.

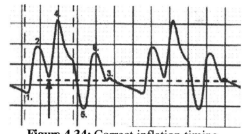

Figure 4.34: Correct inflation timing.
(Courtesy of Arrow International, Inc.)

Early Inflation

- Inflation prior to closure of aortic valve (Figure 4.35).
- Increased aortic pressure causes regurgitation of blood into the LV.
- Rise in aortic pressure prematurely closes the aortic valve and decreases LV emptying.
- Increased end systolic volume and pressure.
- Increased preload.
- Increased MVO_2.
- Increased Stroke Work.
- Decreased SV.
- Decreased CO and systemic perfusion.
- Increased work and oxygen requirements.
- Significantly impaired LV function.

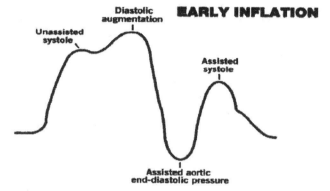

Figure 4.35: Early inflation prior to valve closure.
(Courtesy of Datascope®)

Late Inflation

- Inflation after closure of aortic valve (Figure 4.36).
- PDP (augmentation) is decreased.
- Systolic volume has run off to peripheral circulation.
- Decreased perfusion pressure and volume to coronary arteries.

Deflation

- Decrease in aortic pressure during isovolumetric contraction.

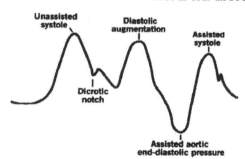

Figure 4.36: Late inflation.
(Courtesy of Datascope®)

- Creates a potential empty space in aorta.
- Allows part of LV stroke volume to be accommodated without resistance.
- The decreased afterload results in increased CO and, therefore, decreased LV filling pressure.
- IAB deflation results in decreased diastolic pressure and decreased assisted systolic pressure.
- Decreased static work:
  - Isometric effort requiring a large amount of energy or myocardial O_2 consumption (MVO_2)
  - Occurs during isovolumetric contraction to develop and maintain ventricular pressure prior to aortic valve opening.
  - Dynamic work: Occurs during ventricular ejection.

Factors Impacting Unloading

- Physical
  - IAB volume: Increased volume produces greater reduction in aortic pressure.
  - Occlusiveness: Goal is 90% occlusiveness.
  - Duration of Inflation: When inflation is maintained into the isovolumetric contraction period, then deflation is more pronounced
- Biological
  - Arterial pressure.
  - Vascular compliance.
    - ★ The greater the compliance, the less the impact of the balloon. A slight decrease in aortic compliance is beneficial.
  - Cardiac reserve.
    - ★ Normal cardiac reserve may result in low afterload reduction. This may occur while weaning.

Deflation Timing Principles

Deflation point is set to achieve two goals:
- BAEDP < PAEDP.
- APSP < PSP.

Note: Deflation, not inflation, affects the assisted pressures.

Early Deflation (Figure 4.37)

- Aortic pressure is allowed to rise to the normal PAEDP.
- Blood fills in the space created by balloon deflation.
- Produces a U-shaped curve.
- APSP = PSP.
- No cardiac unloading.
- No reduction in MVO_2.

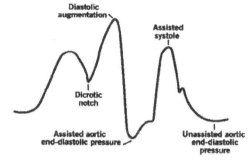

Figure 4.37: Early deflation.
(Courtesy of Datascope®)

Late Deflation (Figure 4.38)

Results in:
- Increased BAEDP.
- Increased workload of LV/increased MVO_2.
- Increased isovolumetric contraction time.
- Decreased CO and SV.
- BAEDP is > PAEDP.

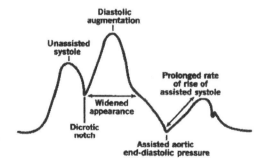

Figure 4.38: Late deflation.
(Courtesy of Datascope®)

Balloon Pressure Waveform

The balloon pressure waveform (Figure 4.39) depicts the movement of helium between the IABP console, through the catheter to the balloon. It is a calibrated, continuous waveform. It provides another measurement of the safety and effectiveness of IABP therapy.

The height of the waveform reflects the pressure in the aorta. The plateau pressure of the waveform should be + or - 20 mm Hg of the peak augmented diastolic pressure.

The width of the waveform reflects the approximate time the balloon is inflated.

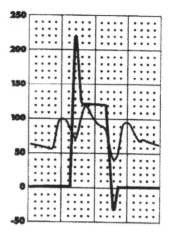

Figure 4.39: Balloon pressure waveform.
(Courtesy of Arrow International, Inc.)

Troubleshooting The Balloon Pressure Waveform

Figure 4.40 shows less than optimal augmentation with a low plateau pressure on the balloon pressure waveform. Assess for:

◆ Low balloon volume.
◆ Balloon too small for patient.
◆ Balloon placement too low in aorta.
◆ Decreased SVR (increased aortic compliance).

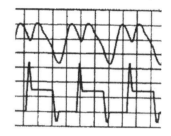

Figure 4.40: Low plateau pressure.
(Courtesy of Arrow International, Inc.)

Figure 4.41 shows very poor augmentation with inflation with balloon pressure waveform artifact. Assess for:

◆ Proximal portion of balloon still in sheath.
◆ Suture too tight around catheter.
◆ Partial kink.
◆ Slow helium shuttle speed.
◆ Very tortuous vessels.

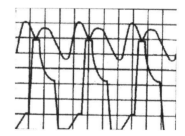

Figure 4.41: Poor augmentation.
(Courtesy of Arrow International, Inc.)

Figure 4.42 shows an elevated baseline in the balloon pressure waveform. Assess for:

◆ Kinked catheter.
◆ Partially wrapped balloon.
◆ Balloon in sheath.
◆ Overfill.
◆ Balloon to low in aorta.
◆ Balloon too large.

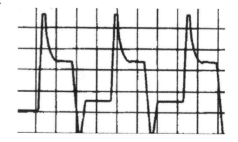

Figure 4.42: Elevated baseline.
(Courtesy of Arrow International, Inc.)

Figure 4.43 shows the baseline of the balloon pressure waveform below zero. Assess for:

◆ Blood in catheter tubing.
◆ Leak in tubing or connections (possible helium loss).
◆ Kinked catheter.
◆ Ectopic beats.

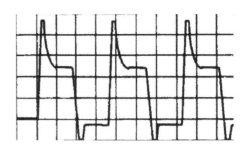

Figure 4.43: Baseline of balloon pressure waveform.
(Courtesy of Arrow International, Inc.)

Figure 4.44 shows a square plateau (can also be rounded) and high pressure. Assess for:

◆ Partially wrapped balloon.
◆ Kink in catheter or tubing.
◆ Balloon in sheath.
◆ Balloon too large for aorta.
◆ Balloon position too high or too low.

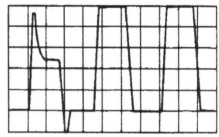

Figure 4.44: Square plateau and high pressure.
(Courtesy of Arrow International, Inc.)

Nursing Considerations

◆ Careful assessment of pressures, including assisted pressures and peak augmented diastolic pressure, are required to assure IABP therapy is being optimized and to assure adequate hemodynamic response to therapy.
◆ Balloon should not be immobile for > 30 minutes to minimize the risk of blood clots forming in folds of the balloon and neurological consequences from cerebral microembolization.
◆ Left radial pulses and urine output should be frequently assessed to assure balloon movement has not occurred and occluded either left subclavian artery or renal artery.
◆ Pedal pulses, color, and temperature of affected leg are carefully assessed for adequate circulation.
◆ The groin insertion site is checked for bleeding, hematoma, and signs of infection. The balloon catheter should be checked with each groin check.
◆ Comfort measures (log rolling and medication) are needed due to immobility.
◆ Platelets and hematocrit should be monitored due to the risk of damage to platelets and red blood cells from balloon inflation.
◆ Another complication is trauma to the aorta, including dissection.

Chapter 4

TEST YOUR KNOWLEDGE

1. The four components of cardiac output are

   a. heart rate, preload, ejection fraction, and contractility.

   b. heart rate, stroke work index, afterload, and contractility.

   c. heart rate, preload, afterload, and contractility.

   d. heart rate, preload, afterload, and stroke work index.

2. The two major determinants of blood pressure are

   a. SVR and cardiac output.

   b. contractility and SVR.

   c. systolic BP x preload.

   d. diastolic BP and cardiac output.

3. The most reliable way to assess right-sided preload without a PA catheter is

   a. lung sounds.

   b. pedal edema.

   c. blood pressure.

   d. JVD.

4. You are caring for a patient post-CABG surgery who is experiencing significant post-operative bleeding. BP is 80/66 mm Hg and HR is 110 bpm. With only this information, what might you assume to be true about this patient's hemodynamic status?

   a. Decreased preload, increased afterload, neutral or decreased contractility

   b. Neutral preload, neutral afterload, neutral contractility

   c. Increased preload, neutral afterload, increased contractility

   d. Increased preload, increased afterload, increased contractility

5. The <u>most likely</u> cause of a PAOP pressure that changes drastically from one reading to the next, with no change in the patient's clinical presentation is

   a. blood in the pressure tubing.

   b. a change in the transducer level from one reading to the next.

   c. the development of asymptomatic pulmonary edema.

   d. a catheter that is no longer in the correct position.

Hemodynamics/Shock States/Intra-Aortic Balloon Pump Therapy

6. On initial insertion of a PA catheter, you obtain the following readings: RA 6 mm Hg, PA 45/25 mm Hg, and PAOP of 12 mm Hg. You know the following to be true:

   a. The patient has pulmonary hypertension.

   b. The PAd pressure cannot be used as a measurement of left ventricular preload.

   c. The patient is fluid overloaded.

   d. a and b.

   e. All of the above.

7. You are caring for a patient with hypovolemic shock. After insertion of a PA catheter you have the following information: BP 80/68 mm Hg, RA 2 mm Hg, PA 20/7 mm Hg, PAOP 4 mm Hg, CI 2.0 L/min/m^2, PVR 150 dynes/sec/cm^{-5} and SVR 1700 dynes/sec/cm^{-5}. Based on the above information, you know the priority treatment is to

   a. add an inotrope to enhance contractility to increase cardiac index.

   b. add a vasopressor to increase blood pressure.

   c. replace volume to increase preload, therefore increasing CI and BP.

   d. insert an IABP to decrease afterload.

8. Your patient with COPD and questionable heart failure on his chest x-ray has a PA catheter placed to monitor fluid status. From previous diagnostic work-ups, your patient has known pulmonary hypertension. Patients with pulmonary hypertension have risk of

   a. left ventricular failure.

   b. right ventricular failure.

   c. aortic valve stenosis.

   d. mitral valve regurgitation.

9. Initial PA catheter readings from the above patient are: RA 14 mm Hg, PA 48/23 mm Hg, PAOP 16mm Hg, PVR 300 dynes/sec/cm^{-5}. What can you conclude from these readings and the patient's history?

   a. The patient is showing signs of right ventricular failure, most likely from underlying pulmonary hypertension.

   b. The patient is showing signs of left ventricular failure.

   c. The patient's elevated PAOP is due to his pulmonary hypertension.

   d. a and b.

   e. All of the above.

Chapter 4

10. You are performing a PAOP measurement and it takes 1.0 cc of air to obtain the occluded waveform. You know

    a. the less air needed to produce an occluded waveform is always better. The ideal goal is to use only 0.5 cc of air.

    b. the ideal amount of air needed to produce a PAOP waveform is between 1.5-1.75 cc.

    c. requiring less than 1.25 cc of air may mean the catheter is too distal, and there is an increased risk of pulmonary artery rupture.

    d. the amount of air used to inflate the balloon does not have any clinical relevance because each manufacturer uses a different sized balloon.

11. You know the formula for delivery of oxygen is cardiac output (or index) x arterial oxygen content. Which of the following has a direct impact on arterial oxygen content?

    a. Hemoglobin

    b. SaO_2

    c. SVO_2

    d. All of the above.

    e. a and b

12. The determinants of <u>delivery</u> of oxygen to the tissues are

    a. cardiac index, BP and LVSWI.

    b. CI, Hgb, and SaO_2.

    c. preload, afterload, contractility, and HR.

    d. Blood gases, blood pressure, and blood viscosity.

13. A patient with an anterior wall myocardial infarction is in cardiogenic shock. You would expect to see what on his hemodynamic profile:

    a. Decreased CI, increased preload, increased afterload, decreased contractility

    b. Decreased CI, decreased preload, increased afterload, decreased contractility

    c. Decreased CI, increased preload, decreased afterload, decreased contractility

    d. Decreased CI, increased preload, increased afterload, neutral contractility

14. You can assume that all patients with a cardiac index < 2.5 have a contractility problem.

    a. True.

    b. False.

Hemodynamics/Shock States/Intra-Aortic Balloon Pump Therapy

15. *A, v* and *c* waves can be found on
    a. arterial waveforms.
    b. PA waveforms.
    c. PAOP waveforms.
    d. RA waveforms.
    e. All of the above.
    f. c and d.

16. The *a* wave on a RA or PAOP, tracing correlates with
    a. closure of the AV valve.
    b. atrial contraction.
    c. ventricular contraction.
    d. closure of semilunar valve.

17. Clinical signs associated with elevated PAOP are
    a. peripheral edema.
    b. crackles in lung bases.
    c. sinus bradycardia.
    d. S3.
    e. All of the above.
    f. b and d.

18. In a non-compliant left ventricle, the PAOP can be elevated without the patient being fluid overloaded.
    a. True.
    b. False.

19. If you do not have a PA catheter in place what is best way to assess SVR?
    a. Diastolic BP
    b. Systolic BP
    c. Heart rate and respiratory rate
    d. Capillary refill

20. What are possible causes of an elevated PAOP?
    a. Increased circulating fluid volume.
    b. Mitral valve regurgitation.
    c. Ischemic left ventricle.
    d. All of the above.

Chapter 4

21. Standards for safe and accurate PA catheter monitoring include all the following, except
    a. obtaining PAOP waveform with 0.5 cc of air.
    b. performing a square wave test at the beginning of each shift to verify accuracy of the patient/transducer interface.
    c. zero and take readings at the level of phlebostatic axis.
    d. correlate RA and PAOP waveforms with the ECG tracing.

22. When assessing a PAOP waveform, you always want to take your measurement
    a. at the end of inspiration.
    b. at the end of expiration.
    c. at the mid-point between inspiration and expiration.
    d. at anytime because the respiratory cycle is not important with PAOP waveforms.

23. A medication that dilates both veins and arteries will have what hemodynamic effect?
    a. Increase preload, decrease afterload
    b. Increase preload, increase afterload
    c. Decrease preload, decrease afterload
    d. Decrease preload, increase afterload

24. You are caring for an acute MI patient with an SVO_2 catheter. The patient's SVO_2 has fallen from 68 to 40% over the last four hours, as the patient has become suddenly and severely hemodynamically unstable. As you attempt to increase the patient's CI, the SVO_2 remains at 40%. From this information you know
    a. you cannot expect to see an increase in SVO_2 for at least one hour from the time of your last intervention.
    b. you have stabilized the patient because the SVO_2 has not fallen below 40%, which is the low normal value.
    c. the SVO_2 is not important in this patient because the patient is a medical, and not a surgical patient.
    d. your patient's oxygen consumption is dependent on delivery, and you are still not delivering enough oxygen to meet the patient's needs.

25. Without a PA catheter, which of the following provide information about the patient's cardiac output?
    a. Blood pressure
    b. Orientation
    c. Urine output
    d. Skin temperature
    e. All of the above.

Hemodynamics/Shock States/Intra-Aortic Balloon Pump Therapy

26. What hemodynamic profile is consistent with a patient when he or she exhibits signs of cardiogenic shock?

    a. CI 2.0 L/min/m² / PAOP 22 mm Hg / SVR 1960 dynes/sec/cm⁻⁵ / LVSWI decreased

    b. CI 2.6 L/min/m² / PAOP 12 mm Hg / SVR 2000 dynes/sec/cm⁻⁵ / LVSWI decreased

    c. CI 2.1 L/min/m² / PAOP 22 mm Hg / SVR 1100 dynes/sec/cm⁻⁵ / LVSWI normal

    d. CI 4.0 L/min/m² / PAOP 6 mm Hg / SVR 2200 dynes/sec/cm⁻⁵ / LVSWI normal

27. You are caring for a patient on anticoagulants with a massive GI bleed. You begin fluid resuscitation after discovering the bleed and a blood pressure of 70/42 mm Hg. A PA catheter is immediately placed to guide fluid replacement. What hemodynamic parameters would you expect?

    a. CI 2.1 L/min/m² / RAP 1 mm Hg / PAOP 3 mm Hg / SVR 2060 dynes/sec/cm⁻⁵

    b. CI 3.5 L/min/m² / RAP 1 mm Hg / PAOP 3 mm Hg / SVR 2060 dynes/sec/cm⁻⁵

    c. CI 2.1 L/min/m² / RAP 5 mm Hg / PAOP 8 mm Hg / SVR 1900 dynes/sec/cm⁻⁵

    d. CI 2.1 L/min/m² / RAP 10 mm Hg / PAOP 2 mm Hg / SVR 1000 dynes/sec/cm⁻⁵

28. You are caring for a patient post CABG with a PA catheter in place. On physical assessment, you notice profound hypotension, distended neck veins and muffled heart sounds. You expect to find the following PA catheter readings:

    a. RAP 18 / PA 35/19 / PAOP 8

    b. RAP 4 / PA 18/5 / PAOP 5

    c. RAP 18 / PA 35/19 / PAOP 18

    d. RAP 10 / PA 25/10 / PAOP 10

29. What do you know to be true regarding independent RV failure?

    a. RA pressures will be low.

    b. RA pressures will be high.

    c. PAOP will be low.

    d. PAOP will be high.

    e. a and d.

    f. b and c.

30. Which of the following statements is true concerning IAB counterpulsation therapy?

    a. It increases coronary artery blood flow by displacing blood retrograde toward the aortic arch, and increasing diastolic coronary perfusion pressure.

    b. It increases blood flow to the kidneys and lower extremities by displacing blood antegrade toward the renal and lower extremity arteries.

    c. It decreases left ventricular afterload via deflation of the balloon.

    d. All of the above.

Chapter 4

31. With optimal timing and balloon function, the following waveform should have the highest pressure reading:

    a. Patient's unassisted systolic pressure.

    b. Peak diastolic augmented pressure.

    c. Patient's assisted systolic pressure.

    d. Balloon assisted end diastolic pressure.

32. Which of the following is not an indication for IAB counterpulsation therapy?

    a. Heart failure from aortic insufficiency.

    b. Post-operative myocardial dysfunction.

    c. Cardiogenic shock.

    d. Mechanical complications of MI.

33. The desired state in IAB counterpulsation therapy is for the patient's unassisted systolic pressure to be lower than the patient's assisted systolic pressure.

    a. True.

    b. False.

34. The patient's MAP should be greater than 40 mg Hg and less than 100 mg Hg in order to achieve optimal balloon augmentation.

    a. True.

    b. False.

35. Important nursing assessment considerations for someone receiving IAB therapy include:

    a. Left radial pulse assessment.

    b. Hourly urine output assessments.

    c. Pulse assessment distal to insertion site.

    d. a and c.

    e. All of the above.

Hemodynamics/Shock States/Intra-Aortic Balloon Pump Therapy

ANSWERS

1.	C	19.	A
2.	A	20.	D
3.	D	21.	A
4.	A	22.	B
5.	B	23.	C
6.	D	24.	D
7.	C	25.	E
8.	B	26.	A
9.	D	27.	A
10.	C	28.	C
11.	E	29.	F
12.	B	30.	D
13.	A	31.	B
14.	B	32.	A
15.	F	33.	B
16.	B	34.	A
17.	F	35.	E
18.	A		

REFERENCES

AACN. (2004). *Practice alert: Pulmonary artery pressure measurement.* Aliso Viejo, CA: American Association of Critical Care Nurses.

Ahrens, T.S. & Taylor, L.A. (1992). *Hemodynamic waveform analysis.* Philadelphia: Saunders.

Arrow International IABP Reference Manual. (2002).

Bloomquist, J. & Love, M.M. (2000). Cardiovascular assessment and diagnostic procedures. In L.D. Urden & K.M. Stacy, (Eds.), *Priorities in critical care nursing* (pp. 99-145). St. Louis: Mosby.

Bojar, R.M.(2005). *Manual of perioperative care in adult cardiac surgery* (4th Ed.). Malden, Massachusetts: Blackwell Publishing.

Bond, E.F. (2005). Cardiac anatomy and physiology. In S.L.Woods, E.S. Froelicher, S.U. Motzer, & E.J. Bridges (Eds.), *Cardiac nursing* (5th ed., pp. 3-48). Philadelphia: Lippincott, Williams and Wilkins.

Bridges, E. J. (2006). Pulmonary Artery Pressure Monitoring. *AACN Advanced Critical Care, 17*(3), 286-303.

Bridges, E.J. (2005a). Systemic circulation. In S.L.Woods, E.S. Froelicher, S.U. Motzer, & E.J. Bridges (Eds.), *Cardiac nursing* (5th ed., pp.49-70). Philadelphia: Lippincott, Williams and Wilkins.

Chapter 4

Bridges, E.J. (2005b). Regulation of cardiac output and blood pressure. In S.L.Woods, E.S. Froelicher, S.U. Motzer, & E.J. Bridges (Eds.) *Cardiac nursing* (5th ed., pp.81-108). Philadelphia: Lippincott, Williams and Wilkins.

Bridges, E.J. (2005c). Hemodynamic Monitoring. In S. L. Woods, E. S. Froelicher, S. U. Motzer & E. J. Bridges (Eds.), *Cardiac nursing* (5th ed., pp. 478-526). Philadelphia: Lippincott, Williams & Wilkins.

Carabello, B.A. and Ganzes, P.C. (2001). *Cardiology pearls* (2nd ed.). Philadelphia: Hanley and Belfus.

Crawford, M.H. (2004). *Essentials of diagnosis and treatment in cardiology*. New York: McGraw-Hill.

Critical care challenges: disorders, treatments and procedures. (2003). Philadelphia: Lippincott, Williams and Wilkins.

Datascope IABP Reference Manual. (2004).

Darovic, G.O. (2002). *Hemodynamic monitoring: invasive and noninvasive clinical application* (3rd ed.). Philadelphia: Saunders.

Dennison, R.D. (2000). *Pass ccrn* (2nd ed.). St.Louis: Mosby.

Ferguson, J.J., Cohen, M., et al. (2001). The current practice of intra-aortic balloon counterpulsation. *J Am College Cardiology, 38*(5), 1456.

Kumar, V., Abbas, A.K., & Fausto, N. (2005). *Pathologic basis of disease* (7th ed.). Philadelphia: Elsevier Saunders.

Martin, G.S. (2006). Pulmonary artery catheterization. *Medscape*. Retrieved March 3, 2007 from http://www.medscape.com/viewprogram/4970_pnt

McGhee, B.H. & Bridges, M.E.J. (2002). Monitoring arterial blood pressure: What you may not know. *Critical Care Nurse, 22*, (5), 60-79.

McLean, B. (2004). Pulmonary artery catheters: And the beat goes on. *Medscape*. Retrieved March 3, 2007 from http://www.medscape.com/viewarticle/497008

Marini, J.J. & Wheeler, A.P. (2006). *Critical care medicine the essentials* (3rd ed.). Philadelphia: Lippincott, Williams and Wilkins.

Medscape Drug Reference (2006). Drug Monograph Albumin. Retrieved July 16, 2006 from http://www.medscape.com/druginfo/monograph?cid=med&drugid=60462&drugname=Albumin+IV&monotype=monograph&secid=2

Medscape Drug Reference (2006). Drug Monograph Dextran 40. Retrieved July 16, 2006 from http://www.medscape.com/druginfo/monograph?cid=med&drugid=16552&drugname=Dextran+40+in+Saline+IV&monotype=monograph

Medscape Drug Reference (2006). Drug Monograph Dextran 70. Retrieved on July 16, 2006 from http://www.medscape.com/druginfo/monograph?cid=med&drugid=16553&drugname=Dextran+75+in+Saline+IV&monotype=monograph&secid=2

Medscape Drug Reference (2006). Drug Monograph Hetastarch. Retrieved July 16, 2006 from http://www.medscape.com/druginfo/monograph?cid=med&drugid=17407&drugname=Hetastarch+in+Lact+Electrolyte+IV&monotype=monograph&secid=4

Melander, S.D. (2004). *Case studies in critical care nursing: A guide for application and review* (3rd ed.). Philadelphia: Saunders.

Morton, P.G., Fontaine, D., Hudak, C.M., & Gallo, B.M. (Eds.). (2005). *Critical care nursing – a holistic approach* (8th edition). Philadelphia: Lippincott, Williams and Wilkins.

Opie, L.H. (2004). *Heart physiology from cell to circulation* (4th ed.). Philadelphia: Lippincott, Williams and Wilkins.

Porth, C.M. (Ed.). (2004). *Essentials of pathophysiology: concepts of altered health states*. Philadelphia: Lippincott, Williams and Wilkins.

Pulmonary Artery Catheter Education Project (PACEP). Accessed from http://www.pacep.org/ on June 29, 2006.

Spyridon, D.M. (2001). Intra-aortic balloon counterpulsation in the treatment of cardiogenic shock: hemodynamic effects and clinical challenges. Retrieved 2/27/2004 from http://www.medscape.com/viewprogram/607_pnt

Thibodeau, G.A. & Patton, K.T. (2003). *Anatomy and physiology* (5th ed.). St. Louis: Mosby.

Wiegand, D.J.L.-M. & Carlson, K.K. (Eds.). (2005). *AACN Procedure Manual for Critical Care* (5th ed.). St. Louis: Elsevier.

CHAPTER 5:
CARDIAC ARRHYTHMIAS

BASICS OF RHYTHM INTERPRETATION
The Cardiac Conduction System

Sinus Node (SA Node) – small group of cells in the high right atrium that functions as the normal pacemaker of the heart because it has the fastest rate of automaticity (60-100 times per minute).

Atrioventricular (AV) Node – small group of cells low in the right atrium near tricuspid valve. The AV node has three major functions:

- It slows conduction of the impulse from the atria to the ventricles to allow time for atrial contribution to ventricular filling (atrial kick).
- Junctional cells surrounding the AV node have automaticity at a rate of 40-60 beats per minute, so it can function as a backup pacemaker in case the sinus node fails.
- It screens out rapid atrial impulses to protect the ventricles from dangerously fast rates.

His Bundle – short bundle of fibers at the bottom of the AV node leading to the bundle branches.

Bundle Branches – bundles of fibers located along the septum that carry the impulse into the right and left ventricles. The right bundle branch travels along the right side of the septum and carries the impulse into the right ventricle. The left bundle branch has two main divisions, the anterior fascicle and the posterior fascicle, which carry the impulse into the large left ventricle.

Purkinje Fibers – hair-like fibers that spread out from the bundle branches along the endocardial surface of both ventricles and rapidly carry the impulse to ventricular muscle cells.

Figure 5.1 illustrates the cardiac conduction system.

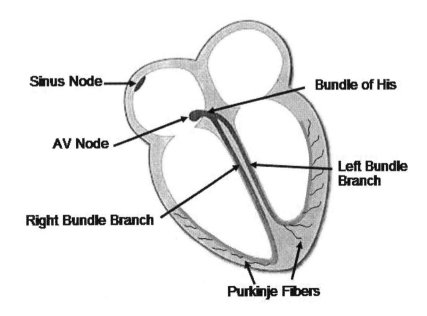

Figure 5.1: Cardiac conduction system.

Chapter 5

Origin and Spread of the Electrical Impulse in the Heart

The impulse originates in the SA node (because it has the fastest rate of automaticity) and spreads through both atria simultaneously. It is delayed for a fraction of a second in the AV node so the atria have time to contract and contribute to ventricular filling before the ventricles contract. As the impulse leaves the AV node, it picks up speed and conducts rapidly down both bundle branches into the ventricles and through the very rapid conducting Purkinje fibers to ventricular myocardium. The first part of the ventricles to depolarize is the septum in a left to right direction, then both ventricles depolarize simultaneously, from endocardium to epicardium. Since the left ventricle is the largest and is posterior to the right ventricle, the main direction of depolarization through the ventricles is downward, leftward, and posterior.

Origin of the ECG Waves and Intervals

P Wave – atrial depolarization as the impulse travels through the atria. Sinus node activity is not recorded because the SA node is too small. P waves may be upright, biphasic, or inverted.

PR Interval – AV conduction time, or the time it takes the impulse to travel through the atria, through the AV node, and down to where the ventricles begin to depolarize. Most of the length of the PR interval is delayed in the AV node.

- Measure from beginning of P wave to beginning of QRS.
  - Normal = .12-.20 sec.

QRS Complex – ventricular depolarization as the impulse travels through both ventricles. The QRS width represents intraventricular conduction time.

- Q wave = first negative deflection from baseline
- R wave = positive deflection from baseline
- S wave = negative deflection following an R wave
- Measure from beginning of Q or R wave to end of complex.
  - Normal = .06-.10 sec.

T Wave – ventricular repolarization as ventricles return to resting electrical state. May be upright, biphasic, or inverted.

ST Segment – early repolarization phase that extends from end of QRS to beginning of T wave. The ST segment should be at the isoelectric line (baseline). ST segment elevation or depression can represent myocardial injury or ischemia.

QT Interval – represents the sum of ventricular depolarization and repolarization and is measured from the beginning of the QRS to the end of the T wave. The QT interval varies with heart rate: at fast rates the QT shortens; at slow rates it lengthens. The QT interval should not exceed half the preceding R-R interval at normal heart rates. Bazett's formula for correcting QT interval is: measured QT (in seconds) divided by the square root of the R-R interval (measured in seconds).

Figure 5.2 shows the waves and intervals of the cardiac cycle.

Steps in Rhythm Interpretation
Regularity

- Regular = equal distance between R waves
- Irregular = varying distances between R waves.

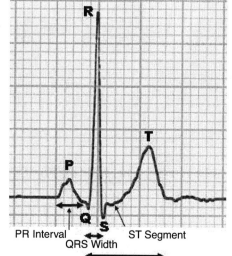

Figure 5.2: Waves and intervals of cardiac cycle.

Cardiac Arrhythmias

Rate (Atrial and Ventricular)

- Count number of R-R intervals (or P-P intervals for atrial rate) in a 6-second strip and multiply by 10 (best method for irregular rhythms).

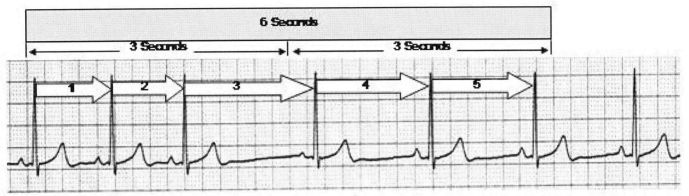

5 R-R intervals x 10 = rate of 50 beats per minute

- Count number of large boxes between R waves and divide into 300:

# boxes	Rate	# boxes	Rate
1	300	6	50
2	150	7	43
3	100	8	37
4	75	9	33
5	60	10	30

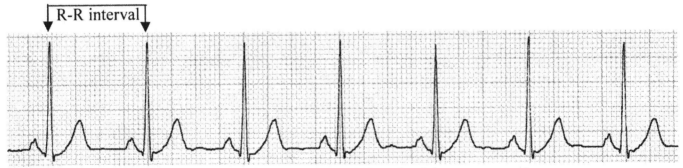

R to R = 4 big boxes = HR of 75 beats per minute

P Waves

- Presence, shape, similarity to each other, relationship to QRS complexes.

PR Interval

- Measure from beginning of P to beginning of QRS.
  - ❖ Normal = .12 -.20 sec.

QRS Width

- Measure from beginning to end of QRS.
  - ❖ Normal = .04 -.10 sec.

Chapter 5

Measurement of the ECG

ECG Paper

The horizontal axis measures time. ECG paper usually moves at a speed of 25 mm/sec. At that speed, these are standard intervals on ECG paper (see Figure 5.3):

- One tiny box = .04 sec. (40 msec).
- One large box (5 tiny boxes) = .20 sec. (200 msec).
- Vertical lines at top edge of paper are 3 seconds apart.
- There are 300 large boxes in a one-minute strip of paper.
- There are 1,500 tiny boxes in a one-minute strip of paper.

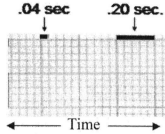

Figure 5.3: Standard intervals on ECG paper.

Practice Strips:

On the following strips, label P waves, QRS complexes, T waves. Measure the heart rate, PR interval, QRS width, and QT interval.

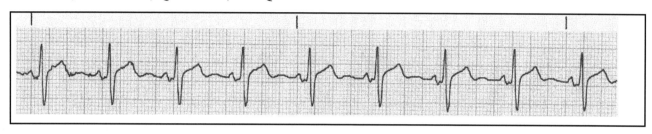

Rate _____ PRI _____ QRS _____ QT _____

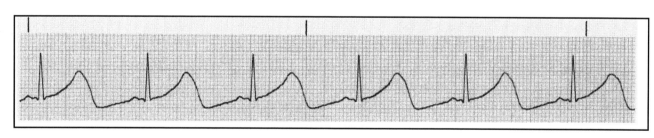

Rate _____ PRI _____ QRS _____ QT _____

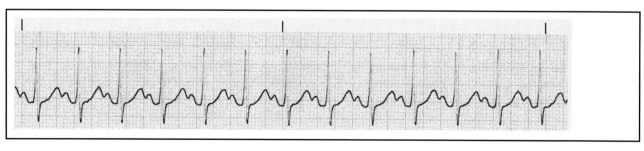

Rate _____ PRI _____ QRS _____ QT _____

Cardiac Arrhythmias

Answers:

1. HR = 80, PR = .12, QRS = .08, QT = .36.
2. HR = 50, PR = .12, QRS = .06, QT = .64.
3. HR = 120, PR = .16, QRS = .08, QT = .32.

If your answers varied a little that is OK. Were you "in the ballpark?"

RHYTHMS ORIGINATING IN THE SINUS NODE

The sinus node is the normal pacemaker of the heart because it has the fastest rate of automaticity of all potential pacemaker sites. The sinus node usually fires regularly at a rate between 60 and 100 beats/minute.

Normal Sinus Rhythm

Regularity: regular.

Rate: 60-100 beats/minute.

P waves: precede every QRS and are consistent in shape.

PR interval: .12-.20 sec.

QRS complex: .04-.10 sec.

Conduction: The impulse originates in the sinus node and conducts through both atria. Conduction is slowed through the AV node, then accelerates through the His Bundle, right and left bundle branches, and both ventricles simultaneously.

Two examples of normal sinus rhythm follow:

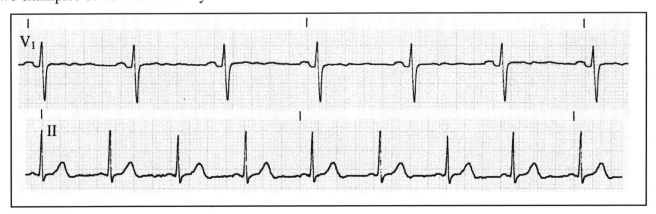

Sinus Tachycardia

Regularity: regular.

Rate: faster than 100 beats/minute; not usually > 150 beats/minute, unless associated with exercise. When rate is ≥ 150 beats/minute, consider other rhythms (i.e. atrial tachycardia). Rate increases and decreases gradually, not suddenly.

P waves: present before every QRS, consistent in shape, may be hidden in preceding T wave if rate is very rapid.

181

PR interval: normal. May be difficult to measure when P waves are buried in T waves.

QRS complex: usually normal.

Conduction: normal. Looks just like NSR but at faster rate.

Significance: Normal in children and a normal response to exercise and emotions in adults. If it persists at rest, it usually indicates some underlying problem like fever, blood loss, anxiety, heart failure, hypermetabolic states, or anemia. Drugs that can cause sinus tachycardia include atropine, isoproterenol, epinephrine, dopamine, dobutamine, norepinephrine, nitroprusside, caffeine. Tachycardia increases the heart's need for O_2, decreases ventricular filling time and decreases coronary artery perfusion time.

Treatment: Treat the cause! Drugs that slow the sinus rate include digitalis, beta blockers, calcium channel blockers, many antiarrhythmics, and sedatives.

Two examples of sinus tachycardia follow:

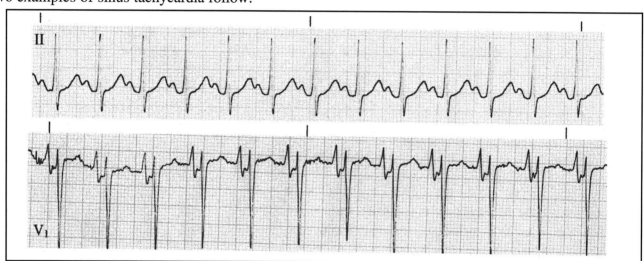

Sinus Bradycardia

Regularity: regular.

Rate: < 50 beats/minute.

P waves: precede every QRS, consistent in shape.

PR interval: usually normal.

QRS complex: usually normal.

Conduction: normal. Looks like NSR but at slower rate.

Significance: Is not normal in children and usually indicates a serious problem that needs treatment. Is a normal variant in adult athletes and during sleep. Can occur in response to vagal stimulation such as carotid sinus massage, ocular pressure, or vomiting. Common in inferior wall MI and can occur with increased intracranial pressure and glaucoma. Drugs such as digitalis, beta blockers, calcium channel blockers, and many antiarrhythmics can slow the sinus rate.

Treatment: In children, treat the cause. No treatment necessary in adults unless it results in symptoms (chest pain, dizziness, hypotension, SOB). Atropine 0.5 mg IV is the drug of choice for symptomatic bradycardia. Transcutaneous pacing can be used in an emergency until a transvenous pacemaker can be inserted. A dopamine drip at 2 to 10 mcg/kg/min or epinephrine drip at 2 to 10 mcg/min can be used to support BP until pacing can be instituted.

Below are two examples of sinus bradycardia:

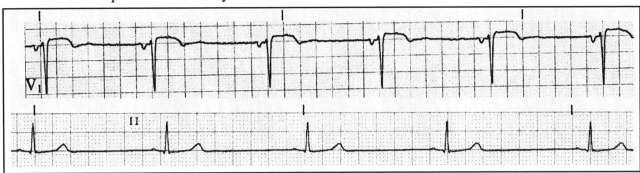

Sinus Arrhythmia

Regularity: irregular, phasic increase and decrease in rate, often varies with respirations.

Rate: usually within normal range but can be bradycardic.

P waves: precede every QRS, consistent in shape, occur irregularly.

PR interval: usually normal.

QRS complex: usually normal.

Conduction: normal.

Significance: not harmful. Common in children; decreases with age.

Treatment: none necessary.

Below are two examples of sinus arrhythmia:

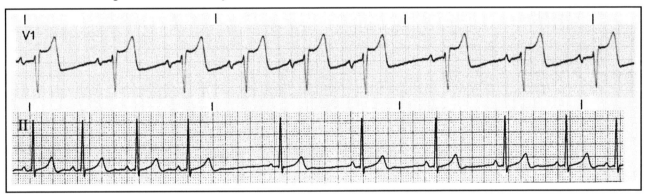

Sinus Arrest (failure of sinus node to fire)

Regularity: irregular due to absence of sinus node discharge.

Rate: atrial – within normal range but may be in bradycardia range if several sinus impulses fail to form. Ventricular – within normal range but may be in bradycardia range if several sinus impulses fail to form and there are no junctional or ventricular escape beats. Ventricular rate may be faster than atrial rate if junctional or ventricular escape beats occur during periods of sinus arrest.

P waves: present when sinus node fires and absent during periods of sinus arrest. When present, they precede every QRS complex and are consistent in shape. Because the sinus node fails to form impulses occasionally, the P-P interval is not an exact multiple of the sinus cycle. If junctional escape beats occur, P waves may be inverted either before or after the junctional QRS.

QRS complex: usually normal when sinus node is functioning and absent during periods of sinus arrest, unless escape beats occur. If ventricular escape beats occur, QRS is wide.

Chapter 5

Conduction: normal through atria, AV node, bundle branches and ventricles when sinus node fires. When sinus node fails to form impulses, there is no conduction through atria. If junctional escape beats occur, ventricular conduction is usually normal; if ventricular escape beats occur, ventricular conduction is abnormally slow.

Significance: sinus arrest occurs when sinus node automaticity is depressed and impulses are not formed when expected. If only one impulse fails to form, the term *sinus pause* is used; if more than one impulse in a row fails to form, the term *sinus arrest* is used. Sinus node depression can occur with vagal stimulation, hypersensitive carotid sinus syndrome, myocardial infarction interrupting blood supply to the sinus node, and with drugs such as digitalis, beta blockers, and calcium channel blockers. If prolonged or frequent periods of arrest occur, the patient may become symptomatic due to bradycardia and decreased cardiac output.

Treatment: treat the cause, if known. Atropine 0.5-1 mg IV may increase sinus rate. Pacemaker therapy may be necessary if other forms of therapy fail.

Two examples of sinus arrest follow:

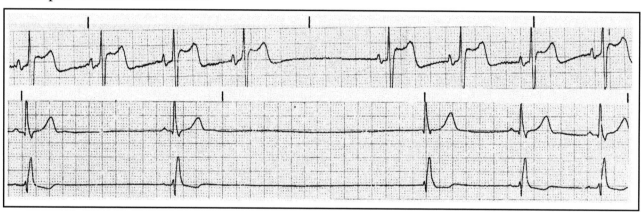

Linking Knowledge to Practice

✔ *It is important to document bradycardia and periods of sinus arrest in the medical record with a rhythm strip that shows how slow the rate gets or how long the pauses are. This can be used to help justify the need for a pacemaker and may facilitate payment from insurance companies by documenting the reason for pacemaker implantation.*

✔ *It is also important to document signs and symptoms that occur with any significant change in heart rate or rhythm. Correlation of symptoms to heart rate and rhythm changes can aid in diagnosing the cause of syncope, palpitations, chest pain, or other symptoms that patients experience with arrhythmias and may facilitate appropriate treatment with drugs or devices (i.e. pacemaker or implantable defibrillator).*

RHYTHMS ORIGINATING IN THE ATRIA

Ectopic foci or reentry circuits can occur in the atrial myocardium, resulting in atrial arrhythmias that take control away from the sinus node.

Premature Atrial Complexes (PACs)

Origin: irritable focus in the atria fires before the next sinus impulse is due.

Regularity: irregular due to early beats. PACs usually have a noncompensatory pause (interval between the beat preceding the PAC, and the beat following the PAC is less that two normal R-R intervals). Premature depolarization of the atria by the PAC also prematurely depolarizes the sinus node and causes it to "reset" itself.

Rate: usually in normal range.

P waves: precede every QRS. P wave of the PAC has a different shape than sinus P waves because the atria depolarize in a different direction. Very early P waves may be buried in the preceding T wave.

PR interval: may be normal or long depending on prematurity of PAC. Very early PACs may find the AV node still partly refractory and unable to conduct normally, resulting in a long PR interval. Very early P waves may not conduct at all (nonconducted PAC).

QRS complex: may be normal, aberrant (wide), or absent, depending on prematurity of PAC. If the ventricles have repolarized completely, they can conduct the PAC normally. If the PAC occurs during the relative refractory period of the bundle branches or ventricles, the impulse conducts aberrantly and the QRS is wide. If the PAC occurs very early during the complete refractory period of the AV node or the bundle branches, the impulse does not conduct to the ventricles, and the QRS is absent.

Conduction: PACs travel through the atria differently from sinus impulses because they originate in a different spot. Conduction through the AV node, bundle branches, and ventricles is usually normal unless the PAC is very early (see above discussion).

Significance: PACs commonly occur in patients who have pulmonary disease, HF, MI, anxiety, hypermetabolic states. Caffeine, nicotine, and alcohol can cause PACs. PACs are not dangerous by themselves but may indicate atrial irritability that can lead to more significant atrial arrhythmias.

Treatment: not necessary unless atrial irritability needs to be suppressed to prevent more serious arrhythmias. Antiarrhythmics including disopyramide, procainamide, flecainide, propafenone can be used to suppress PACs.

PACS (☆) **A:** PACs conduct normally. **B:** nonconducted PAC. **C:** 1st and 5th PACs conduct normally, 2nd and 4th are nonconducted, 3rd conducts with right bundle branch block (RBBB) aberration.

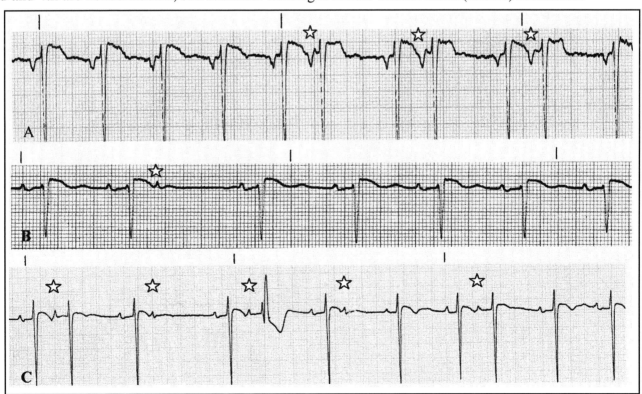

Wandering Atrial Pacemaker (WAP)

Origin: the site of impulse formation shifts within the atria and between the sinus and AV nodes.

Regularity: may be slightly irregular.

Rate: 60-100 beats/minute.

P waves: vary in shape depending on site of impulse origin. May be upright, inverted, biphasic. Must see three different P wave shapes to diagnose WAP.

PR interval: may vary depending on proximity of pacemaker to AV node.

QRS complex: usually normal.

Conduction: variable conduction through atria because impulses originate at different sites. Normal conduction through AV node and ventricles.

Significance: not dangerous.

Treatment: none needed unless rate is slow enough to be symptomatic, then Atropine.

Two examples of WAP follow. Note different shapes of P waves in each strip.

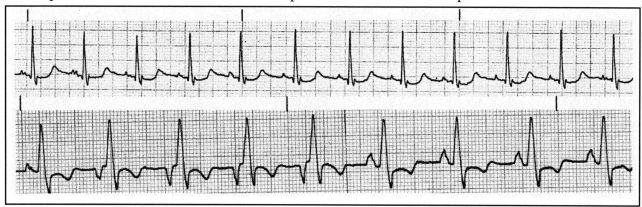

Multifocal Atrial Tachycardia (MAT)

This rhythm is the same as WAP, only the atrial rate is faster than 120 beats/minute. Intra-atrial conduction varies as impulses originate from different spots. Ventricular conduction may be normal or aberrant (wide) if rate is fast. MAT commonly occurs in pulmonary disease and may be due to hypokalemia, hypomagnesemia, and theophylline toxicity. Treating the underlying pulmonary disease and associated hypoxemia, HF, and electrolyte imbalances may convert the rhythm. Calcium channel blockers, beta blockers, or amiodarone may be useful treatments.

Two examples of MAT follow. Note varying shapes of P waves in each strip.

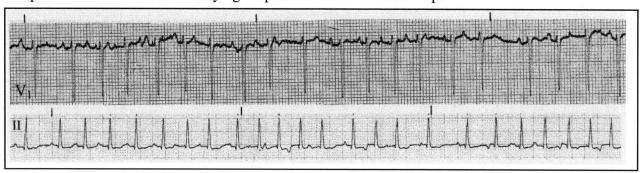

Atrial Tachycardia and Paroxysmal Atrial Tachycardia (PAT)

Origin: rapid firing of ectopic atrial focus or re-entry circuit within atria at rate of 150-250 beats/minute. If the rhythm starts and stops suddenly, it is called *paroxysmal* atrial tachycardia; if it lasts for long periods of time, it is called *sustained* atrial tachycardia.

Regularity: usually regular unless varying AV block is present.

Rate: atrial – 150-250 beats/minute. Ventricular rate varies depending on amount of block at the AV node and may be the same as the atrial rate or slower.

P waves: differ from sinus P waves. Precede each QRS complex, but may be hidden in preceding T wave. When AV block is present, there is more than one P wave before the QRS complex.

PR interval: may be normal, long or short, depending on site of impulse origin in atria.

QRS complex: usually normal but may be wide if aberrant conduction is present.

Conduction: abnormal in atria due to ectopic origin of rhythm. Usually normal through AV node, bundle branches, and ventricles unless impulses enter the AV conduction system during part of its refractory period. In atrial tachycardia with block, some P waves do not conduct to the ventricles.

Significance: rapid ventricular rate may decrease cardiac output and lead to hemodynamic instability, or precipitate HF or angina. Can be caused by digitalis toxicity, MI, HF, hypoxemia, electrolyte imbalances.

Treatment: eliminate underlying cause if possible. Beta blockers, calcium channel blockers, amiodarone, or flecainide may be effective. Catheter ablation of the atrial tachycardia focus is successful in some patients.

Following are two examples of atrial tachycardia. Note sudden onset and termination in top strip, and rate of 214 in second strip (too fast for sinus tachycardia).

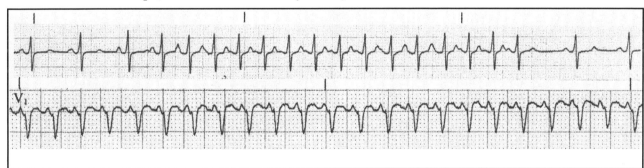

Atrial Flutter

Origin: due to a re-entry circuit in the right atrium around which an impulse "chases" itself at a rapid rate.

Regularity: atrial rhythm is regular; ventricular rhythm can be regular or irregular due to varying AV block.

Rate: atrial — usually 250-350 beats per/minute, most commonly a rate of 300. Ventricular rate varies, depending on amount of block at AV node, commonly 150 beats/minute and very rarely 300 beats/minute. Ventricular rate can be within the normal range when atrial flutter is treated with appropriated drugs.

P waves: F waves (flutter waves) occur and have a "saw-tooth" appearance. One F wave is often hidden in the QRS or T wave, and when 2:1 conduction is present, every other F wave may be hidden.

PR interval (FR interval): may be consistent or may vary. Many F waves are not followed by QRS complexes due to AV block.

QRS complex: usually normal but can be aberrantly conducted when rhythm is very fast or irregular.

Chapter 5

Conduction: because of the extremely rapid atrial rate, the AV node blocks at least every other F wave, and often blocks 2, 3, or more F waves in a row in order to protect the ventricles from the rapid rate.

Significance: rapid ventricular rates and loss of atrial contraction can cause decreased cardiac output and lead to hemodynamic instability. Mural thrombi can form in the atria when they do not contract well and can lead to systemic or pulmonary embolism. Causes include MI, rheumatic heart disease, thyrotoxicosis, HF, ischemia.

Treatment: slow ventricular rate with calcium channel blockers (diltiazem, verapamil), or beta blockers. Flutter can be converted to sinus rhythm by drugs such as amiodarone, flecainide, ibutilide, dofetilide, and procainamide. If ventricular rate is very rapid or if flutter is resistant to drug therapy, electrical cardioversion can be done.

Below are three examples of atrial flutter. There is 4:1 conduction in the first two strips (one flutter wave is hidden in the QRS), and 2:1 conduction in the third strip.

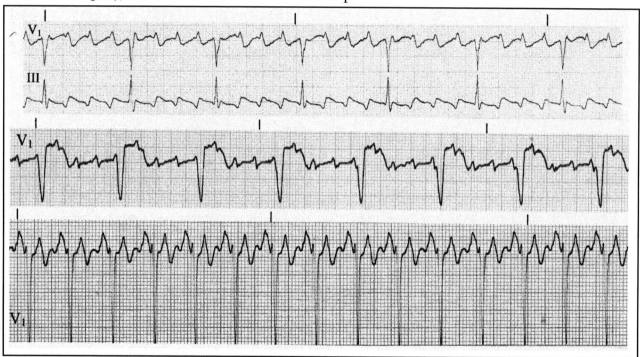

Atrial Fibrillation

Origin: chaotic ectopic or reentrant activity in the atria causing them to quiver rather than contract.

Regularity: irregular. One of the distinguishing features of atrial fib is the marked irregularity of the ventricular response.

Rate: atrial rate is so fast it cannot be counted (400-600). Ventricular rate varies depending on the amount of block at the AV node. New onset atrial fib can be present with ventricular rates from 160-200 beats/minute. Ventricular rate can be maintained within the normal range by appropriate drug therapy.

P waves: not present. Atrial activity is chaotic with no formed atrial impulses visible. Irregular F waves are usually seen and vary from coarse to fine in appearance.

PR interval: none

QRS complex: usually normal, but aberration is common, especially at faster rates.

Conduction: intra-atrial conduction is disorganized and irregular. Most atrial impulses are blocked in the AV node; those that do conduct to ventricles conduct very irregularly, but usually normally through the ventricles. If atrial impulses reach the bundle branch system during part of the refractory period, aberration occurs.

Significance: ventricular rates can be very fast, leading to decreased cardiac output and hemodynamic instability. Mural thrombi are common and can lead to embolization. Loss of atrial contraction contributes to decreased cardiac output. Causes include coronary artery disease, MI, ischemia, valve disease, HF, pulmonary disease, and open heart surgery.

Treatment: slow ventricular rate with calcium channel blockers (diltiazem, verapamil), or beta blockers. Atrial fib can be converted to sinus rhythm by drugs such as amiodarone, flecainide, ibutilide, dofetilide, and procainamide. If ventricular rate is very rapid or if fibrillation is resistant to drug therapy, electrical cardioversion can be done.

Following are two examples of atrial fibrillation:

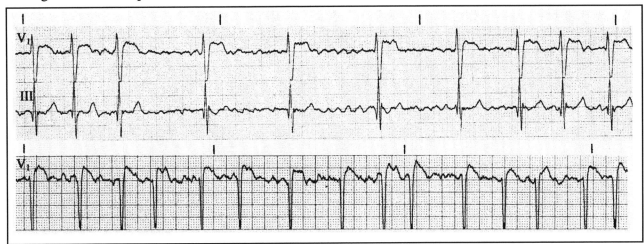

SUPRAVENTRICULAR TACHYCARDIA (SVT)

The term SVT is used to describe a regular, narrow QRS tachycardia in which the exact mechanism cannot be determined from the surface ECG. If P waves can be clearly seen, the mechanism can usually be identified. SVTs can be classified into those that are AV nodal passive and those that are AV nodal active.

AV Nodal Passive SVTs – do not require participation of the AV node for maintenance of the tachycardia.
- Atrial tachycardia
- Atrial flutter
- Atrial fibrillation.

Figure 5.4 illustrates the mechanisms of AV nodal passive SVTs. In atrial tachycardia, a focus in the atrium fires at a rapid rate, and the AV node simply conducts the impulses into the ventricles but does not play an active role in maintaining the atrial tachycardia. In atrial flutter, an impulse circulates around a re-entry circuit in the right atrium. The AV node is not a part of the circuit that maintains the tachycardia, it just conducts the atrial impulses to the ventricles. In atrial fibrillation, multiple foci or re-entry circuits create electrical chaos in the atria, and the AV node conducts some of those impulses into the ventricles, but does not play an active role in maintaining atrial fibrillation.

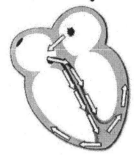 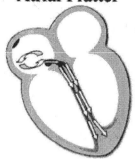 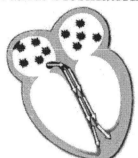

Figure 5.4: AV nodal passive SVTs.

AV Nodal Active SVTs – require participation of the AV node in maintenance of the tachycardia:
◆ AVNRT (AV nodal re-entry tachycardia) – 60% of regular, narrow QRS tachycardias.
◆ CMT (circus movement tachycardia involving an accessory pathway) – 30% of regular, narrow QRS tachycardias. This rhythm is also called AVRT (AV re-entrant tachycardia), but the term CMT is used here.

Figure 5.5 illustrates AV nodal active tachycardias. In AVNRT, an impulse travels around a re-entry circuit that involves two pathways in the AV node. In CMT, the impulse travels around a circuit that involves the atria, the AV node, the ventricles, and the accessory pathway. In both rhythms, the AV node is an active part of the re-entry circuit that maintains the tachycardia, and without the participation of the AV node the arrhythmia cannot continue.

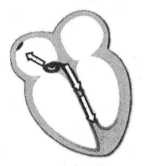 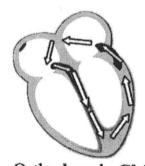 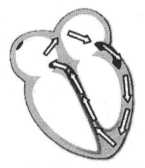

Figure 5.5: AV nodal active SVTs.

Origin: above the ventricles (atria, AV junction). The two most common mechanisms of a regular, narrow QRS tachycardia are AV nodal re-entry (AVNRT) and circus movement tachycardia (CMT), using an accessory pathway in patients with Wolff-Parkinson-White Syndrome.

Regularity: regular.

Rate: 140-300 beats/minute.

P waves: usually not visible. In AVNRT, the P wave is hidden in the QRS or barely peeking out at the end of the QRS. In CMT, the P wave is usually present in the ST segment, but is often not visible.

PR interval: not measurable, since P waves are usually not visible.

QRS complex: usually normal.

Conduction: In AVNRT, the impulse spins around in the AV node and depolarizes the atria in a retrograde direction and the ventricles through the normal conduction system, resulting in a regular narrow QRS tachycardia. In CMT, the impulse follows a re-entry circuit that includes the atria, AV node, ventricles, and accessory pathway. The most common type of CMT is called orthodromic CMT, in which the impulse travels from atria to ventricles through the normal AV node and His-Purkinje system, then back to the atria from the ventricles through the accessory pathway. This results in a regular, narrow QRS tachycardia because the ventricles are depolarized via the normal conduction system. If the circuit reverses direction and the ventricles depolarize via conduction down the accessory pathway, this is called antidromic CMT, and the resulting tachycardia has a wide QRS complex. Figure 5.5 above illustrates these conduction concepts.

Significance: usually well tolerated and often paroxysmal in nature. Can sometimes be easily terminated by a vagal maneuver (breath holding, valsalva, coughing). If rate is very rapid and sustained, cardiac output may be decreased and symptoms can occur.

Treatment: vagal maneuvers or adenosine (6mg, then 12mg rapidly IV) may terminate rhythm. Drugs that slow AV conduction, like calcium channel blockers (diltiazem, verapamil), beta blockers, or digitalis, may either slow rate or convert rhythm to sinus. Radiofrequency ablation offers a cure for AVNRT and CMT.

Below are two examples of SVT. Both are regular, narrow QRS tachycardias at a rate of about 190, with no visible P waves.

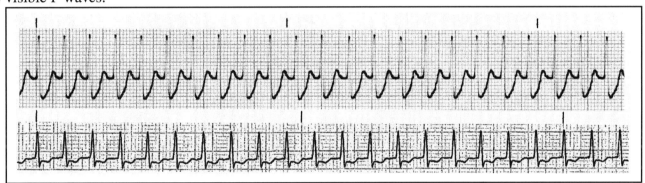

Linking Knowledge to Practice

✔ *Whenever possible, document in the medical record the onset and termination of episodes of SVT, as this can aid in diagnosis of the mechanism of the arrhythmia.*

✔ *Although most SVTs are well tolerated, patients who complain of palpitations or "racing heart" should be referred to a cardiologist or electrophysiologist for evaluation of the cause of these symptoms. Many SVTs can be permanently cured with radiofrequency ablation, but often people who experience symptoms associated with SVT do not receive appropriate follow-up from health care providers who are unfamiliar with these arrhythmias and their treatment.*

Chapter 5

RHYTHMS ORIGINATING IN THE AV JUNCTION

Cells around the AV node have automaticity and are capable of becoming pacemakers when the sinus node fails. Junctional escape beats occur when the sinus node rate falls below the rate of the junctional pacemaker. Junctional rhythm can accelerate above the rate of the sinus node and assume control of the heart's rhythm.

Junctional beats can appear three ways on the ECG (Figure 5.6). If the junctional impulse reaches the atria before it reaches the ventricles, an inverted P wave (indicating retrograde atrial depolarization) precedes the QRS complex, and the PR interval is short (< .12 sec). If the junctional impulse reaches the atria and the ventricles at the same time, the P wave occurs simultaneously with the QRS and only the QRS is seen because it is the largest complex. If the junctional impulse reaches the ventricles before it reaches the atria, the QRS occurs first, followed by a retrograde P wave with a short R-P interval (distance from the beginning of the QRS to the P wave).

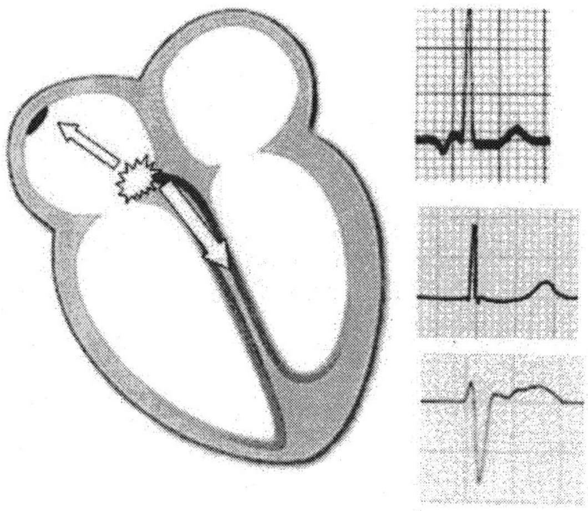

Figure 5.6: Rhythms in AV junction.

Junctional Rhythm, Accelerated Junctional Rhythm, Junctional Tachycardia

Origin: cells in the AV junction surrounding the AV node.

Regularity: regular.

Rate: 40-60 for junctional rhythm, 60-100 for accelerated junctional rhythm, faster than 100 for junctional tachycardia.

P waves: can precede, follow, or be buried in QRS.

PR interval: short, < .12 sec when P waves precede QRS.

QRS complex: usually normal.

Conduction: retrograde through the atria, normal through the ventricles.

Significance: not dangerous when rate is normal. If rate is too fast or too slow, may lead to decreased cardiac output and symptoms. Digitalis toxicity can cause junctional rhythm. This rhythm is common in children.

Treatment: usually not necessary. If rate is slow, atropine 0.5 mg IV may increase sinus rate and overdrive junctional rhythm, or may increase rate of junctional focus. If rate is fast, drugs such as calcium channel blockers, beta blockers, or amiodarone may slow rate or terminate junctional rhythm.

Following are three examples of junctional rhythm. Top strip is junctional tachycardia with an inverted P wave preceding the QRS; second strip shows no P wave; third strip shows retrograde P wave following the QRS.

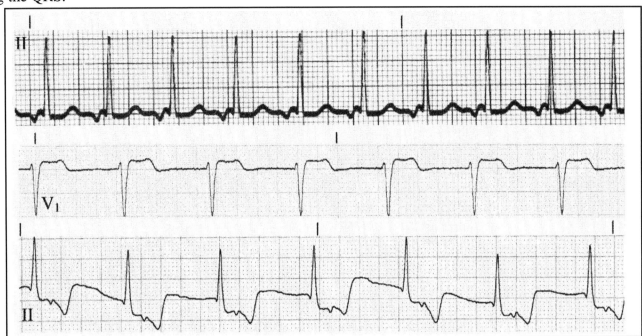

RHYTHMS ORIGINATING IN THE VENTRICLES

Ventricular rhythms originate in ventricular myocardium or in the Purkinje system in the ventricles, and are considered to be more dangerous than supraventricular rhythms because of their greater potential to limit cardiac output. Early ventricular beats are called PVCs; late ventricular beats are *ventricular escape beats*.

Premature Ventricular Complexes (PVCs) and Ventricular Escape Beats

Origin: focus in ventricular myocardium.

Regularity: irregular due to early beats or due to pause, allowing escape beat.

Rate: may occur at any heart rate and with any basic rhythm.

P waves: not related to PVCs. Sinus rhythm often not interrupted by PVCs, so P waves can be seen occurring regularly throughout the rhythm, but are unrelated to PVCs. Retrograde conduction from PVC back through AV node and into atria frequently occurs, and P waves may be seen following the PVC.

PR interval: not present before most PVCs. If end-diastolic PVCs occur, sinus P wave may happen by coincidence to precede PVC, but PR will be shorter than baseline PR interval.

QRS complex: wide, bizarre, usually .12 sec or wider. May vary in shape if they originate from more than one focus in the ventricles (multifocal PVCs).

Conduction: PVCs conduct muscle cell to muscle cell in the ventricles, which is much slower than Purkinje system conduction, resulting in the wide QRS. Many PVCs conduct retrograde to atria, causing an inverted P wave that follows the wide QRS.

Significance: depends on clinical setting in which PVCs occur. PVCs are not dangerous in normal hearts, but may indicate ventricular irritability that can lead to more serious ventricular arrhythmias when the heart is electrically unstable due to ischemia or other reasons. Causes include ischemia, infarction, electrolyte imbalances, hypoxia, drugs, acidosis, increased catecholamine levels, ventricular hypertrophy, cardiomyopathy, and digitalis toxicity. PVCs are considered more dangerous when they follow MI or occur in cardiomyopathy and when they are frequent (> 10/hour) or repetitive (pairs of two, or runs of three or more in a row). *Ventricular escape beats* are a protection against asystole and are a blessing!

Treatment: PVCs are not usually treated unless they occur in the presence of acute ischemia or infarction and are frequent or occur in runs. Many physicians do not treat PVCs at all, while others choose to treat them for up to 24 hours following acute MI or following open heart surgery. If PVCs are frequent or occur in runs, they can be treated with amiodarone or lidocaine. *Ventricular escape beats* are not treated—the reason for escape beats is treated. If a slow, underlying rhythm or AV block is the reason for escape beats, atropine may increase the rate and eliminate the need for escape beats.

Examples of PVCs follow. Top strip is sinus bradycardia with a PVC; second strip is NSR with unifocal PVCs; third strip is NSR with multifocal PVCs; bottom strip is atrial fibrillation with a ventricular escape beat.

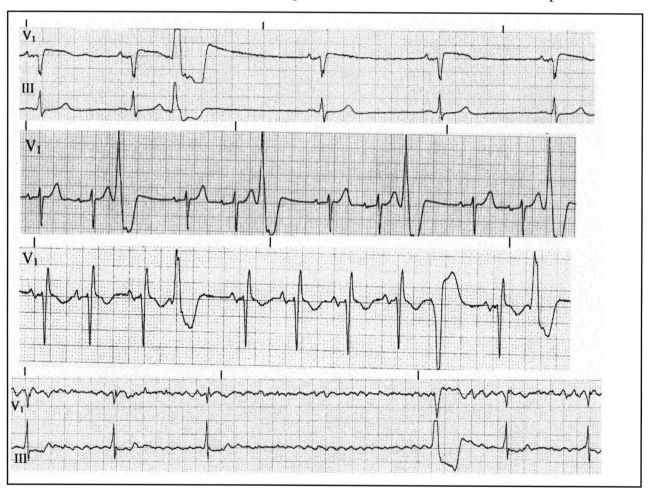

Idioventricular Rhythm and Accelerated Ventricular Rhythm

Cells in the ventricle have automaticity at a rate of 20-40 beats/minute and, therefore, can function as an escape pacemaker if all other pacemaker sites fail. When the rate of the ventricular pacemaker is 20-40, the term *idioventricular rhythm* is used; when the rate is > 40 but < 100, the term *accelerated ventricular rhythm* is used.

Origin: ventricular focus.

Regularity: usually regular.

Rate: 20-40 beats/minute for idioventricular rhythm; 40-100 beats/minute for accelerated ventricular rhythm.

P waves: may be present if sinus node is working, but not related to QRS complexes.

PR interval: not measured, since P waves are unrelated to QRS.

QRS complex: wide and bizarre, > .12 sec.

Conduction: muscle cell-to-cell within ventricles.

Significance: an idioventricular rhythm is slow and usually results in symptoms related to decreased cardiac output (hypotension, cool, clammy skin, dizziness, syncope, chest pain, SOB). If the ventricular rate is within a normal range, the patient may be asymptomatic. Loss of atrial kick can contribute to decreased cardiac output. Idioventricular rhythm is often the last stage before asystole in a very sick heart and may not respond to treatment. Accelerated ventricular rhythm occurs with inferior MI, and is the most common reperfusion arrhythmia in patients receiving fibrinolytic therapy for acute MI.

Treatment: idioventricular rhythm usually requires ventricular pacing. Drug therapy with epinephrine, dopamine, or isoproterenol can be used in an attempt to increase the ventricular rate and support blood pressure until a pacemaker can be inserted or external pacing can be instituted. Accelerated ventricular rhythm is often temporary and harmless and does not require treatment unless it results in symptoms. Atropine can be used to speed up an underlying sinus bradycardia and overdrive the ventricular pacemaker. Suppressive therapy with lidocaine or other drugs is not recommended. (See example below.)

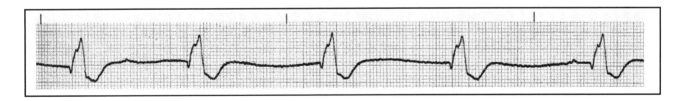

Idioventricular rhythm at rate of about 40.

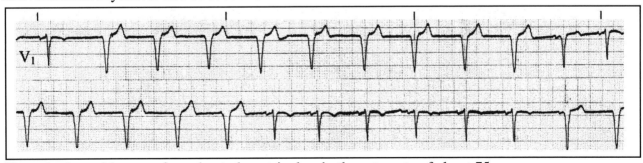

Sinus rhythm with runs of accelerated ventricular rhythm at a rate of about 75.

Chapter 5

Ventricular Tachycardia (VT)

VT is a ventricular rhythm at a rate faster than 100 beats/minute. VT can be either *monomorphic*, meaning all QRS complexes look alike, or *polymorphic*, in which QRS complexes change shape and do not look alike. A special type of polymorphic VT, called *torsades de pointes* ("twisting of the points") occurs in the presence of a long Q-T interval, indicating abnormally prolonged repolarization.

Origin: ectopic focus or re-entry circuit in ventricle.

Regularity: usually regular.

Rate: faster than 100 beats/minute. A rate faster than 200 is often called *ventricular flutter.*

P waves: not related to QRS complexes. May be seen occurring independently of QRS (AV dissociation). If one-to-one retrograde V-A conduction is present, P waves may be seen following each QRS.

PR interval: not measurable, since P waves are unrelated to QRS.

QRS complex: wide, bizarre, > .12 sec.

Conduction: slow through ventricle due to muscle cell-to-cell conduction. There may be retrograde conduction through the atria, but more often the sinus node continues to fire regularly and conduction through the atria is normal. If a sinus beat happens to be able to conduct through the AV node and depolarize the ventricle normally before the next ventricular beat is due, the resulting normal QRS complex is called a *capture beat.* If the sinus impulse conducts through the AV node and meets with the ventricular focus, the resulting complex looks different from both the sinus and the ventricular QRS, and is called a *fusion beat.*

Significance: depends on the rate of the VT and underlying ventricular function. If VT occurs at a relatively slow rate in a heart with good function, it can be well tolerated for long periods of time. If the rate is very fast, cardiac output is decreased and hemodynamic instability can occur. Patients with poor LV function do not tolerate <u>any</u> tachycardia well, including VT. Sometimes VT is so poorly tolerated that unconsciousness results, and the rhythm results in death if not treated immediately. Causes of VT are the same as causes of PVCs.

Treatment: if VT is stable, drug therapy is used first. Amiodarone 150 mg IV over 10 minutes, followed by an infusion at 1 mg/min for 6 hours, then 0.5 mg/min for 18 hours is often the drug of choice. Lidocaine, 1-1.5 mg/kg IV initial bolus, followed in 10 minutes by half that amount, followed by a continuous infusion at 2-4 mg/min can also be used, as can procainamide, up to 17 mg/Kg loading dose, followed by a drip at 2 mg/min. Drugs used to treat VT on a long-term basis include amiodarone, sotalol, and beta blockers. In any VT that is poorly tolerated, cardioversion is done emergently and drug treatment is used later. If VT is pulseless, immediate defibrillation is the treatment (see treatment of ventricular fibrillation).

Cardiac Arrhythmias

Monomorphic VT

Following are three examples of monomorphic VT. Top strip is NSR with onset of VT at a rate of 150; second strip illustrates VT with AV dissociation (P waves are seen but are unrelated to QRS complexes); bottom strip shows two leads of NSR with a 9-beat run of VT.

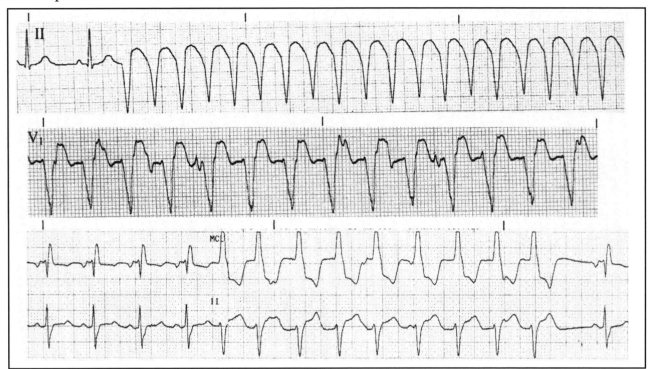

Polymorphic VT

The term "polymorphic" refers to VT in which the QRS complexes have different shapes because multiple foci are involved or re-entry occurs over different pathways within the ventricle. This type of VT is often very rapid and results in hemodynamic instability if it is sustained. Polymorphic VT can occur with acute ischemia or infarction and can be due to drugs. If the QT interval is normal, polymorphic VT can be treated with beta blockers, lidocaine, amiodarone, procainamide or sotalol.

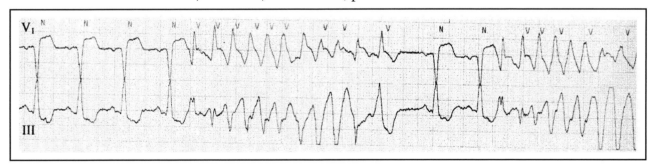

Torsades de pointes

Torsades de pointes (TdP) is a polymorphic VT that occurs in the presence of a long QT interval, which indicates a ventricular repolarization abnormality. QT prolongation can occur in certain congenital abnormalities and secondary to drugs that prolong repolarization, such as quinidine, procainamide, disopyramide, sotalol, amiodarone, ibutilide, tricyclic antidepressants, certain antibiotics, and many others. Electrolyte imbalances, especially low K+ and Mg++, subarachnoid hemorrhage, and right radical neck

Chapter 5

dissection can also prolong the QT interval and lead to TdP. TdP can occur in short bursts that are self terminating or can become sustained and lead to VF.

Two examples of torsades de pointes follow. Note the long QT interval in both strips.

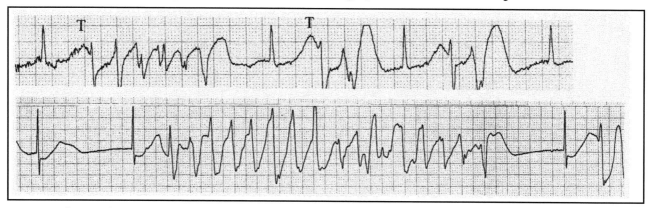

Treatment of torsades

- ◆ Defibrillate if sustained and loss of consciousness occurs.
- ◆ Correct abnormal electrolytes and discontinue any causative drugs.
- ◆ Start IV magnesium 1-2 Gm IV followed by a drip until the cause is corrected.
- ◆ Overdrive pacing at rates of 100-110 to shorten the QT interval until cause is corrected.

Linking Knowledge to Practice

✔ *It is important to differentiate polymorphic VT from torsades de pointes because the treatment is different for the two rhythms. Many practitioners look at the "twisting" nature of the QRS complexes and assume the rhythm is torsades, but the QRS complex can appear to twist in both types of polymorphic VT. The QT interval must be evaluated in order to differentiate regular polymorphic VT (normal QT interval) from torsades de pointes (long QT interval). Remember: All torsades is polymorphic VT, but not all polymorphic VT is torsades!*

Ventricular Fibrillation (VF)

VF is chaotic electrical activity in the ventricles that results in quivering of the ventricles and total loss of cardiac output. VF is always fatal unless treated immediately.

Origin: rapid, disorganized electrical activity within the ventricles.

Regularity: chaotic, irregular.

Rate: unable to measure due to rapid, uncoordinated activity.

P waves: none.

PR interval: none.

QRS complex: none. No formed complexes are seen, just rapid, irregular, uncoordinated electrical activity. VF can be coarse or very fine, looking almost like asystole.

Conduction: multiple ectopic foci conducting chaotically through ventricles.

Significance: VF is always fatal due to loss of ventricular contraction and must be treated immediately. Causes include ischemia, infarction, severe electrolyte imbalances, acidosis, hypoxia, end-stage cardiac disease.

Treatment: CPR until defibrillator is available, then immediate defibrillation at 360 joules with monophasic defibrillator or manufacturer's recommended energy level for biphasic defibrillators (usually

120-150 j). Resume CPR for 2 minutes (about 5 cycles) after each shock before checking for a pulse unless the patient is on a monitor and a rhythm is visible. If VF continues, initiate drug therapy during CPR with epinephrine 1 mg IV every 3-5 minutes during resuscitation, or vasopressin 40 units IV can be used in place of the first or second dose of epinephrine. Attempt defibrillation again after 2 minutes of CPR. Antiarrhythmic drugs can be used to treat VF and pulseless VT, but ACLS guidelines stress the importance of choosing one agent rather than using multiple drugs, as was previously recommended. Antiarrhythmic agents used to treat VF or pulseless VT include:

1) Amiodarone 300 mg IV bolus; may repeat 150 mg IV bolus in 3-5 minutes if VF continues. Maximum cumulative dose is 2.2 Gm in 24 hours.
2) Lidocaine 1-1.5 mg/kg IV, repeat in 8-10 minutes if VF continues.

Once conversion has occurred, a continuous infusion of whatever agent facilitated conversion of the rhythm is initiated.

Following are two examples of VF:

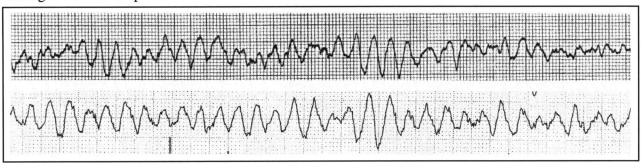

AV BLOCKS

The term AV block is used when there is delayed or failed conduction of impulses from the atria to the ventricles. AV blocks are classified according to the location of the block and the severity of the conduction abnormality. The following classification is used here:

- First Degree AV Block
- Second Degree AV Block
  - Type I
  - Type II
- High-grade (Advanced) AV Block
- Third Degree AV Block.

First Degree AV Block

Regularity: usually regular.

Rate: can occur at any sinus or atrial rate, usually atrial rate within normal range.

P waves: normal, precede every QRS.

PR interval: longer than .20 sec. PR intervals up to 0.80 sec. have been reported.

QRS complex: usually normal unless bundle branch block is present.

Conduction: normal through the atria, delayed in the AV node longer than normal, normal through the ventricles unless bundle branch block is present.

Significance: not dangerous because every impulse gets through to the ventricles, and ventricular rate is usually normal. May progress to higher degrees of block. Occurs commonly with inferior MI, coronary disease, rheumatic heart disease, and drugs that slow AV conduction, like beta blockers, calcium channel blockers, and digitalis.

Treatment: discontinue causative drugs. No specific treatment necessary. Watch for progression to higher degrees of block.

Following are two examples of first degree AV block. In the top strip, the PR interval is 0.28 sec; in the second strip the PR interval is 0.52 sec.

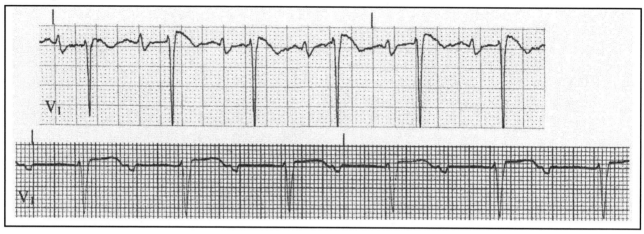

Second Degree AV Block

In second degree block, one atrial impulse at a time fails to conduct to the ventricles. If the block occurs in the AV node, it is Type I; if block occurs below the AV node, it is Type II. Figure 5.7 illustrates the site of Type I and Type II AV block.

Second Degree AV Block - Type I (Wenckebach)

There is a progressive slowing of conduction from the atria to the ventricles until one impulse fails to conduct. Wenckebach appears on the ECG as progressively longer PR intervals on consecutively conducted atrial impulses until one P wave fails to conduct and is not followed by a QRS. The block occurs in the AV node, so unless there is coincidental bundle branch block, the QRS is narrow.

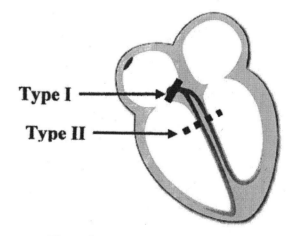

Figure 5.7: Second degree AV block.

Regularity: irregular due to blocked P waves. Appears as "group beating." Is regular when 2:1 conduction occurs.

Rate: can occur at any sinus or atrial rate. Ventricular rate depends on atrial rate and conduction ratio.

P waves: normal, regular. Some P waves do not conduct to ventricles (they are blocked in the AV node).

PR interval: gradually lengthens on consecutively conducted beats. The PR interval preceding the pause produced by the blocked P wave is longer than the PR following the pause. If a 2:1 conduction ratio is present, all PR intervals are the same.

QRS complex: usually normal unless there is associated bundle branch block.

Conduction: Normal through atria, progressively delayed throughout the AV node until one impulse fails to conduct. Ventricular conduction is normal. Conduction ratio is expressed as the number of P waves to QRS complexes; there is always one more P wave than QRS in a Wenckebach cycle. Conduction ratios can vary, with ratios as low as 2:1 (every other P wave blocked) to high ratios like 15:14 (15 P waves to 14 QRS complexes).

Significance: Type I block is usually not symptomatic unless conduction ratios are low enough to result in bradycardia and decreased cardiac output. Causes include coronary artery disease, inferior MI, aortic valve disease, mitral valve prolapse, and drugs that slow AV conduction (beta blockers, calcium channel blockers, and digitalis).

Treatment: If symptomatic bradycardia occurs, atropine 0.5 mg IV is the drug of choice to increase the sinus rate and speed conduction through the AV node. Temporary pacing (either transcutaneous or transvenous) may be necessary if ventricular rate is very slow. No treatment is necessary if ventricular rate is within normal range and patient tolerates the rhythm.

Below are two examples of Type I second degree AV block (Wenckebach). Note progressive prolongation of PR intervals on consecutively conducted P waves. Top strip shows 3:2 conduction; bottom strip shows 4:3 and 5:4 conduction.

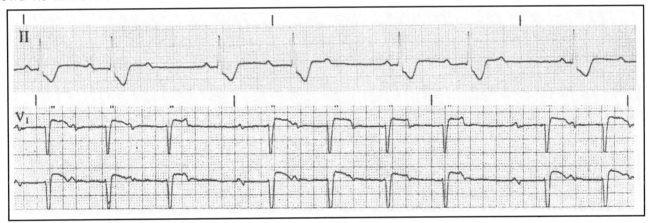

Second Degree AV Block - Type II

Type II second degree block is sudden failure of conduction of an atrial impulse without progressive conduction delay of consecutively conducted P waves. Type II block occurs below the AV node, usually in the bundle branches and very rarely in the His Bundle. Because the pathology is in the bundle branch system, intraventricular conduction is slow and the QRS is wide. (Very rarely the QRS in Type II block can be normal if the block occurs in the His Bundle.) This type of block appears on the ECG as blocked P waves, not preceded by progressively prolonging PR intervals.

Regularity: irregular due to blocked beats. Is regular when 2:1 conduction occurs.

Rate: can occur at any sinus rate. Ventricular rate depends on atrial rate and conduction ratio.

P waves: normal and precede each QRS. Some P waves are not followed by QRS complexes.

PR interval: constant before conducted beats. The PR interval preceding the pause is the same as that following the pause.

QRS complex: almost always wide due to associated bundle branch block.

Conduction: normal through atria and AV node, but intermittently blocked in bundle branch system, so impulse fails to reach ventricles. Intraventricular conduction is abnormally slow due to bundle branch block. Conduction ratios can vary from 2:1 to only occasionally blocked P waves.

Significance: more serious than Type I, with higher incidence of progression to symptomatically slow rates or third degree block. This type of block tends to be permanent and does not usually get better like Type I block does. If conduction ratio is low (2:1), it can result in symptomatic bradycardia. If only occasional beats are blocked, the ventricular rate remains adequate and no symptoms result. Causes include acute anterior wall MI, chronic conduction system disease, and rheumatic heart disease.

Treatment: acute treatment depends on ventricular rate and patient's tolerance of arrhythmia. Symptomatic bradycardia requires temporary, and often permanent, pacing. Atropine is not recommended because it may increase the number of impulses coming through the AV node to the sick bundle branch system and result in even less conduction. External pacing is recommended for symptomatic Type II block until a transvenous or permanent pacemaker can be inserted.

Below are two examples of Type II second degree AV block. Note constant PR intervals.

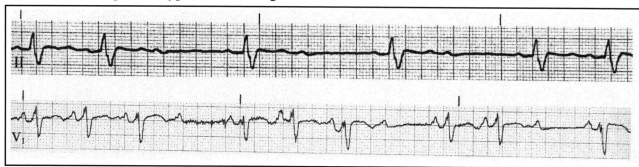

High-grade (Advanced) AV Block

High-grade block is present when two or more consecutive P waves are blocked and the atrial rate is reasonable (< 135 beats/minute). The atrial rate of 135 is an arbitrary rate that is meant to prevent misdiagnosing "high-grade block" when the AV node screens out two or more very rapid atrial impulses, as in atrial flutter where the atrial rate is 300 beats per minute. In that case, the AV node is doing its job protecting the ventricles from excessively fast rates, and therefore cannot be blamed for "high-grade block." If high-grade block occurs in the AV node, it is Type I; if it occurs below the AV node, it is Type II.

Regularity: regular or irregular, depending on conduction pattern.

Rate: atrial rate < 135, ventricular rate depends on conduction ratio.

P waves: normal, present before every conducted QRS.

PR interval: may be normal or long, but constant before conducted beats.

QRS complex: usually normal in Type I and wide in Type II.

Conduction: normal through atria. Impulses block in the AV node in Type I and block in the bundle branch system in Type II. Intraventricular conduction usually normal in Type I and slow in Type II.

Significance: often results in very slow ventricular rates which decrease cardiac output and cause hemodynamic instability. Causes include coronary artery disease, chronic conduction system disease, MI, and drugs that slow AV conduction.

Treatment: atropine 0.5 mg IV can be given and tends to work best in Type I block. Transcutaneous pacing is the treatment of choice for symptomatic bradycardia due to high-grade block until a transvenous pacemaker can be inserted.

Below are two examples of high-grade AV block. Top strip shows 3:1 conduction and ventricular rate of 30 with RBBB; bottom strip shows 4:1 conduction and ventricular rate of 25.

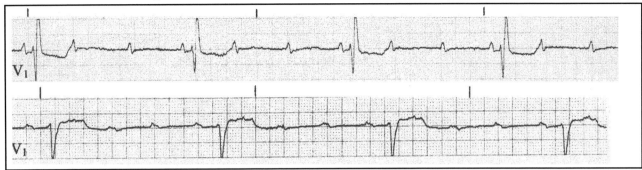

Third Degree AV Block

In third degree AV block, all atrial impulses are blocked in the AV node or bundle branch system, resulting in dissociation between the sinus or atrial rhythm and a junctional or ventricular escape rhythm controlling the ventricles.

Regularity: usually regular.

Rate: atrial rate can be any sinus or atrial rate. Ventricular rate should be less than 45 in order to be called third degree block.

P waves: normal but dissociated from QRS complexes.

PR interval: no relationship between P waves and QRS complexes, so no consistent PR intervals.

QRS complex: normal if junctional rhythm is in control of ventricles; wide if ventricular escape rhythm is present.

Conduction: no AV conduction takes place. Normal conduction through the atria, no conduction through the AV node. Intraventricular conduction usually normal in junctional escape rhythm and wide in ventricular escape rhythm.

Significance: depends on resulting ventricular rate and patient's tolerance. Since ventricular rates tend to be slow (< 45), symptoms of decreased cardiac output may occur. Third degree AV block can be asymptomatic if block develops gradually and the heart has time to compensate for the slow rate. Causes include MI, chronic conduction system disease, congenital heart disease, open heart surgery, digitalis toxicity.

Treatment: pacing is the treatment of choice, either temporary or permanent. If block occurs in the presence of MI, temporary pacing may only need to be done for a few days. When block results from conduction system disease, permanent pacing is required. Transcutaneous pacing can be done on an emergency basis until a transvenous pacemaker can be inserted.

Three examples of third degree AV block follow. In the top strip there is a junctional pacemaker controlling the ventricles at a rate of about 36. In the second strip, a ventricular pacemaker controls the ventricles at a rate of 40. The bottom strip is atrial fibrillation with third degree block and a junctional pacemaker controlling the ventricles at a rate of about 40.

Chapter 5

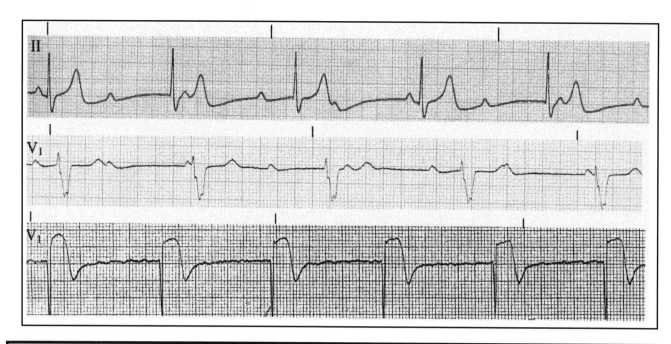

Table 5.1 AV Blocks			
Type of Block	**Number of P Waves Blocked**	**PR Interval**	**QRS Complex**
First Degree	None	Long, constant.	Narrow unless bundle branch block is present.
Second Degree Type I	One at a time	Progressive increase on consecutively conducted P waves. Constant when 2:1 conduction occurs.	Narrow unless bundle branch block is present.
Second Degree Type II	One at a time	Constant, usually normal.	Usually wide (unless block is in His Bundle – rare).
High Grade	Two or more in a row	Constant on conducted beats, may be normal or long.	Narrow in Type I unless bundle branch block is present. Wide in Type II.
Third Degree (Complete)	All P waves are blocked	No relationship between P and QRS.	Narrow if junctional escape pacemaker; wide if ventricular escape pacemaker.

Cardiac Arrhythmias

Linking Knowledge to Practice

✔ *It is important to document in the medical record episodes of AV block that result in symptomatic bradycardia with a rhythm strip that shows the effect of the block on ventricular rate. This can be used to help justify the need for a pacemaker and may facilitate payment from insurance companies by documenting the reason for pacemaker implantation.*

ASYSTOLE

Asystole is total loss of ventricular electrical activity resulting in no ventricular contraction and no cardiac output. Asystole is always fatal unless it can be corrected immediately. If atrial activity is present but there is no ventricular activity, the term *ventricular standstill* is sometimes used.

Regularity: none, there is no ventricular activity.

Rate: none.

P waves: may be present if sinus node is working and atria are capable of depolarizing.

PR interval: none.

QRS complex: none. Very fine VF can look like asystole and should be verified in more than one lead before treatment is started.

Conduction: none in ventricles. If sinus node is working, atrial conduction may be normal.

Significance: always fatal unless immediately corrected. Causes can include end-stage cardiac disease, ischemia, infarction, severe electrolyte imbalances, acidosis, hypoxia. Asystole is often the result of end-stage disease and cannot be treated.

Treatment: immediate CPR, epinephrine 1 mg IV, atropine 1 mg IV. Transcutaneous pacing should be instituted ASAP and used until a transvenous pacemaker can be inserted. The cause of asystole should be determined and treated as rapidly as possible to improve the chance of survival.

Below are three examples of asystole. In the bottom strip, ventricular tachycardia stops suddenly, leaving nothing but P waves –"ventricular standstill."

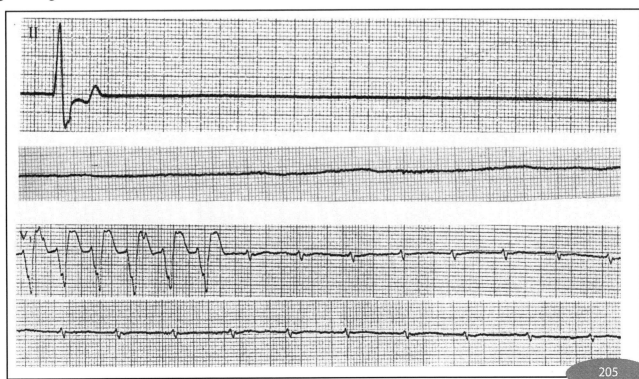

Chapter 5

BUNDLE BRANCH BLOCK

Normal intraventricular conduction results in a narrow QRS complex because both ventricles are activated simultaneously by the impulse traveling down both the right and left bundle branches at the same time. In bundle branch block there is a delay in excitation of one ventricle due to failure of conduction through the blocked bundle. This causes one ventricle to depolarize ahead of the other. The ventricle whose bundle is blocked is depolarized via muscle cell-to-cell conduction, which is much slower than conduction through the Purkinje system. The result is a widening of the QRS to .12 sec. or more.

The best lead for recognizing bundle branch block is V_1, with V_6 being the next best.

Normal Conduction in V_1 and V_6 (Figure 5.8):

QRS is .04-.10 sec.

V_1 = rS complex

V_6 = qR complex or R wave.

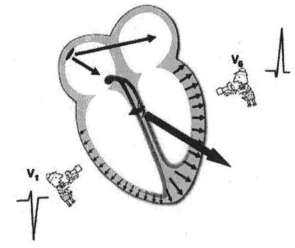

Figure 5.8: Normal conduction in V_1 and V_6.

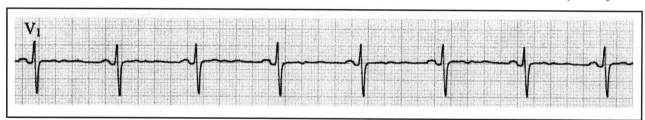

NSR with normal intraventricular conduction in lead V_1.

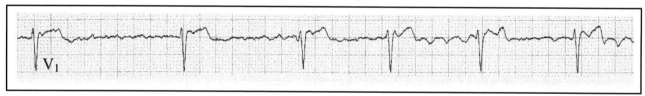

Atrial fibrillation with normal intraventricular conduction in V_1.

Right Bundle Branch Block (RBBB)

In RBBB, there is delayed depolarization of the right ventricle and abnormal spread of the electrical impulse through the right ventricle. The impulse travels down the left bundle into the left ventricle and depolarizes the left ventricle normally. Then the impulse travels via muscle cell-to-cell conduction through the right ventricle, causing the QRS to widen to 0.12 sec or more.

RBBB (Figure 5.9):

QRS is .12 sec. or greater

V_1 = rSR' (or qR or wide R)

V_6 = qRs complex (wide S wave).

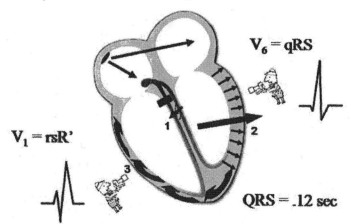

Figure 5.9: RBBB.

Cardiac Arrhythmias

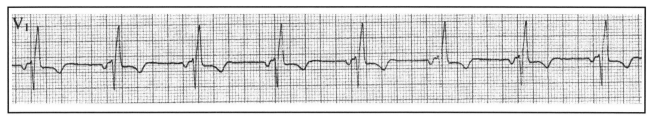

NSR with RBBB (rsR' pattern) in lead V_1.

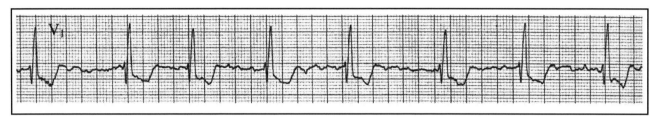

Atrial fibrillation with RBBB in lead V_1.

Left Bundle Branch Block (LBBB)

In LBBB, there is delayed depolarization of the left ventricle and abnormal spread of the electrical impulse through the left ventricle. The impulse travels down the right bundle into the right ventricle and depolarizes it normally, then spreads via muscle cell-to-cell conduction through the thick left ventricle, causing the QRS to widen to 0.12 sec or more.

LBBB (Figure 5.10):

QRS is .12 sec. or greater
V_1 = QS or rS complex
V_6 = wide R wave.

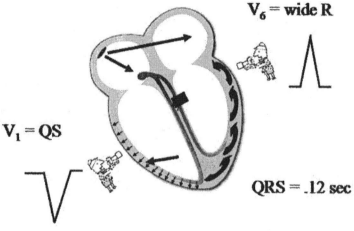

Figure 5.10: LBBB.

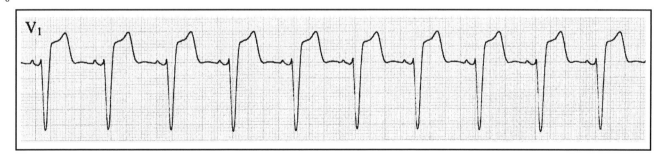

NSR with LBBB in lead V_1.

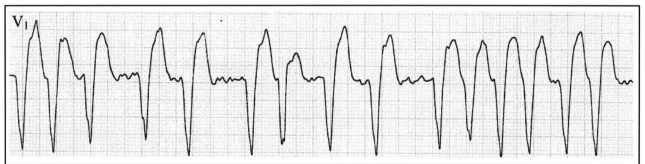

Atrial fibrillation with LBBB in lead V_1.

Table 5.2 illustrates normal QRS complexes compared to QRS complexes of RBBB and LBBB in leads V_1 and V_6.

Table 5.2 Normal Conduction and Bundle Branch Block Conduction	V_1	V_6
Normal Conduction QRS = 0.06-0.10 V_1 = rS V_6 = qR or R		
RBBB QRS = 0.12 or more V_1 = rsR' V_6 = qRs (wide S wave)		
LBBB QRS = 0.12 or more V_1 = QS V_6 = wide R wave		

DIFFERENTIAL DIAGNOSIS OF WIDE QRS BEATS AND TACHYCARDIAS

There are three major causes of wide QRS beats or tachycardias: 1) ventricular origin of the beat or rhythm; 2) conduction of a supraventricular beat or tachycardia into the ventricle with bundle branch block; 3) pre-excitation of the ventricle through an accessory pathway. Other conditions that can also cause the QRS to be wide include ventricular paced rhythms, antiarrhythmic drugs, and electrolyte abnormalities, especially hyperkalemia. Figure 5.11 illustrates the causes of a wide QRS complex (WCT = wide complex tachycardia).

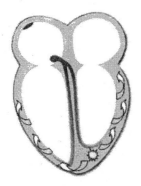
Ventricular origin:
80% of WCT

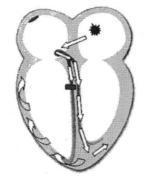
Aberrant conduction:
15-30% of WCT

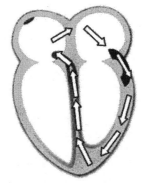
Accessory pathway
conduction: 1-5% of WCT

Figure 5.11: Causes of wide QRS complex.

Mechanisms of Aberration

Aberrancy is defined as abnormal intraventricular conduction of a supraventricular impulse. Aberration can occur if the bundle branch system is still partly or completely refractory when a supraventricular impulse attempts to travel through it. The refractory period of the bundle branches is directly proportional to preceding cycle length. Long cycles (slow heart rates) are followed by long refractory periods, whereas short cycles (fast heart rates) are followed by short refractory periods. Supraventricular beats that occur early in the cycle, like PACs, may enter the conduction system during its refractory period and be conducted aberrantly. Similarly, beats that follow a sudden lengthening of the cycle may be conducted aberrantly because of the increased length of the refractory period that occurs when the cycle lengthens.

There are three situations in which aberration is likely to occur:

◆ Early supraventricular beats (e.g., PACs or PJCs).
◆ Rapid heart rates in which the supraventricular focus conducts into the intraventricular conduction system so rapidly that the bundle branches do not have time to repolarize completely.
◆ Irregular rhythms whereby cycle lengths are constantly changing (e.g., atrial fibrillation).

Since the right bundle branch has a longer refractory period than the left, aberrant beats tend to be conducted most often with an RBBB pattern. Figures 5.12A and 5.12B illustrate these concepts.

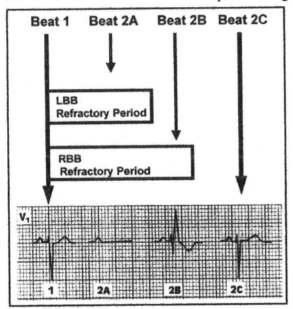

Figure 5.12A

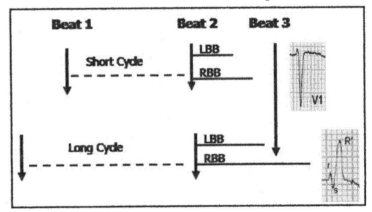

Figure 5.12B

In Figure 5.12A, beat 1 conducts normally into the ventricles, as illustrated by the normal QRS below beat 1. If a PAC occurs very early (beat 2A), it encounters refractoriness in both bundle branches and fails to conduct. If a PAC occurs a little later (beat 2B), it conducts through the left bundle but not the right, resulting in aberrant conduction with RBBB. If the PAC occurs even later (beat 2C), it is able to conduct through both bundles and results in another normal QRS.

In Figure 5.12B, beat 3 following a short cycle is able to conduct normally, but the same beat following a long cycle is aberrantly conducted with RBBB.

Chapter 5

ECG Criteria for Differentiating Wide QRS Beats and Rhythms

P Waves

To make the distinction between aberrancy and ventricular ectopy, a helpful first step is to search for P waves and note their relation to QRS complexes. Atrial activity (represented by a P wave), preceding an early wide beat or a run of tachycardia, strongly favors a supraventricular origin of that beat or tachycardia (see next two strips).

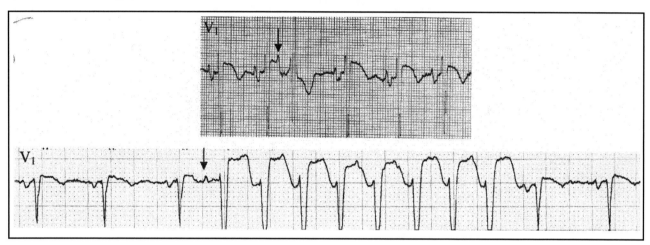

An exception to the preceding P wave rule is the case of end-diastolic PVCs that occur after the sinus P wave has occurred. The following strip shows sinus rhythm with an end diastolic PVC occurring immediately after the sinus P wave. In this case, the P wave preceding the wide QRS is merely a coincidence and does not represent aberrant conduction; the PR interval is much too short to have conducted that beat. In addition, the P wave preceding the wide QRS is not early; it is the regularly scheduled sinus beat coming on time.

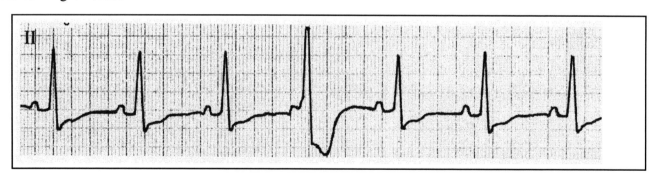

P waves seen during a wide-complex tachycardia can be very helpful in making the differential diagnosis between SVT with aberration and VT. It is common for the sinus node to continue to fire regularly and independently of the ventricular focus when VT occurs. By noting the relationship between P waves and QRS complexes, it is sometimes possible to demonstrate AV dissociation, which means that the atria and ventricles are under the control of separate pacemakers. The presence of independent P waves in a wide QRS tachycardia indicates AV dissociation and is diagnostic of VT, whereas P waves seen before each QRS complex indicate a supraventricular origin of the rhythm. The following strips illustrate how P waves can be useful in differentiating two similar wide QRS tachycardias due to two different mechanisms.

The following strip shows P waves dissociated from wide QRS complexes, indicating that the rhythm is VT.

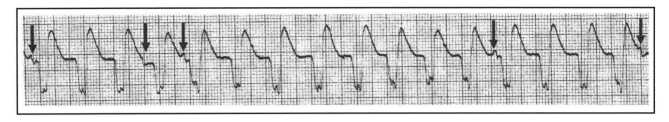

The strip below shows a wide QRS tachycardia that looks almost identical to the one above. However, this one has P waves in front of each QRS complex, indicating the supraventricular origin of this rhythm. This is sinus tachycardia with LBBB.

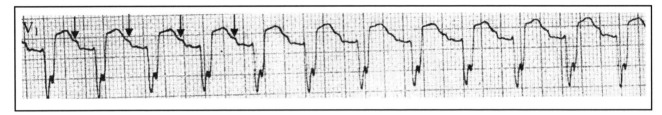

QRS Morphology

The shape of the QRS complexes in a WCT can be helpful in determining the mechanism of the arrhythmia. Whenever possible, a 12 lead ECG should be obtained during the tachycardia, since many of the morphology clues used for differentiating the origin of the tachycardia are present in multiple leads.

The first step in using morphology clues is to look at lead V1 and determine if the tachycardia is shaped like RBBB or like LBBB. Then use the clues in the Figure 5.13 and 5.14 to help determine whether the morphology favors a ventricular origin or a supraventricular origin with aberrant conduction.

Right Bundle Branch Block Pattern (QRS wide and upright in V1) (Figure 5.13)

A wide QRS complex with a triphasic pattern of RBBB in lead V1 (rsR') strongly favors aberrancy. A monophasic or biphasic complex of RBBB type in lead V1 with a taller left "rabbit ear" favors a ventricular origin, whereas a taller right "rabbit ear" favors neither. Often V6 is as helpful as V1; a triphasic qRs complex in V6 favors RBBB aberration, whereas a monophasic QS complex or a biphasic rS complex favors ventricular ectopy.

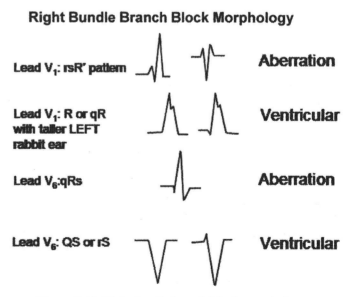

Figure 5.13: Right bundle branch block morphology.

In the following ECG, look at lead V₁ and determine if this tachycardia is shaped like RBBB or LBBB. (The QRS is wide and upright, indicating RBBB morphology.) Use the RBBB morphology clues in Figure 5.13 to determine the origin of the tachycardia.

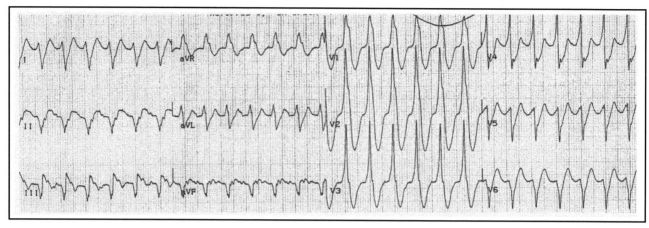

(Lead V₁ is monophasic with a taller left "rabbit ear" – favors VT. Lead V₆ is a rS complex – favors VT. There is also an indeterminate QRS axis which favors VT.) This is VT!

Left Bundle Branch Block Pattern (QRS wide and negative in V1) (Figure 5.14)

Four characteristics of the QRS complex in V₁ or V₂, and V₆ favor a ventricular origin of a wide QRS tachycardia with LBBB morphology:

Left Bundle Branch Block Morphology

- ◆ A wide initial R wave of greater than 0.03 second in V₁ or V₂.

- ◆ Slurring or notching on the downstroke of the S wave in V₁ or V₂.

- ◆ A delay of 0.06 second or more from the beginning of the QRS to the nadir (deepest part) of the S wave in V₁ or V₂.

- ◆ Any q wave (qR or QS) in V₆ favoring a ventricular origin.

In Leads V1 or V2:
Wide r wave (>.03 sec)
Slurred downstroke
>.06 sec to nadir of S wave — Ventricular

In Leads V1 or V2:
Narrow r wave (≤.03 sec)
Straight downstroke
<.06 sec to nadir of S wave — Aberration

In Lead V6:
Any q (QS or qR) — Ventricular

Figure 5.14: Left bundle branch block pattern.

In the following ECG, look at V1 and determine if it is RBBB or LBBB morphology. (The QRS is wide and negative, indicating a LBBB morphology.) Use the LBBB morphology clues in Figure 5.14 to determine the origin of the tachycardia.

Cardiac Arrhythmias

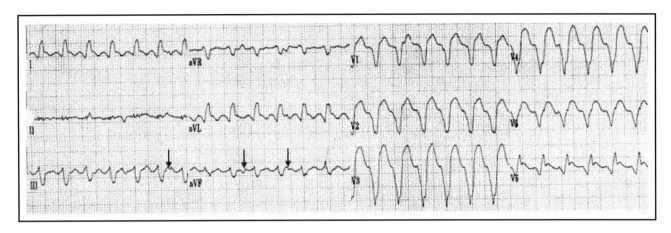

(In V_1 and V_2, there is slurring on the downstroke of the QRS, and the delay from the beginning of the QRS to the nadir of the S wave is > 0.06 sec, both favoring VT. In V_6 there is a Q wave. There is no "r" wave in V_1 or V_2, but there is evidence of dissociated P waves, as indicated by the arrows in III and AVF. This is VT!

Fusion and Capture Beats
Ventricular fusion beats are produced when a supraventricular impulse and an ectopic ventricular impulse both contribute to ventricular depolarization (Figure 5.15). The resulting QRS complex does not look like a normally conducted beat or like the pure ventricular ectopic beat because it is formed by a combination of both depolarization waves (e.g. a "hybrid" morphology). The shape and width of fusion beats vary depending on the relative contributions of both the supraventricular and the ventricular impulses. The presence of fusion beats indicates AV dissociation; the atria and the ventricles are under the control of separate pacemakers. Capture beats occur when, in the presence of AV dissociation, a supraventricular impulse manages to conduct into the ventricles and "capture" them, resulting in a normally conducted QRS complex. The presence of fusion or capture beats in a run of wide QRS tachycardia is diagnostic of VT, but, unfortunately, capture beats are rare and cannot be counted on to make the diagnosis.

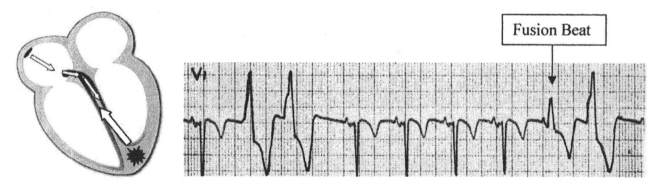

Figure 5.15: Ventricular depolarization.

In the above strip, the basic rhythm is NSR with a pair of PVCs at the beginning and at the end of the strip. The fusion beat is the result of the sinus impulse colliding with the PVC in the ventricle, resulting in a beat that does not look like either of its "parent" beats.

Chapter 5

In the strips below, two fusion beats (☆) are seen and there is evidence of AV dissociation (arrows pointing to P waves). This is VT.

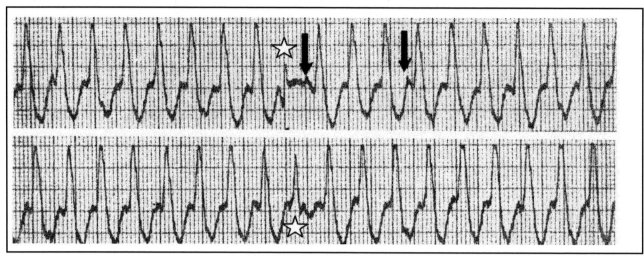

Linking Knowledge to Practice

✔ *Correct diagnosis of the cause of a wide QRS tachycardia is critical to safe and effective therapy. Some drugs that are effective in the treatment of SVT, such as verapamil or adenosine, can be harmful and even fatal if given to a patient who is in VT. Mistakes in making the correct diagnosis are often related to the following:*

  1. Lack of knowledge about the ECG clues (e.g. P waves, QRS morphology) that are so useful in helping make the correct diagnosis.

  2. The belief that if a patient is tolerating a wide QRS tachycardia then it must not be VT.

✔ *The most important things that determine if a patient tolerates any tachycardia, whether the QRS is wide or narrow, are ventricular rate and left ventricular function (ejection fraction). Faster rates are not tolerated as well as slower rates, so a tachycardia at a rate of 130 beats per minute is better tolerated than one at a rate of 180 beats per minute, regardless of the origin of the tachycardia. Similarly, tachycardia is better tolerated when LV function is good than when LV function is poor. Patients with good LV function can often tolerate rapid rates for long periods of time, while patients with reduced ejection fractions may not even tolerate sinus tachycardia very well.*

ACCESSORY PATHWAY CONDUCTION

Conduction of impulses from the atrium to the ventricle via an accessory pathway (AP), also called a *bypass tract,* is another cause of wide QRS rhythms. Two wide QRS tachycardias resulting from AP conduction are antidromic circus movement tachycardia and atrial fibrillation conducting through an AP. Figure 5.16 illustrates these two mechanisms. See Chapter 6 for more information on accessory pathways.

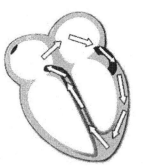
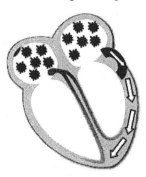
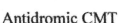

Antidromic CMT presents as a regular, wide QRS tachycardia that looks like VT, and it is often impossible to differentiate the two without an electrophysiology study. One helpful clue is that in antidromic CMT, it is not possible to have AV dissociation, since both the atria and the ventricles are involved in the arrhythmia circuit; therefore, the presence of AV dissociation is proof of VT.

Antidromic CMT   Atrial fibrillation conducting through an AP

Figure 5.16: Accessory pathway conduction.

The ECG below illustrates antidromic CMT.

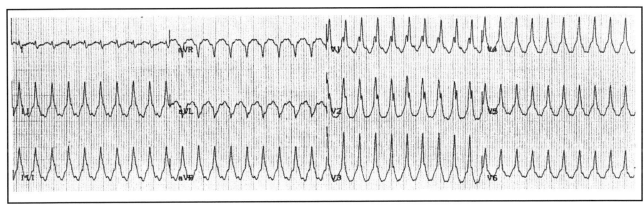

Atrial fibrillation and atrial flutter that occur in the presence of an accessory pathway are particularly dangerous because of the extremely rapid ventricular rate that can result from conduction of the atrial impulses directly into the ventricle through the bypass track. The ventricular rate can be as fast as 250 to 300 beats/min and can deteriorate into ventricular fibrillation, resulting in sudden death. Atrial fibrillation with anterograde conduction over an accessory pathway presents on the ECG as a very rapid, irregular, wide QRS rhythm. The irregularity of the ventricular response helps to differentiate this rhythm from other wide QRS tachycardias.

The ECG characteristics of atrial fibrillation with anterograde conduction through an accessory pathway are as follows:

Rate: Ventricular rates up to 300 beats/min.

Rhythm: Irregular. Often appears as groups of very short R-R intervals alternating with groups of longer R-R intervals. The longest R-R intervals are often more than twice the shortest R-R intervals.

P waves: None because atria are fibrillating.

PR interval: None.

QRS complex: Wide, bizarre due to abnormal depolarization of ventricles through AP.

Conduction: Disorganized and chaotic through atria. Atrial impulses conduct into ventricles through AP, resulting in muscle cell-to-cell conduction through ventricles.

Treatment: Immediate treatment of atrial fibrillation with anterograde conduction through an AP depends on ventricular rate and the patient's tolerance of the arrhythmia. Cardioversion is the treatment of choice when severe hemodynamic impairment occurs. Drug treatment is directed at slowing conduction through the AP to control ventricular rate. Drugs that increase the refractory period and depress conduction in the bypass tract include procainamide, flecainide, propafenone, amiodarone, and sotalol. Many of these drugs are also effective in preventing recurrences of atrial fibrillation. Digoxin and calcium channel blockers, commonly used to treat atrial fibrillation that conducts through the AV node, are contraindicated when the tachycardia is due to anterograde conduction through an AP, because they shorten the refractory period and accelerate conduction through the bypass tract.

The following ECG illustrates atrial fibrillation conducting down an AP. Note the wide, irregular, and very rapid QRS complexes and the occasional narrow QRS that results when the AP tires and gives the normal AV node a chance to conduct an impulse. Remember that no "self-respecting" AV node will allow a ventricular rate to approach 300 beats per minute, so when you see ventricular rates this fast, suspect an AP.

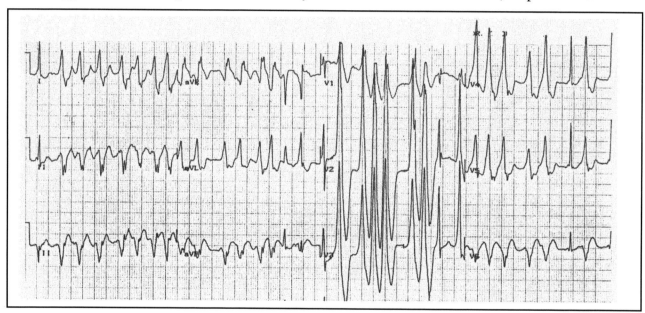

Cardiac Arrhythmias

PRACTICE STRIPS

1.
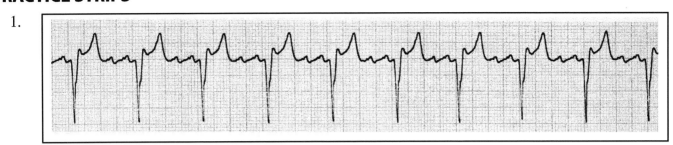

2.
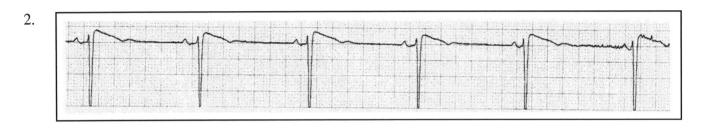

3.
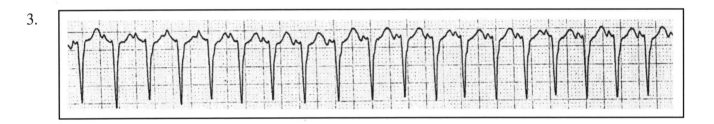

4.
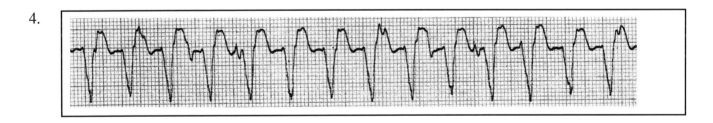

5.
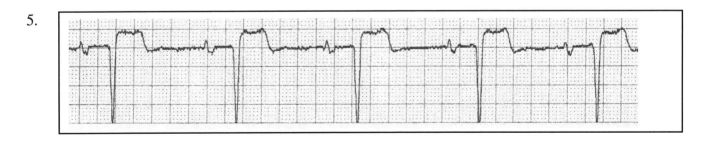

6.
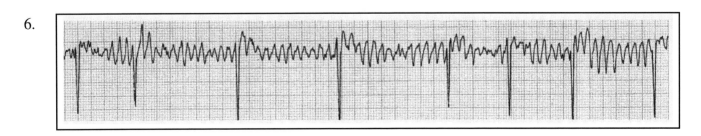

217

Chapter 5

7.
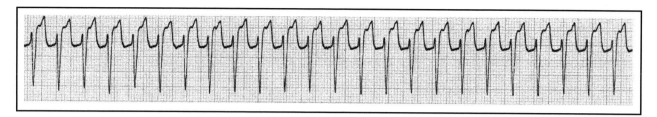

8.
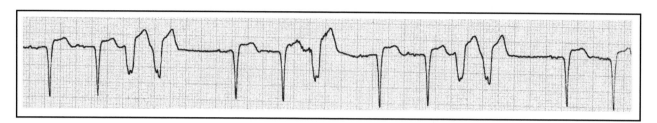

9.
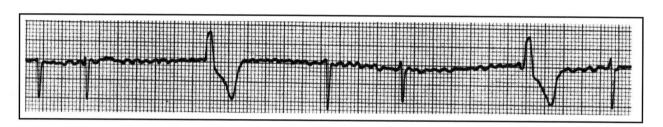

10.
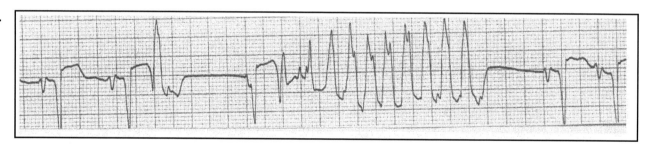

11.
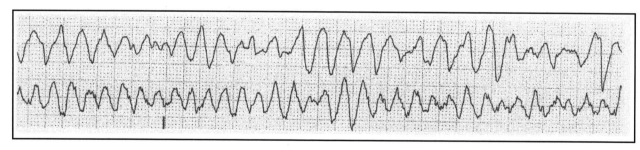

12.
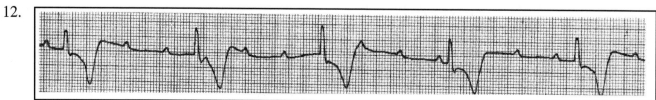

Cardiac Arrhythmias

13.
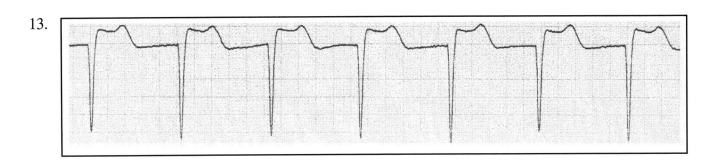

14.
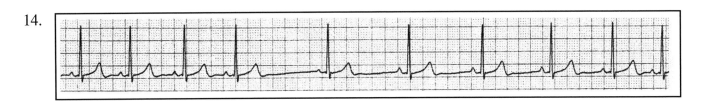

15.
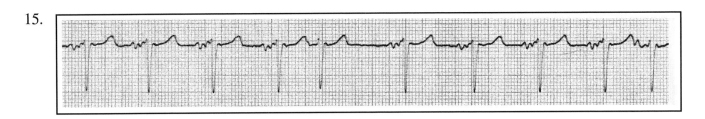

16.
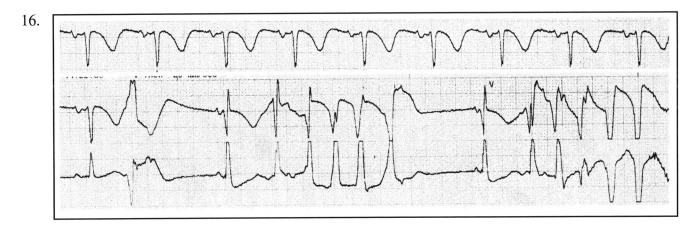

17.
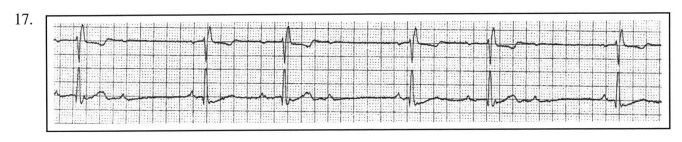

18.
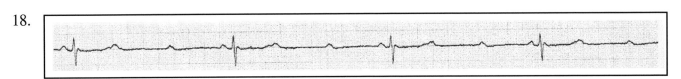

Chapter 5

19.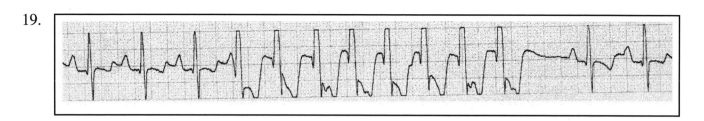

20.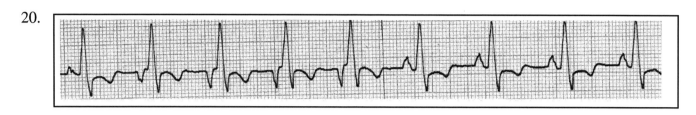

21.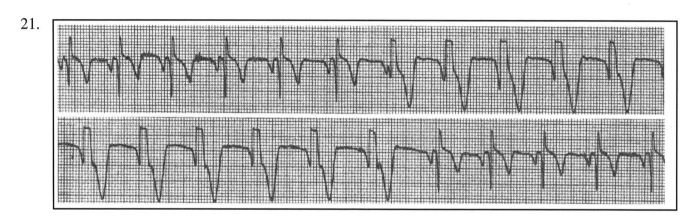

22.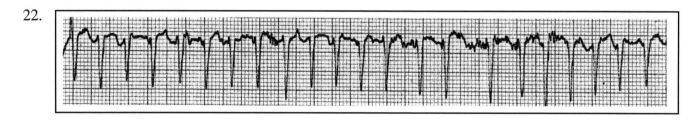

23.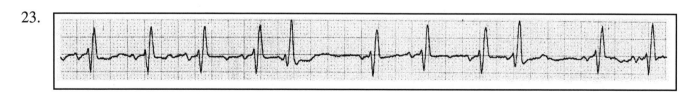

24.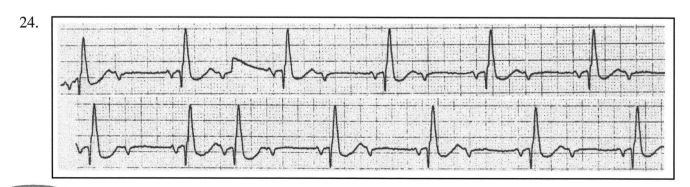

Cardiac Arrhythmias

PRACTICE STRIP ANSWERS

1. Atrial flutter with 4:1 conduction (there is an F wave in the T wave)
2. Sinus bradycardia
3. Atrial tachycardia
4. VT – note independent P waves indicating AV dissociation
5. First degree AV block
6. Atrial fibrillation
7. SVT
8. NSR with multifocal PVCs
9. Atrial fibrillation with ventricular escape beats
10. NSR with polymorphic VT (QT interval appears normal)
11. VF
12. Third degree AV block
13. Junctional rhythm
14. Sinus arrhythmia
15. NSR with two PACs
16. NSR with long QT interval and torsades de pointes in same patient
17. Second degree AV block, Type I (Wenckebach)
18. High grade AV block with 4:1 conduction
19. NSR with run of VT
20. WAP
21. NSR with accelerated ventricular rhythm
22. Atrial fibrillation with rapid ventricular response
23. NSR with 2 PJCs
24. Second degree AV block, Type II

REFERENCES

Arnsdorf, M. F. & Podrid, P. J. (2005). Tachyarrhythmias associated with the Wolff-Parkinson-White syndrome. *UpToDate*. Retrieved July 9, 2005, from www.uptodate.com

Arnsdorf, M. F. & Verdino, R. (2001). Atrioventricular nodal conduction abnormalities. In P. J. Podrid & P. R. Kowey (Eds.), *Cardiac Arrhythmias: Mechanisms, Diagnosis & Management* (2nd ed., pp. 671-691). Philadelphia: Lippincott Williams & Wilkins.

Arnsdorf, M. F. & Wilber, D. (2004). Atrioventricular nodal reentrant tachycardia (junctional reciprocating tachycardia). *UpToDate*. Retrieved July 9, 2005, from www.uptodate.com

Chapter 5

Buxton, A. E. & Duc, J. (2001). Ventricular premature depolarizations and nonsustained ventricular tachycardia. In P. J. Podrid & P. R. Kowey (Eds.), *Cardiac Arrhythmia: Mechanisms, Diagnosis & Treatment* (2nd ed., pp. 549-572). Philadelphia: Lippincott, Williams & Wilkins.

Conover, M. B. (2003). *Understanding Electrocardiography* (8th ed.). St. Louis: Mosby.

Ellenbogen, K. A. & Wood, M. A. (2004). Atrial Tachycardia. In D. P. Zipes & J. Jalife (Eds.), *Cardiac Electrophysiology: From Cell to Bedside* (4th ed., pp. 500-511). Philadelphia: W.B. Saunders.

El-Sherif, N. & Turitto, G. (2004). Torsade de Pointes. In D. P. Zipes & J. Jalife (Eds.), *Cardiac Electrophysiology: From Cell to Bedside* (4th ed., pp. 687-699). Philadelphia: W.B. Saunders.

Epstein, A. E. & Ideker, R. E. (2000). Ventricular fibrillation. In D. P. Zipes & J. Jalife (Eds.), *Cardiac Electrophysiology: From Cell to Bedside* (3rd ed., pp. 677-683). Philadelphia: W.B. Saunders.

Garcia, T. B. & Miller, G. T. (2004). *Arrhythmia Recognition: The Art of Interpretation.* Boston: Jones & Bartlett.

Goldberger, J. J. & Kadish, A. H. (2001). Sinoartrial/atrial tachyarrhythmias. In P. J. Podrid & P. R. Kowey (Eds.), *Cardiac Arrhythmia: Mechanisms, Diagnosis & Management* (2nd ed., pp. 411-431). Philadelphia: Lippincott, Williams & Wilkins.

Grimm, W. & Marchlinski, F. E. (2004). Accelerated Idioventricular Rhythm and Bidirectional Ventricular Tachycardia. In D. P. Zipes & J. Jalife (Eds.), *Cardiac Electrophysiology: From Cell to Bedside* (4th ed., pp. 700-704). Philadelphia: W.B. Saunders.

Hamdan, M. H., Dorostkar, P., & Scheinman, M. M. (2000). Junctional tachycardia and junctional rhythm. In D. P. Zipes & J. Jalife (Eds.), *Cardiac Electrophysiology: From Cell to Bedside* (3rd ed., pp. 482-488). Philadelphia: W. B. Saunders.

Hohnloser, S. H. (2001). Polymorphous ventricular tachycardia, including torsades de pointes. In P. J. Podrid & P. R. Kowey (Eds.), *Cardiac Arrhythmia: Mechanisms, Diagnosis & Management* (2nd ed., pp. 604-619). Philadelphia: Lippincott, Williams & Wilkins.

Hudson, K. B., Brady, W. J., Chan, T. C., Pollack, M., & Harrigan, R. A. (2003). Electrocardiographic manifestations: ventricular tachycardia. *The Journal of Emergency Medicine, 25*(3), 303-314.

Huzar, R. J. (2002). *Basic Dysrhythmias: Interpretation and Management* (3rd ed.). St. Louis: Mosby.

Jacobson, C. (2005). Arrhythmias and conduction disturbances. In S. L. Woods, E. S. Froelicher, S. U. Motzer & E. J. Bridges (Eds.), *Cardiac Nursing* (5th ed., pp. 361-424). Philadelphia: Lippincott, Williams & Wilkins.

Jacobson, C. (2006). Interpretation and management of basic cardiac arrhythmias. In M. Chulay & S. M. Burns (Eds.), *AACN Essentials of Critical Care Nursing* (pp. 37-63). New York: McGraw-Hill.

Jahangir, A., Munger, T. M., & Packer, D. L. (2001). Atrial fibrillation. In P. J. Podrid & P. R. Kowey (Eds.), *Cardiac Arrhythmia: Mechanisms, Diagnosis & Management* (2nd ed., pp. 457-499). Philadelphia: Lippincott, Williams & Wilkins.

Lin, D. & Callans, D. F. (2004). Sinus Rhythm Abnormalities. In D. P. Zipes & J. Jalife (Eds.), *Cardiac Electrophysiology: From Cell to Bedside* (4th ed., pp. 479-484). Philadelphia: W.B. Saunders.

Marinchak, R. A. & Rials, S. J. (2001). Tachycardias in Wolff-Parkinson-White syndrome. In P. J. Podrid & P. R. Kowey (Eds.), *Cardiac Arrhythmia: Mechanisms, Diagnosis & Management* (2nd ed., pp. 517-548). Philadelphia: Lippincott, Williams & Wilkins.

Marriott, H. J. L. (1988). *Practical Electrocardiography* (8th ed.). Baltimore: Williams & Wilkins.

Marriott, H. J. L. & Conover, M. B. (1998). *Advanced Concepts in Arrhythmias* (3rd ed.). St. Louis: Mosby.

Martin, D. & Wharton, J. M. (2001). Sustained monomorphic ventricular tachycardia. In P. J. Podrid & P. R. Kowey (Eds.), *Cardiac Arrhythmia: Mechanisms, Diagnosis & Management* (2nd ed., pp. 573-601). Philadelphia: Lippincott, Williams & Wilkins.

Miller, J. M., Das, M., Arora, R., Alberte-Lista, Cesar, & Wu, J. (2004). Differential Diagnosis of Wide QRS Complex Tachycardia. In D. P. Zipes & J. Jalife (Eds.), *Cardiac Electrophysiology: From Cell to Bedside* (4th ed., pp. 747-757). Philadelphia: W.B. Saunders.

Nattel, S. & Ehrlich, J. R. (2004). Atrial Fibrillation. In D. P. Zipes & J. Jalife (Eds.), *Cardiac Electrophysiology: From Cell to Bedside* (4th ed., pp. 512-522). Philadelphia: W.B. Saunders.

Oral, H. & Strickberger, S. A. (2004). Junctional Rhythms and Junctional Tachycardia. In D. P. Zipes & J. Jalife (Eds.), *Cardiac Electrophysiology: From Cell to Bedside* (4th ed., pp. 523-527). Philadelphia: W.B. Saunders.

Podrid, P. J. (2004). Approach to wide QRS complex tachycardias. *UpToDate.* Retrieved January 8, 2006, from www.uptodate.com

Reiffel, J. A. (2001). Sinus node function and dysfunction. In P. J. Podrid & P. R. Kowey (Eds.), *Cardiac Arrhythmia: Mechanisms, Diagnosis & Management* (2nd ed., pp. 653-670). Philadelphia: Lippincott, Williams & Wilkins.

Schwartzman, D. (2004). Atrioventricular Block and Atrioventricular Dissociation. In D. P. Zipes & J. Jalife (Eds.), *Cardiac Electrophysiology: From Cell to Bedside* (4th ed., pp. 485-489). 2004: Philadelphia: W.B. Saunders.

Waldo, A. L. (2004). Atrial flutter: Mechanisms, Clinical Features, and Management. In D. P. Zipes & J. Jalife (Eds.), *Cardiac Electrophysiology: From Cell to Bedside* (4th ed., pp. 490-499). Philadelphia: W.B. Saunders.

Zipes, D. P., Camm, J. A., Borggrefe, M., Buxton, A. E., Chaitman, B., Fromer, M., et al. (2006). ACC/AHA/ESC 2006 guidelines for management of patients with ventricular arrhythmias and the prevention of sudden cardiac death–executive summary: A report of the American College of Cardiology/American Heart Association Task Forc and the European Society of Cardiology Committee for Practice Guidelines. *Circulation, 114,* 1088-1132.

CHAPTER 6:
12 LEAD ELECTROCARDIOGRAPHY

INTRODUCTION

The electrocardiogram (ECG) is a graphic record of the electrical activity of the heart. The spread of the electrical impulse through the heart produces electrical signals that can be detected and amplified by the ECG machine and recorded on calibrated graph paper. These amplified signals form the ECG tracing, consisting of P waves (atrial depolarization), QRS complexes (ventricular depolarization), and T waves (ventricular repolarization).These waveforms are recorded on grid paper that moves beneath the recording stylus (pen) at standard speed of 25 mm/sec. The grid on the paper consists of a series of small and large boxes, both horizontally and vertically; horizontal boxes measure time, and vertical boxes measure voltage. Each small box horizontally is equal to 0.04 second, and each large box horizontally is equal to 0.20 second. On the vertical axis, each small box measures 1 mm and is equal to 0.1 mV; each large box measures 5 mm and is equal to 0.5 mV. In addition to the grid, most ECG paper places a vertical line in the top margin at 3-second intervals or places a mark at 1-second intervals. The standard 12-lead ECG simultaneously records 12 different views of electrical activity as it travels through the heart and displays all 12 views on a full-page layout using the same grid (see Figure 6.1).

The 12-lead ECG records electrical activity as it spreads through the heart from 12 different leads that are recorded through electrodes placed on the arms, legs, and specific spots on the chest. Each lead represents a different view of the heart and consists of two electrodes with opposite polarity (bipolar) or one electrode and a reference point (unipolar). A *bipolar* lead has a positive pole and a negative pole; a *unipolar* lead has one positive pole and a reference pole in the center of the chest that is algebraically determined by the ECG machine. The standard 12-lead ECG consists of 6 limb leads that record electrical activity in the frontal plane-traveling up/down and right/left in the heart; and 6 precordial leads (also called chest leads) that record electrical activity in the horizontal plane-traveling anterior/posterior and right/left. The ECG records three bipolar frontal plane leads: lead I, lead II, and lead III; three unipolar frontal plane leads: AVR, AVL, and AVF; and six unipolar precordial leads: V_1, V_2, V_3, V_4, V_5, and V_6. Limb leads are recorded by electrodes placed on the arms and legs, whereas precordial leads are recorded by electrodes placed on the chest. For convenience in continuous bedside monitoring, arm electrodes can be placed on the shoulders and leg electrodes on the lower part of the rib cage or hips rather than on the limbs, without significantly altering the signals recorded.

A camera analogy makes the 12-lead ECG easier to understand. Each lead of the ECG represents a picture of the electrical activity in the heart taken by the camera. In any lead, the positive electrode is the recording electrode or the camera lens. The negative electrode (or the reference pole in a unipolar lead) tells the camera which way to "shoot" its picture. If the positive electrode is positioned so that electrical activity in the heart travels toward it, it records an upright deflection on the ECG. If the positive electrode is positioned so that electrical activity travels away from it, it records a negative deflection. If the electrical activity travels perpendicular to a positive electrode, no activity is recorded.

Chapter 6

Anatomy of a 12 Lead ECG

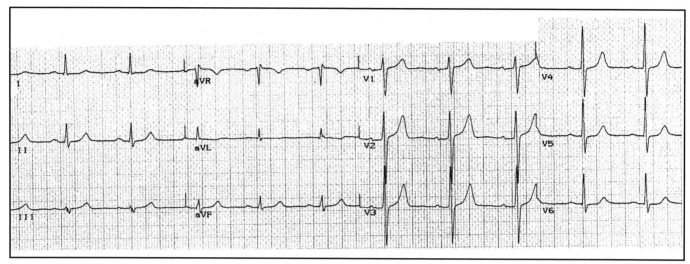

Figure 6.1: Normal ECG.

A 12 Lead ECG records a 10 second "snapshot" of electrical activity in the heart. Leads I, II, and III are recorded simultaneously for 2.5 seconds, then leads AVR, AVL, and AVF are recorded simultaneously for 2.5 seconds, then leads V_1-V_3 are recorded simultaneously for 2.5 seconds, and finally leads V_4-V_6 are recorded simultaneously for 2.5 seconds. Figure 6.1 is a normal ECG.

Lateral Leads = I, AVL, V_5, V_6
Inferior Leads = II, III, AVF
Anterior Leads = V_1-V_4

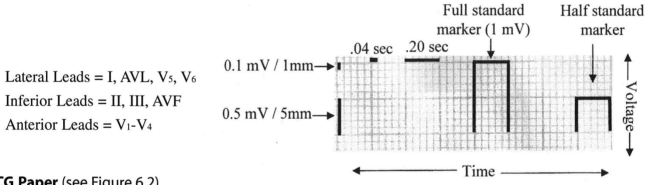

Figure 6.2: ECG paper.

ECG Paper (see Figure 6.2)

- ♦ Horizontal axis = time
- ♦ Vertical axis = voltage
- ♦ ECG is standardized to 1 mV. If QRS voltage is large; ECG may be standardized to 0.5 mV. Be sure to check standardization marker.
- ♦ 0.1 mV = 1 mm. ST segment elevation or depression is measured in mm.

NORMAL AND ABNORMAL ECG WAVEFORMS AND INTERVALS

P Wave

- ◆ Represents atrial depolarization.
- ◆ Normally upright in Lead I, II, AVF, and V$_{4-6}$; can be biphasic or inverted in Lead III. Normally inverted in AVR. Usually biphasic in V$_1$ but can be upright or inverted.
- ◆ No taller than 2.5 mm or wider than .11 sec.
- ◆ Should be symmetrically rounded.

Left atrial enlargement: P wave wider than .12 sec and M shaped in limb leads; larger negative component in V$_1$.

Right atrial enlargement: P wave taller than 2.5 mm and pointed in limb leads; larger initial positive component in V$_1$.

Retrograde conduction: P waves are inverted in leads II, III, and AVF when the atria depolarize from bottom to top (retrograde) rather than from top to bottom. This occurs with junctional or low atrial rhythms or when PVCs conduct backward through the AV node to the atria.

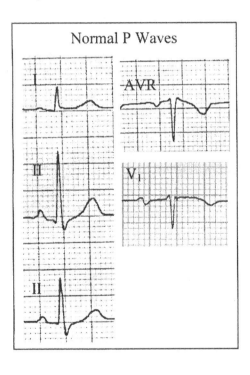
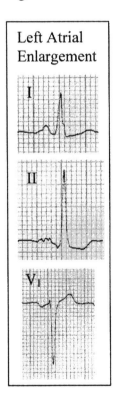
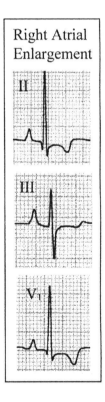
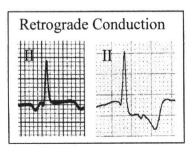

Chapter 6

QRS Complex

- Represents ventricular depolarization.
- Q wave is an initial negative deflection from baseline.
- R wave is a positive deflection from baseline.
- S wave is a negative deflection that follows an R wave.
- QRS width measures intraventricular conduction time and is normally 0.04 to .10 sec.

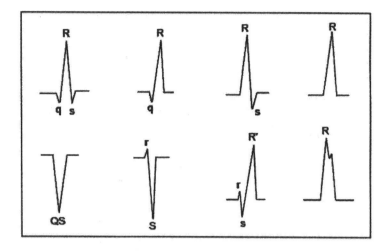

ST Segment

- ST segment begins at end of QRS complex (J point) and ends at beginning of T wave.
- Should be at baseline (isoelectric interval between T wave and next P wave).
- Should not stay on baseline for longer than .12 sec. If it hugs baseline for longer than .12 sec, it can indicate ischemia or hypocalcemia.
- Should curve smoothly up into ascending limb of T wave. A sharp angle can be a sign of ischemia.
- ST elevation of 1mm or more above baseline may indicate myocardial injury.
- ST depression 1mm or more below baseline can indicate ischemia or may be a reciprocal change in MI.

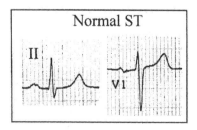

Normal ST

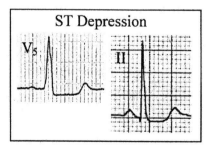

ST Depression

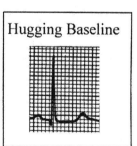

Hugging Baseline

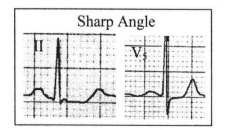

Sharp Angle

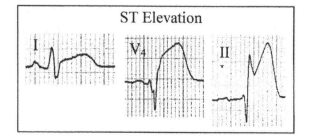

ST Elevation

12 Lead Electrocardiography

T Wave

- Represents ventricular repolarization.
- Is usually upright in Leads I, II, V$_{3-6}$ and inverted in AVR. May vary in other leads. It is preferable to have a slightly inverted T wave in V$_1$.
- Normally asymmetrically rounded with ascending limb more gradual than descending limb.
- Height should not exceed 5 mm in a limb lead or 10 mm in a precordial lead.
- T wave inversion is a sign of ischemia and can occur with evolving MI.
- Tall pointed T waves can indicate ischemia, early infarction, or hyperkalemia.

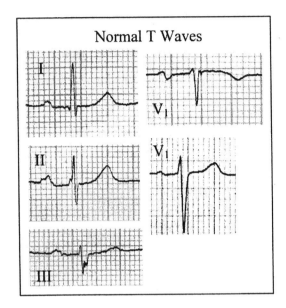

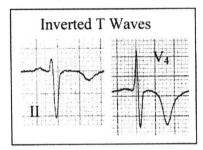

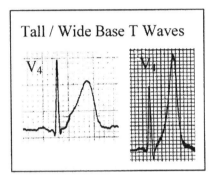

U Wave

- Small rounded wave sometimes seen following the T wave.
- Probably represents repolarization of the terminal Purkinje network or some part of ventricles.
- U wave polarity should be the same as the T wave. Otherwise, inverted U waves can indicate ischemia.
- Large U waves can occur in hypokalemia and with certain drugs (i.e. quinidine).

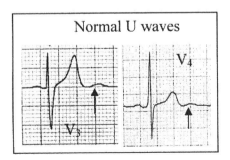
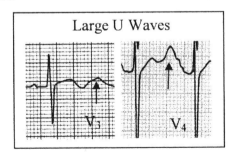
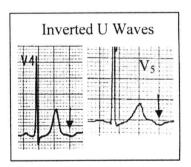

QT Interval

- Measured from beginning of QRS to end of T wave.
- Represents total duration of ventricular depolarization and repolarization.
- QT prolongation indicates a repolarization abnormality which can occur with drugs, including many antiarrhythmics, antipsychotics, antibiotics, and many others; and with electrolyte imbalances, especially hypokalemia and hypomagnesemia.
- QT prolongation can lead to ventricular arrhythmias and torsades de pointes.
- The QT interval is heart rate dependent: it shortens at faster rates and can be longer at slow rates.
- Rule of thumb is that QT interval should be no longer than half the preceding R-R interval at normal heart rates. The best way to determine QT interval is to use a chart that corrects for heart rate (QTc).
- Normal QTc for men = 0.42 sec; for women = 0.43 sec.

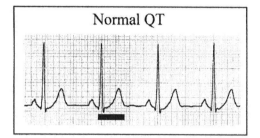
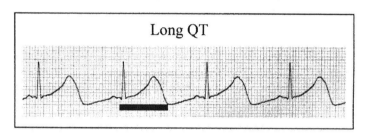

ECG LEADS

The electrocardiogram consists of 12 leads all recording the spread of electrical activity through the heart from different viewpoints. Think of the 12 leads as cameras taking 12 different pictures of the same object from different spots. Each lead of the 12-lead ECG represents a picture of the electrical activity in the heart taken by the camera.

How Leads Record (see Figure 6.3)

- In any lead system, the positive electrode is the recording electrode (or cameral lens).
- The negative electrode tells the camera which way to look and determines the direction in which the positive electrode records.
- Depolarization traveling toward the positive electrode is recorded as a positive deflection.
- Depolarization traveling away from the positive electrode is recorded as a negative deflection.
- Depolarization traveling perpendicular to the lead is not recorded at all.
- If a lead sees depolarization traveling toward it and then away from it, it records a biphasic complex.

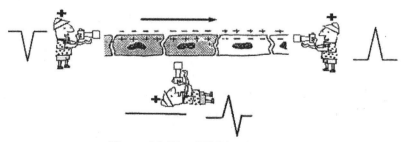

Figure 6.3: How ECG leads record.

Frontal Plane Leads (Limb Leads): I, II, III, AVR, AVL, AVF

These six leads view electrical activity traveling right and left or up and down in the frontal plane. The frontal plane represents two dimensions: up/down and right/left (like a stick figure with no third dimension). Leads I, II, and III are *bipolar* leads – they have a positive and negative pole and record the difference in electrical potential between the two poles. Leads AVR, AVL, and AVF are *unipolar* leads – they have a positive pole located on the right shoulder (AVR), left shoulder (AVL) or left leg (or foot – AVF), and the negative pole is a calculated reference point in the center of the chest. Frontal plane leads are obtained by attaching the limb electrodes from the ECG machine to the arms and legs. The positive pole in each lead is the recording electrode or camera lens and does the actual recording of electrical activity. Figure 6.4 shows where recording electrodes are placed on the body. Figure 6.5 shows how each frontal plane lead records electrical activity.

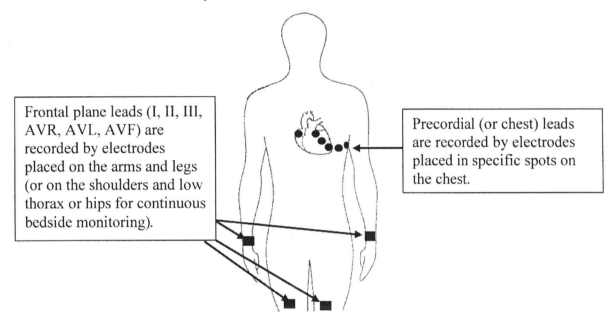

Figure 6.4: Placement of recording electrodes.

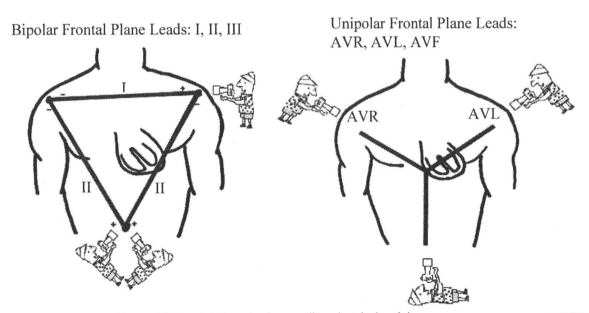

Figure 6.5: Frontal plane leads recording electrical activity.

Precordial (Chest) Leads: V₁ - V₆

- Six unipolar precordial leads record electrical activity in the horizontal plane.
- The positive pole is placed at specific locations across the left chest, and the negative pole is the center of the chest (Figure 6.6).
    - V_1 = 4th intercostal space, right sternal border.
    - V_2 = 4th intercostal space, left sternal border.
    - V_3 = midpoint between V_2 and V_4.
    - V_4 = 5th intercostal space, left midclavicular line.
    - V_5 = left anterior axillary line, same level as V_4.
    - V_6 = left midaxillary line, same level as V_4 and V_5.

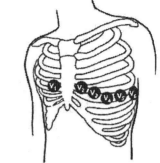

Figure 6.6: Precordial chest leads: V_1-V_6.

NORMAL CARDIAC DEPOLARIZATION

The impulse normally originates in the SA node, high in the right atrium, and spreads leftward through the left atrium and downward toward the AV node low in the right atrium, as indicated in Figure 6.7. The electrical impulse then enters the ventricles via the AV node, passes through the His bundle and into both bundle branches simultaneously. The left bundle branch sprouts some Purkinje fibers high in the left side of the septum and begins activating the septum from left to right. Then the impulse spreads through the Purkinje system of both ventricles simultaneously and activates them from endocardium to epicardium. The base portion of both ventricles depolarizes last in a superior direction.

1. Septum activated from left to right.
2. Both ventricles activated from endocardium to epicardium.
3. Basal portion of both ventricles activated in superior direction.

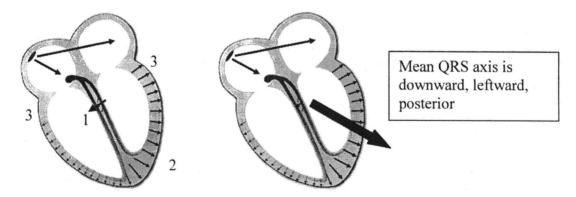

Figure 6.7: Mean QRS axis.

Mean QRS Axis

A vector is an electrical force that has both magnitude and direction. The millions of electrical forces in the heart travel in three dimensions simultaneously, and about 85% of them cancel each other by traveling in opposite directions. If all the forces that travel through the ventricles (represented by small arrows in Figure 6.7) are averaged together, they travel downward, leftward, and posterior – resulting in a mean electrical axis represented by the large arrow.

12 Lead Electrocardiography

THE 12 VIEWS OF THE HEART

The normal sequence of depolarization through the heart and the resulting P, QRS, and T waves for each frontal plane lead are illustrated in Figure 6.8. Leads I and AVL, with their positive electrode (camera lens) on the left side of the body, record leftward electrical activity as an upright P wave because the positive electrode sees atrial depolarization coming toward it. Leads II, III, and AVF, with their positive electrode at the bottom of the heart, record the downward spread of atrial activity as upright P waves for the same reason. Lead AVR, with its positive electrode on the right shoulder, sees the electrical activity moving away from it and records a negative P wave.

The QRS complex is recorded as the ventricles depolarize. Leads I and AVL, with their positive electrodes on the left side of the body, see the septum depolarizing away from them in a left-to-right direction and record a small negative deflection (Q wave). They then see the large left ventricular free wall depolarizing toward them and record an upright deflection (R wave). Leads II, III, and AVF, with their positive electrodes at the bottom of the heart, may not see septal activity at all and not record any deflection as the septum depolarizes. If these leads see septal activity coming slightly toward them, they record a positive deflection. They all then see the forces moving downward through the left ventricle toward them and record an upright deflection (R wave). Lead AVR, positive on the right shoulder, sees all activity moving away from it and records a negative deflection (QS complex).

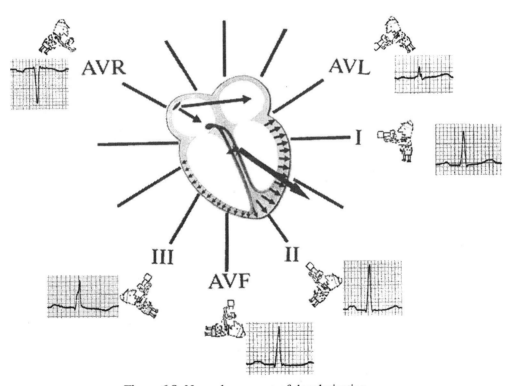

Figure 6.8: Normal sequence of depolarization.

The six precordial leads record electrical activity traveling in the horizontal plane. Figure 6.9 illustrates the position of the precordial leads and how they record electrical activity as it spreads through the ventricles in the horizontal plane. Lead V_1 is located on the front of the chest and records a small R wave as the septum depolarizes toward it from left to right. It then records a deep S wave as depolarization spreads away from it through the thick left ventricle. As the positive electrode is moved across the precordium from the V_1 to the V_6 position, it records progressively more left ventricular forces, and the R wave gets progressively larger. Lead V₆ is located on the left side of the chest and usually records a small Q wave as the septum depolarizes from left to right away from the positive electrode, and a large R wave as electrical activity spreads toward the positive electrode through the thick left ventricle. Normal R wave progression means that the R wave gets progressively larger from V₁ to V₆, or that V₆ is predominantly an R wave compared with V₁, which is predominantly an S wave. Sometimes the largest precordial R wave is recorded in lead V₄ or V₅, which is a normal variant.

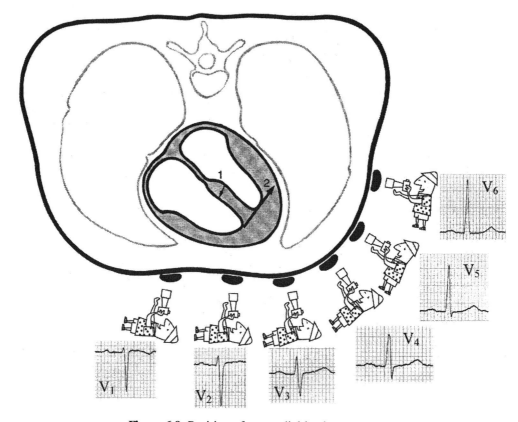

Figure 6.9: Position of precordial leads.

FRONTAL PLANE AXIS

All six frontal plane leads intersecting in the center form the *hexaxial reference system* that is used to describe the mean electrical axis. In Figure 6.10, each lead is labeled at its positive end to make it easy to remember where the positive electrode is. The hexaxial reference system (also called the "axis wheel") forms a circle with 180 positive degrees and 180 negative degrees divided into 30 degree increments. The heart's electrical axis is described in terms of degrees for the sake of consistency.

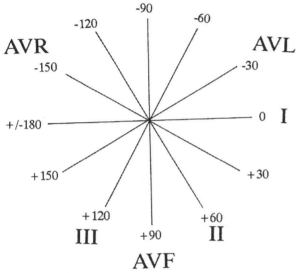

Figure 6.10: Hexaxial reference system.

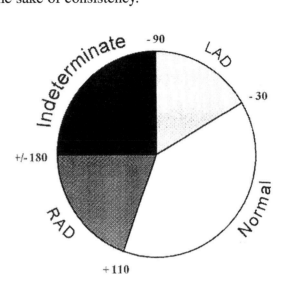

Figure 6.11: Definitions of QRS axis.

The *normal QRS axis* is defined as -30 to +110 degrees because most of the electrical forces in a normal heart are directed downward and leftward toward the large left ventricle. *Left axis deviation* is defined as -31 to -90 degrees and occurs when most of the forces move in a leftward and superior direction. *Right axis deviation* is defined as +110 to +180 degrees and occurs when most of the forces move rightward. When most of the forces are directed superior and rightward between -90 and -180 degrees, the term *indeterminate axis* is used. Figure 6.11 illustrates these definitions of QRS axis.

Potential Causes of Axis Deviation
- Bundle branch block.
- Ventricular hypertrophy.
- Myocardial infarction.
- Dextrocardia.
- Ventricular rhythms.
- WPW syndrome.
- FASCICULAR BLOCKS (always cause axis deviation).

Determining the QRS Axis

The mean frontal plane QRS axis can be determined in a number of ways. The most accurate method is to average the forces moving right and left with those moving up and down because this represents the frontal plane. Because lead I is the most direct right/left lead and lead AVF is the most direct up/down lead, it is easiest to use these two perpendicular leads to calculate the mean axis. On the axis wheel in

Figure 6.12, lead I and AVF are marked with small lines that represent the small 1 mV boxes on the vertical axis of the ECG paper.

The QRS axis is the average of the electrical forces traveling right-left and those traveling up-down.

Lead I is the pure right-left lead.
AVF is the pure up-down lead.

It is easiest to use these two leads to calculate the QRS axis.

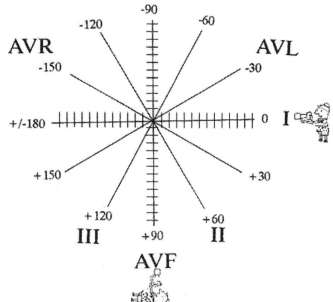

Figure 6.12: QRS axis.

To determine the QRS axis, follow these steps: (use the frontal plane leads shown in Figure 6.13 on the next page).

1. Look at lead I – count the number of positive and negative boxes on the QRS complex. Mark the net vector along the appropriate end of the lead I axis on the axis wheel (toward the positive end if the QRS is mainly upright; toward the negative end if it is mainly negative).
2. Look at lead AVF and repeat the above process. Note that if the QRS is upright in AVF you need to count boxes <u>down</u> (toward the positive end) on AVF. If the QRS is negative in AVF, you count boxes <u>up</u> on AVF.
3. Draw a perpendicular line from the marked spots on the leads I and AVF axis.
4. Draw a line from the center of the reference system to the spot where the two perpendicular lines meet. This is the QRS axis.

> Don't worry about being off by a box or so when you count those tiny little boxes. It won't change the axis significantly. However, you do need to count toward the correct pole on the lead (positive end if the QRS is mostly upright, negative end if the QRS is mostly negative) because if you go the wrong way, the axis will be WAY OFF!

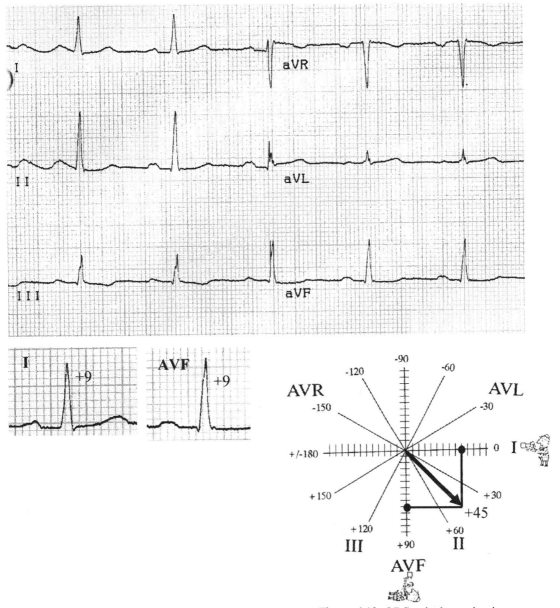

Figure 6.13: QRS axis determination.

In this example (Figure 6.13), lead I has an R wave that is 9 mm tall and such a tiny S wave that we won't even count it. The net vector is plus 9, so count 9 boxes towards the positive end of lead I on the axis wheel and place a dot there.

AVF also has an R wave that is 9 boxes tall and a tiny Q wave that we will ignore. The net vector is plus 9, so count 9 boxes toward the positive end of AVF and place a dot there.

Draw a perpendicular line down from the dot on lead I and across from the dot on AVF. Connect the center of the axis wheel to the place where those two lines meet – that is the axis. Is an axis of +45 degrees normal? (Yes).

Chapter 6

Using the same method, calculate the axis on the ECG in Figure 6.14.

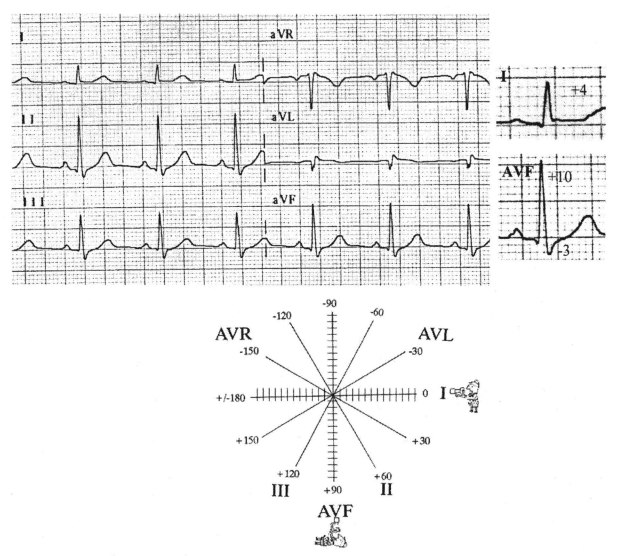

Figure 6.14: QRS axis determination.

> *Don't read the answer until you have tried it yourself!*
>
> In this example (Figure 6.14), lead I has an R wave that is about 4 boxes tall and no negative component at all. So count 4 boxes toward the positive end of lead I and place your dot.
>
> AVF has a Q wave that is 1 box deep and an S wave that is 2 boxes deep, so add them together and call it a -3. There is also an R wave that is 10 boxes tall, so the net vector is +7. Count 7 boxes toward the positive end of AVF and place your dot.
>
> Draw your perpendicular lines and connect the center of the wheel to the place where the two lines meet. Did you get close to +60 degrees? Is that normal? (Yes).
>
> *Pretty simple, isn't it?*

Let's do one more *(no cheating! Do it before you read the answer!)*:

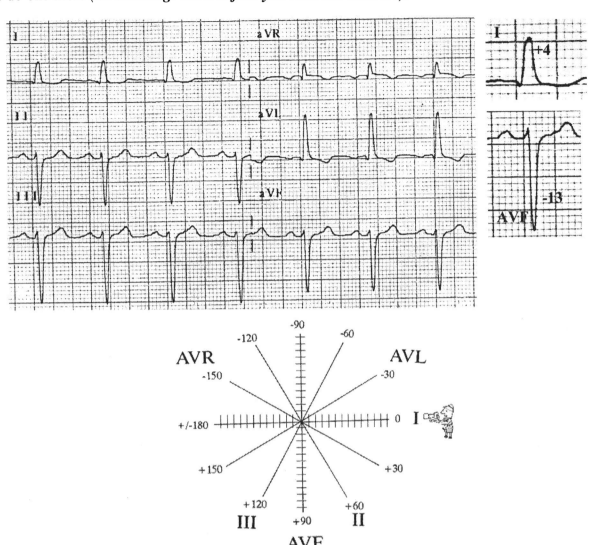

Figure 6.15: QRS axis determination.

This one (Figure 6.15), is a little trickier. Lead I has a small Q wave that is 1 box negative and an R wave that is 5 boxes tall, so the net vector is +4. Count 4 boxes toward the positive end of lead I on the wheel and place your dot.

AVF has a small R wave that is barely over 1 box tall, so let's call it +1. There is also an S wave that is 14 boxes deep, so the net vector is -13 (+1 -14 = -13). Count 13 boxes toward the negative end of AVF (that's UP) and place your dot.

Draw your perpendiculars and connect their meeting place with the center of the wheel. Did you get about -70 degrees or so? This is left axis deviation (LAD) due to anterior fascicular block (you'll learn about that later).

239

Chapter 6

Quick Method of Axis Determination ("Cheating 101")

Figure 6.16 illustrates a quick way to place the axis in the appropriate quadrant. This method is not as accurate as counting boxes, but it is good enough for most situations.

- Look at lead I and AVF and mentally place Lead I on top of AVF.
- If both QRS complexes are upright, the axis is normal.
- If the QRS complexes point together (I is negative and AVF is positive), the axis is in the right quadrant.
- If the QRS complexes point apart (I is positive and AVF is negative), the axis is in the left quadrant.
- If both QRS complexes are negative, the axis is in the indeterminate zone.

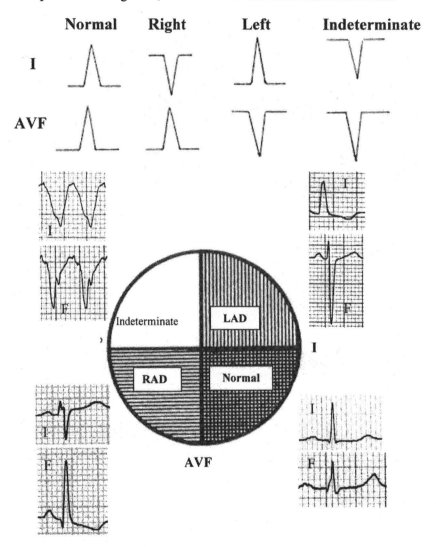

Figure 6.16: Axis determination.

Linking Knowledge to Practice

✔ *The ability to quickly determine QRS axis can help in the differential diagnosis of wide QRS tachycardias. An indeterminate QRS axis strongly favors VT as the cause of a wide QRS tachycardia. If you have the ability to monitor multiple leads at the bedside, using leads I and aVF allows you to quickly recognize axis deviations.*

AXIS PRACTICE *(answers at end of chapter)*

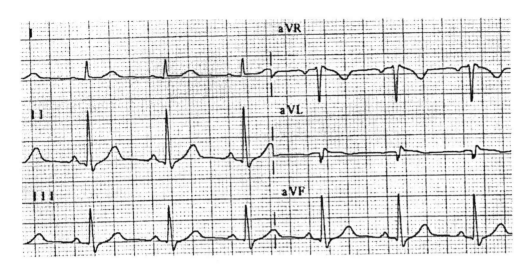

Axis Practice 1

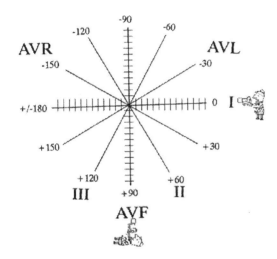
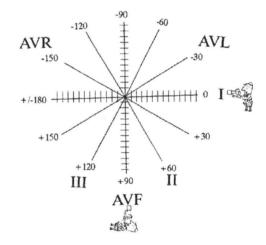

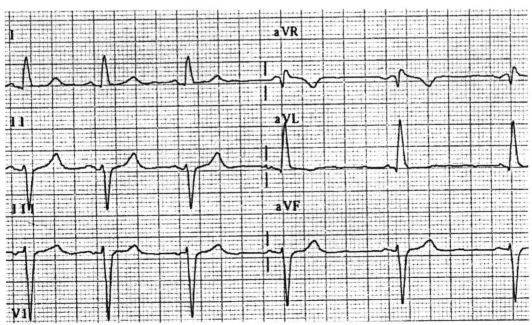

Axis Practice 2

Chapter 6

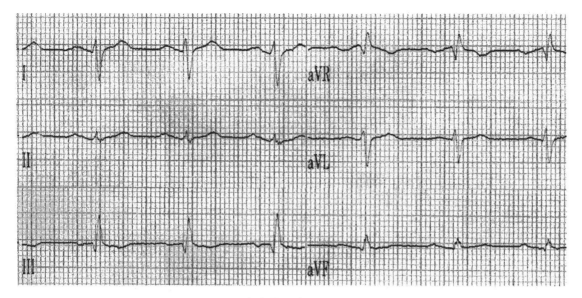

Axis Practice 3

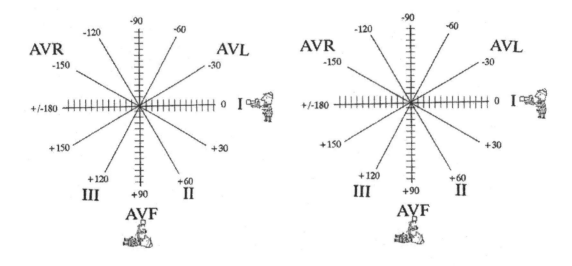

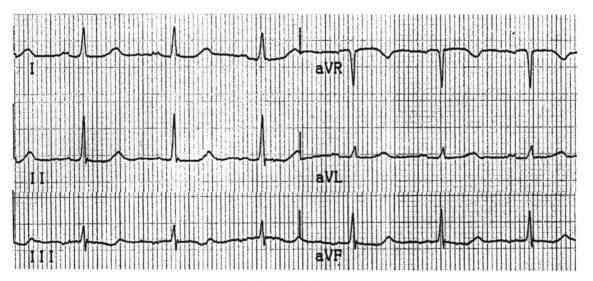

Axis Practice 4

242

BUNDLE BRANCH BLOCK

Bundle branch block is characterized by delay of excitation to one ventricle and abnormal spread of excitation through the ventricle whose bundle is blocked.

ECG characteristics of bundle branch block:

- V_1 and V_6 are the most useful chest leads.
- I and AVL are the most useful limb leads.
- QRS duration .12 sec or more.
- T waves should be directed opposite terminal QRS vector.

Normal ventricular depolarization as recorded by leads V_1 and V_6 is illustrated in Figure 6.17. The positive electrode for V_1 is located on the front of the chest at the fourth intercostal space to the right of the sternum, close to the right ventricle. The positive electrode for V_6 is located in the left mid-axillary line at the fifth intercostal space, close to the left ventricle. Lead V_1 records a small R wave as the septum depolarizes from left to right toward the positive electrode. It then records a negative deflection (S wave) as the main forces travel away from the positive electrode toward the left ventricle, resulting in the normal rS complex in V_1. Lead V_6 may record a small Q wave as the septum depolarizes left to right away from the positive electrode. It then records a tall R wave as the main forces travel toward the left ventricle, resulting in the normal qR complex in V_6. When both ventricles depolarize together, the QRS width is less than 0.12 second.

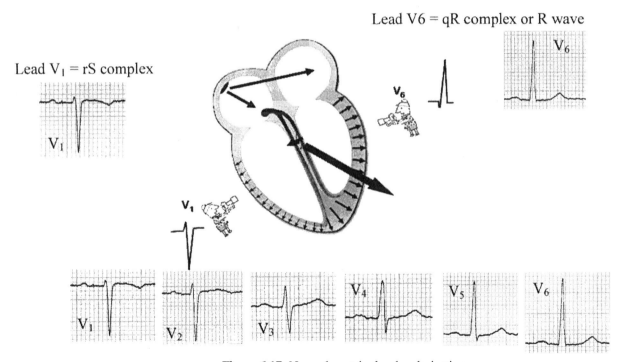

Figure 6.17: Normal ventricular depolarization.

Normal R wave progression across the precordium = r wave gradually gets larger as leads move closer to left ventricle.

Right Bundle Branch Block

Figure 6.18 illustrates the spread of electrical forces in the ventricles when the right bundle branch is blocked. Three separate forces occur:

1. Septal activation occurs first from left to right, resulting in the normal small R wave in V_1 and small Q wave in V_6.
2. The left ventricle is activated next through the normally functioning left bundle branch. Depolarization spreads normally through the Purkinje fibers in the left ventricle, causing an S wave in V_1 as the impulse travels away from its positive electrode, and an R wave in V_6 as the impulse travels toward the positive electrode in V_6.
3. The right ventricle depolarizes late and abnormally as the impulse spreads by cell-to-cell conduction through the right ventricle. This abnormal activation causes a wide second R wave (called R') in V_1 as it travels toward the positive electrode in V_1, and a wide S wave in V_6 as it travels away from the positive electrode in V_6. Because muscle cell-to-cell conduction is much slower than conduction through the Purkinje system, the QRS complex widens to 0.12 second or greater.

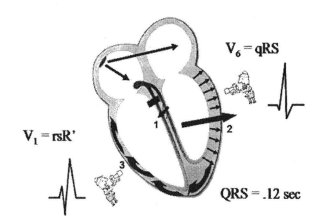

Figure 6.18: Electrical forces in blocked right bundle branch.

- Lead V_1 = rsR' complex (or a variant):
- r = septum.
- s = left ventricle.
- R' = late right ventricular depolarization.

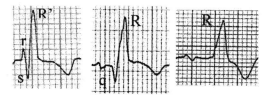

- Lead V_6 = qRS complex:
- Q = septum (not always present).
- R = left ventricle.
- S = late right ventricular depolarization.

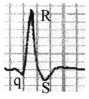

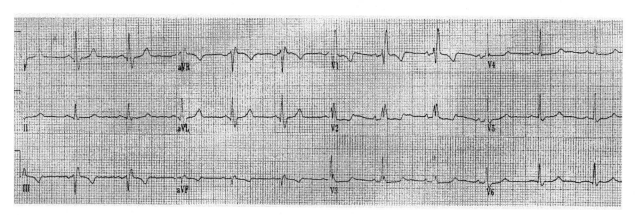

Left Bundle Branch Block

Figure 6.19 illustrates the spread of electrical forces through the ventricles when the left bundle branch is blocked. In LBBB, the septum does not depolarize in its normal left-to-right direction because the block occurs above the Purkinje fibers that normally activate the left side of the septum. This causes the loss of the normal small R wave in V_1 and loss of the Q wave in V_6, lead I, and AVL. Two main forces occur in LBBB:

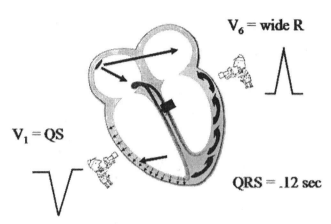

Figure 6.19: Electrical forces in blocked left bundle branch.

1. The right ventricle is activated first through its Purkinje fibers. Because the right ventricular free wall is so much thinner than the left ventricle, forces traveling through it are often not recorded in V_1. Sometimes a small, narrow R wave is recorded in V_1 during LBBB, and this is most likely the result of forces traveling through the right ventricular free wall.
2. The left ventricle depolarizes late and abnormally as the impulse spreads by cell-to-cell conduction through the thick left ventricle. This causes V_1 to record a wide negative QS complex as the impulse travels away from its positive electrode. The lateral leads V_6, I, and AVL record a wide R wave as the impulse travels through the large left ventricle toward their positive electrodes. The QRS widens to 0.12 second or greater due to the slow cell-to-cell conduction in the left ventricle.

◆ Lead V_1 = QS complex (may see rS complex)

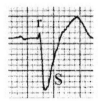

◆ Lead V_6 = wide R

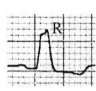

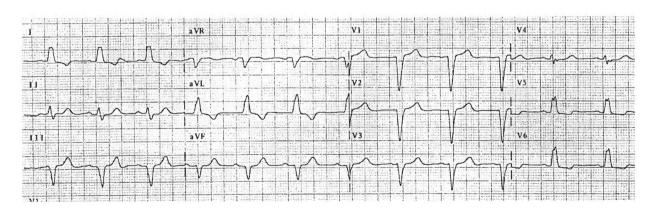

Chapter 6

Bundle Branch Block Practice *(answers at end of chapter)*

1.
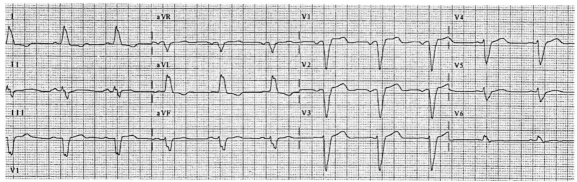

2.
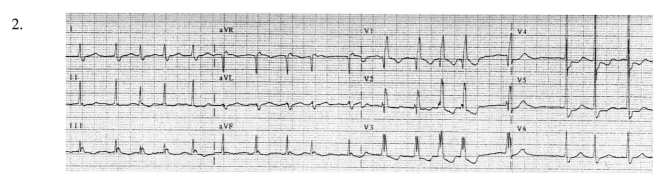

3.
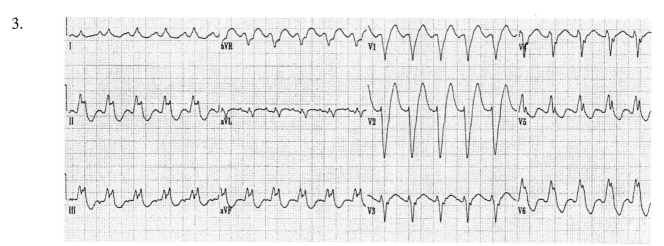

4.
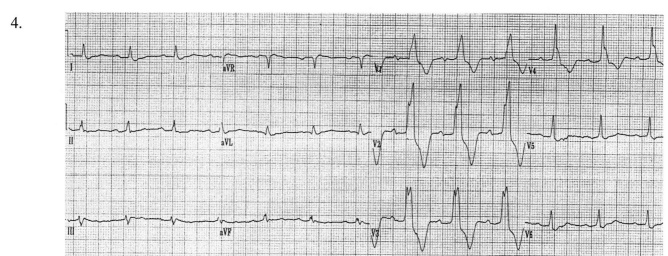

Fascicular Blocks (Hemiblocks)

The term *fascicular block* or *hemiblock* is used to describe block in either division of the left bundle branch. In fascicular block, both ventricles depolarize simultaneously so the QRS remains narrow, but the direction of left ventricular depolarization is altered. The most useful ECG leads for recognizing fascicular block are leads I and AVF for the axis, and leads I and III for the typical pattern of fascicular block.

Figure 6.20 illustrates the normal intraventricular conduction system and the relationship between the anterior and posterior divisions of the left bundle. The posterior fascicle is much thicker than the anterior fascicle and has two blood supplies, making it much more difficult to block. Anterior fascicular block is much more common than posterior fascicular block.

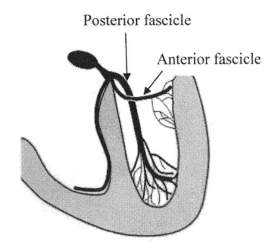

Figure 6.20: Normal intraventricular conduction system.

Figure 6.21 illustrates normal left ventricular activation through both fascicles simultaneously. When the left ventricular free wall is activated normally, the anterior fascicle carries the electrical impulse in a superior and leftward direction and the posterior fascicle carries it downward and rightward (dark arrows in Figure 6.21). Because free wall activation proceeds in both directions simultaneously, most of the forces cancel each other and result in the normal QRS shape seen in leads I and III and a normal QRS axis, as the combined forces proceed downward and leftward through the left ventricle (white arrow in Figure 6.21). When fascicular block occurs, left ventricular activation proceeds from one site instead of both simultaneously, removing the cancellation and altering the shape of the QRS in leads I and III. Because the left ventricle is depolarized in an abnormal direction, an axis deviation always results from fascicular block.

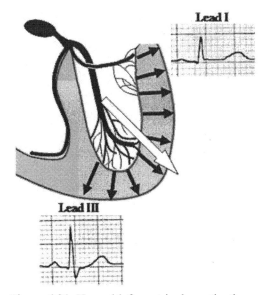

Figure 6.21: Normal left ventricular activation through both fascicles.

Left Anterior Fascicular Block (LAFB)

In LAFB (also called *anterior hemiblock*), the impulse conducts through the posterior fascicle and begins depolarizing the ventricle in an inferior and rightward direction, as illustrated by the dark arrows in Figure 6.22. It then travels through the left ventricular free wall in a superior and leftward direction (white arrows), resulting in a left axis deviation. The degree of left axis deviation required to diagnose LAFB is controversial, but most sources state that the axis should be at least -45 degrees. The initial forces are directed inferiorly and rightward, resulting in a small Q wave in lead I and a small R wave in lead III. The forces then travel superiorly and leftward, causing a normal R wave in lead I and an abnormally deep S wave in lead III. There may or may not be a Q wave in lead I.

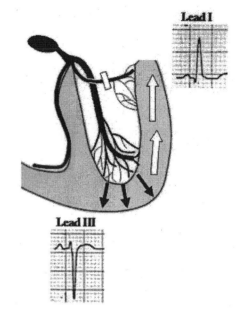

The ECG characteristics of LAFB are:

- Left axis deviation (-45 degrees or more).
- Small Q in lead I, large S in lead III (QI, SIII), or an rS pattern in II, III, AVF.
- QRS duration not prolonged more than 0.11 second.
- Increased QRS voltage in limb leads due to loss of cancellation of forces in left ventricle.

Figure 6.22: Left anterior fascicular block (LAFB)

Below is an illustration of frontal plane leads showing left axis deviation (-70). There is a tiny Q in lead I, a deep S in lead III (QI, SIII), and an rS complex in II, III, and AVF. This is LAFB.

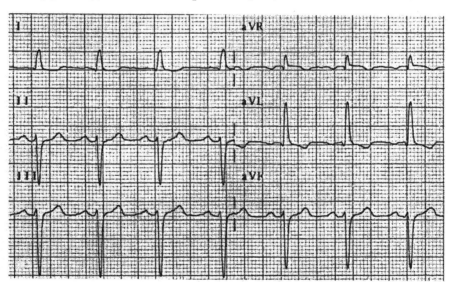

Left Posterior Fascicular Block (LPFB)

In LPFB (also called *posterior hemiblock*), the impulse conducts through the anterior fascicle and begins depolarizing the ventricle in a superior and leftward direction (Figure 6.23). It then travels through the left ventricular free wall in an inferior and rightward direction, resulting in a right axis deviation. The initial forces are directed superiorly and leftward, causing a small R wave in lead I and a small Q wave in lead III. The forces then travel inferiorly and rightward, causing a deep S wave in lead I and a tall R wave in lead III. Before diagnosing LPFB, we must rule out right ventricular hypertrophy (RVH) because RVH can cause the identical frontal plane picture.

The ECG characteristics of LPFB are:

- Right axis deviation (>110 degrees).
- Small R in lead I and AVL, small Q in II, III, AVF (SI, QIII), or an rS pattern in leads I and AVL.
- Normal QRS duration (not >0.11 second).
- Increased QRS voltage due to loss of cancellation of QRS forces.
- No evidence of RVH (this is discussed later in the chapter).

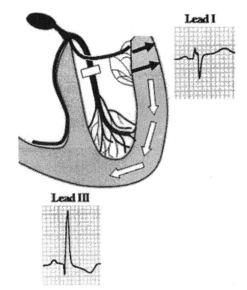

Figure 6.23: Left posterior fascicular block (LPFB).

In this ECG, there is right axis deviation (about +130 degrees). There is an rS in lead I and a tiny Q in lead III (SI, QIII). There is no R wave in V$_1$ or V$_2$, probably due to prior septal infarction, but R wave progression across the rest of the precordial leads is normal, ruling out RVH. This is LPFB.

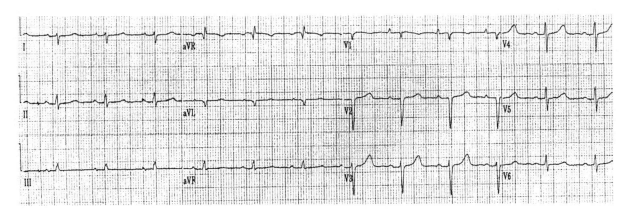

Linking Knowledge to Practice

✔ *Hemiblock always causes an axis deviation but does not widen the QRS complex. Bundle branch block always widens the QRS but rarely causes an axis deviation. If you see a wide QRS and an axis deviation together, suspect RBBB with a hemiblock (called bifascicular block). This combination can indicate more serious conduction system disease with the potential for development of complete heart block. Be prepared to pace!*

Chapter 6

CHAMBER ENLARGEMENT

Atria and ventricles can enlarge due to either dilation (response to volume overload) or hypertrophy (response to pressure overload). Both conditions result in chamber enlargement which can be recognized on the ECG, but the ECG changes do not differentiate between dilation and hypertrophy. Therefore, the term "enlargement" is usually used rather than the older term "hypertrophy."

Atrial enlargement is reflected on the ECG as changes in P wave size and morphology. Normal P waves are no wider than 0.11 second or taller than 2.5 mm. They are usually upright in leads I, II, and V_{4-6}, and biphasic with the initial portion upright and the terminal portion negative in V_1. Right atrial depolarization forms the first half of the P wave; left atrial depolarization forms the second half.

Normal P Wave (Figure 6.24)

- Upright in I, II, AVF, V_{4-6}.
- Inverted in AVR.
- May be biphasic or inverted in other leads.
- Width 0.11 sec or less.
- Height 2.5 mm or less.

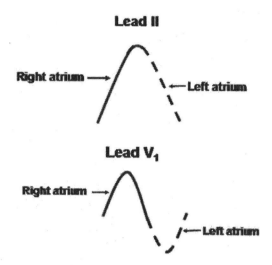

Figure 6.24: Normal P wave.

Right Atrial Enlargement (P Pulmonale)

Right atrial enlargement (RAE) is commonly caused by conditions that increase the work of the right atrium, such as pulmonary hypertension, pulmonary or tricuspid stenosis or regurgitation, and congenital heart disease. P waves in RAE have the following characteristics (Figure 6.25):

- Taller than 2.5 mm in II, III, AVF (taller in III than in I).
- Peaked or pointed.
- Width is normal.
- Biphasic with increased voltage of initial component in V_1, V_2.

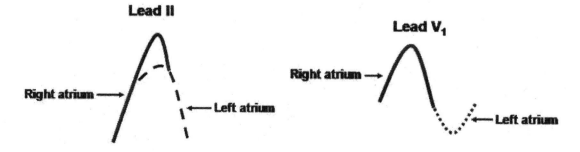

Figure 6.25: Right atrial enlargement (RAE) (P Pulmonale).

Left Atrial Enlargement (P Mitrale)

Left atrial enlargement (LAE) is caused by conditions that increase pressure or volume in the left atrium, such as mitral stenosis, mitral regurgitation, systemic hypertension, and left heart failure. P waves in LAE have the following characteristics (Figure 6.26):

◆ Notched or M shaped in several leads (taller in I than in III).
◆ Interval between the notches is .04 sec or more.
◆ Wider than 0.11 sec.
◆ Biphasic in V_1 with deep terminal component.

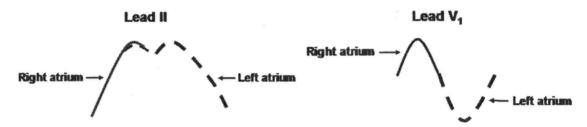

Figure 6.26: Left atrial enlargement (LAE) (P Mitrale).

Biatrial enlargement occurs when both atria become enlarged. It is sometimes seen in mitral valve disease, atrial septal defect, multiple valvular defects, and biventricular failure. Biatrial enlargement is manifested on the ECG in the following ways:

◆ The P wave is taller than 2.5 mm and wider than 0.11 second in lead II.
◆ P waves may be notched.
◆ Both the positive and negative components of the P wave in V_1 may be enlarged.

Figure 6.27 compares normal and abnormal P waves due to atrial enlargement.

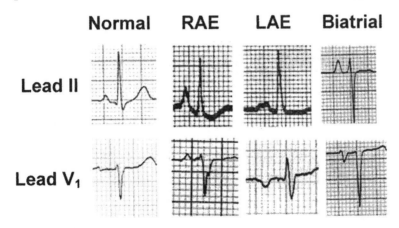

Figure 6.27: Normal and abnormal P waves in atrial enlargement.

Chapter 6

Ventricular Enlargement

The ventricles can enlarge because of increased pressure or volume in the chamber. Ventricular enlargement affects the size of the QRS complex and often causes ST segment and T wave changes and axis deviation as well.

ST-T "Strain" Pattern

In ventricular hypertrophy, leads facing the enlarged ventricle often show ST-T wave changes described as a "strain" pattern. The ST segment may become depressed with an upward convexity, and T waves invert asymmetrically. This "strain" pattern can be seen in leads I, AVL, V_5, V_6 with left ventricular hypertrophy (LVH), and in leads V_1 and V_2 with RVH (Figure 6.28).

Intrinsicoid deflection (measured from beginning of QRS to peak of R wave) is a measure of ventricular activation time and reflects the time required for peak voltage to develop under a lead. A normal intrinsicoid deflection (ID) is less than 0.04 sec. In ventricular hypertrophy, the ID is prolonged to 0.05 sec or more in leads facing the large ventricle (V_{5-6} in LVH; V_{1-2} in RVH).

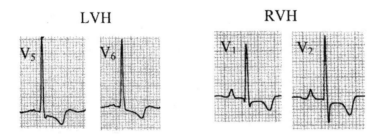

Figure 6.28: ST-T "Strain" pattern (LVH and RVH).

Left Ventricular Enlargement

When the left ventricle hypertrophies, the thicker wall causes increased amplitude (voltage) of the R wave in leads facing the left ventricle (I, AVL, V_5, V_6), and a corresponding increase in the S wave in leads closest to the right ventricle (V_1, V_2). The axis is often, but not always, deviated toward the left. Causes of LVH include chronic hypertension (most common), aortic stenosis or insufficiency, and hypertrophic cardiomyopathy.

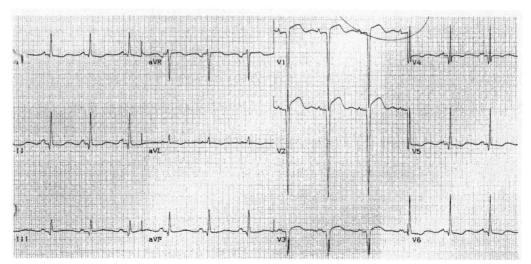

12 Lead Electrocardiography

Right Ventricular Enlargement

When the right ventricle enlarges, normal left ventricular dominance is decreased, and eventually if the RV becomes larger than the left, rightward forces predominate in the precordial leads. This results in a reversal of the normal precordial R wave pattern, causing large R waves in V_1 and V_2 and deep S waves in the LV leads (V_5, V_6). The axis is often deviated to the right (greater than +110 degrees). Causes of RVH include mitral valve disease, COPD, Cor Pulmonale, pulmonic stenosis, and tricuspid insufficiency.

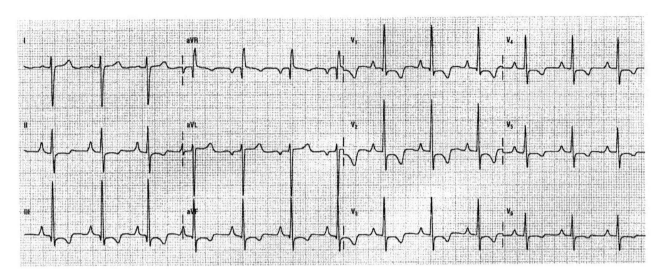

Figure 6.29 compares the normal QRS to changes that occur with RVH and LVH.

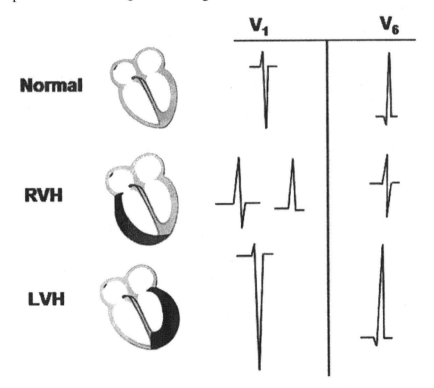

Figure 6.29: Comparison of normal QRS to changes with RVH and LVH.

Chapter 6

CHAMBER ENLARGEMENT PRACTICE

On the following ECGs, can you identify enlargement of any of the chambers? (Answers at end of chapter.)

1.
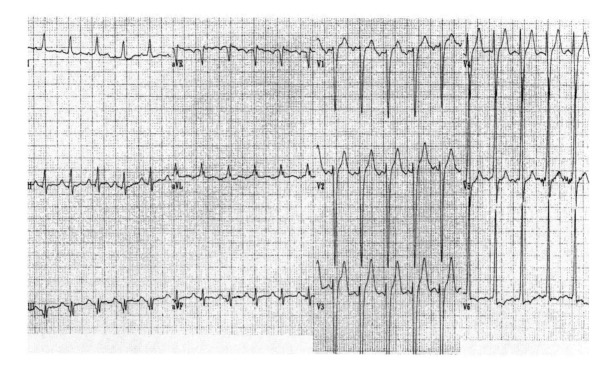

2.
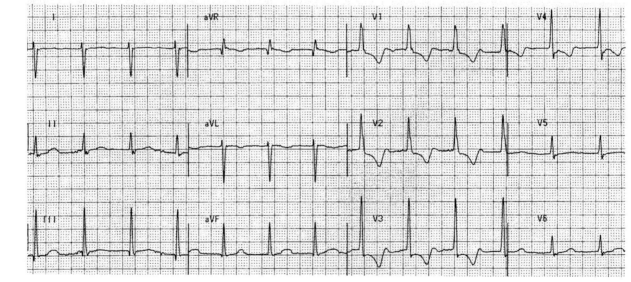

12 Lead Electrocardiography

3.

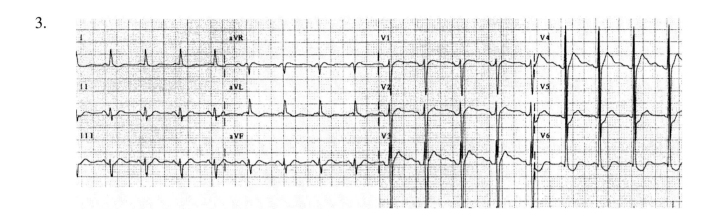

4.

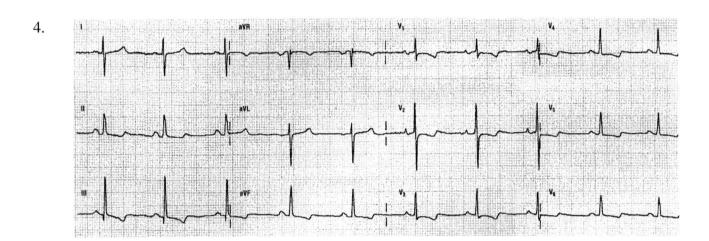

5.

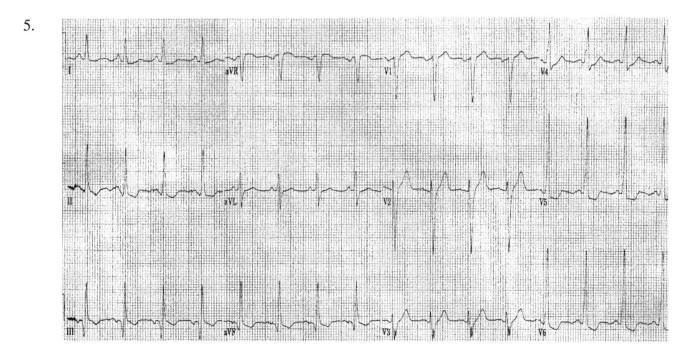

Chapter 6

PREEXCITATION SYNDROMES

Preexcitation refers to early activation of the ventricular myocardium by a supraventricular impulse entering the ventricles through an accessory pathway (AP). An AP (also called a *bypass tract*) is a tract of tissue that is capable of carrying the impulse from the atrium directly into the ventricle, bypassing all or part of the normal AV conduction system. The most common AP is an AV bypass tract, the bundle of Kent, which originates in the atrium and inserts in the ventricle, bypassing the entire conduction system. These pathways can be located anywhere around the tricuspid or mitral valve ring; the most frequent location is left lateral free wall. Other accessory pathways include AV nodal bypass tracts, which carry the impulse from the atrium into the distal AV node or from the atrium to the His bundle (*James fibers*), and nodoventricular connections, which originate in or below the AV node and carry the impulse directly into the ventricular myocardium (*Mahaim fibers*). All of these bypass tracts have the potential to cause atrioventricular re-entrant tachycardias (AVRT). The most common type of preexcitation syndrome is Wolff-Parkinson-White (WPW) syndrome, in which the impulse is transmitted down the bundle of Kent directly from the atrium into the ventricles, bypassing the AV node.

Wolff-Parkinson-White Syndrome

In WPW, during sinus rhythm, the ventricle is stimulated prematurely through the Kent bundle while the impulse is simultaneously conducted through the normal AV node and His-Purkinje system (see Figure 6.30A). Impulses travel faster down the AP because they bypass the normal AV node delay. Part of the ventricle receives the impulse early through the accessory pathway and begins to depolarize before the rest of the ventricle is activated through the normal conduction system. Early stimulation of the ventricle results in a short PR interval and a widened QRS complex as the impulse begins to depolarize the ventricle through muscle cell-to-cell conduction. Premature ventricular stimulation forms a characteristic slurring of the initial portion of the QRS complex, called a *delta wave*. The remainder of the QRS complex is normal because the rest of the ventricle is then activated normally through the Purkinje system. This type of preexcitation results in ventricular fusion beats as the ventricles are depolarized simultaneously by the impulse coming through the AP and through the AV node.

The degree of preexcitation varies depending on the relative rates of conduction through the AP and the AV node. Maximal preexcitation (Figure 6.30B) occurs when the ventricles are activated totally by the AP, resulting in an extremely short PR interval and uniformly wide QRS complex. Less than maximal preexcitation occurs when the impulse enters the ventricle through both pathways simultaneously, and the length of the PR interval and size of delta wave depend on how much of the ventricle is depolarized through the AP. A concealed pathway (Figure 6.30C) is present when the ventricles are depolarized exclusively through the normal conduction system, even though a bypass tract exists. In this case, the PR interval and QRS complex are normal because the AP is not being used for anterograde conduction.

256

12 Lead Electrocardiography

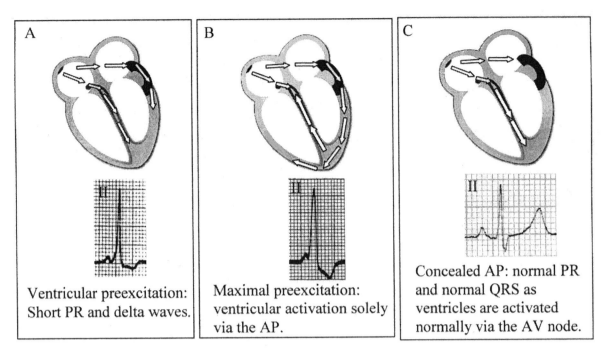

Figure 6.30: Wolff-Parkinson-White Syndrome.

The following ECG illustrates WPW with short PR interval and delta waves in most leads. The delta wave is negative in III, AVR, and V_1. A negative V_1, previously called Type B WPW, indicates a right-sided or anteroseptal AP.

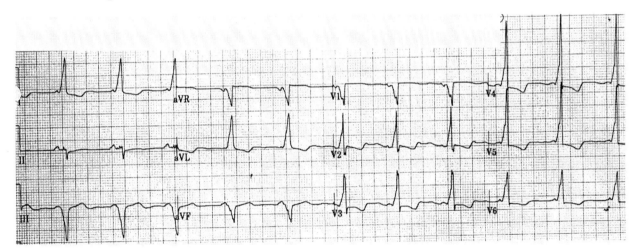

In this ECG, short PR and delta waves are present in most leads. A positive V_1, once called Type A WPW, indicates a left-sided or posterior AP.

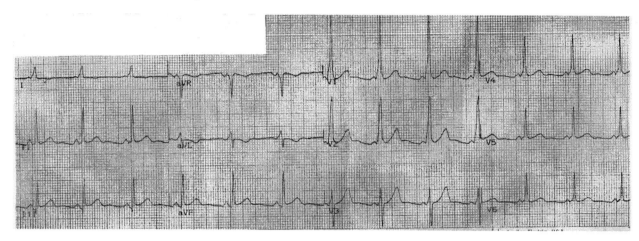

WPW is clinically significant because the presence of two pathways provides the opportunity for re-entry of the impulse and may result in rapid re-entrant tachycardias. When tachycardias accompany the WPW pattern described above, the term WPW Syndrome is used. The most commonly occurring tachy-arrhythmia in WPW is atrioventricular re-entrant tachycardia (AVRT), also called circus movement tachycardia (CMT) by some authors, and accounts for about 80% of tachycardias in patients with WPW syndrome. Refer to Chapter 5 for more information on SVTs seen with WPW.

Atrial fibrillation and atrial flutter that occur in the presence of an AP are particularly dangerous because of the extremely rapid ventricular rate that can result from conduction of the atrial impulses directly into the ventricle through the bypass track. The ventricular rate can be exceptionally fast and can deteriorate into ventricular fibrillation, resulting in sudden death. Atrial fibrillation conducting to the ventricle over an AP presents as a rapid, irregular, wide QRS rhythm and must be differentiated from the usual atrial fibrillation that conducts through the AV node. The following ECGs show atrial fibrillation conducting to the ventricle over an AP. The irregular ventricular response helps to differentiate this from VT. Note that occasional narrow beats are present when the AP tires and gives the AV node a chance to conduct. See Chapter 5 for more information about atrial fibrillation and WPW.

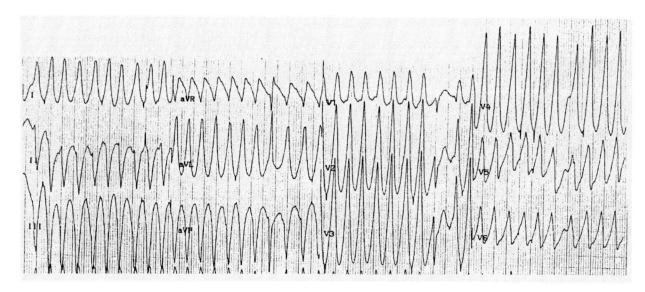

Whenever the ventricular rate approaches 300, as it does in these two examples, suspect an AP.

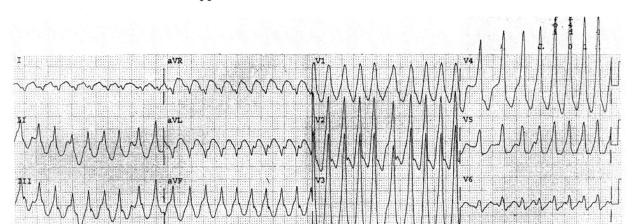

ISCHEMIA, INJURY AND INFARCTION

Myocardial ischemia is the result of an imbalance between myocardial O_2 supply and demand and is a reversible process if blood flow is restored before permanent cellular damage occurs. If blood flow is not restored in a timely manner, cellular injury and eventually necrosis (cell death) result. The term Acute Coronary Syndrome (ACS) is used to refer to the pathophysiological continuum that begins with plaque rupture in a coronary artery and eventually results in permanent cell damage (infarction) if the process is not arrested. ACS encompasses three distinct phases of this continuum: 1) unstable angina (UA), 2) non-ST elevation MI (NSTEMI), and 3) ST elevation MI (STEMI). Once an infarction has occurred, as indicated by elevated biochemical cardiac markers, it is classified electrocardiographically as either a Q wave or a non-Q wave MI based on the presence or absence of Q waves on the ECG.

The degree of cell damage in MI ranges from ischemia to injury to cell death (necrosis). This has traditionally been described as three "zones" of tissue damage, each of which produces distinctive changes on the ECG, as illustrated in Figure 6.32. *Transmural MI* means that the entire thickness of the wall from endocardium to epicardium is involved, and *subendocardial MI* means that only the endocardial area is affected. In transmural MI, ST segment elevation, Q waves, and T wave inversion are recorded in leads facing the damaged myocardium, and are called the *indicative changes* of infarction. Other leads not facing the involved tissue are often affected by the loss of electrical forces in damaged tissue and record mirror-image changes called *reciprocal changes.*

Subendocardial infarction, also called non-Q wave myocardial infarction, has traditionally been considered to involve necrosis of the subendocardial layer of the ventricle and not the entire thickness of the ventricular wall. Necrosis of sufficient myocardium can lead to loss of R wave amplitude rather than to development of Q waves in leads facing the infarcted area. A non-Q wave MI usually presents with ST depression and T wave inversion in leads facing the infarcted area.

Most patients who present with ischemic chest pain and ST elevation ultimately develop a Q wave MI, while most patients with no ST elevation are experiencing either unstable angina or a NSTEMI. The distinction between UA and NSTEMI is made based on elevated cardiac markers in the blood. Most patients with NSTEMI do not develop Q waves on the ECG and are diagnosed as having a non-Q wave MI.

Serial ECGs reflect the progression of the infarction from the acute stage through the fully evolved stage. Very early MI often causes peaking and widening of the T waves, followed within minutes by ST segment elevation. ST segment elevation can persist for hours to several days but resolves more quickly with successful reperfusion. Once the ST segment has returned to baseline, ECG evidence of the acute stage is lost. Q waves appear within hours of pain onset and usually remain forever. T wave inversion occurs within hours after infarction, and T waves often return to their previous upright position within a few months after acute MI. An *evolving infarct* is one in which serial ECGs show ST segments returning toward baseline, the development of Q waves, and T wave inversion. The term *old infarction* or *infarct of undetermined age* is used when the first ECG recorded shows Q waves, ST segment at baseline, and T waves either inverted or upright, indicating that an MI occurred at some time in the past.

Distribution of Coronary Arteries

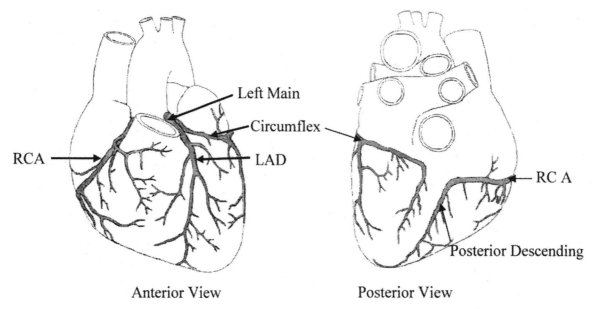

Figure 6.31: Distribution of coronary arteries.

Right Coronary Artery (RCA) supplies the following areas:
- Atria.
- Right ventricle.
- Inferior and posterior wall of left ventricle in 90% of people (right dominant circulation).
- Septum – posterior 1/3.
- Sinus node in 55-60% of people.
- AV node in 90% of people.
- His bundle in 90% of people.
- Right bundle branch – proximal few mm.
- Left bundle branch – part of posterior fascicle.
- Posterior papillary muscle – shares with LAD.

Left Anterior Descending (LAD) supplies the following areas:

- Anterior wall of left ventricle.
- Septum – anterior 2/3.
- Right bundle branch.
- Left bundle branch – anterior fascicle and part of posterior fascicle.
- Anterior papillary muscle.
- Posterior papillary muscle – shares with RCA.

In about 10% of people, the circumflex supplies the posterior and inferior walls of the left ventricle. This is called *left dominant circulation.*

Circumflex Artery supplies the following areas:

- Lateral wall of left ventricle.
- Sinus node in 40-45% of people.
- AV node in 10% of people.
- Posterior wall of left ventricle in 10% of people.

ECG Changes with Infarction

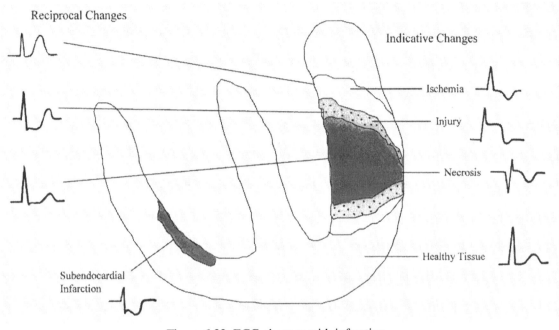

Figure 6.32: ECG changes with infarction.

Indicative changes are seen in leads facing injured myocardium:

- *Ischemia* = T wave inversion.
- *Injury* = ST elevation (1mm in two contiguous leads is significant).
- *Necrosis* = Q waves if transmural infarction (.04 sec duration and/or 25% of the height of the QRS complex).
- *Subendocardial infarction* = ST depression, T wave inversion, and loss of R wave height.
- *Right ventricular infarction* = indicative changes in right chest leads, especially V$_{4R}$.

Reciprocal changes are mirror image changes seen in leads not directly facing injured area.

- *Ischemia* = tall, wide-based T waves.
- *Injury* = ST depression.
- *Necrosis* = tall R waves.

Progressive changes of infarction:

◆ ST elevation usually seen first - appears within minutes of pain and can last 3-4 days. If ST elevation persists for weeks, it may indicate ventricular aneurysm.

◆ Q waves can appear immediately, but more commonly appear within hours of pain. Usually remain permanently.

◆ T wave inversion occurs within hours and can last for months. Can return upright or remain permanent.

Patterns of Ischemia:

The most familiar pattern of ischemia is T wave inversion, although T wave inversion is often a nonspecific finding and can be due to a variety of causes other than ischemia. Other indicators of ischemia include down sloping or horizontal ST segment depression of 0.5 mm or more; an ST segment that remains on the baseline longer than 0.12 second; an ST segment that forms a sharp angle with the upright T wave; tall, wide-based T waves; and inverted U waves. Figure 6.33 illustrates patterns of ischemia.

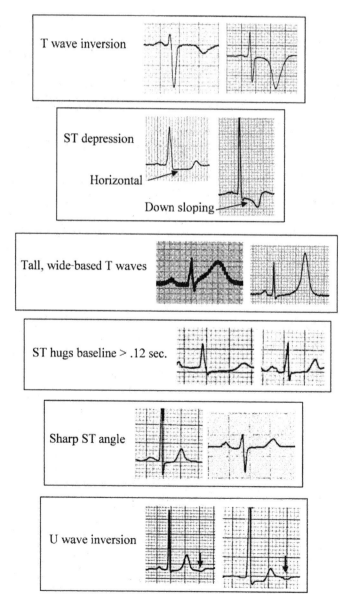

Figure 6.33: Patterns of ischemia.

Acute Injury Patterns:

Myocardial injury is most often indicated by ST segment elevation of 1 mm or more above the baseline. Other signs of acute injury include a straightening of the ST segment that slopes up to the peak of the T wave without spending any time on the baseline; tall, peaked T waves; and symmetric T wave inversion. Figure 6.34 illustrates patterns of injury.

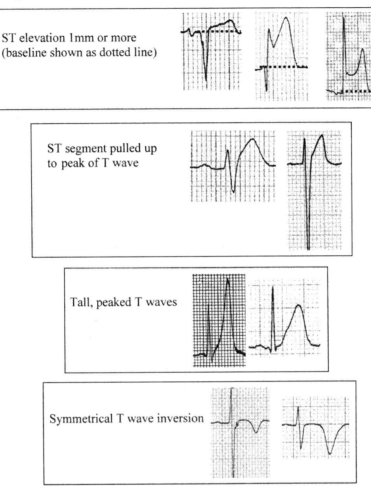

Figure 6.34: Patterns of injury.

Other causes of ST elevation or depression:

Bundle branch block	Myocardial metastases
Fascicular block (hemiblock)	Pancreatitis or acute abdomen
Early repolarization	Pericarditis
Hyperkalemia	Printzmetal's angina
Hypoglycemia	Cocaine vasospasm
Hyperventilation in patient with CAD	Ventricular hypertrophy
Hypothermia	WPW syndrome
Intracranial hemorrhage	Paced rhythm
Ventricular rhythms	Aberrancy
Ventricular aneurysm	Drugs (quinidine, digitalis)

Chapter 6

LOCATING THE INFARCTION ON THE 12 LEAD ECG

12 Lead Views of the Heart

- Lateral wall = I, AVL, V5-6 (high lateral = I, AVL; low lateral = V5, V6).
- Inferior wall = II, III, AVF.
- Anterior wall = V1-V4.
- Septum = V1, V2.
- Posterior wall = reciprocal changes in V1-V2 (sometimes to V4).
- Right ventricle = right chest leads, especially V4R. Suggested by ST elevation in inferior leads and V1 together.

Figure 6.35 shows each area of the heart as a different pattern, with the leads on the 12-lead ECG that face that area in the same pattern. Since V1 and V2 can show changes of both septal and anterior wall MI, they display the patterns of both areas.

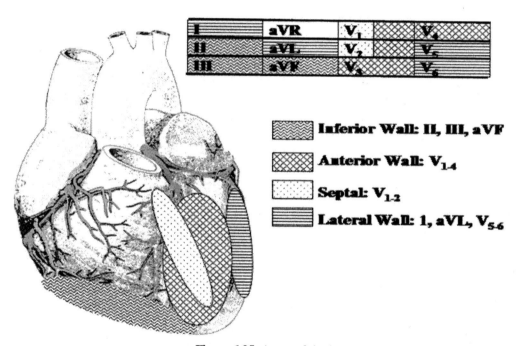

Figure 6.35: Areas of the heart.

Linking Knowledge to Practice

✔ *When caring for patients post acute MI or following a coronary artery interventional procedure, choose a bedside monitoring lead that can show ST segment deviation if reocclusion of the artery occurs. Continuous 12 lead ECG monitoring is the best, but if the bedside monitor limits you to only two leads, make sure that one of those leads looks at the wall of the heart supplied by the culprit artery or can show reciprocal ST segment depression if that artery reoccludes. Leads III and aVF are good ST segment monitoring leads because they show ST elevation with RCA occlusion and can show reciprocal ST depression with LAD or circumflex occlusion.*

Anterior Wall Myocardial Infarction

Anterior wall MI is due to occlusion of the left anterior descending coronary artery and is recognized by indicative changes in leads facing the anterior wall (V_1-V_4). Reciprocal changes are often recorded in the lateral leads I and AVL, and the inferior leads II, III, and AVF. Loss of normal R wave progression or development of Q waves and ST elevation in V_1-V_4 are seen in anterior infarction. If only the septum is infarcted, changes occur only in leads V_1-V_2, but if the entire anterior wall is involved, changes are seen in V_1-V_4. Anterior wall infarction that extends laterally and involves leads I and AVL, or V_5 and V_6, is often referred to as extensive anterior or anterolateral infarction.

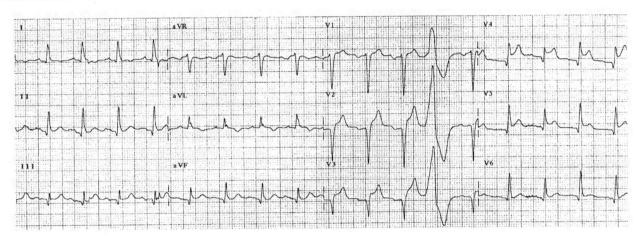

Anterior wall MI: ST elevation in V_2-V_5, and Q waves in V_2-V_4. Q waves in II, III, and AVF indicate probable old inferior wall MI.

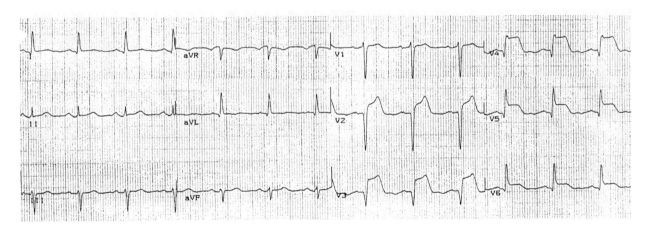

Acute anterior wall MI: ST elevation in leads V_2-V_6, and Q waves in V_2-V_4. There is low lateral wall injury as well, indicated by ST elevation in V_5-V_6.

Chapter 6

Inferior Myocardial Infarction

Inferior wall MI is usually due to occlusion of the right coronary artery and is diagnosed by indicative changes in leads II, III, and AVF. Reciprocal changes are often seen in leads I, AVL, or the V leads. In people with left dominant coronary circulation, the circumflex artery supplies the inferior surface of the heart, and circumflex occlusion is the cause of inferior MI. Lead III can have a Q wave normally, but if the Q wave is large and accompanied by Q waves in leads II or AVF, it is considered indicative of inferior MI.

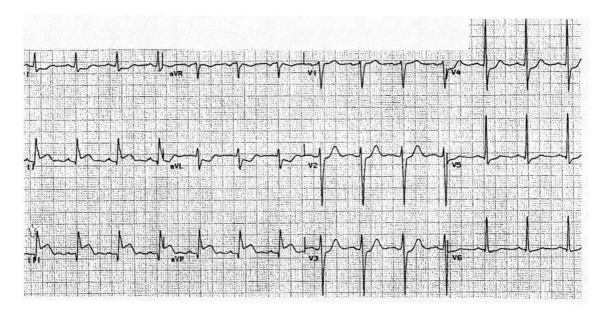

Acute inferior wall MI: ST elevation in leads II, III, AVF. Reciprocal ST depression in leads I, AVL, V_2-V_6. The ST depression in V_1 and V_2 can indicate posterior wall injury.

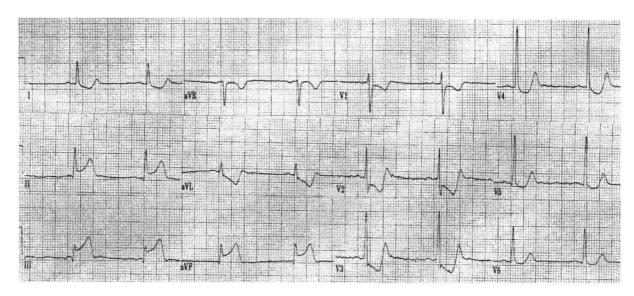

Acute inferior wall MI: ST elevation in leads II, III, AVF with reciprocal ST depression in I, AVL, and all V leads. Tall R waves and ST depression in V_1 and V_2 indicate posterior wall involvement.

12 Lead Electrocardiography

Lateral Wall Myocardial Infarction

Lateral wall MI is due to circumflex artery occlusion and presents with indicative changes in leads I, AVL, V_5 and V_6, with reciprocal changes in inferior or anterior leads. Indicative changes seen only in leads I and AVL indicate involvement of the high lateral wall, while changes seen only in V_5 and V_6 indicate involvement of the low lateral wall. Lateral wall MI does not often occur alone but commonly accompanies anterior MI and may also accompany inferior and posterior wall MIs.

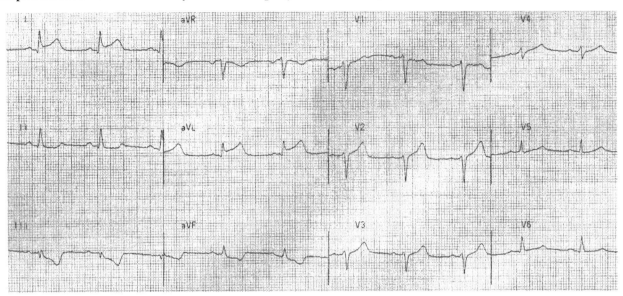

Lateral wall MI: ST elevation in leads I and AVL with reciprocal ST depression in II, III, and AVF.

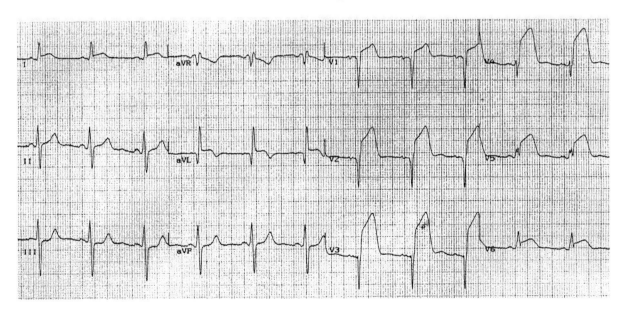

Anterolateral MI: ST elevation in Leads V_1-V_4 (anterior wall) and in leads I, AVL, V_5, V_6 (lateral wall). Q waves are present in AVL and V_1-V_3.

Posterior Wall Myocardial Infarction

Posterior wall MI is usually due to right coronary artery occlusion and usually occurs in conjunction with inferior MI. In a left dominant circulation, circumflex occlusion can cause posterior MI. ECG changes of posterior MI are less obvious because in the standard 12-lead ECG, there are no leads that face the posterior wall, and, therefore, there are no indicative changes recorded. The diagnosis is made by observing reciprocal changes in the anterior leads, especially V_1 and V_2, but often all the way to V_4. Reciprocal changes seen in these leads include a taller R wave than normal (mirror image of the Q wave that would be recorded over the posterior wall), ST segment depression (mirror image of the ST segment elevation from the posterior wall), and upright, tall T waves (mirror image of the T wave inversion from the posterior wall). The diagnosis can be confirmed by recording posterior leads and observing ST elevation and Q waves in those leads. Posterior leads should also be obtained when ST depression occurs in V_1-V_4 with no ST elevation in other leads, as this could be a reciprocal change due to posterior MI.

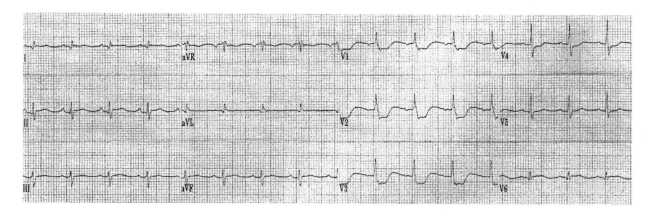

Inferior, lateral, and posterior MI. Note minimal ST elevation in leads II, III, AVF, and lead I. The large R wave and ST depression in leads V_1-V_3 indicate posterior involvement.

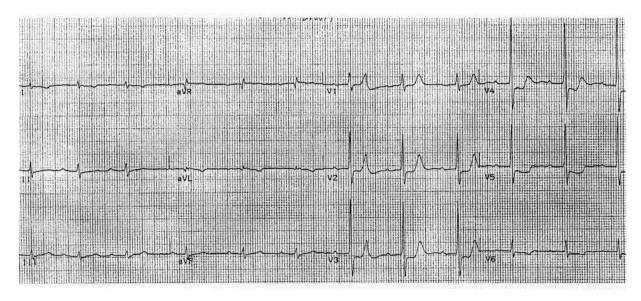

Posterior wall MI: note larger than normal R waves in V_1 and V_2; ST depression in V_1-V_5.

12 Lead Electrocardiography

Right Ventricular Myocardial Infarction

Right ventricular MI occurs in up to 45% of inferior MIs, and, therefore, it usually is associated with indicative changes in the inferior leads II, III, and AVF. There is often ST segment elevation in V_1 as well, because V_1 is the chest lead that is closest to the right ventricle. ST segment elevation in V_1, together with ST segment elevation in the inferior leads, is suspicious for RVMI. Another clue is discordance between the ST segment in V_1 and the ST segment in V_2. Discordance means that the ST segments do not point in the same direction: V_1 shows ST segment elevation, whereas V_2 is either normal or shows ST segment depression. There is often reciprocal ST depression in V_4-V_6 as well. When RVMI is suspected, right-sided chest leads should be obtained as soon as possible since the changes seen in right-sided leads may disappear within 24 hours. Leads V_3R through V_6R develop ST segment elevation when acute RVMI is present. Lead V_4R is the most sensitive and specific lead for recognition of RVMI.

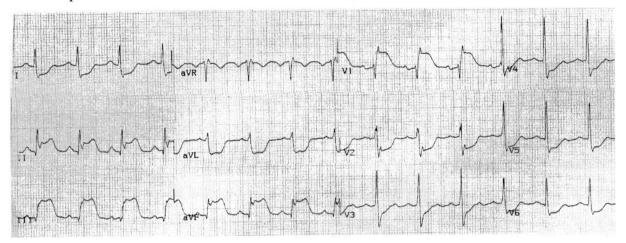

Acute inferior and right ventricular MI: ST elevation in II, III, AVF, and V_1. Note discordant ST segments in V_1-V_2, and reciprocal ST depression in V_2-V_6.

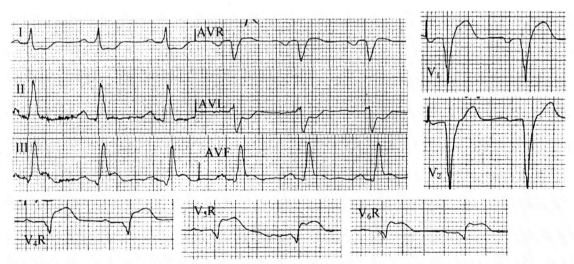

RVMI and right-sided V leads. Limb leads show slight ST elevation in leads III, AVF. Note ST elevation in lead V_1 and relatively normal ST in V_2. Right-sided leads V_4R-V_6R show ST elevation, indicating RVMI.

Chapter 6

Obtaining Right Ventricular and Posterior Leads

To record right ventricular and posterior chest leads, take the standard precordial leads V_4, V_5, and V_6 and move them to their corresponding positions on the right side of the chest (Figure 6.36A). This will record V_4R, V_5R, and V_6R. Take the standard precordial leads V_1, V_2, and V_3 and continue them around to the left side of the back in a straight line from V_6, placing V_1 at the posterior axillary line, V_2 at mid-scapula, and V_3 at the left side of the spine (Figure 6.36B). This will record V_7, V_8, and V_9. With the chest leads in this position, record the ECG again, and be sure to label the V leads as described above and illustrated in the table below.

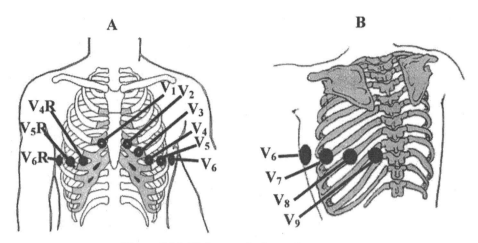

Figure 6.36: Right ventricular and posterior leads.

Table 6.1 Right Side and Posterior Leads	
With chest leads placed for right-sided and posterior leads, this is how the V leads should be labeled on the ECG:	
Standard Placement	New Placement Labeled as:
V_1	V_7
V_2	V_8
V_3	V_9
V_4	V_4R
V_5	V_5R
V_6	V_6R
When to obtain right side and posterior leads	
Right side leads	• ST elevation in II, III, AVF, and V_1. • Discordant ST segments in V_1 and V_2. • Some recommend getting right side leads in all patients with ST elevation in II, III, AVF.
Posterior leads	• Tall R waves in V_1, V_2. • ST depression in V_1-V_4 with no ST elevations anywhere else. • Patients presenting with typical chest pain and normal ECG.

12 Lead Electrocardiography

MYOCARDIAL ISCHEMIA VERSUS NON-ST ELEVATION MYOCARDIAL INFARCTION

Both ischemia and NSTEMI can present with ST segment depression and T wave inversion. The diagnosis of MI is confirmed by elevated cardiac biomarkers. Refer to the previous section of Patterns of Ischemia for other ECG signs of ischemia.

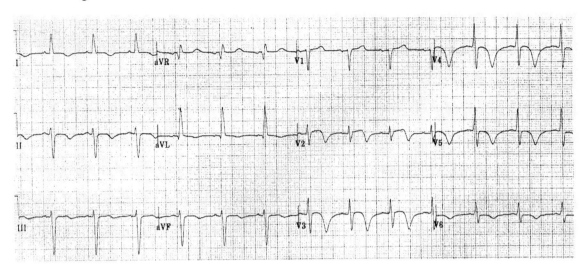

Deep, symmetrical T wave inversion can indicate myocardial ischemia or be a sign of NSTEMI. T wave inversion is present in all leads except AVR and V_1.

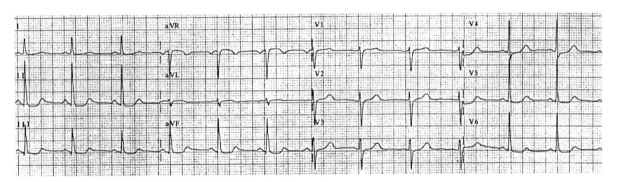

Horizontal ST depression in leads II, III, AVF, V_3-V_6, indicating either ischemia or NSTEMI.

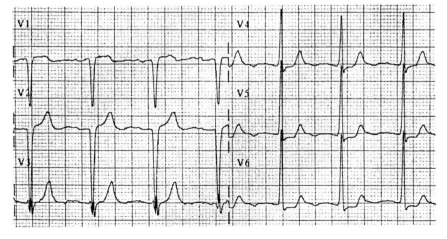

V leads showing U wave inversion in V_4-V_6, a subtle sign of ischemia.

Chapter 6

ISCHEMIA AND MI PRACTICE

Don't forget to look at the axis and check for bundle branch block and hemiblock in addition to signs of ischemia or infarction in these ECGs! *Answers at end of chapter.*

1. Limb Leads

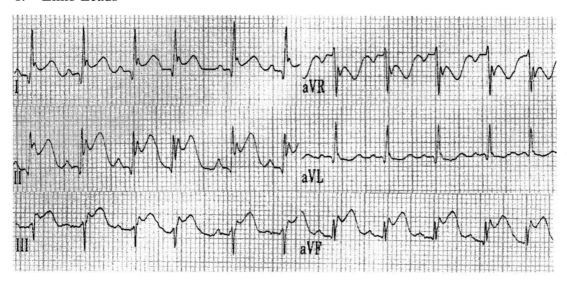

V Leads

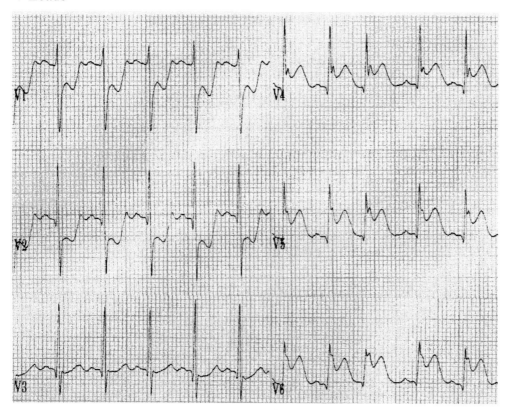

272

2. Limb Leads

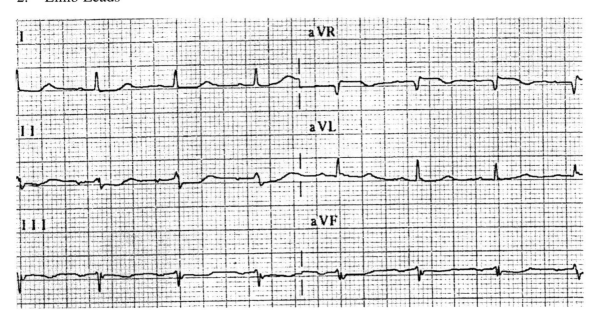

V Leads

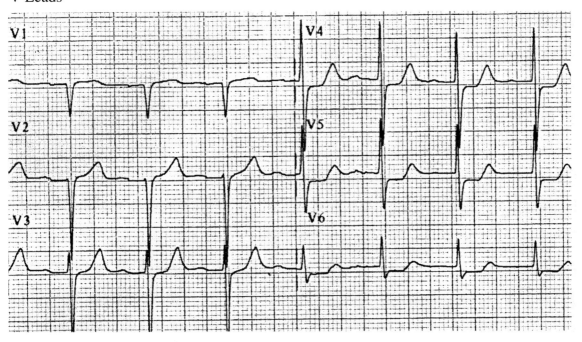

Chapter 6

3. Limb Leads

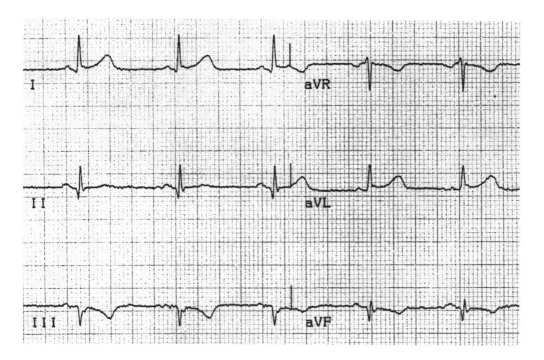

V Leads

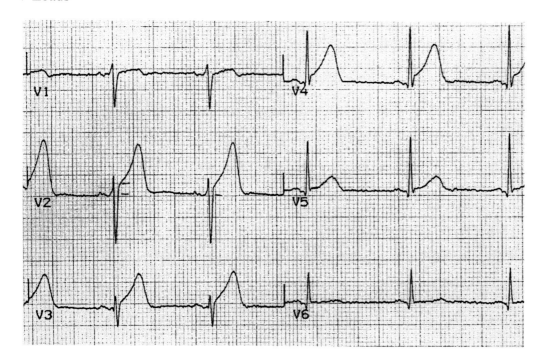

4. Limb Leads

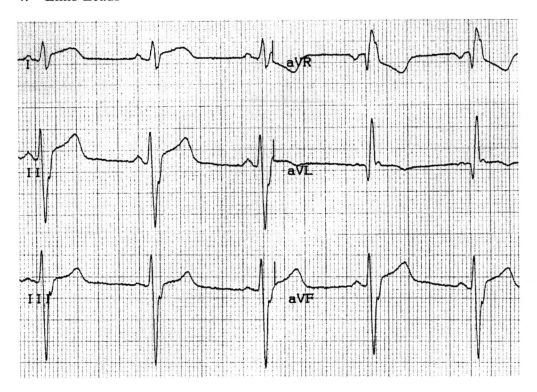

V Leads

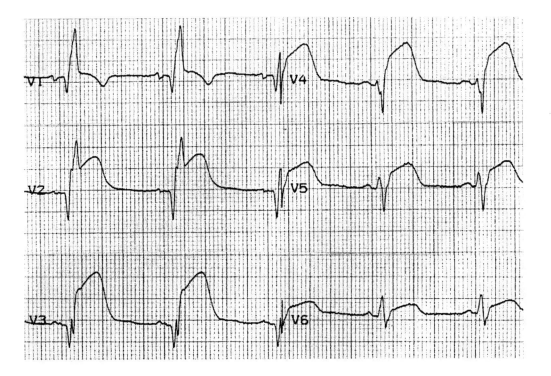

Chapter 6

5. Limb Leads

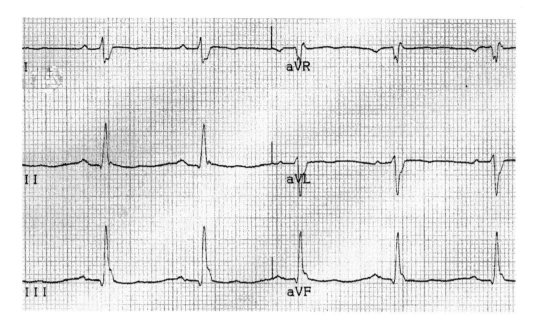

V Leads

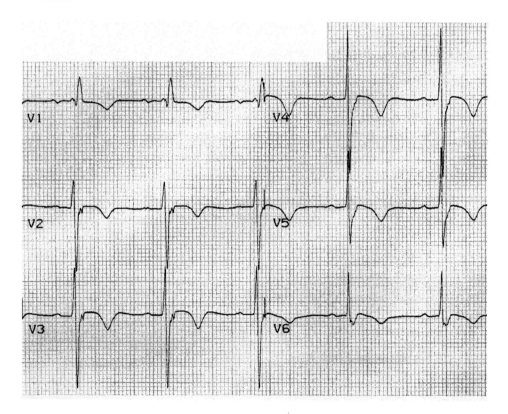

6. Limb Leads

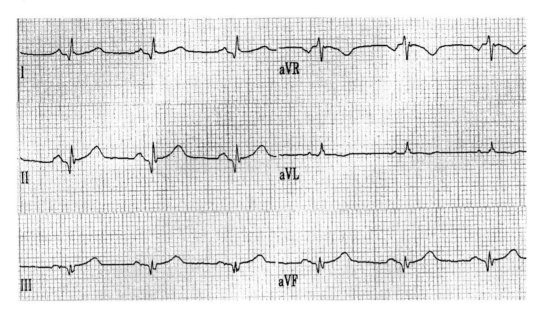

V Leads

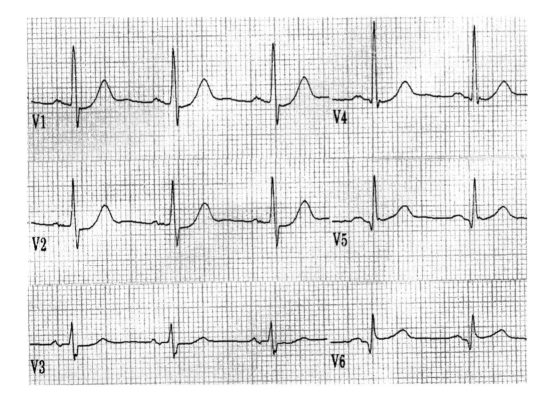

Chapter 6

7. Limb Leads

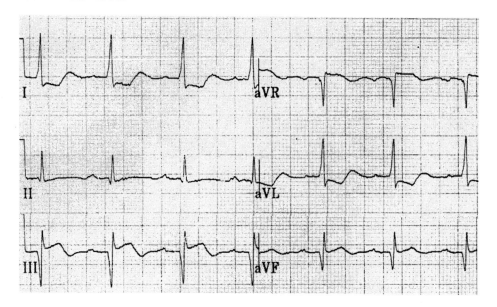

V Leads

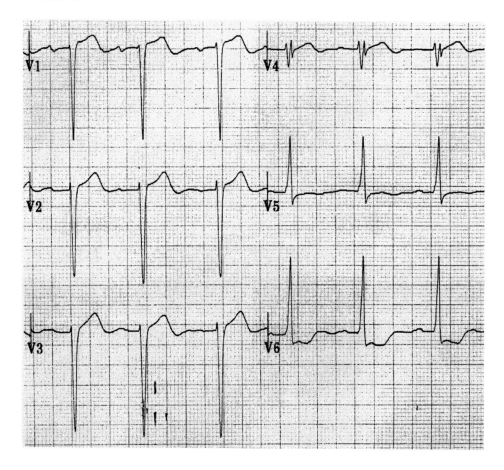

8. Limb Leads

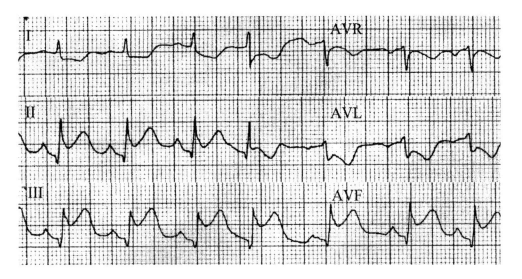

V Leads

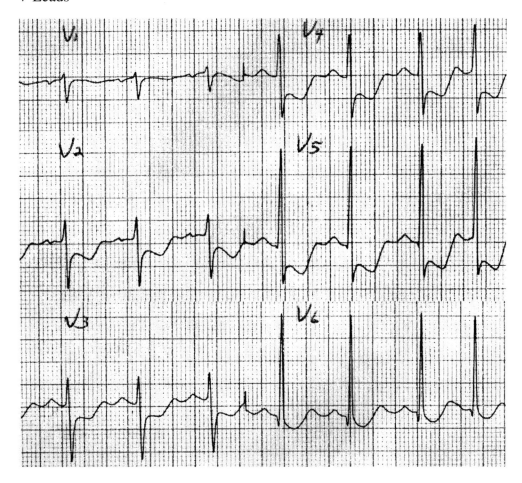

Chapter 6

9. Admission ECG

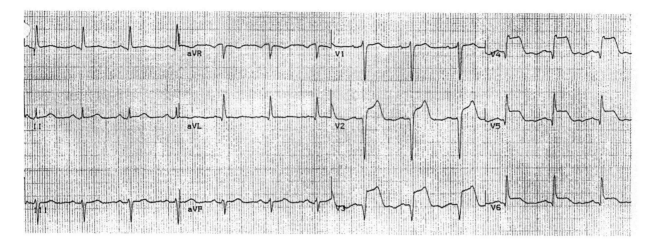

Same patient 3 days later

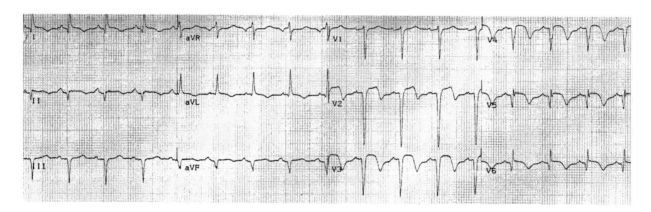

10.

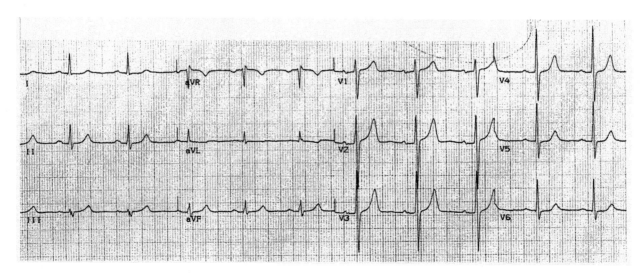

12 Lead Electrocardiography

PRACTICE STRIP ANSWERS

Axis Practice

1. +60
2. -60
3. +150
4. +45.

Bundle Branch Block

1. Sinus rhythm with LBBB, axis -60
2. Atrial fibrillation with RBBB, axis +60
3. Sinus rhythm with LBBB, axis +60
4. Sinus rhythm with RBBB, axis +30.

Chamber Enlargement Practice

1. LAE, LVH, axis -10
2. RVH, axis +120
3. LAE, LVH, axis 0 degrees
4. RVH, axis +100
5. LAE, LVH, axis +60.

Ischemia and MI Practice

1. Acute inferior, lateral, and probably posterior MI. ST elevation in II, III, AVF (inferior), I, V_4, V_5, V_6 (lateral). Larger than normal R waves in V_1 and V_2 indicate possible posterior involvement. ST depression in V_1 and V_2 might be part of posterior MI or reciprocal change. Axis is normal and there is no BBB. Probably a left dominant circumflex artery.

2. Anterior and lateral wall ischemia (ST depression in I, V_3 - V_6). Axis is normal (about 0 degrees), and there is no BBB.

3. Acute anterolateral MI (ST elevation in I, AVL, V_2-V_4). Axis is normal (about 0 degrees); there is no BBB.

4. Acute anterolateral MI (ST elevation in I, V_1 - V_6). Left axis deviation (about -60) indicates LAFB, and there is RBBB as well (bifascicular block). This patient needs to be watched closely for development of third degree block, since only the posterior fascicle of the left bundle branch is working.

5. Anterior and lateral ischemia (flat T waves in I, AVL; T wave inversion in all V leads). Axis is normal (about +90), and RBBB is present.

6. Acute posterior wall MI (large R waves and big upright T waves in V_1, V_2; slight ST depression V_1 - V_4). Q waves in II, III, AVF, V_5, V_6 indicate inferior and lateral MI, but age is uncertain since ST segments do not appear to be acutely elevated.

7. Inferior and probably right ventricular MI (Q waves and ST elevation in III, AVF; ST elevated in V_1 but normal in V_2). Unfortunately, no right-sided leads are available. Reciprocal ST depression in I, AVL, V_6. Axis is normal; no BBB present.

Chapter 6

8. Acute inferior MI (ST elevation II, III, AVF). Reciprocal ST depression in most other leads. Axis is normal; no BBB present.

9. Admission ECG shows acute anterolateral MI (ST elevation V_2-V_6, Q waves already present in V_2 - V_4). Axis is about -20 degrees (normal), and there is no BBB. Three days later, ECG shows evolution of MI with ST segments returning toward baseline, T waves inverting, and significant Q waves from V_2-V_6.

10. Normal ECG. Just checking to make sure you still recognize normal after learning about all these abnormal things!!

REFERENCES

Beasley, B.M. (2006). *Understanding 12 Lead EKGs* (2nd ed.). Upper Saddle River, NJ: Pearson Prentice Hall.

Braunwald, E., Antman, E.M., Beasley, J.W., Califf, R.M., Cheitlin, M.D., Hochman, J.S., Jones, R.H., Kereiakes, D., Kupersmith, J., Levin, T.N., Pepine, C.J., Schaeffer, J.W., Smith, E.E., Steward, D.E., & Theroux, P. (2002). ACC/AHA 2002 Guideline update for the management of patients with unstable angina and non-ST-segment elevation myocardial infarction: a report of the American College of Cardiology/American Heart Association Task Force on Practice Guidelines (Committee on the Management of Patients With Unstable Angina). Available at: http://www.acc.org/clinical/guidelines/unstable/unstable.pdf

Castellanos, A., Interian, I., & Myerburg, R.J. (2001). The resting electrocardiogram. In V. Fuster, R.W. Alexander, & R.A. O'Rourke, (Eds.), *Hurst's The Heart* (10th ed.). New York: McGraw-Hill.

Chan, T.C., Brady, W.J., Harrigan, R.A., Ornato, J.P., & Rosen, P. (2005). *ECG in Emergency Medicine and Acute Care*. Philadelphia: Elsevier/Mosby.

Conover, M.B. (2003). *Understanding Electrocardiography* (8th ed.). St. Louis: Mosby.

Crawford, M.H. & Dimarco J.P. (Eds). (2001). *Cardiology*. New York: Mosby.

Dubin, D. (1988). *Rapid Interpretation of EKGs* (3rd ed.). Tampa, FL: Cover.

Ferry, D.R. (2001). *Basic Electrocardiography in Ten Days*. New York: McGraw-Hill.

Fuster, V., Alexander, R.W., & O'Rourke, R.A., (Eds). (2001). *Hurst's The Heart* (10th ed.). New York: McGraw-Hill.

Garcia, T.B. & Holtz, N.E. (2001). *12 Lead ECG: The Art of Interpretation*. Sudbury, MA: Jones and Bartlett.

Goldberger, A.L. (2006). Electrocardiogram in the diagnosis of myocardial ischemia and infarction. *UpToDate*. Retrieved April 15, 2006, from www.uptodate.com

Goldschlager, N. & Goldman, M.J. (1989). *Principles of Clinical Electrocardiography* (13th ed.). Norwalk, CT: Appleton & Lange.

Jacobson, C. (1997). Advanced ECG Concepts. In M. Chulay, C. Guzzetta, & B. Dossey, (Eds), *AACN Handbook of Critical Care Nursing* (pp. 415-454). Stamford, Connecticut: Appleton & Lange.

Jacobson, C. (2005). Electrocardiography. In S.L. Woods, E.S. Froelicher, S. Motzer, & E.J. Bridges, (Eds.), *Cardiac Nursing* (5th ed., pp. 326-360). Philadelphia: Lippincott.

Jaffe, A.S. & Davidenko, J. (2001). Diagnosis of acute myocardial ischemia and infarction. In M.H. Crawford & J.P. Dimarco, (Eds.), *Cardiology*. New York: Mosby.

Marriott, H.J.L. (1988). *Practical Electrocardiography* (8th ed.). Baltimore: Williams & Wilkins.

Mirvis, D.M. & Goldberger, A.L. (2001). Electrocardiography. In E. Braunwald, D.P. Zipes, P. Libby, (Eds.), *Heart Disease: A Textbook of Cardiovascular Medicine* (6th ed., pp. 82-128). Philadelphia: W.B. Saunders.

Mirvis, D.M. (1993). *Electrocardiography: A Physiologic Approach.* St. Louis: CV Mosby.

Surawicz, B. & Knilans, T.K. (2001). *Chou's Electrocardiography in Clinical Practice* (5th ed.). Philadelphia: W.B. Saunders.

Wagner, G.S.M. (2001). *Marriott's Practical Electrocardiography* (10th ed.). Philadelphia: Lippinicott Williams & Wilkins.

Wellens, H.J.J. & Conover, M.B. (2006). *The ECG in Emergency Decision Making* (2nd ed.). St. Louis: Saunders.

CHAPTER 7:
RISK FACTORS AND PREVENTION OF CORONARY ARTERY DISEASE

OVERVIEW

Definitions

A cardiovascular risk factor is a characteristic found in a healthy person that independently increases the risk of coronary artery disease (CAD). The risk factor can be a lifestyle habit, an environmental factor, or an inherited characteristic. Cardiovascular risk factors are classified as modifiable and non-modifiable.

Risk Factor Statistics

◆ About 90% of CAD patients have prior exposure to at least 1 of these major risk factors, which include high total blood cholesterol levels or current medication with cholesterol-lowering drugs, hypertension or current medication with blood pressure-lowering drugs, current cigarette use, and clinical report of diabetes.

◆ Nine easily measured and potentially modifiable risk factors account for over 90% of the risk of an initial acute MI. The effect of these risk factors is consistent in men and women, across different geographic regions, and by ethnic group. These 9 risk factors include cigarette smoking, abnormal blood lipid levels, hypertension, diabetes, abdominal obesity, a lack of physical activity, low daily fruit and vegetable consumption, over consumption of alcohol, and psychosocial index.

◆ Taking into account CAD risk factors in combination provides a very potent predictor of 10-year risk of CAD compared with individual risk factors.

(Thom et al., 2006).

Prevention of CAD

◆ Primary prevention is defined as reducing risk in people without known CAD to prevent the development of the disease in the future. Atherosclerosis begins early in life, often before the age of 20.

◆ Secondary prevention is defined as reducing risk in people with known CAD to prevent a future event.

◆ The lines between primary and secondary prevention are merging, with the increased understanding of the progression of coronary atherosclerosis.

Risk Equivalents

Those at greatest risk for developing new coronary artery atherosclerotic plaque are people with a history of CAD. Those with a *risk equivalent* for CAD have the same risk for having a cardiac event as someone with a history of CAD.

There are three CAD risk equivalent groups:

◆ People with other forms of atherosclerotic vascular disease (peripheral vascular disease, abdominal aortic aneurysm, or symptomatic carotid disease).

◆ People with type II diabetes.

◆ People with two or more CAD risk factors who score at the equivalent risk on the Framingham risk tool (a mathematical health risk appraisal model in which points are assigned to each risk factor in order to calculate the probability of developing CAD in a 2-year period).

Chapter 7

NONMODIFIABLE RISK FACTORS
Previous Cardiac Event

History of past CAD is the most powerful risk factor for a future event. People with known CAD, or a CAD risk equivalent, have a 20% risk of having a cardiac event within the next 10 years (Levine, 2002).

Family History

◆ Family history refers to the presence of CAD in a first-degree relative.

◆ A first-degree relative is defined as mother, father, brother, or sister.

◆ Premature is considered the development of CAD in men < age 55 and in women < age 65.

◆ A history of myocardial infarction (MI) in a first degree relative doubles the risk for CAD (Newton & Froelicher, 2005). The risk is greater when the myocardial infarction occurs at a premature age.

Age

◆ Eighty-five percent of people who die from CAD are older than age 65.

◆ The lifetime risk of developing CAD after age 40 is almost 50% for men and approximately 30% for women (Levine, 2002).

◆ Women generally lag behind men in the initial presentation of heart disease by about 10 years (Newton & Froelicher, 2005).

Gender

Men are generally considered to be at a higher risk for CAD than women until women reach menopause. After this time, the risk begins to equalize. In general, men between ages 35 and 65 have a higher risk of CAD than women. For this reason, historically, many women have not believed that they are vulnerable to heart disease. In addition, women commonly present with different symptoms (more nausea and fatigue) and have less documented disease on cardiac catheterization (angiography) than men. For these reasons, women have historically been misdiagnosed and under treated. In recent years, however, a major initiative has been underway to educate health care providers and women about the realities of women and heart disease.

This educational movement is getting important messages out to women, including these facts:

◆ CAD is the single largest killer of women, killing more women than all cancers combined.

◆ A woman's lifetime risk of developing CAD after age 40 is 32%.

◆ 38% of women die within one year after a myocardial infarction.

◆ 64% of women who die suddenly of CAD had no previous symptoms of the disease.
(American Heart Association, 2006)

Despite the information known today about women and heart disease, misconceptions still exist, leading people to believe heart disease is not a real problem for women.

Women often experience prodromal symptoms such as:

◆ Unusual fatigue

◆ Shortness of breath

◆ Pain in shoulder/upper back

◆ Indigestion
(McSweeney et al., 2001).

286

Risk Factors and Prevention of Coronary Artery Disease

Guidelines for risk factor reduction in women are consistent with the general risk factor recommendations discussed in this chapter. Special considerations for women include:

◆ Hormone replacement therapy and selective estrogen receptor modulators (SERMS) are not indicated for primary or secondary prevention of CAD. Additional information on hormone replacement therapy is discussed at the end of this chapter.

◆ Routine use of aspirin for the prevention of MI is not indicated in healthy women under the age of 65 years

(Mosca et al., 2007).

Linking Knowledge to Practice

✔ *Some providers may label prodromal symptoms experienced by women as "atypical" symptoms. However, these symptoms are not necessarily atypical for women. Any woman with discomfort from the nose to the navel, especially those with risk factors for CAD, should be carefully evaluated for CAD.*

Socioeconomic Factors and Ethnicity

In developed countries, CAD is concentrated in the lower socioeconomic, less educated portion of society. In less developed countries, CAD is a disease of the middle and upper classes. Coronary disease is virtually nonexistent in traditional tribal villages (Levine, 2002). Coronary heart disease death rates are higher in both black men and women, as compared with white men and women (American Heart Association, 2007).

TOBACCO USE

Smoking is the single most important modifiable cardiovascular risk factor. In 2004, the prevalence of tobacco use was 44,300,000 in the United States. This represents approximately 21% of the population. The most common age for smoking initiation is between the ages of 14 and 15 years. From 1997-2001, there were an estimated 437,902 deaths each year from smoking related illnesses, and greater than 1/3 of those smoking related deaths were from cardiovascular disease. There is tremendous cardiovascular risk associated with tobacco use. Those who smoke are 2-4 times more likely to develop CAD and 10 times more likely to develop peripheral arterial disease. Smoking also doubles the risk for stroke (American Heart Association, 2006). The risk associated with smoking is strongly dose related. In addition to increasing the risk for CAD, smoking increases the risk for cancer and lung disease. Smoking with oral contraceptive use increases the risk of MI and stroke in women. Box 7.1 outlines the cardiovascular effects of the substances found in tobacco.

Cigarettes are the delivery system for nicotine. Nicotine and carbon monoxide are the two most important chemicals in cigarette smoke. It is important to treat smoking as an addictive disorder. Nicotine activates the α4β2 nicotinic receptors in the ventral tegmental area of the brain. This causes a release of dopamine. The dopamine release is believed to be responsible for the feeling of satisfaction achieved with smoking. The effect of nicotine on the brain is very rapid and short acting, and smoking must be repeated to maintain a steady state and to avoid symptoms of withdrawal. Nicotine withdrawal can cause irritability, anxiety, depression, anger, inability to focus, insomnia, and increased appetite (Fiore et al., 2000). These symptoms are commonly observed in smokers who are admitted for acute coronary events. It is important to recognize and treat these symptoms of withdrawal in patients who are hospitalized.

Smoking low-tar, low-nicotine, or filtered cigarettes does not decrease the risk for CAD. In addition to personal tobacco use, exposure to environmental smoke is considered a risk. Guidelines for the secondary prevention of cardiovascular disease now include the recommendation of no exposure to environmental smoke (Smith et al., 2006). In addition, smokeless tobacco is not a safe alternate to cigarette smoking. Smokeless tobacco has been linked to several types of cancer involving the mouth, pharynx, larynx, and esophagus.

Chapter 7

Box 7.1
Cardiovascular Effects of Tobacco: Nicotine and Carbon Monoxide

◆ Endothelial dysfunction: increased arterial wall stiffness with increased coronary vasoconstriction.

◆ Increased catecholamine release: increased incidence of cardiac arrhythmias.

◆ Enhanced oxidation of LDL-C.

◆ Lowered HDL-C.

◆ Enhanced hypercoagulability and thrombus formation: increased C-reactive protein and fibrinogen, increased platelet aggregation.

◆ Increased blood viscosity: increased hematocrit.

◆ Decreased oxygen carrying capacity of the blood: Increased blood carboxyhemoglobin levels .

Net effect: accelerates development of atherosclerosis <u>and</u> increases risk for acute cardiac events.

Source: Adapted from: Fiore et al., 2000 & Martin et al., 2005).

Smoking Cessation Interventions

Smoking prevalence decreased substantially in the 1980s until about 1990 (Fiore et al., 2000). However, since that time, no further substantial decrease in smoking has occurred. Smoking cessation is a safe and cost-effective risk factor intervention for all patients. Although smoking cessation counseling is effective, safe, and cost effective, it is still highly underutilized (Fiore et al., 2000). Some studies have shown that despite the available information about the effects of nicotine, up to one half of smokers have not been advised by their health care providers to quit smoking (Fiore et al., 2000).

◆ Patients who have had an acute cardiac event or are experiencing symptoms from CAD are often receptive to smoking cessation counseling.

◆ Smoking cessation advice given by physicians and other health care workers increases the likelihood of cessation.

◆ Structured programs can be very beneficial for the success of smoking cessation, which is critical in achieving risk reduction for CAD. Structured programs can include nurse-led cessation counseling beginning in the hospital and continuing after discharge with follow-up telephone calls, or they can be part of a comprehensive cardiac rehabilitation program. Referral to a formal nurse led smoking cessation program can improve the effectiveness of smoking cessation counseling, by up to 61% (Gibbons et al., 2002).

◆ Although structured, group-cessation programs can be very effective, the majority of smokers prefer to quit on their own or with individual counseling. In addition, the majority of people who have achieved cessation have done so on their own. Most smokers who successfully quit have 3 to 4 unsuccessful attempts before achieving success (Fiore et al., 2000). It is crucial for nurses not to under estimate the importance of individualized education and support in the success of smoking cessation.

Benefits of Smoking Cessation

Benefits of cessation begin almost immediately:

◆ Blood reduction and a drop in blood levels of carbon monoxide are among the first changes (American Cancer Society, 2003).

◆ A rapid and substantial reduction in coronary risk occurs when smoking cessation is achieved. The risk of myocardial infarction begins to decline within 24 hours (American Cancer Society, 2003).

Risk Factors and Prevention of Coronary Artery Disease

◆ The CAD risk for a former smoker approaches that of a nonsmoker, after 15 years of smoking cessation (Martin & Froelicher, 2005). Cessation of smoking after an initial MI reduces CAD mortality rates by 50% (Martin & Froelicher, 2005).

◆ Smoking cessation also reduces the risk for stroke and several types of cancers (American Cancer Society, 2003).

Factors Critical to Achieving Smoking Cessation:

◆ Brief counseling sessions by multiple health care providers during every patient encounter, including relapse prevention counseling.

◆ Individual or group counseling strategies.

◆ Use of pharmacotherapies, including nicotine replacement therapy and antidepressant therapy (Gibbons et al., 2002).

Practical Guidelines for Smoking Cessation Counseling in Any Setting

◆ Ask the patient if he or she uses tobacco.

◆ Assess the patient's interest in quitting.

◆ Inform the patient about the importance of quitting.

◆ Assist the patient by helping him or her pick resources that can provide counseling and pharmacotherapy.

◆ Arrange a follow-up phone call with the patient

(Fiore et al., 2000).

When providing smoking cessation counseling, it is important to remember the addictive nature of tobacco. All patients should be treated with respect. Cessation counseling efforts will be more effective when the health care provider develops a relationship of collaboration with the patient. The patient's readiness and willingness to discuss smoking cessation should be assessed. According to the transtheoretical model for change, there are five phases:

◆ Precontemplation

◆ Contemplation

◆ Preparation

◆ Action

◆ Maintenance

Supporting a patient as he or she moves through phases is an important part of effective smoking cessation.

Pharmacotherapy for Smoking Cessation

Nicotine replacement therapy. The use of nicotine-replacement therapy can double smoking cessation success rates (Fiore et al., 2000). However, nicotine replacement therapies are often underutilized in smoking cessation efforts. Historically, there has been concern about the use of nicotine replacement therapy in any patient with cardiovascular disease. Although nicotine replacement therapy should be used with caution in patients with very recent MI (within 2 weeks), worsening angina, or serious arrhythmias, its effects on the cardiovascular system are no worse than cigarette smoking (Martin & Froelicher, 2005).

Nicotine replacement therapy comes in several forms, including a patch, gum, inhaler, nasal spray, or lozenge. The patch, gum, and lozenge can be purchased over the counter. Nicotine replacement therapy works by supplying the patient with either a bolus or continuous dose of nicotine. Some patients who are highly addicted to nicotine may require two forms of replacement therapy. Nicotine replacement therapy is not recommended for people who smoke less than 10 cigarettes per day.

Chapter 7

Bupropion SR (Zyban, Wellbutrin). Another pharmacotherapy used in smoking cessation is the oral agent bupropion. Bupropion had been used for many years in the treatment of depression and was the first non nicotine agent approved by the FDA for use in smoking cessation. Bupropion's exact mechanism of action in achieving smoking cessation is not fully understood. Like nicotine replacement therapy, the use of bupropion can double the rate of cessation success (Fiore et al., 2000). Unlike nicotine replacement therapy, bupropion is initiated while the patient is still smoking. Therapeutic blood levels are achieved in approximately 1 week. Patients are usually instructed to pick a quit date during the second week of therapy.

Therapy is generally continued for 7 to 12 weeks. If the patient has not stopped smoking by the seventh week, then therapy is discontinued (Martin & Froelicher, 2005). Bupropion is contraindicated in patients who have the following conditions: seizure disorder, past or present diagnosis of bulimia or anorexia nervosa, use of MAO inhibitors, or are in the active process of discontinuing alcohol or sedative use.

Varenicline (Chantix). A new pharmacotherapy has been available since the fall of 2006. Varenicline (Chantix) is not a nicotinic agent, but rather is both a partial nicotine receptor agonist as well as an antagonist. The partial agonist effect results in a partial release of dopamine, while the antagonist effect prevents nicotine from binding at the receptor sites. Chantix has been shown in clinical trials to reduce the urge to smoke. It has also been shown to be superior to both placebo and to buproprion for smoking cessation.

Chantix is started one week prior to an established quit date. Chantix is dosed in a first month starting kit that contains special dosing for the first week titration. Monthly maintenance packs are also available. Starting the medication one week prior to an established quit date allows the medication to be titrated up to a full therapeutic dose prior to the patient quitting. The maintenance dose of Chantix is 1 mg twice daily.

Chantix is prescribed for a minimum of 12 weeks. For patients who have successfully stopped smoking after 12 weeks, an additional 12 weeks is considered to improve the chance of continued cessation. There is no evidence that patients develop tolerance to this medication. The most common side effect is nausea. Starting at a low dose and titrating up, taking after eating, and taking with a full glass of water can decrease nausea. Dose adjustments are required for patients with advanced renal dysfunction.

Patients who are prescribed Chantix are also offered enrollment in a behavior modification program sponsored by the manufacturers of the medication. Many insurance companies are now covering pharmacotherapy, as well as smoking cessation counseling.

Barriers to Smoking Cessation

Issues that negatively affect cessation include depression and weight-management concerns. The average weight gain associated with smoking cessation is 6 to 10 lb (Martin and Froelicher, 2005). Weight gain is caused by the metabolic changes associated with smoking cessation. If depression is associated with smoking cessation, then weight gain can increase. Weight gain is particularly a concern among female smokers. Premenstrual stress can also play a role in the smoking-cessation efforts of women. Planning a smoking cessation date to avoid the peak of premenstrual stress is an important consideration.

Relapse Prevention

Because the rate of relapse in smoking cessation efforts is high, especially early in cessation efforts, relapse prevention is an important aspect of smoking cessation counseling and education. Relapse prevention counseling includes helping patients identify high-risk situations and providing coping skills to deal with those high-risk situations. When patients achieve smoking cessation, health care providers should congratulate them and encourage them during each visit to remain nonsmokers. Depression is a complicating factor with smoking cessation efforts and should be evaluated and treated as part of the relapse prevention plan. It is important to understand relapse as a component of this chronic addictive medical condition rather than as a failure on the part of the patient. It takes many patients multiple attempts to successfully stop smoking. Therefore, relapse is only a failure if the patient does not try again to stop smoking.

Internet Resources Available for Patients

◆ American Heart Association: www.americanheart.org

◆ American Cancer Society: www.cancer.org

◆ American Lung Association: www.lungusa.org

◆ Agency for Healthcare Research and Quality: www.ahcpr.gov.

Support for Smoking Cessation

◆ National Cancer Institute Toll Free Smoking Quit Line **1-877-448-7848 (1-877-44U-QUIT)**.

◆ On line instant messaging www.smokefree.gov.

◆ American Lung Association Freedom from Smoking On-Line Clinic www.lungusa.org.

Linking Knowledge to Practice

✔ *Most all patients know that in general smoking has negative health consequences. However, most patients do not know the specific effects of each cigarette or the immediate benefits of cessation. Smoking cessation counseling efforts can be improved by providing concrete facts regarding the benefits of cessation. This information may help move the patient to the next phase of change.*

✔ *Smoking cessation is significantly more effective with the use of pharmacotherapy. It is important that healthcare providers have adequate and accurate information regarding available pharmacotherapies.*

HYPERTENSION

Hypertension is a major risk factor for CAD, including MI and sudden cardiac death. Those with hypertension have double the risk for CAD than those who have normal blood pressure (Cunningham, 2005). Hypertension can cause direct vascular injury and also increase myocardial oxygen demand. Hypertension increases the work of the left ventricle, causing left ventricular hypertrophy. Increased wall thickness puts patients at risk for subendocardial ischemia and diastolic dysfunction. Left ventricular hypertrophy can lead to left ventricular dilatation and, eventually, systolic dysfunction and heart failure. Hypertension is also an important risk factor for stroke.

Hypertension is defined by 1 of the 3 criteria below:

◆ Systolic pressure of 140 mm Hg or higher, or diastolic pressure of 90 mm Hg or higher.

◆ Taking antihypertensive medicine.

◆ Being told at least twice by a physician or other health professional hypertension is present.

"Prehypertension" is systolic pressure of 120-139 mm Hg, or diastolic pressure of 80-89 mm Hg, To be considered prehypertensive, one cannot be taking antihypertensive medication or have been told twice that hypertension is present.

High Blood Pressure Statistics

◆ Approximately one in three adults has high blood pressure.

◆ Additionally, about 28% of American adults age 18 and older have "prehypertension."

Chapter 7

♦ Thirty percent of people with high blood pressure don't know they have it. This is why hypertension is called the "silent killer."

♦ Those with hypertension, approximately 63.4%, are aware of their condition; 45.3% are under current treatment; 29.3% have it under control; and 70.7% do not have it controlled

(Thom et al., 2006).

Systolic and Diastolic Blood Pressure

There is a greater than 25% increase in risk for every 7 mm Hg increase in diastolic blood pressure (U.S. Department of Health and Human Services [DHHS], 2003). As a person ages, however, systolic blood pressure becomes a more important indicator of cardiovascular risk. In people older than age 50, a systolic blood pressure greater than 140 mm Hg is a more important indicator of cardiovascular risk than diastolic hypertension (DHHS, 2003). Although systolic blood pressure continues to rise with age, diastolic blood pressure begins to decline at age 60. Systolic hypertension is more difficult to control than diastolic hypertension.

Isolated systolic hypertension is defined as a systolic blood pressure greater than 160 mm Hg with a normal diastolic blood pressure. Isolated systolic hypertension increases the risk of nonfatal MI and cardiovascular death in low-risk patients and the general population. Isolated systolic hypertension accounts for 70% of cases of hypertension in the elderly (DHHS, 2003).

Primary or Essential Hypertension

In adults, 90% to 95% of hypertension is known as *primary*, or *essential*, hypertension. Essential hypertension is characterized by the existence of hypertension with no known cause. *Secondary hypertension* refers to hypertension with an identifiable cause that can be corrected. The vast majority of hypertension in children is secondary. The exact pathophysiology involved in essential hypertension is not fully understood. Possible contributing factors in essential hypertension include:

♦ Excessive salt and water retention from impaired ability of the kidneys to excrete sodium and water.

♦ Dysfunction of the autonomic nervous system with increased sympathetic nervous system stimulation.

♦ Stimulation and higher levels of circulating norepinephrine, resulting in increased vasoconstriction.

♦ Impaired endothelial dysfunction with decreased production of nitric oxide.

♦ Dysfunction of the renin-angiotensin aldosterone system (RAAS).

♦ Coexisting risk factors are also associated with essential hypertension including hyperlipidemia, diabetes, and obesity.

Secondary Hypertension

Although the majority of hypertension in adults is essential, health care providers should always assess for identifiable causes of secondary hypertension. The most common causes of secondary hypertension in adults include:

♦ Chronic renal disease

♦ Renovascular disease

♦ Primary aldosteronism

♦ Oral contraceptive use.

Other possible causes of secondary hypertension include a variety of renal, endocrine, neurologic, and cardiac disorders. For example, coarctation of the aorta is a cardiac cause of secondary hypertension. Genetic disorders, pregnancy, and exposure to exogenous materials can also cause secondary hypertension. Sleep apnea is increasingly being studied for its role as a cause of secondary hypertension. Certain clinical findings provide clues to the cause of secondary hypertension:

◆ Abdominal or renal bruits are associated with renovascular disease.

◆ Unexplained hypokalemia can be associated with primary aldosteronism. (Aldosterone promotes retention of sodium and water and excretion of potassium.)

◆ Decreased blood pressure in the legs compared to the arms is associated with aortic coarctation.

Treatment of Hypertension

The Joint National Committee on Prevention, Detection, Evaluation and Treatment of High Blood Pressure is a coalition of leaders from 46 health care agencies that establishes guidelines for treating hypertension. The most recent guidelines (JNC 7), released in May 2003, contain seven key points:

◆ A systolic blood pressure greater than 140 mm Hg in people over age 50 is a more important cardiovascular risk factor than a high diastolic blood pressure.

◆ People with normal blood pressure at age 55 have a 90% lifetime risk of developing hypertension.

◆ Blood pressure is considered normal only if it is less than 120 mm Hg systolic and less than 80 mm Hg diastolic. People who are considered prehypertensive (systolic pressure between 120 and 139 mm Hg, and diastolic pressure between 80 and 89 mm Hg) require lifestyle modification to prevent cardiovascular disease.

> There are two stages of hypertension:
> *Stage 1: Systolic 140 to 159 mm Hg or diastolic 90 to 99 mm Hg.*
> *Stage 2: Systolic 160 mm Hg or greater or diastolic of 100 mm Hg or greater.*

◆ Thiazide diuretics can be used as first-line treatment in uncomplicated hypertension. Other agents may be used as first-line treatment in patients with preexisting conditions, such as diabetes or coronary artery disease. These other first line agents may include beta blockers or ACE inhibitors in coronary artery disease and ACE inhibitors in diabetes.

◆ Two or more medications are usually required to effectively treat hypertension in the majority of patients.

◆ When initial blood pressure assessment is more than 20 mm Hg systolic, or greater than 10 mm Hg diastolic above the blood pressure goal, then initiation of therapy with two medications should be considered. One of the two medications should be a thiazide diuretic.

◆ Patient motivation is critical in the effective treatment of hypertension. Empathy is a powerful motivator, and motivation improves when patients have a positive relationship with their health care providers (DHHS, 2003).

Pharmacological treatment of blood pressure has been shown to protect against stroke, coronary events, heart failure, and progression of renal disease, as well as reduce all-cause mortality. Effective antihypertensive therapy reduces CAD risk, but it does not reduce the risk back to baseline. Blood pressure treatment goal should be < 140 mm Hg systolic and < 90 mm Hg diastolic in all patients. For patients with diabetes, heart failure, or chronic kidney disease, blood pressure treatment goal should be < 130 mm Hg systolic and < 80 mm Hg diastolic (Smith & Allen et al., 2006).

Goals of hypertension management include the prevention of target organ damage:

◆ Heart: Hypertension is associated with the development of left ventricular hypertrophy, coronary artery disease, MI, and heart failure.

◆ Brain: Hypertension increases the risk of transient ischemic attacks and ischemic or hemorrhagic stroke. Malignant hypertension can also cause cerebral encephalopathy when blood pressure is so high that the brain can no longer maintain autoregulation.

◆ Kidneys: Hypertension causes nephropathy through the production of atherosclerotic renal lesions. Chronic renal disease causes hypertension, and hypertension accelerates the progression of chronic renal disease to end-stage disease.

Chapter 7

◆ Peripheral arteries: Hypertension produces vascular damage that impairs endothelial vasodilation and accelerates atherosclerosis in the peripheral arteries, as well as in the coronary and cerebral arteries.

◆ Eyes: Vessel damage to the retina caused by hypertension is called *hypertensive retinopathy*.

Lifestyle Interventions

Several lifestyle interventions have been shown in clinical trials to delay or prevent the onset of hypertension:

◆ Weight Reduction
A BMI < 25 kg/mm² is an effective strategy to both prevent and treat high blood pressure (Appel et al., 2005). The more the weight loss, the greater reduction in blood pressure. In addition, weight loss can be used as a strategy to reduce or eliminate the need for antihypertensives (Appel et al., 2006).

◆ Increased Physical Activity
For effective blood pressure management, patients should engage in physical activity almost every day for 30 to 45 minutes.

◆ Sodium Reduction
Blood pressure rises as sodium intake rises. Lowering sodium can be an effective strategy for both preventing and treating hypertension. In addition, decreasing sodium intake can reduce the risk of cardiovascular events and heart failure (Appel et al., 2006). However, not all individuals have the same blood pressure response to a decrease in sodium. Sodium reduction is generally more effective in blacks, older adults, and in patients with hypertension, diabetes, or chronic kidney disease. In addition, dietary intake of potassium and certain genetic factors can also impact the blood pressure response to a sodium reduction (Appel et al., 2006). The recommended upper limit for daily sodium intake is 2.3 g/d (Appel et al., 2006). It is important for patients with hypertension to understand that 75% of sodium intake comes from processed food, not from added salt.

◆ Increase in Potassium Intake
A higher potassium intake is associated with a reduction in blood pressure. The American Heart Association recommends an increased potassium intake to 4.7 g/d, which is the approximate level provided in the DASH diet. The recommended method for increasing potassium intake is by eating fruits and vegetables rich in potassium (Appel et al., 2005). There are many websites that list foods high in potassium, including the website for the National Kidney Foundation, www.kidney.org. The effect of potassium on blood pressure is related to the patient's sodium intake. An increase in potassium will have a greater effect on lowering blood pressure when the patient has a high sodium intake. In contrast, a reduction in sodium will have the greatest impact on blood pressure when the potassium intake is low (Appel, 2006).

In healthy people excess potassium is excreted in the urine. However, an increased potassium intake must be used cautiously in patients taking ACE inhibitors, angiotensin receptor blockers, aldosterone blockers, and non-steroidal antiinflammatory agents because these medications impair the excretion of potassium. Patients with diabetes, renal disease, adrenal insufficiency, and advanced heart failure will also have an impaired ability to excrete potassium. Patients with advanced stages of chronic kidney disease will need to adhere to a potassium restricted diet (Appel et al., 2006).

◆ Whole Dietary Patterns
    ❖ The DASH diet
    ❖ Vegetarian diet.
After weight loss, the DASH diet is the second most effective lifestyle intervention. DASH stands for Dietary Approaches to Stop Hypertension. The DASH diet manipulates potassium, calcium, and magnesium, while holding sodium constant. Low calcium consumption is associated with hyperten-

Risk Factors and Prevention of Coronary Artery Disease

sion; high potassium consumption is associated with lower blood pressure in people with hypertension. The DASH diet is high in fruits, vegetables, and low-fat dairy products. It is low in both saturated fat and total fat and rich in potassium and calcium. This diet has been found to reduce both systolic and diastolic blood pressure. The DASH diet can reduce blood pressure by 8 to 14 mm Hg (DHHS, 2003). Vegetarian diets are also associated with lower blood pressures (Appel et al., 2006).

◆ Moderation of Alcohol
For those who drink, moderation is recommended. Moderate alcohol intake is defined as no more than two servings of alcohol per day for men, and no more than one serving per day for women. A serving of alcohol is defined as 12 ounces of regular beer, 4 to 5 ounces of wine, or 1.5 ounces of 80 proof distilled spirits.
(DHHS, 2003; Appel et al., 2006).

◆ Fish oil supplementation
◆ High fiber
◆ Calcium
◆ Magnesium
(Appel et al., 2006)

Specific recommendations also do not exist regarding types of carbohydrates or fats, amount of protein intake, or vitamin C (Appel et al., 2006).

Linking Knowledge to Practice

✔ *Tremendous work needs to be done in the arena of hypertension education and achievement of target blood pressure goal of < 130/80 mm Hg in high risk patients. Relating the physiological impact of hypertension on myocardial performance to future health status is one strategy to impact compliance and follow through.*

Special Considerations for the Elderly

Target blood pressure goals are the same for the elderly as for younger adults. The elderly can show substantial benefits when hypertension is adequately treated. Systolic pressure, rather than diastolic, is a better predictor of events among this group of patients. Pseudo hypertension may occur in the elderly due to excessive vascular stiffness. Thiazide diuretics are also the preferred first-line treatment in the elderly. Long-acting dihydropyridine calcium channel blockers can also be used.

Assessment for orthostatic hypotension is particularly important in elderly patients being treated for hypertension. Their risk for orthostatic hypotension is greater because the percentage of water as body weight declines with aging.

Special Considerations for African-Americans

African-Americans have the highest prevalence and severity of hypertension (Levine, 2002). Hypertension also develops earlier in life among this population. African-Americans produce less renin and are therefore not as receptive to beta blockers or medications that block the RAAS (DHHS, 2003). These patients respond more favorably to thiazide diuretics or calcium channel blockers. Due to these variations in response to medication, BiDil, a combination drug containing isosorbide dinitrate and hydralazine hydrochloride, was approved by the FDA in 2005 for the treatment of heart failure in black patients who are already being treated with standard therapy. Approval for this medication was based on results from the African American Heart Failure Trial (A-HeFT).

Chapter 7

Special Considerations for Patients with Diabetes

An angiotensin-converting enzyme (ACE) inhibitor (or angiotensin II receptor blocker) is usually the first-line agent in diabetic patients. Medications that interrupt the RAAS reduce microvascular and macrovascular complications in both type I and type II diabetes. ACE inhibitors reduce end-organ damage in diabetic patients, even without the presence of hypertension. The blood pressure goal for effective management of hypertension in diabetic patients is below 130/80 mm Hg. Diabetic patients commonly require two or more medications to keep blood pressure within this limit (DHHS, 2003).

Special Considerations for Patients with Renal Disease

Three or more medications are generally needed to keep blood pressure below 130/80 mm Hg and reduce the decline of renal function (DHHS, 2003). Medications that interrupt the RAAS are effective in decreasing renal disease in patients with diabetic and nondiabetic renal disease. Most patients with renal disease also need to be on a loop diuretic.

Resistant Hypertension

A patient is considered to have resistant hypertension if he or she is on full-dose therapy, including a diuretic. Patients with resistant hypertension should be referred to a hypertension specialist if the cause of resistance cannot be determined or corrected. Reasons for resistant hypertension are listed in Box 7.2.

Box 7.2
Causes of Resistant Hypertension

- Volume Overload
- Non steroidal anti-inflammatory drugs
- Cocaine, amphetamines
- Decongestants
- Oral contraceptives
- Adrenal corticosteroids
- Erythropoietin supplementation
- Cyclosporin and tacrolimus
- Licorice (some chewing tobacco)
- Over the counter dietary supplements
- Excessive alcohol intake

Source: Adapted from: JNC 7 Guidelines.

Patient Education and Long-Term Management Issues

Patient compliance is an important part of therapy, thus the costs and side effects of medication should be carefully considered and discussed with the patient. Self-monitoring of blood pressure by patients has been shown to improve compliance because patients receive timely feedback from their therapy. Patients need to be instructed to avoid over-the-counter medications, such as decongestants. They need to receive information regarding the risk of untreated hypertension. Aggressive risk-factor modification is also indicated in any patient with coexisting risk factors. Patients should have monthly follow-up blood pressure checks, with medication adjustments, until target results are achieved. More frequent follow-up is indicated for patients with stage 2 hypertension and for those with cardiovascular disease, renal disease, or diabetes.

After blood pressure goals are achieved, follow-up should continue at 3- to 6-month intervals. Serum potassium and creatinine levels should be evaluated twice annually to assess renal function. Dose reduction of medications should be attempted after 1 year of controlled therapy.

DYSLIPIDEMIA

Approximately 50% of the adult population and 10% of teenage children have abnormal lipid profiles (Levine, 2002). Elevated levels of cholesterol impact the function of the endothelium, resulting in impaired vasodilation, increased platelet aggregation and monocyte adhesion, and increased thrombus formation. Lipid levels may be affected by preexisting conditions, such as renal disease, hypothyroidism, and genetic lipoprotein disorders. Children of parents with premature heart disease need to undergo early diagnostic testing for lipid disorders.

Low-density lipoprotein cholesterol (LDL-C), high-density lipoprotein cholesterol (HDL-C), and triglycerides are all independent risk factors for cardiovascular disease. Hyperlipidemia includes elevated total cholesterol (hypercholesterolemia), elevated LDL-C, or elevated triglycerides. Dyslipidemia includes not only hyperlipidemia, but also the existence of a low HDL-C level. Normal and abnormal lipid levels are defined in Table 7.1.

Table 7.1 Lipid Levels			
Total Cholesterol	LDL-C	HDL-C	Triglycerides
< 200 desirable	< 100 goal for those with CAD < 70 optional goal	< 40 low	< 150 Normal
200-239 borderline	100-129 above optimal	≥ 60 desirable	150 to 499 borderline high to high
> 240 high	130-159 borderline high 160-189 high ≥ 190 very high		≥ 500 very high

Source: NCEP ATP III Guidelines

Hypercholesterolemia

Twenty percent of adults, or approximately 37 million Americans, have cholesterol levels greater than 240 mg/dL, and 50% percent of adults, or 105 million Americans, have cholesterol levels greater than 200 mg/dL (Levine, 2002). There is a 20% to 30% increase in CAD risk for each 10% percent increase in serum cholesterol. There is also a corresponding 2% to 3% risk reduction for each 1% reduction in total cholesterol (Gibbons et al., 2002). A single high-fat meal also transiently impairs endothelial function.

Elevated LDL-C

LDL-C is very important in both primary and secondary prevention of CAD. It is LDL-C that is thought to oxidize and play an important role in the development of atherosclerotic plaque. The size of LDL-C particles is also important. Smaller, denser particles are associated with a higher incidence and accelerated progression of coronary artery disease (Fair & Berra, 2005). Smaller particles might also be better able to enter the subendothelial space and be more prone to oxidation. LDL particle size can be measured directly by several methods including LDL-C gradient gel electrophoresis and nuclear magnetic resonance.

For primary prevention in healthy people, a LDL-C less than 130 mg/dL is considered optimal. Many experts believe the normal value should be lowered to less than 130 mg/dL for all people. LDL-C levels should be less than 100 mg/dL for those with known CAD or a risk equivalent, according to the current published guidelines of the third Adult Treatment Panel (ATP-III) from the National Cholesterol Education Program (DHHS, 2001). Since the publication of these guidelines, however, new research has

Chapter 7

been published, showing improved risk reduction when LDL-C goals of less than 70 mg/dL were met (Grundy et al., 2004). The most recent report of the National Cholesterol Education Program (2004) define an LDL-C goal of less than 100 mg/dL as the minimal treatment goal for those with coronary artery disease. Setting an LDL-C goal of less than 70 mg/dL is a therapeutic option for high-risk patients.

VLDL

VLDL represents very low-density lipoproteins. Normal VLDL is 30 mg/dL.

Non HDL-C

Non HDL-C is defined as LDL-C plus VLDL. Lowering non HDL-C is a secondary treatment goal in patients with elevated triglycerides. If triglycerides are > 200 mg/dL, the non HDL-C should be < 130 mg/dL (Smith & Allen et al., 2006).

Hypertriglyceridemia

Borderline-high or high triglyceride levels are now considered independent risk factors for CAD.

Borderline-high to high levels are 150 to 500 mg/dL. Alcohol and estrogen use can contribute to hyper-triglyceridemia.

Low HDL-C

HDL-C facilitates the transport of excess cholesterol back to the liver. This role helps explain the protection HDL-C provides against the development of heart disease. The lower the concentration of HDL-C, the higher the risk of CAD:

> HDL-C < 40 mg/dL low
> HDL-C > 60 mg/dL high

High levels of HDL-C are associated with a decreased risk of CAD. A 2% to 3% reduction in risk is associated with a 1 mg/dL increase in HDL-C (Newton & Froelicher, 2005). In general, women typically have higher HDL-C levels than men. Estrogen tends to raise HDL-C levels and might explain why premenopausal women are usually protected from heart disease.

Treatment of Hyperlipidemia

The ATP-III guidelines of 2001 were the first updated management guidelines since 1993. With these new guidelines, the number of people eligible for cholesterol-lowering medications tripled. These guidelines recommend a screening with a fasting lipid profile once every 5 years, beginning at age 20. Table 7.1 defines cholesterol values according to the ATP-III guidelines.

LDL-C Treatment Goals

In the Lipid Treatment Assessment Project, only 38% of the persons were at target goals after treatment, and only 18% of patients with CAD were at LDL treatment goals (DHHS, 2001). Treatment goals for LDL-C are defined in Table 7.2.

Risk Factors and Prevention of Coronary Artery Disease

Table 7.2
LDL-C Treatment Goals in Different Patient Populations

Patient Populations	LDL-C Goal
CAD or CAD risk equivalent	< 100 mg/dL < 70 mg/dL optional goal
Moderately high risk	< 130 mg/dL < 100 mg/dL optional goal
Moderate risk	< 130 mg/dL
Lower risk	< 160 mg/dL

Source: NCEP ATP III Guidelines.

For healthy people with high total cholesterol and high LDL-C, the following therapeutic lifestyle changes within the ATP-III guidelines are recommended:

◆ Reduce intake of saturated fats: less than 7% calories from saturated fat and less than 200 mg/day of cholesterol.

◆ Allow monounsaturated fats to be up to 20% of calories. Choose fats and oils with less than 2 g of saturated fat per tablespoon. Use canola oil or olive oil. Avoid tropical oils and hydrogenated vegetable oils.

◆ Increase soluble fiber to at least 10 to 25 grams per day by eating oats, legumes, grains, vegetables, and fruits.

◆ Follow a healthy eating plan. Obtain carbohydrates primarily from whole grains, fruits, and vegetables. Include five servings of fruits and vegetables daily with six servings of whole grains. Low-fat dairy products should be included and proteins should come from fish, legumes, skinless poultry, and lean meats. Foods high in calories and low in nutrition should be limited. These include candy and soft drinks containing high amounts of sugar. Limit sodium intake and alcohol intake to a moderate amount. These guidelines do not need to be applied to every meal, but rather to an overall eating pattern over several days.

◆ Achieve a caloric balance between intake and expenditure, and increase physical activity to achieve weight loss if needed. To balance the number of calories consumed with the number expended each day, multiply the pounds you weigh by 15 calories. This is the typical number of calories used per day by a person who is moderately active. If someone is less active, he or she requires fewer calories.

◆ Increase physical activity and exercise.

◆ Use 2 grams of plant sterols or stanols per day. Sterols are a group of compounds found in the cell membranes of plants and animals. Cholesterol is a sterol found in animal cells. Plant sterols, however, are poorly absorbed and not synthesized by the human body; they can be used to help lower cholesterol levels. Some sterols are saturated to form a stanol derivative. Spreads fortified with plant sterols or stanols are available commercially. Soybeans and sesame and sunflower seeds also contain plant sterols. Sterols or stanols are added after 6 weeks if total cholesterol and LDL-C goals are not met.

◆ Add pharmacological agents if target levels are not met at 12 weeks.

◆ Follow an interdisciplinary approach to lowering lipids involving physicians, dieticians, nurse experts, exercise specialists, and pharmacists. (DHHS, 2001)

An additional recommendation from the American Heart Association includes severely limiting foods containing trans fatty acids. Trans fatty acids are now listed on food labels. Food choices should be evaluated for both saturated fat and trans fatty acids.

Chapter 7

If a person has CAD or a risk equivalent, then secondary prevention guidelines are used.

◆ A lipid profile should be obtained within 24 hours of admission for hospital inpatients.

◆ Lipid-lowering therapy should be initiated prior to discharge.

◆ If LDL-C is not < 100 mg/dL on medications, then therapy should be intensified or combination therapy initiated.

◆ If the patient's initial LDL-C is between 70 and 100 mg/dL then treatment is initiated to achieve LDL-C < 70 mg/dL.

◆ Patients should continue lifestyle interventions while on medication therapy.

In addition, the American College of Cardiology/American Heart Association (ACC/AHA) guidelines for secondary prevention recommend an increased consumption of omega-3 fatty acids. Omega-3 fatty acids inhibit the synthesis of VLDL-C in the liver. Omega-3 fatty acids can also be used to supplement treatment to reduce triglycerides. Approximately 1 gram of omega-3 fatty acids (eicosapentaenoic acid (EPA) and docosahexaenoic acid (DPA) are recommended for patients with CAD. The preferred source of omega-3 fatty acids is oily fish; however, supplements are an acceptable alternative. Two to 4 grams per day are used in the treatment of elevated triglycerides (Fletcher et al., 2005).

Clinical trials have shown that reducing cholesterol reduces the risk of MI, stroke, and death for people with and without a history of CAD. A large meta-analysis evaluating 38 cholesterol-lowering trials demonstrated that for every 10% reduction in total cholesterol, there was a 15% reduction in death related to CAD (DHHS, 2001). Results have been shown to be effective regardless of age, sex, or diabetes status. Newer trials have shown that high-risk groups benefit from statins even when they have normal LDL-C levels, and outcomes are improved when LDL-C levels are taken below current recommended guidelines (Grundy et al.,2004). For most patients with existing coronary artery disease, treatment is indicated (Gibbons et al., 2002).

Diabetics are considered a risk equivalent to those with known CAD and, therefore, should have the same target LDL-C goals as those patients with coronary artery disease. Most diabetic patients are prescribed lipid-lowering drugs to achieve an LDL-C reduction of 30% to 40%, regardless of baseline LDL-C levels (Fonseca et al., 2005). As with all high-risk cardiovascular patients, an LDL-C goal of less than 70 mg/dL is a therapeutic option. The LDL-C goal is a primary treatment goal in secondary prevention. Table 7.3 outlines the effects of cholesterol-lowering medications on LDL-C levels.

Decreasing triglycerides and normalizing insulin sensitivity can reduce the small, dense LDL-C particles. Certain lipid-lowering medications also have a favorable impact on LDL-C particle size. These medications include bile acid sequestrants, nicotinic acid, and fibrates (Fair & Berra, 2005).

Secondary Treatment Goals

Treatment of triglycerides and HDL-C levels are considered secondary to treatment of LDL-C. In patients who have a triglyceride level ranging from 200 to 499 mg/dL, the goal is for the non HDL-C to be < 130 mg/dL. Niacin or fibrates may need to be added to LDL-C lowering therapy to achieve a non HDL-C < 130 mg/dL (Smith et al., 2006). When a patient's triglycerides are greater than 500 mg/dL, then triglyceride reduction is considered before LDL-C reduction in order to prevent pancreatitis. In this case fibrates and niacin may be used prior to LDL-C lowering therapy (Smith et al., 2006). Table 7.4 outlines the effects of cholesterol-lowering medications on triglycerides and HDL-C.

Risk Factors and Prevention of Coronary Artery Disease

Exercise and Lipid Lowering

In general regular aerobic exercise has the following positive impact on lipid levels:

◆ Decreases triglycerides

◆ Increases HDL-C

◆ Increases LDL-C particle size

(Fletcher et al., 2005).

Lipid Lowering Medications
(Chapter 14 contains additional information on lipid lowering medications.)

LDL-C

Of the available lipid-lowering drugs, the HMG CoA reductase inhibitors (statins) are the most potent for reducing LDL-C. Other agents that substantially lower LDL-C are the bile acid resins and nicotinic acid. All three of these drug classes have a dose dependent effect on LDL-C.

In contrast, the effect of fibrates on LDL-C depends not on dose but on the patient's triglyceride level. If triglyceride level is normal, fibrates decrease LDL-C; however, if triglyceride level is elevated, fibrates can potentially increase LDL-C level (Levine, 2002). Among the fibrates, fenofibrate has a greater effect on LDL-C reduction than clofibrate or gemfibrozil. However, fibrates tend to normalize LDL-C particle composition, changing the small, dense, atherogenic LDL particles to a larger, less dense, less atherogenic type. This increase in LDL particle size may contribute to an increase in LDL-C level, while still reducing the risk of coronary atherosclerosis (Clinical Pharmacology Database, 2004). The impact of lipid lowering therapy on LDL-C levels is described in Table 7.3.

| Table 7.3 | | |
| Effect of Lipid Lowering Drugs on LDL-C Levels | | |
Class of Drugs		**% Reduction**
HMG CoA RI (stains)	▼	18-60%
Bile acid resins	▼	15-30%
Nicotinic acid	▼	15-30%
Fibrates	▼	5 - 20%
Intestinal absorption inhibitors	▼	18%

Source: NCEP ATP III Guidelines & Fair et al., 2005.

Triglycerides and HDL-C

The most effective agents for improving triglyceride and HDL-C levels are nicotinic acid (niacin) and the fibrates. Nicotinic acid has a dose-dependent effect; however, side effects may prevent patients from taking a sufficient dose. Fibrates have a fixed dose effect and are without the irritating side effects associated with nicotinic acid. Statins, especially simvastatin and atorvastatin, also lower triglycerides and increase HDL-C. Bile acid resins increase HDL-C but may also increase triglycerides. Table 7.4 describes the impact of lipid lowering medication on HDL-C and triglyceride levels.

301

Chapter 7

Table 7.4
Effect of Lipid Lowering Drugs on HDL-C Levels and Triglycerides

Class of Drugs	HDL-C % Reduction		Triglyceride % Reduction	
Nicotinic acid	▲	15-35%	▼	20-50%
Fibrates	▲	10-20%	▼	20-50%
HMG CoA RI (statins)	▲	5-15%	▼	7-37%
Bile acid resins	▲	3-5%	➤▲	0% or increase
Intestinal absorption inhibitors	▲	1%	▲	8% increase

Source: NCEP ATP III Guidelines & Fair et al., 2005.

HMG-CoA Reductase Inhibitors

Also known as *statins*, HMG-CoA reductase inhibitors have been widely studied in various clinical trials. Statins have been shown to decrease mortality and reduce the risk of major coronary events by 30% (Levine, 2002). They work by stimulating plaque regression.

HMG-CoA reductase inhibitors include:

◆ lovastatin (Mevacor)
◆ simvastatin (Zocor)
◆ pravastatin (Pravachol)
◆ fluvastatin (Lescol)
◆ atorvastatin (Lipitor)
◆ rosuvastatin (Crestor).

Lovastatin was the first HMG-CoA reductase inhibitor introduced (Clinical Pharmacology Database, 2002). Both lovastatin and simvastatin are administered in an inactive form and require hydrolysis to be activated. The mechanism of action of statins involves the inhibition of HMG-CoA reductase. HMG-CoA reductase catalyzes an early step in cholesterol synthesis. These inhibitors reduce the quantity of mevalonic acid, a precursor to cholesterol. Cholesterol levels in liver cells are reduced, and the body responds with increased hepatic uptake of LDL-C from the circulation. The result is a decrease in total cholesterol, LDL-C, and triglycerides.

The effect of HMG-CoA reductase inhibitors is dose dependent. The most active time for cholesterol biosynthesis is during the very early morning hours. For this reason, it is generally recommended to give statins late in the evening, prior to bedtime. However, not all medications in this group are clinically affected by the administration time. For example, the effects of atorvastatin on LDL-C reduction are not impacted by the time of day it is adminstered (Clinical Pharmacology Database, 2004). Higher doses of the most potent statins are generally needed to decrease triglyceride levels.

All medications in this group have been shown to reduce the risk of cardiovascular disease in clinical trials. In the 5-year Heart Protection Study, simvastatin was associated with a decrease in stroke, MI, and all-cause mortality. Benefits occurred regardless of initial cholesterol levels. This study also showed that diabetic patients had a lower rate of first-time vascular events (Grundy et al., 2004; Clinical Pharmacology Database, 2004).

Atorvastatin at the maximal dose has the greatest LDL-C lowering effect of all the HMG-CoA reductase inhibitors. Atorvastatin has a longer half life and greater hepatic selectivity than the other HMG-CoA reductase inhibitors, which might explain its greater LDL-C lowering ability. At maximal doses, LDL-C can be lowered by 60% (Clinical Pharmacology Database, 2004). Clinical benefits of atorvastatin have been seen in patients with acute coronary syndrome, high-risk hypertensive patients, and patients with type II diabetes. Fluvastatin has some properties that differ from other medications in its class. For example, it has a short half-life, is highly bound to proteins, and does not cross the blood-brain barrier. Some researchers claim that fluvastatin is less likely to cause systemic side effects than other HMG-CoA reductase inhibitors (Clinical Pharmacology Database, 2004).

Side effects of HMG-CoA reductase inhibitors range in their severity. Minor effects include:

◆ Headache
◆ GI effects
◆ Potential worsening of cataracts.

Serious effects include:

◆ Myopathy or rhabdomyolysis (both associated with myalgia and fatigue)
◆ Hepatic failure.

Grapefruit juice contains an agent that slows the activity of the liver enzyme that metabolizes some of the agents in this class, particularly simvastatin and atorvastatin. Therefore, grapefruit juice consumption can increase the expected drug levels for a given dose and increase the risk of rhabdomyolysis. Patients should be instructed not to consume large quantities of grapefruit juice.

Coadministration of certain medications with HMG-CoA reductase inhibitors can also cause rhabdomyolysis. Instruct patients to report all medications they are taking to each prescribing physician.

Rhabdomyolysis can result in acute renal failure and even death. Patients must be instructed to immediately report the following signs and symptoms to their physician:

◆ Any muscle aching or weakness
◆ Decreased or brown urine
◆ Fever, blistering or loosening of the skin
◆ Skin rash or itching
◆ Yellowing of the skin or eyes.

Statins are contraindicated in patients with acute or chronic liver disease. Liver enzymes should be assessed after 6 weeks of therapy and every 6 months thereafter. Statins can be combined with nicotinic acid, fibrates, and bile acid sequestrants, if necessary. Caution must be used, however, due to the increased risk of rhabdomyolysis with certain drug combinations. For example, statins combined with gemfibrozil (a fibrate), increase the risk of rhabdomyolysis. Overall, the HMG-CoA reductase inhibitors are the best tolerated and most effective agents used to lower lipid levels.

Bile Acid Sequestrants
Bile acid sequestrants, also called *resins,* include:

◆ Cholestyramine (Questran)
◆ Colestipol (Colestid)
◆ Colesevelam (WelChol).

These drugs combine with bile acids in the intestine and form an insoluble complex that is excreted in feces (Levine, 2002). The low level of bile acids provides feedback to the hepatic circulation to stimulate the production of more bile acids. Because cholesterol is used in the production of bile acids, the liver is also stimulated to produce more cholesterol. Cholesterol, specifically the oxidation of cholesterol from LDL-C, is a major precursor for the formation of bile acids. The body breaks down cholesterol to make bile acids, then compensates by increasing LDL-C receptors to remove LDL-C from circulation

(Fair & Berra, 2005). Although the liver is stimulated to produce more cholesterol, this new cholesterol is used to produce more bile acids. A net decrease in total cholesterol and LDL-C results. Bile acid sequestrants have minimal effects on HDL-C and can actually increase triglyceride levels.

Bile acid sequestrants should be taken with the largest meal of the day because intestinal bile acids are greatest at this time. The cholesterol-lowering effects usually begin in 24 to 48 hours, and peak effects are achieved within a 2 to 4 week time period (Clinical Pharmacology Database, 2004).

Cholestyramine is one of the older medications used to treat hyperlipidemia; the U.S. Food and Drug Administration (FDA) first approved it in 1966 (Clinical Pharmacology Database, 2004). Colesevelam is approved for use with statins and produces a synergistic effect. Side effects of bile acid sequestrants include gastrointestinal (GI) distress and constipation. Constipation is the most common and troublesome side effect. Bile acid sequestrants can bind with other substances (including other medications) in addition to bile acids. Because of this binding potential, bile acid sequestrants interfere with the absorption of fat-soluble vitamins (A, D, and K). It may also accelerate their clearance and lower their effective plasma levels. Because of their binding property, bile acid sequestrants should not be taken at the same time as other medications. Advise patients to take other medications 1 hour before or 4 hours after taking bile acid sequestrants.

The use of these medications is contraindicated in patients with biliary obstruction or abnormal intestinal function. Because bile acid sequestrants can increase triglyceride levels, they are also contraindicated in patients with elevated triglycerides. The powder forms of bile acid sequestrants should be mixed with fluids. Bile acid resins are insoluble and form a gritty solution. This may not be pleasing to some patients and can affect compliance with the therapeutic regime. Tablets should not be cut, chewed, or crushed because they are designed to break down in the GI track. Colestipol is not absorbed and therefore has less toxic potential, making it safer for use in children and pregnant women (Clinical Pharmacology Database, 2004).

Niacin (Nicotinic Acid)
Nicotinic acid – related agents include:
◆ Niacor
◆ Slo-Niacin
◆ Niaspan.

Also called niacin, nicotinic acid is a B complex vitamin. Because niacin is used in the enrichment of refined flour, niacin deficiency is rare in our country today. Dietary requirements for niacin can be met by the intake of either nicotinic acid or nicotinamide. As vitamins, both of these substances have identical functions. However, as pharmacological agents, they are very different. In addition to being a vitamin, niacin has additional dose-related pharmacological effects not seen with nicotinamide (Clinical Pharmacology Database, 2004).

In peripheral circulation, niacin dilates the cutaneous blood vessels and increases blood flow to the face, neck, and chest. Niacin may cause a release of histamine or prostacyclin that is responsible for this vasodilation and the classic "flush" associated with niacin use. This vasodilation can also produce pruritus, headaches, or other pain. Histamine can also increase gastric acid secretion, increasing the likelihood of GI side effects. Niacin was the first lipid-lowering agent shown to decrease mortality in myocardial infarction (MI) patients (Clinical Pharmacology Database, 2004). Decreased very-low-density lipoprotein cholesterol (VLDL-C) production is one of the primary actions of niacin (Fair & Berra, 2005). One explanation for this result is that niacin decreases the lipolysis of triglycerides in adipose tissue, thereby reducing the transport of free fatty acids to the liver and decreasing hepatic triglyceride synthesis (Clinical Pharmacology Database, 2004).

Decreased triglyceride synthesis results in a reduction of VLDL-C production. Lowered LDL-C cholesterol can be a result of decreased VLDL-C production; alternatively, niacin may promote increased clearance of LDL-C precursors. Niacin also raises HDL-C levels through a mechanism that is not fully understood but is related to increased levels of Apo A-I and lipoprotein A-I and a decrease in levels of Apo-B. Women may have better results than men when taking niacin at the same dose (Clinical Pharmacology Database, 2004.)

The effects of niacin on the reduction of cholesterol are unrelated to its role as a vitamin. Therapeutic dosing is 1 to 2 g of niacin per day; therefore, the amount of niacin in vitamin supplements does not affect lipid levels (Levine, 2002). Side effects of niacin include flushing, GI distress, hyperglycemia, gout, and liver toxicity. Flushing and dyspepsia are likely to limit compliance with therapy. Flushing usually subsides within 2 weeks on a stable dose. When given 30 minutes before niacin, aspirin may also blunt the flushing response (Fair & Berra, 2005). Niacin should be administered with food to minimize GI side effects.

The combination of a statin and nicotinic acid produces excellent reduction in LDL-C with simultaneous excellent rise in HDL-C. Combination statin and nicotinic acid therapy is commercially available.

Fibrates
Also called *fibric acid agents*, fibrates include:
◆   clofibrate (Atromid-S)
◆   fenofibrate (Tricor)
◆   gemfibrozil (Lopid).

Fibrates reduce the risk of coronary heart disease in patients with high triglycerides and low HDL-C. The mechanism of action for these medications is complex and not fully understood. However, they stimulate lipoprotein lipase activity, which increases catabolism and clearance of triglycerides. They also decrease hepatic triglyceride production. In addition, they may also decrease cholesterol synthesis, increase the mobilization of cholesterol from tissues, enhance the removal of cholesterol from the liver, and increase cholesterol excretion in feces. They decrease VLDL-C synthesis and significantly reduce triglycerides. Fibrates also raise HDL-C levels (Clinical Pharmacology Database, 2004). Fibrates are the drug of choice for type III hyperlipidemia and hypertriglyceridemia (NIH, ATP-III Guidelines, 2001). They decrease triglycerides by 25% to 50% and increase HDL-C in the presence of hypertriglyceridemia. However, they have variable effects on LDL-C. Despite this, fibrates, particularly fenofibrate, may increase the production of larger, less dense LDL particles, which help promote LDL metabolism and reduce the number of smaller, more dense particles associated with atherosclerosis.

Fenofibrate also reduces lipoprotein (a) and serum fibrinogen, which is an independent risk factor for thrombosis (Clinical Pharmacology Database, 2004). Serum triglyceride levels begin to fall within 2 to 5 days, with maximal effects achieved within 3 weeks (Clinical Pharmacology Database, 2004.) Side effects of fibrates include dyspepsia, rash, alopecia, fatigue, headache, impotence, anemia, myositis flu-like syndrome, cholelithiasis, and abnormal liver function test results (Levine, 2002). Because fibrates are renally excreted, they are contraindicated in patients with severe renal disease. They are also contraindicated in patients with hepatic disease or preexisting gallbladder disease. Combining a fibrate with a statin raises safety concerns because of the potential for myopathy and overt rhabdomyolysis. One fibrate, fenofibrate, however, does not interfere with the catabolism of statins (DHHS, 2001). Concomitant use of gemfibrozil with a statin increases the risk of rhabdomyolysis (Levine, 2002). However, almost all reports of such adverse effects have occured in situations in which the drug combination should have been avoided.

Chapter 7

Fibrates and statins should not be combined in the following situations:

◆ When high doses of statins, particularly simvastatin 80 mg per day or atorvastatin 80 mg per day, are used.

◆ In patients with renal insufficiency because fibrates are renally excreted and plasma levels are increased in patients with renal insufficiency, thereby increasing the risk for drug-drug interactions.

◆ In patients taking any agent that interferes with clearance of statins (for example, the immunosuppressive agent tacrolimus has this effect).

◆ In patients older than age 70 because of general increased problems with renal and hepatic function (DHHS, 2001).

Intestinal Absorption Inhibitors

Intestinal absorption inhibitors are the newest class of lipid lowering medications. These medications can be used alone or in combination with HMG-CoA reductase inhibitors. In 2002, Ezetimibe was the first intestinal absorption inhibitor to be approved by the FDA. Ezetimibe blocks the absorption of cholesterol in the small intestine and, therefore, decreases the delivery of intestinal choelsterol to the liver. This results in a decrease of cholesterol stores in the liver and a subsequent increase in blood clearance of cholesterol (Clinical Pharmacology, 2004).

Box 7.3 summarizes key nursing considerations related to the administration of lipid lowering medications.

Box 7.3
Key Points Regarding Administration of Lipid Lowering Drugs

HMG CoA Reductase Inhibitors

◆ Most statins are taken at bedtime because cholesterol biosynthesis is most active in the early morning hours.

◆ Patients should not consume large quantities of grapefruit juice because it can increase the circulating drug levels by interfering with metabolism.

Bile Acid Sequestrants

◆ Take with the largest meal of the day.

◆ Do not take at the same time as other medications (take other medications one hour before or 4 hours after bile acid sequestrants).

◆ Powder forms should be mixed with fluids to form a gritty solution.

◆ Tablets should not be cut, crushed, or chewed.

Niacin

◆ Give aspirin 30 minutes prior to niacin to blunt flushing.

◆ Administer with food to minimize GI side effects.

Linking Knowledge to Practice

✔ *Helping patients understand the expected, quantifiable improvements in lipid levels associated with drug therapy may encourage compliance with the therapeutic regime.*

DIABETES MELLITUS

The American Diabetes Association has established the criteria for diagnosis of diabetes mellitus as a random glucose of > 200 mg/dL or a fasting glucose of > 126 mg/dL (Newton & Froelicher, 2005). Both types I and II diabetes mellitus increase a person's risk for CAD because of the accelerated atheromatous process associated with diabetes. The absolute risk for CAD is lower in patients with type I diabetes because these patients are younger and have fewer co-existing risk factors (Buse et al., 2007). Approximately 17 million people in the United States have diabetes mellitus (Wallhagen & Nolte, 2005), with an increasing number of cases being diagnosed each year. Type II diabetes, or adult onset diabetes, accounts for 90% to 95% percent of all diabetes and it is therefore considered a modifiable risk factor. Diabetes increases the risk of all forms of cardiovascular disease, including stroke and peripheral vascular disease. Diabetes doubles the CAD risk for men and increases it five to seven times for women (Newton & Froelicher, 2005). Underlying causes of type II diabetes include obesity, physical inactivity, and genetics.

The onset of diabetes can be postponed or prevented with aggressive lifestyle modification, including weight loss and increased levels of physical activity. Long-term glycemic control is an important measurement of risk and is assessed using hemoglobin (Hb)/A1C level. An Hb/A1C level greater than 6% indicates uncontrolled glucose levels. The goal for primary and secondary prevention of CAD is an A1C level < 7% but as close to normal (< 6%) as possible without causing hypoglycemia (Buse et al., 2007).

Diabetes is associated with both microvascular and macrovascular complications. Microvascular complications include vision loss, nephropathy, neuropathy, and amputation. Macrovascular complications include CAD and stroke. Tight glycemic control reduces the risk of microvascular complications of diabetes (Gibbons et al., 2002). To reduce the risk of macrovascular complications, diabetic patients need a comprehensive plan for risk reduction, in addition to tight glycemic control. Hypertension in diabetic patients increases the risk of both microvascular and macrovascular complications (Buse et al., 2007).

Eighty percent of all diabetes-related deaths result from atherosclerotic disease, with CAD accounting for 75% of those deaths (Gibbons et al., 2002). In addition to having a higher risk for the development of cardiovascular disease, diabetic patients who suffer MIs also have a higher rate of complications, including increased heart failure, postinfarction angina, and mortality (Newton & Froelicher, 2005).

Many of the modifiable risk factors for coronary artery disease are also risk factors for the development of type II diabetes, including obesity, physical inactivity, hypertension, HDL-C level less than 35 mg/dL or triglyceride levels more than 250 mg/dL.

Low HDL-C and high triglyceride levels are the common pattern of dyslipidemia in people with type II diabetes. Moderate weight loss, increased physical activity, tight glycemic control, and modest replacement of carbohydrates with polyunsaturated or monounsaturated fat improve triglycerides and HDL-C (Buse et al., 2007).

LDL-C levels may be only modestly elevated but diabetic patients have an increased level of small low-density particles. The Heart Protection Study showed a 22% reduction in major cardiovascular events in diabetics taking simvastatin (a statin lipid-lowering medication). This study also showed that diabetics over age 40 with total cholesterol levels greater than or equal to 135 mg/dL may benefit from statin therapy regardless of baseline LDL-C (Grundy et al., 2004; Fonseca et al., 2005). In diabetic patients combination therapy of a statin and either a fibrate or niacin may be needed to manage the dyslipidemia associated with diabetes.

Aspirin therapy of 75 to 162 mg is recommended for primary prevention in diabetic patients over the age of 40 years or in diabetic patients with additional risk factors for CAD (Buse et al., 2007).

Chapter 7

Linking Knowledge to Practice

✔ *Diabetic patients without coronary artery disease may need special instructions regarding their goals for LDL-C and blood pressure. Diabetes is considered a risk equivalent for CAD; therefore, patients with diabetes should have an LDL-C level less than 100 mg/dL (or less than 70 mg/dL based on newest research) and blood pressure less than 130/80 mm Hg.*

OBESITY

Obesity adversely affects most other risk factors for CAD, including hypertension and type II diabetes mellitus. It also increases myocardial oxygen demand in patients with CAD. Obesity is likewise independently associated with left ventricular hypertrophy. Abdominal obesity (determined by waist-to-hip ratio) is an independent risk factor for vascular disease in women and older men (Levine, 2002). Body mass index (BMI) is commonly used to define overweight and obesity. The BMI measurement is limited because it does not take into account distribution of body fat.

Distribution of fat tissue around the abdomen increases CAD risk more than the distribution of fat tissue around the hip and pelvic area. Waist-to-hip ratio provides information about the distribution of fat tissue. A waist-to-hip ratio less than 0.8 for women and less than 1.0 for men is considered normal. Waist circumference is another way to evaluate body fat distribution around the abdomen. Waist circumferences greater than 35 inches for women and greater than 40 inches for men are considered criteria for abdominal obesity (Smith et al., 2006). BMI less than 25 is considered healthy for all adults, regardless of age. A BMI of 25 relates to approximately 110% of ideal body weight. A healthy diet and an exercise program designed for weight loss are recommended for people with BMI of 25 to 30. Box 7.4 defines calculation and normal values for BMI.

A healthy diet and exercise program should strive for 1 lb per week of weight loss. A negative caloric balance of 400 calories per day produces a weight loss of 1 lb per week. Pharmacological agents may be considered in high risk patients with BMI greater than 30. The achievement of weight loss is especially important for people with hyperlipidemia, hypertension, or elevated blood glucose levels. Achievement of weight loss has the following beneficial effects:

◆ Improved lipid levels
◆ Improved insulin resistance
◆ Lowered blood pressure.

Obesity is associated not only with the risk of cardiovascular disease, but also with many other comorbidities. Although the benefits of weight loss are clear and significant, weight loss goals are difficult to achieve. Both hereditary and environmental factors play a role in weight management. Secondary prevention guidelines for CAD recommend an initial weight loss goal of 10% from baseline (Smith et al., 2006). Box 7.5 includes the American Heart Association Healthy Lifestyle Guidelines.

Risk Factors and Prevention of Coronary Artery Disease

Box 7.4
Body Mass Index

Estimated BMI calculation:

Weight in pounds divided by height in inches squared and multiply by 704.5.

$$\frac{\text{Weight in lbs.}}{\text{Height in inches}^2} \times 704.5$$

BMI measurements

Healthy 18.5 to 24.9

Overweight 25.0 to 29.99

Obesity > 30

BMI Goal: < 25

Box 7.5
American Heart Association Recommendations for Healthy Eating and Lifestyle Choices

◆ Balance calorie intake and physical activity to achieve or maintain a healthy body weight.

◆ Consume a diet rich in vegetables and fruits.

◆ Choose whole-grain, high-fiber foods.

◆ Consume fish, especially oily fish, at least twice a week.

◆ Limit intake of saturated fat to < 7% of total calories, trans fat to < 1% of total calories, and cholesterol to < 300 mg per day by:
  ❖ Choosing lean meats and vegetable alternatives;
  ❖ Selecting fat-free (skim), 1%-fat, and low-fat dairy products; and
  ❖ Minimizing intake of partially hydrogenated fats.

◆ Minimize intake of beverages and foods with added sugars.

◆ Choose and prepare foods with little or no salt.

◆ Consume alcohol in moderation or not at all.

(Lichtenstein et al., 2006).

METABOLIC SYNDROME

Metabolic syndrome represents a grouping of lipid and nonlipid risk factors of metabolic origin. Metabolic syndrome is present in 20% to 25% of the population (Levine, 2002). This represents approximately 48 million people. Metabolic syndrome is closely linked to the generalized disorder of insulin resistance. Excess body fat and physical inactivity promote the development of insulin resistance. Abdominal obesity in particular is a risk factor for metabolic syndrome.

Those with metabolic syndrome without type II diabetes have a five-fold increase in risk for the development of type II diabetes (Grundy & Cleeman et al., 2005)

Chapter 7

Metabolic syndrome abnormalities include:
◆ Defective glucose uptake by skeletal muscle.
◆ Increased release of free fatty acids by adipose tissue.
◆ Overproduction of glucose by the liver.
◆ Hypersecretion of insulin by beta cells in the pancreas.

These abnormalities result in the following clinical manifestations:
◆ Dyslipidemia
   ❖ Elevated triglycerides
   ❖ Elevated apoprotein B
   ❖ Small LDL particles
   ❖ Low HDL-C.
◆ Elevated blood pressure
◆ Elevated glucose
◆ Proinflammatory state
◆ Prothrombotic state.

A diagnosis of metabolic syndrome is made when three or more of the following indicators are present:
◆ Waist circumference greater than 40 inches for men and greater than 35 inches for women. Asian Americans are more prone to insulin resistance, and a lower threshold for waist circumference should be used.
◆ Triglyceride level ≥ 150 mg/dL or drug treatment for high triglycerides.
◆ HDL-C level less than 40 mg/dL for men and less than 45 mg/dL for women, or drug treatment for low HDL-C levels.
◆ Blood pressure greater than 135 mm Hg systolic or greater than 85 mm Hg diastolic or drug treatment for hypertension.
◆ Elevated fasting glucose level greater than 100mg/dL or drug treatment for elevated glucose levels (Grundy & Cleeman et al., 2005).

Treatment goals for metabolic syndrome include treating the underlying cause, such as obesity, and also aggressively treating all lipid and non-lipid risk factors.

PHYSICAL INACTIVITY

Like obesity, physical inactivity is associated with other cardiovascular risk factors. Modest amounts of exercise can result in important health benefits. Higher levels of activity and fitness are associated with decreased risk of CAD (Newton & Froelicher, 2005). People who are overweight but fit have a risk similar to those without CAD risk factors. Exercise is recommended for primary and secondary prevention of cardiovascular disease.

Benefits of exercise include:
◆ Lowered blood pressure
◆ Decreased platelet aggregation
◆ Increased HDL-C
◆ Improved glucose metabolism
◆ Decreased depression and anxiety.

310

Risk Factors and Prevention of Coronary Artery Disease

For primary prevention, healthy people should exercise at a moderate level for 30 minutes per day, on most, if not all, days of the week. Additional benefits can be gained by increasing duration or intensity of exercise. Intensity can be measured by breathlessness or by onset of fatigue.

The American Heart Association and American College of Cardiology recommend 30 to 60 minutes per day of moderate intensity aerobic activity for secondary prevention. This activity should be performed between 5 and 7 days each week. In addition, resistance training should be encouraged 2 days per week (Smith et al., 2006). Walking, as a component of secondary prevention, has been shown to increase survival, decrease reoccurrence rates, and also slow progression of CAD (Gibbons et al., 2002). High-risk patients (acute coronary syndrome, post revascularization, and heart failure) should exercise as part of a medically supervised program (Smith et al., 2006).

STRESS AND OTHER PSYCHOSOCIAL RISK FACTORS

The body has a physiologic response to psychological stress. Stress can cause coronary vasoconstriction. A release of catecholamines in response to stress also promotes alterations in thrombosis and coagulation to favor clot formation. The number of MIs in the early morning hours are higher than during other times of the day due to morning increases in levels of circulating catecholamines. Exposure to acute stress or highly stressful life events can also increase the risk of an acute cardiac event (Maden & Froelicher, 2005). Depression, anxiety, anger, and hostility are other psychosocial risk factors associated with the development of CAD. Hostility is the most powerful of these risk factors (Gibbons et al., 2002). There are two theories used to explain the increased risk of CAD related to psychosocial factors. The first theory is based on the physiological neuroendocrine response to psychosocial stress. The second theory is related to poor health behaviors of people with these psychosocial risk factors (Maden & Froelicher, 2005).

ALCOHOL

Moderate alcohol intake can produce protective cardiovascular effects by increasing HDL-C, lowering platelets, and enhancing fibrinolysis. Light drinkers have lower blood pressures than both nondrinkers and those who drink in excess. Excessive alcohol intake can lead to hypertension and increase the risk of sudden cardiac death, in addition to other ill effects associated with high alcohol consumption. The AHA recommends moderate alcohol consumption for appropriate individuals. Appropriate individuals include those with no contraindications to moderate alcohol consumption and those with no cultural or religious beliefs against alcohol use. Moderate alcohol consumption is defined as no more than one alcoholic beverage per day for women and no more than two alcoholic beverages per day for men. A serving of alcohol is defined as 12 ounces of regular beer, 4 to 5 ounces of wine, or 1.5 ounces of 80 proof distilled spirits.

EMERGING RISK FACTORS

In recent years, much information has developed on what have been termed "emerging risk factors." Some of these emerging risk factors are discussed here.

Hyperhomocysteinemia

Increased homocysteine levels are independently associated with increased risk of cardiovascular disease. Elevated homocysteine levels are responsible for producing endothelial toxicity, accelerating the oxidation of LDL-C, impairing endothelial-derived relaxation factor, and impairing arterial vasodilatation (Levine, 2002; Newton & Froelicher, 2005). Deficiencies in folate and vitamins B6 and B12 lead to elevated serum levels of homocysteine. Supplementation with folic acid and B vitamins decreases homocysteine levels. However, there is currently no evidence that lowering homocysteine levels decreases cardiovascular mortality and morbidity.

Chapter 7

There is current research evaluating the relationship between homocysteine, vitamin therapy, and cardio-vascular outcomes (Newton & Froelicher, 2005). The current guidelines for secondary prevention and for prevention of CAD in women do not include recommendations for folic aid supplementation with or without vitamin B6 and B12.

Hypercoagulability

Increased concentrations of fibrinogen are associated with:
◆ Increased age
◆ Obesity
◆ Smoking
◆ Diabetes
◆ Elevated LDL-C and triglyceride levels.

Fibrinogen concentration is inversely associated with:
◆ High levels of HDL-C
◆ High alcohol intake
◆ Increased levels of physical activity and exercise
(Levine, 2002).

Smoking cessation can also favorably alter fibrinogen levels. People in the top one third of baseline fibrinogen concentrations have almost two times the relative risk for cardiovascular events (Levine, 2002). Although antiplatelet and anticoagulant therapy do not directly alter fibrinogen levels, they are prescribed to reduce the risk of cardiac events in patients with elevated levels.

Apoprotein B

Lipids (cholesterol, triglycerides) are insoluble in plasma. Lipids combine with special proteins called apoproteins to form lipoproteins. Lipoproteins provide a transport system for lipids and allow them to be soluble in plasma. Apoprotein B is produced in the liver and is a component of VLDL and LDL-C. It contributes to peripheral and hepatic uptake of LDL-C. Elevated levels of apoprotein B may be an independent marker for cardiovascular risk.

Lipoprotein a Level

Lipoprotein (a) (Lp[a]) has been shown to be an independent factor in cardiovascular risk (Fair & Berra, 2005). Lp(a) contains apolipoprotein(a), which is structurally similar to plasminogen and it also contains a particle of low-density lipoprotein cholesterol (LDL-C). It is proposed that Lp(a) can promote cardiovascular disease in two ways: its apolipoprotein(a) component is considered thrombogenic, and its LDL-C component is considered atherogenic.

There is currently a lack of standardization for Lp(a) testing, and more research is needed to fully understand its role. High dose niacin lowers Lp (a) (Gibbons et al., 2002). In clinical practice, reduction in LDL-C is used to reduce any adverse hazard associated with Lp(a) (Levine, 2002).

Oxidative Stress

Although much has been written about the harmful effects of oxidative stress, the AHA discourages the use of antioxidant vitamin supplements, such as vitamin E, vitamin C, and selenium, and recommends dietary changes instead to increase antioxidant intake. Increased consumption of fruits and vegetables increases antioxidant consumption. Cruciferous vegetables and blueberries are particularly high in antioxidants. Cruciferous vegetables include but are not limited to: brocolli, cauliflower, brussels sprouts, cabbage, watercress, bok choy, turnip greens, mustard greens, and collard greens, rutabaga, Napa (Chinese cabbage), horseradish, radishes, turnips, kohlrabi, and kale.

Left Ventricular Hypertrophy

Left ventricular hypertrophy increases with age, obesity, and hypertension, and is independently associated with increased risk of cardiovascular disease, including an increased risk for the development of MI, heart failure (HF), and sudden cardiac death (Gibbons et al., 2002). When associated with a reduction in blood pressure, a decrease in left ventricular mass can reduce a person's risk of cardiovascular disease. Reduction of left ventricular (LV) mass can be achieved with effective treatment of hypertension.

Inflammation

Atherosclerosis is a diffuse inflammatory process. Extravascular sources of chronic infection such as gingiva, bronchi, urinary tract, prostate, and diverticula are thought to be possible culprits. Infectious agents being evaluated as contributors to vascular inflammation and injury include cytomegalovirus, *Chlamydia pneumoniae, Helicobacter pylori,* and herpes simplex virus (Levine, 2002).

The following inflammatory markers are released during the acute phase of a coronary event.
- High-sensitivity C-reactive protein (hs-CRP)
- Intercellular adhesion molecule (ICAM-1)
- Interleukin-6 (IL-6) (cytokine)
- Tumor necrosis factor (cytokine).

hs-CRP is a marker of cardiovascular risk with elevated levels increasing the relative risk for vascular events by three to four times (Levine, 2002). Elevated levels are found in smokers and in healthy men with other cardiovascular risk factors. The association of hs-CRP with atherosclerosis does not appear to be independent of other risk factors and, therefore, is not considered an independent marker of risk.

Obstructive Sleep Apnea

Obstructive sleep apnea can result in episodes of upper airway obstruction during sleep. Patients with obstructive sleep apnea also experience daytime drowsiness. The effect of obstructive sleep apnea is altered cardiopulmonary function, which places patients at risk for:
- Diurnal hypertension.
- Nocturnal dysrhythmias.
- Pulmonary hypertension.
- Hypoxemia.
- Hypercapnia.
- Right and left ventricular failure.
- MI.
- Stroke.

OTHER ISSUES IN RISK FACTOR MODIFICATION

Soy Protein and Soy Isoflavones

The benefits of soy protein on cardiovascular risk factors have not been firmly established. Research does suggest that very large amounts of soy protein may lower LDL-C by a few percentage points when the soy protein replaces dairy and animal protein. Soy protein rather than soy isoflavones are thought to

Chapter 7

be responsible for the LDL-C lowering. There has been no other proven benefit for other lipid levels or for blood pressure. In addition, soy protein or soy isoflavones have not been shown to improve symptoms of menopause, and results are not conclusive regarding the effect on slowing of bone loss post menopause. The use of soy isoflavones to prevent or treat endometrial, breast, or prostate cancer is also not recommended due to insufficient evidence and concern of possible adverse side effects. For all of the above reasons, soy isoflavone supplements are not recommended (Sacks et al., 2006).

However, soy food products are thought to be beneficial to cardiovascular health because they are high in polyunsaturated fats, fiber, and vitamins and minerals. Using these food products in place of foods with high content of animal fat (high in saturated fat and high cholesterol) is considered an option in promoting cardiovascular health. Caution should be used to assure the soy food products replace other foods high in protein. The impact of a high protein diet on cardiovascular health has not been determined (Sacks et al., 2006).

Hormone Replacement Therapy (HRT)

Hormone replacement therapy was once thought to protect women from heart disease after menopause. Early observational studies and smaller clinical trials suggested that hormone replacement therapy would decrease the risk of cardiovascular disease in women taking therapy. However, the landmark Heart and Estrogen/Progestin Replacement Study concluded that hormone replacement therapy should not be initiated in women with heart disease. In addition, the Women's Health Initiative clinical trial arm that examined the effects of continuous combined HRT (estrogen-progestin [Prempro],) was stopped in July 2002, when the risks associated with this therapy were shown to outweigh the benefits (Newton & Froelicher, 2005). This large study demonstrated a substantial increase in cardiovascular risk among women taking this form of HRT. The study showed an increased risk of heart disease, stroke, breast cancer, and dementia in women older than age 65. There was a relative risk reduction for hip fracture and colorectal cancer (Newton & Froelicher, 2005). The estrogen-alone arm of the Women's Health Initiative was stopped in March 2004. Again, the risks of therapy were felt to exceed the benefits. The study showed a neutral impact on heart disease and breast cancer, but an increased risk of stroke and dementia in women over age 65. There was also a decreased risk for hip fracture with this therapy (Newton & Froelicher, 2005). The Women's Health Initiative demonstrated that HRT should not be used for the primary prevention of CAD in women. Evidence-based guidelines for cardiovascular disease prevention in women recommend combined estrogen plus progestin hormone therapy should not be initiated to prevent CAD in postmenopausal women, and combined estrogen plus progestin hormone therapy should not be continued to prevent CAD in postmenopausal women (Mosca et al, 2004).

The results of the Women's Health Initiative have been challenged because the mean age of women enrolled in the study was 63 years, and this age does not reflect the typical HRT candidate today. In addition there was a difference in response to HRT between younger and older women in the study. Researchers are now questioning if hormone replacement therapy initiated close to the time of menopause may have a cardiovascular protective effect. (Salpeter et al., 2004; Manson et al., 2005). The KEEPS (Kronos Early Estrogen Prevention Study) is currently in process to evaluate the potential HRT benefits in women aged 45 to 54.

Risk Factors and Prevention of Coronary Artery Disease

CONCLUSION

The burden of cardiovascular disease is great, thus the opportunity for prevention is also great. Risk factors associated with CAD are on the increase in the United States. However, the majority of cardiovascular risk factors are considered modifiable and even small changes in risk factors can have significant results. Risk factor reduction, including smoking cessation, reduction of LDL-C, and effective treatment of hypertension, have been proven to reduce the risk of cardiac events. It is also likely that control and reduction of other risk factors, including diabetes mellitus, HDL-C, triglycerides, obesity, depression, and physical inactivity, also reduce the risk of cardiac events (Gibbons et al., 2002). Cardiovascular nurses must see risk factor modification as a primary goal for all patients, even healthy ones, in all settings. Through education, motivation, support, and referral, nurses can use their knowledge of cardiovascular risk and risk reduction to make an impact on this devastating disease.

TEST YOUR KNOWLEDGE

1. The vast majority of patients with diabetes have type I diabetes.
    a. True.
    b. False.

2. Type II diabetes mellitus is considered a non-modifiable risk factor.
    a. True.
    b. False.

3. A patient who is a smoker and hypertensive with no known CAD has a greater risk for a future coronary event than the patient post PTCA /stent who has no known major risk factors.
    a. True.
    b. False.

4. When taking a cardiac history and assessing for nonmodifiable risk factors, you know the following premature family history to be considered a very high risk:
    a. All males in the family have died of CAD between the ages of 70 and 75.
    b. A brother with an MI and PTCA/stent at age 66 and a father with CABG at age 69.
    c. A sister who died suddenly of an MI at the age of 62.
    d. All of the above.

5. Dyslipidemia includes
    a. total cholesterol of 245 mg/dL.
    b. HDL < 40 mg/dL.
    c. LDL cholesterol of 162 mg/dL.
    d. triglycerides of 350 mg/dL.
    e. All of the above.

315

Chapter 7

6. The appropriate definition of isolated systolic hypertension is
   a. an elevated systolic BP in the presence of a normal diastolic BP.
   b. a systolic BP that has been elevated only during an isolated time period.
   c. hypertension where the systolic BP increases at least 75% above the normal.
   d. None of the above.

7. When caring for a diabetic patient with an anterior MI what do you know to be true?
   a. The diabetic patient tolerates the MI better because his/her body has adapted to the atherosclerotic disease process.
   b. The diabetic patient has a higher mortality rate.
   c. The diabetic patient has an increased risk of developing heart failure.
   d. b and c.

8. What patient below can be said to have the diagnosis of metabolic syndrome?
   a. Black male > 65 with a total cholesterol of 230 mg/dL who is smoking.
   b. An obese white female age 40 with a BP of 149/100 and an LDL-C of 145.
   c. A 32-year-old male with a 42-inch waist, a BP of 138/86 and a fasting BS of 137.
   d. An elderly patient with known CAD and severe hypertension.

9. Obese patients have been shown to have an actual increase in left ventricular size.
   a. True.
   b. False.

10. The release of catecholamines in stress
    a. causes vasoconstriction.
    b. causes alterations in thrombosis and coagulation promoting clot formation.
    c. decreases contractility.
    d. All of the above.
    e. a and b.

11. Elevated homocysteine levels are responsible for
    a. production of endothelial toxicity.
    b. accelerated oxidation of LDL-C.
    c. diminished endothelial derived relaxation factor.
    d. All of the above.
    e. a and c.

Risk Factors and Prevention of Coronary Artery Disease

12. The American Heart Association recommends the use of supplemental antioxidant therapy (in the form of capsules) to slow the oxidation of LDL-C.

    a. True.

    b. False.

13. Increased concentrations of fibrinogen are associated with

    a. obesity, increased HDL-C, and smoking.

    b. high alcohol intake, advanced age, and smoking.

    c. diabetes, smoking, and increased LDL-C.

    d. exercise, obesity, and advanced age.

14. All patients with type II diabetes should be treated as aggressively with risk factor modification as those with known CAD.

    a. True.

    b. False.

15. Hypertension is a risk factor for ischemic stroke, but provides a protective effect for hemorrhagic stroke.

    a. True.

    b. False.

16. When providing information to an interested patient during a smoking cessation counseling session, you would share that it takes a minimum of 10 years of smoking cessation to reap any health benefits.

    a. True.

    b. False.

17. Hormone replacement therapy is a recommended risk factor modification strategy for women to significantly reduce the risk of CAD and stroke.

    a. True.

    b. False.

18. In a patient with triglycerides > 500 mg/dL the primary goal of therapy is reduce the LDL-C to < 70 mg/dL.

    a. True.

    b. False.

19. Waist circumference is preferred to body mass index to determine abdominal obesity.

    a. True.

    b. False.

Chapter 7

20. CAD death rates are higher in both black men and women, as compared with white men and women.
    a. True.
    b. False.

21. Pharmacotherapy is an important component of smoking cessation efforts and will improve the chances of achieving cessation.
    a. True.
    b. False.

22. The answer that best describes the action of Varenicline (Chantix):
    a. Provides a synthetic form of nicotine to replace nicotine in tobacco.
    b. Provides sedation to patients experiencing withdrawal from nicotine.
    c. Acts as a partial agonist and also an antagonist on nicotine receptors.
    d. Acts as an antidepressant to help patients who are trying to quit smoking.

23. All of the life style choices are effective in lowering blood pressures except
    a. reduction in sodium.
    b. increase in potassium.
    c. weight loss.
    d. smoking cessation.

24. All the following are important instructions for a patient taking a statin, except:
    a. Report any muscle weakness to your physician immediately.
    b. Large quantities of grapefruit juice should be avoided.
    c. Some statins are more effective when taken at bedtime.
    d. Statins will block cholesterol from being absorbed in the GI tract, so it is not important to limit dietary cholesterol.

25. The following statement is true regarding physical activity, except:
    a. Moderate aerobic activity is recommended for 30 to 60 minutes per day, 5 to 7 days per week.
    b. High risk patients should exercise in a medically supervised setting.
    c. Resistance training is contraindicated in all patients with CAD.
    d. Overweight persons who are fit have a risk advantage compared to overweight persons who are not fit.

Risk Factors and Prevention of Coronary Artery Disease

ANSWERS

1.	B	14.	A
2.	B	15.	B
3.	B	16.	B
4.	C	17.	B
5.	E	18.	B
6.	A	19.	A
7.	D	20.	A
8.	C	21.	A
9.	A	22.	C
10.	E	23.	D
11.	D	24.	D
12.	B	25.	C
13.	C		

REFERENCES

American Cancer Society. (2003). *When smokers quit.*

American Heart Association. (2007). *Heart Disease and Stroke Statistics.*

Anthem, E.M., Anbe, D.T., Armstrong, P.W., Bates, E.R., Green, L.A., Hand, M., Hochman, J.S., Krumholz, H.M., Kushner, F.G., Lamas, G.A., Mullany, C.J., Ornato, J.P., Pearle, D.L., Sloan, M.A., & Smith, S.C. Jr. (2004). ACC/AHA guidelines for the management of patients with ST-elevation myocardial infarction: executive summary: Q report of the ACC/AHA task force on practice guidelines (Committee to Revise the 1999 Guidelines on the Management of Patients with Acute Myocardial Infarction). *Journal of the American College of Cardiology, 44,* 671-719.

Appel, L.J., Brands, M.W., Daniels, S.R., Karanja, N., Elmer, P.J., & Sacks, F.M. Dietary approaches to prevent and treat hypertension: A scientific statement from the American Heart Association. *Hypertension, Feb 2006*; 47: 296-308.

Arauz-Pacheco, C., Parrott, M.A., & Raskin, P. (2004). Hypertension management in adults with diabetes. *Diabetes Care, 27,* Supplement 1, S65-S67.

Artificial Pacemaker (n.d.). Retrieved January 3, 2005 from Wikipedia Web site: http://en.wikipedia.org

Bond, E.F. & Heitkemper, M.M.. (2005). Complementary and alternative medicine in cardiac and vascular disease. In S.L.Woods, E.S. Froelicher, S.U. Motzer, & E.J. Bridges (Eds.), *Cardiac nursing* (5th ed., pp. 974-985). Philadelphia: Lippincott, Williams and Wilkins.

Chapter 7

Braunwald, E., Antman, E.M., Beasley, J.W., Califf, R.M., Cheitlin, M.D., Hochman, J.S., Jones, R.H., Kereiakes, D., Kupersmith, J., Levin, T.N., Pepine, C.J., Schaeffer, J.W., Smith, E.E., III, Steward, D.E., & Thoroux, P. (2002) ACC / AHA 2002 guideline update for the management of patients with unstable angina and non ST elevation myocardial infarction: A report of the American College of Cardiology / American Heart Association Task Force on Practice Guidelines (Committee on the Management of Patients with Unstable Angina). Retrieved from: http://www.acc.org/clinical/guide lines/unstable/unstable.pdf

Burke, L.E. & Cartwright, M.A. (2005). Obesity: An overview of assessment and treatment. In S.L.Woods, E.S. Froelicher, S.U. Motzer, and E.J. Bridges (Eds.), *Cardiac nursing* (5th ed., pp.937-947). Philadelphia: Lippincott, Williams and Wilkins.

Buse, J.B., Ginsberg, H.N., Bakris, G.L., Clark, N.G., Costa, F., Eckel, R., et al. (2007). Primary prevention of cardiovascular diseases in people with diabetes mellitus. *Circulation, 115*, 114-126.

Clinical Pharmacology Database. (2004). Gold Standard Multimedia. www.gsm.com

Cunningham, S. (2005). Hypertension. In S.L.Woods, E.S. Froelicher, S.U. Motzer, & E.J. Bridges (Eds.), *Cardiac nursing* (5th ed., pp. 856-896). Philadelphia: Lippincott, Williams and Wilkins.

Davis, M.M., Taubert, K., Benin, A.L., Brown, D.W., Mensah, G.A., Baddour, L.M., et al. (2006). Influenza vaccination as secondary prevention for cardiovascular disease. *Circulation, 114,* 1549-1553.

Deedy, M.G. (2002). Coronary artery disease. Cleveland Clinical Disease Management Medical Education. Retrieved September 26, 2004 from http://www.clevelandclinicmeded.com/disease management/cardiology/cad

Dietary guidelines. Retrieved August 21, 2004, from American Heart Association Web site: http://www.americanheart.org

Fair, J.M. & Berra, K.A. (2005). Lipid management and coronary artery disease. In S.L.Woods, E.S. Froelicher, S.U. Motzer, & E.J. Bridges (Eds.), *Cardiac nursing* (5th ed., pp.897-915). Philadelphia: Lippincott, Williams and Wilkins.

Fiore, M.C., Bailey, W.C., Choen, S.J., et al. (2000). Treating tobacco use and dependence: Clinical practice guideline. Rockville, MD: U.S. Department of Health and Human Services. Public Health Service. June 2000.

Fletcher, B., Berra, K., Ades, P., Braun, L.T., Burke, L.E., Durstine, J.L., Fair, J.M., Fletcher, G.F., Goff, D., Hayman, L.L., Hiatt, W.R., Miller, N.H., Krauss, R., Kris-Etherton, P., Stone, N., Wilterdink, J., & Winston, M. Managing abnormal blood lipids: A collaborative approach. *Circulation, Nov 2005*; 112: 3184-3209.

Fonsecca, V. Bakris, G.L., Benjamin, E.M., Blonde, L., & Boucher, J. (2005). Summary of revisions for the 2005 clinical practice recommendations. [Electronic Version]. *Diabetes Care, 28* (1), S3.

Gibbons, R.J., Abrams, J., Chatterjee, K., Daley, J., Deedwania, P.C., Douglas, J.S., Ferguson, T.B. Jr., Fihn, S.D., Fraker, T.D.Jr., Gardin, J.M., O'Rourke, R.A., Pasternak, R.C., & Williams, S.V. (2002) Guidelines update for the management of patients with chronic stable angina: A report of the American College of Cardiology / American Heart Association Task Force on Practice Guidelines (Committee to Update the 1999 Guidelines for the Management of Patients with Chronic Stable Angina). 2002. Available at www.acc.org/clinical/guidelines/stable/stable.pdf

Risk Factors and Prevention of Coronary Artery Disease

Giles, T. (2004). Hypertension – unique phenotypes and antihypertensive treatment: One size does not fit all. Medscape. *Cardiology, 8* (2). Retrieved October 11, 2004, from http://www.medscape.com

Grady, D., McDonald, K., Bischoff, K., Cabou, A., Chaput, L., Hoerster, K., Kristof, M., Shahpar, C., & Walsh, J. (2003). Results of systematic review of research on diagnosis and treatment of coronary heart disease in women. Agency for Healthcare Research and Quality. (AHPRQ Publication No. AHRQ 03-E035.)

Grundy, S.M., Cleeman, J.I., Bairey Merz, C.N., Brewer, B. Jr., Clark, L.T., Hunninghake, D.B., Pasternak, R.C., Smith, S.C., & Stone, N.J. (2004). Implications for recent clinical trials for the national cholesterol education program adult treatment panel III guidelines. *Circulation, 110*, 227-239.

Grundy, S.M., Cleeman, J.I., Daniels, S.R., Donato, K.A., Eckel, R.H., Franklin, B.A., Gordon, D.J., Krauss, R.M., Savage, P.J., Smith, S.C. Jr, Spertus, J.A., & Costa, F. Diagnosis and management of the metabolic syndrome: An American Heart Association/National Heart, Lung, and Blood Institute Scientific Statement: Executive summary. *Circulation, Oct 2005*; 112: e285-e290.

Haffner, S.M. (2004). Dyslipidemia management in adults with diabetes. *Diabetes Care, 27,* Supplement 1, S68-S71.

Haire-Joshu, D., Glasgow, R.E., and Tibbs, T.L. (2004). Smoking and diabetes. *Diabetes Care, 27,* Supplement 1, S74-S75.

Leon, A.S., Franklin, B.A., Costa, F., Balady, G.J., Berra, K.A., Stewart, K.J., Thompson, P.D., Williams, M.A., & Lauer, M.S. Cardiac rehabilitation and secondary prevention of coronary heart disease: An American Heart Association Scientific Statement from the Council on Clinical Cardiology (Subcommittee on Exercise, Cardiac Rehabilitation, and Prevention) and the Council on Nutrition, Physical Activity, and Metabolism (Subcommittee on Physical Activity), in Collaboration with the American Association of Cardiovascular and Pulmonary Rehabilitation Circulation, Jan 2005; 111: 369-376.

Levine, B.S. (2002). *Cardiac vascular nursing review and resource manual.* Washington, DC: American Nurses Credentialing Center.

Lichtenstein, AH, Appel, LJ, Brands, M, Carnethon, M, Daniels, S, Franch, HA, Franklin, B, Kris-Etherton, P, Harris, WS, Howard, B, Karanja, N, Lefevre, M, Rudel, L, Sacks, F, Van Horn, L, Winston, M, & Wylie-Rosett, J. Diet and lifestyle recommendations Revision 2006. A Scientific Statement From the American Heart Association Nutrition Committee. *Circulation. 2006*;114:82-96.

Maden, S.K., & Froelicher, E.S.(2005). Psychosocial risk factors: assessment and management interventions. In S.L.Woods, E..S. Froelicher, S.U. Motzer, and E.J. Bridges (Eds.), *Cardiac nursing* (5th ed., pp.825-837). Philadelphia: Lippincott, Williams and Wilkins.

Manson, J.E., Hsia, J., Johnson, K.C., et al. Estrogen plus progestin and the risk of coronary heart disease. *New England Journal of Medicine 2003* Aug 7; 349(6):523-34.

Martin, K., & Froelicher, E.S. (2005). Smoking cessation: a systematic approach to managing patients with heart disease. In S.L.Woods, E.S. Froelicher, S.U. Motzer, & E.J. Bridges (Eds.), *Cardiac nursing* (5th ed., pp.838-855). Philadelphia: Lippincott, Williams and Wilkins.

Chapter 7

Mosca, L. Appel, L.J., Benjamin, E.J., Berra, K. Chandra-Strobes, N., et al. (2004). Evidence based guidelines for cardiovascular disease prevention in women. *Journal of American College of Cardiology, 43,* 900-921.

Mosca, L., Banka, C.L., Benjamin, E.J., Berra, K., Bushnell, C., Dolor, R.J., et al. (2007). Evidence-based guidelines for cardiovascular disease prevention in women: 2007 update. *Circulation.* Retrieved on March 16, 2007, from http://circ.ahajournals.org/cgi/reprint/CIRCULATIONAHA.107.181546

Myers, J. (2005). Exercise and activity. In S.L.Woods, E.S. Froelicher, S.U. Motzer, & E.J. Bridges (Eds.), *Cardiac nursing* (5th ed., pp.916-936). Philadelphia: Lippincott, Williams and Wilkins.

National Vital Statistics Reports, Vol. 53, No. 15, February 28, 2005. Retrieved March 21, 2005 from http://www.cdc.gov/nchs

Newton, K.M. & Froelicher, E.S. (2005). Coronary heart disease risk factors. In S.L.Woods, E.S. Froelicher, S.U. Motzer, & E.J. Bridges (Eds.), *Cardiac nursing* (5th ed., pp.809-824). Philadelphia: Lippincott, Williams and Wilkins.

Opie, L.H. & Gersh, B.J. (2005). *Drugs for the heart* (6th ed.). Philadelphia: Elsevier Saunders.

Sacks, F.M., Lichtenstein, A., Van Horn, L., Harris, W. Kris-Etherton, P., & Winston, M. (2006). Soy protein, isoflavones, and cardiovascular health. *Circulation, 113,* 1034-1044.

Salpeter, S.R., Walsh, J.M.E., Greyber, E., et al. Mortality associated with hormone replacement therapy in younger and older women. *J Gen Intern Med 2004*; 19:791-804.

Smith, S.C. Jr., Allen, J., Blair, S.N., Bonow, R.O., Brass, L.M., Fonarow, J.C., Grundy, S.M., Hiratzka, L., Jones, D., Krumholz, H.M., Mosca, L., Pasternak, R.C., Pearson, T., Pfeffer, M.A., & Taubert, K.A. AHA/ACC guidelines for secondary prevention for patients with coronary and other atherosclerotic vascular disease: 2006 update: Endorsed by the National Heart, Lung, and Blood Institute. *Circulation, 113:* 2363-2372.

Smith, S.C. Jr., Blair, S.N., Bonow, R.O., Brass, L.M., & Cerqueira, M.D., et al. (2001). ACC/AHA guidelines for preventing heart attack and death in patients with atherosclerotic cardiovascular disease: 2001 update. *Circulation, 104,* 1577-1579.

Thom, T., Haase, N., Rosamond, W., Howard, V.J., Rumsfeld, J., Manolio, T., Zheng, Z.J., Flegal, K., O'Donnell, C., Kittner, S., Lloyd-Jones, D., Goff, D.C., Jr., Hong, Y., Members of the Statistics Committee and Stroke Statistics Subcommittee, Adams, R., Friday, G., Furie, K., Gorelick, P., Kissela, B., Marler, J., Meigs, J., Roger, V., Sidney, S., Sorlie, P., Steinberger, J., Wasserthiel-Smoller, S., Wilson, M., & Wolf, P. Heart disease and stroke statistics—2006 update: A report from the American Heart Association Statistics Committee and Stroke Statistics Subcommittee. *Circulation, Feb 2006*; 113: e85-e151.

U.S. Department of Health and Human Services. (2003). The seventh report of the Joint National Committee on prevention, detection, evaluation, and treatment of high blood pressure (NIH publication No. 03-5233). Washington, DC: U.S. Government Printing Office.

U.S. Department of Health and Human Services. (2001). Third report of National Cholesterol Education Program (NCEP) Expert Panel on detection, evaluation, and treatment of high blood cholesterol in adults (Adult Treatment Panel III) (NIH publication No. 01-3670). Washington, DC: U.S. Government Printing Office.

Risk Factors and Prevention of Coronary Artery Disease

Veerakul, G. (2001). Coronary risk factors and modification. In A.V. Adair (Ed.), *Cardiology secrets* (pp. 118-123). Philadelphia: Hanley and Belfus, Inc.

Wallhagen, M.I., Nolte, M.S. (2005). Diabetes mellitus. In S.L.Woods, E.S. Froelicher, S.U. Motzer, & E.J. Bridges (Eds.), *Cardiac nursing* (5th ed., pp.948-960). Philadelphia: Lippincott, Williams and Wilkins.

Women and coronary heart disease. Retrieved August 21, 2004, from American Heart Association Web site: http://www.americanheart.org

Woods, S.E., Smith, J.M., Sohail, S., Sarah, A., & Engle, A. (2004). The influence of type 2 diabetes mellitus in patients undergoing coronary artery bypass graft surgery: An 8-year prospective cohort study [Electronic Version]. *Chest, 126,* 1789-1793.

CHAPTER 8:
ACUTE CORONARY SYNDROME

INTRODUCTION

Facts About Cardiovascular Disease

- An estimated 700,000 Americans will have a new coronary attack and about 500,000 will have a recurrent attack annually.
- The average age of a person having a first myocardial infarction (MI) is 65.8 for men and 70.4 for women.
- Coronary Artery Disease (CAD) is the single largest killer of American males and females. About every 26 seconds an American will suffer a coronary event, and about every minute someone will die from one. About 40% of the people who experience a coronary attack in a given year will die from it.
- From 1993–2003, the death rate from CAD declined 30.2%; however, the actual number of deaths declined only 14.7% because the total number of people with CAD increased.
- The estimated average number of years of life lost due to a heart attack is 14.2 years.
- Within 1 year after having an initial recognized MI, 25% of men and 38% of women will die. This death rate is due in part because women have MIs at older ages than men, and women are more likely to die from MIs within a few weeks of the infarction. Almost half of men and women under age 65 who have an MI die within 8 years.
- From 1990-1999, in-hospital acute MI (AMI) mortality declined from 11.2% to 9.4%.

(Thom et al., 2006).

Overview of CAD and Acute Coronary Syndrome (ACS)

CAD is the presence of atherosclerosis or atherosclerotic plaque in the epicardial coronary arteries. As atherosclerotic plaque progresses, the lumen of the coronary artery can become narrowed and blood flow can be impaired. Reduced blood flow can lead to ischemia, which is a lack of oxygen to the myocardium. Prolonged ischemia can result in injury, and ultimately necrosis of myocardial tissue. The presentation of CAD ranges from stable angina to AMI (Table 8.1). The term acute coronary syndrome (ACS) is used to describe the presentation of CAD in the form of unstable angina, non-ST-segment elevation MI (non-STEMI), and ST-segment elevation MI (STEMI).

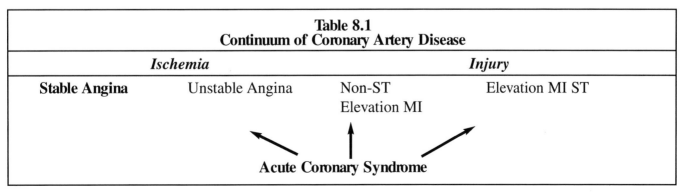

Table 8.1
Continuum of Coronary Artery Disease

Chapter 8

PATHOPHYSIOLOGY OF CORONARY ARTERY DISEASE

Overview

◆ The development of CAD begins in adolescence and continues throughout life. Symptoms may not manifest until decades after the development begins.

◆ Cardiac risk factors accelerate the development process.

◆ CAD is considered a chronic condition.

◆ Atherosclerosis involves the deposit of lipids, calcium, fibrin, and other cellular substances within the lining of the arteries. This deposit initiates a progressive inflammatory response in an effort to heal the endothelium.

◆ The end result of this inflammatory process is the production of a fibrous atherosclerotic plaque. This plaque can partially or totally occlude blood flow.

Steps in the Development of Atherosclerotic Plaque

◆ Macrophage foam cells rich in lipids accumulate on the intimal layer of the arterial wall.

◆ Smooth muscle cells become involved and accumulate intracellular lipids.

◆ Fatty streaks form between the endothelium and the intima of the artery (Aouizerat, 2005; Deedy, 2002).

◆ The inflammatory process is activated and immune cells, such as T lymphocytes and mast cells, begin to invade the lesion (Aouizerat, 2005).

◆ As the lesion progresses, extracellular lipids are deposited among the layers of smooth muscle cells.

◆ The integrity of smooth muscle cells is destroyed.

◆ An extracellular lipid core (atheroma) develops as the lesion becomes clinically significant. The lipid core may contain calcium deposits (Deedy, 2002).

◆ Foam cells die and contribute their necrotic components to the growth of the lipid core.

◆ The lipid core thickens the external edge of the arterial wall, but does not greatly narrow the lumen.

◆ Fibrous tissue, mainly collagen, ultimately forms a fibrous cap that covers the lipid core (fibrous atheroma) (Aouizerat, 2005; Deedy, 2002).

◆ More noticeable vessel narrowing occurs and lesions are prone to ulcerations and sudden rupture.

◆ Mechanical and inflammatory vascular changes impact the vulnerability of plaque (Gardner & Altman, 2005). The release of enzymes from immune response cells contributes to the vulnerability of rupture by weakening the collagen matrix of the fibrous cap.

◆ Plaque rupture exposes the core of the lipid to circulating blood.

◆ Exposure results in platelet adherence, activation, and aggregation and activation of the coagulation pathway, which results in thrombus formation.

◆ After rupture, reparative cells respond, incorporating existing thrombi into the expanding lesion as new fibrous tissue is formed to repair the lesion (Aouizerat, 2005).

◆ The lumen of the vessel is thus further narrowed.

Stable Versus Vulnerable Plaque

Stable plaques have thick fibrous caps that separate the lipid core from the endothelium. Stable plaques are less complicated than vulnerable plaques and tend to have smooth outlines. More vulnerable plaques have thinner caps. The edge of the fibrous cap, called the shoulder, is a particularly vulnerable area and is commonly the location of ruptured plaque (Deedy, 2002). A comparison of stable and vulnerable plaque is seen in Figure 8.1

Both mechanical features and inflammatory responses impact the vulnerability of a lesion. The role of the inflammatory response in ACSs has been the focus of new, emerging risk factors that measure levels and risk of vascular inflammation. Biomarkers for this inflammation include high-sensitivity C-reactive protein, fibrinogen, homocysteine, lipoprotein A, serum amyloid A, and interleukin-6 (Gardner & Altman, 2005).

Rupture of a coronary plaque produces an acute coronary event and increases the short-term risk of cardiac death or nonfatal MI. (Braunwald et al., 2002). It is important to know that most vulnerable plaques identified during cardiac catheterization (angiography) are not found in tightly stenotic vessels. Patients can have plaque in the coronary arteries that does not cause lumen stenosis. It is this plaque that is usually most vulnerable and the cause of acute coronary syndromes.

In most patients, MI results from atheromas that produce less than 50% narrowing of the vessel lumen (Gardner & Altman, 2005). Plaques that cause greater than 75% stenosis, and therefore angina, are usually more stable plaques and less likely to rupture. Because vulnerable plaque typically does not produce symptomatic stenotic disease, stress testing has a limited ability to detect vulnerable plaque. Vulnerable plaque may not be visible as a stenotic lesion, but may be visualized using intracoronary ultrasound during cardiac catheterization. Patients with minimal stenotic disease on cardiac catheterization may still have a substantial plaque burden and may be at high risk for vulnerable plaque rupture. Aggressive risk factor modification is as important in these patients as in patients with stenotic disease.

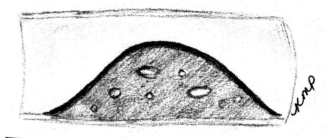
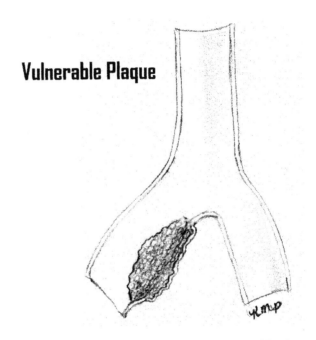

Figure 8.1: Comparison of stable and vulnerable plaque.

CLINICAL SIGNS AND SYMPTOMS OF CORONARY ARTERY DISEASE

Angina pectoris is the clinical symptom that results from decreased blood flow to the myocardium. It usually occurs in patients with coronary heart disease involving 70% or more stenosis and at least one major epicardial artery (Gibbons et al., 2002). Decreased blood flow results in ischemia or a temporary lack of oxygen to the heart muscle. Although typically caused by coronary artery disease, angina can also be caused by other cardiac conditions, such as coronary artery spasm, valvular heart disease, uncontrolled hypertension, and hypertrophic cardiomyopathy. Approximately one half of patients with AMI have had preceding angina (Gibbons et al., 2002).

Characteristics of Angina Pectoris

- ◆ Sensation of pressure, tightness, heaviness, burning, or squeezing.
  - ❖ Rarely described as a sharp or stabbing pain.

Chapter 8

❖ Should not worsen with changes in position or respiration.
◆ Can be located behind the sternum, in the upper back, shoulder, arm, jaw, or epigastric area.
   ❖ Not usually located in the middle to lower abdomen and does usually not radiate to the lower extremities.
◆ May be associated with symptoms (or stand alone symptoms) of dyspnea, nausea, palpitations, or diaphoresis.
◆ Duration of discomfort is typically defined in minutes.
   ❖ Not typically defined in seconds or hours.

Assessment of Angina Pectoris

◆ Quality of discomfort
   ❖ It is important to use the word "discomfort" when assessing patients with potential angina. Many patients with dyspnea or chest pressure deny the presence of pain.
◆ Location of discomfort including radiation
   ❖ Time of onset and duration of symptoms.
   ❖ Aggravating and alleviating factors.

The assessment of angina and chest pain is discussed in full detail in Chapter 2.

CLASSIFICATION AND SPECIAL FEATURES OF ANGINA PECTORIS

Stable Angina

Stable angina pectoris typically occurs with physical exertion or emotional stress and is relieved by rest or sublingual nitroglycerin. Angina is considered stable when its pattern is predictable over several weeks. To be considered predictable, angina should be triggered by the same amount of physical or emotional stress and should be easily relieved by rest or sublingual nitroglycerin.

Unstable Angina

Angina is considered unstable when it occurs with minimal exertion or when an increased dose of nitroglycerin is required to achieve relief. Prolonged rest angina is also considered unstable angina. Any angina that increases in severity or is very severe on first presentation is considered unstable. Unstable angina is caused by unstable or ruptured plaque that causes abrupt complete or partial closure of a coronary artery. It is treated very differently than stable angina. This treatment will be discussed later in this chapter, in the section on non-STEMIs.

Angina in Women

Many women, and even some health care providers, do not consider heart disease a major health risk for women. For this reason, many women delay seeking healthcare and may attribute their symptoms to other non-cardiac causes. Although heart disease kills more women than all cancers combined, many women still fear breast cancer and other forms of cancer as their primary health risk.

Angina frequently presents different in women than in men. Substernal chest pressure radiating to the arm or jaw, often described as a typical symptom, is less common in women than in men. Women may complain of more generalized epigastric discomfort or present with less specific complaints, such as dyspnea or fatigue. These symptoms are often prodromal. Women presenting with symptoms of discomfort from their nose to their navel should be evaluated for the presence of coronary heart disease.

328

Coronary spasm, mitral valve prolapse, and microvascular disease are more likely to be the cause of symptoms in women than in men. Women presenting with anginal symptoms who proceed to cardiac catheterization have less documented stenotic disease of major epicardial coronary arteries. Women are also more likely to have unstable angina than AMIs (Braunwald et al., 2002). Older women who present with ACS have a higher incidence of complications, including the development of heart failure (Braunwald et al., 2002). Women are also prescribed less intensive pharmacological regimes for CAD than men, including less frequent prescription of aspirin (Braunwald et al., 2002).

Before menopause, women appear to have a protective mechanism in place against CAD. However, after menopause, the risk of CAD in women begins to approach that of men. Women lag behind men in their presentation of CAD by about 10 years. Despite the premenopausal protective benefits seen in women, hormone replacement therapy is no longer a recommended strategy to reduce the risk of heart disease in postmenopausal women, based on the results of the Women's Health Initiative (Newton & Froelicher, 2005).

Angina in the Elderly

The elderly with angina pectoris often present with more generalized symptoms, such as weakness, dyspnea, and confusion. These symptoms are often attributed to the aging process, and the potential diagnosis of angina may be overlooked. The elderly have more cardiac and non-cardiac co-morbidities that complicate the diagnosis of ACS and increase the risk.

Cardiac co-morbidities associated with the elderly include:

◆ Decreased response to beta sympathetic stimulation.

◆ Increased afterload due to decreased arterial compliance and systemic hypertension.

◆ Left-ventricular hypertrophy.

◆ Diastolic dysfunction.

The elderly also face special challenges in the medical treatment of angina. In many cases the elderly are on multiple medications and have co-existing conditions, such as renal insufficiency, that complicate the administration of cardiovascular drugs. Many medications need to be started at lower doses, particularly those that produce a hypotensive response.

Angina in Diabetics

Autonomic dysfunction occurs in about one-third of patients with diabetes and can affect the symptoms they experience with angina. Diabetic patients may be less likely to experience pain. Up to 25% of all patients presenting with ACS are diabetic (Braunwald et al., 2002). Diabetic patients frequently have severe multivessel disease and higher rates of complications after acute cardiac events. Diabetic patients have a greater proportion of ulcerated plaques resulting in intracoronary thrombi. This fact places diabetic patients at risk for instability.

Beta blockers are used with caution, but not withheld in the treatment of ACS in diabetic patients. Beta blockers may mask the symptoms of hypoglycemia and may blunt the hyperglycemic response.

DIAGNOSIS OF CORONARY ARTERY DISEASE

History and Physical

Assessment information also includes the presence of cardiovascular risk factors or history of CAD, cerebral vascular disease, or peripheral vascular disease. A history of CAD, cerebral vascular disease, or peripheral vascular disease increases the likelihood that the presentation of symptoms is related to myocardial ischemia. Pulmonary disorders, gastrointestinal disorders, chest wall pain, and sometimes psychiatric conditions can have symptoms similar to those of angina.

Chapter 8

12-Lead ECG

The 12-lead ECG can be normal in up to 50% of patients with chronic stable angina (Gibbons et al., 2002); therefore, a normal ECG does not exclude coronary heart disease. However, an abnormal ECG or the presence of a cardiac arrhythmia increases the likelihood that coronary artery disease is the cause of the symptoms.

Patients with chronic stable angina who have an abnormal resting ECG are at a higher risk for adverse outcomes. The following ECG findings indicate higher risk and poorer prognosis:

- Evidence of prior MI.
  - ❖ Q waves in multiple leads.
  - ❖ Large R wave in V_1 (evidence of old posterior MI).
  - ❖ Loss of R wave progression in leads V_1-V_6.
- Persistent T wave inversions in V_1-V_3.
- Left bundle branch block
- Bifasicular block (Right Bundle Branch Block with Left Anterior Hemiblock).
- 2° or 3° AV block.
- Atrial fibrillation.
- Ventricular arrhythmias.
- Left-ventricular hypertrophy.
- Left-atrial enlargement (indicating mitral regurgitation or pulmonary venous congestion).

Chest Radiograph

The presence of cardiomegaly, pulmonary venous congestion or left-ventricular aneurysm also indicated a higher risk and poorer prognosis.

Laboratory Studies

A variety of laboratory studies may provide some information that may assist in the diagnosis of CAD.

- Hemoglobin and hematocrit to assess for anemia (decreased oxygen carrying capacity).
- Fasting blood sugar level to assess for diabetes.
- Fasting lipid profile to assess for hyperlipidemia.
- Thyroid studies to assess thyroid function.
- Cardiac biomarkers to assess for myocardial damage (discussed later in this chapter).

Stress Testing

Stress testing can be done using exercise or chemicals. During a stress test, the 12-lead ECG is evaluated for changes in response to stress. In addition to the stress component, stress testing is often accompanied by some form of myocardial imaging. Certain patients require the use of myocardial imaging with their stress test because the ECG component of the test will not provide an accurate diagnosis. Patient conditions requiring myocardial imaging with stress testing, due to lack of reliable ECG interpretation include:

- Left bundle branch block.
- > 1 mm ST-segment depression at rest.
- Paced ventricular rhythm.
- Wolf-Parkinson-White syndrome (Gibbons et al., 2002).

Acute Coronary Syndrome

Exercise Stress Testing

Treadmills or bicycles are used for exercise stress tests. When patients are able to exercise on a treadmill for 6 to 12 minutes, exercise stress testing is generally performed instead of chemical stress testing. During exercise, myocardial oxygen demand increases and coronary arteries dilate in response to this increased demand. In a patient with coronary artery disease, the coronary arteries are not able to adequately dilate to meet the needs of the increased myocardial oxygen demand, and abnormalities occur on the 12-lead ECG or associated imaging studies. An exercise stress test can be conducted with or without myocardial imaging. Patients on beta blockers who are scheduled to undergo exercise stress testing should have these medications held for approximately 48 hours prior to testing. During exercise stress testing, the achievement of a predicted heart rate is important for good test results. If beta blockers are not held, it may be difficult to achieve an adequate heart rate. There is the rare occasion that a patient being treated medically is ordered a stress test to assess the patient's exercise tolerance while taking the beta blocker to assure the patient is being adequately treated. In these situations it is important to give the beta blocker. Nurses should seek out an order to hold the beta blocker before an exercise stress test. Exercise stress testing is less sensitive in women than in men (Gibbons et al., 2002).

Exercise Changes with Bundle Branch Blocks

◆ Exercise-induced ST depression usually occurs with LBBB and is not associated with ischemia.

◆ Exercise-induced ST depression usually occurs in RBBB in leads V_1-V_3 and is not associated with ischemia. However, exercise-induced ST depression with RBBB is significant when it occurs in the low lateral or inferior leads.

(Gibbons et al., 2002).

Chemical Stress Testing

Three pharmacological agents are used in chemical stress testing: dobutamine, dipyridamole, and adenosine. All pharmacological stress testing is done in conjunction with myocardial imaging. Both dipyridamole and adenosine cause coronary microvascular dilatation similar to the coronary artery vasodilation that occurs with exercise. Dipyridamole is an indirect coronary vasodilator, whereas adenosine causes direct coronary vasodilation.

These medications commonly cause chest pain because vasodilation pulls blood away from compromised areas of the myocardium. Another common side effect of these medications is flushing caused by vasodilation. Adenosine can also cause brief episodes of heart block due to its ability to slow or stop conduction through the atrioventricular (AV) node. A rare but severe side effect of both medications in patients with asthma or other lung disease is bronchospasm. Any patient with severe lung disease or active wheezing prior to stress testing is not a candidate for use of these medications. Aminophylline can be given as an antidote to both medications, but is seldom needed with adenosine due to its short half-life. Patients who are currently taking aminophylline-containing medications should not undergo these chemical stress tests because aminophylline counteracts the medications being administered for the stress test.

Dobutamine works differently than the other two agents. During a dobutamine stress test, high-dose dobutamine is used to increase contractility and heart rate, thereby increasing myocardial oxygen demand. Dobutamine stress testing more closely mimics exercise stress testing in that high-dose Dobutamine is used to increase myocardial oxygen demand by increasing heart rate and contractility. In response to this increased myocardial oxygen demand, normal coronary arteries dilate. Coronary arteries do not, however, dilate to the extent they do with agents that produce more direct coronary vasodilation. A potential side effect of dobutamine that is not present with dipyridamole or adenosine is cardiac tachyarrhythmias.

Chapter 8

Cardiac Imaging With Stress Testing

Exercise or chemical stress testing is combined with pretest cardiac imaging, such as cardiac echocardiography or radionuclide imaging; pre-test and post-test cardiac images are compared. When echocardiography is used, coronary artery disease is suspected when echocardiography images show a new wall motion abnormality after exercise or after the administration of high-dose dobutamine. Echocardiography is not used as the imaging modality with dipyridamole or adenosine stress testing.

When radionuclide imaging is used, the peak stress images are compared to the resting images. An area of relative hypoperfusion on the peak stress images is suspicious for coronary artery disease. Radioisotopes are taken up by myocardial tissue in proportion to blood flow to the area. The imaging portion of a stress test provides information about the extent, severity, and location of ischemia. Radionuclide studies can differentiate areas of necrosis from ischemic but viable tissue.

Nuclear scan results reflect perfusion at the time of injection. Patients can be injected during an episode of pain and scanning can be delayed for several hours after the injection.

Prognostic Information From Stress Testing

The exercise portion of a stress test (excluding dipyridamole and adenosine testing) can provide prognostic information (Gibbons et al., 2002). One example of prognostic information obtained from exercise stress testing is the heart rate recovery score. This score is calculated by taking the heart rate at peak exercise and subtracting the heart rate at 1-minute after exercise. A normal score is a heart rate difference greater than 12 beats per minute. A normal score is associated with a low risk of death. A low score is considered less than 8 beats per minute and is associated with a high risk of death. A score of 8 to 12 is considered an intermediate risk (Gibbons et al., 2002).

Contraindications To Stress Testing

There are certain absolute contraindications to stress testing in high-risk patients. High-risk patients include those with:

◆ Acute MI $\leq$ 2 days old.
◆ Acute myocarditis or pericarditis.
◆ Acute pulmonary embolism.
◆ Acute aortic dissection.
◆ Symptomatic heart failure.
◆ Severe aortic stenosis.
◆ Symptomatic arrhythmias.
◆ High-risk unstable angina.
(Gibbons et al., 2002)

Cardiac Catheterization

Cardiac catheterization, or angiography, is currently the gold standard for determining the presence, location, and extent of obstructive coronary heart disease. Cardiac catheterization is an invasive procedure that has a small but serious risk of severe adverse outcomes, including stroke, MI, and even death. For this reason, patients are chosen carefully and must meet certain criteria. The American Heart Association and American College of Cardiology have very specific guidelines, stating indications for cardiac catheterization. Patients for whom cardiac catheterization is an indication include:

◆ Patients with disabling angina despite medical treatment.
◆ Patients with high-risk criteria for CAD on non-invasive testing.

Acute Coronary Syndrome

◆ Patients who have survived sudden cardiac death.
◆ Patients with angina and clinical signs of CAD.
◆ Patients with low ejection fraction and ischemia on non-invasive testing.
◆ Patients with inadequate information obtained from non-invasive testing.

(del Bene & Vaughan, 2005)

In addition to determining the location and severity of lesions, cardiac catheterization can evaluate intracardiac pressures and left-ventricular function. Cardiac catheterization is also done to evaluate patients with possible vasospastic angina who have chest pain at rest. Provocative testing can be done in the cardiac catheterization laboratory using ergonovine maleate. If needed, intracoronary vasodilators can be given to treat the induced spasm. If femoral artery access cannot be used, then radial or brachial access is an alternative approach for cardiac catheterization.

Cardiac Computed Tomography (CT)

Cardiac CT is an emerging diagnostic testing option. Cardiac CT has a high negative predictive value and may be a useful tool for ruling out the presence of CAD in patients presenting with chest pain in the emergency department or in other settings. Coronary artery calcium scoring shows calcified plaque, which may also be a predictor of non-calcified plaque. A calcium score of greater than 400 in an intermediate risk patient may indicate a risk equivalent for CAD comparable to a patient with diabetes or peripheral arterial disease. Calcium scoring in low-risk and high-risk patients seems to be of less benefit (Greenland et al., 2007). In addition, a calcium score of 0 does not rule out soft plaque, but does help rule out significant stenotic disease. Cardiac CT is less useful in obtaining physiological information, such as myocardial viability in patients with known CAD. Cardiac CT is an evolving image modality, and active research regarding its role remains in process.

CARDIAC ISCHEMIA

Aggravating Conditions

Patients with CAD develop symptoms due to an imbalance between myocardial oxygen supply and demand. Certain conditions can upset the balance between myocardial oxygen supply and demand. Conditions that can increase myocardial oxygen demand include hyperthermia, hypertension, tachycardia, and conditions that produce over stimulation of the sympathetic nervous system, such as cocaine use and hyperthyroidism. Certain co-existing cardiac conditions can also increase myocardial oxygen demand and reduce supply, including aortic stenosis and hypertrophic cardiomyopathy. Non-cardiac conditions that decrease the delivery of oxygen to tissues can also exacerbate angina. These include conditions that decrease hemoglobin or oxygen saturation levels, such as anemia and pulmonary disease.

Complications of Chronic Ischemic Heart Disease

The extent of ischemia and its impact on left ventricular function determine the outcome in patients with angina (Gibbons et al., 2002). Complications of ischemia include the development of mitral regurgitation or left-ventricular thrombi. These complications are a result of left-ventricular dilatation and dysfunction.

TREATMENT OPTIONS FOR STABLE ANGINA

Stable patients who are diagnosed with greater than 70% stenosis during cardiac catheterization have three primary treatment options: medical treatment, primary percutaneous coronary intervention (PCI), or coronary artery bypass grafting (CABG). Lifestyle modification and aggressive risk factor reduction is included in all three treatment arms. The goals of treatment in CAD are to reduce symptoms (improve quality of life) and

Chapter 8

prevent complications (improve quantity of life). Complications include disease progression, MI, and death. The highest priority of treatment is to reduce death. When treatment decisions are made, first preference is given to those treatments proven to reduce the risk of death (Gibbons et al., 2002).

Pharmacological Management

Treatment of angina usually begins with medical therapy. Medical management of patients with CAD includes the use of a combination of medications from the following list:

◆ Antiplatelet therapy.
◆ Antianginal therapy.
◆ Lipid-lowering therapy.

Antiplatelet Therapy

Antiplatelet therapy is prescribed for all patients. Aspirin is the primary antiplatelet agent used for patients with known CAD or those with symptoms suggestive of CAD. For patients with known CAD, peripheral vascular disease, or stroke, aspirin in doses from 75 to 325 mg has been shown to reduce the risk of MI, stroke, and vascular death by approximately 33% (Gibbons et al., 2002). Clopidogrel is more effective than aspirin in reducing the risk of MI, stroke, and death in patients with atherosclerotic vascular disease (Deedy, 2002). However, there is a dramatic cost difference between aspirin and clopidogrel that prevents clopidogrel from being more widely used as a primary antiplatelet agent. Administration of clopidogrel with aspirin adds an additional 20% risk reduction in patients with unstable angina or non-STEMI (Deedy, 2002).

Antianginal Agents

Patients with coronary heart disease are also prescribed antianginal agents. These agents include beta blockers, nitrates, and calcium channel blockers. The goals of antianginal therapy are to reduce symptoms and improve activity tolerance, thereby improving quality of life.

Beta Blockers

Beta blockers are the first-line agents in the treatment of stable angina. Beta blockers are very effective in controlling angina brought on by physical exertion. The initial target heart rate goal is 55 to 60 beats per minute at rest for patients with stable angina (Gibbons et al.,2002). Resting heart rate may need to be lowered if angina cannot be controlled. Patients can experience side effects that limit dosing. Beta blockers are not used to treat vasospastic angina. Beta blockers are the one class of antianginal medications that have survival benefit in certain groups of patients, such as those patients who have had a recent MI (Antman et al., 2004).

Nitrates

Nitrates improve exercise tolerance and prolong the time to onset of angina. For nitrates to remain effective, patients need to have an 8- to 10-hour nitrate-free period each day. Headache is the most common side effect of nitrate use. Headaches associated with nitroglycerin administration should be treated because pain activates the sympathetic nervous system, which increases myocardial oxygen demand and, potentially, myocardial ischemia. Headaches usually subside over time in patients taking long-acting nitrates. Patients with a history of angina should always carry sublingual nitroglycerin.

Calcium Channel Blockers

Calcium channel blockers or long-acting nitrates are used as first-line agents for vasospastic angina because they are direct coronary vasodilators. These medications can also be added to beta blocker therapy when angina is not controlled. Calcium channel blockers must be used very cautiously in patients with impaired systolic left-ventricular dysfunction. Amlodipine and felodipine, newer dihydropyridine calcium channel blockers, are more selective coronary arterial vasodilators and are better tolerated than other calcium channel blockers in patients with left-ventricular dysfunction (Gibbons et al., 2002).

Lipid-lowering Therapy

Lipid lowering therapy is discussed in Chapters 7 and 14.

Nonpharmacological Treatment Options

PCI and CABG are two nonpharmacological treatment options in patients with CAD that are discussed in detail in Chapters 15 and 16. External counterpulsation is another non-pharmacological treatment option for patients with debilitating angina on maximal medical therapy; this option is used for patients who are not candidates for revascularization. During this therapy, a series of cuffs are wrapped around the patient's legs. Compressed air is used to apply pressure in the cuffs in synchronization with the cardiac cycle. The cuff pressure results in an increased arterial pressure that is used to increase retrograde aortic blood flow into the coronary arteries during diastole. Patients receive 35 hours of treatment over a 4- to 7-week period (Gibbons et al., 2002).

Long-Term Management

For patients with stable angina, it is important to evaluate the effectiveness of risk factor reduction with each follow-up. An assessment of the patient's anginal symptoms, functional capacity, and tolerance to medications is also important. The patient should know to report worsening angina or rest angina. Follow-up office visits are usually scheduled every 4 to 6 months during the first year after initiation of antianginal therapy. Long-term follow-up is generally based on the patient's other existing medical conditions, but should occur at least annually. Patients with conditions that exacerbate angina require more frequent follow-up. Follow-up visits can be alternated between the primary care physician and cardiologist.

ACUTE CORONARY SYNDROME OVERVIEW

CAD presents in a continuum, as seen in Table 8-1. Patients presenting with an ACS are treated differently than patients presenting with stable angina. With ACS there is an urgency for treatment to preserve myocardial function. Acute myocardial ischemia develops when oxygen supply is insufficient to meet the metabolic demands of cardiac cells. When cells are deprived of oxygen, ischemia occurs within 10 seconds. Myocardial function is affected after 1 minute of ischemia, and cells begin to swell after just a few minutes. After 20 minutes of oxygen deprivation, irreversible cellular injury begins to occur (Gardner & Altman, 2005).

ACS includes unstable angina, non-STEMI, and STEMI. The rupturing of unstable vulnerable plaques is a frequent cause of ACS. When vulnerable plaques rupture, thrombi form at the site of injury, blocking blood flow and causing ischemia or injury to myocardial cells. Patients with a longer history of ischemic heart disease may have collateral circulation that provides protection during the occlusion of a coronary vessel. Collateral vessels are those that connect major branches of coronary arteries. As luminal narrowing gradually occurs, pressure changes promote the development and use of these collateral vessels to supply oxygen to ischemic areas. New capillaries can grow in response ischemia.

Chapter 8

Younger patients without collateral circulation are more vulnerable to extensive damage from an occluded coronary artery. When an ACS begins, the endocardial region is the first to become ischemic and is also the first area where tissues begin to die. As ischemia continues and the injury extends, the middle myocardium (or subendocardium) is affected. If left untreated and MI continues, the injury can extend toward the epicardium, affecting the full thickness of the myocardium. A full-thickness MI is commonly referred to as a transmural MI.

Classifications of Myocardial Infarction

MIs are now classified by their initial presentation as either STEMI or non-STEMI. Patients presenting with STEMI are candidates for reperfusion therapy. Early in an STEMI, the ST-segment will lift off baseline to form a hyper acute T wave. Hyper acute T waves may form as early as 2 minutes after occlusion of a coronary artery. The hyper acute T wave can be formed by an oblique straightening of the ST segment. There may also be subtle enlargement of the T wave. The size of a T wave should always be assessed in relation to the size of the QRS complex. T waves should not appear to dominate over the QRS complex. T waves may also appear bulky and wide, forming a broad base. QT interval is usually prolonged in a hyper acute T wave. The hyper acute T wave will be present before any J point elevation is evident. J point may actually be slightly depressed initially, with the T wave appearing to have its take off below the isoelectric line.

See Figure 8.2 below. Early hyper acute T waves best seen in leads V_2, V_3, and V_4. Note the depressed J points in leads V_3 and V_4.

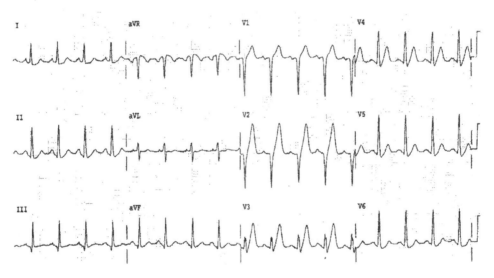

Figure 8.2: Early hyper acute T waves best seen in leads V_2, V_3, and V_4.
Note the depressed J points in leads V_3 and V_4.

See Figure 8.3 below. Post hyper acute T waves in leads V₂, V₃, and V₄. Note the change in the J points in leads V₃ and V₄ as they begin to elevate.

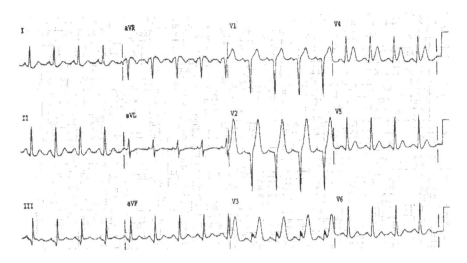

Figure 8.3: Post hyper acute T waves in leads V₂, V₃, and V₄.
Note the change in the J points in leads V₃ and V₄ as they begin to elevate.

The hyper acute T waves of a STEMI need to be differentiated from T waves of early repolarization (a normal variant) and T waves of hyperkalemia.

Keys to Differentiating Hyper Acute T Waves

- Early Repolarization
  - More upward concavity.
  - Asymmetric (steeper down slope).
- Hyerkalemia
  - More narrow based.
  - More peaked.
  - Short QT interval in the absence of a wide QRS.

If the initial ECG is not diagnostic of STEMI, but the patient remains symptomatic with clinical suspicion for STEMI, then serial ECGs and ST-segment monitoring are indicated.

STEMI and non-STEMI can both produce either a Q wave or non-Q wave MI. Non-Q wave MIs are usually associated with damage that has not extended through the full thickness of the myocardium. Myocardial damage progresses from the subendocardium to the epicardium. A Q wave MI is diagnosed by the presence of a pathological Q wave in the leads of infarction on a 12-lead ECG. This type of MI is usually associated with full thickness damage of the myocardium. Q waves are the first negative deflection of the QRS complex; when they are too large, they represent altered depolarization due to necrotic tissue. Q waves are more common with STEMI. A 12-lead ECG is used to differentiate STEMI from non-STEMI. However, a 12-lead ECG cannot distinguish between non-STEMI and unstable angina. Cardiac biomarkers help differentiate between these two conditions.

Chapter 8

Cardiac Biomarkers

Cardiac biomarkers are released into the blood when necrosis occurs as a result of membrane rupture of the myocytes. Cardiac biomarkers used in the evaluation of ACS includes myoglobin, creatine kinase (CK), CK-MB, and troponin I or T.

Myoglobin is the biomarker that rises the earliest, within 2 hours after myocardial damage. Although it is a very sensitive biomarker, it is not specific to myocardial damage. CK is an enzyme present in the heart, brain, and skeletal muscle, so elevations are not specific to myocardial damage. CK-MB is more specific to the heart. Therefore, CK-MB measurements are helpful in identifying more than minor amounts of myocardial damage. CK-MB rapidly rises in the presence of myocardial damage.

Troponin I is found only in cardiac muscle. It is the most sensitive indicator of myocardial damage. Approximately 30% of patients with non ST elevation and normal CKMB levels will test positive for a non-STEMI based on troponin results (Braunwald, 2002). Troponin I and T are of equal sensitivity and specificity. Because troponin I remains elevated for a long period, with a gradual return to normal, it is a beneficial indicator in patients presenting late after symptom onset. Troponin levels are capable of diagnosing small amounts of myocardial necrosis not measured by rises in CK-MB levels. Table 8.2 summarizes the cardiac biomarkers.

Table 8.2
Cardiac Biomarker Summary

Cardiac Biomarker	Specificity/Sensitivity	Rise	Peak	Duration
Myoglobin	Sensitive but not specific	Within 2 hours	4 to 10 hours	< 24 hours
CK-MB	Highly specific	4 to 6 hours	18 to 24 hours	2 to 3 days
Troponin I or T	Highly specific and sensitive	4 to 6 hours	18 to 24 hours	10 or more days

Biomarker results are not needed to proceed with reperfusion in STEMI. Cardiac biomarkers are also limited in the diagnosis of reinfarction within 18 hours after the onset of STEMI because initial biomarker elevation can still exist.

ST-SEGMENT ELEVATION MI

An estimated 500,000 STEMIs occur each year (Antman et al., 2004). Complete occlusion of a vessel by a thrombus (Figure 8.4) produces a STEMI. Patients with STEMIs are classified more specifically by the portion of the left ventricle suffering injury. Mortality is greatest within the first 24 to 48 hours of symptom onset (del Bene & Vaughn, 2005).

Inferior Wall MI

Coronary Artery Distribution

- The inferior wall of the left ventricle is fed by the right coronary artery (RCA) in 80-85% of the population.
- The circumflex artery feeds the inferior wall in the remainder of the population.
- The marginal branch of the RCA supplies the right ventricle.

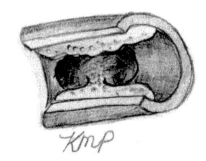

Figure 8.4: Thrombus formation caused by plaque rupture resulting in complete occlusion of coronary artery.

- The posterior descending artery is a branch of the RCA in most people and supplies the posterior wall of the left ventricle.
- Inferior MIs frequently involve a concurrent right-ventricular MI and/or posterior wall MI.
- Infarction of the right ventricle occurs in anywhere from one-third to one-half of inferior MIs. (del Bene & Vaughan, 2005).
- A proximal RCA occlusion will result in an infarct of both the inferior wall of the left ventricle and the right ventricle.
- An occlusion distal to the marginal branch of the RCA will spare the right ventricle.
- An occlusion proximal to the posterior descending artery will result in an inferior posterior MI.
- A very large RCA or circumflex artery may supply both the inferior and lateral walls of the left ventricle.

12-lead ECG Changes

- ST-segment elevation in leads II, III, and aVF. (Figure 8.5 shows a 12-lead ECG representation of an inferior wall MI with J point elevation in leads II, III, and aVF.)
- ST elevation ≥ 0.5mm in inferior leads should be considered abnormal until proven otherwise.
- Lead III typically elevates sooner and more prominently than the other inferior leads.
- When lead II elevation is greater than lead III elevation, the circumflex is suspected as the culprit vessel.
- Reciprocal depression, particularly in lead aVL (Note: Leads 3 and aVL are the most reciprocal to each other. ST depression seen in lead aVL in Figure 8.5.)
- A right-sided and posterior ECG should be performed on all patients with inferior wall MIs to assess for involvement of the right ventricle and posterior wall. Patients with right-ventricular involvement have different treatment considerations, as discussed later in this chapter. The proper lead placement for right-sided and posterior leads is discussed in Chapter 6.

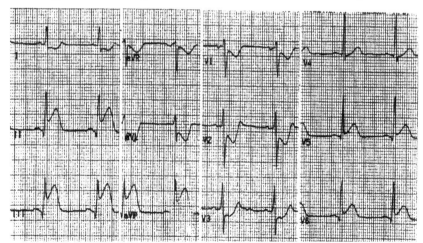

Figure 8.5: Acute J point and ST segment elevation in the inferior leads with reciprocal depression in the high lateral leads, particularly lead aVL. ST segment depression in leads V_1-V_3 represent reciprocal changes related to co-existing posterior wall injury.

Chapter 8

Complications

◆ Bradycardia and first- and second-degree heart block are common because the RCA also feeds the sinoatrial (SA) node and AV node in the majority of people. First- and second-degree heart block with an inferior MI usually do not progress to complete heart block because the His bundle and bundle branches are not fed by the RCA.

◆ Increased parasympathetic activity associated with inferior MIs causes nausea and vomiting.

◆ Right-ventricular involvement increases the short-term mortality associated with an inferior MI.

◆ Patients with inferiorposterior MIs are also at risk for the development of papillary muscle rupture. Papillary muscle rupture results in acute mitral regurgitation and usually occurs 48-72 hours after the onset of the MI.

Anterior Wall MI

Coronary Artery Distribution

◆ The left anterior descending artery (LAD) supplies blood to the anterior portion of the septum and the anterior wall of the left ventricle.

◆ An occlusion of the mid-LAD produces an anterior MI.

◆ A proximal LAD occlusion prior to first diagonal branch produces an anterolateral MI.

◆ A proximal LAD occlusion prior to first septal perforator artery produces an anteroseptal MI.

◆ On rare occasions, a patient has a wrap around LAD vessel that also feeds the inferior wall. An occlusion of this vessel produces an anteroinferior MI and may mimic pericarditis.

12-Lead ECG Changes

◆ An infarct of the anterior wall of the left ventricle produces ST-segment elevation in leads V_3 and V_4 on a 12-lead ECG.

◆ ST-segment elevation occurs in leads V_1 through V_4 if the septum is involved (Figure 8.6).

◆ ST elevation occurs in lead I and aVL if there is high lateral wall involvement and in leads V_5 and V_6 if there is low lateral wall involvement.

◆ Inferior depression in anterior MI typically indicates high lateral wall involvement because the inferior leads are most reciprocal to the high lateral wall. (Note: Lead III and lead aVL have the most reciprocal relationship.) Note the depression in leads II, III, and aVF representing reciprocal changes to the ST elevation seen in leads and I and aVL in Figure 8.6.

◆ Inferior ST depression in anterior MI is highly predictive of LAD occlusion prior to the first diagonal, which produces a co-existing high lateral wall infarction.

◆ Associated inferior depression is associated with higher precordial elevation and a worse prognosis.

Complications

◆ Anterior MIs have the greatest amount of myocardium at risk, and the highest mortality and complication rates.

◆ Post MI ejection fraction is worse than other MI types even when controlled for CKMB levels.

◆ A large anterior MI can result in profound left-ventricular dysfunction, leading to heart failure and cardiogenic shock.

◆ The bundle branches of the conduction system run through the septum; therefore, patients with occlusion of the LAD are at risk for the development of bundle branch blocks and complete heart blocks.

Acute Coronary Syndrome

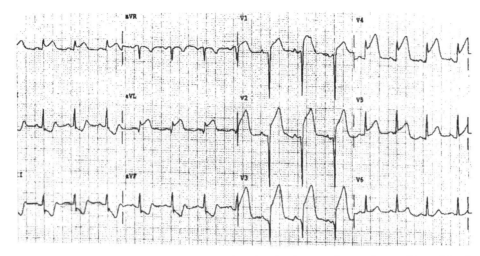

Figure 8.6: Acute J point and ST segment elevation in the septal, anterior, and lateral leads. Reciprocal ST segment depression in the inferior leads from the high lateral wall injury.

- A patient who develops a right bundle branch block (RBBB) as a complication of an acute anterior MI should be carefully observed for the development of a left anterior hemi-block (LAHB). Patients with RBBB and LAHB in the presence of an acute anterior MI are at high risk for the development of complete heart block and potential cardiogenic shock.
- Patients with septal involvement are also at risk for ventricular septal rupture. A ventricular septal rupture produces a holosystolic murmur. This medical emergency requires prompt afterload reduction and emergency surgery to repair the rupture.

Lateral Wall MI

Coronary Artery Distribution

- The circumflex artery off the left main coronary artery supplies blood to the lateral wall of the left ventricle.
- A large portion of the myocardium is supplied by the circumflex artery, and a stand-alone lateral wall MI should be treated as aggressively as other MIs.
- Other coronary branches also supply portions of the lateral wall.
  - ❖ First diagonal branch of LAD.
  - ❖ Obtuse marginal branches of circumflex.
- Lateral wall MIs are frequently associated with inferior or posterior wall MIs.
- Posterior lateral MIs are usually due to circumflex occlusion, but may be due to RCA lesion with occlusion of the posterior lateral branches.

12-Lead ECG Changes

- Leads I and aVL view the high lateral wall of the left ventricle and leads V₅ and V₆ view the low lateral wall. Figure 8.7 shows a high lateral wall MI.
- The myocardium supplied by the circumflex artery is less represented on a 12-lead ECG than the myocardium supplied by the RCA or LAD. For this reason, occlusions of the circumflex artery may be less visible on a 12-lead ECG than occlusions of the LAD and RCA.
- The sensitivity of ST elevation for detection of lateral MI is lower because the circumflex supplies an electrographically silent area of the myocardium.
- An isolated lateral wall MI is frequently missed.

- ST elevation may be < 1 mm in the high lateral leads due to the low voltage of these leads.
- ST elevation may only be in aVL.
- New ST elevation in aVL is significant, especially if there is reciprocal depression in lead III. These patients should be considered for reperfusion. Note: If only one lead demonstrates ST elevation, then angiography with PCI is the preferred method of reperfusion.

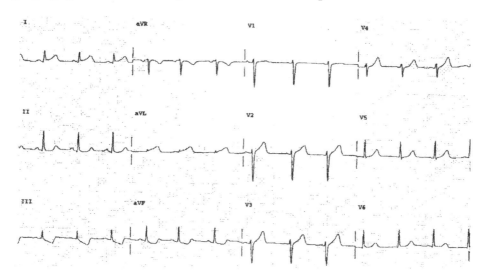

Figure 8.7: Subtle ST segment elevation in leads I and aVL representing high lateral wall injury. Reciprocal ST segment depression in the inferior leads.

Complications

- The circumflex artery supplies the AV node, His bundle, and papillary muscles in about 10% of people. Therefore, conduction abnormalities and papillary muscle dysfunction with resultant mitral regurgitation are potential complications of lateral wall MIs.
- The amount of myocardium at risk varies widely. The mean size of a lateral wall MI is larger than inferior MI.

Posterior Wall MI

Coronary Artery Distribution

- Posterior wall MIs are caused by obstruction of the posterior descending artery, usually originating from the RCA, and thus commonly occurring in conjunction with inferior wall MIs.
- The posterior descending artery in some patients can originate from the circumflex artery; in these patients, a posterior MI may occur in conjunction with lateral wall MI.

12-Lead ECG Changes

- ST elevation is seen in leads V_7-V_9 when a posterior ECG is done.
- A true isolated posterior MI does not produce ST-segment elevation on a standard 12-lead ECG because no electrodes are placed directly over the posterior wall of the left ventricle. However, the ACC/AHA recommend fibrinolytics if the physician can interpret the ECG correctly.
- 3.3-8.5% of all MIs are posterior MIs without ST elevation on standard 12-lead ECG (Smith et al., 2002).
- A posterior wall MI may show ST-segment depression on the standard 12-lead ECG in the leads reciprocal to the posterior wall, including leads V_1 to V_4. See Figure 8.5 with a posterior MI (ST depression in V_1-V_3) in the presence of an acute inferior wall MI.

Acute Coronary Syndrome

- Some ST elevation in V_1-V_4 can be normal in up to 90% of the population; therefore, any ST depression can be significant.
- Maximal ST depression ≥ 2 mm in leads V_1-V_3 may be 90% specific for posterior MI (Smith et al., 2002). T waves in the reciprocal V leads usually remain upright and enlarged.
- Persistent ST depression in leads V_1-V_3 is more commonly due to posterior STEMI than to ischemia of LAD disease. However, with deep symmetrical T wave inversion, anterior unstable angina or non-STEMI is most likely.
- In a non-reperfused posterior MI, tall R waves develop in the reciprocal leads of V_1-V_3.

Complications

Posterior wall involvement predisposes patients to papillary muscle ischemia and rupture leading to acute mitral valve regurgitation.

Right Ventricular MI

Coronary Artery Distribution

- The marginal branch of the RCA feeds the right ventricle; therefore, an occlusion of the RCA proximal to this branch infarcts the right ventricle.
- Marginal branch occlusion causes independent RV infarct (not common).
- The medial RV may also be partially supplied by small branches of the LAD, so small RV infarct may occur with LAD occlusion, but not significant.

12-Lead ECG Changes

- > 1 mm ST elevation in right-sided precordial leads, especially in V_4R. Figure 8.8 demonstrates ST elevation in the right precordial leads in the presence of a co-existing posterior MI. Note ST depression in V_1R and V_2R.
- ST elevation as high as 0.6 mm can be seen in V_4R in normal population.
- In context of an inferior MI, ST elevation > 0.5 mm in V_4R is generally interpreted as a RV infarct.
- Isolated ST elevation in lead V_1 with no ST elevation in lead V_2. Lead V_1 is the closest lead on the standard 12-lead ECG to the right ventricle. Note: Co-existing posterior wall injury may cause ST-segment depression in V_1 and mask any sign of an RV infarct on the standard 12-lead ECG. This is why it is important to assess right precordial leads.

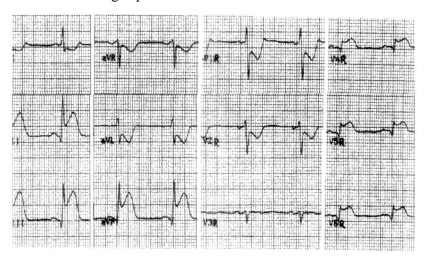

Figure 8.8: ST segment elevation in V_4R, V_5R, and V_6R confirming a right ventricular infarct in the presence of an inferior and posterior wall MI.

Chapter 8

♦ Reciprocal changes (ST depression) associated with an RV infarct can often be seen in the low lateral leads (V_5 and V_6).

Complications

♦ The right ventricle supplies preload to the left ventricle. When the right ventricle fails, the left ventricle does not receive adequate preload and, therefore, cardiac output decreases.

♦ Patients with right-ventricular infarct may show clinical signs of right-sided heart failure, such as increased jugular venous pressure. However, the lungs remain clear because left-sided preload is low. RV infarcts resulting in significant hemodynamic changes occur in less than 10% of patients with an inferior MI (del Bene & Vaughn, 2005).

♦ RV involvement with an inferior MI increases patient mortality. However, if the patient survives to 10 days, then the RV recovers well with little excess long term mortality and morbidity (Smith et al., 2002).

Special Treatment Considerations

♦ Intravenous (IV) fluids are indicated in the treatment of these patients to help assure adequate preload. Caution must be used when administering fluids because excessive volume can result in leftward displacement of septum during diastolic filling.

♦ Venous vasodilators and diuretics are avoided because they decrease preload.

♦ Inotropic medications, such as dobutamine, may be needed if fluid administration (500 to 1000 cc) is ineffective in supplying adequate preload to the left side of the heart.

♦ Bradycardic rhythms should be corrected.

♦ The RV becomes distended in a fixed pericardial space. Patients needing coronary artery bypass surgery (CABG) should wait 4 weeks if possible until the RV heals before having surgery to assure that the distended RV does not interfere with closing the chest.

♦ Patients with right-ventricular infarctions are at higher risk for the development of atrial fibrillation because the right atrium can stretch from volume overload due to right-ventricular failure and infarct. The presence of atrial fibrillation can further complicate a right-ventricular infarct because the loss of atrial kick further decreases right ventricular preload. Patients who are hemodynamically unstable require emergency cardioversion. If pacing is required, AV pacing is optimal.

ECG Changes in Right Bundle Branch Block (RBBB)

♦ The presence of a RBBB causes altered T waves because altered depolarization results in altered repolarization. In the presence of a RBBB, the T wave is expected to be in the opposite direction of the terminal part of the QRS complex. This is called discordance.

    ❖ T wave is typically inverted in leads with rSR' pattern (V_1, V_2, V_3).

    ❖ T wave is typically upright in leads with a terminal S wave.

♦ When the T wave is in the same direction as the terminal part of the QRS complex, it is called concordance, and usually indicates injury or ischemia.

♦ RBBB alone does not affect (cause elevation or depression) the actual ST-segment and, therefore ST-segment elevation and depression can be assessed in the presence of a RBBB.

♦ J points are usually not deviated except for frequent depression (1mm) in leads V_1-V_3 (especially V_1).

♦ ST elevation is usually due to injury. Note ST-segment elevation in Figure 8.9 below in leads I, aVL, V_1, V_2, V_3, V_4, and V_5. ST-segment elevation is easiest to see in V_4. Also note depression in inferior leads.

Acute Coronary Syndrome

Identifying ST elevation in RBBB

◆ Measure QRS in easiest identified lead. Apply this QRS measurement to any lead to find the J point.
◆ Atrial depolarization is complete at the end of the QRS in a RBBB.
◆ Assess ST-segment relative to the TP-segment.

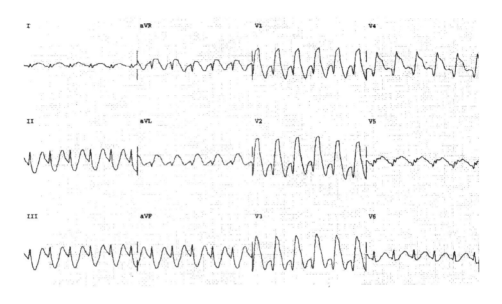

Figure 8.9: ST elevation in leads 1, aVL, and V_1-V_5 in the presence of a RBBB.

Left Bundle Branch Block (LBBB) and Acute MI (Figures 8.10 and 8.11)

◆ LBBB is a common reason for delayed or withheld reperfusion
◆ Only 8.4% to 16.6% of patients with LBBB and AMI receive reperfusion therapy (Smith et al., 2002).
◆ Patients with AMI and LBBB have a higher mortality than those with AMI with no LBBB (Smith et al., 2002).
◆ New LBBB and clinical signs of AMI is an indication for reperfusion therapy.
◆ Old LBBB with increased ST elevation or specific clinical signs should receive reperfusion.
◆ History of heart failure, low EF and dilated cardiomyopathy indicate the LBBB is most likely not new.

ECG Changes and LBBB

◆ LBBB typically manifests J point and ST elevation in the precordial leads in the absence of AMI, so specificity of ST elevation for AMI in the presence of LBBB is much less than in the presence of normal conduction.
  ❖ LBBB without ST elevation in the precordial leads may represent relative ST depression. A posterior MI should be considered when a LBBB is present with no ST elevation in leads V_1-V_4.
◆ ST-segments and T waves are normally directed opposite the terminal portion of the QRS complex (discordance) in LBBB. When T waves are in the same direction of the terminal QRS, suspect ischemia or infarction.
◆ ST-segments and T waves are expected to be discordant; however, the magnitude of the discordance should be in proportion to the voltage of the QRS. For example V_1 to V_3 can have up to 5 mm ST elevation normally in the presence of a LBBB; however, ST elevation > 5 mm should be considered

a sign of injury. Discordant ST elevation of > 5 mm and disproportionate with the QRS voltage is 85-90% specific for AMI (Smith et al., 2002).

- Concordant ST elevation > 1 mm in leads where the terminal QRS is positive (V$_5$, V$_6$, I, aVL, II) should be considered a sign of injury.
- Concordant ST depression > 1 mm in leads where the terminal QRS is negative (V$_1$-V$_4$) is 90% specific for AMI due to posterior injury (Smith et al., 2002).

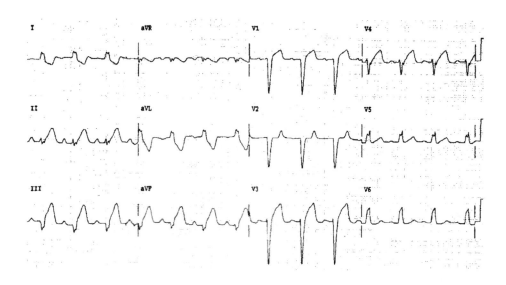

Figure 8.10: Inferior posterior MI in presence of LBBB

Reperfusion and STEMI

STEMI patients meet criteria for immediate reperfusion. Reperfusion is defined as the restoration of oxygen to ischemic tissue. Two methods of reperfusion are available: Administration of fibrinolytics and PCI. If a patient is receiving a fibrinolytic, the drug should be administered within 30 minutes of arrival in the emergency department (ED) or on first contact with the paramedics. If a patient is receiving PCI, balloon inflation should occur within 90 minutes of arrival in the ED or on first contact with the paramedics.

PCI is the preferred method of reperfusion when an experienced operator can promptly treat patients within 90 minutes in a facility with experienced cardiac catheterization personnel. Fibrinolysis is the preferred method of reperfusion when there is a delay to PCI or if PCI is not an option. If any contraindications to fibrinolytic therapy exist, the patient should be transferred directly to a facility capable of performing PCI. PCI is also the preferred option for safety reasons if the onset of symptoms is longer than 3 hours, if there is any question as to the diagnosis of STEMI, and if patient is in shock or presents with severe congestive heart failure (Antman et al., 2004).

Many patients delay seeking treatment at the onset of symptoms. There is an increased overall mortality rate associated with those who delay seeking treatment (del Bene &Vaughn, 2005).

Criteria and Assessment for Reperfusion

- ST-segment elevation in 2 contiguous leads on a standard 12-lead ECG.
- New (or presumably new) left bundle branch.
- Evidence of posterior wall MI.

Acute Coronary Syndrome

An initial ECG should be completed within 10 minutes of arrival to the hospital, if not already completed by EMS in route. If the initial ECG is not diagnostic of ST-segment elevation and the patient remains symptomatic, then serial ECGs should be done at 5- to 10-minute intervals until a diagnosis is made or until symptoms resolve (Antman et al., 2004). Imaging studies such as echocardiography to detect a wall motion abnormality can also be done in the ED if the patient's symptoms are suspicious of acute MI, but the ECG is not clearly demonstrating ST-segment elevation. An echocardiogram may be particularly helpful in assessing patients presenting with possible acute posterior MI or those with LBBB. Fibrinolytics remain underutilized in the treatment of STEMI due in part to the challenge of ECG assessment.

A targeted history and physical should be completed, focusing on the goal of early reperfusion for STEMI patients. Special attention should be paid to contraindications to fibrinolytic therapy and assessment of possible myocardial mimics, such as aortic dissection (pain mimic) and pericarditis (ECG mimic). There is an increasing focus on pre-hospital care of STEMI patients, including the ability of advanced cardiac life support (ACLS) providers to identify STEMI on a 12-lead ECG, and complete a reperfusion checklist prior to arrival in the hospital.

Myocardial Mimics

The pain of aortic dissection can mimic the pain of MI, and intracranial hemorrhage can cause ECG changes consistent with injury or ischemia. ECG changes and pain associated with pericarditis can also mimic the ECG changes seen in acute MI. It is key in both of these circumstances to differentiate these diagnoses from acute MI because treatment with fibrinolytic therapy could be devastating in either case. Figure 8.11 is an ECG showing the ST-segment elevation of pericarditis. More information about pericarditis is discussed in Chapter 12.

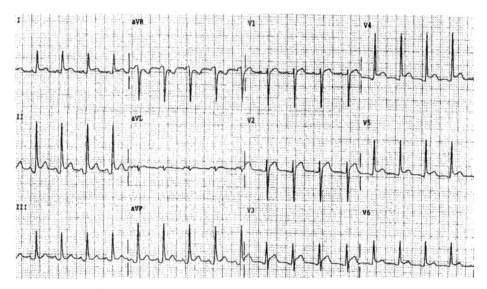

Figure 8.11: Diffuse ST elevation of classic pericarditis.
Also note ST segment depression in lead aVR.

Fibrinolytic Therapy Criteria for Administration

◆ Symptom onset within 12 hours of administration (ideally within 3 hours).
◆ ST-segment elevation of greater than 1 mm in two leads evaluating the same wall of the myocardium or the presence of a new left bundle branch block.
◆ ECG and other findings consistent with a true isolated posterior wall MI.

Chapter 8

Contraindications to the Administration of Fibrinolytics

◆ Prior intracranial hemorrhage.

◆ Known structural cerebral vascular lesion.

◆ Malignant intracranial neoplasm.

◆ Significant closed-head injury within last 3 months.

◆ Ischemic stroke within last 3 months (unless within last 3 hours).

◆ Suspected aortic dissection.

◆ Active bleeding or bleeding diathesis (excluding menses).

◆ Severe uncontrolled hypertension.

◆ Recent cardiac or thoracic surgery.

◆ Symptoms greater than 24-hours old.

◆ ST-segment depression (unless indicative of a true posterior wall MI).
(Antman et al., 2004).

◆ In addition to these absolute contraindications, there are multiple other relative contraindications.

There are several fibrinolytic agents. Some are fibrin selective and, therefore, clot specific; others are non-fibrin selective and, therefore, create more systemic effects. Fibrinolytics are discussed in more detail in Chapter 14.

Intracranial hemorrhage is a potential complication of fibrinolytic therapy, and any STEMI patient at substantial risk for intracranial hemorrhage should be treated with PCI rather than fibrinolytic therapy. Any change in neurological status within 24 hours of administration of a fibrinolytic is considered an intracranial hemorrhage until proven otherwise. All fibrinolytic, anticoagulation, or antiplatelet therapy should be immediately discontinued when a change in neurological status occurs until intracranial hemorrhage is ruled out. Patients with intracranial hemorrhage receive fresh frozen plasma and cryoprecipitate for clotting factors, platelets, and protamine. Blood pressure and blood sugar should be optimized. Mannitol may be given to reduce intracranial pressure. Patient may need to be intubated and prepared for possible evacuation of intracranial hematoma.

Successful Reperfusion with Fibrinolytics

◆ Relief of presenting symptoms.

◆ Reduction of at least 50% of initial ST-segment elevation on repeat ECG.

◆ Hemodynamic stability.

◆ Reperfusion arrhythmias such as accelerated idioventricular rhythm should be transient and not result in an unstable rhythm.

◆ Early peaking of the CKMB or excessively high levels may also be associated with reperfusion.

Reasons for Delayed or Missed Reperfusion Therapy

◆ Missed performance of unequivocal ECG due to atypical symptoms.

◆ Unrecognized unequivocal ECGs.

◆ Delay in diagnosis of subtle ECGs/failure to perform serial ECGs.

◆ Delay in administration of therapy.

◆ Abortion of treatment.

Resolution of pain alone is not indication for aborting therapy. With a 50-100% resolution of ST-segment elevation, it is appropriate to suspend reperfusion therapy based on further assessment.

STEMI patients who are not reperfused can be treated with IV unfractionated heparin or SQ low molecular weight heparin for at least 48 hours.

Comparison of Reperfused and Non-reperfused STEMI

Evolution of Non-Reperfused Complete Coronary Occlusion

- T wave enlargement: T wave enlarges in height and width, sometimes with depressed ST takeoff (hyper acute T waves).
- ST elevation.
- Q wave formation or loss of R wave amplitude: Q wave may form in less than 1 hour, be reversible for up to 6 hours and completely formed by 12 hours.
- ST stabilization: ST stabilization (often with persistent ST elevation) within the first 12 hours.
- T wave inversion before ST resolution: T wave inverts within 72 hours.
- ST resolution: ST resolution over 12 to 72 hours, or may never completely resolve.
- Normalization of T waves: T waves may normalize in days, weeks to months, or never completely normalize.
- Possible disappearance of Q waves: Established Q waves disappear in days, weeks or months in up to 30% of AMI.

(Smith et al., 2006)

Evolution of Reperfused Coronary Occlusion

- Earlier ST normalization and stabilization.
- T wave inversion may accelerate.
- Terminal T wave inversion initially: Because T wave inversion begins while the ST remains elevated, the early morphology is a terminal T wave. T waves deepen symmetrically over time. Figure 8.12 shows early terminal T wave inversion and symmetrical T wave inversion after reperfusion in an acute anteroseptal MI.
- Q wave development is less pronounced or even absent.

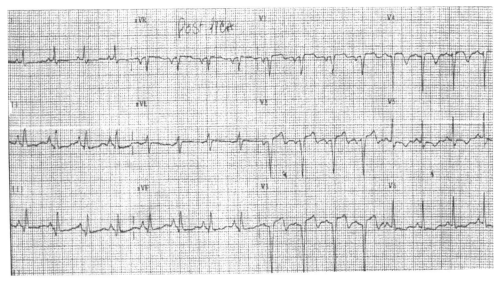

Figure 8.12: Terminal T wave inversion in leads V_2 and V_3 and symmetrical T wave inversion in lead V_4 showing the evolution of an ST segment elevation MI after an interventional procedure.

Chapter 8

Pharmacological Treatment for Acute STEMI

Aspirin

Initial treatment of all patients presenting with ACSs includes aspirin immediately on arrival, if not already taken at home or given by EMS. Nonenteric coated aspirin, in the dose range of 162 to 325 mg, should be chewed by the patient.

Oxygen

Oxygen is used in patients with an arterial oxygen saturation less than 90%. Oxygen can also be administered to patients with STEMI during the first 6 hours. After the first 6 hours, oxygen is not indicated unless the patient's oxygen saturation is below normal limits.

Nitroglycerin

Up to three doses of sublingual nitroglycerin, 0.4 mg, can be given every 5 minutes. If ischemic discomfort continues after sublingual nitroglycerin and beta blocker administration, an intravenous nitroglycerin drip can be started at 5 to 10 mcg/min and titrated in increments of 5 to 10 mcg every 5 to 10 minutes. Sublingual nitroglycerin and high-dose intravenous nitroglycerin dilate arteries and veins. In addition to management of ischemic symptoms, intravenous nitroglycerin can be used in patients who are hypertensive or who have signs of pulmonary congestion. Nitroglycerin should not be used in hypotensive patients, patients who are bradycardic or tachycardic, patients who have taken sildenafil (Viagra) or similar medication, or in those with right-ventricular infarct. If blood pressure is a limiting factor, beta blockers should be given priority for administration over nitrates.

Morphine Sulfate

Morphine sulfate is the pain reliever of choice for ischemic cardiac pain. The initial dose is usually 2 to 4 mg intravenously. Morphine can be repeated at 5-minute intervals in increments of 2 to 8 mg (Antman et al., 2004). Morphine is a predominant preload reducer. It also reduces anxiety and limits activity of the sympathetic nervous system, thereby reducing myocardial oxygen consumption.

Beta Blockers

Oral beta blockers should be administered promptly if no contraindications exist. Beta blockers may be given intravenously initially, especially if the patient is tachycardic or hypertensive or if pain persists. Calcium channel blockers (diltiazem or verapamil) can be used if beta blockers are not effective in controlling ischemia or if patient cannot tolerate beta blockers. Beta blockers are preferred over calcium channel blockers because of the associated mortality benefits. Calcium channel blockers are contraindicated in congestive heart failure or severe LV dysfunction.

ACE Inhibitors

ACE inhibitors are given within the first 24 hours of an acute MI in the following circumstances: anterior wall MI, presence of pulmonary congestion, or left-ventricular ejection fraction less than 40% (Antman et al., 2004).

Anticoagulants

Heparin or low-molecular-weight heparin (LMWH) is indicated for 48 hours in STEMI in the following circumstances: Large MI or anterior wall MI, presence of atrial fibrillation, previous embolus, known presence of thrombus, or current cardiogenic shock (Antman et al., 2004).

Acute Coronary Syndrome

Pathophysiology of Ventricular Remodeling after STEMI

Acute Period

◆ Cellular edema produces an inflammatory response.

◆ Recruitment of some stem cells leads to some tissue regeneration.

◆ Damaged tissue is bruised and cyanotic.

◆ Catecholamines are released from myocardial cells, thus increasing the risk of arrhythmias. Note: Beta blockers are particularly important in suppressing cardiac arrhythmias in ischemic tissue because they suppress catecholamine release.

◆ Cardiac biomarkers are released.

◆ White blood cells invade the necrotic tissue within 2 to 3 days.

◆ Scavenger cells release enzymes to break down necrotic tissue.

◆ The necrotic wall can become very thin during this phase, and the patient is at risk for cardiac rupture. (Gardner & Altman, 2005).

Weeks Following Acute Event

◆ A weak collagen matrix forms by second week, but the myocardium is still vulnerable to reinjury.

◆ Scar formation has started by third week

◆ Necrotic area is completely replaced with scar tissue by week 6 (Gardner & Altman, 2005). Note: Although scar tissue is very strong, it does not contribute to the contractile function of the myocardium.

◆ Surviving myocytes hypertrophy in an attempt to compensate for damaged tissue.

◆ Excessive non-contractile collagen is present in the newly hypertrophied myocardium, leading to a ventricle that is stiff and noncompliant.

Hemodynamic Alterations after STEMI

When myocardial function is impaired as a result of MI, stroke volume decreases. To compensate for decreased stroke volume, heart rate increases. If myocardial function is impaired to the point that adequate stroke volume cannot be maintained, diastolic filling pressures increase and pulmonary edema results. Tachycardia is a poor prognostic sign in the presence of an acute MI because it is a compensatory mechanism for decreasing stroke volume due to a failing left ventricle.

Hemodynamic alterations depend on the size and location of the infarction. A large MI affecting more than 40% of the myocardium can result in circulatory collapse and cardiogenic shock. The prognosis of patients in cardiac shock remains very poor unless successful revascularization can occur in a timely fashion. Long-term hemodynamic alterations from left ventricular dysfunction result in chronic heart failure. With current reperfusion technology, many patients with MIs are left with no clinical evidence of left-ventricular dysfunction.

A pre-shock state of hypoperfusion with a normal blood pressure may develop before circulatory collapse. Signs and symptoms of hypoperfusion in this pre-shock state include:

◆ Cold extremities.

◆ Cyanosis.

◆ Oligurua.

◆ Decreased mentation.

The initial intervention is Dobutamine to improve inoptropic function. An intra aortic balloon pump should be placed and if blood pressure is adequate, a pharmacological agent should be used to reduce afterload. Revascularization to reduce ischemia and improve mortality should be attempted.

Chapter 8

Cardiogenic Shock

◆ Beta blockers and calcium channel blockers not used in acute period if patient is experiencing signs of cardiogenic shock.

◆ Intra aortic balloon pump to help stabilize the patient.

◆ Prompt revascularization efforts to salvage myocardium.

◆ Echocardiography to rule out mechanical complication.

◆ Arterial line and PA catheter to guide therapy.

Ventricular Arrhythmias after STEMIs

Ventricular fibrillation is a major cause of preventable death in the early period after MI. Many episodes of prehospital sudden death are caused by untreated ventricular fibrillation. During MI, arrhythmias are caused by ischemia to the electrical conduction system, catecholamine release, and electrolyte imbalances. Hypokalemia and hypomagnesia increase the risk of ventricular fibrillation. Routine magnesium sulfate is not administered in STEMI; however, any magnesium deficiency should be corrected. Magnesium sulfate is also considered the treatment of choice for torsades de pointes in a STEMI, even if hypomagnesemia is not present.

Accelerated idioventricular rhythm (AIVR) may be commonly seen after reperfusion. It is usually transient and does not require treatment. Sinus tachycardia and atrial arrhythmias can increase myocardial oxygen demand and ischemia.

Mechanical Complications of STEMI

Septal Rupture

Septal rupture is most common with a large anteroseptal infarction. It most commonly occurs 3 to 7 days after an infarct.. The patient experiences sudden and severe left-ventricular failure. Blood is shunted from the left side of the heart back to the right side through the ruptured area. This shunting of blood results in poor systemic perfusion. The rupture also produces a very loud holosystolic murmur. Emergency measures to reduce afterload are indicated while the patient is prepared for surgical repair with a patch. If CABG is indicated, it is done at the time of septal repair.

Papillary Muscle Dysfunction or Rupture

Papillary muscle dysfunction or rupture results in acute mitral valve regurgitation. This complication occurs most frequently with inferior-posterior wall MIs and usually occurs within the first week after infarction. As with septal ruptures, emergency measures to reduce afterload are indicated while preparing the patient for emergency surgery. Inotropic support may also be needed to assist with forward flow.

Free Wall Rupture with Cardiac Tamponade

At least 10% of all deaths from AMI are due to myocardial rupture (Smith et al., 2002). Although perceived to be a sudden event, it is often due to an infiltrating hemorrhage and a slow tear that occurs over 24 hours or more. Free wall rupture causes hemopericardium and death due to tamponade. It is associated with late fibrinolytics (12 to 24 hours after symptom onset) and delayed hospital admission (more than 24 hours after onset of symptoms). A rupture requires emergency surgical intervention to suture or patch the perforated area.

Other Complications of Acute MI

Pericarditis

Pericarditis caused by inflammation of the pericardial sac can occur immediately after an MI or several weeks later. If pericardial effusion develops, anticoagulation should be discontinued. When pericarditis occurs several weeks after an infarction, it is called Dressler's syndrome. When it occurs acutely, it is usually caused by a transmural infarct extending to the epicardium and causing an inflammatory response. Pain associated with pericarditis is sharp and severe. It is worse with inspiration and relieved by sitting up and leaning forward. A pericardial friction rub may be heard during auscultation of the heart. As with many complications of MI, the incidence of pericarditis has decreased significantly due to reperfusion therapy.

Aspirin therapy is recommended for treatment of pericarditis after STEMI. Doses as high as 650 mg of enteric coated aspirin every 4-6 hours can be used. If pain is not controlled with aspirin, then colchicine or acetaminophen can be used. Nonsteroidal anti-inflammatory medication should not be used for extended periods due the increased risk of myocardial scar thinning. Ibuprofen also blocks the antiplatelet effects of aspirin. Corticorsteroids also have an increased risk for myocardial scar thinning (Antman et al., 2004). Myocardial scar thinning can increase the risk for myocardial rupture.

Left-Ventricular Aneurysms

Localized myocardial wall thinning and bulging of the left ventricle at the site of infarction can cause a ventricular aneurysm. Aneurysms can be classified as true or false. A true aneurysm is a localized outpouching of ventricular wall. True aneurysms can be a source of ventricular arrhythmias that originate from the tissue at the junction of the aneurysm. The mouth of the aneurysm is typically wide. These aneurysms typically do not rupture but can be associated with ventricle dysfunction, in addition to ventricular arrhythmias. True ventricular aneurysms can also contain thrombi that can emobolize. This type of aneurysm is associated with the anterior, lateral, and apical walls of the left ventricle. Patients can be considered for left-ventricular aneurysmectomy.

False aneurysms or pseudoaneurysms occur when the ventricular wall ruptures into the pericardial sac and adhesions contain the rupture. False aneurysms are associated with the posterior lateral wall of the left ventricle. These aneurysms can continue to grow, and there is a high risk for delayed rupture of the false aneurysm. Rupture of these aneurysms results in death. If identified, these aneurysms require immediate surgical repair.

ST elevation can persist indefinitely after an MI. Persistent ST elevation occurs in up to 60% of anterior MIs but is much less frequent with inferior MIs. Persistent ST elevation may also be associated with systolic dyskinesis, akinesis, or a large area of necrosis, even in the absence of anatomic aneurysm. Persistent ST elevation after a MI is called ventricular aneurysm, even when anatomic aneurysm may be absent.

Key Nursing Considerations Post Reperfusion of STEMI

◆   Assure immediate and uninterrupted cardiac monitoring for minimum of first 24 hours. (Drew et al., 2004). Sudden onset ventricular fibrillation is the major preventable cause of death during the early period.

◆   Assure aspirin was administered.

◆   Assess that response to beta blocker therapy is adequate enough to control heart rate and arrhythmias. No other prophylactic antiarrhythmic therapy is indicated.

◆   Assess the need for continued antianginal therapy, including the need for intravenous nitroglycerin during the first 48 hours. Intravenous nitroglycerin can also be used for patients who are hypertensive or have pulmonary congestion. Oral or topical agents can be used after 24 hours, if needed.

◆   Morphine sulfate can be given for pain that does not respond to antianginal therapy.

- Note: If a patient has low blood pressure, life-saving treatments such as beta blocker and ACE inhibitor administration should occur before nitrate administration.
- Initiate ACE inhibitor, as ordered, within the first 24 hours for patients with anterior STEMIs, heart failure, or ejection fractions less than 40%.
- Reassess oxygen saturation after 6 hours of supplemental oxygen and discontinue if saturation is more than 90%.
- Administer anxiolytics, as needed, to reduce anxiety. Control of pain and anxiety is key not only for patient comfort but also to reduce myocardial oxygen demand. Pain and anxiety activate the sympathetic nervous system and increase myocardial oxygen demand.
- Assess heart sounds for new holosystolic murmurs.
- Restrict activity for at least the first 12 hours, then begin a step approach to activity progression (phase I cardiac rehabilitation exercises). An uncomplicated MI patient does not need bed rest > 12 hours.
- Provide back support while patient is eating to reduce energy requirements in the initial post MI period. There is no support for not allowing caffeine (del Bene & Vaughn, 2005). Moderate caffeine does not increase ventricular arrhythmias, and withdrawal of caffeine may cause headache and increase heart rate.
- Assess fasting lipid panel if not available from previous records.
- Utilize cardiac monitoring and ST-segment monitoring to assess for recurrent ischemia and the presence of arrhythmias. Observe for pseudo-normalization of the T wave after reperfusion. The T wave should evolve from terminal T wave inversion to symmetrical T wave inversion. T waves that quickly resume their upright position after reperfusion of a STEMI are not normal. Figure 8.13 shows the pseudo-normalization of T waves after reperfusion in a STEMI.
- Intravenous insulin may be indicated in first 24 to 48 hours after STEMI to tightly control blood sugars.
- Observe for signs of left ventricular dysfunction, including hypotension or clinical signs of heart failure.
- Hemodynamic monitoring may be indicated in the following situations:
  - Hypotension not corrected by volume, or hypotension associated with congestive heart failure.
  - Hemodynamic instability requiring titration of vasoactive drugs or intra aortic balloon pump.
  - Mechanical complications.
- Intra-arterial monitoring may be indicated in the following situations:
  - Severe hypotension (systolic BP < 80 mm Hg).
  - Cardiogenic shock.
  - Titration of vasoactive drugs.
- Include the family. Family visits do not have a negative impact on vital signs or cardiac rhythm. (Antman et al., 2004)

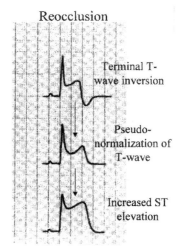

Figure 8.13: Pseudo normalization of a T wave after a ST segment elevation MI, representing reocclusion of a vessel.

Echocardiography can be used post-STEMI to assess left- and right-ventricular function and detect mechanical complications, intracardiac thrombus, and pericardial effusion. Left-ventricular function should be documented in all STEMI patients.

When hemodynamic stability is achieved, patients can be transferred to a step-down unit. With successful reperfusion, some patients can transfer to a step-down unit within 24 hours. Post-PCI care is discussed in Chapter 15.

Discharge Criteria From the CCU Includes

◆ Free of acute cardiac arrhythmias: sinus tachycardia, atrial fibrillation or flutter, heart block, ventricular arrhythmias.
◆ Stable blood pressure.
◆ Absence of heart failure or mechanical complications.
◆ Free of ischemia.

NON-ST-SEGMENT ELEVATION MI

Non-STEMI and unstable angina are usually caused by a ruptured plaque that causes a partially occluded vessel. The partial occlusion is generally caused by incomplete thrombosis. A non-STEMI cannot be differentiated from unstable angina at the time of presentation because the 12-lead ECG findings, such as ST-segment depression and T wave inversion, may be similar (Figure 8.14). In unstable angina, these ECG changes are usually more transient; in non-STEMI, they are usually more persistent.

Patients with a normal initial ECG should have serial ECGs or ST-segment monitoring in the emergency department. There is an approximate 6% rate of non-STEMI in patients presenting with a normal ECG (Gibler et al., 2005).

Approximately 50% of patients with ST depression will be positive for an MI within hours of presentation (Gibler et al., 2005). Any patient with ST depression in the anterior chest leads needs to have posterior leads recorded to rule out a posterior STEMI.

Cardiac biomarkers are used to differentiate between non-STEMI and unstable angina. If initial biomarkers drawn within 6 hours of pain onset are normal, another set of biomarkers should be drawn in the window of 6 to 12 hours from pain onset. Approximately 40% of all MIs are non-STEMIs (del Bene & Vaughan, 2005). Patients in this category are at an increased risk for recurrent ischemia, MI, and death. The risk is highest during the first 2 months after the acute event (Braunwald et al., 2002).

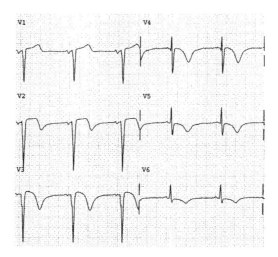

Figure 8.14: Deep symmetrical T wave inversion of a non STEMI confirmed by positive cardiac biomarkers. Note: T wave inversion can also represent reversible ischemia when cardiac biomarkers are within normal limits.

Chapter 8

Causes of Non-STEMI/Unstable Angina

Non-STEMI or unstable angina is caused by altered myocardial oxygen supply and demand. A decreased supply is the most common cause. A decrease in supply can be caused by:

◆ Non-occlusive thrombus on a disrupted plaque (most common cause).

◆ Focal spasm (Prinzmetal's angina).

◆ Severe narrowing of coronary arteries with spasm or thrombus further interfering with blood flow.

◆ Arterial inflammation, constriction of small vessels, or endothelial dysfunction can also decrease supply.

◆ Factors outside the coronary system such as anemia, hypoxemia, or decreased cardiac output.

An increase in myocardial oxygen demand can also cause an imbalance in patients who have existing coronary artery narrowing. Fever and tachycardia are two common causes of increased myocardial oxygen demand.

Pharmacological Treatment of Non-STEMI

All patients with ACS, including non-STEMI and unstable angina, should initially be treated with aspirin, oxygen, nitroglycerin, and morphine (for pain not relieved by nitroglycerin). Patients should also receive beta blockers unless contraindicated. ACE inhibitors are given if hypertension is present after nitroglycerin and beta blocker administration.

Other special pharmacological considerations for this group of patients are listed here.

Clopidogrel

◆ As soon as possible in patients receiving non-interventional treatment strategies (continued for ≥ 1 month).

◆ Also used in patients with planned interventional treatment strategies.

◆ Held for 5 to 7 days in patients undergoing CABG surgery.

Unfractionated heparin (UFH) or LMWH

UFH preferred in patients likely to have CABG surgery within 24 hours.

Glycoprotein IIb/IIIa Inhibitor

◆ In addition to aspirin and heparin when an interventional treatment strategy is planned.

◆ May also be used in patients with continuing ischemia or elevated troponin levels when an interventional procedure is not planned (Braunwald et al., 2002).

Additional Treatment Considerations

The two treatment arms for patients with unstable angina and non-STEMI include the early conservative arm and the early invasive arm. The early invasive treatment arm involves cardiac catheterization and revascularization within 24 hours.

Recent clinical trials have shown a significant reduction in adverse cardiac events with an early invasive strategy after non-ST-segment ACS (Cantor et al., 2005). In the current published guidelines, early invasive treatment recommended for high-risk patients, including those with:

◆ Age > 70 years.

◆ Prior MI.

◆ Recent PCI or history of CABG.

  ❖ Native CAD progression versus graft occlusion is difficult to determine with noninvasive testing.

Acute Coronary Syndrome

◆ Recurrent ischemia at rest or low-level activity.

◆ Depressed left-ventricular function or clinical signs of heart failure.

◆ Sustained ventricular arrhythmias or hemodynamic instability.

◆ Significant ST-segment changes (including new or presumably new ST-segment depression) on a 12-lead ECG or high-risk findings on other noninvasive testing.

◆ Positive troponins.

(Braunwald et al., 2002)

When patients are treated conservatively, non-invasive testing is indicated to assess for areas of ischemia and the need for revascularization. Approximately 50% of patients presenting with unstable angina or non-STEMI have three vessel disease or left main disease, and are therefore candidates for revascularization (Braunwald et al., 2002).

Patients with unstable angina and non-STEMI usually have complex plaques that have irregular borders and are prone to rupture. Rupture causes platelet aggregation and intracoronary thrombi. These patients have an increase risk for recurrent ischemia, MI, and death. Highest risk for complications is within 2 months following the event ((Braunwald et al., 2002).

SPECIAL CONSIDERATIONS

Treatment of Cocaine-Induced Chest Pain

Cocaine produces excess concentrations of neurotransmitters at the post synaptic receptors by blocking pre-synaptic uptake. This leads to sympathetic nervous system activation and direct stimulation of vascular smooth muscle, resulting in vasoconstriction and increased coronary vascular resistance.

Cocaine also promotes platelet aggregation and thrombus formation by increasing thromboxane A2 production and reducing protein C and antithrombin III. Chronic cocaine use accelerates the process of atherosclerosis. Cocaine-induced ischemic chest discomfort cannot be distinguished from unstable angina and non-STEMI caused by coronary heart disease.

Nitroglycerin or calcium channel blockers are used to treat cocaine-induced chest pain. If ST-segment elevation is present, then calcium channel blockers are administered intravenously. Angiography is indicated if ST-segment elevation does not resolve with nitroglycerin and calcium channel blockers. A small percentage (6%) of cocaine users develop MIs as a result of cocaine use (Braunwald et al., 2002).

Other complications of cocaine use include:

◆ Aortic or cornary artery dissection.

◆ Myocarditis.

◆ Cardiomyopathy.

Variant (Vasospastic/Prinzmetal's) Angina

Variant angina is caused by spasm of the coronary arteries. This type of angina usually occurs spontaneously, but can be triggered by exercise, hyperventilation, and cold. The majority of episodes occur in the early morning hours and appear to be under the influence of a circadian rhythm. The only associated risk factor for variant angina is smoking. Patients can have long asymptomatic periods between episodes.

The pathophysiology of variant angina is not fully understood. One possible explanation is that endothelial dysfunction causes an imbalance between local vasodilatory and local vasoconstrictive factors. The autonomic nervous system may also play a role in variant angina with decreased parasympathetic tone and reactivity of alpha receptors.

Chapter 8

Transient ST-segment elevation usually occurs with variant angina, but usually does not result in MI if the spasm occurs in a nonstenotic vessel. However, if the patient has spasms in vessels that are already stenosed, MI can occur.

Provocative testing can be done to induce spasm which is visible during angiography. Methylergonovine, acetylcholine, and methacholine can be used to induce coronary spasm. Nitrates and calcium channel blockers are stopped prior to angiography.

Variant angina is treated with high dose calcium channel blockers. If symptoms are not controlled, long acting nitrates can be added. Alpha-blockers may need to be added if symptoms are not controlled with calcium channel blockers and nitrates.

Syndrome X

Syndrome X is the presence of stable angina symptoms, or, at times, unstable angina symptoms in the absence of epicardial coronary artery disease. Patients have chest discomfort or related symptoms with exercise and ST-segment depression with stress testing.

This syndrome is more common in women (post menopausal) than in men. The exact cause of chest pain and ST-segment depression is not fully understood. Patients may have decreased nitric oxide production from endothelial dysfunction. They may also have increased sensitivity to sympathetic nervous system stimulation. Syndrome X may be caused by microvascular angina. In microvascular angina the capillaries constrict and cause decreased blood flow.

There is an excellent prognosis with Syndrome X so medications are used for symptom control. Nitrates are typically used as first-line treatment. Beta blockers and calcium channel blockers may also be used.

Tako Tsubo Syndrome or Tako Tsubo Cardiomyopathy

This syndrome presents with transient left-ventricular (LV) apical ballooning. LV contractility recovers in several days. Myocardial stunning is a state of diminished contractility in non-infarcted myocardium. Stunning is caused by an excess production of free radicals.

This syndrome usually affects elderly women, frequently preceded by emotional/physical stress. These patients present with chest pain and ECG abnormalities mimicking an acute anterior wall MI, yet obstructive coronary artery disease has been ruled out as the cause.

The exact mechanism is unknown, but microvascular dysfunction is suspected. Simultaneous multi-vessel spasm is also considered as possible etiology (Upadya, 2004).

LONG TERM MANAGEMENT OF ACS

Medical Management

After an acute event, most patients resume a medical management course similar to patients with stable angina. Post-ACS patients continue a daily dose of aspirin aspirin (typically 81 to 162 mg) indefinitely. Clopidogrel is used if a patient is unable to take aspirin. Higher doses of aspirin may be indicated, especially for a period of time after stent placement.

Clopidogrel is also continued post discharge in patients with ACS who have undergone PCI.
- Clopidogrel is prescribed for at least one month in patients with bare metal stents.
- Clopidogrel is prescribed for at least one year in patients with drug eluting stents.
- Clopidogrel may also be continued indefinitely in some patients.

Beta blockers initiated in the acute phase of ACS and are continued indefinitely after discharge.

ACE inhibitors should be given within the first 24 hours to patients with anterior wall MIs, pulmonary congestion, or left-ventricular ejection fraction less than 40%. In addition, ACE inhibitors are indicated in patients with hypertension, diabetes and chronic kidney disease. ACE inhibitors can be considered for secondary prevention in all patients post ACS (Smith & Allen et al., 2006). ACE inhibitors are continued indefinitely. An angiotensin II receptor blocker may be used as an alternative for patients unable to tolerate ACE inhibitors.

Aldosterone blockers are given after MI to patients with ejection fractions less than 40% and who have clinical heart failure or diabetes. Aldosterone blockers are added to therapy for patients who are already on ACE inhibitor and beta blocker therapy. Aldosterone blockers cannot be added to therapy for patients with renal dysfunction or hyperkalemia (Smith et al., 2006).

Discharge medications should include a lipid-lowering agent (statin) and should be initiated 24 to 96 hours after admission (Braunwald et al., 2002).

Warfarin is used in patients with persistent atrial fibrillation or flutter, and in those with left-ventricular thrombus or extensive regional wall motion abnormalities. Risk of left-ventricular thrombus is the highest the first few weeks after myocardial infarction. Apical akinesis at 10 days post infarct is a predictor for the development of left-ventricular thrombus (Eagle et al., 2004). Warfarin can also be used in patients allergic to aspirin.

Patients should not take ibuprofen for pain after STEMI because it interferes with healing and can cause thinning of the scarred area.

Discharge medical management includes three main objectives:
1) Improve prognosis.
2) Control ischemia.
3) Achieve risk reduction and secondary prevention.

Medications to Improve Prognosis

◆ Aspirin.
◆ Clopidogrel.
◆ Beta blockers.
◆ Lipid-lowering drugs (statins).
◆ ACE inhibitors.
◆ Aldosterone antagonists

(Smith et al., 2006).

Medications to Control Ischemia

◆ Beta blockers.
◆ Nitrates (all patients should be given sublingual nitroglycerin).
◆ Calcium channel blockers.

Secondary Prevention Through Risk Factor Reduction

◆ Smoking cessation.
◆ Reduction of hyperlipidemia.
◆ Hypertension control.
◆ Diabetes control.

Chapter 8

Medical Follow-Up

Patients should be instructed on the importance of physician follow-up. High-risk patients should be seen in 1 to 2 weeks after discharge, and low-risk patients within 6 weeks. The patient should be instructed to notify the physician any time there is a change in condition, such as a change in activity tolerance or perceived medication side effects. Repeat angiography is indicated in recurrent unstable angina, positive stress test, development of heart failure, or survival of sudden cardiac death.

Influenza Vaccine As Component of Secondary Prevention

Influenza can exacerbate chronic medical conditions and can also result in viral or bacterial pneumonia. Influenza related death is more common in patients with cardiovascular disease than in patients with other chronic medical conditions. The hypothesis for the more profound impact in patients with cardiovascular disease is related to the inflammatory response. The inflammatory response is thought to initiate a chain of events, resulting in the progression of atherosclerotic vascular injury. There is evidence that the influenza vaccine is protective against cardiovascular events in patients with known CAD or other forms of atherosclerotic disease. In addition, there is no evidence that the vaccine is harmful (Davis et al., 2006).

Risk Factor Reduction

A major focus of patient education for any patient with coronary heart disease is secondary prevention by aggressive reduction of cardiac risk factors. The reduction of cardiac risk factors is discussed in detail in Chapter 7.

Recognition of Signs and Symptoms and Emergency Response

Another focus is the recognition of and response to symptoms of an acute coronary event.

Patients should know how to activate the EMS, as well as the location of the nearest hospital with 24-hour cardiac care.

Patients should be instructed in the use of sublingual nitroglycerin or nitroglycerin spray, in addition to how to activate the EMS if symptoms do not improve after 5 minutes or after one sublingual nitroglycerin. Patients with a history of stable angina should be instructed to rest with the onset of angina and to take up to three sublingual nitroglycerin.

Patients with signs and symptoms of ACS should also be instructed to take an aspirin (if not already taken) while awaiting the arrival of EMS.

Family members who are appropriate candidates may be given resources to learn about cardiopulmonary resuscitation and the use of automated external defibrillators.

Medication Adherence

Barriers to Compliance

◆ Chronic medical conditions.
◆ Multiple medications.
◆ Revascularization resulting in improvement of cardiac symptoms.
◆ Fixed or low incomes.

Noncompliance with medications is associated with increased adverse outcomes in the cardiac population. Compliance with clopidogrel is of particular concern in patients post PCI. Noncompliance results in an increased risk for subacute instent thrombosis.

Acute Coronary Syndrome

Activity and Cardiac Rehabilitation

Exercise in the Early Recovery Period

◆ The goal of rehabilitation in the early recovery period is to counteract the negative effects of deconditioning. Three percent of total body muscle mass deconditions per every day of bed rest. Bed rest also results in altered distribution of body fluids and can cause orthostatic intolerance and increase the risk of venous thrombosis. Early activity progression in stable patients improves outcomes.

◆ Initiation of Phase I cardiac rehabilitation:
  ❖ Initiated in a post MI patient as soon as the patient is medically stable and after evaluation for orthostatic hypotension.
  ❖ Phase I exercises usually begin on day 1 for an acute MI patient who is hemodynamically stable.
  ❖ Phase I rehabilitation is typically initiated on post op day 1 for CABG patients.

◆ Contraindications to beginning or continuing exercise include:
  ❖ Unstable angina.
  ❖ Complete heart block.
  ❖ Uncontrolled tachyarrhythmias.
  ❖ Uncontrolled hypertension.
  ❖ Decompensated heart failure.

◆ Signs of activity intolerance:
  ❖ Increase of 20 beats per minute above resting heart rate, or a heart rate more than 110 beats per minute, demonstrates an inappropriate chronotropic response.
  ❖ Failure of systolic blood pressure to increase or decrease in systolic blood pressure of 20 mm Hg also indicate activity intolerance (Levine, 2002).

◆ Patients with post myocardial infarction are more likely to experience angina, ST depression, BP abnormalities (drop in systolic blood pressure with exercise), or serious arrhythmias with exertion, and therefore should be monitored and assessed during activity periods in the early recovery phase (Nadel, 2006). Activity in post MI patients is advanced more cautiously and at a slower rate than in patients post intervention or bypass surgery who have not had an MI.

◆ Only non-resistive range-of-motion (ROM) exercises should be done because resistive exercises increase afterload. The best exercises involve flexion and extension of arms and legs. Internal and external rotation and abduction of legs should be avoided because these exercises can also increase afterload (Levine, 2002).

◆ The majority of patients begin with a 1.5 to 2.0 MET (metabolic equivalent) level of exercise (using bedside commode, transferring to a chair, feeding self, washing face and hands), progressing to 2 to 3 MET of activity (sitting up longer, walking to bathroom, showering).

◆ The goal is for patients to be at a rehabilitation level of activity equivalent with activities of daily living by the time of discharge. With shorter hospital stays, the steps involved in inpatient rehabilitation programs have been modified to allow for more rapid progression.

◆ After the patient achieves a rehabilitation level equivalent with activities of daily living, he/she can begin a walking program. In the early recovery period, patients should walk 5 to 10 minutes at a time.

Exercise in the Later Recovery Period

◆ Walking and secondary prevention have been shown to increase survival, decrease reoccurrence rates, and possibly slow progression of CAD. Post MI, there is a 20-30% reduction in cardiac deaths with exercise training (Gibbons et al., 2002). In addition, a regular walking program after an acute

Chapter 8

cardiac event improves the patient's perception of quality of life. Exercise as part of cardiac rehabilitation limits disability and improves the physical function of participants (Myers, 2005).

◆ The same heart rate guidelines are used as with activity progression early in the recovery period. Activity that is well tolerated is accompanied by no adverse symptoms, arrhythmias or excessive tachycardia.

◆ Exercise later in recovery should be guided by a symptom-limited stress test, which can typically be done at 10 to 14 days post MI.

◆ Low-risk patients can implement an exercise prescription at home or in a community setting. Low-risk patients include those with absence of ischemia or arrhythmias on a stress test. The majority of patients exercising for secondary prevention are classified as low risk.

◆ High-risk patients should be in medically supervised exercise programs. They are defined as patients with ischemia or serious arrhythmias on a stress test.

Specific Home-Going Guidelines

◆ Most patients should be at a 3 to 4 MET level of activity by the time of discharge. Patients should keep activity at this MET level for the first 3-4 weeks (Nadel, 2006). Box 8.1 lists safe activities of daily living that are 3 MET levels or less.

◆ Patients should be instructed to monitor their response to activity. Shortness of breath means overexertion. Other signs of activity intolerance include: Angina, dizziness, diaphoresis, prolonged fatigue, and nausea.

◆ In general, patients should rate their level of exertion as moderate (Nadel, 2006). Patients should be able to talk while exercising if the intensity is appropriate. However, they should not have enough breath to sing a song. Patients may also use a scale, such as the Borg scale, that allows them to rate their perceived level of exertion.

◆ Patients should be instructed on pulse-taking prior to discharge. The heart rate should not increase by more than 30 beats above resting during the six-week period after discharge, or until the patient begins a formal phase II cardiac rehabilitation program.

◆ Patients should lower activity if breathing and heart rate do not return to normal within 10 minutes of stopping exercise.

◆ Patients should wait 1-2 hours after a meal before doing any exercise (Nadel, 2006).

◆ After a steady state of activity is well tolerated at home, the duration of activity may be increased in 1-minute increments each day or 5-minute increments each week, up to a maximum 30 minutes per session.

◆ Aerobic activity sessions should be done at least 5 times per week and may be done up to 7 times per week. Intensity may also be increased as activity progresses.

◆ Exercises should involve large muscle groups and include a warm-up and cool-down. The warm-up should be active, such as slow walking, and the cool-down should include stretching.

◆ Isometric activities should be limited due to their potential to increase afterload. Isometric exercises involve the contraction of a muscle with no movement of the joint.

◆ Most patients will be discharged with a lifting restriction of no greater than 10 pounds. High-risk patients should not lift greater than 5 pounds. Box 8.2 provides more details regarding weight lifting restrictions.

Acute Coronary Syndrome

Box 8.1
Safe Activities (3 MET) During the Immediate Post Discharge Period

◆ Light housekeeping (no vacuuming).
◆ Light gardening.
◆ Walking speed of 2 mph or less on flat surface (treadmill or outside).
   ❖ No dog walking
   ❖ No outside walking in temperatures less than 30 degrees or greater than 80 degrees
◆ Stationary biking at 50 watts or less.
(Nadel, 2006)

Box 8.2
Weight Lifting Restriction Guidelines

◆ Weights of common items
   ❖ Gallon of milk = 8 pounds
   ❖ Large basket of laundry = 20 to 30 pounds
   ❖ One bag of groceries = 5 to 10 pounds.
◆ Carrying objects while walking distance or upstairs increases the MET level of the activity.
◆ Using force to open windows or stuck jar lids should be avoided in patients with lifting restrictions.

Special Activities

◆ Driving
   ❖ Requires only 1.5 to 3.0 METS.
   ❖ Most patients with an uncomplicated hospital course can drive about 1 week after discharge (Braunwald et al., 2002). However, driving regulations may also vary between states.
   ❖ MI patients do not drive until they return to work.
   ❖ Many post CABG patients postpone driving due to the fear of injuring the sternum.
◆ If stable, patients can usually travel by air in 2 weeks if accompanied by a travel companion, and if the patient has SL nitroglycerin. The patient should also have assistance to avoid excessive amounts of walking in the airport. Patients should also take precautions when traveling to avoid the development of deep vein thrombosis. Interventions include wearing compression stockings, moving feet and legs during the flight (including getting up and walking), and staying well hydrated.
◆ Sexual relationships
   ❖ Patients are uncomfortable asking about resuming sexual relationships, so instructions regarding sexual activity should be included as a routine part of all discharge instructions.
   ❖ Patients with a history of angina during sexual relationships may be instructed by their physician to take nitroglycerin prior to engaging in sexual activities.
   ❖ The average intimate session ranges from 2.5-4 METS for most people. Walking at 2 mph on level ground is 2.5 METS. Mowing the lawn with a power mower or walking at 3.5 mph is 4 METS. Climbing up a flight of stairs is 8 METS. With this information, patients can compare their ability to perform day-to-day activities to having sex. Research has shown that the mild spike in blood pressure and heart rate associated with sex are short lived, lasting 3-5 minutes on average. The biggest risk with sex in the cardiac patient is the possibility of arrhythmias, which is associated

Chapter 8

with sympathetic activity increased during arousal. Patients with uncontrolled or untreated hypertension need to discuss specific guidelines with their physician (Sotile & Cantor-Cooke, 2003).

Formal Cardiac Rehabilitation

◆ A formal cardiac rehabilitation program involves medically supervised exercise after an acute cardiac event.

  ❖ It usually begins 1 to 2 weeks after discharge and involves exercise 3 times weekly for a period of 4 to 12 weeks.

  ❖ The program is multi-disciplinary and requires physician referral.

  ❖ Patients enrolled in a formal cardiac rehabilitation program have baseline exercise testing and annual follow-ups.

  ❖ Exercise prescription is guided by exercise physiologists, and the patient's plan of care is directed by a registered nurse.

  ❖ Aerobic exercise and resistive training are components of the exercise program.

  ❖ Risk factor counseling, patient education regarding signs, symptoms and medications, and psychosocial support are also components of a comprehensive program.

◆ Health insurance generally covers formal cardiac rehabilitation programs during the immediate recovery period after admission for MI, PCI, CABG, valve surgery, and chronic stable angina.

◆ All appropriate candidates should be referred to a formal cardiac rehabilitation program.

◆ Pooled data from a meta-analysis of studies involving cardiac rehabilitation in secondary prevention show a benefit of reduced cardiovascular mortality of approximately 25% at 1 and 3 years (Gibbons et al., 2002; Myers, 2005). Participation in formal exercise training is safe, and patients benefit from increased functional capacity and exercise tolerance (Gibbons et al., 2002).

◆ Those with decreased exercise tolerance at baseline can benefit the most from participation, but are often among those not referred. Cardiac rehabilitation exercises are safe and beneficial in clinically stable coronary patients. Unfortunately, only approximately 20% of appropriate cardiac candidates participate in outpatient cardiac rehabilitation (Levine, 2002).

Psychosocial Issues

Anxiety and Stress

Anxiety is common during and immediately after the acute phase of a cardiac event. Assisting the patient gain accurate perceptions of the recovery process can reduce anxiety. The use of relaxation techniques and methods of worry control can also help reduce anxiety. Patient and family education are important in relieving stress when the patient and family are ready to receive information. If they are not ready, providing information can actually increase stress. In post MI patients, interventions to reduce stress can reduce recurrent cardiac events by as much as 35-75% (Gibbons et al., 2002).

Interventions to reduce stress include:

◆ Relaxation training.

◆ Behavior modification.

◆ Psychosocial support.

Depression

Approximately 1 in 5 patients hospitalized with MI have major depression. There is also evidence that depression continues for several months after discharge (Bush et al., 2005). There is strong evidence that patients who are depressed post MI have a higher rate of mortality from both cardiac and non-cardiac causes (Bush et al., 2005). Patients who have major depression post MI are less adherent to prescribed medications and lifestyle modifications (Bush et al., 2005). Depression also affects quality of life post discharge; therefore, assessment and treatment of depression should be a routine component of treating patients with ACS.

Selective serotonin reuptake inhibitors (example: citalopram (Celexa)) can be useful in treating depression during the first year after an acute MI or in other cardiac patients with co-existing depression. This group of medications is generally considered safer than other antidepressant medications for use in the cardiac population (Maden & Froelicher, 2005). There is evidence that both psychosocial intervention and selective serotonin reuptake inhibitor antidepressants improve depression in MI patients. However, additional evidence is needed to demonstrate whether effective treatment improves mortality and other outcomes (Bush et al., 2005).

Principles of Patient Education

The key to effective patient education is to individualize the approach and take advantage of every patient encounter. Many patients are afraid or have anxiety or depression after an acute cardiac event. Patients must be allowed to express concerns and have questions answered before they are able to accept new information. Patients should be active participants in the education process. Adult patients need to be in control of their learning; therefore, it is critical to assess the patient's readiness and desire for information. In many cases, sharing scientific information about the value of the treatment or risk factor plan increases motivation and compliance. Patients who are engaged should be encouraged to seek out additional information and resources from the library or on the internet.

Family, as defined by the patient, should be included in education. When providing patient education, it is helpful to individualize the information to the patient. For example, discuss the patient's individual risk factors, type of coronary heart disease, area of infarction, or specific ejection fraction. This allows the patient to assimilate and take ownership of the information being provided. Effective patient education requires a great deal of time and is often neglected. However, the rewards of effective patient education can be tremendous. Patients can benefit from improved physical functioning and quality of life, even improve survival from increased adherence to the medical regime.

During post discharge follow-up or cardiac rehabilitation, the patient's psychosocial status should be evaluated. Many patients with left-ventricular dysfunction as a result of acute MI experience role identity crisis after their acute event. They miss a great deal of work and must alter their work roles if high levels of physical exertion and stress are involved. Altered work roles may add family and financial stresses. Patients may also experience anxiety and sleep disorders.

An assessment of the patient's support system is an important part of the psychosocial assessment. Social isolation is a predictor of worse outcomes after an acute cardiac event, such as MI (Maden & Froelicher, 2005). Depression is not uncommon after an acute cardiac event. Patients with depression are three to four times more likely to die within the first year following an MI (Maden & Froelicher, 2005). Depression also impacts participation in exercise, medication compliance, seeking attention for symptoms, and return to work. Minor depression may respond to increased accomplishment and association with others. Exercise can also improve minor depression so patients should be referred to formal cardiac rehabilitation programs for the social support, as well as the exercise component. Mended Hearts is an organization for those who have survived a cardiac event. Referral to Mended Hearts is another option for social support for those who are depressed or who have limited social support.

Chapter 8

Linking Knowledge to Practice

✔ *Patients admitted with symptoms suspicious for ACS but with a normal initial ECG should have serial ECG, continuous ST-segment monitoring, and a right-sided and posterior ECG.*

✔ *Patients admitted with chest pain with a LBBB should have old medical records assessed to determine if LBBB is new. If old records are not available and clinical presentation is consistent with ACS, the patient meets criteria for reperfusion.*

✔ *Patients admitted with acute anterior MI with RBBB should be monitored for the development of a left anterior hemiblock. These patients are at high risk for the development of complete heart block.*

✔ *Patients intolerant of beta blockers (decreased blood pressure or heart rate) should be assessed for tolerance to a lower dose before a decision is made to discontinue a medication. Beta blockers have mortality benefit in the management of ACS.*

✔ *Patients need to be educated in the critical need to continue clopidogrel as prescribed, especially after the placement of a drug eluting stent. They should be instructed not to stop their clopidogrel for elective surgeries or procedures without the permission of their cardiologist. Stopping clopidogrel increases the risk for sub acute instent thrombosis. Cost is a barrier for compliance with clopidogrel, so patient financial concerns need to be addressed prior to discharge.*

✔ *Nurses can make an impact on patient outcomes by improving referral and enrollment rates for phase II cardiac rehabilitation. Patients need to understand the importance of aggressive risk factor modification in impacting the underlying disease process.*

TEST YOUR KNOWLEDGE

1. Stable angina is best defined as angina that
   a. increases in severity.
   b. is new.
   c. occurs at rest.
   d. has a predictable pattern over time.

2. The gold standard diagnostic procedure to definitively diagnose the presence, location, and severity of coronary artery disease (CAD) is
   a. stress testing with nuclear imaging.
   b. stress echocardiography.
   c. cardiac catheterization.
   d. spiral computed tomography (CT).

Acute Coronary Syndrome

3. Vulnerable plaque and acute coronary syndromes (ACS) are related in what way?

    a. The rupture of vulnerable plaque is the most frequent cause of ACS.

    b. They are not related in any way.

    c. The episode of an ACS causes plaque to become vulnerable.

    d. They are only related in men with ACS.

4. Goals of medical treatment for CAD include

    a. providing surgical revascularization for all patients.

    b. reducing symptoms, preventing complications, and reducing the risk of death.

    c. placing all patients on antiarrhythmic drugs to prevent sudden cardiac death.

    d. placing all patients on warfarin to reduce the risk of stroke.

5. Risk factor modification is important for all patients with CAD because

    a. risk factor modification can eliminate all possible chance of developing CAD.

    b. CAD only occurs in patients with three or more risk factors.

    c. although it does not benefit patients with CAD, risk factor modifications set a good example for their children.

    d. CAD is a systemic and progressive disease.

6. Which of the following patients is a candidate for reperfusion therapy?

    a. A patient with a 5-year history of stable angina who develops chest pain with extreme exertion.

    b. A patient with a history of CAD who develops shortness of breath with exertion after he/she stopped taking cardiac medications.

    c. A patient with no history of CAD who presents with ST-segment elevation MI (STEMI).

    d. A patient who underwent coronary artery bypass grafting (CABG) surgery who presents for the second time with a non-STEMI.

7. During an acute myocardial infarction (MI), the medication that is not routinely administered prior to reperfusion is

    a. morphine.

    b. lipid-lowering agent.

    c. aspirin.

    d. nitroglycerin.

8. A potential mechanical complication of acute MI that requires surgical repair is

    a. reinfarction.

    b. death.

    c. pericarditis.

    d. papillary muscle rupture.

Chapter 8

9. Which of the following cardiac enzymes is highly sensitive but has low specificity?
    a. CPK-MB
    b. LDH
    c. Myoglobin
    d. Troponin

10. A non-STEMI is definitively differentiated from unstable angina by
    a. location of chest pain.
    b. cardiac biomarkers.
    c. ECG changes.
    d. extent of cardiac history.

11. You are assessing your patient who had an inferior MI yesterday. When listening to his heart, you notice a new murmur that was not present during your last assessment. You note it occurs between S1 and S2 and it is best heard in the 5th intercostal space, mid-clavicular line. You suspect the patient has developed a
    a. ventricular septal rupture.
    b. cardiac tamponade.
    c. papillary muscle rupture.
    d. None of the above.

12. You are caring for a patient admitted with an extensive anteroseptal MI. You know this patient to be at high risk for
    a. development of heart failure.
    b. septal rupture.
    c. complete heart block.
    d. All of the above.

13. True ventricular aneurysms are more likely to rupture and cause death than false or pseudoaneurysms.
    a. True.
    b. False.

14. Aldosterone blockade is indicated post MI in patients
    a. with an EF < 40% and heart failure or diabetes.
    b. as an alternative to ACE-I and beta blocker therapy.
    c. with renal failure.
    d. as a strategy to protect against hyperkalemia.

368

Acute Coronary Syndrome

15. Medications used in secondary prevention to improve prognosis include
    a. aspirin.
    b. beta blockers.
    c. nitrates.
    d. a and b only.

16. Patients with a new RBBB meet criteria for immediate reperfusion, regardless of ECG assessment.
    a. True.
    b. False.

17. The following is true regarding patient management during a right-ventricular infarct:
    a. An increased amount of venous vasodilation is needed to reduce preload and restore hemodynamic balance.
    b. Inotropes should be considered only after maximal dose vasopressors fail to raise blood pressure.
    c. Venous vasodilators and diuretics are used with caution.
    d. CABG is urgently indicated to avoid complications.

18. A patient presents to the ED with chest pain. Initial ECG shows ST-segment depression in leads V_1-V_4. An appropriate intervention is:
    a. Perform an ECG that evaluates leads V_7-V_9 to assess for posterior ST elevation.
    b. Plan for an immediate stress test to confirm anterior ischemia.
    c. Assure the patient that he cannot be having a myocardial infarction based on his ECG.
    d. None of the above.

19. Patients with acute STEMI should have uninterrupted cardiac monitoring for the first 24 hours due to the high risk of ventricular fibrillation.
    a. True.
    b. False.

20. Home-going activities that are safe for the first several weeks post MI (prior to starting Phase II Cardiac Rehab) include:
    a. Walking the dog around the block as long as there are no steep hills.
    b. Vacuuming the house as long as there are no more than 10 stairs.
    c. Walking on a flat outside surface at a slow speed as long as the wind chill factor is not less than minus 10 degrees.
    d. Riding a stationary bike at 50 watts or less.

Chapter 8

ANSWERS

1.	D	11.	C
2.	C	12.	D
3.	A	13.	B
4.	B	14.	A
5.	D	15.	D
6.	C	16.	B
7.	B	17.	C
8.	D	18.	A
9.	C	19.	A
10.	B	20.	D

REFERENCES

Antman, E.M., Anbe, D.T., Armstrong, P.W., Bates, E.R., Green, L.A., Hand, M., Hochman, J.S., Krumholz, H.M., Kushner, F.G., Lamas, G.A., Mullany, C.J., Ornato, J.P., Pearle, D.L., Sloan, M.A., & Smith, S.C. Jr. (2004). ACC/AHA guidelines for the management of patients with ST-elevation myocardial infarction: executive summary: A report of the ACC/AHA task force on practice guidelines (Committee to Revise the 1999 Guidelines on the Management of Patients with Acute Myocardial Infarction). *Journal of the American College of Cardiology, 44*, 671-719.

Braunwald, E., Antman, E.M., Beasley, J.W., Califf, R.M., Cheitlin, M.D., Hochman, J.S., Jones, R.H., Kereiakes, D., Kupersmith, J., Levin, T.N., Pepine, C.J., Schaeffer, J.W., Smith, E.E., III, Steward, D.E., & Thoroux, P. (2002). *ACC/AHA 2002 guideline update for the management of patients with unstable angina and non ST elevation myocardial infarction: A report of the American College of Cardiology/American Heart Association Task Force on Practice Guidelines* (Committee on the Management of Patients with Unstable Angina). Retrieved from: http://www.acc.org/clinical/guidelines/unstable/unstable.pdf

Bush, D.E., Ziegelstein, R.C., Patel, U.V., Thombs, B.D., Ford, D.E., Fauerbach, J.A., et al. (2005). *Post-Myocardial Infarction Depression. Summary*, Evidence Report/Technology Assessment: Number 123. AHRQ Publication Number 05-E018-1. Agency for Healthcare Research and Quality, Rockville, MD. http://www.ahrq.gov/clinic/epcsums/midepsum.htm

Cantor, W.J., Goodman, S.G., Cannon, C.P., Murphy, S.A., Charlesworth, A., Braunwauld, E., & Langer, A. (2005). Early cardiac catheterization is associated with lower mortality only among high-risk patients with ST- and non-ST-elevation acute coronary syndromes: Observations from the OPUS-TIMI 16 Trial. *American Heart Journal, 149*(2), 275-283.

Carabello, B.A. & Ganzes, P.C. (2001). *Cardiology pearls* (2nd ed.). Philadelphia: Hanley and Belfus.

Conover, M.B. (2003). *Understanding electrocardiography* (8th ed.). St. Louis: Mosby.

Davis, M.M., Taubert, K., Benin, A.L., Brown, D.W., Mensah, G.A., Baddour, L.M., et al. (2006). Influenza vaccination as secondary prevention for cardiovascular disease. *Circulation, 114*, 1549-1553.

370

Deedy, M.G. (2002). Coronary artery disease. *Cleveland Clinical Disease Management Medical Education*. Retrieved September 26, 2004 from http://www.clevelandclinicmeded.com/disease management/cardiology/cad

del Bene, S. & Vaughan, A. (2005). Acute coronary syndrome. In S.L.Woods, E.S. Froelicher, S.U. Motzer, & E.J. Bridges (Eds.), *Cardiac nursing* (5th ed., pp. 550-584). Philadelphia: Lippincott, Williams and Wilkins.

Drew, B.J., Califf, R.M., Funk, M., Kaufman, E.S., Krucoff, M.W., Laks, M.M., Macfarlane, P.W., Sommargren C, Swiryn, S., & Van Hare, J.F. (Oct 2004). Practice Standards for Electrocardiographic Monitoring in Hospital Settings: An American Heart Association Scientific Statement From the Councils on Cardiovascular Nursing, Clinical Cardiology, and Cardiovascular Disease in the Young: Endorsed by the International Society of Computerized Electrocardiology and the American Association of Critical-Care Nurses. *Circulation*, 110, 2721-2746.

Fenton, D.E. (2004). Acute coronary syndrome. Retrieved on December 31, 2004 from http://www.emedicine.com/emerg/topic31.htm

Gardner, P., & Altman, G. (2005). Pathophysiology of acute coronary syndrome. In S.L.Woods, E.S. Froelicher, S.U. Motzer, & E.J. Bridges (Eds.), *Cardiac nursing* (5th ed., pp. 541-549). Philadelphia: Lippincott, Williams and Wilkins.

Gibler, W.B., Cannon, C.P., Blomkalns, A.L., Char, D.M., Drew, B.J., Hollander, J.E. (2005). Practical implementation of the guidelines for unstable angina / non-st-segment elevation myocardial infarction in the emergency department. *Circulation*, 111, 2699-2710.

Greenland, P., Bonow, R.O., Brundage, B.H., Budoff, M.J., Eisenberg, M.J., Grundy, S.M., Lauer, M.S., Post, W.S., Raggi P., Redberg, R.F., Rodgers, G.P., Shaw, L.J., Taylor, A.J., Weintraub, W.S. (2007). ACCF/AHA 2007 clinical expert consensus document on coronary artery calcium scoring by computed tomography in global cardiovascular risk assessment and in evaluation of patients with chest pain: A report of the American College of Cardiology Foundation Clinical Expert Consensus Task Force (ACCF/AHA Writing Committee to Update the 2000 Expert Consensus Document on Electron-Beam Computed Tomography). *Circulation*, 115, 402-426.

Leon, A.S., Franklin, B.A., Costa, F., Balady, G.J., Berra, K.A., Stewart, K.J., Thompson, P.D., Williams, M.A., & Lauer, M.S. (Jan. 2005). Cardiac rehabilitation and secondary prevention of coronary heart disease: An American Heart Association scientific statement from the council on clinical cardiology (Subcommittee on Exercise, Cardiac Rehabilitation, and Prevention) and the Council on Nutrition, Physical Activity, and Metabolism (Subcommittee on Physical Activity) in Collaboration with the American Association of Cardiovascular and Pulmonary Rehabilitation. *Circulation*, 111, 369-376.

Marriott, H.J.L., (1999). *Board review manual of electrocardiography* (2nd ed.). Riverview, FL: Marriott Foundation/ACCN.

Marriott, H.J.L. (1997). *Emergency electrocardiography*. Naples, FL: Trinity Press.

Mendoza, R. & Trujillo, N. (2001). Complication and care following myocardial infarction. In A. V. Adair (Ed.), *Cardiology secrets* (pp. 113-117). Philadelphia: Hanley and Belfus, Inc.

Nadel, S. (2006). *Get Physical: The Basics of Exercise for the Heart Patient*. Presentation at Aultman Heart Center Patient Education Symposium, February 2006, Canton, Ohio.

Chapter 8

Smith, S.C. Jr, Allen, J., Blair, S.N., Bonow, R.O., Brass, L.M., Fonarow, J.C., Grundy, S.M., Hiratzka, L., Jones, D., Krumholz, H.M., Mosca, L., Pasternak, R.C., Pearson T., Pfeffer, M.A.,& Taubert, K.A. (2006). AHA/ACC Guidelines for Secondary Prevention for Patients With Coronary and Other Atherosclerotic Vascular Disease: 2006 Update: Endorsed by the National Heart, Lung, and Blood Institute. *Circulation, 113,* 2363-2372.

Smith, S.W., Zvoxec, D.L., Sharkey, S.W., & Henry, T.D. (2002). *The ECG in acute MI: An evidence-based manual of reperfusion therapy.* Philadelphia: Lippincott, Williams and Wilkins.

Sotile, W.M. & Cantor-Cooke, R. (2003). *Thriving with heart disease.* New York: Free Press.

Stahmer, S. (2004). Myocardial infarction. E-medicine. Retrieved on December 31, 2004 from http://www.emedicine.com/emerg/topic327.htm

Trujillo, N.P. & Lindenfeld, J. (2001). Myocardial infarction. In A.V. Adair (Ed.), *Cardiology secrets* (pp. 105-112). Philadelphia: Hanley and Belfus, Inc.

Upadya, S.P., Hoq, S.M., Pannala, R., Alsous, F., Tuohy, E., & Zarich, S. (2004). Tako-Tsubo Cardiomyopathy (Transient Left Ventricular Apical Ballooning) – A Myocardial Perfusion Echocardiogram Study. *Chest, 126,* 933-934.

Wellens, H.J.J., & Conover, M. (2006). *The ECG in Emergency Decision Making* (2nd ed.). St. Louis: Saunders Elsevier.

CHAPTER 9:
HEART FAILURE

INTRODUCTION

Understanding heart failure and its management is very important in cardiovascular nursing. Approximately 5 million Americans live with heart failure today, and 550,000 new cases are diagnosed annually. Moreover, 300,000 patients die each year of heart failure-related causes. Once diagnosed with heart failure, approximately 50% of patients die within 5 years (Hunt et al., 2005). Heart failure is the single most common cause of hospitalization in the United States for people older than age 65, and one third of hospitalized patients are readmitted within 90 days due to further decompensation (Hobbs & Boyle, 2004). In addition, another 20 million people with asymptomatic cardiac impairment are likely to develop heart failure symptoms within a 5-year period (Laurent, 2005).

The increasing number of people with heart failure is attributed to several factors, including the aging population, improved short-term survival of myocardial infarction (MI) patients (placing this group in the high-risk category for development of heart failure in the future), and an increased awareness of heart failure and established guidelines, resulting in increased diagnosis and management of the syndrome (Hunt et al., 2005).

Update 2007 statistics regarding the incidence of heart failure include:
- ◆ Heart failure incidence approaches 10 per 1000 population after age 65.
- ◆ At age 40, the lifetime risk of developing HF for both men and women is 1 in 5.
- ◆ The lifetime risk doubles for people with BP greater than 160/90 mm Hg versus those with BP less than 140/90 mm Hg

(Rosamond et al., 2007).

Definition

Heart failure is a complex clinical syndrome that can develop from any cardiac disorder that impairs the ability of the ventricle to either fill properly or eject optimally. This syndrome results in a pathologic state in which the heart is unable to pump enough oxygenated blood to meet the metabolic needs of the body. Patients with heart failure present with one or both of the hallmark manifestations of heart failure:
- ◆ Dyspnea and fatigue, which may impact exercise tolerance.
- ◆ Extracellular fluid (ECF) retention, which can cause peripheral edema and pulmonary congestion (Hunt et al., 2005).

Patients may have only one of the two manifestations of heart failure at any given time. For this reason, the term "heart failure" is more accurate than "congestive heart failure." With either dyspnea and fatigue or ECF retention, the patient's functional capacity and quality of life are affected.

The terms, backward and forward failure, are also used to describe the two distinct components of heart failure.

Chapter 9

Forward Failure

◆ Ventricles fail to pump well in a forward direction
  ❖ Left ventricular forward failure results in end organ hypoperfusion.
  ❖ Right ventricular forward failure results in failure to adequately fill the left ventricle.

Backward Failure

◆ Ventricular pressure rises
  ❖ High left ventricular pressure is transmitted backwards into lungs.
  ❖ High right ventricular pressure is transmitted backwards into venous system.

CLINICAL PRESENTATION

Dyspnea, Fatigue and Exercise Intolerance

Most patients with heart failure present with decreased exercise tolerance due to dyspnea or fatigue. Because these presenting symptoms are non-specific, many patients are not readily diagnosed with heart failure. These symptoms are sometimes attributed to deconditioning associated with the aging process. Many heart failure patients also have coexisting conditions, such as pulmonary disease, which also contribute to exercise intolerance and make differential diagnosis challenging. Symptom assessment is more difficult in elderly patients who often do not experience exertional dyspnea because they have developed more sedentary lifestyles to accommodate their decreased functional capacity.

Linking Knowledge to Practice

✔ *When assessing for exertional dyspnea, remember to do so within the context of the patient's activity level. The nurse must not only ask the patient about dyspnea with exertion, but must also assess the degree to which the patient has been exerting himself or herself. For example: A patient who sits in a chair for the majority of the day may not complain of dyspnea on exertion because they are not routinely engaging in activities that are considered exertional.*

Volume Overload

Patients may also present with extracellular fluid overload, manifested as peripheral edema or abdominal swelling. Anorexia commonly accompanies abdominal swelling. Additional findings during physical exam that indicate fluid overload are the presence of a third heart sound (S3), hepatic tenderness, and jugular venous distention. Patients with pulmonary congestion present with dyspnea on exertion, cough, orthopnea, and paroxysmal nocturnal dyspnea. Pulmonary congestion usually occurs when the ventricle rapidly fails. Many patients with left ventricular end stage heart failure have no signs of pulmonary congestion due to the efficiency of the lymphatic system in removing excess volume. Regardless of initial presentation, progressive changes in symptoms over time are common to most heart failure patients.

374

ETIOLOGY

A variety of cardiac disorders can cause heart failure, but the most common cause is left ventricular dysfunction (Hobbs & Boyle, 2004; Hunt et al., 2005). The most common cause of left ventricular dysfunction is ischemic coronary heart disease (CAD), followed by hypertension and dilated cardiomyopathy. Dilated cardiomyopathy is discussed in detail in Chapter 10.

Heart failure is not equivalent to cardiomyopathy or left ventricular dysfunction, although these may be common reasons for the manifestation of heart failure. Heart failure is rather a clinical syndrome with specific symptoms.

The American Heart Association (AHA) reports that up to 75% of patients with heart failure have hypertension (Hunt et al., 2005). Because coronary artery disease (CAD) and hypertension increase the risk of heart failure, strategies to reduce risk and control disease progression in these disorders are also key in reducing heart failure risk.

Other causes of left ventricular dysfunction include:

◆ Valvular disease.
◆ Hyperthyroidism or hypothyroidism.
◆ Infection.
◆ Alcohol or drug abuse.
◆ Cardiotoxic agents such as chest irradiation, certain chemotherapy agents, and other cardiotoxic drugs or poisons.
◆ Certain antiarrhythmic and anesthetic agents.
◆ Chronic tachyarrhythmias.
◆ Congenital or mechanical cardiac defects.
◆ Connective tissue disorders.
◆ Peripartum cardiomyopathy.
◆ Idiopathic.

INITIAL EVALUATION

Recommendations from the American College of Cardiology (ACC) and AHA Guidelines for the Management of Heart Failure and from the Heart Failure Society of America include:

◆ Thorough history and physical to identify cardiac and non-cardiac conditions that contribute to the development and acceleration of heart failure.
◆ Initial diagnostic tests to include electrocardiogram (ECG), chest x-ray, and two-dimensional echocardiogram with Doppler to assess the function of the left ventricle.
◆ Initial laboratory evaluation to include complete blood count, electrolytes, blood urea nitrogen, creatinine, blood glucose, thyroid-stimulating hormone, liver function studies, and urinalysis.
◆ Assessment of functional capacity based on the patient's ability to perform routine ADLs and / or based on a 6-minute walk test.
◆ Assessment of fluid volume status.
◆ Assessment of risk for life-threatening arrhythmias.
◆ Identification of exacerbating factors.
◆ Identification of barriers to understanding of and adherence to treatment plan.
  ❖ Financial limitations.
  ❖ Lack of family and social support.

Chapter 9

- ❖ Illiteracy.
- ❖ Depression.
- ❖ Multiple medications.
- ❖ Transportation difficulties.
- ❖ Multiple co-morbidities.

Because of the high association between ischemic CAD and heart failure, most patients with chest pain of unknown etiology, presenting with the clinical syndrome of heart failure also undergo cardiac catheterization (Hobbs & Boyle, 2004; Hunt et al., 2005).

Echocardiography

Two-dimensional echocardiography with Doppler flow studies is the most frequently used diagnostic test in evaluating patients with the clinical syndrome of heart failure. A non-invasive, cost-effective diagnostic tool, the echocardiogram, can identify systolic and diastolic dysfunction, including a measurement of ejection fraction. When systolic dysfunction is identified, the echocardiogram can assist in determining the etiology. Regional wall-motion abnormalities indicate ischemic CAD as the cause, whereas global dysfunction usually indicates a non-ischemic origin. An echocardiogram can also identify other causes of heart failure, such as valvular or pericardial disease. Although an echocardiogram can provide essential information regarding the possible cause of heart failure, it cannot identify the exact cause.

CLASSIFICATIONS OF HEART FAILURE

Staging of Heart Failure

The AHA/ACC staging system (see Table 9.1) classifies heart failure as a progressive disorder. In this model of progression, left ventricular dysfunction begins with an initial insult to the myocardium. Even without further identifiable insults, left ventricular dysfunction continues to progress.

<table>
<tr><th colspan="4">Table 9.1
Stages of Heart Failure</th></tr>
<tr><th>Stage A</th><th>Stage B</th><th>Stage C</th><th>Stage D</th></tr>
<tr>
<td>High risk for developing HF.

No identified structural or functional abnormalities.

No signs or symptoms of HF.</td>
<td>Presence of structural heart disease strongly associated with development of HF.

No signs or symptoms of HF</td>
<td>Past or present symptoms of HF associated with underlying structural heart disease.</td>
<td>Advanced structural heart disease.

Specialized interventions required.

Marked symptoms of HF at rest, despite maximal medical therapy.</td>
</tr>
<tr><td colspan="4">Source: Hunt et al., 2005.</td></tr>
</table>

Left ventricular dysfunction can range from predominantly diastolic dysfunction to predominant systolic dysfunction. Patients with heart failure can also have a combination of both systolic and diastolic dysfunction. Patients with combined systolic and diastolic dysfunction have a worse prognosis than those with isolated systolic or diastolic dysfunction (Hobbs & Boyle, 2004).

Systolic versus Diastolic Dysfunction

In the 2007 American Heart Association updated statistics for heart failure, one prevalence study of asymptomatic individuals showed the prevalence of left ventricular diastolic dysfunction was 21% for mild diastolic dysfunction and 7% for moderate or severe diastolic dysfunction. The prevalence of systolic dysfunction was 6%, with 2% having moderate or severe systolic dysfunction (Rosamond et al., 2007).

Systolic Dysfunction

In systolic dysfunction, the left ventricular wall thins and the cavity dilates (eccentric hypertrophy, Figure 9.1). A thin, dilated ventricle is unable to contract effectively and the ejection fraction (percent of blood the ventricle ejects per beat relative to the total amount of blood in the ventricle) decreases. A normal ejection fraction is greater than or equal to 55%. An ejection fraction less than 40% generally defines systolic dysfunction (Laurent, 2005). Systolic dysfunction is found in two thirds of patients with heart failure (Hunt et al., 2005). Patients with systolic dysfunction also have low cardiac output. As a result, left ventricular end diastolic volume (preload) increases, leading to pulmonary congestion.

Systolic dysfunction can be regional (as in MI) or global. Dilated cardiomyopathy is a common cause of systolic dysfunction. However, cardiomyopathy should not be used interchangeably with systolic heart failure. Cardiomyopathy is a structural disorder associated with the development of heart failure, but heart failure is a clinical syndrome characterized by the presentation of certain symptoms. Cardiomyopathy is discussed in detail in Chapter 10.

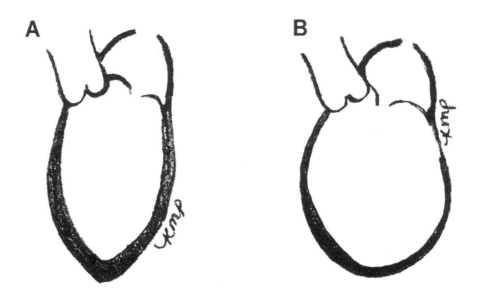

Figure 9.1: Normal left ventricle (A), ventricle with systolic dysfunction and eccentric hypertrophy (B).

Physiologic Change	Signs & Symptoms
↓ Ability of left ventricle to pump blood	Fatigue, chest pain if coronaries underperfused
↓	
↑ LVEDV & ↑ LVEDP (volume & pressure)	S3, S4, ↑ PAOP
↓	
↑ Left atrial pressure	Atrial arrhythmias
↓	
↑ Pressure in pulmonary capillaries & pulmonary artery	↑ PAP, ↑ PAD
↓	
Leaking of fluid from pulmonary capillaries into lungs	Crackles (rales), SOB, cough, orthopnea, wheezing, hypoxia
↓	
↑ Right ventricular pressure	Sternal heave, RV S3
↓	
↑ Right atrial pressure	↑ CVP ↑ neck veins
↓	
Backup of blood into systemic veins	Peripheral edema + adominojugular test

Figure 9.2: Relationship of pathophysiology of left ventricular systolic failure to clinical presentation

Diastolic Dysfunction

In diastolic dysfunction, the ventricular muscle thickens (concentric hypertrophy), and the cavity size may remain normal or become smaller. Ejection is not impaired, and the ejection fraction remains within normal limits. In diastolic dysfunction, ventricular relaxation is impaired and the ventricle does not fill properly. The presence of diastolic dysfunction has been shown to be predictive of all-cause mortality (Rosamond et al., 2007).

Diastolic dysfunction is commonly associated with chronic systemic hypertension with left ventricular hypertrophy. The aging process affects the elastic properties of the heart, and elderly women are at an especially high risk for diastolic dysfunction. Ischemic heart disease and restrictive or hypertrophic cardiomyopathy can also cause diastolic dysfunction. In these conditions, the ventricle can become stiff or noncompliant. Other causes of diastolic dysfunction include hypertrophic cardiomyopathy, infiltrative diseases (sarcoidosis, amyloidosis), and aortic stenosis.

A noncompliant ventricle is unable to completely relax during diastole, impairing filling (see Figure 9.3). In diastolic dysfunction, end-diastolic pressures are elevated; however, volumes remain low to normal. To increase diastolic filling, the pressure in the left atria increases. When increased left atrial pressure rises above the pres-

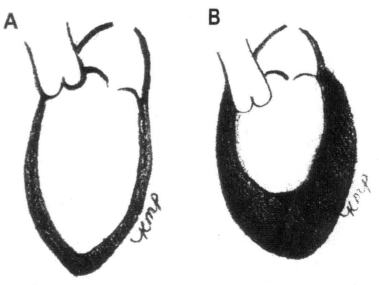

Figure 9.3: Normal left ventricle (A), ventricle with diastolic dysfunction and concentric hypertrophy (B).

sure in the pulmonary capillaries, pulmonary edema can result.

Patients with diastolic dysfunction commonly become symptomatic with exertion when heart rate is increased. With faster heart rates, ventricular filling time is reduced and cardiac output is impaired. Increased levels of circulating catecholamines also increase heart rate and worsen diastolic dysfunction. Flash pulmonary edema can develop during periods of ischemia due to increased noncompliance of the ventricle.

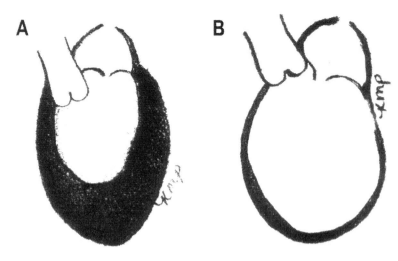

Figure 9.4: Concentric hypertrophy (A), Eccentric hypertrophy (B).

Three conditions are required for diagnosis of diastolic dysfunction: 1) signs and symptoms of heart failure, 2) normal or only slightly decreased ejection fraction, 3) increased diastolic filling pressure and abnormal relaxation of the left ventricle (Hunt et al., 2005). For practical purposes, the diagnosis of diastolic heart failure is made in patients presenting with the clinical syndrome of heart failure with no evidence of systolic dysfunction. Table 9.2 summarizes the comparison between systolic and diastolic heart failure. Figure 9.4 compares the concentric hypertrophy of diastolic heart failure with the eccentric hypertrophy of systolic heart failure. Remember that patients can have coexisting systolic and diastolic dysfunction.

Table 9.2
Summary Comparison of Systolic and Diastolic Dysfunction

Systolic Dysfunction	2/3 of symptomatic heart failure patients	Decreased left-ventricular contractility and ejection fraction	Most common cause is coronary artery disease, resulting in myocardial infarction or chronic ischemia
Diastolic Dysfunction	1/3 of symptomatic heart failure patients	Impaired left-ventricular relaxation and abnormal filling	Usually related to chronic hypertension or ischemic heart disease

Left- and Right-Ventricular Failure

The left and right ventricles are part of a closed circulatory system. Right-ventricular failure usually results from prolonged left-ventricular failure. Isolated right-ventricular failure can occur with right-ventricular MI, primary pulmonary hypertension, acute or chronic lung disease, or chronic severe tricuspid regurgitation. Comparison of signs and symptoms of right- and left-sided heart failure are outlined in Table 9.3.

Chapter 9

Table 9.3 Comparison of Right- and Left-Sided Heart Failure	
Right-Sided Backward Failure	**Left-Sided Backward Failure**
Elevated CVP	Dyspnea, tachypnea
Jugular venous distention	Orthopnea
+ abdominojugular reflux	Cough
Peripheral edema	Wheezes, rhonchi
Weight gain	Crackles
Sternal heave	Respiratory alkalosis
Abdominal distention	Hypoxemia, hypoxia
Liver engorgement	S3 extra heart sounds
Anorexia, nausea	Systolic murmur of mitral regurgitation
Right-Sided Forward Failure	**Left-Sided Forward Failure**
Decreased Pulmonary Perfusion (Forward Failure)	Fatigue, weakness, poor exercise tolerance
Dyspnea	Chest pain, arrhythmias
Tachypnea	Exertional dyspnea
Hypoxia	Tachycardia
Cyanosis	Narrow pulse pressure
Decreased Left Ventricular Filling	Cool, pale diaphoretic
	Decreased urine output
	Decreased mentation

NEUROHORMONAL RESPONSES IN HEART FAILURE

Neurohormonal responses are activated as the body's response to decreased cardiac output and poor organ perfusion. Initially, these responses are helpful in improving cardiac output and organ perfusion. Over time, however, these responses actually lead to clinical deterioration. Several neurohormonal responses have been identified in the progression of left-ventricular dysfunction.

Among the most important and well-understood of these responses are SNS stimulation and activation of the renin-angiotensin-aldosterone system (RAAS). Other neurohormonal responses to heart failure include increased circulating levels of endothelin, vasopressin (also known as *antidiuretic hormone*), and cytokines (Hunt et al., 2005). The same compensatory mechanisms that initially help preserve cardiac output and blood pressure actually cause progressive deterioration of myocardial function in the long term.

Sympathetic Nervous System

One of the first responses to failing left ventricle is activation of the SNS. As the left ventricle begins to fail, cardiac output and blood pressure decrease. This fall in blood pressure activates the baroreceptors and vasomotor regulatory centers in the medulla. The result is an increased level of circulating cate-cholamines, which stimulates alpha- and beta-adrenergic receptors to increase heart rate, peripheral vasoconstriction (increase afterload), and contractility. Figure 9.5 shows the cardiovascular effects of SNS stimulation.

In chronic heart failure, beta-receptors are less able to respond to circulating catecholamines. This decreased response to circulating catecholamines is called *beta-receptor down regulation* and is an attempt to protect the failing heart from chronic over stimulation of the SNS (Laurent, 2005). Beta-receptor down regulation contributes to the exercise intolerance associated with heart failure.

Chronic stimulation of the SNS also accelerates the ventricular remodeling process (discussed later in this chapter). Increased heart rate, afterload, and contractility not only help maintain cardiac output and blood pressure, but also have the negative effect of increasing myocardial oxygen demand. Over time, this increased stimulation of the SNS can worsen ischemia and cause cardiac arrhythmias and even sudden cardiac death. In addition, norepinephrine, one of the circulating catecholamines, has direct cardiotoxic properties (Hobbs & Boyle, 2004) that are responsible for the beta-receptor down regulation seen with chronic heart failure.

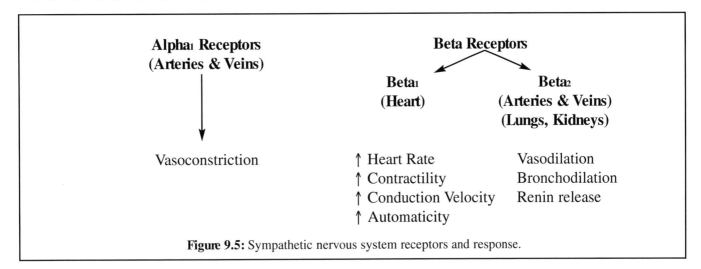

Figure 9.5: Sympathetic nervous system receptors and response.

Renin-Angiotensin-Aldosterone System

Activation of the RAAS is another compensatory neurohormonal response to a failing heart. The RAAS is activated as the kidneys respond to decreased renal perfusion. It is also activated by an increase in SNS activity. When the RAAS is activated, circulating levels of renin, angiotensin II, and aldosterone increase. Angiotensin II is a potent vasoconstrictor, thus there is systemic vascular resistance and afterload increase. Aldosterone is a mineralocorticoid responsible for sodium and water retention, which increases preload. Enhanced preload increases end-diastolic volume, which further dilates the ventricle and enhances the ventricular remodeling process. If the left ventricle becomes overstretched, contractility is depressed. Figure 9.6 shows the effects of RAAS stimulation.

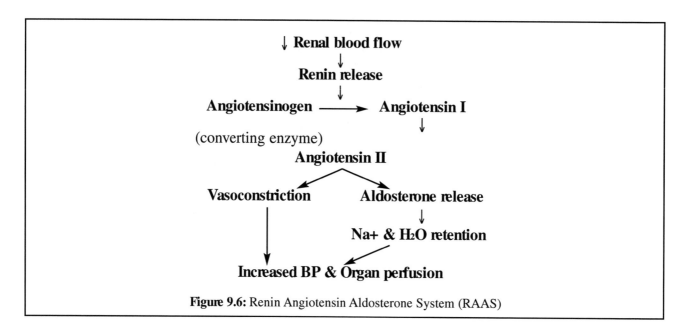

Figure 9.6: Renin Angiotensin Aldosterone System (RAAS)

Vasopressin and Endothelin

In chronic heart failure, angiotensin II and osmotic stimuli produce an increase in vasopressin release, causing a reabsorption of water and additional vasoconstriction. Levels of endothelin, an endogenous hormonal vasoconstrictor, are elevated in heart failure in response to angiotensin II, vasopressin, and circulating catecholamines (Laurent, 2005).

Linking Knowledge to Practice

✔ *Current treatment of heart failure involves inhibition of neurohormonal systems with beta blockers and angiotensin-converting enzyme (ACE) inhibitors. Patients typically do not understand the neurohormonal blockade associated with these medications or the importance they play in stopping disease progression. If patients think these medications are only used to treat hypertension and their blood pressures are normal, they may be less compliant because they do not fully understand the impact of therapy.*

Inflammatory Response

Cytokine levels are also elevated in heart failure, producing both local and systemic inflammatory responses. Local inflammatory responses occur early in the course of the disease; systemic responses occur later in the course. Cytokines promote cell growth (hypertrophy) and cell death (apoptosis) (Laurent, 2005; Opie, 2004). Hypertrophy and apoptosis are seen in the ventricular remodeling process. Figure 9.7 shows the vicious cycle of heart failure caused by uninterrupted neurohormonal responses.

Positive Neurohormonal Response

The release of the hormones atrial natriuretic peptide and brain natriuretic peptide (BNP) from cardiac myocytes is the one beneficial neurohormonal response in heart failure. These hormones have the positive effect of systemic and pulmonary vasodilatation and also enhance sodium and water excretion. Other substances, such as nitric oxide, bradykinin, and some prostaglandins work to counteract the vasoconstrictive effects of the SNS and RAAS stimulation. However, the vasoconstrictive effects of neurohormonal activation commonly overpower these counter efforts. Table 9.4 summarizes the results of neurohormonal responses to heart failure.

Heart Failure

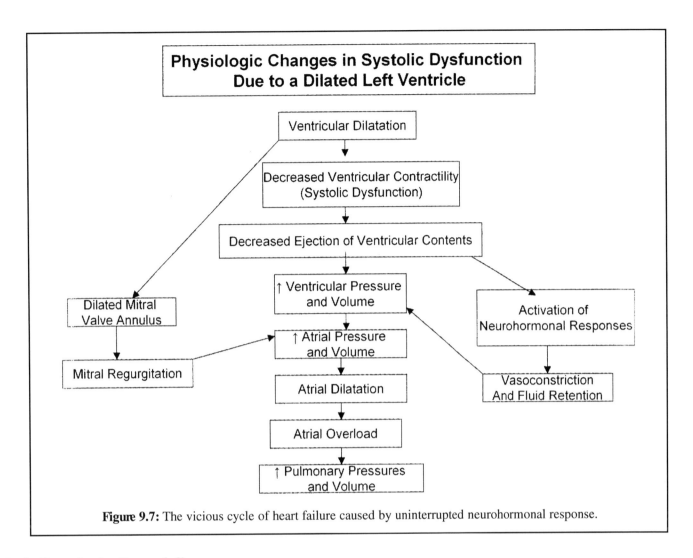

Figure 9.7: The vicious cycle of heart failure caused by uninterrupted neurohormonal response.

Left-Ventricular Remodeling

Left-ventricular remodeling is another response to the initial left-ventricular injury. Remodeling is a process of pathological growth whereby the ventricle hypertrophies, then dilates. Ventricular remodeling occurs in response to both pressure and volume overload in the ventricles. When pressure overload occurs, the myocytes thicken and concentric hypertrophy results. When volume overload occurs, the myocytes elongate and eccentric hypertrophy results (Laurent, 2005; Opie, 2004). Concentric and eccentric hypertrophy are shown in Figure 9.4.

The process of ventricular remodeling is very complex at the cellular level. Concentric hypertrophy causes left-ventricular wall thickening and leads to an increased risk of subendocardial ischemia. Eccentric hypertrophy and eventual dilatation can cause regurgitation of the mitral valve and elevated left atrial pressures. In eccentric hypertrophy, the ventricle changes from its natural "football-like" shape to a more "basketball-like" shape. The development of concentric and eccentric hypertrophy further accelerates the remodeling process.

Another component of ventricular remodeling includes necrosis and apoptosis of cardiac myocytes. Necrosis, accidental cell death, occurs in response to deprivation of oxygen. Apoptosis, programmed cell death, is stimulated by several factors, including angiotensin II and cytokines (Laurent, 2005). Myocyte loss in either form can facilitate slippage of myocytes. In response to slippage, a reparative fibrosis

Chapter 9

occurs that makes the ventricle stiffer. This process of ventricular remodeling is complicated by other physiological responses beyond the scope of this chapter.

Remodeling is also enhanced by the prolonged activation of the SNS, RAAS, and other neurohormonal responses, including endothelin production (Opie, 2004). In addition to norepinephrine, other substances produced in the activation of neurohormonal responses may have direct cardiotoxic effects.

Table 9.4
Summary of Results of Neurohormonal Stimulation in Heart Failure

Sympathetic Nervous System Stimulation	◆ Stimulation of RAAS and endothelin. ◆ Vasoconstriction (increased afterload), increased heart rate, increased contractility. ◆ Aggravation of ischemia. ◆ Potentiation of arrhythmias. ◆ Acceleration of ventricular remodeling. ◆ Direct toxicity to cardiac myocytes.
Renin Angiotensin Aldosterone System	◆ Arterial vasoconstriction from angiotensin II. ◆ Stimulation of vasopressin and endothelin. ◆ Sodium and water retention from increased aldosterone. ◆ Endothelial dysfunction from increased aldosterone. ◆ Organ fibrosis from increased aldosterone.
Vasopressin	◆ Reabsorption of water. ◆ Vasoconstriction.
Endothelin	◆ Vasoconstriction. ◆ Fluid retention. ◆ Increased contractility. ◆ Hypertrophy.
Cytokines	◆ Pro-inflammatory response. ◆ Contribution to apoptosis (programmed cell death). ◆ Contribution to cardiac cachexia (systemic inflammatory response).
Natriuretic Peptides*	◆ Systemic and pulmonary vasodilation. ◆ Increased sodium and water excretion. ◆ Suppression of other neurohormones.
Nitric oxide,* bradykinin,* some prostaglandins	◆ Arterial smooth muscle relaxation and vasodilation.
*Neurohormonal response with positive benefit in heart failure.	

ONGOING ASSESSMENT IN HEART FAILURE MANAGEMENT

Functional Capacity

The New York Heart Association (NYHA) classification is the most commonly used system to assess functional capacity (see Table 9.5). Patients classified as NYHA class IV have 20% overall annual mortality (Hunt et al., 2005). The NYHA classification system has limitations due to the subjectivity involved in the assessment process. In addition, NYHA functional capacity class assessment does not always progress in a systematic way. Patients can move between classes throughout the progression of

384

Heart Failure

their disease. NYHA classifications do not correspond with the ACC/AHA stages of heart failure progression. In addition, the degree of left-ventricular systolic dysfunction does not correlate well with the degree of activity intolerance (Adams et al., 2006).

Other tools that are used to assess functional capacity include the 6-minute walk test, maximal exercise testing, and peak oxygen consumption (Hobbs & Boyle, 2004; Hunt et al., 2005).

Table 9.5
New York Heart Association Functional Classifications

Class I	Class II	Class III	Class IV
Cardiac disease with no resulting limitation in physical activity.	Cardiac disease with slight limitation of physical activity.	Cardiac disease with marked limitation on physical activity.	Cardiac disease resulting in inability to carry out any physical activity without discomfort.
Ordinary activity free of fatigue, palpitation, dyspnea or anginal pain.	Comfortable at rest, but ordinary activity results in fatigue, palpitations, dyspnea, or anginal pain.	Comfortable at rest, but less than ordinary activity results in fatigue, palpitations, dyspnea, or anginal pain.	May have symptoms of cardiac insufficiency at rest.

Source: Hunt et al., 2005

Linking Knowledge to Practice

✔ *Because patients commonly decrease their activity levels to adjust to declining functional capacity, it is important to ask specific questions regarding the level of activity the patient is able to tolerate. For example, ask, "Is there any leisure activity you are no longer able to do that you wish you still could do?"*

Fluid Volume Status

Several ongoing physical parameters are assessed to determine ECF volume status, including;

◆ Weight.
◆ Amount of jugular venous distention.
◆ Edema of legs, abdomen, sacral area, or scrotum.
◆ Presence of organ congestion: hepatomegaly or crackles.

The most reliable sign of ECF overload is jugular venous distention (Hunt et al., 2005). Most patients with peripheral edema also have ECF overload; however, peripheral edema also has noncardiac causes. Most patients with compensated chronic heart failure do not have audible crackles in their lung fields on physical examination. Crackles are generally a sign of rapid onset of heart failure. Therefore, the absence of pulmonary crackles should not be considered an adequate measure of optimal fluid volume status. Short-term assessment of ECF volume status is best measured by a change in daily weight.

Linking Knowledge to Practice

✔ *Patients should be instructed to weigh themselves daily first thing in the morning, after urinating, and prior to eating. They should be instructed to use the same scale and wear the same amount of clothing. A weight gain of more than 2 lb in 24 hours, or more than 3 lb in a week, should be reported to the physician. Remember that 1 lb of weight = 1 pint of fluid.*

Chapter 9

Many physicians have patients adjust their diuretic doses at home based on daily weights. With the assessment of daily weights and appropriate intervention, ECF volume can be managed on an outpatient basis, and many hospital admissions can be avoided.

Laboratory Values

Monitoring potassium levels is particularly important in heart failure patients. Diuretics can cause hypokalemia. Many heart failure patients are also on digoxin, and hypokalemia increases the risk of digoxin toxicity. In contrast, other medications used in the treatment of heart failure, such as ACE inhibitors, angiotensin II receptor blockers (ARBs), and aldosterone antagonists, can predispose patients to hyperkalemia. Patients taking loop diuretics who experience the expected side effect of hypokalemia and who also take one or more medications that can predispose patients to hyperkalemia, are unlikely to be ordered potassium supplements.

Using laboratory values to monitor renal function and anemia is also important in heart failure management.

Exacerbating or Complicating Factors

Hypertension, ischemia, and new or worsening valve disease can exacerbate heart failure. In addition, the development of arrhythmias can exacerbate heart failure or can represent a complication of heart failure. Patients should be assessed for any history of palpitations, known arrhythmias, pre-syncope, or syncope.

Self Care Abilities and Adherence to Treatment Plan

Functional capacity and fluid volume status will provide information regarding the patient's response to the treatment plan. A complete review of additional signs and symptoms should be done with each follow-up including an assessment of the patient's ability to recognize and report subtle changes. Special attention should also be given to the patient's adherence to a low sodium diet and to all prescribed medications.

TREATMENT GOALS

The majority of major clinical trials performed have evaluated treatment strategies for systolic dysfunction. Few large-scale clinical trials have evaluated the treatment of isolated diastolic dysfunction. Clinical practice guidelines exist for the treatment of systolic dysfunction; these guidelines are addressed in this section. However, many patients with diastolic dysfunction are on many of the same medications. Treatment goals in diastolic dysfunction aim to control hypertension, heart rate, and blood volume.

Risk Control in Patients with Structural Heart Disease (Stage B)

Once a patient has evidence of structural heart disease, aggressive measures should be put in place to reduce risk. Strict control of blood pressure, both systolic and diastolic, should be maintained in patients with hypertension. Blood pressure targets of less than 130/80 mm Hg should be established for patients with diabetes and renal disease. When combination drug therapy is required to manage hypertension, those medications effective in treating both heart failure and hypertension become the preferred medications. These include diuretics, ACE inhibitors or angiotensin II receptor blockers, and beta blockers. Optimal control of blood pressure reduces the risk of new onset heart failure by approximately 50% (Hunt et al., 2005; Adams et al., 2006). In patients with prior MI, the risk can by reduced by approximately 80% (Adams et al., 2006). ACE inhibitors are recommended to reduce risk in all high-risk groups, including those with vascular disease in the coronary arteries, carotid arteries, or peripheral arteries. ACE inhibitors and beta blockers are indicated for prevention of heart failure in all patients with prior MI.

Diabetes not only increases the risk of heart failure but also worsens outcomes for those with heart failure. ACE inhibitors have been shown to limit end-organ damage in diabetic patients, even if hypertension is not present (U.S. Department of Health and Human Services, 2003). Angiotensin II receptor blockers have also been shown to prevent heart failure in high-risk patients, including those with vascular disease, hypertension, and diabetes (Hunt et al., 2005).

Any patient with CAD should have aggressive control of risk factors to decrease the risk of future coronary events and the risk of heart failure development. Treatment of hyperlipidemia in patients with previous MI has been shown to reduce the risk of heart failure (Braunwald et al., 2002).

After an MI, all patients should be started on a beta blocker and ACE inhibitor. Aldosterone antagonists are also indicated in a subset of post MI patients. These medications help reduce left-ventricular remodeling after MI. Aggressive efforts to reperfuse patients during acute MI are important in preserving myocardial function in the short-term and preventing heart failure in the long-term.

Patients with contributing lifestyle habits, such as smoking, illicit drug use, or excessive alcohol consumption, should be counseled regarding the impact of these habits on the development of heart failure. Coexisting noncardiac disorders, such as thyroid disease, should be treated because untreated tachycardia associated with hyperthyroidism can cause cardiomyopathy.

Asymptomatic Chronic Left-Ventricular Systolic Dysfunction (Stage B)

Patients with asymptomatic chronic left ventricular systolic dysfunction should be managed with ACE inhibitors, or angiotensin II receptor blockers, and beta blockers because these two classifications of medications have been proven to slow the progression of left-ventricular dysfunction. There are no data to support the use of digoxin in these patients because digoxin has minimal impact on disease progression (Hunt et al., 2005). Diuretics are not indicated because these patients show no signs or symptoms of fluid overload.

Aggressive efforts at secondary prevention, cardiac revascularization, and treatment of valvular heart disease should be undertaken.

Symptomatic Left-Ventricular Dysfunction (Stage C)

Patients with symptomatic left ventricular dysfunction are generally considered as having active heart failure. These patients are managed with ACE inhibitors or angiotensin II receptor blockers and beta blockers to slow disease progression.

In addition, they are placed on diuretics and moderate sodium restrictions to control extra cellular fluid volume status. Daily weight can be used to guide diuretic therapy. Diuretic therapy can also improve symptoms, increase cardiac function, and improve exercise tolerance (Hunt et al., 2005); however, diuretics do not improve survival and may cause renal and metabolic side effects (Hobbs & Boyle, 2004).

Patients may also be on digoxin to improve symptoms and exercise tolerance. Physical activity should be encouraged in all heart failure patients, except those in an acute decompensated state. Physical activity is encouraged to prevent deconditioning, which contributes to exercise intolerance.

Chapter 9

PHARMACOLOGICAL TREATMENT OF HEART FAILURE

ACE Inhibitors and Angiotensin II Receptor Blockers

ACE inhibitors interfere with the conversion of angiotensin I to angiotensin II in the RAAS system. In addition, they enhance the action of kinins, which promote a positive vasodilatory effect in heart failure. Both actions are responsible for their positive impact in heart failure. These medications interfere with the ventricular remodeling process, slow disease progression, and reduce the risk of death (Calclasure, Kozlowski, & Highfill, 2001; Hobbs & Boyle, 2004; Hunt et al., 2005; Laurent, 2005). ACE inhibitors also improve symptoms and contribute to a sense of well-being.

Benefits are seen in all stages of heart failure, although it may take several weeks to months for the effects to be seen. ACE inhibitors are used for mortality benefits, even when no improvement in symptoms is noted. ACE inhibitors should be titrated to target doses based on patient tolerance. ACE inhibitor dosing guidelines are included in Table 9.6.

ACE inhibitors should be used cautiously in the following situations:

◆ Systolic blood pressure < 80 mm Hg.

◆ Creatinine > 3 mg/dL.

◆ Bilateral renal artery stenosis.

◆ Elevated serum potassium.

ACE inhibitors are contraindicated in:

◆ Angioedema.

◆ Pregnancy.

◆ Anuric renal failure.

Table 9.6 ACE Inhibitor Dosing in Heart Failure		
Drug	**Starting Dose**	**Maximum Dose**
Captopril	6.25 mg TID	50 mg TID
Enalapril	2.5 mg BID	10 to 20 mg BID
Fosinopril	5 to 10 mg daily	40 mg daily
Lisinopril	2.5 to 5 mg daily	20 to 40 mg daily
Perindopril	2 mg daily	8 to 16 mg daily
Quinapril	5 mg BID	20 mg BID
Ramipril	1.25 to 2.5 mg daily	10 mg daily
Trandolapril	1 mg daily	4 mg daily
(Hunt et al., 2005).		

The positive effects of ACE inhibitors are diminished in fluid overload states. Non-steroidal anti-inflammatory medications can block favorable and enhance adverse effects of ACI inhibitors. Aspirin may also interfere with effectiveness of ACE inhibitors because aspirin blocks kinin-mediated prostaglandin synthesis (Hunt et al., 2005).

ACE inhibitors remain the first choice for interuption of the RAAS in chronic heart failure.

Angiotensin II receptor blockers directly block angiotensin II. In addition to being an acceptable first-line agent in some patient sub groups (those at risk for heart failure), angiotensin II receptor blockers are

Heart Failure

indicated in chronic heart failure patients who cannot tolerate an ACE inhibitor due to cough or angioedema. Candesartan was the first angiotensin II receptor blocker to be approved by the FDA for the treatment of heart failure (Hunt et al., 2005). Guidelines for angiotensin II receptor blocker dosing is included in Table 9.7.

Table 9.7 Angiotensin II Receptor Blockers Dosing in Heart Failure		
Drug	**Starting Dose**	**Maximum Dose**
Losartan	25 to 50 mg daily	50 to 100 mg daily
Valsartan	20 to 40 mg BID	160 mg BID
Candesartan	4 to 8 mg daily	32 mg daily
(Hunt et al., 2005).		

Linking Knowledge to Practice

✔ *Always assess creatinine and potassium level before administering ACE inhibitors and angiotensin II receptor blockers.*

✔ *Assure that the presence of a cough with an ACE inhibitor is related to the ACE inhibitor and not a sign of worsening heart failure.*

✔ *Assess for exaggerated hypotensive response when giving with diuretics.*

✔ *The blood pressure hold criteria for these medications may be much lower in patients with chronic heart failure than in patients taking these medications only for hypertension.*

Hydralazine and Nitrate Combination

A combination of hydralazine and a nitrate may used for afterload and preload reduction in patients who cannot tolerate an ACE inhibitor due to renal insufficiency or hyperkalemia (Adams et al., 2006). In addition, a combination of hydralazine and a nitrate may be added to patients who are taking an ACE inhibitor and a beta blocker and who still have symptoms.

Hydralazine and isosorbide dinitrate is recommended in addition to an ACE inhibitor in African Americans with systolic dysfunction and NYHA Class II-IV heart failure (Adams et al., 2006).

Beta Blockers

Beta blockers are indicated in heart failure to block the neurohormonal responses of chronic SNS stimulation. Multiple studies have proven a mortality benefit in patients treated with beta blockers. Beta blockers have several beneficial effects, including favorably affecting ventricular remodeling and apoptosis. Beta blockers can decrease arrhythmias and ischemia by decreasing heart rate and contractility, thereby decreasing myocardial oxygen consumption. Beta blockers in heart failure patients are initiated in low doses and titrated upward slowly. Titrations are usually made at intervals of two or more weeks with the goal to reach target dose in 8-12 weeks. Referral to a heart failure specialist is suggested when upward titration is difficult (Adams et al., 2006). Dosage guidelines for beta blockers are included in Table 9.8.

Beta blockers are not initiated when the patient is fluid overloaded or in a decompensated state. Prior to initiating a beta blocker, the patient's fluid status should be optimized and the patient should not require IV diuretics or IV vasodilators (Adams et al., 2006). ACE inhibitors are initiated first in new onset heart

Chapter 9

failure, and a beta blocker is started prior to full titration of the ACE inhibitor (Hunt et al., 2005). Whenever possible, beta blockers should be started at low doses prior to hospital discharge. Beta blocker administration in heart failure is a core quality assurance measure. If a beta blocker cannot be initiated or tolerated then the medical record must contain documentation related to the contraindication.

Patients who show signs of decompensation after a maintenance dose of beta blocker therapy has been administered, generally do not have the beta blocker therapy discontinued. In some cases of decompensation the beta blocker dosage may need to be temporarily reduced. Abrupt discontinuation of beta blockers should be avoided.

Table 9.8
Beta Blocker Dosing in Heart Failure

Drug	Starting Dose	Maximum Dose
Metoprolol succinate extended release	12.5 to 25 mg daily	200 mg daily
Bisoprolol	1.25 mg daily	10 mg daily
Carvedilol	3.125 mg BID	25 mg BID (can use 50 mg BID for patients > 85 kg)
(Hunt et al., 2005).		

Linking Knowledge to Practice

✔ *Cardvedilol has alpha blocking properties in addition to beta blocking properties, and therefore patients may demonstrate a more pronounced hypotensive response.*

✔ *Many patients think they are taking ACE inhibitors and beta blockers for blood pressure control. Patients need to understand that although these medications lower blood pressure, they are indicated in heart failure for their interruption of the neurohormonal responses of the RAAS and the sympathetic nervous system. Patients need to know that these medications have a positive impact on ventricular remodeling and also reduce the risk for mortality. For these reasons patients need to understand the importance of compliance with these medications even in the absence of hypertension.*

✔ *Many patients with heart failure have co-existing chronic lung disease. Patients should be observed for the potential side effect of bronchospasm when initiating a beta blocker that blocks beta 2 in addition to beta 1 receptors.*

Diuretics

Loop diuretics work at the ascending loop of Henle to excrete 20-25% of the filtered sodium. These are the diuretics of choice and are usually initiated in the management of heart failure, beginning with the presentation of fluid overload. Rapid onset of action is seen with IV administration. After fluid overload has been resolved, diuretics are usually continued orally to maintain fluid volume status.

Few heart failure patients are able to maintain optimal extra cellular fluid balance without the use of a diuretic. Diuretics improve symptoms more rapidly than any other drug and can also increase cardiac function and improve exercise tolerance.

The goal of diuretic therapy is to eliminate signs of fluid retention. Diuresis can continue with mild hypotension and azotemia if the patient remains asymptomatic. If the patient develops hypotension and azotemia with no signs of fluid retention, then volume depletion is most likely the cause; the dosing of diuretics will need to be decreased.

Electrolytes (potassium and magnesium) should be carefully assessed and abnormalities rapidly corrected so diuresis can continue, if needed. Diuretics are usually used in conjunction with a moderate sodium restriction.

Examples of loop diuretics:

◆ Torsemide.

❖ Torsemide is a loop diuretic with anti-aldosteronergic properties. This loop diuretic may have benefits in heart failure due to the positive influence on ventricular remodeling.

◆ Furosemide.

◆ Bumetanide.

Thiazide diuretics can be added to loop diuretics, if needed. Thiazide diuretics are not used alone or as a first-line agent. Thiazide diuretics work in the distal tubule and only excrete 5-10% of filtered sodium. Examples of thiazide diuretics include:

◆ Hydrochlorothiazide.

◆ Chlorothiazide.

◆ Metolazone.

◆ Chlorthalidone.

◆ Indapamide.

Potassium sparing diuretics can also be used in heart failure:

◆ Amiloride.

◆ Spironolactone, Eplerenone.

◆ Triamterene.

Aldosterone antagonists are discussed in more detail below.

Diuretic dosing can be adjusted on an outpatient basis based on daily weights. Optimal use of diuretics is also key to the effectiveness of ACE inhibitor and beta blocker therapy. ACE inhibitor therapy is less effective and patients are less likely to tolerate beta blocker therapy if the diuretic dose is too low and ECF overload is present. The risk of hypotension and renal insufficiency are increased with ACE inhibitor use if diuretic dose is too high.

As heart failure progresses, patients may need higher doses of diuretics for several reasons:

◆ Absorption is decreased due to intestinal edema or hypoperfusion.

◆ Decreased renal perfusion may impair delivery of the drug to the renal tubules.

◆ High sodium intake and use of non-steroidal anti-inflammatory agents can also decrease the response to diuretics.

Patients who become resistant to diuretic therapy may require the use of IV agents or dual agents.

Chapter 9

Linking Knowledge to Practice

✔ *Congested patients receiving diuresis should be observed for signs and symptoms of over diuresis. These signs and symptoms include excessive urine output, decreased potassium, magnesium, or sodium, worsening renal function, and hypotension.*

✔ *Diuresis may make some patients more sensitive to the hypotensive effects of vasodilator therapy, especially to the hypotensive effect of ACE inhibitors. Diuretics may also increase the incidence of digitalis toxicity either due to associated electrolyte disturbances or due to a decrease in glomerular filtration rate.*

✔ *In patients who develop resistance to loop diuretics, metolazone may be added intermittently to the therapy to produce a synergistic effect on diuresis. In this situation metolazone should be administered approximately 60 minutes before the loop diuretic to produce optimal results. A daily dose of metolazone is usually avoided due to the increased risk of hypokalemia and hyponatremia.*

Aldosterone Antagonists

An aldosterone antagonist, such as spironolactone or eplerenone, can be beneficial in heart failure patients who experience symptoms at rest (NYHA Class IV Heart Failure). In a large scale, long-term trial, low-dose spironolactone reduced the risk of death in patients already taking ACE inhibitors. The greatest benefit was seen in those patients who were also taking beta blockers and digoxin (Hunt et al., 2005). Aldosterone antagonists are indicated for NYHA Class IV patients with systolic dysfunction and an ejection fraction ≤ 35% who are on standard medical therapy, including a diuretic (Adams et al., 2006). Aldosterone antagonists have also been shown to have benefit in post-MI patients and should be considered when a MI patient has clinical heart failure, an ejection fraction < 40%, or diabetes (Adams et al., 2006).

Hyperkalemia is a potential side effect, especially when patients are already on ACE inhibitors. Creatinine and potassium levels should be evaluated prior to initiation and monitored carefully throughout therapy. Aldosterone antagonists should not be used when the creatinine is greater than 2.5 mg/dL or when the potassium is > 5.0 mEq/L. Potassium levels are reassessed at one week and one month after initiation, then every three months on an ongoing basis (Adams et al., 2006).

Digoxin

Digoxin is a weak inotropic agent, but its benefits in heart failure come from its other effects, including reducing sympathetic outflow and suppressing renin secretion. Digoxin can improve symptoms and decrease the rate of hospitalization, but has not been proven to reduce mortality (Hobbs & Boyle, 2004). A dose of 0.125 mg per day, lower than once thought necessary to be effective, is recommended in most patients (Hunt et al., 2005). There is no need for a loading dose. Digoxin is recommended for heart failure patients who remain symptomatic despite treatment with ACE inhibitors, beta blockers, and diuretics. These patients are typically in Stage 3 heart failure. Digoxin is not recommended in patients with structural heart disease and no symptoms of heart failure (Hunt et al., 2005). Assessment for signs and symptoms of toxicity are important because toxicity may be seen with serum levels in the normal range.

Medications used in the treatment of heart failure are summarized in Table 9.9. Specific medications by class are listed in Table 9.10. Additional details regarding the pharmacological agents presented in this chapter are discussed in Chapter 14.

Heart Failure

Table 9.9 Summary of Heart Failure Medications by Class	
Ace Inhibitors	Interrupt the neurohormonal response of the renin-angiotensin-aldosterone system and favorably impact disease progression. Reduces mortality and morbidity.
Beta blockers	Interrupts the neurohormonal response of the SNS and favorably impact disease progression. Reduces arrhythmias Reduces mortality and hospitalizations. * Not initiated in acute decompensated state.
Diuretics	Decrease extracellular fluid load and improve symptoms in an overload state, Maintain extracellular fluid volume status and sodium balance, No mortality impact, Loop diuretics with addition of thiazide diuretic, if needed,
Digoxin	Improves symptoms, exercise tolerance and quality of life, Used in patients symptomatic on above three medications, No mortality impact, *Dosage is usually 0.125 mg; toxicity can occur with normal serum levels,*
Aldosterone Antagonists	Reserved for patients with moderate to severe heart failure *Cannot be used if creatinine > 2.5 mg/dL due to risk of hyperkalemia,*

Table 9.10 Specific Medications By Class				
ACE Inhibitors		**Beta Blockers**	**Loop Diuretics**	**Aldosterone Antagonists**
Captopril	Fosinopril	Carvedilol	Furosemide	Spironolactone
Enalapril	Perindopril	Metoprolol	Torsemide	*(non selective)*
Lisinopril	Quinapril	Bisoprolol	Bumetanide	Epleranone
Ramipril	Trandolapril			*(selective)*

Medications to Avoid In Heart Failure

Certain medications should be avoided in patients with heart failure. Most antiarrhythmics are poorly tolerated in heart failure patients due to their proarrhythmic and cardiodepressant effects. Amiodarone is the only antiarrhythmic that does not adversely affect survival in heart failure patients (Hunt et al., 2005).

Calcium channel blockers, with the exception of amlodipine, adversely affect survival in patients with systolic dysfunction. Amlodipine has a neutral effect in heart failure and can be used if needed to treat coexisting angina or hypertension.

Avandia (Rosiglitasone Maleate) can cause fluid retention that may exacerbate or lead to heart failure. This medication is not recommended for patients with known heart failure and particularly in those with NYHA Class III or IV. Patients with NYHA class I or II being treated with avandia have an increased risk of cardiovascular events. All diabetics taking avandia should be carefully monitored for signs and symptoms of fluid retention. If fluid retention occurs the medication should be discontinued.

Chapter 9

Patients with heart failure should be instructed to avoid the use of non-steroidal anti-inflammatory drugs (NSAIDs). These medications increase the risk of fluid retention and renal failure. Due to these effects, NSAIDs diminish the efficacy of diuretics and ACE inhibitors. The risk of renal failure is also increased when used in the presence of ACE inhibitors, or in the presence of existing renal insufficiency (Adams et al., 2006).

NONPHARMACOLOGICAL TREATMENT STRATEGIES FOR HEART FAILURE

Exercise Training

Controlled trials have shown that exercise training improves symptoms, quality of life, and exercise capacity in patients with heart failure. This beneficial effect is additive to the effects of optimal medical therapy (Hunt et al., 2005; Myers, 2005). Exercise training in heart failure patients is best accomplished in a formally structured program, such as cardiac rehabilitation. Although many studies have demonstrated the short-term benefits of exercise training, there has been a lack of randomized clinical control trials evaluating the long-term outcomes of rehospitalization and mortality. The HF-Action study is ongoing to evaluate the long-term effects of exercise rehabilitation in heart failure patients. Caution must still be used in recommending exercise training to heart failure patients because patient characteristics may not match those of patients enrolled in clinical trials (Adams et al., 2006).

The physiological benefits of exercise training in chronic heart failure include:

◆ Improved changes in skeletal muscle metabolism.

◆ Improved heart rate variability.

◆ Decreased resting plasma norepinephrine levels.

◆ Increased exercise cardiac output.

◆ Increased endothelium dependent vasodilation.

◆ Increased coronary blood flow reserve in patients with CAD

(Adams et al., 2006).

Resynchronization Therapy

Resynchronization therapy is indicated in patients with moderate to severe heart failure and those with bundle branch block (typically left bundle branch block) who are symptomatic, despite optimal medical therapy. Dysynchrony is common in heart failure because many patients have bundle branch block that causes the right and left ventricles to depolarize at different times. When this occurs, the walls of the right and left ventricles do not contract simultaneously.

Clinical Implications of Dysynchrony

◆ Contractility problems

❖ Septum depolarizes before LV.

❖ Late activation of LV = LV pressure after septum has finished repolarizing, causing septum to move away from LV instead of contributing to LV ejection.

❖ Results in decreased contribution of septum to LV ejection and contributes to reduced LV stroke volume.

◆ Mitral Regurgitation

❖ Late activation of LV causes lateral papillary muscle to depolarize and contract late.

❖ Late papillary muscle contraction allows mitral leaflets to enter into left atrium during ventricular systole.

❖ Contributes to decreased stroke volume from LV.

394

◆ Reduced LV filling
  ❖ Late LV activation = late LV filling and decreases preload.

Criteria for Resynchronization Therapy in Heart Failure

◆ Symptomatic despite stable, optimal medical therapy.
◆ Moderate to severe heart failure (NYHA Class III/IV).
◆ LV ejection fraction ≤ 35%.
◆ QRS ≥ 120 ms.
◆ Sinus Rhythm

(Adams et al., 2006).

Mechanics of Resynchronization

A biventricular pacemaker is used to improve synchrony and is placed with leads in both the right and left ventricles. A lead is also implanted in the right atrium to allow for atrial pacing. Standard atrial and right-ventricular pacing leads are inserted transvenously. The left-ventricular lead is placed in a left-ventricular vein via the coronary sinus.

Resynchronization therapy with a bi-ventricular pacemaker allows the right and left ventricles to contract simultaneously, thereby improving cardiac performance. Figure 9.8 shows the placement of the left-ventricular lead. Figure 9.9 shows a rhythm strip from standard RV pacing, creating a LBBB pattern that can cause dyssynchrony, and a strip of a biventricular paced rhythm.

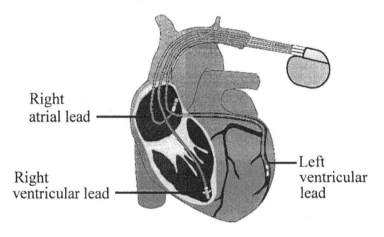

Figure 9.8: Placement of the left ventricular lead in resynchronization therapy.

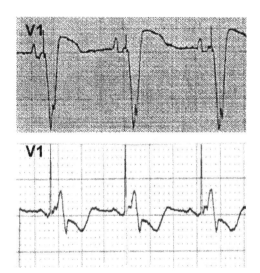

Figure 9.9: Paced complex with standard right ventricular pacing (top) compared to biventricular pacing (bottom). Note the biphasic component to the paced QRS complex in biventriuclar pacing representing a more synchronous contraction.

Results of Resynchronization

◆ Improved coordination of contraction of LV and septum.
  ❖ Pacing of both RV and LV together.
◆ Improved AV timing to optimize LV filling.
  ❖ Atrial synchronized ventricular pacing (dual chamber pacing to control AV interval).

Studies show clinical improvement in exercise tolerance and quality of life after resynchronization therapy in patients with moderate to severe heart failure.(Hunt et al., 2005; Jacobson & Gerity, 2005). Improvement in NYHA class is also an expected outcome. In addition, reduction in hospitalizations and mortality have also been demonstrated.

Chapter 9

SPECIAL ISSUES IN HEART FAILURE

Nutritional Needs

◆ Patients with advanced heart failure can develop cardiac cachexia. The support of a nutritionist to help with caloric supplementation is beneficial.

◆ Daily multivitamin and mineral supplementation is recommended for heart failure patients (Adams et al., 2006).

Ventilation and Oxygenation

◆ Continuous positive airway pressure (CPAP) is recommended in patients with obstructive sleep apnea. The use of CPAP has been shown to improve functional capacity and quality of life in this group of patients.

◆ Patients with hypoxemia (resting or exertional) should be evaluated for residual fluid overload or coexisting pulmonary disease. The routine use of supplemental oxygen is not indicated (Adams et al., 2006).

Psychosocial Issues

◆ Heart failure patients should be screened for depression at regular intervals. Selective serotonin reuptake inhibitors are preferred over tricyclic anti-depressants in this population. Tricyclic anti-depressants are associated with ventricular arrhythmias.

◆ Sexual dysfunction may be a contributor to poor quality of life for both men and women. Sildenafil may be used for sexual dysfunction in men who have chronic heart failure. Sildenafil should not be prescribed to patients taking nitrates.

◆ The maintenance of employment or retraining for another employment opportunity should be encouraged in heart failure patients whenever possible (Adams et al., 2006).

Anemia Management

Anemia has been associated with poor outcomes in heart failure. Some research has demonstrated potential clinical benefits in heart failure by augmenting hemoglobin. However, augmenting hemoglobin in heart failure also has potential risks, including the increased viscosity of blood. Clinical trials are currently being conducted to evaluate the safety and efficacy of augmenting hemoglobin in heart failure patients (Adams et al., 2006).

Sudden Death in Heart Failure

Patients with heart failure are at high risk for sudden cardiac death. They can also die from progressive pump failure and congestion or end-organ failure from systemic hypoperfusion. Although more than 50% of heart failure patients have episodes of nonsustained ventricular tachycardia, it is not necessarily the simple progression to sustained ventricular tachycardia that increases the risk of sudden death (Hunt et al., 2005). Sudden death in heart failure patients is commonly associated with an acute ischemic event or even bradyarrhythmias. For this reason, interventions in heart failure are aimed at preventing sudden death rather than treating asymptomatic ventricular arrhythmias.

Heart Failure

Linking Knowledge to Practice

✔ *Always consider electrolyte abnormalities (low potassium and or low magnesium) and digitalis toxicity as the etiology of arrhythmias in patients with heart failure.*

Interventions in heart failure to decrease the risk of sudden cardiac death include:

◆ Beta blockers

◆ Amiodarone

◆ Implantable cardioverter-defibrillators (ICDs).

Most antiarrhythmic drugs are poorly tolerated in heart failure patients. Amiodarone, although a class III antiarrhythmic, also has vasodilatory properties and is generally well tolerated in heart failure patients. Because of the toxicity associated with amiodarone, it is not routinely used in the treatment of heart failure. However, it is used in patients with a history of sudden cardiac death, ventricular fibrillation, or sustained unstable ventricular tachycardia (Hunt et al., 2005).

Prophylactic ICD therapy is considered in heart failure patients who have been on optimal medical therapy for 3 to 6 months. It is also considered in conjunction with resynchronization therapy for patients who meet criteria (Adams et al., 2006).

ICDs are indicated in the following heart failure patients:

◆ Survivors of cardiac arrest.

◆ Sustained ventricular tachycardia.

◆ Inducible ventricular tachycardia during an ectrophysiology study.

◆ Ejection fraction less than 30% > 40 days after an MI.

◆ Ejection fraction less than 30% with no ischemic heart disease.

◆ Reasonable expectation of survival and good functional status for at least one year (Jacobson & Gerity, 2005).

See Chapter 17 for more information on ICDs.

Acute Decompensated Heart Failure

BNP Levels

BNP is used as a diagnostic indicator in patients presenting with signs of decompensation. The cardiac ventricles are the major source of plasma BNP. Elevated plasma levels support the diagnosis of reduced left-ventricular function or other hemodynamic alterations, causing symptomatic heart failure. This diagnostic tool is also helpful when a patient's primary complaint is shortness of breath, yet the etiology is unclear. BNP levels can be elevated in other situations, such as pulmonary embolism and chronic lung disease, so the BNP result cannot be used as a definitive diagnostic tool. A BNP level of less than 100 pg/mL has a high negative predictive value; therefore, it can be helpful in eliminating heart failure as the cause of dyspnea. BNP levels greater than 500 pg/mL at the time of discharge are highly associated with readmission within 30 days. BNP levels can remain chronically elevated in end-stage heart failure (Hunt et al., 2005).

Signs and Symptoms of Acute Decompensation and Appropriate Treatment

Patients with acute decompensated heart failure commonly present with signs of fluid overload, and need to be treated based on assessment of both fluid status and hypoperfusion. Table 9.11 describes four clinical subsets of patients in decompensated heart failure, based on the presence or absence of both pulmonary congestion and signs of hypoperfusion.

Chapter 9

Table 9.11 Clinical Presentation in Decompensated Heart Failure	
Warm and Dry: No Congestion Normal Perfusion	**Warm and Wet:** Congestion Normal Perfusion
Cold and Dry: No Congestion Low Perfusion	**Cold and Wet:** Congestion Low Perfusion

Linking Knowledge to Practice

✔ *Patients with congestion and adequate perfusion need to be treated with IV diuretics and venous vasodilators to reduce preload.*

✔ *Patients with inadequate perfusion will benefit from arterial vasodilators to reduce afterload and improve forward flow. Patients may also need inotropic support. However, inotropic therapy is not used as first line treatment because it increases myocardial oxygen demand.*

Patients with volume overload have different signs and symptoms than those with hypoperfusion. Signs of hypoperfusion occur when cardiac output decreases significantly or abruptly. Table 9.12 lists clinical signs of fluid overload and hypoperfusion.

Table 9.12 Clinical Signs of Fluid Overload and Hypoperfusion	
Clinical Signs of Fluid Overload	**Clinical Signs of Hypoperfusion**
Weight gain	Narrow pulse pressure
Peripheral edema	Resting tachycardia
Jugular venous distention	Cool skin
SOB	Altered mentation
Crackles in lungs	Decreased urine output
	Increased BUN/creatinine
	Cheyne Stokes respirations

Diuretics

IV loop diuretics are commonly used in acute decompensated heart failure. The goal is to relieve symptoms of congestion without producing an excessive reduction in circulating intravascular volume. A rapid reduction in circulating volume can produce hypotension and also worsen renal function.

When a patient does not respond to initial therapy with IV loop diuretics, the following options should be considered:

◆ Sodium and fluid restriction.

◆ Increase in the dose of loop diuretics (increased number of doses is preferable to a very large single dose).

◆ Continuous infusion of a loop diuretic.

◆ Addition of a second type of diuretic: oral metolazone or spironolactone, or IV chlorothiazide (Adams et al., 2006).

Heart Failure

Ultrafiltration

Ultrafiltration (mechanical diuresis) is another treatment option in acute decompensated heart failure when congestion does not respond to loop diuretics (Adams et al., 2006). Ultrafiltration can provide clinical benefit in diuretic-resistant patients and help restore sensitivity to loop diuetics (Hunt et al., 2005).

Vasodilator Therapy

Patients in acute decompensated heart failure usually need vasodilator therapy to help reduce preload and/or afterload. Nesiritide, a synthetic BNP, is one vasodilator used in the treatment of acute decompensated heart failure. It is not indicated for planned intermittent or continuous infusions in patients with chronic heart failure.

Nesiritide is a venous and arterial vasodilator, so it reduces both preload and afterload. Careful monitoring for hypotension is required with nesiritide therapy. Nesiritide will also cause diuresis so electrolytes should be carefully monitored. BNP lab test is not recommended for 48 hrs after infusion is discontinued.

Other vasodilators used in acute decompensated heart failure include nitroglycerin and nitroprusside. Intravenous nitroglycerin is usually given in low doses as a venous vasodilator, and nitroprusside is predominantly an arterial vasodilator .

Inotropic Therapy

Patients in acute decompensated heart failure may require intravenous administration of a positive inotrope. Vasodilator therapy, however, should always be considered before the administration of inotropic therapy (Adams et al., 2006). Dobutamine, a sympathomimetic, and milrinone, a phosphodiesterase inhibitor, are the commonly used intravenous inotropes. Milrinone has vasodilator properties in addition to inotropic properties and can cause hypotension as a side effect. Inotropic medications also have the potential side effect of ventricular arrhythmias.

IV inotropic therapy is used to relieve symptoms and improve end-organ function. Inotropic therapy is only indicated in acute decompensated heart failure in patients with advanced disease. Inotropic therapy is not indicated unless filling pressures are known to be elevated (Adams et al., 2006). Chronic intermittent use is not recommended (Hunt et al., 2005).

Other

A fluid restriction of < 2 liters/day should be initiated in patients not responsive to diuretic therapy and in those with a sodium level < 130 mEq/L. A fluid restriction can also be considered in other patients who are in a congested state (Adams et al., 2006).

The routine use of oxygen in the absence of hypoxemia is not indicated (Adams et al., 2006).

Discharge Criteria

◆ Patients should be stable on an oral regime and free from required IV therapy for at least 24 hours prior to discharge.

◆ Fluid volume status should be near optimal prior to discharge.

◆ Any exacerbating factors contributing to decompensation should be addressed and resolved prior to discharge:

❖ Atrial or other arrhythmias.

❖ Exacerbation of hypertension.

❖ Ischemia.

Chapter 9

❖ Thyroid disease.

❖ Anemia.

❖ Drug interactions.

❖ Worsening renal function.

◆ Patients should be ambulated prior to discharge to assess for functional capacity.

◆ Assessment of patient home scale should be complete, and patients should be educated on self-care skills. These skills are discussed in the patient education section below.

◆ All patients should have a follow up healthcare provider visit scheduled for within 7 to 10 days of discharge. Patients with advanced heart failure or recurrent admissions should have a scheduled home care visit or telemanagement phone call within 3 days of discharge.

◆ Advanced heart failure patients should be considered for referral to a comprehensive disease state management program

(Adams et al., 2006).

End-Stage Heart Failure

Patients with end-stage refractory heart failure have special management issues. These patients need very careful control of their extra cellular fluid volume status because many of their symptoms are related to sodium imbalances caused by extra cellular fluid overload. ACE inhibitors and beta blockers are effective in patients with end-stage refractory heart failure; however, these patients may not tolerate these medications well and lower doses may need to be used. Patients should not receive these medications if systolic blood pressure is less than 80 mm Hg or if they show signs of hypoperfusion. Patients should not be initiated on beta blockers if they have symptomatic extra cellular fluid retention or require intravenous inotropic support.

End-stage heart failure patients often decompensate frequently and may need to be admitted for intravenous inotropic or vasodilator therapy. After the patient is stabilized and oral medications are resumed, the patient must be observed to assure the oral regime is sufficient to avoid further decompensation. Patients unable to be weaned from intravenous inotropic support may be candidates for at-home continuous inotropic support. This measure is a final option, used only for palliative relief in end-stage disease. Because inotropic therapy is associated with an increased risk of sudden death and there is a lack of research supporting the benefit, intermittent inotropic therapy is not indicated in the management of chronic heart failure (Hunt et al., 2005).

Transplantation

Cardiac transplantation is the only established surgical treatment for refractory heart failure. Unfortunately, this treatment option is available only to a small group of patients each year. Evaluation for transplantation is indicated only for patients with refractory heart failure, refractory angina, or refractory ventricular arrhythmias who are not controlled, despite optimal medical therapy, device therapy, and alternative surgical therapy (Adams et al., 2006). Candidates need to be otherwise healthy. The survival rate at 1 year is 85%, with a decline of approximately 4% each year thereafter (LeDoux & Luikart, 2005). After transplantation, patients remain on lifelong immunosuppression therapy, placing them at risk for further complications.

Left-ventricular Assist Devices

Left-ventricular assist devices can be used to provide hemodynamic support to failing hearts for patients waiting for cardiac transplantation as well as those who are not candidates for transplantation. Patients who are not transplant candidates will be considered for surgically implanted assist devices. Complications with left-ventricular assist devices are common and have the potential to be life threatening. For this reason, the use of these devices is evolving and remains limited.

Alternative Surgical Procedures

◆ Partial left-ventricular resection ("Batista" procedure) is not indicated in non-ischemic cardiomyopathy.

◆ Infarct exclusion surgeries and passive restraint surgeries are currently being evaluated as potential surgical options for patients with heart failure.

❖ Infarct exclusion surgeries involve removing all the akinetic or dyskinetic myocardium from the left ventricle and septum. An endoventricular circular patch plasty (using a tight circumferential suture) is used to reduce the left-ventricular volume and return the left-ventricular shape to near normal.

❖ Passive restraint surgery involves the application of an epicardial prosthetic wrap that provides a positive impact on ventricular remodeling.

Prognosis and Hospice Referral

Physicians should discuss end-of-life care issues with patients with end-stage heart failure while they are still able to participate in the decision-making process. Hospice care is one option for end-stage disease management that is often underutilized. Hospice services traditionally require a prediction of death within 6 months as criteria for admission to the program. Because sudden cardiac death is one of the major reasons for death in heart failure, the time of death is difficult to predict. Many patients with end stage heart failure have periods of good quality of life during the final 6 months. Hospice admission policies need to be flexible enough to allow end-stage heart failure patients to participate in these palliative programs when appropriate. Heart failure health care providers also need to be more attentive to end-of-life care in this population, and initiate more patient dialogue and appropriate hospice referrals.

PATIENT EDUCATION

Heart failure is the final pathway for many cardiac disorders. Heart failure care is complex and involves continuity across the continuum. Research shows that careful monitoring and follow-up make a difference. Nurses play an important role in the monitoring and follow-up of heart failure patients. Nurses also contribute substantially to patient and family education. Teaching the patient and family self-management strategies is key in the effective management of heart failure. Through discharge education, post-discharge telephone follow-up, and nurse-led heart failure clinics, nurses are making a difference in the management of heart failure.

Recognition of Signs and Symptoms

Patients need to understand how to recognize the signs and symptoms of worsening heart failure. Recognizing changes in activity tolerance is key. Some patients and families find it helpful to keep an activity diary so a more objective assessment of their activities and tolerance is recorded.

Daily weights are important in accurately assessing extracellular fluid volume status. Patients should weigh themselves first thing in the morning after emptying the bladder. Patients should also wear the same amount of clothing for each weight. A scale with large numbers for visibility is important for elderly patients. Some patients require family assistance in weighing because they cannot independently step on and off a scale. Scales with grab bars are beneficial, but due to their cost, may not be an option for all patients.

Nurses should instruct patients to keep a chart of daily weight and to take the chart with them to their physician office visits. Patients should also be instructed to report any gain of greater than 2 lb in 24

Chapter 9

hours, or greater than 3 lb in 1 week, even if no other symptoms are present. Some hospitals have programs that allow patients to call in and report their weights each day to a nurse or a computer system. Patients with weight gain and patients who do not call in are identified to receive further follow-up.

Linking Knowledge to Practice

✔ *Self-care requires skills in addition to knowledge. Nurses should assure patients have the skills necessary to engage in self-care. Having patients weigh themselves, record the data, and determine if the weight change requires physician notification can be practiced while in the hospital prior to discharge.*

Medication Compliance

Medication compliance is critical to the effective management of heart failure. Patients are more compliant when they fully understand the benefits of therapy. Heart failure patients are on multiple medications, and this can cause a variety of compliance issues. A careful assessment of any financial concerns regarding prescribed medications is important. Nurses should discuss any financial concerns with physicians so that every effort can be made to prescribe the most cost-effective, yet appropriate medication regime. Social services should be consulted to assure that patients receive all available health care support services.

Physical limitations affecting compliance include poor vision and poor dexterity. Nurses should assess ability to read the small print on labels, open vials, and divide pills, if necessary. Nurses should also instruct patients to report any perceived side effects to their physician prior to stopping any medications.

Because of the effects of NSAIDs on diuretic and ACE inhibitor therapy, nurses should instruct patients to avoid the use of these medications. Patients should always carry with them a complete list of medications and their doses, especially to every physician office visit. Nurses can facilitate this practice by providing a comprehensive, legible list of medications with a current date printed on a wallet card. Nurses should review all admission and discharge medications to ensure all necessary medications are ordered and that different providers have not prescribed duplicate medications. Instructing patients to always use the same pharmacy will also help in avoiding duplicate prescriptions.

Linking Knowledge to Practice

✔ *It is important for patients to fully understand the purpose and benefit of medications in order to improve compliance. Patients should be asked to explain the purpose of each medication prior to administration in the hospital. Asking the patient to provide the explanation helps the nurse to assess the patient's level of understanding.*

✔ *Many heart failure patients are elderly and have co-existing co-morbidities, including arthritis. NSAIDs are commonly used in the treatment of arthritis. Alternatives to NSAID use, as well as the risk and benefits of therapy for patients with heart failure, need to be addressed by the prescribing provider.*

Sodium Restriction

Heart failure patients also need information regarding adherence to a sodium restriction. In many cases, patients do not realize the hidden sodium content in processed foods. Fresh foods are the best choice for low sodium content. Frozen foods are better than canned foods, which contain high amounts of sodium. Because high amounts of sodium are already in most of the foods that are currently available, patients, or those responsible for grocery shopping, will need to learn how to read the sodium content on food labels.

Patients with heart failure should limit their sodium intake to 2 to 3 grams of sodium per day. Patients with moderate to severe heart failure may require a further sodium restriction of < 2 grams per day (Adams et al., 2006).

Linking Knowledge to Practice

✔ *Prior to discharge patients and families should demonstrate the proper reading of food labels to assess their ability to determine the sodium content per serving. Special attention should be given to the number of servings in the product.*

Physical Activity and Socialization

Physical activity should be promoted in all heart failure patients to prevent deconditioning. If exercise training is prescribed, patients should be referred to a medically supervised program, such as a cardiac rehabilitation program. Participation in a cardiac rehabilitation program also provides interaction with other people and the opportunity for a health care provider to assess the patient at regular intervals. Heart failure patients are at risk for isolation and depression if they have limited activity tolerance. Many hospitals and communities have support groups for patients and families living with heart failure. Nurses should carefully assess support systems and opportunities for socialization in heart failure patients who are home bound.

Additional Risk Factor Modification

In addition to heart failure specific education, patients should receive risk factor counseling related to the modification of all cardiovascular risk factors. This information is discussed in detail in Chapter 7. In addition, all heart failure patients should be instructed to receive the pneumococcal and annual influenza vaccines.

Follow-Up

Close physician or nurse practitioner follow-up is critical to the successful management of heart failure. Patients need to understand the importance of keeping all scheduled appointments, even when they are feeling well. Many medications are titrated to optimal doses on an outpatient basis. Nurses need to assess for any barriers to keeping office appointments, such as lack of transportation or conflicting work schedules of family members. Key components of patient education for heart failure patients are summarized in Table 9.13. Additional resources for patient education can be found through the Heart Failure Society of America at www.hfsa.org.

Chapter 9

Table 9.13
Patient Education Checklist

◆ Recognition of signs and symptoms
   ❖ Activity intolerance: Activity diary
   ❖ Extracellular fluid retention: Daily weight
     ★ Assess for home scale.

◆ Medication compliance
   ❖ Review benefits of therapy
   ❖ Provide wallet card with current medication list
   ❖ Assess for and eliminate barriers to accurate and consistent administration
   ❖ Encourage use of one consistent pharmacy.

◆ Sodium limitation
   ❖ Label reading
   ❖ Avoid processed and canned foods.

◆ Physical activity plan.
◆ Support system and socialization opportunities.
◆ Pneumococcal vaccine and annual influenza vaccine.
◆ Follow-up with heart failure provider.
◆ Printed educational resource materials or referral to www.hfsa.org for patient education modules.

CONCLUSION

Heart failure is a chronic condition in which nurses play an important role in patient management. Nurses have a tremendous opportunity to collaborate with physicians and other members of the health care team to maximize patient outcomes. Research regarding the management of heart failure is ongoing, and practice guidelines are works in progress. New pharmacological agents involved in blocking various inflammatory and neurohormonal responses are being studied. In addition, gene therapy offers exciting hope regarding the possibility of preventing the loss of, or restoration of the function of left-ventricular myocytes (Laurent, 2005). The role of nurses in the management of heart failure will continue to expand.

Future treatment options currently under investigation include:

◆ Vasopressin receptor antagonists.

◆ Implantable hemodynamic monitoring devices.

◆ Internal cardiac support devices.

◆ External counterpulsation.

◆ Treatments for sleep-related breathing disturbances.

◆ Myocardial growth factors.

◆ Stem cell transplantation.

◆ Alternative surgical therapies.

Heart Failure

TEST YOUR KNOWLEDGE

1. You are caring for a patient admitted with heart failure. The patient had an anterior MI three months ago. On admission, the patient has crackles in both lung bases, an audible S3, and is dyspneic with any exertion. You expect the patient to have heart failure from diastolic dysfunction.
    a. True.
    b. False.

2. Cardiac resynchronization therapy is used in heart failure to
    a. restore sinus rhythm in patients with atrial fibrillation.
    b. defibrillate patients out of life-threatening arrhythmias.
    c. restore synchrony between right and left ventricle depolarization by pacing both ventricles at the same time.
    d. restore synchrony between the heart and lungs by dilating the pulmonary artery.

3. The hallmark manifestations of heart failure are
    a. rapid heart rate with syncope.
    b. chest pain with positive myocardial enzymes.
    c. dangerously low heart rate requiring a pacemaker.
    d. dyspnea and fatigue or fluid retention.

4. Heart failure is most commonly a result of
    a. digoxin toxicity.
    b. ischemic coronary heart disease.
    c. an untreated viral infection.
    d. renal failure.

5. Systolic left ventricular dysfunction is best defined as
    a. impaired ability of the left ventricle to contract and effectively eject blood.
    b. impaired ability of the left ventricle to relax and fill.
    c. heart failure with an elevated systolic blood pressure.
    d. heart failure in which the heart stops beating during systole.

6. Neurohormonal responses in heart failure with long-term negative consequences include
    a. activation of the liver to release glycogen stores.
    b. increased production of cholesterol to make more needed hormones.
    c. activation of the SNS and RAAS.
    d. increased production of hemoglobin to increase oxygen capacity.

Chapter 9

7. The one positive neurohormonal response in chronic heart failure, which results in vasodilation, is

    a. increased release of endothelin.

    b. increased release of cytokines.

    c. increased release of natriuretic peptides.

    d. increased release of vasopressin.

8. Medications commonly used in the treatment of heart failure to interrupt neurohormonal responses, reduce ventricular remodeling, and decrease mortality include

    a. ACE inhibitors and beta blockers.

    b. ACE inhibitors and calcium channel blockers.

    c. calcium channel blockers and nitrates.

    d. beta blockers and nitrates.

9. Which of the following statements is true concerning the use of diuretics in heart failure?

    a. Diuretics have common life-threatening side effects and are only used in severe decompensation.

    b. Diuretics are used in patients with past and present signs of fluid overload.

    c. Diuretics are used because they reduce mortality.

    d. Diuretics should only be used in patients who cannot tolerate ACE inhibitors.

10. A true statement regarding end-stage heart failure is:

    a. All patients die within 6 months from the time of diagnosis of end-stage disease.

    b. Most patients are candidates for and receive cardiac transplantation.

    c. Most patients come to the hospital once a week for an intermittent infusion of an intravenous inotrope.

    d. Many patients can have periods of good quality of life, even after they are diagnosed as having end-stage disease.

11. Optimal control of blood pressure has the potential to reduce new onset heart failure by

    a. approximately 50% in the general population.

    b. approximately 80% in patients post MI.

    c. Both a and b.

    d. Neither a nor b.

12. Patient self-care strategies in heart failure include

    a. the ability to accurately determine the sodium content per serving from a food label.

    b. the ability to accurately weigh oneself each morning, record the results, and report abnormal weight gain to the healthcare provider.

    c. the ability to recognize and report subtle changes in activity tolerance.

    d. All of the above.

Heart Failure

13. Hydralazine and isordil (oral nitrate) combination is a therapeutic option in the following situation:
    a. In a patient who cannot tolerate an ACE inhibitor or ARB because of renal dysfunction.
    b. In an African American male in place of ACE inhibitors and beta blockers.
    c. In all heart failure patients who have diastolic dysfunction.
    d. None of the above.

14. Inotropic therapy is indicated in heart failure in the following situations:
    a. For routine prevention of fluid overload by providing scheduled intermittent infusions.
    b. In patients with acute decompensated heart failure in which vasodilator therapy has failed or is contraindicated, and filling pressures are known to be elevated.
    c. As the first-line treatment option in acute decompensated heart failure.
    d. There are no indications for inotropic therapy in patients with heart failure.

15. Hemoglobin augmentation is the current standard of care for any heart failure patient with a hemoglobin level below normal.
    a. True.
    b. False.

16. End-organ hypoperfusion is a direct result of
    a. genetic abnormalities in kidney and brain tissue.
    b. backward failure as a component of heart failure.
    c. an increase in lactic acid.
    d. forward failure as a component of heart failure.

17. Aldosterone antagonists are contraindicated in the following conditions:
    a. A serum potassium of 2.9 mEq/dL
    b. A creatinine of 1.5 mg/dL
    c. A creatinine of 4.0 mg/dL
    d. A glucose of 200 mg/dL

18. The sodium restriction for most heart failure patients who are not in advanced stages should be
    a. 2 to 3 grams per day.
    b. 1 to 2 grams per day.
    c. < 1 gram per day.
    d. 3 to 5 grams per day.

Chapter 9

19. Intravenous vasodilators used in the treatment of acute decompensated heart failure include

    a. nitroglycerin only to prevent ischemia.

    b. nitroglycerin and dobutamine.

    c. nitroglycerin, nitroprusside, and nesritide.

    d. dobutamine and milrinone.

20. Ultrafiltration is an option for fluid removal only in patients with acute decompensated heart failure who have not responded to diuretic therapy, due to end stage renal disease.

    a. True.

    b. False.

ANSWERS

1.	B	11.	C
2.	C	12.	D
3.	D	13.	A
4.	B	14.	B
5.	A	15.	B
6.	C	16.	D
7.	C	17.	C
8.	A	18.	A
9.	B	19.	C
10.	D	20.	B

REFERENCES

Adair, O.V. & Fuenzalida, C.E. (2001). Beta-adrenegereic receptor blockers. In A.V. Adair (Ed.), *Cardiology secrets* (pp. 257-263). Philadelphia: Hanley and Belfus, Inc.

Adams, K.F., Lindenfield, J., Arnold, J.M.O., Baker, D.W., Barnard, D.H., Baughman, K.L. (2006). HFSA 2006 comprehensive heart failure practice guideline. *Journal of Cardiac Failure, 12*(1), 1-86.

Albert, N.M. (2003). Cardiac resynchronization therapy through biventricular pacing in patients with heart failure and ventricular dyssynchrony. *Critical Care Nurse,* Supplement June 2003.

Bozkurt, B. & Mann, D.L. (2000). Dilated cardiomyopathy. In J.T. Willerson, & J.N. Cohn, (Eds.), *Cardiovascular medicine* (2nd ed., pp. 1034-1053). New York: Churchill Livingston.

Braunwald, E., Antman, E.M., Beasley, J.W., Califf, R.M., Cheitlin, M.D., Hochman, J.S., Jones, R.H., Kereiakes, D., Kupersmith, J., Levin, T.N., Pepine, C.J., Schaeffer, J.W., Smith, E.E., III, Steward, D.E., & Thoroux, P. (2002). *ACC/AHA 2002 guideline update for the management of patients with unstable angina and non ST elevation myocardial infarction: a report of the American College of Cardiology/American Heart Association Task Force on Practice Guidelines* (Committee on the Management of Patients with Unstable Angina). Retrieved from: http://www.acc.org/clinical/guide lines/unstable/unstable.pdf

Bridges, E.J. (2005). Regulation of cardiac output and blood pressure. In S.L.Woods, E.S. Froelicher, S.U. Motzer, & E.J. Bridges (Eds.) *Cardiac nursing* (5th ed., pp. 81-108). Philadelphia: Lippincott, Williams and Wilkins.

Calagan, J.L., Schachter, D.T., Kruger, M., Cameron, R.W. & Loghin, C. (2001). Diuretics and nitrates. In A.V. Adair (Ed.), *Cardiology secrets* (pp. 270-274). Philadelphia: Hanley and Belfus, Inc.

Calclasure, T.F., Kozlowski, C.M., Highfill, W.T. & Loghin, C. (2001). Angiotensin-converting enzymes and other vasodilators. In A.V. Adair (Ed.), *Cardiology secrets* (pp. 275-279). Philadelphia: Hanley and Belfus, Inc.

Chebaclo, M. & Loghin, C. (2001). Digoxin and other positive inotropes. In A.V. Adair (Ed.), *Cardiology secrets* (pp. 280-284). Philadelphia: Hanley and Belfus, Inc.

Clinical Pharmacology Database (2004). Gold Standard Multimedia. www.gsm.com

Fischbach, F. (2004). *A manual of lab and diagnostic test* (7th ed.). Philadelphia: Lippincott, Williams and Wilkins.

Havranek, E.P. & Giuglian, G. R. (2001). Congestive heart failure. In A.V. Adair (Ed.), *Cardiology secrets* (pp. 124-128). Philadelphia: Hanley and Belfus, Inc.

Hobbs, R. & Boyle, A. (2004) Heart failure. Retrieved September 25, 2004 from Cleveland Clinic Web site: http://www.clevelandclinicmeded.com

Hunt, S.A., Abraham, W.T., Chin, M.H., Feldman, A.M., Francis, G.S., Ganiats, T.G., Jessup, M., Konstam, M.A., Mancini, D.M., Michl, K., Oates, J.A., Rahko, P.S., Silver, M.A., Stevenson, L.W., &Yancy, C.W. *ACC/AHA 2005 guideline update for the diagnosis and management of chronic heart failure in the adult: a report of the American College of Cardiology/American Heart Association Task Force on Practice Guidelines* (Writing Committee to Update the 2001 Guidelines for the Evaluation and Management of Heart Failure). American College of Cardiology Web Site. Available at: http://www.acc.org/clinical/guidelines/failure//index.pdf

Jacobson, C. & Gerity, D. (2005). Pacemakers and implantable defibrillators. In S.L.Woods, E.S. Froelicher, S.U. Motzer, & E.J. Bridges (Eds.), *Cardiac nursing* (5th ed., pp. 709-755). Philadelphia: Lippincott, Williams and Wilkins.

Jessup, M. (2004). Resynchronization therapy is an important advance in the management of congestive heart failure; view of an antagonist. [Electronic version]. *Journal of Cardiovascular Electrophysiology, 14*(9) S30-S34.

Kavinsky, C.J. & Parrillo, J.E. (2000). Severe heart failure in cardiomyopathy: pathogenesis and treatment. In A. Grenvik, S.M. Ayers, P.R. Holbrook & W.C. Shoemaker (Eds.), *Textbook of critical care* (4th ed., pp. 1105-1116). Philadelphia: W.B. Saunders Company.

Chapter 9

Laurent, D. (2005). Heart failure. In S.L.Woods, E.S. Froelicher, S.U. Motzer, & E.J. Bridges (Eds.) *Cardiac nursing* (5th ed., pp. 601-627). Philadelphia: Lippincott Williams and Wilkins..

LeDoux, D. & Luikart, H. (2005). Cardiac surgery. In S.L.Woods, E.S. Froelicher, S.U. Motzer, & E.J. Bridges (Eds.) *Cardiac nursing* (5th ed., pp. 628-658). Philadelphia: Lippincott Williams and Wilkins.

Loghin, C. (2001). Dilated cardiomyopathy. In A.V. Adair (Ed.), *Cardiology secrets* (pp. 156-160). Philadelphia: Hanley and Belfus, Inc.

Mendoza, R. & Trujillo, N. (2001). Complication and care following myocardial infarction. In A.V. Adair (Ed.), *Cardiology secrets* (pp. 113-117). Philadelphia: Hanley and Belfus, Inc.

Miller, N.H. & Froelicher, E.S. (2005). Disease management models in cardiovascular care. In S.L.Woods, E.S. Froelicher, S.U. Motzer, & E.J. Bridges (Eds.), *Cardiac nursing* (5th ed., pp. 986-996). Philadelphia: Lippincott, Williams and Wilkins.

Murphy-Lavoie, H. & Preston, C.P. (2004). *Cardiomyopathy, dilated.* Retrieved November 11, 2004 from hhtp://www.emedicine.com/emerg/topic80.htm

Myers, J. (2005). Exercise and activity. In S.L.Woods, E.S. Froelicher, S.U. Motzer, & E.J. Bridges (Eds.), *Cardiac nursing* (5th ed., pp. 916-936). Philadelphia: Lippincott, Williams and Wilkins.

New York Heart Association Classification. (n.d.). Retrieved February 2, 2005, from http://www.hcoa.org

Opie, L.H. (2004). *Heart physiology from cell to circulation* (4th ed.). Philadelphia: Lippincott, Williams and Wilkins.

Opie, L.H. & Gersh B.J. (2005). *Drugs for the Heart* (6th ed.). Philadelphia: Elsevier Saunders.

Rosamond, W., Flegal, K., Friday, G., Furie, K., Go, A., Greenland, K., et al. (2007). Heart Disease and Stroke Statistics-2007 Update: A Report From the American Heart Association Statistics Committee and Stroke Statistics Subcommittee. *Circulation, 115,* 69-171.

Saxon, L.A. & DeMarco, T. (n.d.). *Resynchronization therapy for heart failure.* Retrieved December 16, 2004, from www.HRSonline.org/professional_education_/learning_categories/articles.htm

Shelelle, P., Morton, S., Atkinson, S., Suttorp, M. Tu, W., Heidenreich, P., Gubens, M., Maglione, M., Jungvig, L., Roth, E., & Newberry, S. (2003). Pharmacological management of heart failure and left ventricular systolic dysfunction: effect in female, black, and diabetic patients, and cost-effectiveness. *Agency for Healthcare Research and Quality.* (AHPRQ Publication No. AHRQ 03-E045).

Smith, S.C. Jr, Allen J., Blair, S.N., Bonow, R.O., Brass, L.M., Fonarow, J.C., Grundy, S.M., Hiratzka, L., Jones, D., Krumholz, H.M., Mosca, L., Pasternak, R.C., Pearson T., Pfeffer, M.A.,& Taubert, K.A.AHA/ACC Guidelines for Secondary Prevention for Patients With Coronary and Other Atherosclerotic Vascular Disease: 2006 Update: Endorsed by the National Heart, Lung, and Blood Institute. *Circulation, 113,* 2363-2372.

Thom, T., Haase, N., Rosamond, W., Howard, V.J., Rumsfeld, J., Manolio, T. et al. (2006). Heart Disease and Stroke Statistics – 2006 Update: A Report From the American Heart Association Statistics Committee and Stroke Statistics Subcommittee. *Circulation, 113,* e85-e151.

Trupp, Robin, J. (2004) Cardiac resynchronization therapy. [Electronic Version]. *Journal of Cardiovascular Nursing, 19*(4) 223-233.

Heart Failure

Vesty, J., Rasmusson, K.D., Hall, J., Schmitz, S., & Brush, S. (2004). Cardiac resynchronization therapy and automatic implantable cardiac defibrillators in the treatment of heart failure: a review article. [Electronic Version]. *Journal of the American Academy of Nurse Practitioners, 16,* 441-450.

CHAPTER 10:
CARDIOMYOPATHY

INTRODUCTION

Cardiomyopathy is a disease of the heart muscle that affects primarily the myocardial layer of the heart. The endocardium and pericardium may also be involved. Maron et al., in a scientific statement released by the American Heart Association in March of 2006, defines cardiomyopathy as follows:

> Cardiomyopathies are a heterogeneous group of diseases of the myocardium associated with mechanical and/or electrical dysfunction that usually (but not invariably) exhibit inappropriate ventricular hypertrophy or dilation and are due to a variety of causes that frequently are genetic. Cardiomyopathies either are confined to the heart or are part of generalized systemic disorders, often leading to cardiovascular death or progressive heart failure-related disability. (p. 1809)

Classification of Cardiomyopathy

Cardiomyopathies are classified as either primary or secondary cardiomyopathies. Primary cardiomyopathy was once also referred to as idiopathic cardiomyopathy because the cause of the disease process was unknown. Current literature now identifies primary cardiomyopathy as a process that is confined to the heart muscle. Recent research, especially in the area of genetics, has identified more causes of cardiomyopathy. Many of these causes are rare and not seen in large populations. Secondary cardiomyopathies were considered diseases of the heart muscle that result from another disease process. It is difficult at times to clearly classify a cardiomyopathy as primary or secondary, so the AHA Scientific Statement on the Classification of Cardiomyopathies now classifies cardiomyopathy as:

◆ Primary (genetic).
◆ Mixed (genetic and nongenetic).
◆ Acquired.
◆ Secondary.

Disease processes that fall into the above classification of cardiomyopathies are:
◆ Primary (Genetic)
  ❖ Hypertrophic cardiomyopathy.
  ❖ Arrhythmogenic right-ventricular cardiomyopathy/dysplasia.
  ❖ Left-ventricle noncompaction.
  ❖ Conduction system disease.
  ❖ Ion channelopathies:
    ☆ Long-QT syndrome.
    ☆ Brugada syndrome.
    ☆ Catecholaminergic polymorphic ventricular tachycardia.
    ☆ Short-QT syndrome.
    ☆ Idiopathic ventricular fibrillation.

Chapter 10

- ◆ Mixed (Genetic and Nongenetic)
  - ❖ Dilated cardiomyopathy.
  - ❖ Primary restrictive nonhypertrophied cardiomyopathy.
- ◆ Acquired
  - ❖ Myocarditis (inflammatory cardiomyopathy).
  - ❖ Stress cardiomyopathy ("Tako-Tsubo").
  - ❖ Others
    - ☆ Peripartum (postpartum) cardiomyopathy.
    - ☆ Alcoholic-dilated cardiomyopathy.
- ◆ Secondary
  - ❖ Infiltrative disorders
  - ❖ Storage disease
  - ❖ Toxicity
  - ❖ Endomyocardial disorders
  - ❖ Inflammatory disorders
  - ❖ Neuromuscular/neurological disorders
  - ❖ Nutritional deficiencies
  - ❖ Autoimmune/collagen disorders
  - ❖ Electrolyte imbalances
  - ❖ Consequences of cancer therapy.

In this new classification system, disease processes that were once classified as causes of secondary cardiomyopathy are no longer included. Disease processes such as valvular heart disease, systemic hypertension, congenital heart disease, and atherosclerotic coronary artery disease producing ischemic myocardial damage secondary to impairment in coronary flow (ischemic cardiomyopathy) have been eliminated from the cardiomyopathy definition (Maron et al., 2006).

This chapter focuses on the functional classifications of cardiomyopathy that are common in the literature. The functional classification identifies the pathological situation that occurs, regardless of the causes, and provides a discussion that is based on patient presentation and related pathology, as often times in clinical practice the cause is unknown. The functional classification of cardiomyopathy describes the ventricular changes that occur.

Three primary types of cardiomyopathy are discussed (Figure 10.1):

- ◆ Dilated Cardiomyopathy (DCM)
  - ❖ Enlargement of the left ventricular chamber.
  - ❖ Systolic dysfunction.
  - ❖ Most common type of cardiomyopathy.
- ◆ Hypertrophic Cardiomyopathy (HCM)
  - ❖ Changes in the myocytes with thickening of the ventricular wall.
- ◆ Restrictive Cardiomyopathy (RCM)
  - ❖ Interstitial fibrosis limiting myocardial stretch.
  - ❖ Diastolic dysfunction.
  - ❖ Least common type of cardiomyopathy.

Cardiomyopathy

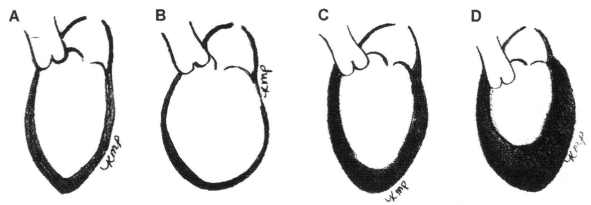

Figure 10.1: Comparison of the normal left ventricle (A) with the abnormal left ventricle. in DCM (B), RCM (C) and HCM (D)

DILATED CARDIOMYOPATHY

An enlarged, dilated cardiac chamber is the hallmark characteristic of DCM. This dilation can affect one or all four cardiac chambers. As the chamber enlarges, its ability to contract becomes impaired, resulting in systolic dysfunction (see Figure 10-1).

Prevalence

Dilated cardiomyopathy is the most common form of cardiomyopathy and represents the primary pathology for heart failure cases (O'Neill & Bott-Silverman, 2003). It is often referred to as congestive cardiomyopathy. Although the exact number of people with DCM is difficult to determine, the population is large. The American Heart Association and the American College of Cardiology (ACC) stage heart failure into four categories (see Table 10.1). Most people who fall into stage B, C, or D have one type of cardiomyopathy. African Americans have an increased risk of developing DCM due to increased presence of risk factors. African Americans with DCM also have a higher mortality rate than white Americans (Bozkurt & Mann, 2000). DCM is more prevalent in men than women and in those over the age of 65.

	Table 10.1 American Heart Association / American College of Cardiology Staging of Heart Failure
STAGE	**DESCRIPTION**
A	Patients at risk of heart failure, with no structural heart disease
B	Patients with structural heart disease, without symptoms of heart failure
C	Patients with past or present heart failure symptoms
D	Patients with advanced disease

(Hunt et al, 2001).

Causes

Idiopathic DCM still represents a fair number of cases of DCM, but more and more causes are being identified. Approximately 25-30% of the cases of DCM can be related to a genetic cause (Kumar et al, 2005). Myocarditis is one of the major causes of DCM; alcohol and drug abuse have also been identified as causes of DCM. Regardless of the cause (see Table 10.2), a variety of disease processes are involved that result in damage to the myocardial fibers, with the end result being dilation of the cardiac chambers.

Chapter 10

Table 10.2 Causes of Dilated Cardiomyopathy
Idiopathic
Genetic Disorders
Myocarditis (Infections)/Inflammatory
Chemotherapy
Peripartum Syndrome Related to Toxemia
Cardiotoxic Effects of Drugs or Alcohol

Pathophysiology

The primary dysfunction in DCM involves ventricular dilation and a decreased ability of the ventricle to contract. As the ventricular chamber enlarges, the myocardial fibers become overstretched and can no longer forcefully contract. This loss of contractile function is referred to as systolic dysfunction. As contractile function is lost, the ventricle is unable to eject its contents and ejection fraction decreases, as does stroke volume. As a result, volume in the ventricle at the end of systole increases. When the left atrium empties into the left ventricle during diastole, the increased residual volume in the ventricle prevents the atrium from emptying completely. The increased volume in the left atrium subsequently increases the pressure in the left atrium, resulting in dilation. Left atrial dilation can provide adequate compensation for some time. Ultimately, however, this compensation fails and the increased volume and pressure in the atrium are reflected back into the pulmonary system. Pulmonary failure occurs and symptoms of left-sided heart failure develop. As left ventricular function deteriorates, the right ventricle ultimately fails as well, resulting in right-sided heart failure. Many compensatory mechanisms occur in response to ventricular dilation. Normally, as the ventricular wall dilates, it becomes thinner. In some instances, the ventricular wall may actually increase in thickness to help maintain cardiac contraction, as seen with aortic regurgitation. This compensatory mechanism, although helpful initially, eventually results in diastolic dysfunction.

The mitral valve develops a "functional" regurgitation as the left ventricle becomes larger. The valve opening (annulus) dilates with the dilating left ventricle, resulting in an inability of the leaflets to come together completely and impairing the ability of the valve to close normally. Papillary muscle dysfunction may also occur, as dilation of the ventricular walls disrupts normal function of these muscles.

The neurohormonal system becomes activated in response to the decrease in forward ejection of blood. As ejection fraction decreases, the body responds to the decrease in cardiac output (CO). The renin-angiotensin-aldosterone system (RAAS) activates, causing vasoconstriction (increased afterload) and retention of fluids and sodium (increased preload). The vasoconstriction increases afterload and causes an already poorly contracting ventricle to pump harder, as it attempts to overcome vasoconstriction and eject its contents. Fluid retention places an increased burden on the already overloaded system, and heart failure develops. A full discussion of the response of the neurohormonal system is covered in Chapter 9.

Heart rate normally increases when CO decreases. In the early stages of DCM, this response is adequate to maintain perfusion. However, as the disease process progresses, this response is no longer enough to compensate for the contractile defect. A diagram of the basic physiologic changes in DCM is presented in Figure 10-2.

Cardiomyopathy

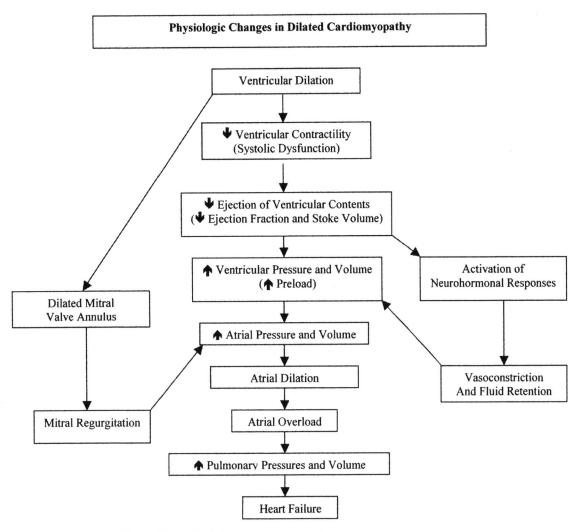

Figure 10.2: Physiologic changes in dilated cardiomyopathy.

Symptoms

Symptoms of DCM are directly related to the severity of the disease process and generally develop over time. Symptoms reflect inadequate CO and perfusion, along with fluid overload of the pulmonary and venous circulatory system. Weakness, fatigue, and decreased activity tolerance are hallmark signs of dilated cardiomyopathy. Because symptoms develop slowly, patients make adjustments in activity levels to compensate for the changes, commonly without being aware that they are doing so. It is important to question patients about their normal level of activity to determine exercise intolerance. Those having symptoms with minimal activity are more seriously ill than those who can participate in activities on a regular basis.

Shortness of breath, dyspnea on exertion, and orthopnea occur as pulmonary edema develops. Left-sided heart failure symptoms appear before right-sided symptoms, and include dyspnea and paroxysmal nocturnal dyspnea. Symptoms of right-sided failure are usually a late development. The predominant symptoms of right-sided failure include dependent edema, enlarged, tender liver (right upper quadrant pain), ascites, and nausea secondary to gastrointestinal congestion. Some conditions, such as right-ventricular infarctions can cause direct damage to the right ventricle. In these cases, right-ventricular failure may occur without any damage to the left ventricle.

Chapter 10

Physical Examination

Findings during the physical examination vary depending on the severity of the disease. The severity of DCM depends on the degree of systolic dysfunction. Patients are usually alert until the end stages of the disease process, when perfusion is not adequate to support cerebral perfusion.

- Skin
    - Cool and pale.
    - Cyanosis (late in the disease process).
- Pulsus alternans (Figure 10.3)
    - Alternation between weak and strong pulse amplitude.

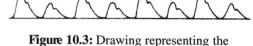

Figure 10.3: Drawing representing the alternating pulse amplitude with pulsus alternans.

- Elevated heart rate
    - Rises in an attempt to compensate for decreased stroke volume.
    - Rates of 120 to 130 beats per minute may be tolerated.
    - Sustained heart rates greater than 140 beats per minute usually result in rapid decompensation.
    - Rate may also be irregularly irregular if in atrial fibrillation, which is not uncommon.
- Blood pressure
    - Generally low, with a narrowed pulse pressure.
    - Orthostatic hypotension may also be present.
- Displaced apical impulse
    - Normally palpable at the fourth or fifth intercostal space, at the left mid-clavicular line.
    - Left-ventricular dilation moves the location of the apex to the left and downward.
    - Decreases in force of apical impulse may also be present.
- S3 (Ventricular Gallop) (Figure 10.4)
    - Third heart sound.
    - Due to atria passively emptying into a fluid overloaded ventricle.
    - Should resolve when fluid overload state resolves.
    - Best heard with patient in left lateral position.
    - Timing: Early diastolic filling sound, just after S2.
    - Location: Mitral Area (5th intercostal space, mid-clavicular line).
    - Intensity: Loudest during expiration.
    - Duration: Short.
    - Quality: Dull, thud-like.
    - Pitch: Low.
    - Best heard with bell of stethoscope.

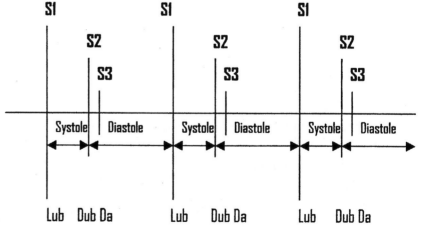

Figure 10.4: Drawing indicating the location of an S3 in relation to a normal S1 and S2.

- Systolic Murmur (Figure 10.5)
  - Dilation of left ventricle causes dilation of the mitral valve annulus, resulting in mitral regurgitation.
  - Timing: Early, mid- or late-systole or may be holosystolic.
  - Location: Best heard at 5th intercostal space, mid-clavicular line.
  - Radiation: Towards the axilla or posteriorly over the lung bases.
  - Configuration: Plateau.
  - Pitch: Medium to high.
  - Quality: Blowing.
- Lung sounds
  - Clear early in the disease process.
  - Crackles develop indicating pulmonary edema.
  - Dullness to percussion or diminished breath sounds could indicate pleural effusion.
- Jugular venous distension
- Hepatomegaly
- Peripheral Edema
- Ascites.

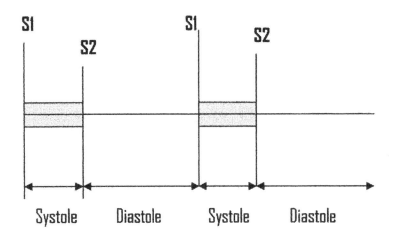

Figure 10.5: Drawing demonstrating the holosystolic plateau murmur of mitral regurgitation.

Diagnosis

- *Chest x-ray*
  - Enlarged cardiac silhouette.
  - Pulmonary congestion if in failure.
  - Pleural effusion may also be present.
- *Cardiac Echocardiogram*
  - Very useful in the diagnosis of DCM.
  - Evaluates left ventricular size.
    - ★ Chamber enlargement may be present in all four chambers or only the left ventricle.
  - Evaluates ventricular wall thickness.
    - ★ Chamber walls are normal and often thin.
  - Evaluates left-ventricular function by determining ejection fraction.
    - ★ Normal ejection fraction is 55-65%.
    - ★ Ejection fraction < 40% is consistent with DCM (Kumar, Abbas, & Fausto, 2005).
  - Evaluates valve function
    - ★ Assessment for mitral regurgitation with left-ventricular dilation.
    - ★ Assessment for tricuspid regurgitation with right-ventricular dilation.
  - Demonstrates presence of thrombi in the ventricular cavity.
  - Demonstrates regional wall motion abnormalities.

Chapter 10

- *Cardiac catheterization*
  - Beneficial only to determine the presence of coronary artery disease (CAD). Although catheterization provides information about wall motion and ejection, non-invasive cardiac echocardiography is a better choice.
- *Electrocardiogram*
  - ECG changes are neither sensitive nor specific to mitral regurgitation and always require other testing for confirmation
  - Sinus tachycardia
  - Arrhythmias
    - ★ Atrial fibrillation not uncommon.
    - ★ Ventricular ectopy may be present.
  - Left bundle branch block
    - ★ Dilated ventricle may cause changes in the conduction pattern through the bundle branches.
  - Left-ventricular hypertrophy
    - ★ ST-T wave changes associated with "strain" pattern.

Medical Treatment

If the cause of the DCM can be identified, then treatment should be focused on eliminating the cause. In addition to focusing on the cause, medical therapy for DCM is essentially the same as therapy for heart failure. The chapter on heart failure covers the treatment options in full detail. Long-term survival rates for patients with DCM remain low, with approximately 50% alive 5 years after diagnosis. Medical therapy has three primary goals while trying to provide symptom relief: 1) preload reduction, 2) afterload reduction, and 3) increased contractility.

Preload Reduction

- Diuretics
- Venous vasodilators
  - Nitrates
    - ★ Dilate veins, allowing more blood to remain in the vascular system and sending less to the heart.
  - Angiotensin-converting enzyme (ACE) inhibitors
    - ★ Interferes with the RAAS effect of reabsorption of sodium and water.
    - ★ Effect on preload: decreases volume overload.
  - Aldosterone antagonists
    - ★ Spironolactone and eplerenone.
    - ★ Added if the patient continues to have symptoms at rest to help with the diuretic effect.
    - ★ Studies show that the addition of this class of medication can reduce mortality, especially in patients with ejection fractions less than 35% (Loghin, 2001).

Afterload Reduction

- Arterial Vasodilators
  - ACE Inhibitors
    - ★ Interferes with RAAS effect of vasoconstriction.
    - ★ Enhances the action of kinins, which promote a positive vasodilatory effect.

420

Cardiomyopathy

❖ Angiotensin Receptor Blockers

  ☆ Angiotensin II receptor blockers directly block angiotensin II, which results in a vasodilitory effect.

  ☆ In addition to being an acceptable firstline agent in some patient sub groups (those at risk for heart failure), angiotensin II receptor blockers are indicated in chronic heart failure patients who cannot tolerate an ACE inhibitor due to cough or angioedema.

❖ Hydralazine and Nitrate Combination

  ☆ Hydralazine is an arterial vasodilator (afterload reduction).

  ☆ Oral nitrates are venous vasodilators (preload reduction).

  ☆ A combination of hydralazine and a nitrate may used for afterload and preload reduction in patients who cannot tolerate an ACE inhibitor due to renal insufficiency or hyperkalemia. (Adams et al., 2006).

Contractility

◆ Increased contractility is achieved first by decreasing afterload. Usually, as afterload decreases, contractility increases.

◆ Digoxin

  ❖ Oral medication of choice to assist with contractility.

  ❖ No effect on mortality, but does improve exercise capacity and quality of life, and decreases hospitalizations.

  ❖ Most effective in patients who have low ejection fractions.

Other Considerations in Medical Therapy

◆ Beta blockers

  ❖ Block the neurohormonal responses of chronic SNS stimulation.

  ❖ Have several beneficial effects, including favorably affecting ventricular remodeling and apoptosis.

  ❖ Can decrease arrhythmias and ischemia by decreasing heart rate and contractility, thereby decreasing myocardial oxygen consumption.

  ❖ Not initiated when the patient is fluid overloaded or in a decompensated state.

  ❖ Initiate after fluid status is optimized – no longer requiring IV diuretics or IV vasodilators.

  ❖ Carvedilol (Coreg), metoprolol (Lopressor), and bisoprolol (Zebeta) have been found in multiple studies to decrease mortality and morbidity in heart failure (Kavinsky & Parrillo, 2000; Loghin, 2001).

◆ Antiarrhythmic Therapy

  ❖ Medication choices should be made carefully because some medications can cause further depression of the myocardium.

  ❖ Amiodarone is the antiarrhythmic medication of choice.

  ❖ Attempts should be made to convert patients from atrial fibrillation by either mechanical or pharmacological options. If conversion cannot be achieved, then rate control is essential. Digoxin and beta blockers can be helpful in rate control.

◆ Anticoagulation therapy

  ❖ DCM patients are at increased risk for embolization due to the insufficient contraction of the large ventricular chambers.

  ❖ Also at high risk for the development of atrial fibrillation.

Chapter 10

- ❖ Recommended for patients with:
  - ★ evidence of a left ventricular thrombus
  - ★ a previous embolic event
  - ★ atrial fibrillation
  - ★ some literature supports anticoagulation for any patient with an ejection fraction less than 30% (Loghin, 2001).
- ◆ Dietary Restrictions
  - ❖ Excessive salt leads to retention of extracelluar fluid.
  - ❖ A salt restriction of 2 to 4 g per day, depending on the severity of the disease process.
  - ❖ Fluid restrictions are only necessary in late stages of the disease process, when medical therapy is no longer effective in controlling volume.
- ◆ Exercise
  - ❖ Should be encouraged.
  - ❖ Cardiac rehabilitation programs can be very beneficial in helping develop appropriate exercise programs.
- ◆ Daily Weights
  - ❖ Necessary for monitoring of fluid status.
  - ❖ Report weight gains of 2 pounds in one day or 3-5 pounds in one week.
- ◆ Home infusion therapy
  - ❖ Routine intermittent infusion of positive inotropic agents are not recommended for patients with refractory end-stage heart failure as it has been shown to decrease life expectancy (Hunt et al., 2005).

Surgical Treatment

Cardiac Resynchronization Therapy (CRT or bi-ventricular pacing)

- ◆ Goal: Modification of native interventricular, intraventricular and atrial-ventricular activation sequences to improve outcomes.
- ◆ Improves right and left ventricular synchrony, increasing right-ventricular stroke volume and left-ventricular filling.
- ◆ Criteria for implantation:
  - ❖ New York Heart Association (NYHA) heart failure class III or IV.
  - ❖ Maximum medical therapy without relief of symptoms.
  - ❖ Ejection fraction less than 35%.
  - ❖ Normal Sinus Rhythm.
    - ★ Patients with atrial fibrillation do not have results that are as favorable to those in sinus rhythm.
    - ★ Atrial ablation prior to placement of the CRT device has demonstrated an improvement in outcomes.
  - ❖ QRS width > 0.12 sec.
    - ★ Provides evidence the right and left ventricles are not contracting at the same time.
- ◆ Anatomical location of pacemaker wires:
  - ❖ Standard pacing wire in right atrium for atrial pacing.
  - ❖ Standard pacing wire (usually with defibrillation lead) in right ventricle for right-ventricular pacing.

Cardiomyopathy

❖ Special left-ventricular lead placed via the coronary sinus into the left-ventricular cardiac vein to pace the lateral wall of the left ventricle.

◆ Resynchronization of the right and left ventricle.
  ❖ Improvement in exercise tolerance.
  ❖ Improves quality of life.
  ❖ Decreased hospitalization.

Implantable Cardioverter-Defibrillators (ICD)

◆ High incidence of sudden death from ventricular arrhythmias in patients with DCM.

◆ Patients with ejection fractions less than 35% and a history of MI are candidates for ICD placement (Ganz, 2004).

◆ ICDs are commonly implanted as part of the procedure for CRT.

Other Surgical Procedures

◆ Mitral Valve Repair/Replacement
  ❖ Replacement of regurgitant mitral valve may provide some clinical improvement.
  ❖ Effect on improved survival is undocumented.

◆ Battista Procedure (Partial Left Ventriculectomy)
  ❖ Also referred to as heart reduction surgery.
  ❖ Triangular portion of lateral wall of left ventricle is removed.
  ❖ Goal is to reduce the size of the dilated left ventricle.

◆ Cardiomyoplasty
  ❖ Latissimus dorsi muscle (skeletal muscle) in the back is dissected and wrapped around the left ventricle.
  ❖ Cardiomyostimulator stimulates the newly resected muscle graft to contract in synchrony with the myocardium to provide support for the weak and dilated left ventricle.
  ❖ Entire procedure takes several surgeries.
  ❖ Requires a patient who is able to tolerate several surgeries and the emotion and physical demands of this procedure.
  ❖ Originally met with enthusiasm, it is rarely utilized today.

◆ Left-Ventricular Assist Devices
  ❖ Generally considered a bridge to transplantation.

◆ Acorn Cardiac Support Device
  ❖ Investigational treatment device for treating moderate heart failure.
  ❖ Use as an adjunctive therapy with standard treatment for heart failure.
  ❖ Biocompatible, mesh-like jacket placed around the ventricles of the heart during surgery.
  ❖ Provides support and relieves the stress to the myocardial walls.
  ❖ Diastolic support device which supports the heart to reduce myocardial stretching during diastole.
  ❖ Intended to reverse dilation of the heart and return the heart to its normal shape.

◆ Cardiac Transplantation
  ❖ Only established surgical approach to refractory heart failure (Hunt et al., 2005).
  ❖ Many more patients waiting for heart transplant than hearts available.
  ❖ Many die before transplantation.

Chapter 10

Outcomes

DCM is the final disease process for many other disorders and diseases that affect the myocardium. Once diagnosed, 50% of patients with heart failure die within 5 years (Loghin, 2001). Death is usually due to progressive heart failure, but can also be caused by sudden cardiac death, pulmonary emboli, or embolic stroke. The lower the ejection fraction, the poorer the prognosis. Patient follow-up and compliance with treatment regimes seem to impact the outcomes. Patient understanding impacts compliance and outcomes in this disease process.

Linking Knowledge to Practice

✔ *Confusion and disorientation should be carefully evaluated because patients with DCM commonly develop atrial fibrillation and are at high risk for the development of cerebral emboli.*

✔ *Asking patients to tightly squeeze your hand while listening to their hearts enhances murmurs and the additional heart sound in DCM. Hypertrophic changes on the ECG may cause ST- and T wave changes that mimic myocardial ischemia. Careful patient assessment and ECG analysis is needed to differentiate between ischemia and these changes.*

✔ *Arterial vasodilators decrease blood pressure. Patients on arterial vasodilators should be instructed to report any symptoms of low blood pressure, such as dizziness, when standing up.*

✔ *Patients with DCM are commonly prescribed multiple medications. It is essential to ensure that the patient understands the importance of each medication and the value of compliance.*

RESTRICTIVE CARDIOMYOPATHY

Restrictive cardiomyopathy (RCM) is characterized by rigidity of the myocardial wall that causes a decreased ability of the chamber walls to expand during cardiac filling, resulting in diastolic dysfunction (Figure 10.1).

Prevalence

RCM is the least common form of cardiomyopathy and accounts for approximately 5% of all primary heart muscle diseases (Goswami & Reddy, 2003). Men and women are equally affected. This process can be seen in children as well as adults; however, it appears to be better tolerated by adults.

Causes

As with other cardiomyopathies, RCM has both primary and secondary causes (see Table 10.3). Each cause results in different processes that restrict the myocardium. Some patients present with hemodynamics representative of RCM, but no cause can be determined. Amyloidosis is responsible for 90% of RCM cases in North America (Darovic, 2002). This disease process deposits protein fibrils (amyloid) in tissues of the body and impairs organ function. These protein fibrils are deposited throughout the myocardium, resulting in a firm, rubbery heart with thick, but not dilated, ventricular walls. Not all patients with amyloidosis develop cardiac involvement; however, amyloid heart disease has a very poor prognosis. Although not prevalent in North America, endomyocardial fibrosis is relatively common in children and young adults in Africa and the tropics. Fibrosis of the ventricular endocardium and subendocardium that extends to the mitral and tricuspid valves greatly decreases ventricular chamber function. Patients who have undergone radiation treatments may develop radiation-induced myocardial fibrosis that is not evident for several years after treatment.

424

Cardiomyopathy

Table 10.3 Causes of Restrictive Cardiomyopathy

Primary Causes
 	
◆ Endomyocardial Diseases
   ❖ Eosinophilic Endomyocardial Fibrosis
   ❖ Endocardial Fibrosis
   ❖ Cardiac Transplant
   ❖ Anthracycline Toxicity
◆ Loeffler's Endocarditis
◆ Idiopathic

Secondary Causes
 	
◆ Infiltrative Disorders
   ❖ Amyloidosis
   ❖ Sarcoidosis
   ❖ Radiation Carditis
◆ Storage Diseases
   ❖ Hemochromatosis
   ❖ Glycogen Storage Disease
   ❖ Fabry's Disease

(From O'Neill & Bott-Silverman, 2003).

Pathophysiology

Normally, as ventricular diastole begins, the atrioventricular valves open and the contents of the atria passively empty into the ventricles. At the end of ventricular diastole, the atria contract and add an additional volume of blood to the ventricles. During ventricular filling, the ventricular walls expand, stretching the cardiac muscle fibers and allowing for adequate filling. In patients with RCM, the ability of the ventricular walls to expand is limited due to the disease process occurring in the myocardium. This limitation in chamber expansion results in impaired diastolic filling. Decreased diastolic filling results in a decrease in the volume of blood available for ejection during systole; therefore, stroke volume is decreased. Systolic function is usually not effected. If the disease process is an infiltrative type disorder, contractile function can become impaired as the disease progresses. The ventricles are unable to accept all the contents from the atria, resulting in increased volume and pressure in the atria. Blood backs up into the lungs (left-sided failure) and ultimately the venous circulation (right-sided failure), resulting in heart failure. Both ventricles are involved as the disease process affects both ventricles. The size of the ventricular cavity usually remains the same or may be slightly decreased. With endomyocardial fibrosis, there is usually fibrosis of the endocardium as well as the cardiac valves.

Symptoms

◆ Fatigue and weakness
   ❖ Symptoms of fatigue and weakness are due to decreased stroke volume and an inability to compensate for the increased metabolic demands of activity. Normally, any increase in activity causes the heart rate to increase. This increase in heart rate provides an increase in circulating blood volume to support the increase in demand. For patients with RCM, who already have decreased ventricular filling, an increase in heart rate decreases CO because it decreases the amount of time the ventricles have to fill during diastole. Decreased CO results in symptoms of fatigue and weakness.

- Syncope
  - May be present in patients with amyloidosis.
  - Due to the development of SA node disease from the amloyd infiltrates.
- Other symptoms related to heart failure
  - Biventricular failure.
    - ★ Right-sided failure may be more prominent early, as the impaired function of the right ventricle helps decrease the load on the left side of the heart, therefore decreasing the left-sided failure.
  - Palpitations may be present and are caused by atrial fibrillation, which is common with RCM.
  - Disturbances in cardiac conduction are not uncommon in infiltrative disorders.

Physical Examination

- Signs of right- and left-sided failure (see discussion in DCM section).
- Signs of low CO.
  - Cool extremities
  - Hypotension (not uncommon in amyloidosis)
  - Lethargy
  - Peripheral pulses – decreased and become weaker as the disease progresses and stroke volume continues to decrease.
- S4 (Atrial Gallop) (Figure 10.6)
  - Fourth heart sound.
  - Result of decreased compliance of the ventricle.
  - Best heard with patient in left lateral position.
  - Timing: Late diastolic filling sound, just before S1.
  - Location: Mitral area (5th intercostal space, mid-clavicular line)
  - Intensity: Loudest during expiration.
  - Duration: Short.
  - Quality: Dull, thud-like.
  - Pitch: Low.
  - Best heard with bell of stethoscope.

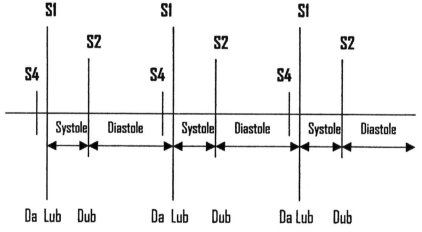

Figure 10.6: Drawing indicating the location of an S4 in relation to a normal S1 and S2.

- Systolic murmurs
  - Mitral or tricuspid insufficiency (regurgitation) murmurs (Figure 10.4).
  - Fluid overload state causes atrial dilation, resulting in a dilated valve annulus and regurgitation.
  - Amyloidosis may infiltrate the papillary muscles, resulting in regurgitation of the mitral or tricuspid valve.
  - Fibrosis may affect the cardiac valves, as well as the endocardium.
- Elevation of pulmonary artery pressures if pulmonary hypertension has developed

Diagnosis

Aortic stenosis, cardiac tamponade, HCM, and hypertensive heart disease should all be ruled out when considering a diagnosis of RCM (Goswami & Reddy, 2003). The most important process that must be differentiated is constrictive pericarditis because this disease process can mimic RCM, and the clinician must differentiate these two processes so appropriate intervention can be initiated (see Table 10.4).

Table 10.4
Clinical Features of Constrictive Pericarditis and Restrictive Cardiomyopathy

Clinical Features	Constrictive Pericarditis	Restrictive Cardiomyopathy
History	Prior history of pericarditis or condition that causes pericardial disease.	History of systemic disease (eg. Amyloidosis, Hemochromatosis).
Heart Sounds	Pericardial knock, high frequency sound.	Presence of loud diastolic filling sound S4, low frequency sound.
Murmurs	No murmurs.	Murmurs of mitral and tricuspid insufficiency.
Cardiac Pressures	Left (PAWP) and right (CVP) filling pressures are elevated and equal.	Left-sided filling pressures generally > right-sided filling pressures by 5 mm Hg or >.
Chest X-ray	Visual pericardial calcification.	Atrial dilation with normal ventricular size.
CT Scan/MRI	Pericardial thickening.	No pericardial thickening.
Echocardiogram	Normal ventricles and atria Pericardial thickening.	Atrial dilation with normal ventricular size. If amyloid infiltration of the heart – speckled texture of myocardium.

◆ Chest x-ray
  ❖ Ventricular size appears normal.
  ❖ Atrial dilation may be present.
  ❖ Pulmonary congestion if in failure.
◆ Echocardiogram
  ❖ Very useful in the diagnosis of RCM.
  ❖ Most helpful in differentiating constrictive pericarditis from RCM (Table 10.5).
  ❖ Evaluation of ventricular size
    ★ Usually normal.
    ★ Chamber size may be slightly diminished.
  ❖ Evaluation of atrial size
    ★ Enlarged.
  ❖ Evaluation of ventricular wall thickness
    ★ Normal unless an infiltrative disease process is present.
  ❖ Evaluation of left ventricular function
    ★ Normal contractility (systolic function).
    ★ Diastolic dysfunction.

Chapter 10

- ❖ Evaluation of valve function
  - ★ Mitral or tricuspid regurgitation.
- ❖ Amyloid heart
  - ★ Abnormal myocardial textures.
  - ★ Speckled appearance of the myocardium may be noted (Carroll & Crawford, 2003).
- ◆ Cardiac catheterization
  - ❖ Complete cardiac catheterization may not be necessary unless CAD is suspected.
  - ❖ Invasive hemodynamic measurements may be valuable.
    - ★ Elevated right and left ventricular end diastolic pressures.
    - ★ Elevated pulmonary artery occlusive pressure.
    - ★ Elevated right atrial pressure.
  - ❖ Differentiation between constrictive pericarditis (CP) and RCM.
    - ★ RCM: right- and left-sided ventricular filling pressures are increased; however, left-sided filling pressures are generally higher than those of the right side by 5 mm Hg or greater.
    - ★ CP: Filling pressures are generally equal.
- ◆ Endomyocardial biopsy
  - ❖ Obtained from the septal wall of the right ventricle.
  - ❖ Essential for the diagnosis of RCM for a variety of disease processes, including amyloidosis, hemochromatosis, and sarcoidosis.
  - ❖ Multiple specimens obtained from multiple sites because many of these disease processes spread in a patchy, scattered pattern.
  - ❖ Can positively identify infiltrative disorders and provide a definitive diagnosis of RCM.
- ◆ Electrocardiogram
  - ❖ ECG changes are neither sensitive nor specific to cardiomyopathy and always require other testing for confirmation.
  - ❖ QRS voltage is low.
  - ❖ Nonspecific ST-segment and T wave changes.
  - ❖ Large P waves indicative of atrial enlargement.
  - ❖ Cardiac conduction abnormalities occur as the infiltrative disease infiltrates the conduction system.
  - ❖ Atrial fibrillation is common in patients with RCM.
  - ❖ Ventricular arrhythmias are common in patients with cardiac amyloidosis.

Medical Treatment

Treatment for RCM is supportive and aimed at the reduction of symptoms. Treatment focuses on:

- ◆ Reduction of diastolic dysfunction
  - ❖ No medication directly affects restriction.
  - ❖ Treatment aimed at reducing the effects of the restriction.
    - ★ Increased ECF volume.
      - ✱ Diuretics are the medication of choice to reduce ECF volume.
      - ✱ Careful assessment of volume status is essential in the treatment of RCM. Reduction of ECF volume is necessary to prevent symptoms of heart failure; however, over reduction of volume further decreases the already decreased filling of the ventricle. Patients with severe RCM have a very narrow range of acceptable volume.

Cardiomyopathy

* ☆ Decreased stoke volume.
  * ✱ Arterial vasodilators, such as ACE inhibitors, may be useful in decreasing afterload, allowing for a more effective contraction by the ventricle.
  * ✱ ACE inhibitors contribute to diuresis, so volume status must be considered when utilizing ACE inhibitors with diuretics.
  * ✱ Any vasodilator that produces venous vasodilation decreases the volume entering the heart (preload) and further decreases ventricular filling.
  * ✱ Treatment should be initiated with very low doses, with the patient being carefully monitored.
* ◆ Treatment of Arrhythmias
  * ❖ Atrial fibrillation is the most common arrhythmic complication in RCM (Carroll & Crawford, 2003).
    * ☆ Loss of atrial contraction can contribute to a decrease in ventricular filling; therefore, a normal sinus rhythm is preferable to atrial fibrillation.
    * ☆ Digoxin:
      * ✱ Used cautiously for ventricular rate control.
      * ✱ Patients with amyloidosis are particularly susceptible to digoxin-induced arrhythmias and heart blocks (Carroll & Crawford, 2003).
  * ❖ Heart blocks, including complete heart blocks, may develop, resulting in the need for a permanent atrioventricular pacemaker.
  * ❖ Ventricular arrhythmias may also develop.
    * ☆ Treatment of these arrhythmias is based on the patient's hemodynamic response and whether the arrhythmias are sustained or life threatening.
* ◆ Treatment of thromboembolic complications
  * ❖ At risk for thrombus formation (Carroll & Crawford, 2003).
  * ❖ In atrial fibrillation, clots can form in the enlarged atrium, usually in the left atrial appendage.
  * ❖ Thrombi are also a concern in patients with low CO states and mitral or tricuspid valve regurgitation.
  * ❖ Anticoagulation with warfarin is recommended unless contraindicated.
* ◆ Treatment of Underlying Disease Process
  * ❖ Amyloidosis.
    * ☆ No cure.
    * ☆ Steroids and chemotherapy may be helpful in slowing the progression of the disease.
    * ☆ Cardiac transplantation has limited benefits in amyloidosis because the amyloid infiltrates the transplanted organ.
  * ❖ Hemochromatosis.
    * ☆ Chelation therapy or phlebotomy may be beneficial, depending on the cause of the iron overload (Grenvick et al., 2000).

Surgical Treatment

Cardiac transplant is beneficial in idiopathic and familial restrictive cardiomyopathy (Goswami & Reddy, 2003). Transplant of both the heart and liver is indicated in hemochromatosis. Its usefulness in infiltrative disorders, such as amyloidosis and sarcoidosis, is questionable because these disorders affect the new organ once transplant is completed. In fibrotic endocarditis, excision of the fibrotic endocardium may provide symptomatic relief. Replacement of regurgitant valves may also provide symptomatic relief; however, both of these procedures have a fairly high mortality rate.

Outcomes

Prognosis is poor in patients with RCM with a 90% mortality rate at 10 years (Kavinsky & Parrillo, 2000). Amyloidosis carries the highest mortality, with a 2-year mortality rate being greater than 80% (Darovic, 2002).

Linking Knowledge to Practice

- ✔ *Anything that would normally cause the heart rate to increase, including activity, decreased blood pressure, fever, shivering, and low blood volume, results in a further decrease in stroke volume in patients with RCM.*
- ✔ *Patients with RCM should be closely monitored for signs of decreased CO that may result from overdiuresis. Signs include hypotension, especially orthostatic hypotension, lethargy, increased heart rate, and increased blood urea nitrogen levels.*

HYPERTROPHIC CARDIOMYOPATHY

HCM is characterized by hypertrophy of the myocardium (Figure 10.1). Associated with the increase in muscle mass is a decrease in ventricular filling (diastolic dysfunction) and a decrease in CO. Other causes of ventricular hypertrophy, including long-standing hypertension and aortic stenosis, must be ruled out before a diagnosis of HCM can be made. This disease process has had many names in the past, including idiopathic hypertrophic subaortic stenosis (IHSS). The World Health Organization's recommendation of "hypertrophic cardiomyopathy" as the correct terminology for this disease process has been widely accepted. HCM is a general term that covers all cases; however, a subgroup of patients with HCM develop HCM with obstruction. Once obstruction develops, the process is referred to as hypertrophic obstructive cardiomyopathy or HOCM.

Prevalence

HCM is found in one in every 500 people and affects women and men equally (Maron et al., 2003). It is the most common reason for sudden cardiac death in young adults.

Causes

The cause of HCM is unknown; however, over 50% of HCM cases are transmitted genetically (Kavinsky & Parrillo, 2000). An abnormal sympathetic nervous system response or abnormal catecholamine levels may cause the other half of the cases (Shah, 2003).

Pathophysiology

In HCM, a generalized disarray of the cardiac myofibrils occurs, along with hypertrophy of the myocytes (Figure 10.7). Cardiac cells take on a variety of shapes, and myocardial scarring and fibrosis occur. These changes result in myocardial walls that become very thick and stiff. The left ventricle is usually affected, with little effect on the right ventricle. The changes may be symmetrical; however, in many cases, asymmetrical septal hypertrophy is the most common finding (Figure 10.8). In asymmetrical hypertrophy, the ventricular septum experiences the greatest increase in wall thickness, often up to twice its normal size.

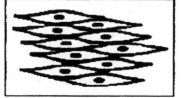 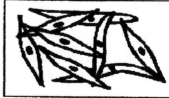

Figure 10.7: The difference between normal myocardial cells and the myocardial disarray with HCM.
Courtesy of the Hypertrophic Cardiomyopathy Association www.4hcm.org

Involvement of the septum may be limited to the upper one third, the lower two thirds, or the entire length of the septum (Figures 10.8 and 10.9). Ventricular chamber size decreases as the enlarging ventricular walls close in on the ventricular chamber. The thick, stiff walls resist filling. The most prominent hemodynamic effect is decreased ventricular filling, or diastolic dysfunction. As ventricular diastole begins, the mitral valve opens and the contents of the left atrium passively empty into the left ventricle. Normally 70-75% of left-ventricular filling occurs during this passive stage.

In the presence of HCM, early passive filling is slowed due to the stiff, small left ventricle. The second part of diastole is atrial contraction (atrial kick), which delivers an additional 25-30% more volume to the ventricle. A normal ventricle can hold approximately 150 ml of volume and normally ejects 55-65% of that volume with each beat. A stiff, noncompliant ventricle can neither hold 150 ml of volume nor accept the amount of volume (70-75% of total) normally provided during passive filling, due to the high pressure in the left ventricle. Therefore, atrial kick becomes essential in delivering the volume needed to fill the ventricle.

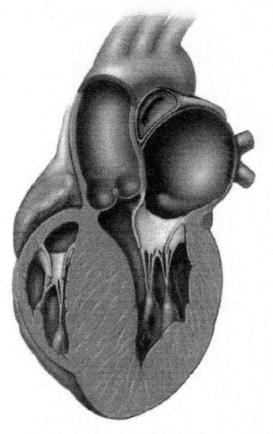
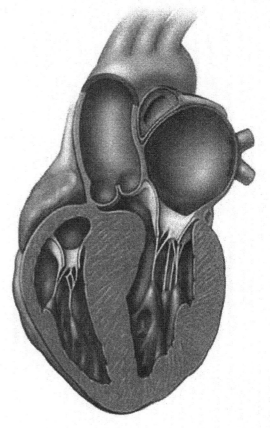

Figure 10.8: Asymmetrical HCM. Note: The septal wall hypertrophy is greater than the lateral wall of left ventricle.
© 2007. All rights reserved.

Figure 10.9: Asymmetrical septal hypertrophy involving the upper portion of the septal wall.
© 2007. All rights reserved.

To compensate for the decreased volume in the ventricle, systolic function becomes hyperdynamic. The ejection fraction that is normally 55-65% rises, and a greater portion of the ventricular contents are ejected. Ejecting 70-80% of a smaller volume helps maintain normal stroke volume.

Hypertrophic obstructive cardiomyopathy (HOCM) occurs when the upper one-third of the intraventricular septum becomes hypertrophied and partially obstructs the left-ventricular outflow tract (Figure 10.10). The left-ventricular outflow tract is the path the blood in the ventricle must follow when ejected from the ventricle. Obstruction occurs due to a combination of events. The septal wall enlarges into the ventricular cavity, including the outflow tract area. Additionally, the anterior leaflet of the mitral valve can be drawn toward the septum as the hyperdynamic ventricular contraction produces high-velocity blood flow. The rapid current of blood pulls the anterior leaflet toward the outflow tract as it passes the leaflet, resulting in early closure of the aortic valve with a greatly decreased ejection fraction (Figure 10.10). Referred to as SAM (systolic anterior motion), this obstruction by the anterior leaflet can be life threatening. It is estimated that 30-50% of patients with HCM have obstruction (Nishimura & Holmes, 2004).

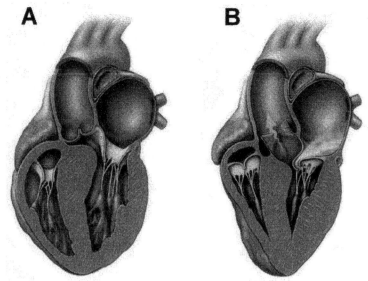

Figure 10.10: Hypertrophic obstructive cardiomyopathy during ventricular diastole (A) and ventricular systole (B).
© 2007. All rights reserved.

Mitral valve regurgitation develops as HCM progresses. As papillary muscles become hypertrophied, valve leaflets may also become thick and the annulus calcified. As the left atrium dilates to compensate for the increased pressure and volume in the atrium, the mitral valve ring enlarges as well. These processes contribute to a valve that does not close properly, and regurgitation occurs. Atrial dilation occurs in an attempt to compensate for the increased volume and pressure in the atrium that result from decreased left-ventricular filling. As hypertrophy of the left ventricle increases, forward flow decreases, resulting in decreased CO. Additionally, fluid overload occurs with a backup of the additional volume in the lungs.

Summary of Primary Pathophysiologic Changes in Hypertrophic Cardiomyopathy

Thick and Stiff Ventricular Walls
With Decreased Ventricular Chamber Size

Passive Atrial Emptying Slows
Decrease in Ability to Empty Atrial Contents
↓
↑ Left Atrial Volume and Pressure
↓
Left Atrial Dilation
↓
Stretching of Mitral Valve Annulus
↓
Mitral Valve Regurgitation

Decreased Left-Ventricular Filling
Diastolic Dysfunction
↓
Decreased Stroke Volume
↓
Development of
Hyperdynamic Systolic Dysfunction
↓
Improved Stroke Volume

Cardiomyopathy

Symptoms

Many patients with HCM remain asymptomatic for years. In many cases, HCM is first identified during routine screening of relatives of a known HCM patient. Symptoms usually develop as the disease progresses. The severity of the hypertrophy does not always relate to the severity of symptoms. Symptoms may be closer related to the severity of the diastolic dysfunction or mitral regurgitation. An episode of sudden death is frequently the first clinical presentation in children and young adults. The most common symptoms are dyspnea, chest pain, syncope or presyncope, and sudden death.

◆ Dyspnea
  ❖ Ninety percent of patients presenting with symptoms cite dyspnea as the most prevalent problem (Loghin, 2001).
  ❖ Rising left atrial pressures result in left atrial dilation in an attempt to compensate for the increased volume in the atrium. The increase in pressure is ultimately referred back to the pulmonary system. As pulmonary pressures increase, the patient is predisposed to bouts of pulmonary congestion, resulting in dyspnea.
  ❖ Dyspnea is commonly related to activity. Any increase in activity normally increases heart rate to provide an increase in circulating blood volume to support the increase in demand. As with RCM, the normal cardiac response of an increase in heart rate with activity is detrimental to patients with HCM. Increased heart rate decreases diastolic filling time in a patient who already has impaired diastolic filling.
  ❖ The hyperdynamic walls of the heart continue to eject a larger-than-normal percentage of the volume in the ventricle, which is helpful to a point. As left-ventricular filling decreases, so does the total volume available for ejection. Ultimately stroke volume will decrease, resulting in decreased perfusion.

◆ Chest Pain
  ❖ Chest pain is caused by an imbalance in myocardial oxygen supply and demand.
  ❖ Increased myocardial oxygen demand is due to:
    ☆ Increased left-ventricular wall mass.
    ☆ Hypercontractile state of the left ventricle.
  ❖ Decreased myocardial oxygen supply due to:
    ☆ Decreased left-ventricular filling.
    ☆ Increased myocardial mass requires more oxygenated blood due to its size.
    ☆ Coronary arteries are small and have difficulty dilating due to the sheer mass of the myocardium.
  ❖ At rest, blood supply may be adequate to meet the body's needs.
  ❖ Angina results when stress or exercise increases myocardial oxygen demand, and the needs of the thickened ventricular wall can no longer be met.
  ❖ Angina can be caused by coronary artery disease in addition to increased wall mass, but coronary artery disease does not usually occur in HCM.

◆ Syncope
  ❖ Normal response to exercise
    ☆ Arterial blood vessels dilate to increase blood flow to the system.
    ☆ Blood pressure decreases.
    ☆ Heart rate increases to increase forward flow and compensate for decreased blood pressure.
    ☆ Provides increased CO to meet the myocardial demands of activity.

Chapter 10

- ❖ Patient with HCM – response to exercise
  - ✦ Myocardial oxygen demand increases with exercise.
  - ✦ Arterial blood vessels dilate (reduced afterload) in response to increased myocardial oxygen demand to allow improved forward flow with each contraction.
  - ✦ Heart rate increases to improve cardiac output (CO = HR x SV).
  - ✦ Increased heart rate decreases diastolic filling time. Decreased diastolic filling time results in decreased preload. A decrease in preload will decrease stroke volume (components of stroke volume = preload, afterload and contractility). If the diastolic dysfunction is severe enough the increase in heart rate will not be enough to compensate for the decreased afterload and decreased preload. Cardiac output will actually decrease instead of the normal increase with activity.
  - ✦ Dizziness, light-headedness, and syncope may occur.
  - ✦ Exercising can also cause ventricular or atrial arrhythmias which may result in syncope as well.
- ◆ Sudden Death
  - ❖ Often the first indication of HCM.
  - ❖ Degree of hypertrophy generally correlates to the incidence of arrhythmias.
  - ❖ Ventricular wall thickness of 30 mm or greater is associated with an increased risk of sudden death arrhythmias (Maron et al., 2003).
  - ❖ Ventricular wall thickness less than 15 mm is associated with no risk of sudden death arrhythmias.
  - ❖ Life threatening arrhythmias tend to occur in patients under 40 years of age.
  - ❖ Undiagnosed HCM is one of the most common causes of sudden death in young adults.
  - ❖ Life-threatening arrhythmias generally occur when the young adult engages in strenuous activity.
- ◆ Other Symptoms
  - ❖ Fatigue.
  - ❖ Activity intolerance.
  - ❖ Palpitations due to the hyperdynamic contraction of the heart.
  - ❖ Atrial fibrillation due to atrial dilation.
    - ✦ Results in a loss of atrial kick.
    - ✦ Atrial kick provides active filling during ventricular diastole.
    - ✦ Hypertrophic ventricle counts on atrial kick for ventricular filling.
    - ✦ Atrial fibrillation is poorly tolerated.

Physical Examination

- ◆ Bisferous Carotid Pulse (Pulsus Bisferiens) (Figure 10.11)
  - ❖ Characteristic of patients with HOCM.
  - ❖ Initial upstroke of the carotid pulse is brisk because there is initially no difficulty ejecting blood through the outflow tract.

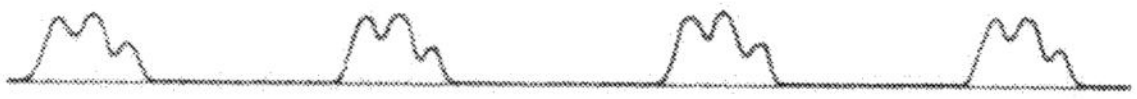

Figure 10.11: The early collapse and the secondary rise of impulse that is characteristic of Pulsus Bisferiens in the patient with HOCM.
(Note: The third rise in this drawing depicts the normal dicrotic notch noted in the arterial pressure trace.)

  - ❖ As systole progresses and the left-ventricular walls come closer together, left-ventricular outflow tract obstruction may occur. This obstruction results in a collapse of the pulse and then a secondary rise.
  - ❖ Because hypertrophic cardiomyopathy may be confused with aortic stenosis, it is important to note that in aortic stenosis, the carotid pulse has a delayed upstroke and amplitude.

434

- Forceful and brisk PMI (located at apex of heart).
- S4 (Atrial Gallop)
  - Fourth heart sound.
  - Caused by atrial contraction and the propulsion of blood into a stiff, noncompliant ventricle.
  - Best heard with patient in left lateral position.
  - Timing: Late diastolic filling sound, just before S1.
  - Location: Mitral area (5th intercostal space, mid-clavicular line).
  - Intensity: Louder during expiration.
  - Duration: Short.
  - Quality: Thud-like.
  - Pitch: Low.
  - Best heard with bell of stethoscope.
  - Not audible in patients in atrial fibrillation.
- Subvalvular Left Ventricular Outflow Obstruction Systolic Murmur (Figure 10.12)
  - Timing: Midsystolic.
  - Location: Best heard along left sternal boarder.
  - Radiation: Usually does not radiate.
  - Configuration: Crescendo-decrescendo.
  - Intensity: Grade 3/6 to 4/6.
  - Pitch: Medium.
  - Quality: Harsh or rough.
  - Heard equally well with bell or diaphragm of stethoscope.
  - Must differentiate between aortic stenosis (AS) and HCM.
    - ☆ The HCM murmur becomes louder during Valsalva's maneuver.
      - ∗ Decreases venous return to the heart (preload).
      - ∗ Decreased preload results in decreased left-ventricular filling.
      - ∗ Decreased left-ventricular filling results in increased obstruction.
      - ∗ Any factor that decreases venous return to the heart increases the murmur in HCM (Table 10.5).
    - ☆ Aortic stenosis murmur becomes quieter during Valsalva's maneuver.

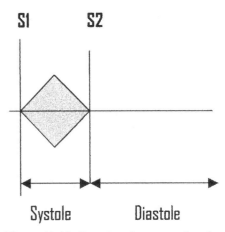

Figure 10.12: Drawing demonstrating the subvalvular left-ventricular outflow obstruction systolic murmur of HOCM

Table 10.5 Maneuvers Decreasing Venous Return to the Heart
Valsalva
Arising from squatting to standing
Tachycardia
Venodilating drugs (Nitroglycerine)
Decreased volume from blood loss or diuretics
Developed by Author.

Chapter 10

- ◆ Systolic Murmur of Mitral Regurgitation
  - ❖ Timing: Early, mid- or late-systole, or may be holosystolic.
  - ❖ Location: Best heard at 5th intercostal space, mid-clavicular line.
  - ❖ Radiation: Towards the axilla or posteriorly over the lung bases.
  - ❖ Configuration: Plateau.
  - ❖ Pitch: Medium to high.
  - ❖ Quality: Blowing.
  - ❖ Does not change in the way a left-ventricular outflow obstruction murmur does.
  - ❖ Careful assessment for murmur of MR is essential, as murmur may help in identifying SAM (systolic anterior motion of the anterior leaflet of the mitral valve) and with HOCM.
- ◆ Other Finding on Physical Exam
  - ❖ Heart Failure.
    - ★ Signs of heart failure will be present if in failure.
    - ★ Right-sided heart failure is a late sign because left-sided failure generally occurs first.

Diagnosis

- ◆ Chest X-ray
  - ❖ Not often helpful.
  - ❖ HCM does not usually increase ventricular size.
  - ❖ Heart generally appears normal in size.
  - ❖ Left atrium may be slightly larger than normal and increased in size as the disease progresses.
  - ❖ Signs of pulmonary congestion if in failure.
- ◆ Cardiac Echocardiogram
  - ❖ Diagnosis is easily established utilizing echocardiography.
  - ❖ Gold standard diagnosing HCM.
  - ❖ A wide variety of information can be obtained during echocardiography that leads to a diagnosis of HCM.
  - ❖ Evaluation of Wall Thickness
    - ★ Wall thickness increased.
    - ★ Septal wall usually greater than rest of left-ventricular walls.
  - ❖ Evaluation of Ventricular Size
    - ★ Outer dimensions of left-ventricular wall usually unchanged.
    - ★ Left-ventricular chamber size diminished.
  - ❖ Evaluation of Atrial Size
    - ★ Usually dilated.
  - ❖ Evaluation of Mitral Valve
    - ★ Identification of systolic anterior motion of anterior leaflet of mitral valve.
    - ★ Dilation of mitral annulus from dilated left atrium.
    - ★ Thickened and fibrotic leaflets from primary disease process.
  - ❖ Evaluation of Left-Ventricular Outflow
    - ★ Obstruction may be present and noted during systole.
  - ❖ Evaluation for Obstruction
    - ★ Administration of amyl nitrate during echocardiography will increase severity of obstruction, or may demonstrate an obstruction when an obstruction is not noted at rest.

436

Cardiomyopathy

◆ Cardiac catheterization
  ❖ Provides little or no additional information for the diagnosis of HCM.
  ❖ Most patients with HCM do not have coronary artery disease.
  ❖ May identify small vessels due to the increased muscle mass.
  ❖ Ventricular cavity size and left-ventricular outflow tract gradient can be assessed.
◆ Electrocardiogram
  ❖ ECG changes are neither sensitive nor specific to cardiomyopathy and always require other testing for confirmation.
  ❖ Changes consistent with left-ventricular hypertrophy.
    ☆ Deep S waves in leads V_1 and V_2 with tall R waves in leads V_4, V_5 and V_6.
    ☆ Strain Pattern in leads with tall R waves.
      ✱ Deep inverted T waves.
      ✱ In patients experiencing chest pain, T wave inversions need to be carefully evaluated because these changes may indicate myocardial ischemia.
    ☆ The lack of QRS complexes with an increase in size does not rule out HCM.
    ☆ Bundle branch blocks, including left anterior hemi-block, right bundle branch block, or left bundle branch block may be present, but are not specific to HCM.
    ☆ Arrhythmias
      ✱ Atrial fibrillation or ventricular arrhythmias may be present, but are not specific to HCM.

Medical Treatment

Treatment for HCM is aimed at relieving symptoms, preventing complications and/or reducing the risk of sudden death. No clinical evidence supports treating nonsymptomatic patients. The data for this population are small because many patients are unaware of the disease process until symptoms appear.

◆ Beta blockers
  ❖ First-line therapy for symptomatic patients with or without obstruction.
  ❖ Provides symptomatic improvement.
  ❖ Can increase exercise tolerance.
  ❖ Greatest benefit seen in patients experiencing symptoms with exertion or exercise.
  ❖ Blocks normal beta responses of increased contractility, increased heart rate, and increased conduction of impulses from the atrium to the ventricle.
  ❖ Slower heart rate increases diastolic filling time.
  ❖ Limits the ability of the heart rate to increase in response to stimulation, such as exercise.
  ❖ Allows for relaxation of ventricular walls.
    ☆ Improves ventricular filling, especially passive filling.
  ❖ Decreases myocardial oxygen demand.
◆ Calcium Channel Blockers
  ❖ Second-line therapy for symptomatic patients with or without obstruction.
  ❖ Shown to decrease symptoms, particularly chest pain.
  ❖ Exerts a negative inotropic effect (decreasing contractility).
  ❖ Verapamil is the calcium channel blocker of choice because it decreases ventricular contractility and improves myocardial relaxation, resulting in increased ventricular filling.
  ❖ Verapamil should not be used in the presence of severe pulmonary hypertension.

Chapter 10

* May develop excessive vasodilation that increases left-ventricular outflow obstruction which decreases CO.
* Pulmonary edema could develop.
❖ Nifedipine, amlodipine, and felodipine should be avoided due to their vasodilatory effects.
* Decreased left-ventricular filling.
* Worsening of outflow tract obstruction.

Generally, a beta blocker is the first medication of choice. If the beta blocker does not provide symptom relief, a calcium channel blocker is substituted for the beta blocker. There is currently no evidence that supports utilizing a beta blocker with a calcium channel blocker.

◆ Disopyramide (Norpace)
  ❖ Useful in patients with obstructive HCM.
  ❖ Negative inotrope.
  ❖ Decreases SAM.
  ❖ Decrease outflow obstruction.
  ❖ Decreases mitral regurgitant volume.
  ❖ May induce accelerated AV nodal conduction and consequently heart rate, so should be administered with a beta blocker.
  ❖ QT Interval should be monitored to assess for prolongation.
◆ Atrial fibrillation
  ❖ Most common arrhythmia associated with HCM.
  ❖ Attempts should be made to convert atrial fibrillation to normal sinus rhythm.
  ❖ Loss of atrial contraction and potentially high ventricular heart rates contribute to decreased ventricular filling and, quite often, rapid hemodynamic deterioration.
  ❖ Pharmacologic or mechanical cardioversion are acceptable.
  ❖ Beta blockers help control ventricular rate.
  ❖ Amiodarone is also useful in both obstructive and non-obstructive disease with ventricular or atrial arrhythmias.
  ❖ Digoxin should be avoided in patients with HOCM because it increases contractility, thereby increasing the obstruction.
  ❖ Anticoagulation protocol should be followed, as with anyone who may have atrial fibrillation.
◆ Other Medications
  ❖ Diuretics
    * Used cautiously in patients with HCM.
    * Volume status is very important.
    * Preload is already decreased due to the ventricle's inability to expand during filling. Any further loss of filling can result in a decrease in CO.
  ❖ ACE inhibitors and nitroglycerin preparations
    * Avoid in patients with HOCM.
    * Vasodilation causes a decrease in preload.
    * Can increase the outflow obstruction and greatly decrease CO.

- ❖ *Special Note:* Any medication that increases contractility should be strictly avoided in patients with HOCM. An increase in contractility increases the outflow obstruction and greatly decreases CO. This effect can be life threatening. Examples of drugs that increase contractility include digoxin, dobutamine, dopamine, epinephrine, and norepinephrine.
- ◆ Endocarditis Prophylaxis
  - ❖ Infective endocarditis prophylaxis is recommended by the ACC in patients with evidence of outflow obstruction, both resting and with exercise, before dental work or surgical procedures (Maron et al., 2003).
  - ❖ No evidence supporting the use of prophylaxis in non-obstructive disease.

Some patients never develop obstructive disease. These patients can be more difficult to treat, and therapy may be less effective in providing symptom relief. Beta blockers and calcium channel blockers are beneficial in decreasing heart rate and improving diastolic function. However, over time, the hypertrophic heart evolves into a dilated myocardium and the clinical picture becomes similar to DCM with the development of systolic dysfunction. As patients develop symptoms of heart failure, diuretics, ACE inhibitors, and digoxin may be helpful. Ultimately, cardiac transplant may be considered as the heart deteriorates.

Many patients with HCM are young and wish to become pregnant. According to the ACC and European Society of Cardiology (ESC) Clinical Expert Consensus Document on Hypertrophic Cardiomyopathy (Maron et al., 2003), there is currently no evidence that pregnancy should be avoided in patients with HCM. Mortality risk may be slightly higher; however, that risk is generally associated with women who are already at high risk for other reasons. Normal vaginal deliveries can occur without difficulties.

Surgical Treatment

- ◆ Cardiac Pacemakers
  - ❖ Dual-chamber cardiac pacing has been utilized to assist in symptom relief.
  - ❖ Not a primary treatment for HCM.
  - ❖ Some patients report improvement in symptoms with cardiac pacing.
  - ❖ Particular benefit noted for elderly patients older than age 65 (Maron et al., 2003).
  - ❖ Allows for more aggressive treatment with medications that can decrease heart rate.
- ◆ Ventricular Septal Myectomy
  - ❖ Indicated in marked outflow obstruction.
  - ❖ Surgical removal of a portion of the hypertrophied septum to enlarge the outflow tract (Figure 10.13)
  - ❖ Reserved for those patients on maximum medical therapy who continue to experience severely limiting symptoms and are classified as NYHA functional class III or IV (Maron et al., 2003).
  - ❖ Immediately decreases outflow tract obstruction and SAM of the anterior leaflet of the mitral valve.
  - ❖ Immediate improvement in symptoms.

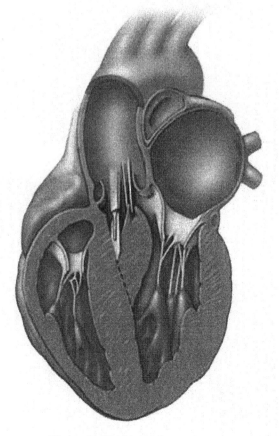

Figure 10.13: Surgical myectomy.
© 2007. All rights reserved.

- Improvements are sustained and may last as many as 30 years.
- Most patients improve from NYHA class III or IV to class II or III.
- Survival rates greater than 83% at 10 years (Salberg, 2004).
- Mitral valve replacement or repair may also occur during the procedure.
- Myectomy without valve replacement is becoming a low-risk procedure with a relatively low operative mortality rate with all age groups (Maron et al., 2003).
- May develop left bundle branch block as a result of the procedure, but pacemakers are rarely necessary.
- Open heart surgery procedure

◆ Percutaneous Alcohol Septal Ablation (PASA) (Figure 10.14)
- Nonsurgical alternative to septal myectomy.
- Indicated for symptomatic patients with obstruction who are NYHA class III or IV on maximum medical therapy (Maron et al., 2003).
- If mitral valve involvement is advanced and requires repair or replacement, then surgery is the preferable option.
- Less invasive procedure without the risks associated with a major surgery.
- May be appropriate for elderly patients who are not good operative candidates.
- Performed in the cardiac catheterization laboratory.
- Catheter is placed in the left anterior descending coronary artery. The catheter is then advanced into one of the septal perforator branches, which provides blood flow to the septum. Once the appropriate septal perforator is located, ethyl alcohol is injected (Figure 10.15). The alcohol infiltrates the surrounding myocardial tissue as a toxic agent and a controlled myocardial infarction occurs.
  ★ Infarcted septum does not contract, so outflow obstruction is reduced.

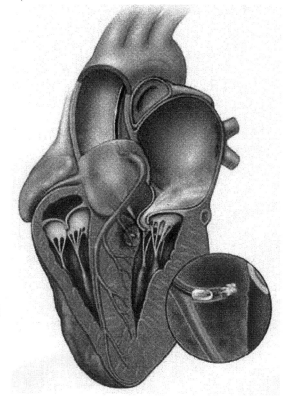

Figure 10.14: Alcohol septal ablation.
© 2007. All rights reserved.

- The enlarged septal tissue eventually shrinks and the outflow obstruction is relieved.
- Reduction in tissue size does not occur immediately and may actually continue to occur for up to 1 year after the procedure.
- In young patients, the benefits of the surgical procedure outweigh the post-procedure arrhythmia risk of PASA.
- A larger percentage of patients require permanent pacing after PASA than after myectomy.

Sudden Cardiac Death

On the whole, life expectancy in patients with HCM is normal; however, sudden cardiac death is the most serious complication of HCM. In most cases, sudden cardiac death is the event that leads to a diagnosis of HCM. Sudden cardiac death occurs most frequently in young people (less than age 35) who are asymptomatic or mildly symptomatic. However, the risk is not limited to this age group. Researchers continue to attempt to predict the HCM population that is at high risk for sudden cardiac death so that ICDs can be implanted. As risk criteria continues to be evaluated, most literature agrees that ICDs should be placed in any patient with an episode of sudden cardiac death, sustained ventricular tachycardia, or a family history of sudden cardiac death. Patients with other risk factors should not be eliminated from ICD consideration because multiple risk factors may warrant placement of a device. Medication to treat the ventricular arrhythmias should be utilized in conjunction with the ICD; amiodarone is the drug of choice.

Risk Factors for Sudden Cardiac Death In HCM/HOCM

- One or more 1st degree relative with an episode of SCD.
- Left-ventricular wall thickness greater than 35 mm.
- Prolonged or repetitive non-sustained ventricular tachycardia on Holter monitor.
- Hypotensive BP response to exercise.
- Syncope or near syncope.

Activity Recommendations

- Restricted from intense competitive sports.
- HCM is the most common cause of sudden cardiac death in young athletes, especially in football and basketball.
- Not all sudden cardiac death occurs with intense activity; in fact, sudden cardiac death can occur with rest. However, the incidence of sudden cardiac death increases with the intensity of the activity in the presence of HCM.
- Routine activity does not need to be avoided but should avoid "burst" exertion, such as sprinting, and isometric exercises, such as heavy lifting.
- Patient response to activity provides a guide for determining the level of activity that is acceptable. Development of chest pain, overt shortness of breath, and syncope may indicate that the activity is too strenuous.
- No evidence supports the exclusion from competitive sports of athletes with a family history of HCM, but no personal evidence of the disease.

Family Evaluation for HCM

HCM is largely a genetic disease process. If HCM is diagnosed or an HCM-related death occurs, all first-degree relatives should be screened for the disease and other blood relatives should be encouraged to undergo screening. The ACC/ESC Clinical Expert Consensus Document on Hypertrophic Cardiomyopathy recommends genetic testing, if available. If genetic testing is not feasible, a history and physical, 12-lead ECG and echocardiogram can be utilized for screening. These screenings should occur annually from ages 12 through 18. Delayed adult onset is also possible; therefore, relatives with normal studies through age 18 should have an evaluation every 5 years. Children under age 12 need not undergo evaluation unless there is a high-risk family profile, or the child is involved in intense competitive sports.

Chapter 10

Outcomes

The majority of patients with HCM can expect a normal life span if they survive past the age of 35 (Shah, 2003). Once diagnosed with the disease, routine follow-up every 12 to 18 months is recommended. Sudden cardiac death continues to be the primary cause of shortened life spans. Prevention and identification of risk for sudden cardiac death is a major area of focus. Many studies continue to increase the understanding of the genetic code and its impact on the disease process. Hopefully, these studies will provide the key to successful treatment in the future.

Conclusion

Cardiomyopathy impacts millions of people, including those who are diagnosed with these diseases and millions more who are related to them and care for them during debilitating years. Early recognition of the disease process, in conjunction with good medical follow-up and patient compliance with treatment strategies and risk factor adjustments, can improve long-term outcomes. Every health care professional caring for patients will come in contact with someone with cardiomyopathy at some point in his or her career. A good base knowledge of these disease processes helps with early recognition and improves outcomes for such patients.

Linking Knowledge to Practice

✔ *ECF volume balance in patients with HCM is critical. Because the ventricular chamber is no longer able to expand during filling, the ventricle must fill fully in order to produce adequate stroke volume.*

✔ *The development of atrial fibrillation results in a loss of atrial kick. Without atrial kick, ventricular filling (preload) decreases, with an associated decrease in stroke volume.*

✔ *Beta blockers can cause fatigue, impotence, and sleep disturbances, especially with initial dosing. These symptoms generally ease, especially the fatigue, over time as the patient's body adjusts to the medication. Patients should be made aware of these effects and encouraged to continue the medication as the body adjusts to the changes*

✔ *Implantation of an ICD is a very emotional process, and patients should be provided with emotional support. Many facilities that place ICDs are aware of an ICD support group that can be helpful to patients dealing with the emotions associated with sudden death and implantation of this device.*

ARRHYTHMOGENIC CARDIOMYOPATHY

This type of cardiomyopathy is an inherited muscle disorder that may manifest as an arrhythmia, heart failure, or sudden death. In the majority of families, the genetic characteristics include autosomal dominance inheritance with incomplete penetration. This type of cardiomyopathy most frequently affects the right ventricle and is often referred to as arrhythmogenic right-ventricular cardiomyopathy. However, there have been some cases of arrhythmogenic left-ventricular cardiomyopathy.

Pathophysiology

The key pathological findings in arrhythmogenic cardiomyopathy include progressive loss of cardiomyocytes, followed by replacement with fibrofatty tissue. Fibrofatty replacement of muscle tissue is also observed in muscular dystrophies, and arrhythmogenic cardiomyopathy may be associated with some forms of muscular dystrophy. The thinnest portions of the right ventricle are usually affected first. The initial changes usually occur in the inflow, outflow, and apical regions of the right ventricle. This area has been called the triangle of dyplasia. When the left ventricle is involved, the changes usually impact the thinner posterior lateral wall. The thicker wall of the septum is usually not affected.

Cardiomyopathy

There are several factors that contribute to the arrhythmogenic qualities of this type of cardiomyopathy.

◆ Multiple bouts of myocarditis promote arrhythmias. A bout of myocarditis can trigger myocyte loss and inflammation in a previously unaffected area of the myocardium.

◆ Altered mechanical coupling can cause gap junction remodeling. Cardiac myocytes rely on the intercalated discs for both electrical and mechanical coupling. Desmosomes are one of the types of cells within the intercalated discs. Impaired desmosome functioning during mechanical stress is thought to be responsible for myocyte detachment and eventual myocyte death. Arrhythmogenic cardiomyopathy is sometimes called the disease of the desmosome. Athletes usually have more severe forms of the disease, which is attributed to the increased mechanical stress on the heart.

◆ Cardiomyocytes have a poor ability to regenerate; to compensate, fibrofatty tissue is used to replace the lost cells. Fibrofatty infiltrates lead to the development of macro re-entrant circuits.

Aneurysm formation is common in the disease because there is non-uniform mechanical stress on the heart leading to regionally affected areas. As the disease progresses, more diffuse involvement can lead to right-ventricular dilation. In very advanced disease, the left ventricle can also become involved.

Disease Progression

In the most severe form of the disease there are four distinct phases. There are also other common forms of the disease that do not progress through the classic four phases. The classic four phases of severe disease are:

◆ Early: This phase is often called the concealed phase because patients may be asymptomatic. In this phase, however, patients may still be at high risk for sudden death, especially those who engage in intense physical activities.

◆ Overt electrical disorder: During this phase, patients experience symptomatic right-ventricular arrhythmias. They may also experience symptoms ranging from palpitations to syncope. During this phase, changes in the right ventricle can also be seen during imaging studies.

◆ Impaired contractility and right-sided heart failure are the hallmarks of the third phase.

◆ In the fourth and final stage of the disease, both ventricles are involved, and bi-ventricular failure occurs.

Diagnosis

◆ Arrhythmogenic cardiomyopathy is difficult to diagnose in the concealed stage.

◆ The primary diagnostic challenge is making the distinction between arrhythmogenic cardiomyopathy and dilated cardiomyopathy.

◆ Predominant right-ventricular involvement is common with arrhythmogenic cardiomyopathy, but arrhythmogenic cardiomyopathy may affect the left ventricle and, therefore, primary right-ventricular involvement cannot be used as strict diagnostic criteria.

◆ Fibrofatty infiltrates are one of the key pathological findings in arrhythmogenic cardiomyopathy. However, fatty infiltrates may also be seen in relatively healthy hearts in the elderly.

◆ Regional ventricular involvement and aneurysm formation are other assessment-finding characteristic of arrhythmogenic cardiomyopathy.

◆ The key differential factor between arrhythmogenic cardiomyopathy and dilated cardiomyopathy is that those with arrhythmogenic cardiomyopathy are at risk for ventricular arrhythmias and sudden death, even without significant left-ventricular dysfunction. Although sudden cardiac death is a complication in patients with dilated cardiomyopathy, the risk is typically associated with significant left-ventricular dysfunction. Sudden death is rarely the initial presentation of dilated cardiomyopathy. In arrhythmogenic cardiomyopathy, sudden death is the first clinical presentation in more than half of the patients (Sen-Chowdry, Syrris, & McKenna, 2005).

- Not all patients with arrhythmogenic cardiomyopathy will present with ventricular arrhythmias, so familial evaluation is also important in known families.

Clinical Manifestations

- ECG (right precordial leads V_1-V_3)
  - Delayed depolarization.
  - Epsilon waves (notch at the end of the QRS complex).
  - Inverted T waves.
- Imaging Studies
  - RV dilation.
  - Wall motion abnormalities.
  - Systolic dysfunction.
- Right ventricular tachycardia
  - Sustained monomorphic ventricular tachycardia is attributed to the re-entrant circuits created by the fibrofatty infiltrates.
  - A stimulus such as myocarditis may trigger sudden death in a previously silent disease state. Gap junction remodeling may also explain the arrhythmias that cause an episode of sudden death in a patient in the concealed stage of the disease.

Idiopathic right-ventricular outflow tract tachycardia mimics arrhythmogenic right-ventricular cardiomyopathy (Figure 10.15). Idiopathic right ventricular outflow tract tachycardia (Figure 10.16) differs in that it is a relatively benign disorder with no genetic or familial component.

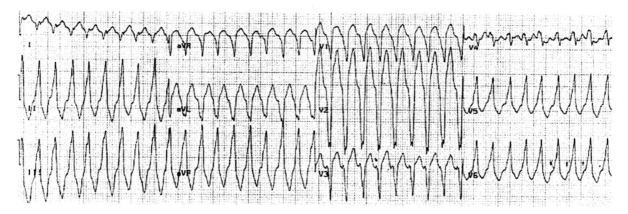

Figure 10.15: Right-ventricular outflow tract tachycardia in a patient diagnosed with arrhythmogenic cardiomyopathy

Cardiomyopathy

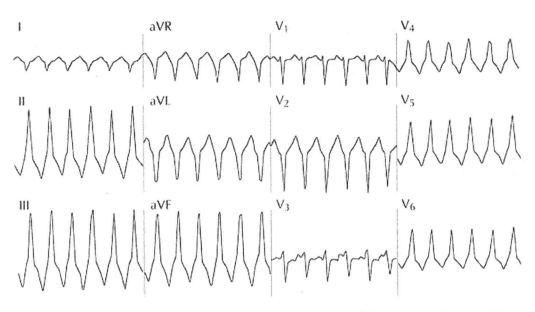

Figure 10.16: Idiopathic right-ventricular outflow tract tachycardia in a structurally normal heart

Treatment

Treatment is aimed at the prevention of sudden cardiac death. Implantation of an implantable cardiovertor-defibrillator is the treatment of choice. Catheter ablation has been found to be unsuccessful in eliminating ventricular arrhythmias due to the progressive nature of the disease process.

TEST YOUR KNOWLEDGE

1. In caring for a patient with hypertrophic cardiomyopathy, you are aware that the following medications may be used in treatment:

    a. Beta blockers

    b. Calcium channel blockers

    c. Digoxin

    d. a and b

    e. All of the above.

2. When caring for a patient with hypertrophic cardiomyopathy you know the following classes of medications need to be avoided or administered with extreme caution:

    a. Venous vasodilators

    b. Antiplatelets

    c. Diuretics

    d. a and c

    e. b and c

Chapter 10

3. The following statements are true regarding dilated cardiomyopathy:
   a. It may be caused by alcoholism or an infectious process.
   b. It has a clinical presentation similar to heart failure.
   c. Atrial fibrillation is common.
   d. All of the above.

4. Restrictive cardiomyopathy mimics this type of heart failure:
   a. Systolic dysfunction
   b. Diastolic dysfunction

5. The primary pathophysiological change associated with dilated cardiomyopathy is
   a. ventricular dilation with decreased ventricular contraction.
   b. decreased ventricular chamber size with decreased ventricular filling.
   c. obstruction of the left ventricular outflow tract.
   d. decreased ventricular filling.

6. The primary treatment goals for dilated cardiomyopathy include treatment of arrhythmias, thromboembolic complications, the underlying disease process, and
   a. reduction of diastolic dysfunction.
   b. reduction of preload.
   c. reduction of contractility.
   d. increased afterload.

7. Which of the following medications should be avoided in the patient with hypertrophic cardiomyopathy who has obstruction (HOCM)?
   a. Beta blockers
   b. Calcium channel blockers
   c. Positive inotropes
   d. Negative inotropes

8. Which of the following disease processes can mimic restrictive cardiomyopathy and should be eliminated as a possible diagnosis when evaluating the patient?
   a. Aortic stenosis
   b. Myocarditis
   c. Constrictive pericarditis
   d. Infective endocarditis

9. This type of cardiomyopathy is characterized by a replacement of cardiomyocytes with fibrofatty tissue:

   a. Arrhythomogenic cardiomyopathy

   b. Hypertrophic cardiomyopathy

   c. Restrictive cardiomyopathy

   d. Dilated cardiomyopathy

10. The primary diagnosis challenge in arrhythmogenic cardiomyopathy is the differentiation from dilated cardiomyopathy. The key differentiating factor is those with arrhythmogenic cardiomyopathy

    a. are at risk for ventricular arrhythmias and sudden cardiac death due to significant left ventricular dysfunction.

    b. are at risk for ventricular arrhythmias and sudden cardiac death even without significant left ventricular dysfunction.

    c. only experience the effects of the disease process in the right ventricle.

    d. only experience the effects of the disease process in the left ventricle.

ANSWERS

1. D
2. D
3. D
4. B
5. A
6. B
7. C
8. C
9. A
10. B

REFERENCES

Bozkurt, B. & Mann, D.L. (2000). Dilated cardiomyopathy. In J.T. Willerson & J.N. Cohn, (Eds.), *Cardiovascular medicine* (2nd ed., pp. 1034-1053). New York: Churchill Livingston.

Carabello, B.A. & Ganzes, P.C. (2001). *Cardiology pearls* (2nd ed.). Philadelphia: Hanley and Belfus.

Carroll, J.D. & Crawford, M.H. (2003). Restrictive myopathy. In M.H. Crawford (Ed.), *Current diagnosis and treatment in cardiology* (2nd ed., pp. 1188-195). New York: McGraw Hill.

Celebi, M. (2004). Cardiomyopathy, dilated. Retrieved December 19, 2004 from http://www.emedicine.com/med/topic289.htm

Chapter 10

Chen, M.S. & Levere, H.M. (2003). *Hypertrophic cardiomyopathy.* Retrieved November 28, 2004, from http://www.clevelandclinicmeded.com

Crawford, M.H. (2004). *Essentials of diagnosis and treatment in cardiology.* New York: McGraw-Hill.

ElSakr, A., Clark, L.T., & Loghin, C., (2001). Hypertrophic cardiomyopathy. In A.V. Adair (Ed.) *Cardiology secrets* (pp.161-165). Philadelphia: Hanley and Belfus, Inc.

Goswami, G., Reddy, S., & Kuwajerwala, N.K. (2003). Cardiomyopathy, restrictive. Retrieved December 19, 2004 from http://www.emedicine.com/med/topic291.htm

Hunt, S.A., Abraham, W.T., Chin, M.H., Feldman, A.M., Francis, G.S., Ganiats, T.G., Jessup, M., Konstam, M.A., Mancini, D.M., Michl, K., Oates, J.A., Rahko, P.S., Silver, M.A., Stevenson, L.W., & Yancy, C.W. ACC/AHA 2005 guideline update for the diagnosis and management of chronic heart failure in the adult: A report of the American College of Cardiology/American Heart Association Task Force on Practice Guidelines (Writing Committee to Update the 2001 Guidelines for the Evaluation and Management of Heart Failure). American College of Cardiology Web Site. Available at: http://www.acc.org/clinical/guidelines/failure//index.pdf

Kavinsky, C.J. & Parrillo, J.E. (2000). Severe heart failure in cardiomyopathy: Pathogenesis and treatment. In A. Grenvik, S.M. Ayers, P.R. Holbrook, & W.C. Shoemaker (Eds.), *Textbook of critical care* (4th ed., pp. 1105-1116). Philadelphia: W.B. Saunders Company.

Loghin, C., (2001). Dilated cardiomyopathy. In A.V. Adair (Ed.), *Cardiology secrets* (pp. 156-160). Philadelphia: Hanley and Belfus, Inc. Aug 7, 349(6), 523-34.

Maron, B.J., McKenna, W.J., Danielson, G.K., Kapperberger, L.J., Kuhn, H.J., Seidman, C.E., Shah, P.M., Spencer, W.H., Spirito, P., Ten Cate, F.J., Wigle, E.D. ACC/ESC clinical expert consensus document on hypertrophic cardiomyopathy: a report of the American College of Cardiology Task Force on Clinical Expert Consensus Documents and the European Society of Cardiology Committee for Practice Guidelines (Committee to Develop an Expert Consensus Document on Hypertrophic Cardiomyopathy). *J Am Coll Cardiol,* 2003, 42, 1687-713.

Maron, B.J., Towbin, J.A., Thiene, G., Antzelevitch, C., Corrado, D., Arnett, D., Moss, A.J., Seidman, C.E., & Young, J.B. Contemporary Definitions and Classification of the Cardiomyopathies: An American Heart Association Scientific Statement From the Council on Clinical Cardiology, Heart Failure and Transplantation Committee; Quality of Care and Outcomes Research and Functional Genomics and Translational Biology Interdisciplinary Working Groups; and Council on Epidemiology and Prevention Circulation, Apr 2006, 113, 1807-1816.

Murphy-Lavoie, H. & Preston, C.P. (2004). Cardiomyopathy, dilated. Retrieved November 11, 2004 from http://www.emedicine.com/emerg/topic80.htm

Nishimura, R.A. & Holmes, D.R., Jr. (2004, March 25). Hypertrophic obstructive cardiomyopathy. *The New England Journal of Medicine, 350,* 1320-1330.

Ommen, S.R. & Nishimura, R.A. (2001). *Treatment of patients with hypertrophic cardiomyopathy: A clinician's guide.* Retrieved 12/31/04 from http://www.mayoclinic.org/hypertrophic-cardiomyopathy/physiciansguide/html

O'Neill, J.O. & Bott-Silverman, C. (2003). *Dilated and restrictive cardiomyopathies.* Retrieved November 11, 2004 from http://www.clevelandclinicmeded.com

Cardiomyopathy

Opie, L.H. (2004). *Heart physiology from cell to circulation* (4th ed.). Philadelphia: Lippincott, Williams and Wilkins.

Porth, C.M. (Ed.) (2004). *Essentials of pathophysiology: Concepts of altered health states*. Philadelphia: Lippincott, Williams and Wilkins.

Salberg, L. (2004). How to choose a septal reduction method. From the Hypertrophic Cardiomyopathy Association. Retrieved December 31, 2004 from http://www.enewsbuilder.net

Sen-Chowdry, S., Syrris, P., & McKenna, W.J. (2005). The genetics of right ventricular cardiomyopathy. *Journal of Cardiovascular Electrophysiology, 16*(8), 927-935.

Shah, P. (2003). Hypertrophic cardiomyopathies. In M. Crawford (Ed.), *Current diagnosis and treatment in cardiology* (2nd ed., pp. 179-187). New York: McGraw Hill.

CHAPTER 11:
VALVE DISEASE

Proper functioning of the cardiac valves allows blood to flow smoothly in a forward direction through the atria and ventricles of the heart. Normal valve function is essential for a normal cardiac output. Impedance of forward flow, or the backward flow of volume that should be moving forward, can greatly decrease cardiac output. Compensatory changes with chronic valve disease occur over many years and in some cases decades before any symptoms develop. Early recognition of cardiac valve disease is the key to treatment. Cardiac auscultation is the primary method used for screening all patients and will alert the practitioner to the development of valve disease. Careful, routine follow up of patients with known cardiac valve disease provides the information needed to determine when valve replacement or repair is appropriate. With a limited lifespan, prosthetic valves should not be implanted until necessary; therefore valves are not generally replaced until the patient develops symptoms of valve disease or has severe disease by echocardiography. However, if the valve disease is not identified early through routine cardiac auscultation the patient cannot be educated on signs and symptoms to look for indicating a worsening of the valve disease, nor will they have the benefit of routine follow up with echocardiography to identify the progression to severe valve disease.

The ACC/AHA 2006 guidelines for the management of patients with valvular heart disease note that murmurs are due to three factors: 1) high blood flow rate through normal or abnormal orifices, 2) forward flow through a narrowed or irregular orifice into a dilated vessel or chamber, and 3) backward or regurgitant flow through an incompetent valve (Bonow et al, 2006). A cardiac murmur may or may not be related to an abnormal cardiac valve. There are many systolic murmurs that are the related to processes other than cardiac valve disease resulting in an increase in blood flow. Cardiac echocardiography is a reliable tool to determine the cause of a cardiac murmur and can be especially useful in the assessment of a systolic murmur. Diastolic murmurs, however, nearly always represent abnormal valve pathology and baseline echocardiography should be obtained so disease progression can be followed.

NORMAL VALVE FUNCTION

There are two atrioventricular (AV) valves and two semilunar valves in the heart. The AV valves are the tricuspid valve located between the right atrium and the right ventricle, and the mitral valve located between the left atrium and the left ventricle. The semilunar valves are the pulmonic valve located between the right ventricle and the pulmonary artery, and the aortic valve located between the left ventricle and the aorta.

Normal Function of the Valves in Relation to the Cardiac Cycle (Figure 11.1)

The normal opening and closing of the valves is dependent on pressure changes in the atria, the ventricles and the circulatory system throughout the cardiac cycle. There are four major components of the cardiac cycle.

◆ Cardiac Diastole (Figure 11.1A): Passive ventricular filling from atria
  ❖ Mitral and tricuspid valves are open and the pulmonic and aortic valves are closed.
  ❖ Blood passively leaves the atria to fill the ventricles.

Chapter 11

- ❖ This part of the cardiac cycle is also referred to as early diastolic filling time or early diastole.
- ❖ 70%-75% of ventricular filling occurs passively during this stage.
- ◆ Atrial Systole and Ventricular Diastole (Figure 11.1B): Active Ventricular Filling with Atrial Contraction – Atrial Kick
    - ❖ During the second part of ventricular diastole, the atria contract to propel the rest of the atrial contents into the ventricle.
    - ❖ Atrial contraction is known as "atrial kick."
    - ❖ This part of the cardiac cycle is also referred to as late diastolic filling time.
    - ❖ 25%-30% of ventricular filling occurs actively during this stage.
    - ❖ The pulmonic and aortic valves remain closed.
- ◆ Early Ventricular Systole (Figure 11.1C): Isovolumic (or Isovolumetric) Contraction
    - ❖ The walls of the ventricle begin to contract, causing an increase in ventricular pressure.
    - ❖ The mitral and tricuspid valves close when pressure in the ventricles becomes greater than pressure in the atria.
    - ❖ This part of the cardiac cycle is referred to as "isovolumic contraction" or "isovolumetric contraction" because there is no change in volume in the ventricles during this part of ventricular systole.
    - ❖ All four cardiac valves are closed.

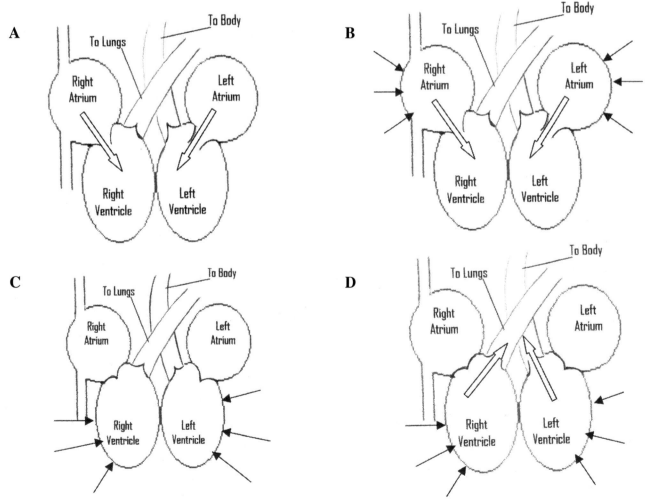

Figure 11.1: The cardiac cycle (A, B, C, D).

- ❖ When pressure in the ventricle becomes greater than the pressure on the other side of its semilunar valve, the valve is forced open.
  - ☆ The right ventricle opposes the pulmonic valve and pulmonary vascular resistance.
  - ☆ The left ventricle opposes the left ventricular outflow track, the aortic valve, aortic pressure and systemic vascular resistance (SVR).
- ❖ 70% of myocardial oxygen consumption occurs during this portion of the cardiac cycle.
- ◆ Ventricular Systole (Figure 11.1D): Ejection
  - ❖ Blood is ejected from the ventricles through the pulmonic and aortic valves into the pulmonary and peripheral vascular systems.
- ◆ Early Ventricular Diastole: Isovolumic Relaxation
  - ❖ Ventricular pressure begins to fall and becomes less than the pressure in the pulmonary arterial system and the systemic arterial system.
  - ❖ Ventricular pressure continues to fall, and for a period of time, all valves are closed.
  - ❖ When ventricular pressure falls below atrial pressure, the tricuspid and mitral valves open and the cycle repeats.

AORTIC VALVE DISEASE

Normal Aortic Valve

Normal Structure (Figure 11.2)

- ◆ Semilunar valve.
- ◆ Located between the left ventricle and the aorta.
- ◆ Three cusps or leaflets open and close based on pressure changes in the aorta and left ventricle.
- ◆ Valve annulus is the cartilaginous "ring" at the base of the valve that helps the valve maintain its shape.
- ◆ Valve Commissures – the point at which the cusps join together at the level of the annulus.

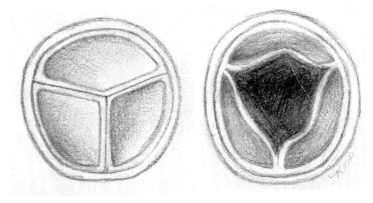

Figure 11.2: Normal aortic valve closed (left) and open (right).

Aortic Recoil and Coronary Artery Perfusion (Figure 11.3).

Ejection of blood from the left ventricle through the aortic valve to the aorta causes the normal compliant aorta to distend as it accepts the volume from the ventricle. At the end of ventricular ejection, the pressure in the aorta becomes greater than the pressure in the left ventricle. Once this pressure gradient occurs, the walls of the distended aorta naturally recoil, displacing blood forward and backward. The forward displacement of

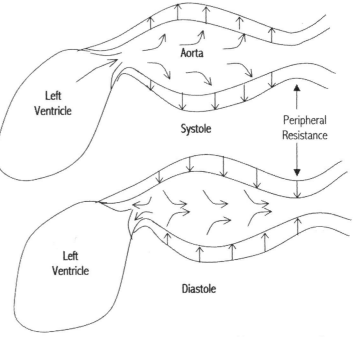

Figure 11.3: Aortic recoil.

blood provides cardiac output to the systemic system. The backward displacement of blood towards the aortic valve forces the normal aortic valve to rapidly close and prevent backflow of blood into the left ventricle. The blood that is displaced backwards collects at the cusps of the aortic valve where the origins to the right and left coronary artery are located (Figure 11.4). This system provides highly oxygenated blood to fill the coronary arteries during diastole.

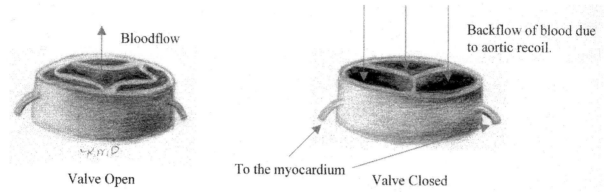

Figure 11.4: Perfusion to the coronary arteries.

Aortic Stenosis (AS)

Aortic stenosis occurs when there is an abnormality impeding the normal flow of blood across the aortic valve. Impedance to normal flow occurs when there is constriction or narrowing of the aortic valve opening.

Classification of Aortic Stenosis

Aortic valve stenosis is classified as congenital or acquired.

- Congenital
  - Most common cause of AS in men under the age of 70.
  - More prevalent in men than women.
  - Abnormal number of valve cusps (unicuspid, bicuspid, tricuspid, or even quadricuspid).
  - Symptoms can appear between ages 40 and 60 in patients who have had murmurs for years (Novaro & Mills, 2004).
- Acquired
  - Most common cause of symptom-producing aortic stenosis in patients over age 70 (Havranek & Adair, 2001).
  - Two causes for acquired aortic stenosis.
    - Rheumatic Heart Disease
      - Fibrosis of valve leaflets with fusion of the commissures present.
      - Occasionally calcification of valve occurs.
      - Fibrotic leaflets are unable to open completely.
      - Accompanied by mitral valve disease – if no mitral valve disease then cause of aortic stenosis considered nonrheumatic.
      - The incidence of rheumatic aortic valve disease has decreased due to decrease in the incidence of rheumatic heart disease in this country.
    - Senile Degenerative Calcification
      - Develop calcified nodules on the valve leaflets.

Valve Disease

✳ Thickened leaflets.
✳ Progressive calcification and thickening results in stiff valve leaflets that do not move easily.
✳ Aortic valve does not open easily or fully.
✳ Development of concomitant aortic regurgitation is not uncommon in late stages.
✳ Most common form of AS in patients > 70 years (Carabello & Crawford, 2003).
✳ More common in men than women.
✳ Most common reason for aortic valve surgery (Carabello & Crawford, 2003).
✳ Higher incidence in the following population (LeDoux, 2005):
  – elevated lipoprotein and low-density lipoprotein cholesterol levels.
  – hypertension.
  – diabetes.
  – elevated serum calcium levels.
  – elevated serum creatinine levels.

Pathophysiology

Blood flow through the abnormal aortic valve becomes turbulent and less efficient. The left ventricle must work harder to eject blood across the stiff, noncompliant valve. As valve compliance decreases, afterload (pressure the left ventricle must overcome to eject blood) increases. In an effort to compensate for the increase in afterload, the left ventricular wall mass (myocardial wall thickness) increases in size, resulting in progressive concentric left ventricular hypertrophy. Concentric hypertrophy is characterized by increasing left ventricular wall mass with no increase in ventricular chamber size. In fact, the increasing muscle mass may begin to encroach on the chamber and ultimately decrease the size of the intraventricular chamber.

As the left ventricular wall becomes thicker, an associated decrease in the ability of the ventricular wall to expand normally during ventricular filling occurs. An inability to expand normally during ventricular filling is referred to as "diastolic dysfunction" and results in decreased ventricular filling during ventricular diastole. With less volume entering the ventricle, there is less volume available for ejection during systole. The ventricle normally ejects 55% to 65% of its contents with each beat. Now, however, the thickened myocardium compensates with a stronger contraction and ejects a larger percentage of the decreased volume, thereby maintaining good cardiac output. As the disease progresses, the left ventricle's attempt to compensate ultimately fails and left ventricular contractile function begins to decrease. This decrease in contractile function results in decreased stroke volume, leaving the ventricle with an excess volume at the end of each contraction. The left ventricle experiences volume overload, the overload is transferred to the left atrium, and ultimately to the lungs, as signs of heart failure begin.

Compensatory Mechanisms In Aortic Stenosis

◆ ↑ Left ventricular afterload
  → ↑ Left ventricular workload
    → ↑ Left ventricular wall mass
      → LV hypertrophy
        → Diastolic dysfunction.
◆ Compensatory system ultimately fails → Left ventricular failure → Heart failure.

Chapter 11

Symptoms

As the obstruction to flow from the left ventricle continues to increase, so does left ventricular mass. This ability to compensate can last many years before symptoms appear. Symptoms generally begin to appear when the valve opening is one-third its normal size. Once symptoms appear, mortality rates rise greatly. The mortality rate in patients with moderate to severe aortic stenosis treated medically is 50% within 2 to 3 years from the onset of symptoms (Darovic, 2002). Generally, after the sixth decade of life, a trio of classic symptoms occurs: angina, syncope, and heart failure.

◆ *Angina.* Angina results from an imbalance in myocardial oxygen supply and demand. The increased left ventricular wall mass (hypertrophy) increases left ventricular myocardial oxygen demand. While the patient is at rest, blood supply may be adequate to meet the body's needs. However, with stress or exercise, the increased myocardial oxygen needs of the thickened ventricular wall are no longer met, resulting in angina. Commonly, angina during exercise is the first presenting symptom in aortic stenosis. Angina can, of course, be caused by coronary artery disease (CAD) in addition to increased wall mass. Approximately one half of aortic stenosis patients presenting with angina also have CAD (Massie & Amiodon, 2004).

◆ *Syncope.* The normal vascular response to exercise is arterial vasodilation with an increase in heart rate. Arterial dilation occurs not only in the large arteries but also in the arterioles to provide adequate perfusion to all tissues and muscles during exercise. Arterial vasodilation causes the blood pressure to decrease. The heart rate increases to provide the cardiac output needed to meet the additional metabolic demands of the body and compensate for the arterial vasodilation. This system keeps blood pressure in a normal range and allows patients to tolerate the exercise while providing the body with an increased flow of oxygenated blood. With the narrowed valve opening, it is essentially impossible to increase cardiac output because the restriction of the valve does not allow for increased blood flow across the valve. Patients with severe aortic stenosis experience decreased blood pressure during exercise, resulting in dizziness, light-headedness, and blackout spells. In patients with aortic stenosis, exercise can also cause ventricular or atrial arrhythmias, resulting in syncopal episodes.

◆ *Heart Failure.* Patients with severe aortic stenosis ultimately develop diastolic and systolic failure. Left ventricular hypertrophy results in diastolic dysfunction as the thick-walled ventricle becomes noncompliant and loses its ability to expand during filling. This inability to expand decreases the amount of blood that can enter the left ventricle from the left atrium, resulting in a back up of blood into the left atrium. The subsequent overload in the left atrium is transferred back to the pulmonary veins, and pulmonary edema results. Additionally, over time, the hypertrophy that has been compensating for the increased afterload causes the myofibrils to stretch beyond the point of returning to a normal state. The ability of the ventricle to contract decreases and ejection fraction begins to decline. This decrease in ejection fraction results in a state of extracellular fluid (ECF) overload because the ventricle is unable to empty properly. The patient experiences dyspnea on exertion, orthopnea, and paroxysmal nocturnal dyspnea, as well as other signs of volume overload.

Physical Examination

◆ Systolic Ejection Murmur (Figure 11.5)

❖ May be present before any significant hemodynamic changes occur.

❖ Intensity (loudness) of murmur does not correspond with severity of aortic stenosis. Intensity increases with the patient sitting up and leaning forward.

❖ As AS becomes more severe the murmur will peak later as well as last longer – S2 may not be audible in severe AS.

- Timing: Midsystolic.
- Location: Best heard over aortic area (2nd intercostal space, right sternal border).
- Radiation: Towards neck, shoulders and carotid areas. May also radiate to apex (5th intercostal space, left midclavicular line), resulting in a misinterpretation of mitral regurgitation.
- Configuration: Crescendo-decrescendo.
- Pitch: Medium to high. Heard equally well with bell or diaphragm of stethoscope.
- Quality: Harsh.

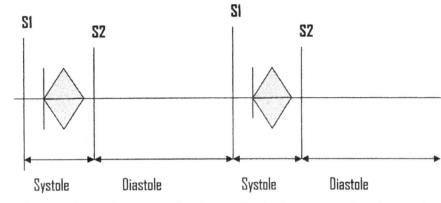

Figure 11.5: Drawing representing the systolic ejection murmur of aortic stenosis.

◆ S4 – Atrial Gallop (Figure 11.6)
- Fourth heart sound.
- Caused by atrial contraction and the propulsion of blood into a noncompliant ventricle.
- Best heard with patient in left lateral position.
- Timing: Late diastolic filling sound, just before S1.
- Location: Mitral area (5th intercostal space, mid-clavicular line).
- Intensity: Louder during expiration.
- Duration: Short.
- Quality: Thud-like.
- Pitch: Low.
- Best heard with bell of stethoscope.

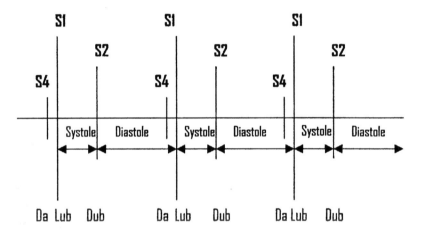

Figure 11.6: Drawing indicating the location of an S4 in relation to a normal S1 and S2.

◆ S3 – Ventricular Gallop (Figure 11.7)
- Third heart sound.
- Caused when atria passively empty into a fluid overloaded ventricle.
- Should resolve when fluid overload state resolves.
- Best heard with patient in left lateral position.
- Timing: Early diastolic filling sound, just after S2.

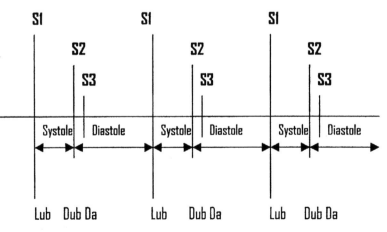

Figure 11.7: Drawing indicating the location of an S3 in relation to a normal S1 and S2.

- Location: Mitral area (5th intercostal space, mid-clavicular line).
- Intensity: Loudest during expiration.
- Duration: Short.
- Quality: Dull, thud-like.
- Pitch: Low.
- Best heard with bell of stethoscope.
- Pulse sharpness
  - Decrease in sharpness of pulse upstroke as aortic stenosis worsens.
  - Due to delay in the rush of blood through the slowly opening aortic valve.

Diagnosis

- Cardiac Echocardiogram
  - Primary tool utilized to confirm the diagnosis of aortic stenosis.
  - Quantifies severity of stenosis.
  - Evaluation of pressure gradient (Bonow et al, 2006) – difference in pressure from one side of the valve to the other.
    - As disease progresses, peak aortic systolic pressure (PASP) becomes lower than peak left ventricular pressure (PLVP).
    - Mild AS   Mean Gradient < 25 mm Hg
    - Moderate AS   Mean Gradient 25-40 mm Hg
    - Severe AS   Mean Gradient > 40 mm Hg (PLVP 40 mm Hg > PASP).
  - Evaluation of Valve Area (Bonow et al., 2006).
    - Normal valve area ranges from 3 cm^2 to 4 cm^2
    - Change in flow across the valve occurs when valve area is one forth the normal size.
    - Normal   Valve area 3.0-4.0 cm^2
    - Mild AS   Valve area >1.5 cm^2
    - Moderate AS   Valve area 1.0 to 1.5 cm^2
    - Severe AS   Valve area <1.0 cm^2
  - Evaluation of Jet Velocity (Bonow et al., 2006).
    - Evaluated with Doppler echocardiography.
    - Directly related to valve gradient and valve area.
    - Increases as gradient increases and valve area decreases.
    - Mild AS   < 3.0 m/second
    - Moderate AS   3.0-4.0 m/second
    - Severe AS   > 4.0 m/second.
  - Evaluation of Valve Leaflets for:
    - Thickening of valve leaflets.
    - Decreased mobility of valve leaflets.
    - Calcification of valve cusps.
  - Evaluation of Left Ventricular Function for:
    - Concentric hypertrophy.
    - Left ventricular chamber size (usually normal).
    - Diastolic dysfunction.

Valve Disease

- Stress Testing
  - May be beneficial to assess for:
    - Limited exercise capacity.
    - Abnormal blood pressure response to exercise.
    - Exercise induced symptoms -angina, ST segment abnormalities (Bonow et al., 2006).
  - **SHOULD NOT** be performed on patients with aortic stenosis who have presented with symptoms or have severe AS by echocardiogram as the patient is at high risk for developing syncope during the stress test (Bonow et al., 2006).
- Cardiac Catheterization
  - Required for patients with symptomatic aortic stenosis.
  - Determine extent, if any, of coronary artery disease prior to valve replacement.
  - The presence of operable coronary artery disease in a patient with asymptomatic aortic stenosis will support a decision to replace the valve in asymptomatic patients.
  - Pressure gradients can also be evaluated to verify echocardiographic results.
  - Injection of dye during cardiac catheterization causes arterial dilation and can result in loss of an adequate blood pressure in the patient with severe AS.
- Electrocardiogram
  - ECG changes are neither sensitive nor specific to aortic stenosis and always require other testing for confirmation.
  - Left ventricular hypertrophy with or without strain may be present.
    - Some patients with severe aortic stenosis do not show clear ECG evidence of hypertrophy.
  - Conduction defects may be present depending on significance of aortic stenosis.
    - 1st degree heart block.
    - Left bundle branch block.
- Chest X-ray
  - Heart: Normal size.
  - Concentric hypertrophy: rounded left ventricular border.
  - Calcification of the valve may be visible on the lateral view.

Medical Treatment

Medical treatment, beyond the occasional need for rate control with atrial fibrillation, is rarely needed early in the disease process. Medications temporarily resolve heart failure; however, if the valve is not replaced, failure worsens, and death is the end result.

- Angiotensin-Converting Enzyme Inhibitors
  - Arterial vasodilator – decreased SVR.
  - Contraindicated in patients with severe aortic stenosis due to the resulting decrease in SVR.
  - Decreased SVR decreases blood pressure. Normal response to decreased SVR is an increase in heart rate to compensate for the decrease in blood pressure. A severely stenotic valve prevents larger volumes of blood from being forced through the valve, resulting in an inability to increase cardiac output. The patient develops hypotension, and syncope could result.
- Nitroglycerin
  - Use nitrates cautiously in severe aortic stenosis.
  - Low-dose nitroglycerin venous vasodilates resulting in a decrease in preload and consequently

Chapter 11

decreased left ventricular filling. In the patient with diastolic dysfunction preload is already compromised due to the decreased ability to stretch during filling. The patient with severe AS is more dependent on preload and even small decreases in filling volumes can result in decreased cardiac output.

❖ Nitroglycerin at high doses (>1mcg/kg/min) causes arterial dilation and decreases SVR with effects similar to the effects of ACE inhibitors (Balentine & Eisenhart, 2005).

◆ Beta blockers

❖ Contraindicated in patients with severe aortic stenosis.

❖ Blocks the normal adrenergic response that occurs to compensate for decreased cardiac output (increased heart rate and contractility) and lessens the ability of the ventricle to overcome the pressure gradient that has developed (LeDoux, 2005).

◆ Antibiotic Prophylaxis to Prevent Endocarditis

❖ This discussion on antibiotic prophylaxis to prevent endocarditis is pertinent to all patients with valve disease.

❖ The blood flow through the abnormal valve results in hemodynamic turbulence of blood across the valve. The hemodynamic turbulence provides an environment that supports the attachment of platelets and fibrin at the valve with the development of a platelet-fibrin thrombus (vegetation) that is prone to the adherence of bacteria if it is introduced into the system.

❖ In April 2007, the American Heart Association published new guidelines for the prevention of endocarditis. These guidelines significantly alter the past practices related to antibiotic administration prior to specific procedures in patients who were felt to be at high risk for the development of infective endocarditis. Within the new guidelines the committee noted that it is no longer reasonable to believe that antimicrobial prophylaxis is effective in the prevention of infective endocarditis associated with dental, GI or GU procedures (Wilson, Taubert, Gewitz, Lockhart, Baddour, Levison, et al., 2007). The guidelines provide the following as rationale for the changes to the guidelines:

1. Infective endocarditis is much more likely to result from frequent exposure to random bacteremias associated with daily activities than from bacteremia caused by a dental, GI tract, or GU tract procedure.

2. Prophylaxis may prevent an exceedingly small number of cases of infective endocarditis, if any, in individuals who undergo dental, GI tract, or GU tract procedures.

3. The risk of antibiotic associated adverse events exceeds the benefit, if any, of prophylactic therapy.

4. Maintenance of optimal oral health and hygiene may reduce the incidence of bacteremia from daily activities and is more important than prophylactic antibiotics for dental procedures to reduce the risk of infective endocarditis (Wilson et al., 2007).

❖ The new guidelines recommend prophylaxis for only those with the highest risk for the development of infective endocarditis. The American Heart Association panel identified the following population as those at the highest risk for the development of infective endocarditis:

1. Prosthetic cardiac valve.

2. Previous infective endocarditis.

3. Congenital heart disease.

4. Cardiac transplant recipients who develop cardiac valvulopathy (Wilson et al., 2007).

Valve Disease

◆ Volume Management
  ❖ Volume balance in patients with severe AS is critical because the ventricular chamber is no longer able to expand during filling due to hypertrophy and diastolic dysfunction.
  ❖ Complete filling of the ventricular chamber (adequate preload) is essential to produce sufficient stroke volume.
  ❖ Monitor volume status carefully.
  ❖ Anything that increases heart rate will decrease ventricular filling time during diastole and therefore decreases preload.

◆ Continuous Follow Up for Asymptomatic Patients with AS
  ❖ Depends on severity of disease process.
  ❖ Occurs more frequently as the disease progresses.
  ❖ Occurs more frequently if other co-morbid conditions exist.
  ❖ Annual physician visit reasonable with focus on:
    ☆ History and physical.
    ☆ Careful assessment for the development of signs and symptoms.
    ☆ Patient education about the importance of reporting:
      ✶ Change in exercise tolerance.
      ✶ Exertional chest discomfort.
      ✶ Shortness of breath.
      ✶ Lightheadedness.
      ✶ Syncope (Bonow et al., 2006).

◆ Serial echocardiography (Bonow et al., 2006)
  ❖ Follow up dependent on severity of disease process.
  ❖ Mild AS   Every 3-5 years.
  ❖ Moderate AS   Every 1-2 years.
  ❖ Severe AS   Annually.

◆ Exercise
  ❖ Asymptomatic patients with mild AS:
    ☆ Not restricted.
    ☆ May participate in competitive sports.
  ❖ Asymptomatic with moderate to severe AS:
    ☆ Avoid competitive sports involving high physical demands.
    ☆ Ability to tolerate an exercise program or become involved in competitive sports program can be best evaluated with stress testing.

Surgical Treatment

The first cardiac valve surgeries completed in the early 1950's consisted of atrial commissurotomy for mitral stenosis. Since that time cardiac valve surgery has advanced rapidly. The introduction of cardiopulmonary bypass in the 1960's opened the door for the surgical valve procedures that are common today.

With the onset of symptoms, mortality rates dramatically increase. Survival rates of patients with symptomatic aortic stenosis without surgical intervention are 50% at 2 to 3 years (Darovic, 2002; Bonow et al., 2006). There is a high incidence of sudden death in patients with severe AS. Once symptoms appear, the need for surgical replacement becomes imminent. The asymptomatic patient with severe AS by

Chapter 11

echocardiography presents a more complex decision making process. According to Bonow et al. (2006) the probability of remaining symptom free in five years without cardiac surgery is less than 50%. Those patients who are at risk for rapid disease progression should be considered for aortic valve replacement (AVR) when the AS is severe by echocardiography. Surgical outcomes improve with early detection; therefore, close follow-up, once symptoms begin, is imperative (see follow-up covered previously). While valve replacement is the treatment of choice, aortic valvotomy (discussed later) may be utilized in rare cases. The American College of Cardiology (ACC) and American Heart Association (AHA) 2006 Guidelines for the Management of Patients with Valvular Heart Disease recommendations for surgical replacement in patients with aortic stenosis are reviewed in Table 11.1. Options for the surgical treatment of a dysfunctional aortic valve include:

◆ AV Replacement with mechanical valve.
◆ AV Replacement with a tissue (bioprosthetic) valve.
◆ Ross Procedure.
◆ Aortic Valve Repair.

Table 11.1 **ACC/AHA Recommendations for Aortic Valve Replacement (AVR) in Aortic Stenosis**
Class I Recommendations
1. AVR is indicated for symptomatic patients with severe AS.
2. AVR is indicated for patients with severe AS undergoing coronary artery bypass graft surgery (CABG).
3. AVR is indicated for patients with severe AS undergoing surgery on the aorta or other heart valves.
4. AVR is recommended for patients with severe AS and LV systolic dysfunction (ejection fraction less than 0.50).
Class IIa Recommendations
1. AVR is reasonable for patients with moderate AS undergoing CABG or surgery on the aorta or other heart valves.
Class IIb Recommendations
1. AVR may be considered for asymptomatic patients with severe AS and abnormal response to exercise.
2. AVR may be considered for adults with severe asymptomatic AS if there is a high likelihood of rapid progression, or if surgery might be delayed at the time of symptom onset.
3. AVR may be considered in patients undergoing CABG who have mild AS when there is evidence, such as moderate to severe valve calcification, that progression may be rapid.
4. AVR may be considered for asymptomatic patients with extremely severe AS when the patient's expected operative mortality is 1.0% or less.
(Bonow et al., 2006).

- Aortic valve replacement
  - Surgical mortality rates increase as left ventricular function decreases.
  - Age is not a contraindication for surgery.
  - Mitral valve evaluation is necessary prior to surgery because quite frequently, mitral regurgitation also exists, and mitral valve replacement may also be necessary.
  - Cardiac catheterization should be performed to determine the need for coronary artery bypass surgery.
  - A preoperative assessment of left ventricular function determines systolic and diastolic dysfunction. Surgical mortality risk is lowest in those with normal left ventricular function and increases as systolic function decreases (Darovic, 2002).
- Types of valve prosthesis
  - This discussion on the types of valve prosthetics is common to all valve surgeries.
  - Determined by the anticipated longevity of the patient and patient's ability to tolerate lifelong anticoagulants.
  - Mechanical Valves.
    - More durable than tissue valves.
    - Require life-long anticoagulation with warfarin (coumadin).
    - Best suited for young patients with no contraindications to anticoagulation.
    - Question young females about future pregnancy desires as anticoagulation during pregnancy increases fetal mortality.
    - Mortality related to mechanical valves centers around thromboembolism, hemorrhage (related to anticoagulation), endocarditis, and periprosthetic leak but not valve failure.
    - Three primary types of mechanical valves.
      - Ball and cage.
        - Noisy.
        - Rarely used.
        - Hemodynamically inefficient.
        - Very stable with some lasting up to 30 years.
      - Single leaflet tilting disc.
        - Superior hemodynamic efficiency.
        - Structurally stable.
        - Severe hemodynamic compromise occurs if thombosed or immobility occurs.
      - Bileaflet valve (Figure 11.8).
        - Quiet.
        - Mechanically stable with failure due to repetitive opening and closing not common.
        - Hemodynamically efficient as the wide opening of the discs result in minimal flow disturbances.

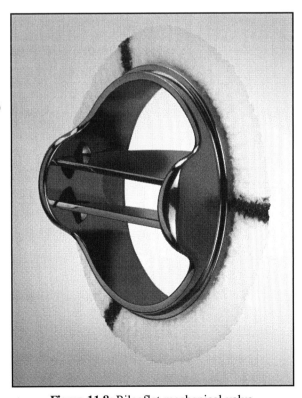

Figure 11.8: Bileaflet mechanical valve.
(Courtesy of St. Jude Medical®)

- Tissue valves (bioprosthetic).
  - Generally less durable than mechanical valves and will need replacement earlier.
  - Lifetime valve expectancy varies with patient age.
    - 7-10 years in younger patients.
    - 15-20 years in those greater than 70 years old.
  - Do not have risk the of mechanical failure that is seen in mechanical valves.
  - No anticoagulation with warfarin required however, a daily aspirin regime is required with all tissue valves.
  - Beneficial in elderly not already on anticoagulation and in women of child bearing age.
  - Homograft or allograft.
    - From human donors.
    - History of early failure rates limits use.
    - Most commonly used in total aortic root replacement.
    - Reoperation is difficult.
  - Heterograft.
    - Transplant of tissue or an organ from one species to another species such as a pig or cow to a human. Heterografts are also referred to as xenografts.
    - Stented heterograft (Figure 11.9).
      - Utilizes bovine (cow) pericardial tissue or porcine (pig) aortic valve tissue arranged over a cloth and metal frame (Bonow et al., 2006).
      - Low thromeombolic rate.
      - Easy to implant and reimplant.
      - Low risk of valve failure.
      - Imperfect hemodynamic efficiency.
    - Stentless heterograft.
      - Utilize porcine aortic valves with a smaller amount of cloth.
      - May be a potential for improved hemodynamic stability over stented grafts as stented heterografts are considered to be partially stenotic due to stents especially in the smaller sizes.
      - Implantation easier than with stented heterograft.
    - Valve replacement easiest with heterograft over homograft or mechanical valve.
- Aortic valve replacement
  - Bileaflet valve is the most common mechanical valve used in the aortic position.
  - Stented heterograft most common aortic valve prosthetic used in the United States (Bonow et al., 2006).
  - Mechanical prosthesis utilized in patients under 65 with no contraindication to anticoagulation.
  - Stented heterograft utilized in patients over 65 not currently on anticoagulation.
  - Homograft most commonly used in total aortic root replacement.
  - Homograft may be utilized in the replacement of a valve with endocarditis.

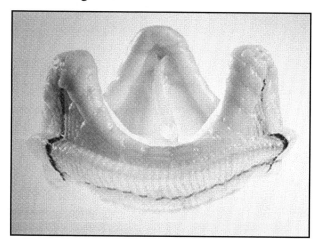

Figure 11.9: Stented heterograft.
(Courtesy of St. Jude Medical®)

Valve Disease

- ◆ Aortic valve repair
  - ❖ Limited use.
  - ❖ Involves decalcification of the valve.
  - ❖ High rate of recalcification and restenosis.
  - ❖ Can be useful when cause of AS is traced to the aortic root and repair of the aortic root results in returning the valve to a functional state.
  - ❖ Prevents the need for anticoagulation.
- ◆ Ross Procedure (autograft): pulmonic valve auto transplantation
  - ❖ Involves placing patient's pulmonic valve in the aortic valve position and placing a tissue valve in the pulmonic valve location.
  - ❖ Not a frequently performed procedure.
  - ❖ Difficult surgery (double valve) with increased mortality and morbidity.
  - ❖ Need for anticoagulation is avoided.
  - ❖ Useful in children as autograft (pulmonic valve) may grow as the child grows.
  - ❖ Autograft is hemodynamically efficient.
  - ❖ Currently no advantage of Ross procedure in adults.
- ◆ Percutaneous balloon valvotomy
  - ❖ Balloon placed across the aortic valve and inflated.
  - ❖ Used to fracture calcium deposits in the leaflets and separate the fused or calcified commissures.
  - ❖ Minor stretching of the aortic annulus may occur as well.
  - ❖ Reasonable procedure in children and young adults with a congenital aortic valve abnormality.
  - ❖ Procedure is considered palliative in adults.
  - ❖ Procedure should be reserved for patients who are not surgical candidates, but are seeking relief from symptoms.
  - ❖ May also be useful as a bridge to valve surgery in high risk, unstable patients.
    - ☆ Allows time for stabilizing and "fine tuning" the patient prior to valve replacement surgery.
  - ❖ All benefits from procedure lost within six months of the procedure in most patients.
  - ❖ Aortic regurgitation is an expected postoperative result after valvuloplasty.
  - ❖ Procedure should not be performed if the patient has 2+ or greater aortic valve regurgitation.
  - ❖ Procedure is associated with a high mortality and morbidity rate.
  - ❖ Should only be completed in centers that are skilled in this procedure
- ◆ Post Operative Care
  After successful aortic valve replacement, decreased left ventricular systolic pressure and decreased afterload results in improved ejection fraction and increased cardiac output. Left ventricular hypertrophy actually regresses, with most of that regression occurring in the first year, but continuing to improve for up to 10 years (Carabello & Crawford, 2003). However, diastolic function most likely never returns to normal due to the increase in collagen content in the myocardial tissue. Patients with a successful aortic valve replacement surgery commonly experience symptom improvement immediately after surgery, especially in cases of severe aortic stenosis.
  - ❖ Post-operative follow-up recommendations include:
    - ☆ This discussion on post operative valve surgery follow-up is common to all valve surgeries.
    - ☆ Often at first post-operative visit 3-4 weeks after surgery and includes:
      - ✳ History and physical.

Chapter 11

* Chest X-ray.
* ECG.
* 2D and Doppler echocardiogram (if not completed in the hospital).
* Lab work as needed including and INR.
* If valve replacement occurred due to infective endocarditis blood cultures would be repeated at this time if one or more weeks have passed since the last dose of antibiotics.

☆ Follow-up visits at 6 and 12 months post operatively and then annually (Bonow et al., 2006).

☆ Annual echocardiograms in patients with bioprosthetic valve replacement even without a change in clinical status may be reasonable after the first 5 years.

☆ Repeat echocardiograms in patients with mechanical valve replacement is required if there is:
* Evidence of prosthetic valve dysfunction.
* Evidence of LV dysfunction.
* Evidence of a new murmur.
* A change in clinical status.

☆ Patients with complications are followed up more closely.

❖ Antibiotic prophylaxis against infective endocarditis.

☆ This discussion on antibiotic prophylaxis is common to all patients after valve replacement surgery. These recommendations are based on the American Heart Association guidelines for the prevention of endocarditis published in April 2007 (Wilson et al,, 2007).

* Endocarditis prophylaxis is appropriate for all patients with a prosthetic valve.
* Procedures requiring endocarditis prophylaxis include all dental procedures that involve manipulation of the gingival tissue or the periapical region of teeth or perforation of the oral mucosa. Procedures that fall within these guidelines include:
  – Biopsies.
  – Suture removal.
  – Placement of orthodontic bands.
* Procedures that do not require prophylaxis include:
  – Routine anesthetic injections through noninfected tissue.
  – Dental X-rays.
  – Placement of removable prosthodontic or orthodontic appliances.
  – Placement of orthodontic brackets.
  – Adjustment of orthodontic appliances.
* Endocarditis prophylaxis may be considered appropriate for patients with a prosthetic valve undergoing an invasive procedure of the respiratory tract involving an incision or biopsy of the respiratory mucosa. This does not include standard endoscopic procedures.
* Endocarditis prophylaxis is no longer recommended for patients with a prosthetic valve undergoing a GU or GI procedure.
* Antibiotics should be administered in a single dose up to two hours prior to the procedure.
* Amoxicillin is the oral antibiotic of choice.
* For those allergic to penicillin or amoxicillin should use a cephalexin or another first-generation oral cephalosporin such as clindamycin, azithromycin or clarithromycin.

Valve Disease

❖ Anticoagulation.
  ☆ This discussion on anticoagulation is common to all patients post valve replacement.
  ☆ These recommendations are adapted from the ACC/AHA 2006 Guidelines for the Management of Patients with Valvular Heart Disease (Bonow et al., 2006).
  ☆ Warfarin therapy is required in all patients with a prosthetic mechanical valve.
  ☆ Aspirin alone is required for all patients with bioprosthetic valves and no risk for thromboembolism (atrial fibrillation, previous thromboembolism, LV dysfunction, and hypercoagulable condition).
  ☆ Combined warfarin and aspirin therapy is recommended in patients with mechanical valves and in patients with a bioprosthetic valve who are high-risk for thromboembolism.
  ☆ Clopidogrel should be considered in combination with warfarin in patients who are unable to take aspirin.
  ☆ Risk for embolism is higher in those patients with a valve in the mitral position (Bonow et al., 2006).
  ☆ Patients with a bioprosthetic valve should be placed on warfarin for up to 3 months after valve replacement, especially those with a bioprosthetic valve in the mitral position.
    ✶ Once the valve is endothelialized the risk of embolization is greatly decreased.
  ☆ INR goals may vary with the type of valve, as different valve types have higher or lower embolic rates.
    ✶ INR levels in patients with mechanical valves should be 2.5 to 3.5.
    ✶ Bioprosthetic valves requiring anticoagulation with warfarin should achieve an INR of 2.0 to 3.0.
  ☆ INR goals may change if the patient experiences an embolic event while on anticoagulation therapy.
    ✶ INR of 2.0-3.0 increases to INR of 2.5 to 3.5.
    ✶ INR of 2.5 to 3.5 increases to INR of 3.5 to 4.5.
    ✶ Add aspirin if not on aspirin.
    ✶ Increase aspirin does if already on aspirin.
  ☆ If anticoagulation therapy must be terminated temporarily for a procedure, some patients may require intravenous or subcutaneous heparin and others may not, depending on the embolic risk and the length of time the warfarin is held.
  ☆ If surgery is required emergently fresh frozen plasma or Vitamin K can be administered for quick reversal of the anticoagulatant.
    ✶ Stop warfarin 48-72 hours prior to procedure so INR can fall to less than 1.5.
    ✶ High risk patients (any mitral valve replacement or mechanical AVR with risk factors) require intravenous heparin after INR is less than 2.0.
    ✶ Warfarin should be restarted within 24 hours after the procedure.

Chapter 11

Linking Knowledge to Practice

✔ *Intravascular fluid balance in patients with severe aortic stenosis is critical because the ventricular chamber is no longer able to expand during filling. In order to produce an adequate stroke volume, complete filling of the ventricular chamber is essential.*

✔ *Patients with little or no CAD may still have angina as a result of a thickened myocardial wall. These patients benefit from the same things that increase supply to the myocardium, such as oxygen and adequate hemoglobin levels.*

✔ *The development of atrial fibrillation results in the loss of atrial kick. A loss of atrial kick results in a decrease in ventricular preload and an associated decrease in stroke volume; therefore, decreased cardiac output and typically an increase in symptoms depending on the degree of AS.*

✔ *Patients should be reminded not to make any sudden position moves. They should be taught to move from a lying to standing position slowly, as well as to be aware that exercise may result in syncope.*

✔ *Patients with aortic valve disease should be aware of signs of decompensation. With early recognition, the appropriate treatment can take place before any permanent damage to the ventricle has occurred.*

Aortic Regurgitation (AR)

Aortic regurgitation (or aortic insufficiency) occurs when the valve leaflets of the aortic valve do not close completely (coapt) to form a tight seal, resulting in backward flow of blood from the aorta to the left ventricle during ventricular diastole.

Classification of Aortic Regurgitation

Aortic regurgitation can be classified as acute or chronic. Both types can further be classified as processes that alter the valve itself or either damage or dilate the aortic root where the valve joins the aorta. Symptoms depend on the severity and rapidity of onset. With the decreased incidence of rheumatic valve disease, chronic non-rheumatic causes now account for the majority of isolated cases of aortic regurgitation.

◆ Chronic Aortic Regurgitation
  ❖ Processes changing the valve itself:
    ☆ Congenital aortic valve (bicuspid instead of tricuspid).
    ☆ Rheumatic Heart Disease.
      ✱ Changes that cause aortic stenosis usually result in a degree of aortic regurgitation.
      ✱ Incidence of rheumatic heart disease greatly decreased since the development of antibiotics.
      ✱ Still prevalent in underdeveloped countries.
    ☆ Infective Endocarditis.
    ☆ Age.
  ❖ Processes that damage or dilate the aortic root:
    ☆ Systemic Hypertension.
    ☆ Reiter's Arthritis.
    ☆ Syphilis.
    ☆ Connective or Collagen Tissue Disorders.
      ✱ Marfan Syndrome.
      ✱ Ankylosing Spondylitis.
      ✱ Systemic Lupus Erythematosus.
      ✱ Ehlers-Danlos Syndrome.

Valve Disease

◆ Acute Aortic Regurgitation
  ❖ Process changing the valve itself.
    ☆ Acute infective endocarditis.
  ❖ Processes that damage or dilate the aortic root.
    ☆ Trauma.
      ✳ Steering wheel trauma to chest.
    ☆ Acute Aortic Dissection.

Because the presentation of acute aortic regurgitation is entirely different from that of chronic aortic regurgitation, the two are discussed separately.

Chronic Aortic Regurgitation
Pathophysiology
In patients with aortic regurgitation, blood enters the left ventricle normally from the left atrium, while blood also enters the left ventricle from the aorta. The backflow (regurgitant flow) from the aorta through the aortic valve into the left ventricle occurs because the aortic valve does not close properly (see concept of aortic recoil discussed at the beginning of the chapter). This results in a larger-than-normal volume in the left ventricle and causes the left ventricle to dilate. Additionally, the left ventricular wall thickness increases (hypertrophy) to maintain normal wall stress. The dilated left ventricle maintains a normal or near-normal preload, and the increase in wall thickness results in increased contractility which helps increase stroke volume (hyperdynamic perfusion). An increased stroke volume is necessary to compensate for the portion of blood ejected into the aorta with each beat that returns to the left ventricle. If the ventricle can eject a larger-than-normal volume with each beat, the cardiac output needs should be met. With the dilation to compensate for the volume and the hypertrophy to assist with increased contractility, forward stroke volume can eventually reach more than two times normal. The heart becomes so large it is often referred to as a "cow's heart." While maintaining preload, normal wall stress, and contractility, ejection fraction remains the same. This phase of the disease process is considered the chronic compensatory phase and lasts for many years or even decades.

As with aortic stenosis, patients remain asymptomatic for years with very low morbidity. Eventually, the compensatory mechanisms begin to fail, and the enlarged heart begins to show signs of decompensation. As the left ventricle continues to dilate, contractility decreases because the myocardium becomes overstretched. Left ventricular ejection fraction decreases, resulting in systolic dysfunction. As ejection fraction decreases, left ventricular volume increases. Afterload increases to compensate for decreased cardiac output. Heart rate also increases to compensate for the decrease in cardiac output; however, this increased rate is often ineffective. After decades without any difficulties, patients begin to develop symptoms of fluid overload and heart failure.

Compensatory Mechanisms In Aortic Regurgitation
◆ ↑ volume in left ventricle (forward filling from left atrium, backward filling from aorta)
  → ↑ left ventricular size (ventricular dilatation)
    → ↑ Left ventricular wall mass → LV hypertrophy (hyperdynamic stroke volume)
      → Increased stroke volume.
◆ Compensatory system ultimately fails → Systolic dysfunction → Heart failure.

Symptoms
The initial symptoms noted most frequently are exertional dyspnea and fatigue. As the disease progresses, complaints of paroxysmal nocturnal dyspnea and orthopnea with pulmonary edema are not unusual. The patient may note an awareness of the heart beating, including a pulsetile sensation in the head that

469

increases when lying down. This is due to the hyperdynamic stroke volume that occurs with aortic regurgitation.

As with aortic stenosis, angina occurs with aortic regurgitation. Angina is the result of an inability of the coronary arteries to supply the volume of oxygenated blood needed for the increased myocardial mass. This type of ischemia without associated coronary artery disease is common in aortic regurgitation. The incidence of concurrent coronary artery disease with aortic regurgitation is less common than with aortic stenosis.

Physical Examination
- Apical Impulse
    - Normally 5th intercostal space, mid-clavicular line.
    - Displaced laterally and inferiorly.
    - Hyperdynamic (strong).
- Diastolic Murmur of AR (Figure 11.10)
    - As the disease progresses, the murmur of aortic regurgitation become more complex, and three different murmurs (other two noted below) may actually occur.
    - The duration of the murmur during diastole correlates with the severity of the AR.
    - Timing: Early diastole.
    - Location: Best heard over 3rd or 4th intercostals space along the left sternal border; may be heard all along the left sternal border.
    - Radiation: Toward the apex (5th intercostals space mid-clavicular line).
    - Configuration: Decrescendo.
    - Pitch: High.
    - Quality: Blowing.
    - Heard best with patient sitting and leaning forward while holding breath at end expiration.
    - Intensity of murmur increases with an increase in peripheral vascular resistance (squatting, exercising, hand gripping).

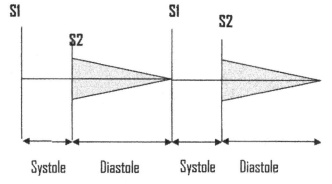

Figure 11.10: Drawing representing the diastolic decrescendo murmur of AR.

- Systolic Flow Murmur
    - Systolic flow murmurs are the result of turbulent blood flow across a valve during systole, and are usually inaudible. In aortic regurgitation, due to the hyperdynamic contraction of the left ventricle, this systolic murmur may be audible as a large amount of blood is ejected rapidly through the aortic valve during systole.
    - Timing: Mid-systolic.
    - Location: Usually heard best along the left sternal border. Best heard 2nd intercostal space, right sternal border.
    - Radiation: Toward the right side of the neck.
    - Configuration: Crescendo-decrescendo.
    - Pitch: Medium pitch, best herd with diaphragm of stethoscope.
    - Quality: Soft.
    - Intensity may be increased by having the patient cough several times or raise his/her legs from a lying position.

Valve Disease

- Austin Flint Murmur
  - During ventricular diastole, the backward flow of blood through the aortic valve presses on the open anterior leaflet of the mitral valve, moving the leaflet toward a closed position, while blood is moving from the left atrium to the left ventricle. This results in a functional murmur of mitral stenosis.
  - Heard in very severe or acute AR.
  - Timing: Mid-diastolic to late diastolic.
  - Location: Best heard at the mitral area – 5th intercostal space, mid-clavicular line.
  - Configuration: Plateau.
  - Pitch: Low pitch, best heard with the bell of the stethoscope.
  - Quality: Rumbling.
  - Intensity: Soft.
- S3 (Ventricular Gallop)
  - Third heart sound.
  - Caused when atria passively empty into a fluid overloaded ventricle.
  - Should resolve when fluid overload state resolves.
  - Best heard with patient in left lateral position.
  - Timing: Early diastolic filling sound, just after S2.
  - Location: Mitral area (5th Intercostal space, mid-clavicular line).
  - Intensity: Loudest during expiration.
  - Duration: Short.
  - Quality: Dull, thud-like.
  - Pitch: Low.
  - Best heard with bell of stethoscope.
- Signs of Hyperdynamic Perfusion
  - The hyperdynamic stroke volume causes a variety of peripheral signs, indicating chronic aortic regurgitation.
    - ☆ Warm skin that may be flushed, reddish mucous membranes.
    - ☆ De Musset's Sign
      - ∗ Visible head bobbing with each heart beat.
    - ☆ Water-Hammer Pulse
      - ∗ Bounding peripheral pulse with a rapid rise, referred to as a "slapping" pulse, with a quick collapse.
    - ☆ Corrigan's Pulse
      - ∗ Large carotid pulsation in the neck.
    - ☆ Traube's Sign
      - ∗ Loud, sharp pistol-shot-like sound heard over the femoral pulse.
    - ☆ Duroziez's Sign
      - ∗ Murmur heard over the femoral artery when compressed.
        - – Systolic murmur heard distal to finger pressure on the artery.
        - – Diastolic murmur heard proximal to finger pressure.
    - ☆ Quinke's Sign
      - ∗ Pulsatile blanching and reddening of the fingernails when light pressure is applied.

Chapter 11

　　★　Widened pulse pressure
　　　　∗　Systolic blood pressure increases abnormally due to the increased stroke volume.
　　　　∗　Diastolic blood pressure decreases abnormally as more blood is returned to the heart with each beat – often less than 60 mm Hg.
　　　　∗　Not unusual to have pulse pressures greater than 100 mm Hg.
　　　　∗　As the aortic regurgitation increases, the pulse pressure widens, which may help determine the extent of the regurgitation.

Diagnosis
◆　Cardiac Echocardiogram
　❖　Primary tool utilized to confirm diagnosis of aortic regurgitation.
　❖　Color Flow Doppler Echocardiography evaluates the regurgitant jet velocity and size.
　❖　Determination of Angiographic Grade of Severity (Bonow et al., 2006).
　　★　Mild AR　　　　　　1+.
　　★　Moderate AR　　　　2+.
　　★　Severe AR　　　　　3-4+.
　❖　Evaluation of Regurgitant Jet Width (Bonow et al., 2006).
　　★　Mild AR　　　　　　Width < 25% of left ventricular outflow track.
　　★　Moderate AR　　　　Width > mild, but no signs of severe AR.
　　★　Severe AR　　　　　Width > 65% of left ventricular outflow track.
　❖　Evaluation of Regurgitant Volume (amount returned to LV each beat) (Bonow et al., 2006).
　　★　Mild AR　　　　　　< 30 ml/beat.
　　★　Moderate AR　　　　30-59 ml/beat.
　　★　Severe AR　　　　　≥ 60 ml/beat.
　❖　Evaluation of Valve Leaflets for:
　　★　Thickening.
　　★　Loss of coaptation (closure) of the commissures.
　　★　Presence of vegetation on valve.
　　★　Dilatation of aortic root (may prevent closure of leaflets).
　❖　Evaluation of Left Ventricular Function for:
　　★　Eccentric hypertrophy – dilated left ventricle.
　　★　Concentric hypertrophy – thickened left ventricular wall.
　　★　Left ventricular ejection fraction – assessment for systolic dysfunction.
◆　Stress Testing
　❖　May be beneficial to assess for functional capacity, symptomatic and hemodynamic response to exercise.
　❖　May be beneficial to assess for exercise tolerance before participating in organized athletics.
　❖　Not needed if clear diagnosis can be made from patient symptoms and echocardiogram.
◆　Cardiac Catheterization
　❖　Echocardiography is usually sufficient to diagnose aortic regurgitation.
　❖　Cardiac catheterization provides an assessment of the absence or presence of coronary artery disease, which is useful when valve replacement is necessary.

Valve Disease

◆ Electrocardiogram
  ❖ ECG changes are neither sensitive nor specific to aortic regurgitation and always require other testing for confirmation.
  ❖ Changes are dependent on the severity of the disease process.
  ❖ Signs of left ventricle hypertrophy with left axis deviation are usually present with moderate to severe aortic regurgitation.
◆ Chest X-ray
  ❖ Enlarged heart – concentric and eccentric hypertrophy.
  ❖ Heart failure in chronic decompensated aortic regurgitation.
  ❖ Heart failure in acute aortic regurgitation.

Medical Treatment
With normal left ventricular function, the asymptomatic patient requires no treatment. Once symptoms begin to occur, surgical replacement should be considered as the treatment of choice. Some medical treatment may be beneficial in easing the amount of regurgitation on a temporary basis.

◆ Arterial Vasodilators
  ❖ Reduce SVR, allowing more blood to flow forward and thereby decreasing the regurgitation.
  ❖ Indicated as a short-term therapy for those awaiting surgery.
  ❖ May be beneficial for those symptomatic patients who are not surgical candidates.
  ❖ Not indicated for long-term therapy in asymptomatic patients with mild to moderate AR and normal left ventricular function.
    ☆ Dihydropyridine calcium channel blockers – specifically nifedipine
      ✳ Depresses contraction of cardiac and vascular smooth muscle.
      ✳ Decreases SVR and increases cardiac output.
      ✳ Diltiazem and verapamil contraindicated due to negative inotropic effect.
    ☆ Hydralazine (Apresoline)
      ✳ Relaxes vascular smooth muscle.
      ✳ Decreases system vascular resistance and increases cardiac output.
    ☆ Felodipine
      ✳ Decreased peripheral vascular resistance.
      ✳ Decreases myocardial contractility.
◆ Angiotensin-Converting Enzyme Inhibitors
  ❖ Decrease afterload but not proven to provide long-term benefits.
  ❖ May be better tolerated in patients who cannot tolerate calcium channel blocker.
◆ Digoxin and Diuretics
  ❖ Helpful with heart failure symptoms.
◆ Antibiotic Prophylaxis Against Infective Endocarditis
  See discussion on antibiotic prophylaxis under aortic stenosis.
◆ Arterial Vasoconstrictors
  ❖ Utilization of vasopressors such norepinephrine (Levophed) or dopamine (Intropin) is contraindicated in aortic regurgitation.
  ❖ Cause increased SVR, which increases the regurgitation.

Chapter 11

- ◆ Intra-aortic Balloon Pump
  - ❖ The utilization of an intra-aortic balloon pump is **absolutely contraindicated** in acute aortic regurgitation and should be avoided in all patients with aortic regurgitation.
- ◆ Continuous Follow Up for Asymptomatic Patients with AR
  - ❖ Depends on severity of disease process.
  - ❖ Occurs more frequently as the disease progresses.
  - ❖ Occurs more frequently if other co-morbid conditions exist.
  - ❖ Annual physician visit with focus on:
    - ☆ History and physical.
    - ☆ Careful assessment for the development of signs and symptoms.
    - ☆ Patient education about the importance of reporting:
      - ✳ Change in exercise tolerance.
      - ✳ Chest discomfort.
      - ✳ Shortness of breath.
  - ❖ Serial echocardiography (Bonow et al., 2006).
    - ☆ Necessary to determine onset of left ventricular dysfunction.
    - ☆ Mortality with valve replacement worsens as ejection fraction worsens; careful assessment of left ventricular function is essential.
    - ☆ Asymptomatic patient with normal left ventricular function with mild AR.
      - ✳ Echocardiography every 2-3 years.
    - ☆ Asymptomatic patients with severe AR.
      - ✳ Echocardiography every 6-12 months.
    - ☆ Echocardiography with onset of any symptoms.
  - ❖ Patients with chronic aortic regurgitation should have regular follow-up serial testing that includes echocardiograms to assess left ventricular function. Asymptomatic patients and those with mild aortic regurgitation may participate in regular activity. Those with moderate to severe aortic regurgitation should not engage in competitive sports or vigorous activity.

Surgical Treatment

Once symptoms begin, patients should be evaluated for surgical repair or replacement of the aortic valve. Left untreated, 50% of the patients with symptomatic aortic regurgitation will not survive more than three to five years after the onset of symptoms. With surgical mortality rates of 1-5%, surgical treatment is the best option for most patients. Those patients with higher surgical risks should be evaluated carefully before ruling out surgical replacement.

Surgical repair is becoming a reasonable alternative to replacement in aortic regurgitation if the cause of the regurgitation is abnormalities involving the valve annulus, not calcification or stiffness of the valve leaflets. Aortic valve repair is successful for this population in surgical centers that are focusing on perfecting the surgical technique, and may be considered in those centers.

Throughout the discussion of surgical treatment of aortic regurgitation, AVR is utilized to refer to aortic valve replacement and aortic valve repair. The determination for surgery should be based on quality of life, not longevity. Symptom relief should be the most important guide in making the decision for aortic valve replacement.

The American College of Cardiology (ACC) and American Heart Association (AHA) 2006 Guidelines for the Management of Patients with Valvular Heart Disease recommendations for surgical replacement

Valve Disease

in patients with aortic regurgitation are reviewed in Table 11.2. Options for the surgical treatment of a dysfunctional aortic valve include:

◆ AVR with mechanical valve.

◆ AVR with a tissue (bioprosthetic) valve.

Table 11.2 ACC/AHA Recommendations for Aortic Valve Replacement / Repair (AVR) in Aortic Regurgitation
Class I Recommendations
1. AVR is indicated for symptomatic patients with severe AR irrespective of LV systolic function.
2. AVR is indicated for asymptomatic patients with chronic severe AR and LV systolic dysfunction (ejection fraction $\leq$ 0.50).
3. AVR is indicated for patients with chronic severe AR while undergoing CABG or surgery on the aorta or other heart valves.
Class IIa Recommendations
1. AVR is reasonable for asymptomatic patients with severe AR with normal left ventricular systolic function, but with severe left ventricular dilatation.
Class IIb Recommendations
1. AVR may be considered in patients with moderate AR while undergoing surgery on the ascending aorta.
2. AVR may be considered in patients with moderate AR while undergoing CABG.
3. AVR may be considered for asymptomatic patients with severe AR and normal left ventricular function at rest when the degree of dilatation exceeds an end-diastolic dimension of 70mm or end-systolic dimension of 50 mm, when there is evidence of progressive left ventricular dilatation, declining exercise tolerance, or abnormal hemodynamic responses to exercise.
(Bonow et al., 2006)

◆ Aortic Valve Repair or Replacement

  ❖ Surgical mortality rates increase as left ventricular function decreases.

  ❖ Age is not a contraindication for surgery.

  ❖ Cardiac catheterization should be performed prior to surgery to determine the need for coronary artery bypass surgery.

  ❖ Surgical intervention is indicated if ejection fraction is abnormal, with or without the presence of symptoms.

  ❖ Types of valves utilized for replacement are the same as with aortic stenosis. (For discussion on types of valves utilized for surgical replacement, see section on aortic stenosis.)

◆ Post Operative Considerations
Left ventricular function generally improves within the first 10-14 days after surgery, but may improve for up to 2 years after surgery, with a gradual decline in ventricular hypertrophy (Zoghbi & Afridi, 2003). These results vary depending on the preoperative condition of the left ventricle.

  ❖ Post-operative follow-up recommendations include:

    ☆ Echocardiogram performed soon after surgery to assess left ventricular size and function, often at first post-operative visit, 3-4 weeks after surgery.

Chapter 11

★ Follow-up visits at 6 and 12 months post-operatively, then annually (Bonow et al., 2006).

★ Patients with complications are followed up more closely.

❖ Antibiotic prophylaxis against infective endocarditis.
See discussion on postoperative antibiotic prophylaxis under aortic stenosis.

❖ Anticoagulation.
See discussion on postoperative anticoagulation under aortic stenosis.

Acute Aortic Regurgitation

Pathophysiology

Acute aortic regurgitation is most noted with trauma, aortic dissection, and acute cases of infective endocarditis. The pathophysiologic changes associated with acute aortic regurgitation are the result of acute decompensation. There is no opportunity for the development of long-term compensatory changes. With the acute damage to the valve, a large volume of blood suddenly returns to the left ventricle from the aorta. The left ventricle is unable to increase stroke volume because it has no time to adapt. Forward flow (stroke volume) dramatically decreases. Much of the blood ejected from the ventricle to the aorta is returned to the ventricle during diastole. The body attempts to compensate for this decrease in cardiac output by an increased heart rate and arterial vasoconstriction. As volume travels to the area of least resistance, the increase in left ventricular afterload results in a worsening of the acute aortic regurgitation. The volume overload is transferred backward to the left atrium and, ultimately, the pulmonary veins, resulting in acute pulmonary edema.

◆ Sudden ↓ cardiac output
→↑ Left ventricular afterload
→ Further ↑ in regurgitation
→ Fluid overload in LV
→ Pulmonary edema and acute decompensation.

Signs and Symptoms

◆ Abrupt onset.
❖ Symptoms may be delayed somewhat if mitral valve is competent.
★ Increase in left ventricular volume and pressure causes the early closure of the mitral valve. This helps protect the pulmonary system against the high pressure of the left ventricle.
❖ Increased heart rate decreases diastolic time, resulting in a decreased time for regurgitation to occur.

◆ Signs of acute pulmonary edema with severe dyspnea and pulmonary congestion.
❖ Auscultation of extra heart sounds.
★ S3.
★ S4.

◆ Signs of cardiogenic shock ultimately develop as forward flow decreases.
❖ Cool, clammy, cyanotic.
❖ Tachycardia.
❖ Hypotensive.

◆ Diastolic murmur as described in chronic aortic regurgitation.

Diagnosis

◆ Echocardiogram.

476

Valve Disease

❖ Utilized for quick confirmation of the diagnosis and determination of the extent of the problem.

❖ Transesophageal echocardiogram may be done if aortic dissection is suspected.

◆ Cardiac Catheterization

❖ Only completed if patient is stable enough to undergo the procedure, or if unable to determine a diagnosis by the noninvasive route.

Medical Treatment

Surgical treatment is the therapy of choice in acute aortic regurgitation. Until the patient is taken to surgery, several non-surgical treatment options may be of some benefit.

◆ Afterload Reduction

❖ May help decrease the regurgitant volume and stabilize the patient before surgery.

❖ Sodium Nitroprusside.

☆ Nitroprusside decreases afterload and preload.

◆ Preload Reduction

❖ May help decrease the fluid overload state.

◆ Beta blockers.

❖ Used with caution.

❖ Block the normal sympathetic response of increased heart rate to compensate for decreased forward flow.

◆ Inotropic Support

❖ Dobutamine assists with ventricular contractility and helps increase cardiac output.

◆ Contraindicated therapies

❖ Intra-aortic balloon pump.

☆ Grossly increases aortic regurgitation.

☆ As the balloon inflates in the aorta during ventricular diastole, blood in the aorta is forced to return to the ventricle through the regurgitant valve.

❖ Arterial vasoconstrictors.

☆ Increased afterload further increases regurgitation.

Surgical Treatment

◆ Urgent surgery is the treatment of choice.

◆ If the patient has developed acute aortic regurgitation as a result of infective endocarditis, 48 hours of antibiotics are preferred if the patient can tolerate the delay in surgery (LeDoux, 2005). However, surgery should not be delayed if the patient is hemodynamically unstable.

Outcomes

Once the patient with acute aortic regurgitation has the valve successfully replaced, outcomes are very good. If left ventricular function was normal prior to the acute event, there should be no long-term effects on the ventricle. Follow-up is the same as with all valve surgeries.

Linking Knowledge to Practice

✔ *Although utilized in acutely ill patients, intra-aortic balloon pumping is contraindicated in patients with aortic regurgitation because it grossly increases aortic regurgitation. As the balloon inflates in the aorta during ventricular diastole, blood in the aorta is forced to return to the ventricle through the regurgitant valve.*

Chapter 11

◆ *Patients with acute aortic regurgitation are acutely ill and generally in a life-threatening situation, especially in the presence of aortic root dissection.*

MITRAL VALVE DISEASE

A normal functioning mitral valve allows one-way flow of blood from the left atrium to the left ventricle. Cardiac output can be greatly affected by the volume of blood in the left ventricle at the end of diastole. A normal functioning mitral valve supports proper filling of the left ventricle. A dysfunctional valve can alter ventricular preload or forward stroke volume and, ultimately, perfusion.

Normal Mitral Valve

Normal Structure (Figure 11.11)

◆ Atrioventricular valve (AV valve).

◆ Located between the left atrium and the left ventricle.

◆ Complex structure referred to as the mitral valve apparatus.

❖ Valve annulus

★ Fibrous valvular "ring" at the top of the valve that helps the valve maintain its shape.

★ Situated between the left atrium and the left ventricle; therefore, its shape and size can be altered by a change in the shape or size of the atrium or ventricle.

❖ Leaflets (cusps)

★ 2 leaflets: one anterior and one posterior.

★ Uppermost portions of the leaflets are joined together by the fibrous ring (annulus) at the top of the valve.

★ Form a funnel shape when open.

❖ Papillary muscles

★ Project from the inner surface of the left ventricular wall and attach to the delicate strands of fibrous material called chordae tendineae.

★ Attachment of the papillary muscle to the wall of the ventricle is important to maintain the normal function of the valve.

❖ Chordae tendineae

★ Fibrous strands of material that attach the valve leaflets to the papillary muscle.

The AV valves open passively during diastole, forming a funnel-like shape and allowing blood to flow from the atria to the ventricles. At the beginning of systole, ventricular pressure rises and forces the valve leaflets to come together and close the valve opening between the atria and the ventricles. As the ventricles contract to eject blood, the papillary muscles contract to prevent the valve leaflets from prolapsing into the atria. The closure of the leaflets prevents the backflow of blood from the ventricles to the atria. At the beginning of diastole, when the ventricle relaxes, the AV valves open again and the cycle is repeated.

Mitral Regurgitation (MR)

Mitral regurgitation occurs when the cusps of the mitral valve do not close properly (coapt) to form a seal, and blood in the left ventricle returns to the left atrium during ventricular systole. Other terms used to refer to a mitral valve that does not close properly are insufficiency or prolapse.

Valve Disease

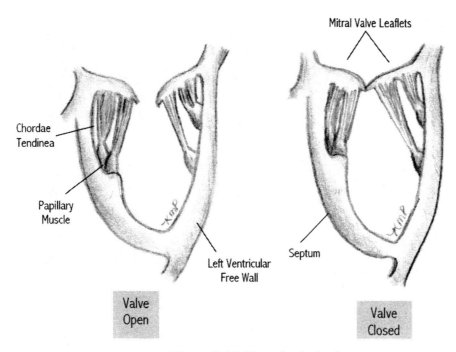

Figure 11.11: Normal mitral valve.

Classification of Mitral Regurgitation

Mitral valve regurgitation can be classified as organic or functional

◆ Normal functioning depends on normal valve leaflets, chordae tendineae and papillary muscles that stretch and contract appropriately, as well as to normal ventricular tissue where the papillary muscle is attached to the ventricular wall.

◆ Organic processes
  ❖ Involve the structure of the valve itself.
  ❖ Mitral Valve Prolapse.
    ☆ Mitral valve prolapse is the most common form of valvular heart disease that can result in regurgitation and occurs in 2% to 6% of the population (Bonow et al., 1998).
    ☆ Most commonly affects young women.
    ☆ Results when changes in valve leaflets and chordae tendineae cause lengthening of the chordae tendineae. The papillary muscle, functioning normally during ventricular systole, contracts. The contraction applies pressure to the chordae tendineae. As contraction occurs, the chordae tendineae "pull" on the valve leaflets to prevent them from prolapsing into the atria as the force of ventricular contraction and ejection pushes against the leaflets. In mitral valve prolapse, the lengthened chordae tendineae cannot keep the valve leaflet in its proper place, so the valve leaflets are forced into the left atrial chamber (Figure 11.12).
    ☆ Not all patients with mitral valve prolapse have regurgitation.
    ☆ Mitral valve prolapse that occurs in young, otherwise healthy women may cause only mild mitral regurgitation with little effect on the heart.

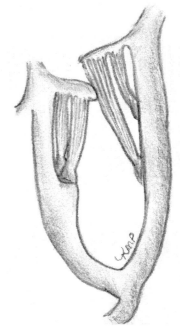

Figure 11.12: Drawing representing the abnormal leaftlet closure in mitral valve prolapse.

479

Chapter 11

- ❖ Rheumatic Heart Disease.
  - ☆ As incidence of rheumatic heart disease in the United States decreases, so does the incidence of mitral regurgitation.
  - ☆ Valve leaflets become fibrotic and shorten.
  - ☆ Calcification may also occur, causing leaflets to become stiff and remain in an open position.
- ❖ Infective Endocarditis.
  - ☆ Vegetation grows on the valve leaflets, preventing proper closure.
- ❖ Collagen Vascular Diseases.
  - ☆ Systemic Lupus Erythematosus.
- ◆ Functional abnormalities
  - ❖ Changes in other structures result in changes in valve function.
  - ❖ Left ventricular or left atrial dilatation resulting in a dilated annulus, preventing leaflets from coapting.
  - ❖ Papillary muscle ischemia prevents papillary muscle from contracting efficiently.
  - ❖ Papillary muscle rupture.
    - ☆ Once the myocardial wall becomes damaged, the attachment of the papillary muscle to that ventricular wall can become weak. As the heart continues to pump, the papillary muscle continues to contract. With each contraction of the papillary muscle, the attachment to the ventricle can weaken. If enough damage to the myocardial wall or papillary muscle has occurred, the papillary muscle can disconnect from the ventricular wall. This results in an acute mitral regurgitation state and the development of pulmonary edema.
    - ☆ Inferior wall myocardial infarctions are particularly susceptible to acute papillary muscle ruptures. Papillary muscle ruptures do not generally occur at the onset of the infarct, but may develop 48 to 72 hours later.
  - ❖ Infective endocarditis.
    - ☆ Bacterial invasion of the heart with the development of endocarditis can cause chordae tendinaea or papillary muscle dysfunction, or papillary muscle rupture.

Chronic Mitral Regurgitation

Mitral regurgitation can occur acutely or chronically. Acute mitral regurgitation provides a much different clinical picture than chronic mitral regurgitation, therefore, they are addressed separately.

Pathophysiology

During ventricular systole, blood flow normally travels from the left ventricle through the aortic valve. In the presence of mitral regurgitation, some of that forward blood flow is diverted retrograde (backward) through the dysfunctional mitral valve. This retrograde flow decreases stroke volume (forward flow) by the percentage of blood that flows backward. That percentage of blood increases the normal volume of blood in the left atrium, resulting in an increase in left atrial pressure. The left atrium responds to this increased volume and pressure by dilating. If this dilatation is not adequate to handle the volume and subsequent pressure increase, the effects are transferred backward to the pulmonary system and pulmonary hypertension develops.

The left ventricle also experiences an increase in filling volume during diastole. During diastole, the ventricle receives the blood that is in the left atrium. The amount of blood in the atrium now includes the volume normally delivered via the pulmonary veins and also the volume that has been returned from the left ventricle via the abnormal mitral valve. The ventricle adjusts to this increased volume by enlarging. Additionally, left ventricular contractions may become stronger for a period. As ejection occurs, normal stroke volume is ejected forward, with the additional volume being returned to the atrium through the regurgitant valve. This compensatory mechanism functions well for many years, until the myocardial fibers have been stretched beyond their physical limitations and systolic ventricular dysfunction occurs.

Compensatory Mechanisms in Mitral Regurgitation
- ◆ Some of blood ejected from left ventricle is diverted retrograde through dysfunctional mitral valve during systole to left atrium
  - → Increased left atrial volume and pressure AND
  - → Stroke volume decreased by percentage of blood returned to atrium
    - → Left atrium responds by dilating
      - → Enlarged atrium sends increased volume to ventricle
        - → LV adjusts to increased volume by enlarging (dilation)
        - → LV increases contractility to assure forward flow.
- ◆ Compensatory system ultimately fails → systolic dysfunction → heart failure.

Symptoms
Patients with chronic mitral regurgitation remain asymptomatic for many years. As symptoms develop, the patient most frequently reports fatigue and dyspnea, initially on exertion. These symptoms progress to include paroxysmal nocturnal dyspnea, orthopnea, and even palpitations from atrial fibrillation. In many cases, the initial diagnosis of mitral regurgitation is made when patients present with new-onset atrial fibrillation. Patients with mitral valve prolapse early on may report symptoms of tachycardia, orthostatic hypotension, or panic attacks.

Physical Exam
- ◆ Systolic Murmur (Figure 11.13)
  - ❖ Timing: Early, mid or late systole or may be holosystolic.
  - ❖ Location: Best heard at 5th intercostal space, mid-clavicular line.
    - ☆ Occasionally, due to the leaflet that is prolapsed, the murmur is louder at the aortic area.
  - ❖ Radiation: Towards the axilla or posteriorly over the lung bases.
  - ❖ Configuration: Plateau.
  - ❖ Pitch: Medium to high.
  - ❖ Quality: Blowing.
- ◆ S3 (Ventricular Gallop)
  - ❖ Third heart sound.
  - ❖ Heard in moderate to severe mitral regurgitation.
  - ❖ Sound is related to increased left ventricular volume in early diastole, not ventricular failure.
  - ❖ Best heard with patient in left lateral position.
  - ❖ Timing: Early diastolic filling sound, just after S2.
  - ❖ Location: Mitral area (5th intercostal space, mid-clavicular line).
  - ❖ Intensity: Loudest during expiration.

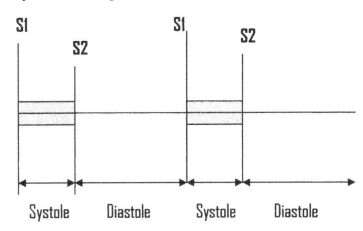

Figure 11.13: Drawing demonstrating the holosystolic plateau murmur of MR.

Chapter 11

- Increased heart rate with atrial fibrillation or heart failure.
  - Atrial fibrillation not uncommon due to dilation of left atrium.
- Pulse pressure narrows with decreased stroke volume.
- Decreased carotid pulse volume.
- Apical impulse displaced due to the dilation of the left ventricle.
- Signs of pulmonary hypertension indicate advanced disease.
- Signs and symptoms of heart failure may be present.

Diagnosis

- Cardiac Echocardiogram
  - Primary tool utilized to confirm diagnosis of mitral regurgitation.
  - Color Flow Doppler Echocardiography evaluates the regurgitant jet velocity and size.
  - Determination of Angiographic Grade of Severity (Bonow et al., 2006).
    - ★ Mild MR   1+.
    - ★ Moderate MR   2+.
    - ★ Severe MR   3-4+.
  - Evaluation of Regurgitant Jet (Bonow et al., 2006).
    - ★ Mild MR   Width < 4cm^2 or < 20% of left atrial area.
    - ★ Moderate MR   Width > mild but no sign of severe MR.
    - ★ Severe MR   Width > 40% of left atrial area or with a wall impinging jet of any size, swirling in left atrium.
  - Evaluation of Regurgitant Volume (amount returned to left atrium each beat) (Bonow et al., 2006).
    - ★ Mild MR   < 30 ml/beat.
    - ★ Moderate MR   30-59 ml/beat.
    - ★ Severe MR   ≥ 60 ml/beat.
  - Evaluation of Valve for:
    - ★ Thickening valve leaflets.
    - ★ Loss of coaptation (closure).
    - ★ Presence of vegetation on valve.
    - ★ Papillary muscle dysfunction.
    - ★ Lengthening of chordae tendineae.
  - Evaluation of Left Ventricle for:
    - ★ Eccentric hypertrophy – dilated left ventricle.
    - ★ Left ventricular ejection fraction – assessment for systolic dysfunction.
      - ★ If contractility is not affected, ejection fraction of 60% or greater is not uncommon.
  - Evaluation of Left Atrium for:
    - ★ Left atrial dilatation.
- Cardiac Catheterization
  - Echocardiography is usually sufficient to diagnose mitral regurgitation.
  - Indicated if non-invasive tests are inconclusive.
  - Provides an assessment of the presence or absence of coronary artery disease which is useful when valve replacement is necessary.
  - Right heart catheterization is helpful in assessing for pulmonary hypertension.

Valve Disease

◆ Electrocardiogram
  ❖ ECG changes are neither sensitive nor specific to mitral regurgitation and always require other testing for confirmation.
  ❖ Changes are dependent on the severity of the disease process.
  ❖ Evidence of left atrial hypertrophy.
    ★ Wide notched P waves in Lead II.
  ❖ Left ventricular hypertrophy.
  ❖ Atrial fibrillation may be present.
◆ Chest X-ray
  ❖ Enlarged left atrium.
  ❖ Enlarged left ventricle.
  ❖ Enlarged right ventricle if pulmonary hypertension is present, as well as an enlarged pulmonary artery.
  ❖ Volume overload if in heart failure.

Medical Treatment
For asymptomatic patients with normal ventricular function, no treatment has been found to decrease the progression of the disease process (Darovic, 2002). After a diagnosis of mitral regurgitation has been made, annual physical exams should be done. Once symptoms occur, surgical replacement should be considered as the treatment of choice.

◆ Angiotensin-Converting Enzyme Inhibitors
  ❖ Originally thought to assist in afterload reduction with subsequent reduction in regurgitation. However, if left ventricular function as normal cardiac output remains normal and afterload is not increased, ACE inhibitors are most likely of no benefit.
  ❖ In the absence of systemic hypertension, there is no known indication for the use of vasodilating drugs in asymptomatic patients with mitral regurgitation (Bonow et al., 2006).
  ❖ ACE inhibitors may be helpful if left ventricular dysfunction is present.
◆ Rhythm Control
  ❖ Atrial fibrillation may occur and heart rate should be controlled.
  ❖ Digoxin, beta blockers or calcium channel blockers may be useful.
◆ Antibiotic Prophylaxis Against Infective Endocarditis
  See discussion on antibiotic prophylaxis under aortic stenosis.
◆ Continuous Follow Up for Asymptomatic Patients with MR
  ❖ Depends on severity of disease process.
  ❖ Occurs more frequently as the disease progresses.
  ❖ Occurs more frequently if other co-morbid conditions exist.
  ❖ Annual physician visit with focus on:
    ★ History and physical.
    ★ Careful assessment for the development of signs and symptoms.
    ★ Patient education about the importance of reporting:
      ✹ Change in exercise tolerance.
      ✹ Shortness of breath.
  ❖ Serial echocardiography (Bonow et al., 2006)
    ★ Necessary to determine onset of left ventricular dysfunction .

Chapter 11

★ Mortality with valve replacement worsens as ejection fraction worsens; careful assessment of left ventricular function is essential.

★ Asymptomatic patient with normal left ventricular function with mild MR.

    ✳ Echocardiography every 2-3 years.

★ Asymptomatic patients with severe MR.

    ✳ Echocardiography every 6-12 months.

★ Echocardiography with onset of any symptoms.

❖ Asymptomatic patients with normal left ventricular function, normal left atrial size and normal pulmonary artery pressures may exercise without restrictions (Bonow et al., 2006). Patients with ventricular enlargement, systolic dysfunction or pulmonary hypertension should avoid competitive sports or vigorous activity.

Surgical Treatment

Once symptoms of heart failure develop, surgery should be considered. With careful monitoring of the patient to assess for development of left ventricular dysfunction, the decision for surgery can be made quickly. If surgical intervention occurs before marked damage, the ventricle can be preserved and pulmonary hypertension should improve. In patients with mitral regurgitation, an ejection fraction less than 60% is considered abnormal because a calculated ejection fraction of 60% does not differentiate between the amount of blood that is moving forward through the aortic valve and the amount of blood that is moving retrograde through the abnormal mitral valve. The ejection fraction is only a calculation of the amount of left ventricular contents that is ejected. As the severity of left ventricular dysfunction increases, so does operative mortality. Options for surgical treatment of a dysfunctional mitral valve include:

◆ Mitral valve repair.

◆ Mitral valve replacement with preservation of part or all of the mitral apparatus.

◆ Mitral valve replacement with removal of the mitral apparatus.

Mitral valve replacement occurs more frequently than mitral valve repair. The Society of Thoracic Surgeons National Cardiac Database (STS DATABASE) reported a 2004 mortality rate of < 2% with isolated mitral valve repair, while the mortality rate associated with isolated mitral valve replacement was greater than 6%. The lower rate of repair versus replacement may be due to the difficulty of the procedure. The decision between repairing or replacing the valve may not be fully decided until after the surgeon has begun the operation and can view the valve and associated structures.

Elderly patients, age 75 and older, have a higher mortality rate with mitral valve surgery than the same age group having aortic valve surgery. Mortality rates for this age group are lower with valve repair surgery than they are with valve replacement surgery. However, many times valve replacement is required due to the valve pathology.

Valve Disease

The ACC/AHA Guidelines for the Management of Patients with Valvular Heart Disease recommendations for surgical treatment of mitral stenosis are reviewed in Table 11.3.

Table 11.3
ACC/AHA Recommendations for
Mitral Valve Repair/Replacement in Mitral Regurgitation

Class I Recommendations

1. Symptomatic patients with acute severe MR.

2. Chronic severe MR and NYHA functional class II, III, or IV symptoms in the absence of severe LV dysfunction (ejection fraction < 30% or end-systolic dimension > 55 mm).

3. Asymptomatic patients with chronic severe MR and mild to moderate LV dysfunction (ejection fraction 30%-60% and / or end-systolic dimension ≥ 40 mm).

4. Repair is recommended over replacement for the majority of patients with severe chronic MR who require surgery, and patients should be referred to surgical centers experienced in MV repair.

Class IIa Recommendations

1. MV repair reasonable in experienced surgical centers for asymptomatic patients with chronic severe MR and preserved LV function (ejection fraction >60% and end-systolic LV dimensions > 40 mm) in whom the likelihood of successful repair without residual MR is > 90%.

2. Asymptomatic patients with chronic severe MR, preserved LV function and new onset atrial fibrillation.

3. Asymptomatic patients with chronic severe MR and preserved LV function and pulmonary hypertension.

4. Chronic severe MR due to a primary abnormality of the mitral apparatus and NYHA functional class III-IV symptoms and severe LV dysfunction (ejection fraction <30% and/or end-systolic dimension > 55 mm in whom MV repair is highly likely.

Class IIb Recommendations

1. Repair may be considered for patients with chronic severe MR due to severe LV dysfunction (ejection fraction <30%) that has persistent NYHA functional class III-IV symptoms, despite optimal therapy for heart failure, including biventricular pacing.

(Bonow et al., 2006)

◆ Mitral valve repair
  ❖ Operation of choice if the valve is suitable for repair.
  ❖ Preserves the native valve and avoids chronic anticoagulation.
  ❖ Preservation of native valve apparatus results in better LV function postoperatively as the mitral apparatus helps preserve the shape, volume and function of the left ventricle.
  ❖ Technically complex surgery.
  ❖ Surgeon expertise very important to the success of the surgery.
  ❖ May require longer cardiopulmonary bypass time.
  ❖ Reoperation rates for repair are similar to those for replacement.
  ❖ Annular ring placement is utilized to support the native annular ring in most mitral valve repairs.

Chapter 11

- Mitral valve replacement with preservation of part or all of the mitral apparatus
  - ❖ Better postoperative valve compliance than with complete replacement.
  - ❖ Helps preserve left ventricular function.
  - ❖ Better survival than with the complete replacement of the valve.
  - ❖ Requires the use of a prosthetic valve (see discussion regarding prosthetic valves in section on aortic stenosis).
- Mitral valve replacement with removal of the mitral apparatus
  - ❖ Required if native apparatus is damaged beyond the ability to repair it (rheumatic heart disease, severe calcification).

Post Operative Considerations

If the timing of surgical treatment occurs prior to the development of left ventricular dysfunction, the patient should experience a decrease in symptoms post operatively. Results will vary dependent on pre-operative left ventricular function and the disease process affecting the valve. Patients who have developed mitral regurgitation due to myocardial ischemia or MI have a poorer prognosis than others (Crawford, 2003). These patients generally have left ventricular dysfunction from the MI. Rheumatic heart disease patients have better results, but those with mitral valve prolapse have the best outcome.

- Post-operative Follow-up Recommendations include:
  - ❖ Echocardiogram performed soon after surgery to assess left ventricular size and function. Often at first post-operative visit 3-4 weeks after surgery.
  - ❖ Follow-up visits at 6 and 12 months post-operatively, then annually (Bonow et al., 2006).
  - ❖ Patients with complications are followed up more closely.
- Antibiotic Prophylaxis Against Infective Endocarditis
  See discussion on postoperative antibiotic prophylaxis under aortic stenosis.
- Anticoagulation
  See discussion on postoperative anticoagulation under aortic stenosis.
- If anticoagulation therapy must be terminated temporarily for a procedure, some patients may require intravenous or subcutaneous heparin, while others may not, depending on the embolic risk and the length of time the warfarin is held.

Acute Mitral Regurgitation
Pathophysiology

In contrast to the progressive development of mitral regurgitation, acute mitral regurgitation occurs when a sudden event causes the immediate development of mitral regurgitation. In acute mitral regurgitation, the body has no time to develop compensatory mechanisms to adjust to the increased volume in the left atrium, and fluid overload occurs rapidly. Acute mitral regurgitation can result from papillary muscle ischemia or when a papillary muscle tears away from the ventricular wall. With the papillary muscle free, the attached valve leaflet does not close, leaving a gaping hole through which blood ejects. With only 50% of the mitral valve area closing, a very large volume of blood is ejected retrograde into the atrium, resulting in increased preload and a decreased stroke volume. Decreased stroke volume and subsequent decreased cardiac output result in increased SVR (afterload). As the vessels constrict in an attempt to compensate for the decreased forward flow of blood, the resistance against which the ventricle must pump increases. With an increase in SVR, even more blood is ejected retrograde into the atrium and less is available for cardiac output (forward flow).

Valve Disease

Pathophysiologic Mechanisms in Acute Mitral Regurgitation

◆ Acute decrease in cardiac output

→ ↑ SVR

→ blood flow to area of least resistance (through non-functional MV)

→ ↓ cardiac output (forward flow) and ↑ atrial volume (fluid overload)

→ ↑ SVR and symptoms of volume overload

→ blood flow to area of least resistance

→ ↓ cardiac output (forward flow) and ↑ atrial volume (fluid overload)

→ acute pulmonary edema.

Signs and Symptoms

With the acute changes, the heart has no time to compensate for the regurgitant flow. With no time for the left atrium to dilate, the pulmonary system quickly becomes overloaded. and pulmonary edema ensues. Other assessment findings may include:

◆ A blood pressure that is initially normal but rapidly deteriorates.

◆ A rapid heart rate with a decreased pulse amplitude.

◆ The development of cardiac arrhythmias as perfusion decreases.

◆ A sudden onset of the same murmur described in chronic regurgitation.

  ❖ A new murmur in an acutely ill patient is a key assessment finding.

◆ Any signs and symptoms related to cardiogenic shock may be present.

Diagnosis

Usually no time for extensive testing. Therefore, the most reliable diagnostic tools should be utilized.

◆ Echocardiogram is the key diagnostic tool.

  ❖ Quickly identifies the primary valve problem.

◆ Cardiac catheterization

  ❖ Indicated when ischemia may be causing the problem.

  ❖ Rarely stable enough to undergo cardiac catheterization.

Medical Treatment

Surgical treatment is the therapy of choice in acute mitral regurgitation. Until the patient is taken to surgery, several non-surgical treatment options are used to stabilize the patient while preparations for emergency surgery take place. Medical treatment goals are aimed at decreasing the amount of mitral regurgitation, increasing forward cardiac output and decreasing pulmonary congestion.

◆ Intra Aortic Balloon Pump

  ❖ Reduces afterload, resulting in less mitral regurgitation and increased forward flow.

  ❖ Increases mean arterial blood pressure.

◆ Sodium Nitroprusside

  ❖ If patient has normal blood pressure.

  ❖ Decreases SVR to improve forward flow and diminish mitral regurgitation.

  ❖ If hypotensive, then used in combination with an inotrope, such as dobutamine, may result in positive benefits.

◆ Antibiotics

  ❖ If the acute mitral regurgitation is the result of endocarditis, the infectious organism must be identified and treated.

Chapter 11

Surgical Treatment
Emergent surgical repair or replacement is the treatment of choice. The patient outcomes are dependent on the pre-operative co-morbidities. Those with acute myocardial infarctions have a higher risk than those with chronic mitral regurgitation.

Linking Knowledge to Practice

✔ *Patients with mitral valve prolapse should avoid caffeine and other stimulants because they can increase the incidence of tachycardia and anxiety attacks.*

✔ *Regular follow-up for patients with mitral regurgitation becomes important in determining the correct timing for valve replacement. Appropriate timing of replacement can prevent irreversible ventricular damage.*

✔ *Post mitral valve replacement for mitral regurgitation the patient often feels "draggy" for the first four to six weeks due to the ventricles sudden increase in workload. These patients may require short term diuretics due to increased left ventricular volume and distension.*

Mitral Stenosis

Mitral stenosis occurs when there is an abnormality impeding the normal flow of blood across the mitral valve. Impedance to normal flow occurs when there is constriction or narrowing of the mitral opening.

Causes of Mitral Stenosis

◆ Rheumatic Heart Disease
  ❖ Most common cause of mitral stenosis (Darovic, 2002).
  ❖ 40% of all patients with rheumatic heart disease have mitral stenosis.
  ❖ 60% of all patients presenting with mitral stenosis have a history of rheumatic heart disease (Bonow et al., 2006).
  ❖ Many patients with rheumatic mitral stenosis have no recollection of having rheumatic fever.
  ❖ Fibrosis and calcification of the valve leaflets present.
  ❖ Valve commissures fuse together.
  ❖ Chordae tendineae thicken and shorten.
  ❖ Combination of some or all of these changes results in a valve orifice that is much smaller than normal.

◆ Other Causes
  ❖ Other causes of mitral stenosis are rare (Swain, 2001).
  ❖ Atrial myxoma.
  ❖ Systemic lupus erythematosus.
  ❖ Bacterial endocarditis.

Pathophysiology

During ventricular diastole, the mitral valve opens and blood moves passively from the left atrium to the left ventricle. As the valve opening becomes smaller, it becomes more difficult for blood to flow passively from the atrium to the ventricle. The only way to maintain filling from the left atrium to the left ventricle is by the development of a pressure gradient referred to as the transmitral gradient. Left atrial pressure rises in an attempt to maintain normal flow across the valve. This increase in left atrial pressure is transferred back to the pulmonary vascular bed, and pulmonary pressure subsequently increases. As the obstruction worsens, the chronic increase in left atrial pressure results in pulmonary hypertension and, ultimately, right ventricular failure. The left atrium dilates in response to the increased pressure and volume, and it becomes increasingly more difficult to empty the atrium.

Compensatory Mechanisms in Mitral Stenosis

◆ Valve opening becomes smaller.
   → More difficult for blood to flow passively from the atrium to the ventricle
      → Left atrial pressure rises in attempt to maintain normal flow across the valve
         → Increased left atrial pressure transferred back to the pulmonary vascular bed
            → Pulmonary pressures subsequently rises
               → Obstruction worsens
                  → Left atrium dilates
                     → More difficult to empty atrium
                        → Chronic increase in left atrial pressure results
                           → Pulmonary hypertension develops.
◆ Compensatory system ultimately fails → Right ventricular failure.

Symptoms

The development of symptoms could begin as long as 40 years after the development of rheumatic fever. After the onset of initial symptoms, another 10 years may pass before symptoms that change the patient's lifestyle occur. With the normal mitral valve area being 4.0 to 5.0 cm^2, symptom development is usually delayed until the valve orifice is < 2.5cm^2 (Bonow et al., 2006). Symptoms at rest are usually absent until the valve orifice is less than 1.5 cm^2 (Griffin & Hayek, 2004). Generally, the valve area is less than half the normal size before any symptoms occur. Once symptoms begin, they develop slowly and patients make adjustments in activity levels to compensate for the changes, often without being aware that they are doing so.

◆ Dyspnea with exertion with no symptoms at rest is the most common initial finding. Conditions that increase heart rate, such as pregnancy, new-onset atrial fibrillation, hyperthyroidism, or fever, commonly result in symptoms that alert the physician to the possibility of mitral stenosis. An increased heart rate shortens diastolic filling time and, therefore, decreases ventricular filling time as well as atrial emptying. Poor atrial emptying results in a fluid overload state and pulmonary edema can occur. Decreased filling time results in decreased stroke volume, which contributes to decreased cardiac output. When cardiac output is insufficient, symptoms of dyspnea and fatigue occur.

◆ Orthopnea and paroxysmal nocturnal dyspnea develop as valve dysfunction increases, and the valve orifice decreases (1 cm^2 to 1.4 cm^2).

◆ Dyspnea at rest develops with a valve orifice less than 1 cm^2.

◆ Cough and hemoptysis develop as the disease progresses.

◆ Ultimately, the failure of the system affects the right side of the heart, and signs of right ventricular failure appear.

◆ Stroke caused by an embolus in many situations is the first indication of mitral stenosis. As the atrium enlarges, the risk of embolization increases.

◆ Atrial fibrillation is noted in more than one half of the patients with mitral stenosis due to atrial enlargement (Massie & Amiodon, 2004).

Physical Examination

- S1 (First Heart Sound)
  - First heart sound (S1, or "lub") is louder than normal,
  - If valve is heavily calcified, then the sound is diminished (Griffin & Hayek, 2004).
- Opening Snap (OS) (Figure 11.14)
  - Opening of stenotic mitral valve.
  - If valve is heavily calcified and the leaflets are not moving well, the opening snap may not be present.
  - Timing: Just after second heart sound (S2, or "dub").
  - Location: Best heard at the apex (5th intercostal space, left mid-clavicular line).
  - Radiation: Often heard across the precordium; often heard in other normal ausculatory areas.
  - Pitch: High pitch, best heard with the diaphragm of the stethoscope.
  - Often confused with S3
    - S3 better heard with bell of stethoscope.
    - S3 not as well heard across the precordium as the OS.
    - S3 louder during expiration than inspiration, while OS does not change in relation to the respiratory pattern.
    - OS occurs earlier in diastole than an S3, so OS should occur closer to the S2.
    - Presence of diastolic murmur helps confirm an OS.

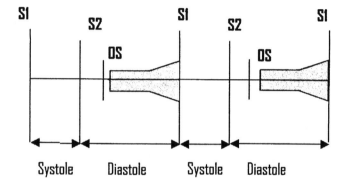

Figure 11.14: Drawing demonstrating the diastolic crescendo murmur of MS with an opening snap (OS).

- Diastolic Murmur (Figure 11.14)
  - Timing: Depends on severity of disease
    - Severe mitral stenosis: Holodiastolic.
    - Moderate mitral stenosis: Early and late diastole.
  - Location: Best heard near the apex (5th intercostal space, left mid-clavicular line).
  - Configuration: Crescendo.
  - Pitch: Low pitch best heard with bell of stethoscope.
  - Quality: Rumble.
  - Best heard with the patient lying on the left side.
  - Increases with isometric exercise, amyl nitrate and expiration.
- Other Heart Sounds
  - Systolic murmur of mitral regurgitation.
    - Presence of mitral regurgitation in the setting of mitral stenosis is not uncommon.
  - Systolic murmur of tricuspid regurgitation.
    - Tricuspid regurgitation may be present if pulmonary hypertension and right ventricular failure is present.
- Signs Of Left-Sided Heart Failure
  - Respiratory distress.
  - Pulmonary edema.

- ◆ Signs Of Right-Sided Heart Failure
  - ❖ May be present if disease progression is severe.
  - ❖ Jugular venous distension.
  - ❖ Hepatomegaly.
  - ❖ Peripheral edema.
  - ❖ Ascites.
- ◆ Mitral Facies
  - ❖ Pinkish purple discoloration of the cheeks that is common in patients with severe mitral stenosis (Darovic, 2002).

Diagnosis

- ◆ Cardiac Echocardiogram
  - ❖ Primary tool utilized to conform the diagnosis of mitral stenosis.
  - ❖ Quantifies the severity of stenosis.
  - ❖ Evaluation of Transmitral Pressure Gradient (Bonow et al., 2006).
    - ☆ Pressure difference between left atrium and left ventricle.
    - ☆ Mild MS   < 5 mm Hg.
    - ☆ Moderate MS   5-10 mm Hg.
    - ☆ Severe MS   > 10 mm Hg.
  - ❖ Evaluation of Valve Area (Bonow et al., 2006).
    - ☆ Normal   4-5 cm^2.
    - ☆ Mild MS   > 1.5 cm^2.
    - ☆ Moderate MS   1.0-1.5 cm^2.
    - ☆ Severe MS   < 1.0 cm^2.
  - ❖ Evaluation of Valve Leaflets.
    - ☆ Important for determination of treatment options.
    - ☆ Mobility.
      - ✶ Minimal to severe disease progression: from restriction of the tips of the leaflets to minimal or no forward movement of the leaflets during diastole.
    - ☆ Calcification.
      - ✶ Minimal to severe disease progression: from minimal calcification as identified by minimal areas of increased echo brightness to highly calcified, with extensive echo brightness indicating calcification.
    - ☆ Valve Thickening.
      - ✶ Minimal to severe disease progression: from minimal leaflet thickening (4-5 mm) to considerable leaflet thickening (greater than 5-8 mm).
    - ☆ Subvalvular (chordae tendineae and papillary muscle) Thickening.
      - ✶ Minimal to severe disease progression: from thickening just below the mitral leaflets to extensive thickening and shortening of the chordae tendineae and the papillary muscles (Wilkens et al., 1988).
  - ❖ Evaluation of Left Atrial Size.
    - ☆ Left atrial size increases with severity of disease.

Chapter 11

- ❖ Evaluation of Pulmonary Artery Pressures (Bonow et al., 2006).
  - ☆ Mild MS   < 30 mm Hg.
  - ☆ Moderate MS   30-50 mm Hg.
  - ☆ Severe MS   > 50 mm Hg.
- ◆ Stress Testing
  - ❖ May be beneficial for:
    - ☆ Determination if symptoms are from MS or other causes in patients with significant symptoms and only mild MS by echocardiogram.
- ◆ Cardiac Catheterization
  - ❖ When noninvasive assessment of severity of disease is inconclusive.
  - ❖ To evaluate for the presence of coronary artery disease when valve replacement surgery is planned.
- ◆ Chest X-ray
  - ❖ The presence of signs of mitral stenosis on chest x-ray film depends on the extent of the disease.
  - ❖ In pulmonary hypertension, pulmonary arteries are more visible on the x-ray film.
  - ❖ Elevation of the left main stem bronchus may be noted with left atrial enlargement.
  - ❖ Signs of pulmonary edema are noted if the patient is in a volume overload state.
- ◆ Electrocardiogram (ECG)
  - ❖ ECG changes are neither sensitive nor specific to mitral stenosis and always require other testing for confirmation.
  - ❖ Signs of left atrial enlargement may be present.
    - ☆ Wide, notched P waves in lead II.
    - ☆ Biphasic P wave in lead V_1 with a wide negative deflection greater than 0.04 seconds.
  - ❖ Signs of severe pulmonary hypertension.
    - ☆ Right-axis deviation.
    - ☆ Right ventricular hypertrophy.
      - ✶ Tall R waves in the V_1, V_2 and V_3.
  - ❖ Atrial fibrillation.
    - ☆ Usually develops with left atrial hypertrophy.

Medical Treatment

Medical management is of limited use in asymptomatic patients with normal sinus rhythm. There is no medical treatment for the fixed obstruction that occurs at the mitral valve. Once symptoms begin, treatment is directed at alleviation of symptoms.

- ◆ Heart Rate Control
  - ❖ Exercise increases the heart rate, which decreases diastolic filling time.
  - ❖ Decreased diastolic filling time increases left atrial pressure and leads to activity intolerance.
  - ❖ Beta blockers or calcium channel blockers that help control heart rate can be useful in patients who have exercise intolerance.
- ◆ Atrial Fibrillation
  - ❖ Over one-third of the patients with MS develop atrial arrhythmias.
  - ❖ Atrial fibrillation with a rapid ventricular response greatly decreases diastolic filling time, which can result in hemodynamic compromise.

Valve Disease

- ❖ Risk of stroke increases in the patient with MS and atrial fibrillation, as does the mortality rate.
- ❖ Because atrial fibrillation is poorly tolerated, it is reasonable to attempt to return the patient to normal sinus rhythm with cardioversion, either electrical or chemical (with medications).
- ❖ According to the ACC/AHA guidelines (Bonow et al., 2006), cardioversion for patients in atrial fibrillation longer than 24-48 hours may occur in one of two manners:
  - ☆ Anticoagulation with warfarin for 3 weeks, then proceed with the cardioversion.
  - ☆ Anticoagulation with heparin and transesophageal echocardiography to assess for left atrial thrombus. If no thrombus is noted, the cardioversion may be performed while continuing heparinization.
- ❖ Continued use of antiarrhythmics after successful cardioversion to sinus rhythm has proven to be helpful in maintaining a normal rhythm.
- ❖ Calcium channel blockers or beta blockers can be useful in the treatment of atrial fibrillation to maintain a ventricular rate of less than 100 beats per minute (Griffin & Hayek, 2004).
- ❖ It is not unusual for MS patients to have recurrent bouts of atrial fibrillation, with rate control of atrial fibrillation being the end goal.

◆ Antibiotic Prophylaxis Against Infective Endocarditis
  See discussion on antibiotic prophylaxis under aortic stenosis.

◆ Anticoagulation
  - ❖ Guidelines for anticoagulation based on the ACC/AHA Practice Guidelines for Valvular Heart Disease appear in Table 11.4.
  - ❖ Risk of embolization increase with age and the presence of atrial fibrillation.
  - ❖ Currently, no clinical trials support the use of anticoagulants in patients without a history of embolic events (Griffin & Hayek, 2004).

Table 11.4 ACC/AHA Recommendations for Anticoagulation in Patients with Mitral Stenosis
Class I Recommendations
1. Patients with mitral stenosis and atrial fibrillation.
2. Patients with mitral stenosis and a prior embolic event.
3. Patients with mitral stenosis and left atrial thrombus.
Class IIb Recommendations
1. Considered in asymptomatic patients with severe mitral stenosis and left atrial dimension > 55 mm by cardiac echo.
2. Considered in patients with severe mitral stenosis, left atrial enlargement and spontaneous contrast on cardiac echo.

◆ Preload Reduction
  - ❖ Diuretics provide symptomatic relief if fluid overload develops.
  - ❖ Sodium restriction may also be helpful in decreasing a fluid overload state.

◆ Continuous Follow Up for Asymptomatic Patients with Mitral Stenosis
  - ❖ Depends on severity of disease process.
  - ❖ Occurs more frequently as the disease progresses.

Chapter 11

❖ Occurs more frequently if other co-morbid conditions exist.
❖ Annual physician visit reasonable with focus on:
 ☆ History and physical.
 ☆ Careful assessment for the development of signs and symptoms.
 ☆ Careful evaluation of heart sounds.
  ✳ Shortening of the time from the second heart sound to the opening snap and/or longer duration of the diastolic murmur could indicate worsening valve disease.
 ☆ Patient education about the importance of reporting:
  ✳ Change in exercise tolerance.
  ✳ Shortness of breath.
❖ Serial echocardiography (Bonow et al., 2006).
 ☆ Mild MS – Every 3-5 years.
 ☆ Moderate MS – Every 1-2 years.
 ☆ Severe MS – Annually.
❖ Exercise.
 ☆ Asymptomatic patients with mild MS.
  ✳ Not restricted.
  ✳ May participate in competitive sports.
 ☆ Asymptomatic with moderate to severe MS.
  ✳ Strenuous exercise can cause an increase in heart rate with a sudden decrease in diastolic filling time, and an increase in pulmonary pressures, resulting in pulmonary edema.
  ✳ Ability to exercise is determined by the development of symptoms.

Surgical Treatment

When the valve area becomes less than 1.5 cm^2, most patients with mitral stenosis begin to experience symptoms at rest and lifestyle is affected. Once these symptoms occur, surgical options should be considered. Several options are available depending on the situation:

◆ Percutaneous mitral balloon valvotomy (PMBV)
◆ Closed surgical commissurotomy
◆ Open surgical commissurotomy
◆ Mitral valve replacement
◆ Percutaneous Mitral Balloon Valvotomy
 ❖ The ACC/AHA guidelines recommend valvotomy as described in Table 11.5.
 ❖ Better long-term results than with aortic valvotomy.
 ❖ Balloon is passed into the right atrium via a femoral approach, then through the atrial septum to the left atrium. The balloon is placed across the mitral valve and inflated, causing the fused leaflets to split apart.
 ❖ Procedure is carried out in the cardiac catheterization laboratory.
 ❖ Has the best results in patients with no valve calcification and strictly a fusion of the commissures.
 ❖ If the left atrium is greatly dilated or the valve is heavily calcified, results are usually suboptimal.
 ❖ Mitral balloon valvotomy should not be performed on patients who also have mitral regurgitation of 2+ or more because the procedure increases the amount of regurgitation (Griffin & Hayek, 2004).

Valve Disease

- ❖ Post procedure complications.
  - ✩ Embolization.
  - ✩ Mitral regurgitation.
  - ✩ Atrial or ventricular septal defects.
  - ✩ Ventricular perforation.
- ❖ Mortality rates as low as < 1% in centers with experienced operators.

Table 11.5 **ACC/AHA Recommendations for** **Percutaneous Mitral Balloon Valvotomy**
Class I Recommendations
1. Symptomatic patients (NHYA functional class II, III, or IV) with moderate or severe MS and valve morphology favorable (non-calcified pliable valves, mild subvalvular fusions and no calcium in the commissures) for PMBV in the absence of left atrial thrombus or moderate to severe MR.
2. Asymptomatic patients with moderate or severe MS and valve morphology that is favorable for PMBV in the absence of left atrial thrombus or moderate to severe MR.
Class IIa Recommendations
1. Moderate or severe MS with a non-pliable calcified valve and NYHA functional class III-IV AND not a surgical candidate.
Class IIb Recommendations
1. Considered for asymptomatic patients with moderate or severe MS and valve morphology favorable for PMBV, with new onset atrial fibrillation in the absence of left atrial thrombus or moderate or severe MR.
2. Considered for symptomatic patients with MV area greater then 1.5 cm,^{2} if evidence of pulmonary hypertension.
3. Considered as an alternative to surgery for patients with moderate or severe MS who have non-pliable calcified valve and are NYHA functional class III-IV.
(Bonow et al., 2006)

- ◆ Mitral Commissurotomy
  As stenosis develops, the commissures (points where valve leaflets come together) begin to fuse together. During mitral commissurotomy, commissures are cut apart to allow for increased movement of the leaflets. This procedure is beneficial to patients with pliable leaflets that have no calcification. The procedure is not recommended in patients with a clot in the left atrium or with moderate or severe mitral regurgitation, as the development of some degree of regurgitation post procedure is not uncommon.
  - ❖ Closed Commissurotomy.
    - ✩ Limited effectiveness due to inability to visualize the valve.
    - ✩ Dilator is introduced via the apex of the left ventricular wall and pass through the mitral valve.
    - ✩ Once across the valve, the dilator is opened to dilate the mitral valve.
    - ✩ Assessment of effectiveness is completed via transesophogeal echocardiography.
    - ✩ No need for cardiopulmonary bypass.
    - ✩ Less expensive than traditional replacement surgery.
    - ✩ No longer the procedure of choice as effects are similar to valvotomy, which is percutaneous.

Chapter 11

- ❖ Open Commissurotomy.
  - ★ Requires a median sternotomy or antero-lateral thoracotomy.
  - ★ Beneficial to patients with pliable leaflets and no calcification.
  - ★ Open repair preferred method.
  - ★ Can visualize and remove calcium deposits and left atrial clots during surgery.
  - ★ Amputation of the left atrial appendage may also occur during surgery.
  - ★ Open chest procedure requires use of cardiac bypass, which increases risk and cost.
- ◆ Mitral Valve Replacement

  Patients with extensive calcification, fibrosis, mitral regurgitation, in addition to stenosis and pulmonary hypertension, are candidates for mitral valve replacement. If the valve is replaced with a mechanical valve, lifelong anticoagulation is required. Anticoagulation is not required if the patient in sinus rhythm receives a bioprosthetic valve. However, a large percentage of patients with MS are already receiving anticoagulation due to atrial fibrillation. The ACC/AHA recommendations for mitral valve replacement are listed in Table 11.6. Mitral valve replacement is not indicated for patients with mild mitral stenosis.

  - ❖ Mitral valve replacement surgery can include replacement of the entire mitral apparatus or replacement of the mitral valve with preservation of the subvalvular apparatus (chordae tendineae, papillary muscles). The latter is often difficult to do as the chordae tendineae and the papillary muscles may also be thickened, fibrotic and calcified.
  - ❖ If the patient has chronic atrial fibrillation a Maze procedure will often be completed at the time of mitral valve replacement.
  - ❖ Amputation of the left atrial appendage may also be done during valve replacement surgery, especially if the patient is not a candidate for the Maze procedure. Removal of the left atrial appendage may help decrease thrombus development.
  - ❖ Surgical risk in the young healthy adult has a relatively low mortality rate. Mortality rates increase with age, co-morbid factors and the presence of pulmonary hypertension.
  - ❖ Surgery should not be delayed until symptoms are severe. Patients with NYHA functional class IV have a higher mortality rate than those with class III failure.
  - ❖ The decision to utilize a mechanical valve versus a tissue valve is similar to any other valve replacement and discussed in the section on aortic stenosis.

Valve Disease

| Table 11.6 |
ACC/AHA Recommendations for Mitral Valve Surgery in Mitral Stenosis
Class I Recommendations
1. Symptomatic patients (NYHA functional class III-IV), moderate or severe MS when PMBV is unavailable, PMBV is contraindicated due to left atrial clot, or the valve morphology is not favorable for PMBV in a patient with acceptable operative risk. Repair over replacement if able.
2. Symptomatic patients with moderate to severe MS who also have moderate to severe MR should receive valve replacement unless repair is possible.
Class IIa Recommendations
1. Replacement for patients with severe MS and severe pulmonary hypertension and NYHA functional class I-II symptoms who are not considered candidates for PMBV or surgical repair.
Class IIb Recommendations
1. Considered for asymptomatic patients with moderate or severe MS who have had recurrent embolic events while receiving adequate anticoagulation, and who have morphology favorable for repair.
(Bonow et al., 2006)

◆ Post Operative Care
As cardiovascular technology and skill continue to advance, patients undergoing valvuloplasty and open-heart commissurotomy continue to experience excellent short- and long-term results (Stoltz & Bryg, 2003). Patients who have the correct valve anatomy should undergo valvuloplasty to avoid the risks associated with bypass surgery. Patients begin to experience an improvement in symptoms as soon as the valve is replaced or repaired.

   ❖ Post-operative follow-up recommendations include:
      ☆ Echocardiogram performed soon after surgery, but no sooner than 72 hours after the procedure, as acute change postoperative affects the reliability of the study.
      ☆ Follow up visits at 6 and 12 months post operatively, and then annually (Bonow et al., 2006).
      ☆ Patients with complications are followed up more closely.
   ❖ Antibiotic prophylaxis against infective endocarditis.
   See discussion on postoperative antibiotic prophylaxis under aortic stenosis.
   ❖ Anticoagulation.
   See discussion on postoperative anticoagulation under aortic stenosis.

Linking Knowledge to Practice

✔ *Patients with severe mitral stenosis may develop acute pulmonary edema with exercise because the narrowed mitral opening cannot handle the increased blood flow produced by the normal increase in heart rate and venous return that occurs with exercise.*

✔ *Although patients with mild to moderate mitral stenosis should be counseled to avoid unusually stressful exercise, they should be encouraged to maintain a low-level aerobic exercise program to maintain cardiovascular fitness. The limits of this exercise should be determined by individual patient tolerance.*

✔ *Patients with mitral stenosis are dependent on atrial contraction for a large portion of ventricular filling because stenosis slows the passive filling phase. Therefore, the development of atrial fibrillation*

497

Chapter 11

in patients with mitral stenosis can quickly result in symptoms of decreased perfusion, because atrial contraction is lost with the onset of atrial fibrillation.

◆ *Clinicians should be particularly alert for the development of atrial fibrillation because the incidence of stroke is high with this rhythm. Many patients are unaware of the development of an irregular heart rhythm, but astute practitioners can recognize the changes of atrial fibrillation and begin appropriate treatment.*

TEST YOUR KNOWLEDGE

1. The primary tool used for the screening of cardiac valve disease is
    a. cardiac echocardiogram.
    b. 12 lead ECG
    c. cardiac auscultation.
    d. chest X-ray.

2. The heart's primary compensatory response to chronic aortic stenosis includes
    a. left atrial hypertrophy.
    b. left ventricular hypertrophy.
    c. left ventricular dilation.
    d. left atrial dilation.

3. The classic trio of symptoms noted in symptomatic patients with aortic stenosis include
    a. angina, syncope, and heart failure
    b. hypotension, palpitations, and angina
    c. murmurs, hypotension, and palpitations
    d. palpitations, syncope, and angina.

4. In the patient with **severe** aortic stenosis, which class of medications is contraindicated due to its primary effect of decreasing SVR?
    a. Beta blocker
    b. ACE inhibitor
    c. Low dose nitrate
    d. Diuretic

Valve Disease

5. In the patient with chronic aortic regurgitation, which of the following physiological change is the direct result of the heart compensating for the regurgitation?
    a. Left atrial enlargement
    b. Aorta enlargement
    c. Decreased contractility
    d. Left ventricular enlargement

6. Which of the following signs and symptoms are specific to the patient with acute aortic regurgitation?
    a. Decreasing activity tolerance
    b. Abrupt onset of shortness of breath
    c. Bradycardia
    d. Water-Hammer Pulse

7. All of the following may be helpful in stabilizing a patient with acute aortic regurgitation until emergency surgery can performed except:
    a. Sodium nitroprusside
    b. Lasix
    c. Dobutamine
    d. Intra Aortic Balloon Pump

8. Patients with mitral valve prolapse should avoid which of the following to help prevent the development of tachycardia and anxiety attacks?
    a. Smoking
    b. Alcohol
    c. Caffeine
    d. Sodium

9. The ultimate response to long term chronic mitral regurgitation includes
    a. decreased left ventricular contractility.
    b. primary pulmonary hypertension.
    c. dilated left atrium.
    d. loss of atrial kick.

Chapter 11

10. Forty-eight hours after admission your patient, who is hospitalized with an inferior myocardial infarction, reports that he suddenly started to have difficulty breathing. During your assessment you notice that the respiratory rate and heart rate are increased. You also discover a new systolic murmur, best heard at the 5th intercostal space, left midclavicular line that was not present during an earlier assessment. As you call the physician, you anticipate these symptoms may be caused by

   a. recurrent myocardial infarction.

   b. pulmonary embolism.

   c. pericardial effusion.

   d. papillary muscle rupture.

11. You are caring for a patient newly diagnosed with atrial fibrillation. On physical assessment you hear a diastolic murmur you would describe as a rumble. The diastolic rumble is the loudest at the cardiac apex. What valvular disease does this patient most likely have that predisposed him to atrial fibrillation?

   a. Mitral stenosis

   b. Mitral regurgitation

   c. Aortic stenosis

   d. Aortic regurgitation.

12. In addition to the above murmur you recognize an additional heart sound that is heard just after S2, does not change in relation to inspiration or expiration and is best heard with the diaphragm of the stethoscope. You recognize this sound as

   a. S3.

   b. S4.

   c. opening snap.

   d. click.

13. The development of high heart rates with exercise in patients with mitral stenosis can be detrimental. Which class of medication may be helpful in keeping the heart rate at a lower rate, even with exercise?

   a. Beta blockers

   b. ACE inhibitors

   c. Angiotensin receptor blockers

   d. Positive inotrope

500

Valve Disease

14. Antibiotics administration for the prevention of infective endocarditis is indicated in all of the following patient populations except
    a. patients with cardiac valve disease.
    b. patients who have had a prosthetic valve implanted.
    c. patients with a previous history of infective endocarditis.
    d. select patients with congenital heart disease.

15. Patients with this type of prosthetic valve implant require lifelong anticoagulation:
    a. Homograft
    b. Stented heterograft
    c. Stentless heterograft
    d. Mechanical valve

ANSWERS

1.	C	9.	C
2.	B	10.	D
3.	A	11.	A
4.	B	12.	C
5.	D	13.	A
6.	B	14.	A
7.	D	15.	D
8.	C		

REFERENCES

Alcomo, I.E. (1996). *Anatomy and physiology the easy way.* Hauppauge, NY: Barrons.

Ballentine, J. & Eisenhart, A. (2002). Aortic stenosis. Retrieved March 3, 2005 from http://www.emedicine.com/emerg/topic40.htm

Bhola, R. & Gill, E.A. (2001). Rheumatic heart disease and mitral stenosis. In A.V. Adair (Ed.). Cardiology secrets (pp. 226-235). Philadelphia: Hanley and Belfus, Inc.

Bojar, R.M.(2005). *Manual of perioperative care in adult cardiac surgery* (4th ed.). Malden, Massachusetts: Blackwell Publishing.

Bonow, R.O., Carabello, B.A., Chatterjee, K., de Leon, A.C. Jr., Faxon, D.P., Freed, M.D., Gaasch, W.H., Lytle, B.W., Nishimura, R.A., O'Gara, P.T., O'Rourke, R.A., Otto, C.M., Shah, P.M., Shanewise J.S. ACC/AHA 2006 guidelines for the management of patients with valvular heart disease: A report of the American College of Cardiology/American Heart Association Task Force on Practice Guidelines (Writing Committee to Develop Guidelines for the Management of Patients With Valvular Heart Disease). American College of Cardiology Web Site. Available at: http://www.acc.org/clinical/guidelines/valvular/index.pdf

Carabello, B.A., & Crawford, M.H. (2003). Aortic stenosis. In M.H. Crawford (Ed.), *Current diagnosis and treatment in cardiology* (2nd ed., pp. 108-120). New York: McGraw-Hill.

Carabello, B.A. & Ganzes, P.C. (2001). *Cardiology pearls* (2nd Ed.). Philadelphia: Hanley and Belfus.

Crawford, M.H. (2003). Mitral regurgitation. In M.H. Crawford (Ed.), *Current diagnosis and treatment in cardiology* (2nd ed., pp. 142-150). New York: McGraw-Hill.

Darovic, G.O. (2002). *Hemodynamic monitoring: invasive and noninvasive clinical application* (3rd Ed.). Philadelphia: Saunders.

Dennison, R.D. (2000). *Pass CCRN* (2nd ed.). St. Louis, Missouri: Mosby.

Griffin, B. & Hayek, E. (2004). *Mitral valve disease*. Retrieved September 9, 2004, from http://www.clevelandclinicmeded.com

Havranek, E.P. & Adair, A.V. (2001). Aortic stenosis and regurgitation. In A.V. Adair (Ed.), *Cardiology secrets* (pp. 237-240). Philadelphia: Hanley and Belfus, Inc.

Hilkert, R.J. & Yoo, H. (2002). Aortic regurgitation. Retrieved May 5, 2003 from http://www.emedicine.com/med/topic156.htm

Kumar, V., Abbas. A.K., & Fausto, N. (2005). *Pathologic basis of disease* (7th ed.). Philadelphia: Elsevier Saunders.

LeDoux, D. (2005). Acquired valve disease. In S.L.Woods, E.S. Froelicher, S.U. Motzer, & E.J. Bridges (Eds.), *Cardiac nursing* (5th ed., pp. 756-775). Philadelphia: Lippincott, Williams and Wilkins.

Lewis, S.M., Heitkemper, M.M., & Dirksen, S.T. (2004) *Medical surgical nursing: assessment and management of clinical problems* (6th ed.). St. Louis, Missouri: Mosby, Inc.

Massie, B.M. & Amiodon, T.M. (2004). Heart. In L.M. Tierney, Jr, S.J. McPhee, & M.A. Papadakis, *Current medical diagnosis and treatment* (43rd ed., pp. 315-400). New York: McGraw-Hill.

Melander, SD. (2004). *Case studies in critical care nursing: A guide for application and review.* Philadelphia: W.B. Saunders Company.

Mills, R.M. & Novaro, G.M. (2004). *Aortic valve disease*. Retrieved September 9, 2004, from http://www.clevelandclinicmeded.com/diseasemanagment/cardiology/aortic_valve/aortic_valve.htm

Moore, K.L. & Dalley, A.F. (1999). *Clinically oriented anatomy* (4th ed.). Philadelphia: Lippincott, Williams and Wilkins.

Morton, P.G., Fontaine, D., Hudak, C.M., & Gallo, B.M. (Eds.). (2005). *Critical care nursing: A holistic approach* (8th ed.). Philadelphia: Lippincott, Williams and Wilkins.

Porth, C.M. (Ed.). (2004). *Essentials of pathophysiology: concepts of altered health states*. Philadelphia: Lippincott, Williams and Wilkins.

Schell, H.M. & Puntillo, K.A. (2001). *Critical care nursing secrets*. Philadelphia: Hanley and Belfus, Inc.

Staab, M. & Krasnow, N. (2001). Prosthetic valves. In A.V. Adair (Ed.), *Cardiology secrets* (pp. 100-104). Philadelphia: Hanley and Belfus, Inc.

Stolrz, C. & Bryg, R.J. (2003). Mitral stenosis. In M.H. Crawford (Ed.), *Current diagnosis and treatment in cardiology* (2nd ed., pp. 131-141). New York: McGraw-Hill.

Swain, D.K. (2001). *Mitral stenosis*. Retrieved May 5, 2003 from http://www.emedicine.com/emerg/top315.htm

Thelan, L.A., Davie, J.K., Urden, L.D., & Lough, M.E. (1994). *Critical care nursing: Diagnosis and management* (2nd ed.). St. Louis, Missouri: Mosby, Inc.

Thibodeau, G.A. & Patton, K.T. (2003). *Anatomy and physiology* (5th ed.). St. Louis, Missouri: Mosby, Inc.

Urden, LD, Stacy, KM (2000). *Priorities in critical care nursing* (3rd ed.). St. Louis, Missouri: Mosby, Inc.

Weinberger, H.D. (2001). Mitral valve prolapse and mitral regurgitation. In A.V. Adair (Ed.), *Cardiology secrets* (pp. 241-243). Philadelphia: Hanley and Belfus, Inc.

White, T.R. & Schwartz, D.E. (2003). Valvular heart disease. In P.E. Parsons & J.P. Wiener-Kronish (Ed.), *Critical care secrets* (3rd ed., pp. 153-162). Philadelphia: Hanley and Belfus, Inc.

Wilson, W., Taubert, K., Gewitz, M., Lockhart, P., Baddour, L., Levison, M., Bolger, A., Cabell, C., Takahashi, M., Baltimore, R., Newburger, J., Strom, B., Tani, L., Gerber, M., Bonow, R., Pallasch, T., Shulman, S., Rowley, A., Burns, J., Ferrieri, P., Gardner, T., Goff, D., & Durack, D. (2007). Prevention of endocarditis guidelines from the American Heart Association: A guideline from the American Heart Association rheumatic fever, endocarditis, and Kawasaki disease committee, Council on cardiovascular disease in the young, and the Council on clinical cardiology, Council on cardiovascular surgery and anesthesia, and the Quality of care and outcomes research interdisciplinary working group. Retrieved from www.circ.ahajournals.org on June 3, 2007.

Zoghbi, W.A. &. Afridi, I. (2003). Aortic regurgitation. In M.H. Crawford (Ed.), *Current diagnosis and treatment in cardiology* (2nd ed., pp. 121-130). New York: McGraw-Hill.

CHAPTER 12:
INFLAMMATORY CARDIOVASCULAR DISEASES: DISEASES INVOLVING THE PERICARDIUM, MYOCARDIUM AND ENDOCARDIUM

PERICARDIAL DISEASES

The pericardium is the outermost layer of the heart. While the pericardium is not essential and can be removed without a functional detriment, it serves many purposes. The outer surface of the pericardium is attached to the diaphragm, sternum, and costal cartilage to help anchor the heart in the chest cavity. The outermost surface of the pericardium is referred to as the fibrous layer or the fibrous pericardium. This layer has a tough fibrous surface that is not easily distensible. The fibrous pericardium helps to maintain the shape and size of the heart, especially in fluid overload situations. The serous layer of the pericardium (serous pericardium) is the inner surface that surrounds the potential space referred to as the pericardial cavity (Figure 12.1). The parietal layer of the serous pericardium is contiguous with the fibrous layer and is the inner wall of this layer of the pericardium. The epicardial layer of the heart is also the visceral layer of the serous pericardium. The serous pericardium protects the heart against inflammation and immunological compromise.

The pericardial cavity contains approximately 15 to 20 ml of serous fluid and functions to reduce friction on the pericardium. The tough fibrous layer of the pericardium does not distend easily; therefore, accumulation of fluid in the pericardial space may or may not result in hemodynamic compromise. Small amounts of fluid accumulated quickly in the pericardial cavity may result in hemodynamic compromise, as the fibrous pericardium cannot quickly expand to adjust for the volume changes. However, large amounts of fluid accumulated gradually over time may be tolerated as the fibrous pericardium has time to adjust to the increase of fluid. The pericardial space is usually able to adapt to acute volume additions up to 100 ml without increased pressure on the heart and hemodynamic compromise. If fluid accumulates slowly, up to 1-2 liters of fluid may be held in the pericardial space (DeCastro & Schwartz, 2003) without hemodynamic compromise.

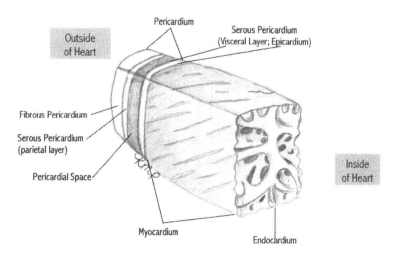

Figure 12.1: Layers of the heart.

Pericarditis

Pericarditis is an inflammatory process involving the visceral or parietal layers of the pericardium.

Causes

There are many causes of pericarditis (Table 12.1), viral infection being the most common (Goyle and Walling, 2002). Echovirus and coxsackievirus A and B are the most common causes of viral pericarditis.

Chapter 12

Human immunodeficiency virus, hepatitis, measles, mumps and vericella viruses are some less common causes of viral pericarditis. Staphylococcus, streptococcus, pneumococci and *Mycobacterium tuberculosis* are the most common causes of bacterial pericarditis. Metastatic cancers and the treatment for some of these cancers can contribute to the development of pericarditis. Tumors of the lung and breast, as well as lymphomas, melanomas and leukemia can all cause pericarditis. Radiation treatments to the chest or thorax may also result in pericarditis. Uremic pericarditis is usually noted in patients with newly diagnosed renal failure prior to the start of dialysis. Some medications have been noted to cause pericarditis, with hydralazine and procainamide being the most frequently cited. Any trauma involving the pericardial layer of the heart may result in pericarditis. Trauma can include traumatic penetrating injuries to the heart, as well as surgical procedures that can involve the heart.

Pericarditis occurring within 24 to 96 hours of a myocardial infarction is referred to as infarction pericarditis. Post myocardial infarction syndrome, also referred to as Dressler's Syndrome, is pericarditis that occurs weeks to months after the myocardial infarction. Since myocardial infarctions begin with the endocardial surface of the heart and expand through the myocardial surface to the epicardial surface, infarction pericarditis generally occurs only with transmural myocardial infarctions that have traversed the entire thickness of the myocardial layers. Both infarction pericarditis and Dressler's Syndrome tend to occur with transmural infarcts, especially anterior infarcts, inferior infarcts with right-ventricular involvement, and myocardial infarctions with complex hospitalizations (Spodick, 2004). The incidence of Dressler's Syndrome has decreased greatly since the development of reperfusion therapies. Infarct pericarditis is thought to be an inflammatory response to the damaged myocardial tissue. The cause of Dressler's Syndrome is unknown, but an autoimmune response is thought to be the cause.

Pericarditis occurring two to ten days after cardiac or thoracic surgery is referred to as post cardiotomy or post thoracotomy syndrome. Pericardial effusions are common in this population as well. This condition may also be referred to as Dressler's Syndrome.

Symptoms

Patients with pericarditis usually present with precordial or retrosternal chest pain that is described as sharp or stabbing. The pain has a pleuritic characteristic and increases with inspiration, cough, or movement. The pain is more intense with the patient in the recumbent position. The discomfort eases when the patient sits up and leans forward. Not all patients with pericarditis present with chest pain, but may complain only of trapezius ridge pain, which is very specific to pericarditis. When presenting with precordial chest pain, the patient should be carefully questioned about the discomfort to differentiate between the pain of angina or acute myocardial infarction and the discomfort of pericarditis. Myocardial pain is usually described as crushing, squeezing, pressure or heaviness that does not change with position or respiratory effort. Many patients presenting with viral pericarditis report a period of "flu-like" symptoms with complaints of malaise and fever. The patient may also report difficulty breathing, as they tend to breathe with a shallow respiratory pattern to ease the discomfort associated with deeper breaths.

Inflammatory Cardiovascular Diseases: Diseases Involving the Pericardium, Myocardium and Endocardium

Table 12.1
Etiologies of Pericarditis

Idiopathic

Infections

Viral	Bacterial	Fungal
Coxsackievirus	*Streptococcus*	*Histoplasmosis*
Echovirus	Staphylococcus	*Aspergillosis*
Human immunodeficiency virus	Pneumococcus	
Mumps virus	*Mycobacterium Tuberculosis*	
Measles virus		
Influenza virus		
Chickenpox virus		

Neoplasm

Metastatic
  Breast
  Lung
  Lymphoma
  Melanoma
  Leukemia

Autoimmune Disorders (Connective Tissue Diseases)

Systemic Lupus Erythematosus
Rheumatoid Arthritis
Scleroderma
Vasculitis

Radiation Therapy

Renal Failure
  Uremia

Acute Myocardial Infarction

Post Myocardial Infarction Syndrome (Dressler's Syndrome)

Post cardiotomy or Post thoracotomy Syndrome

Chest Trauma

Penetrating Injury
Surgical Procedure (e.g. pacemaker insertion)

Dissecting Aortic Dissection

Drug Reaction

Hydralazine (Apresoline)
Procainamide (Pronestyl)
Phenytoin (Dilantin)
Penicillin
Ionized (e.g. Nydrazid)

(Alspach, 2006; Goyle & Wallings, 2002; Marinella, 1998; McNeill, 2005).

Chapter 12

Physical Examination

◆ Tachypnea is noted in patients who have altered their respiratory pattern to ease the discomfort associated with breathing.

◆ Tachycardia may be present with fever or in response to pain.

◆ Low-grade fever is common in pericarditis. High grade fever may be present, but the fever associated with pericarditis is usually low grade (below 39° C).

◆ A pericardial friction rub may or may not be present. The presence of pericardial friction rub confirms the diagnosis of pericarditis, but the absence of a pericardial friction rub does not rule out the diagnosis of pericarditis. A pericardial friction rub is present about 50% of the time (Valley, 2005). Pericardial friction rubs are also transient. A rub that is present during one assessment may not be present at the next, as it may come and go.

   ❖ Timing: Heard throughout the cardiac cycle. The rub may have three components including a late diastolic sound that occurs when the atrium contracts, an early systolic sound when the ventricle contracts, and an early diastolic sound when early ventricular filling occurs. Not all components of the sound may be present. The ventricular filling sound is the sound most commonly identified.

   ❖ Location: Best heard over the lower left sternal boarder.

   ❖ Pitch: High pitch sound best heard with diaphragm of stethoscope.

   ❖ Quality: Grating, scratchy, squeaking, and leathery.

   ❖ Best heard with patient sitting and leaning forward.

   ❖ Tends to be louder during inspiration.

   ❖ To differentiate a pericardial friction rub from a pleural rub:

     ★ Ask patient to hold breath.

     ★ Pericardial rub will continue when no respiratory effort is made.

     ★ Pleural rub will cease when no respiratory effort is made.

Diagnosis

During the diagnosis process, the presence of increased fluid in the pericardial space must be evaluated, as well as the presence of hemodynamic compromise associated with tamponade. Both are discussed in detail later in this chapter.

Electrocardiogram

The 12-lead ECG may or may not be abnormal. Typically, diffuse ST-T wave changes occur as a result of inflammation of the myocardium beneath the inflamed pericardium. A patient may demonstrate ECG changes that occur in a four-stage evolutionary pattern that is diagnostic of pericarditis. Approximately 50% of the patients with pericarditis demonstrate all four stages (Valley, 2005).

◆ Stage 1: ST Elevation with concave upward ST-Segments

   ❖ The ECG of pericarditis shows diffuse ST elevation with upward concavity in nearly all leads. The concavity of the ST-segment is helpful in differentiating the ST elevation of acute myocardial infarction (AMI), which more often has a convex ST-segment elevation (Figure 12.2). The ST elevation is typically greatest in leads II and V5.

   ❖ Another unique ECG finding that is helpful in differentiating ECG changes of pericarditis from AMI is the absence of reciprocal changes. Since most leads demonstrate ST elevation, the reciprocal ST depression typically seen in AMI is not present.

   ❖ ST elevation is never present in lead aVR, but ST depression can be seen in this lead. Lead V1 usually demonstrates a depressed ST-segment.

Inflammatory Cardiovascular Diseases: Diseases Involving the Pericardium, Myocardium and Endocardium

- ❖ PR depression may also be present in pericarditis and is most commonly seen in leads II, aVF and V4-V6 (Smith et al, 2002). PR elevation in lead aVR is also an ECG sign of pericarditis.
- ◆ Stage 2: ST-segment returns to baseline with decreased T wave.
  - ❖ During stage 2,, the ST-segments return to baseline as the T waves decrease in amplitude and begin to flatten.
- ◆ Stage 3: T wave inversion without Q wave formation or loss of R wave.
  - ❖ Inversion of the T wave indicates Stage 3. This progression of the T wave is similar to the normal T wave progression in an ST elevation AMI; however, there is no development of the Q waves that are typical in ST elevation AMI.
- ◆ Stage 4: ECG normalization.
  - ❖ The final stage is the stage of normalization when the ECG returns to the pre-pericarditis ECG. The movement through the stages may occur over hours to weeks. The first two stages usually occur quickly, with the last two stages progressing more slowly.

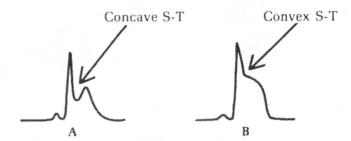

Figure 12.2: **A.** Concave ST seen in pericarditis. **B.** Convex ST seen in acute myocardial infarction.

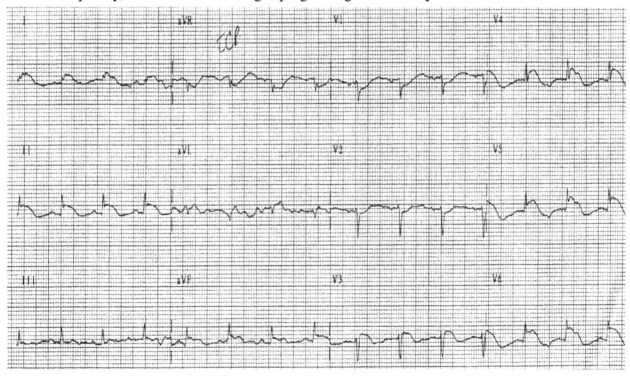

Figure 12.3: ECG of patient presenting with acute chest pain and normal cardiac catheterization. Note the changes consistent with pericarditis: Diffuse ST elevations in leads I, II, III, aVL, aVF and V3-6, with ST depression in leads aVR, V1 and V2.

Laboratory Tests

Abnormal laboratory test may be noted in pericarditis as follows:
- ◆ Elevated erythrocyte sedimentation rate.
- ◆ Elevated C-reactive protein levels.
- ◆ Troponin elevation more often noted than an elevated CK MB.

Chapter 12

- Elevated WBC levels.
- Antinuclear antibody test (ANA) positive if connective tissue disease is present.
- Positive blood cultures if an infective process is present.

Echocardiogram
- The echocardiogram is helpful in determining if there is a fluid accumulation in the pericardial space, but may appear normal without fluid accumulation.

CT Scan
- CT scanning is helpful in ruling out constrictive pericarditis and can determine the thickness of pericardium.
- Able to evaluate entire pericardium with CT scanning.
- Of limited value in diagnosis of pericarditis. Is helpful in other diagnoses related to the pericardium, such as constrictive pericarditis.

MRI
- Provides more detail without the need for contrast.
- Not often used to diagnose pericarditis.
- Useful in other diagnoses related to pericardial disease.

Chest X-Ray
- Pericarditis without fluid accumulation is not evident on routine chest x-ray.

Treatment

Once pericardial effusions, tamponade and constrictive pericarditis have been ruled out, the treatment goals for pericarditis include treating the underlying cause and providing symptomatic relief.

- Non-steroidal anti-inflammatory medications (NSAIDs) are the treatment of choice to decrease the inflammation and relieve pain. Aspirin, ibuprofen or indomethacin (Indocin) are the most commonly used medications in the treatment of pericarditis.
- Corticosteroids may be administered if the patient does not respond to the NSAID.
- Positioning the patient in an upright position while leaning forward seems to be the most comfortable position.
- Pain medication should be provided to keep the patient comfortable. With the pain controlled, the patient is able to breathe normally and should be able to avoid the complications associated with the short rapid respiratory pattern noted in patients with pericarditis. Pericarditis can be very painful, especially in the early stages. Narcotics may be needed initially to alleviate the discomfort from pericarditis.
- Anticoagulants should be discontinued, if possible. If the benefit of anticoagulation therapy outweighs the risk of bleeding, anticoagulation should be continued cautiously. The patient should be assessed carefully for the development of hemodynamic compromise that would indicate bleeding into the pericardial space. Heparin may be the anticoagulant of choice due to its reversibility and short half-life.
- Antibiotic and antifungal medications should be administered to treat the cause if bacterial or fungal.
- Dialysis is the treatment for uremic pericarditis.
- Steroids may be effective in connective tissue disorders.
- Medications causing pericarditis should be discontinued.

Inflammatory Cardiovascular Diseases: Diseases Involving the Pericardium, Myocardium and Endocardium

◆ All patients with pericarditis should be carefully assessed for the development of pericardial effusion that results in hemodynamic compromise.

◆ Pericarditis that is the result of ST elevation AMI requires some adjustments in the standard treatment protocol. The ACC/AHA Guidelines For The Management of Patients With ST-Elevation Myocardial Infarction (Antman et al, 2004) provide the following recommendations:

❖ Enteric coated aspirin up to 650 mg every 4 to 6 hours.

❖ Immediately discontinue anticoagulants if pericardial effusion develops or increases. If the benefits of antithrombotic therapy outweigh the risks of therapy, due diligence should be taken to assess the patient for signs of increasing effusion and hemodynamic compromise.

❖ For pericarditis not controlled with aspirin, colchicine and/or acetaminophen may be added to the treatment regime.

❖ Corticosteroids may be used with caution if other treatment modalities are ineffective. The use of corticosteroids post myocardial infarction has been associated with an increased risk of scar thinning and myocardial rupture.

❖ NSAIDs may be considered for pain relief, but their use should be limited to short-term administration. There is an associated increased risk of myocardial scar thinning and infarct expansion, in addition to their effect on platelet function.

❖ Ibuprofen blocks the antiplatelet effect of aspirin and can cause myocardial scar thinning and infarct expansion; it should not be used for pain relief in the post infarct patient.

Outcomes

Once treatment begins, pain relief usually occurs within the first 24 hours. Outcomes related to pericarditis vary, depending on the cause of the pericarditis. Episodes of idiopathic or viral pericarditis, once treated, rarely reoccur. Pericarditis associated with an underlying disease process may reoccur, depending on the disease process itself. On occasion, pericarditis can lead to pericardial effusion, cardiac tamponade or constrictive pericarditis, depending on the underlying cause. Until the pericarditis is resolved, the patient should be assessed for the development of any of these processes.

Linking Knowledge to Practice

✔ *Patients with pericarditis may have a poor respiratory effort, as breathing causes discomfort, especially deep breaths. Providing comfort relief (pain medication and sitting upright and leaning forward) will allow the patient to inspire and expire normally and avoid the pulmonary complications resulting from rapid, swallow respiratory patterns.*

✔ *Pericardial friction rubs may be transient. The absence of a friction rub does not rule out pericarditis.*

✔ *Many of the disease processes causing pericarditis may also cause pericardial effusions and tamponade. The patient with pericarditis should be monitored for the development of a pericardial effusion and cardiac tamponade (discussed later in this chapter).*

✔ *Patients with acute renal insufficiency or acute renal failure cannot take NSAIDs, only steroids.*

✔ *There is a high risk of gastritis with steroid use; therefore, patients on steroid therapy are usually placed on a proton pump inhibitor for the duration of the therapy.*

Pericardial Effusion

Pericardial effusion occurs when there is an abnormal amount and/or type of fluid in the pericardial space. The increased volume may be in the form of fluid, blood, pus, or a combination of all three.

Chapter 12

Causes

Pericardial effusions can be acute or chronic, and caused by the same variety of disorders resulting in pericarditis. All incidents of pericarditis can progress to develop pericardial effusions. Increased capillary permeability due to inflammation of the pericardial sac may cause a fluid leak into pericardial space. Fluid development is secondary to inflammation, infection, malignancy, or an autoimmune process occurring within the pericardial space. Pericardial effusion is not an uncommon occurrence in patients with heart failure; it is referred to as hydropericardium. Approximately 50% of post cardiac surgery patients have pericardial effusions that usually resolve on their own (Bojar, 2005).

Breast and lung cancer patients have a high incidence of effusion, with 37% of lung cancer patients and 22% of breast cancer patients having malignant pericardial effusions (Strimel, 2005). HIV patients with or without AIDS are noted to have a 41-87% incidence of asymptomatic effusions and a 13% incidence of moderate to severe effusions (Strimel, 2005).

Symptoms

Symptoms vary depending on the volume of fluid accumulated and the ability of the pericardium to make adjustments to the fluid accumulation. If fluid accumulates rapidly, the onset of symptoms occurs relatively quickly. If the fluid accumulation occurs over time, as may be the case with cancer or HIV, the onset of symptoms is gradual, as hemodynamic compromise occurs slowly. Symptoms associated with a rapid accumulation of fluid in the pericardial space causing hemodynamic compromise are discussed in the section on cardiac tamponade.

Small pericardial effusion may not cause any symptoms and may never be noted unless recognized during the evaluation of other symptoms. Patients with a large pericardial effusion that is not compressing on the heart and causing tamponade may have a variety of clinical findings. Symptoms are first related to any underlying disease process. For those with an infective process, it is not unusual for the patient to describe "flu-like" symptoms. Pericarditis may or may not be present with pericardial effusion. If the patient has pericarditis, as well as pericardial effusion, symptoms associated with pericarditis may also be present.

Physical Examination

◆ A pericardial friction rub may or may not be present.

◆ Heart sounds may be diminished as the fluid in the pericardial space muffles the heart sounds.

◆ Decreased breath sounds may be present due to pleural effusions. Some of the disease processes associated with pericardial effusion also result in pleural effusions.

◆ Other physical exam findings noted previously with pericarditis may be present.

Diagnosis

Electrocardiogram

◆ Electrical alternans is a common finding on the ECG when there is a large volume of pericardial fluid. The alternans is an alternating change in the amplitude of the QRS complex (large complex alternating with a small complex) that is caused by a swinging of the heart in the pericardial fluid. The swinging of the heart moves the heart toward and away from the ECG electrodes as it swings in the pericardial fluid. The alternans may only be present in one lead on the 12-lead ECG, so it may not be noted on a bedside monitor.

◆ Diffuse low voltage is present throughout the ECG when there is a large pericardial effusion; however, this change is not specific to pericardial effusion and may be caused by other processes.

◆ ECG changes associated with pericarditis may also be present.

Inflammatory Cardiovascular Diseases: Diseases Involving the Pericardium, Myocardium and Endocardium

Chest X-ray

◆ The cardiac silhouette is enlarged if there is greater than 250 ml of fluid present in the pericardial space (Perea & Sherry, 2001). An enlarged cardiac silhouette does not provide a diagnosis of pericardial effusion, as there are many other causes of an enlarged heart.

◆ Co-existing pleural effusions may be evident on the chest x-ray.

Echocardiogram

◆ The echocardiogram is the most reliable method of diagnosing pericardial effusion. Small amounts of fluid can be detected with two-dimensional echocardiography. On the echocardiogram, pericardial effusion is noted when there is an echo free-space between the walls of the heart and the pericardium. The size of the effusion can be estimated during echocardiography.

◆ Effusions noted in the posterior/lateral pericardium are considered to be early small effusions, as this is where fluid accumulation settles early in the process.

◆ If the effusion is greater than 1 mm thick and surrounds the heart, it is considered to be a large effusion.

◆ The swinging heart can be visualized during echocardiography.

◆ Sometimes loculated effusions are not seen on a routine transthoracic echocardiogram (TTE).

◆ A transesophogeal echocardiogram may provide further diagnostic benefit if there is suspicion of a loculated effusion or clot that is not visible with the transthoracic echocardiogram.

CT Scan

◆ With echocardiography being the diagnostic tool of choice, the CT scan is of limited use. However, a CT scan may be helpful in determining the composition of fluid and can detect small amounts of pericardial fluid.

MRI

◆ MRI, as with CT scan, offers little benefit over the echocardiogram. An MRI can detect small amounts of fluid and help differentiate between hemorrhagic and nonhemorrhagic effusion.

Laboratory Tests

◆ Laboratory test results are primarily based on the underlying cause of the effusions. White blood count is elevated with an infection; renal function tests are abnormal with uremia, etc.

◆ Pericardial Fluid

   ❖ To aid in the diagnosis of a cause for the effusion, a pericardial tap is required to obtain a sample of pericardial fluid. Routine analysis may include viral, bacteria and fungal cultures, total protein, specific gravity and glucose levels to differentiate normal pericardial fluid from abnormal fluid.

Treatment

The primary goal of treatment is to determine and treat the underlying cause of the pericardial effusion. NSAIDs and corticosteroids are helpful in autoimmune processes. Antibiotics are required when there is a bacterial infection.

Pericardiocentesis

Peicardiocentesis may provide diagnostic information as well as a mode of treatment for the pericardial effusion. Pericardiocentesis is not without complications, and rarely does a fluid sample provide the necessary information to make a definitive diagnosis. If a thorough history does not provide a probable cause of the effusion, then a pericardiocentesis may be indicated. Additionally, if the effusions continue after customary treatment strategies, then pericardiocentesis may be helpful. The benefits of pericardiocentesis, both diagnostic and therapeutic, tend to be greater when larger amounts of fluid have accumulated (DeCastro & Schwartz, 2003). In patients with cancer, the rate of reoccurrence of the fluid may be as high as 90% in 90 days (Strimel, 2005).

Chapter 12

♦ Pericardiocentesis may be performed at the bedside in the critical care unit.

♦ The procedure is performed with the head of the bed elevated up to 60 degrees to help bring the heart closer to the anterior chest wall.

♦ Bedside cardiac monitoring is essential during the procedure, which is completed with a local anesthetic as well as sedatives to help relieve anxiety and promote comfort.

♦ Pericardiocentesis is usually completed with echocardiography to assist the physician in locating the pericardial space with the pericardial needle. Some physicians may prefer to use a subxiphoid approach with ECG monitoring. With this approach, one end of an alligator clamp is attached to the pericardiocentesis needle, and the other end attached to a lead wire on the 12-lead ECG machine (most frequently lead V_5). With this approach, ST elevation in the lead with the alligator clamp will occur when the needle comes in contact with the myocardial wall. The echocardiographic approach is more reliable; however, echocardiography may not always be readily available.

♦ During the procedure, fluid may be obtained for diagnostic purposes. Fluid may also be removed to reduce the amount that has accumulated in the pericardial space. In some instances, a catheter with a drainage bag may be left in place indefinitely while fluid is allowed to continue to drain.

♦ The volume, color and consistency of aspirate should be documented. Blood that has accumulated slowly in the pericardial space does not usually clot after it has been aspirated, but blood that has accumulated quickly will clot.

♦ After the procedure the patient's vital signs and heart sounds should be monitored carefully for signs of cardiac tamponade (discussed later in this chapter). A chest x-ray should be performed to assess for pneumothorax or hemothorax. The pericardiocentesis site should be monitored for signs of bleeding, hematoma or infection.

♦ After removal of any significant amount of fluid, the patient may demonstrate some hemodynamic compromise, as the heart may dilate once the fluid is removed.

Subxiphoid Pericardiostomy (Pericardial Window)
A pericardial window may be required for patients with pericardial effusions if the accumulated pericardial contents cannot be removed by pericardiocentesis, as with a loculated effusion or an effusion that is located posteriorly. A pericardial window may also be appropriate when there is reoccurrence of the effusions, as is known to be the case with effusions caused by malignancies.

♦ The procedure is ideally performed with general anesthesia, but can be done under local anesthesia if the patient's condition does not warrant general anesthesia.

♦ The patient is prepped for a full sternotomy in the event more invasive surgery is required.

♦ During surgery, the xiphoid process is removed, as the sternum must be retracted upward to expose the pericardium.

♦ The pericardium is opened and the pericardial contents are drained out of the pericardial space. A sample of the pericardial contents may be obtained to assist with the diagnosis of the effusion, if necessary.

♦ A piece of the pericardium, usually up to 4 cm, is removed and sent for analysis. This area is left open and fluid can continue to drain into the thoracic cavity where it will be absorbed.

♦ If there is a large amount of drainage, a pericardial drain may be placed for several days and removed after drainage is less than 100 ml/day.

♦ Post operative complications are usually minimal, as this procedure is considered to have low risk and low mortality. Complications include bleeding, infection, cardiac perforation and normal complications associated with anesthesia.

Inflammatory Cardiovascular Diseases: Diseases Involving the Pericardium, Myocardium and Endocardium

Thorascopic Pericardiostomy

A pericardiostomy may also be utilized for drainage of pericardial effusions and the creation of a pericardial window. This approach is especially beneficial if pleural effusions requiring drainage are also present. This procedure requires general anesthesia with intubation.

Balloon Pericardiotomy

This procedure has also been utilized to help increase the success rate in patients with a high reoccurrence rate. During this percutaneous procedure, a catheter is placed in the pericardial space. A balloon is then inflated, creating an opening in the pericardium. The opening allows the fluid in the pericardial space to drain into the pleural space where it is reabsorbed. Balloon pericardiotomy is usually performed in the cardiac catheterization laboratory; it is an alternative to a surgical pericardial window.

Outcomes

In patients with viral, idiopathic or post myocardial infarction, pericardial effusions have a good prognosis with a low incidence of recurrence. If the pericardial effusion is the result of HIV/AIDS or cancer, the prognosis is poor with high mortality rates from the disease process. Recurrence of the effusion in these patients is high. There are reports that as many as 55% of these patients will require repeat intervention for recurrent effusions (Meyerson & DiAmico, 2000). The instillation of a sclerosing agent into the pericardial space has been utilized to fuse the two layers of the pericardium together to prevent the development of further effusions in these high-risk patients. This procedure has increased the success rate of pericardiocentesis by as much as 85% (Meyerson & DiAmico, 2000).

Linking Knowledge to Practice

✔ *Patients should be carefully monitored post pericardiocentesis for signs of cardiac tamponade (discussed below).*

✔ *If a large volume of fluid that has been accumulating over time is removed from the pericardial space, the patient may become hemodynamically compromised. Once the fluid is removed, the chambers of the heart can dilate and cardiac output will drop unless volume is increased to fill the dilated chambers.*

If the fluid accumulation begins to interfere with the heart's ability to function, then cardiac tamponade occurs and the urgency for treatment increases.

Cardiac Tamponade

Cardiac tamponade is a clinical syndrome that occurs when the accumulation of pericardial content causes compression of the heart and impedes normal cardiac function. As the compression of the heart increases, cardiac output decreases. It is not the volume of the pericardial content that determines the significance of the tamponade, but the amount of compression. The significance of the tamponade is most often directly proportional to the speed in which the pericardial contents are accumulated.

As the volume in the pericardial space increases for whatever reason, a larger space is required to hold the volume. Since the fibrous pericardium is not easily distensible, the only place for the pericardial space to expand is inward. As the pericardial space expands inward, the heart is compressed. The pericardial space is a continuous space and covers the entire surface of the heart. As volume increases, it is distributed over the entire surface area of the heart, so all areas of the heart are equally compressed. As the intrapericardial pressure increases, the intracardiac pressures all increase. Compression of the heart results in a reduction in filling. The ventricle is unable to expand during diastolic filling, resulting in a decreased stroke volume and cardiac output. Venous return to the heart is also altered, and right atrial collapse occurs. Blood accumulates in the venous system and signs of right-sided failure occur.

Chapter 12

Causes

Tamponade is the result of an increase in volume in the pericardial space that interferes with myocardial function. Therefore, any process that causes pericardial effusion, including infection, malignancies, or uremia, can cause cardiac tamponade. Any intervention involving the heart could result in cardiac tamponade, including coronary interventions (angioplasty), pacemaker insertions, and cardiac surgery. Traumatic accidents involving the heart or acute disease processes, such as post myocardial infarction, free wall rupture, or aortic rupture can also result in cardiac tamponade.

Symptoms

The presenting symptoms are directly related to the degree of cardiac impairment. The patient with acute tamponade may be restless, cool and clammy, while complaining of shortness of breath. They often express a feeling of impending doom. The chest pain of pericarditis may also be present, with the patient feeling better sitting upright and learning forward.

Physical Exam

◆ Beck's Triad of symptoms incorporates the classic signs of pericardial effusion.

❖ Jugular venous distension occurs as the right atrium becomes compressed and venous return to the heart is impeded. In patients without a history of heart failure, there are usually no other signs of right-sided failure, such as edema. Central venous pressures may be a high as 30 mm Hg (Shabetai, 1998).

❖ Hypotension develops due to the decreased cardiac output. While the sympathetic nervous system attempts to compensate with increased heart rate, increased contractility and increased systemic vascular resistance to maintain blood pressure, ultimately cardiac output falls too low and blood pressure cannot be maintained. A narrow pulse pressure is not uncommon.

❖ Muffled heart sounds are noted as the pericardial contents diminish the transmission of the heart sounds.

◆ Pulsus Paradoxus

❖ When tamponade becomes moderate to severe, pulsus paradoxus may develop.

❖ During normal inspiration there is an increase in venous return to the heart. As a result of the increased venous return, the right ventricle distends to accept the additional volume. Additionally, the interventricular septum bulges gently into the left ventricle, resulting in a slightly smaller left ventricular cavity. The slightly smaller left ventricle accepts a smaller filling volume during inspiration, and therefore produces a slightly reduced stroke volume. This decrease in stroke volume is translated into a systemic blood pressure that normally decreases up to 10 mm Hg during inspiration.

❖ The physiologic changes that occur in cardiac tamponade during inspiration and expiration are complex, with multiple suggestions as to why the pulsus paradoxus occurs. One of the more frequently cited causes is explained here. During inspiration, in the patient with cardiac tamponade, the venous return to the heart increases; however, the right ventricle is unable to increase in size due to the tamponade. The interventricular septum is the only part of the right ventricle that is able to make the adjustment, and the adjustment results in a greater bulging of the septum into the left ventricle. This decreases left-ventricular filling more than during the normal inspiratory process and results in a greater decrease in stroke volume. This is noted with a drop in systemic blood pressure during inspiration of greater than 10 mm Hg. It is referred to as a pulsus paradoxus.

Inflammatory Cardiovascular Diseases: Diseases Involving the Pericardium, Myocardium and Endocardium

❖ The skillful measurement of pulsus paradoxus takes practice and patience.
   ✩ The patient should be placed in a semi-recumbent position.
   ✩ The patient must be able to cooperate and breathe regularly and slowly without respiratory distress.
   ✩ Inflate the blood pressure cuff at least 20 mmHg above the systolic blood pressure or after the disappearance of the radial pulse.
   ✩ Begin to very slowly deflate the cuff until the first Korotkoff sounds are heard intermittently (this should be during expiration). If the cuff is not further deflated, there should be no audible Korotkoff sounds during inspiration at that reading. Note the reading.
   ✩ Further deflate the cuff slowly until Korotkoff sounds are heard both during inspiration and expiration. Note the reading.
   ✩ The difference between the first and second sound is the size of the pulsus.
   ✩ If the pulsus is greater than 10 mm Hg, then a pulsus paradoxus is present.
❖ While pulsus paradoxus is a significant finding in cardiac tamponade and present in over 70% of the patients with tamponade, it is not exclusive to cardiac tamponade (DeCastro & Schwartz, 2003). Pulsus paradoxus may also be observed in constrictive pericarditis, severe obstructive pulmonary disease, restrictive cardiomyopathy, pulmonary emboli, and RV infarct with shock.

◆ Equalization of filling pressures occurs in cardiac tamponade. As the intrapericardial pressure increases the right atrial pressure, both the pulmonary artery diastolic pressure and the pulmonary artery occlusive pressure (wedge) all "rise to equalize" and will usually move to within 5 mm Hg of each other.

◆ An evaluation of the venous pressure waveform (CVP) demonstrates a loss of the Y descent that occurs when the tricuspid valve opens and the atrium empties in to the right ventricle. An increased intrapericardial pressure prevents passive diastolic filling, thereby eliminating the Y descent on the CVP pressure waveform. The venous waveform then only has one negative waveform (the X descent) that occurs just after atrial contraction and indicates atrial relaxation. Atrial pressures do fall during systole due to decreased volumes; the X descent is preserved (DeCastro & Schwartz, 2003).

Diagnosis

Cardiac tamponade is usually a medical emergency, and rapid, accurate diagnosis can lead to early successful treatment.

Chest X-ray
◆ Cardiomegaly may be noted on the chest x-ray with a water bottle shaped heart.
◆ Pericardial accumulations greater than 250 ml usually need to be present before visible changes are noted with chest x-ray.

Electrocardigram
◆ Electrical alternans may be present, but this is not specific to cardiac tamponade.
◆ ECG findings may be non-specific and are not usually helpful in the diagnosis of cardiac tamponade.

Echocardiogram
◆ A TTE is the diagnostic tool of choice for the patient with symptoms of cardiac tamponade and can be quickly and easily obtained.
◆ A TTE may provide further diagnostic benefit if there is suspicion of a loculated effusion or clot that is not visible with the transthoracic echocardiogram.
◆ Pericardial effusion appears as an echo-free space with the two-dimensional echocardiogram.

Chapter 12

- ◆ A collapsing right and left ventricle during diastole is diagnostic of cardiac tamponade (Perea & Sherry, 2001).

- ◆ Left atrial and ventricular diastolic compression may also be visible.

- ◆ If the pericardial accumulation is large, a "swinging" heart may be noted as well.

Treatment

In acute situations rapid treatment is essential, with stabilization of the patient as the first goal.

- ◆ Volume expansion is utilized to help in the prevention of collapse of the heart during diastole.

- ◆ Elevation of the legs may help increase venous return.

- ◆ Dobutamine may be helpful in increasing contractility without increasing systemic vascular resistance.

- ◆ Positive pressure mechanical ventilation should be avoided, if possible, as it decreases venous return to the heart and exacerbates the situation.

- ◆ Ultimately, drainage of the pericardial accumulation through pericardiocentesis is necessary to eliminate the tamponade. Either a percutaneous or surgical procedure, as described above with pericardial effusion, may be completed, as determined by the treating physician.

- ◆ If the cause of the tamponade is bleeding, surgical treatment may prove to be the better option. The amount of bleeding may be controlled by the pressure caused with the tamponade; therefore, a skilled surgeon should be available to identify and control the source of the bleeding once the pressure in the pericardium is relieved.

- ◆ Occasionally, a percutaneous pericardiocentesis may be performed to stabilize the patient prior to surgery and a pericardial window.

Outcomes

Early recognition and prompt treatment are the keys to positive outcomes with cardiac tamponade. Following a pericardial window, patients can develop tamponade from accumulation of blood in the mediastinum that compresses the heart, so they should be monitored for returning signs of tamponade. A widened mediastinum on the chest x-ray may be seen.

Linking Knowledge to Practice

- ✔ *Beck's triad, jugular vein distention, hypotension and muffled heart sounds describes the classic presentation of cardiac tamponade. Before the signs of Beck's triad occur the earliest signs of tamponade may be sinus tachycardia and a drop in urine output which are both signs of a decrease in cardiac output.*

- ✔ *Assessing for pulsus paradoxus is a skill that takes time, practice and patience, but can prove to be valuable in the diagnosis of cardiac tamponade.*

- ✔ *Keep in mind not all patients with cardiac tamponade present with acute decompensation. A patient with a developing effusion is more likely to have a gradual onset of symptoms, while the trauma patient or the patient with a cardiac perforation is more likely to develop symptoms quickly. It is the astute clinician who recognizes subtle changes that can make the greatest difference.*

Constrictive Pericarditis

Constrictive pericarditis occurs when the pericardium becomes thickened and fibrotic, impeding normal diastolic filling. The parietal pericardium, and sometimes the visceral layer, is usually involved. Constrictive pericarditis usually begins with an episode of pericarditis that may or may not be clinically significant. The pericarditis developed into pericardial effusion that reabsorbed over time and left the peri-

518

Inflammatory Cardiovascular Diseases: Diseases Involving the Pericardium, Myocardium and Endocardium

cardium with fibrotic scaring. The pericardial space adheres to itself and becomes non-existent, and the fibrotic pericardium restricts the normal expansion of the heart during diastolic filling. The fibrotic tissue calcifies over time, and the restriction on diastolic filling increases until cardiac output is compromised.

Causes

The most common cause of constrictive pericarditis is idiopathic. Pericarditis from any cause can ultimately result in the development of constrictive pericarditis. Other common causes of constrictive pericarditis include those that result in chronic inflammation of the pericardium, including tuberculosis, radiation therapy to the chest, and cardiac surgery.

Symptoms

The most common symptoms of dyspnea and fatigue make the diagnosis of constrictive pericarditis very difficult to determine based on the patient's chief complaint. Symptoms generally occur gradually, as the constriction of the heart occurs over time. Heart failure symptoms are not uncommon, with signs of right-sided heart failure more common than those of left-sided heart failure. Chest pain may be present as the coronary artery perfusion decreases with the lower cardiac output.

Physical Examination

Findings on physical examination are related to a reduced cardiac output with an increase in systemic venous pressure and pulmonary venous congestion. Many of the signs associated with constrictive pericarditis can mistakenly lead to a diagnosis of hepatic failure. As the constriction on the heart becomes greater, many signs and symptoms noted with cardiac tamponade may be present. There are, however, some differences between constrictive pericarditis and cardiac tamponade. Pulsus paradoxus is often not present in constrictive pericarditis, as there is not an associated increase in response to venous return during inspiration in constrictive pericarditis. The constriction in constrictive pericarditis is more symmetrical and results in the elevation of diastolic pressures equally in all chambers. One classic sign differentiating constrictive pericarditis from cardiac tamponade is Kussmaul's sign. Kussmaul's sign is observed in patients with right-ventricular failure, right-ventricular infarct, restrictive cardiomyopathy and tricuspid stenosis, but not in cardiac tamponade. Kussmaul's sign is noted when prominent neck veins do not decrease during inspiration, indicating an elevation of systemic venous pressure.

A pericardial knock may be auscultated in patients with constrictive pericarditis. This early diastolic filling sound is often confused with an audible S_3, but it occurs earlier and has a higher frequency than an S_3. A pericardial knock is best heard along the left sternal border, with the diaphragm of the stethoscope (S_3 better heard with the bell), and represents the sudden cessation of ventricular diastolic filling.

Other signs associated with constrictive pericarditis include:
- Tachycardia
- Hypotension
- Jugular venous distention
- Hepatomegaly
- Ascites
- Edema
- Cough
- Chest Pain.

Chapter 12

Diagnosis

Since the clinical symptoms of constrictive pericarditis and restrictive cardiomyopathy are similar because both are related to a decrease in diastolic filling, it is important to recognize the differences when making a clinical diagnosis. Table 12.2 differentiates the clinical features.

Table 12.2
Clinical Features of Constrictive Pericarditis and Restrictive Cardiomyopathy

Clinical Features	Constrictive Pericarditis	Restrictive Cardiomyopathy
History	Prior history of pericarditis or condition that causes pericardial disease	History of systemic disease (eg. amyloidosis, hemochromatosis)
Heart Sounds	Pericardial knock, high frequency sound	Presence of loud diastolic filling sound S_3, low frequency sound
Murmurs	No murmurs	Murmurs of mitral and tricuspid insufficiency
Cardiac Pressures	Left (PAWP) and right (CVP) filling pressures are elevated and equal	Left-sided filling pressures are > right-sided filling pressures
Chest X-ray	Visual pericardial calcification	Atrial dilation with normal ventricular size
CT Scan/MRI	Pericardial thickening	No pericardial thickening
Echocardiogram	Normal ventricles and atria, pericardial thickening	Atrial dilation with normal ventricular size. If amyloid infiltration of the heart – speckled texture of myocardium

Chest X-ray
◆ Normal or mildly enlarged cardiac silhouette.
◆ Cardiac calcification may be present, but is not diagnostic of constrictive pericarditis.
◆ Pleural effusions are not uncommon in constrictive pericarditis.

Echocardiogram
◆ Used to differentiate between constrictive pericarditis and restrictive cardiomyopathy.
◆ Pericardial thickening may be present with constrictive pericarditis.
◆ Transesophageal echo may provide a better evaluation of the thickened pericardium.
◆ Atrial and ventricular sizes should be normal.
◆ Abnormal diastolic filling patterns related to constrictive pericarditis are noted.

CT Scan
◆ Can visualize pericardial thickness.
◆ Normal pericardial wall thickness is 1-2 mm.
◆ Pericardial wall thickness that is 3-4 mm is considered abnormal.
◆ Thickening of > 4mm supports constrictive pericarditis over restrictive cardiomyopathy.

MRI
◆ MRI is the most sensitive for pericardial thickening.

Inflammatory Cardiovascular Diseases: Diseases Involving the Pericardium, Myocardium and Endocardium

Cardiac Catheterization

◆ Non-invasive testing can provide information to assist with the diagnosis, but findings are not often conclusive, nor can they stand alone to diagnose constrictive pericarditis. A thickened pericardium does not always mean a hemodynamically significant constrictive pericarditis is present. The most reliable diagnosis can be made in the cardiac catheterization laboratory with an evaluation of cardiac pressures.

◆ Findings include:
  ❖ Low resting cardiac output.
  ❖ Elevated pulmonary capillary wedge pressure.
  ❖ Right ventricular end-diastolic pressure that is more than one-third of the systolic pressure.

Myocardial Biopsy

◆ Myocardial biopsy may be necessary to assist in the diagnosis of the disease, especially in the differentiation between constrictive pericarditis and restrictive cardiomyopathy.

Treatment

The treatment of constrictive pericarditis is generally symptom related, as well as treating the cause. Since constrictive pericarditis is a progressive disease, many patients may live many years with minimal hemodynamic compromise. The use of low doses of diuretics may be helpful if there is evidence of elevated volume. Diuretics should be used cautiously, as they may decrease cardiac output, and good filling is important when the heart is unable to expand properly. Beta-blockers are generally avoided, as they block the normal sympathetic response of an increased heart rate, which is a compensatory mechanism in constrictive pericarditis. Clinicians should treat the cause of the constrictive pericarditis, if known, with standard treatment strategies.

Over time, the constriction progresses to the point that hemodynamics are compromised and the patient can become debilitated. Pericardectomy, the surgical removal of the pericardium, is the definitive treatment for constrictive pericarditis. The best results occur when surgery takes place prior to the development of dense pericardial calcifications and debilitation. Close follow-up with the chronic constrictive pericarditis patient should allow for adequate timing of the surgery. Diastolic filling abnormalities tend to remain in those patients who have had a longer history of symptoms pre operatively. The surgery is long and technically difficult, as the entire pericardium is resected. The heart is able to function normally without the pericardium. Complications of surgery include bleeding and atrial or ventricular arrhythmias.

Outcomes

Outcomes post operatively are better in those with fewer symptoms pre operatively. Persistent diastolic filling problems seem to persist in those with greater signs of diastolic dysfunction prior to surgery. Those entering surgery with NYHA Class IV have poorer outcomes as well.

Linking Knowledge to Practice

✔ *It is important to differentiate constrictive pericarditis from restrictive cardiomyopathy, as treatment strategies are different.*

✔ *Pericardial knock may be present with constrictive pericarditis. This sound is similar to an S3. Pericardial knock is heard best with the diaphragm of the stethoscope and is earlier than an S3, which is heard best with the bell of the stethoscope.*

✔ *Patients may live with constrictive pericarditis for years and should be educated to know the signs of impending hemodynamic compromise (heart failure), so appropriate treatment strategies can be implemented before cardiac tamponade occurs.*

Chapter 12

✔ *Constrictive pericarditis results in an inability to expand the ventricles during diastole. Anything that would decrease normal filling (preload), such as loss of atrial kick, tachycardias, and fluid volume deficit states, can result in a decrease in cardiac output.*

MYOCARDITIS

Myocarditis is an inflammatory infiltrate of the myocardium with necrosis and/or degeneration of adjacent myocytes. The inflammation can be caused by a variety of organisms, as well as drugs or chemicals.

Pathophysiology

There is a direct invasion of myocardial tissue by the offending organism, drug, or chemical, causing myocyte destruction and necrosis. The destruction of the myocytes may be global or sporadic. After the initial insult, an autoimmune response to the invasion occurs and further myocyte damage continues as the body, in an attempt to rid itself of the offending agent, not only attacks the offending agent, but also the normal myocardial cells. Microvascular spasm and reperfusion injury, resulting from the viral attack of the vascular endothelium, are thought to produce the myocardial damage that occurs (McNeill, M., 2005). If left untreated, the myocardium expands, and for awhile, contraction increases until the cells become overstretched, and dilated cardiomyopathy ultimately develops. For those with an acute onset, the myocardial damage and dysfunction occurs rapidly and presents as an acute myocardial infarction with a decrease in ejection fraction.

Causes

There is a wide variety of causes of myocarditis. Approximately 50% of the cases of myocarditis are idiopathic (Tang & Young, 2005). Viral myocarditis is the most common type of myocarditis.

- ◆ Viral
  - ❖ Most common cause in North America
  - ❖ Coxsackievirus types A and B (most common)
  - ❖ Cytomegalovirus
  - ❖ HIV
  - ❖ Hepatitis
  - ❖ Mumps
  - ❖ Rubella
  - ❖ Influenza.
- ◆ Bacterial infections
  - ❖ Tuberculosis
  - ❖ Diptheria
  - ❖ Staphylococcal
  - ❖ Pneumococcal
  - ❖ Streptococcal.
- ◆ Parasitic infections
- ◆ Fungal infections
- ◆ Protozoal infections
  - ❖ Chagas disease.
- ◆ Radiation therapy to chest
- ◆ Chronic alcoholism

Inflammatory Cardiovascular Diseases: Diseases Involving the Pericardium, Myocardium and Endocardium

◆ Cardiac toxins (cocaine, inotropes)

◆ Rickettsia

◆ Lyme Disease

◆ Peripartum condition (30 days before to 150 days after delivery) (Stein et al., 2001).

Symptoms

A small percentage of patients present with an acute onset of heart failure and even cardiogenic shock. Unless it is an acute event, patients present with non-specific symptoms, including fatigue, dyspnea, and chest pain. In cases of viral myocarditis, a recent history of a cold, fever, chills, or other flu-like symptoms is reported. The chest pain can be similar to ischemic chest pain, confusing the diagnosis, or it may be pleural or precordial in nature. Chest pain is often described as sharp and stabbing, but may also be described as squeezing. In addition to dyspnea on exertion, respiratory complaints may include paroxysmal nocturnal dyspnea and orthopnea.

Physical Examination

On physical examination, findings are usually consistent with signs of decreased cardiac output. The severity of the symptoms correlates with the severity of the disease process. Fever with tachycardia may be present and the tachycardia may be faster than would be expected with the fever. As the disease progresses and heart failure develops, pulmonary edema, jugular venous distention, a third heart sound, hepatomegaly, and peripheral edema may develop. The development of cardiogenic shock results in hypotension, cool, clammy skin with cyanosis, decreased urine output and a decreased level of consciousness.

Diagnosis

Myocarditis may be difficult to diagnose, but may be diagnosed by ruling out other causes of decreased myocardial function, such as a myocardial infarction. A recent history of infection may be the best indicator of a viral myocarditis with no other cause. Elevated serum viral antibody titers may provide information regarding a viral infection. Elevated white blood cell counts support an infective process. Elevated myocardial biomarkers (CK-MB and Troponin I or T) support myocardial damage. Rheumatoid screening may be helpful in ruling out inflammatory processes.

Chest X-Ray

Findings on the chest x-ray are typically not helpful in diagnosing myocarditis. Signs of heart failure may be present, but these are not specific to myocarditis.

Echocardiogram

The cardiac echo is useful for the assessment of myocardial function. It is sensitive to myocardial dysfunction, but is not specific to a diagnosis of myocarditis. Systolic dysfunction with a decreased ejection fraction and global hypokenesis is not an uncommon finding in myocarditis.

Endomyocardial Biopsy

While endomyocardial biopsy has been the gold standard for the diagnosis of myocarditis, there is some controversy in the literature about its usefulness. This invasive procedure has been noted to have a high rate of false-negative results. Endomyocardial tissue samples are obtained through a percutaneous route in the cardiac catheterization laboratory. Several tissue samples are collected from the right-ventricular septal wall with a specialized biopsy catheter. In cases of myocarditis when the disease presents in a sporadic pattern, it is difficult to assure the specimens obtained are from the invaded site.

Chapter 12

Treatment

Treatment strategies for myocarditis are based on the severity of the disease process. Some patients presenting with only mild symptoms may be managed at home; however, hospitalization offers opportunities to assure support in cases of progressive loss of left-ventricular dysfunction. Withdrawal of the offending agent or elimination of the cause, if known, is an important aspect of treatment. Decreasing myocardial oxygen demand through simple treatment strategies, such as bed rest or limitation of activities, is essential to allow the myocardium to recover and prevent further myocardial damage. Additional treatment is based on the patient presentation. Patients presenting with signs of heart failure and even cardiogenic shock should be treated in the same manner as those disease processes are treated. Mechanical ventilation with sedation is utilized in severe cases. Intra aortic balloon counterpulsation or ventricular assist devices can be employed to improve cardiac output. As with cardiogenic shock, medications to decrease left-ventricular afterload, such as intravenous nitroprusside in severe cases, and ACE Inhibitors in less severe cases, are beneficial in decreasing myocardial oxygen demand. Dobutamine or Milronone (Primacor) are used to improve contractility. Beta blockers may be beneficial in decreasing heart rate and controlling arrhythmias. Fluid status should be monitored and diuretics used as needed. Arrhythmias are usually transient and should resolve; however, those with more severe cases are at high risk for sudden death during the acute process and should be monitored closely. As in all low cardiac output states, anticoagulant treatment is reasonable for the prevention of thrombus development.

The use of immunosuppressive therapy has not been proven to be effective in the treatment of myocarditis, except in a small population of patients (Howes, D.S., 2005; Tang & Young, 2005). Non-steroidal anti-inflammatory drugs are contraindicated in patients with myocarditis, as they have been found to be ineffective, may interfere with myocardial healing, and may actually exacerbate the inflammatory process and increase mortality (Tang & Young, 2005).

Supportive care for the patient and family is important. Activity levels should be gradually increased with continuous evaluation of tolerance. In-hospital cardiac rehabilitation programs are useful in the assessment of cardiac tolerance to exercise. Low sodium diets are beneficial in fluid overload states, along with careful assessment of intake and output.

Outcomes

Repeat echocardiography is utilized to evaluate myocardial function, as it may improve over time, with some patients experiencing full recovery. The long-term survival is based on the extent of permanent myocardial damage. Some patients develop a dilated cardiomyopathy and require treatment.

Linking Knowledge to Practice

✔ *Myocarditis presents as acute cardiogenic shock. Patients should be treated aggressively, as some experience full recovery.*

ENDOCARDIAL DISEASE

The endocardium is the inner most layer of the heart and is contiguous with the vessels and the valves. The endocardium is located where the endothelium and the endothelial cells that line the endocardium of the heart and the vasculature of the entire body are located. The endothelium also covers all the valves and the structures that support the proper functioning of the valves. The integrity of the endothelium is crucial to protecting these surfaces from the invasion of bacteria.

524

Inflammatory Cardiovascular Diseases: Diseases Involving the Pericardium, Myocardium and Endocardium

Infective Endocarditis

Infective endocarditis (IE) occurs when an infective organism invades the endothelial lining of the heart. The infection usually involves one or more valves and their associated structures.

Pathophysiology

Damage to the endothelial surface of the heart from trauma (e.g. indwelling catheter insertion, pacemaker insertion) or hemodynamic abnormalities that occur with valve disease, prosthetic valves, or some congenital heart diseases, provides an environment that supports the attachment of infective organisms. With the endothelium no longer intact, platelets and fibrin collect to develop a platelet-fibrin thrombus that is referred to as a non-bacterial thrombotic endocarditis lesion (vegetation). These lesions are prone to the adherence of bacteria that is introduced into the blood stream through a variety of avenues, including procedures that involve the mouth, gastrointestinal tract, or genitourinary tract, or secondary to the placement of intravenous lines, invasive monitoring devices, wound infections, pneumonia or urinary tract infections. Once bacteria begin collecting, an infective process develops. The colonization of the microorganisms further increases the size of the thrombotic lesions and large vegetations develop on the endocardial surface. If left untreated, the valvular structures are destroyed by the infection. Valvular ring abscesses develop, as well as valve ruptures or ulcerations. If the infection continues it may cause septal abscess resulting in bundle branch block or AV block.

The most commonly found organisms in infective endocarditis include staphylococcus and streptococci. S. *viridans* and S. *aureus* are the most prevalent, but many other organisms may be involved, including those causing fungal infections.

Types of Infective Endocarditis

Endocarditis in years past was referred to as rheumatic valvulitis because the majority of cases involved patients with rheumatic valve disease. As the incidence of rheumatic valve disease decreases, other processes that put the patient at high risk for the development of infective endocarditis are coming to the forefront, such as mitral valve prolapse with regurgitation, aortic stenosis, and bicuspid aortic valve. The most common classification of infective endocarditis involves identifying the affected valve as either being a native valve or a prosthetic valve. Infective endocarditis may also be referred to as nosocomial if the infection is determined to have occurred as the result of hospitalization.

Native Valve Infective Endocarditis

◆ Native valve infective endocarditis usually occurs in patients with an abnormal native valve or congenital heart disease. The most common valve abnormalities include mitral valve prolapse with regurgitation, degenerative aortic or mitral valve disease, especially calcific aortic valve disease, or rheumatic heart disease involving the mitral valve. Congenital heart disease accounts for 10-20% of the cases of native valve infective endocarditis (Einhorn, Adair, & Voorhees, 2001; Marill, 2006). Congenital heart diseases include those associated with areas of high turbulence, such as patent ductus arteriosus, ventricular septal defect, bicuspid aortic valve, coarctation of the aorta, and pulmonic stenosis. Two other disease processes associated with high turbulence and native valve infective endocarditis include hypertrophic obstructive cardiomyopathy and Marfan Syndrome with aortic insufficiency.

◆ Native valve infective endocarditis is also associated with intravenous drug abuse. The majority of this population has a normally functioning valve. Up to half of the cases of native valve infective endocarditis in intravenous drug abusers involve the tricuspid valve. The skin is the most frequent origin of the bacteremia in infective endocarditis with intravenous drug abusers. S. *aureus* is the most common organism found in this group.

Chapter 12

- ◆ Acute and Subacute
  - ❖ The terms acute and subacute are used in relation to native valve infective endocarditis.
  - ❖ Acute infective endocarditis involves normal healthy valves. The development of endocarditis progresses rapidly, and the patient becomes acutely ill.
  - ❖ The acute development of the disease does not allow time for hemodynamic adjustments that normally occur with valve damage from a slower developing disease processes.
  - ❖ Subacute infective endocarditis involves abnormal, previously damaged or diseased valves with the progression of endocarditis occurring over longer periods of time.
  - ❖ With the slow disease process occurring in subacute infective endocarditis, hemodynamic adjustments are made to adapt to the changing valve dynamics, as with other valve disease processes.

Prosthetic Valve Infective Endocarditis
- ◆ Prosthetic valve infective endocarditis occurs more frequently than native valve infective endocarditis. The aortic valve is most frequently involved. There is no appreciable difference in the occurrence of infective endocarditis between a mechanical or bioprosthetic valve.
- ◆ Early prosthetic valve infective endocarditis refers to an infection that is the result of perioperative contamination that occurred directly or through the use of central lines. To be considered perioperative contamination, the infection generally presents itself within 60 days after implant. The organism involved with early prosthetic valve infective endocarditis is most frequently from a staphylococcal origin, with *S. epidermis* being the most frequent.
- ◆ Late prosthetic valve infective endocarditis occurs more than 60 days after implant and is usually associated with bacteremia from procedures such as dental, genitourinary or gastrointestinal procedures. The organism involved with late prosthetic valve infective endocarditis is usually from a streptococcal origin, most frequently *S. viridans,* followed by *S. epidermis* and *S. aureus.*
- ◆ IE that results from the implantation of a permanent pacemaker or implantable defibrillator falls into the same category as prosthetic valve infective endocarditis. Any part of the pacemaker can become infected, including the pacemaker generator in the pocket or the pacemaker lead(s). Once the infection travels to the leads, there is a direct connection to the endocardial wall and endocarditis may occur.

Nosocomial Infective Endocarditis
- ◆ Nosocomial infective endocarditis occurs secondary to invasive procedures, such as line placement or dialysis.
- ◆ Nosocomial infections are infections that present 48 hours after hospital admission or infections that present within four weeks after the completion of a procedure. Early prosthetic valve infective endocarditis and early pacemaker infections are considered nosocomial infective endocarditis.

Right-Sided Infective Endocarditis
- ◆ Occurs when a valve on the right side of the heart is affected.
- ◆ Usually involves a nosocomial infective endocarditis that occurs when an invasive line, such as a pulmonary artery catheter, injures the valve during insertion.
- ◆ Is more common in intravenous drug abusers.
- ◆ May result in embolization to the lung.
- ◆ Fewer peripheral signs of infective endocarditis occur with right-sided infective endocarditis than with left-sided infective endocarditis.
- ◆ Patients with right-sided infective endocarditis are more likely to have negative blood cultures than those with left-sided infective endocarditis.

Inflammatory Cardiovascular Diseases: Diseases Involving the Pericardium, Myocardium and Endocardium

◆ Patients with right-sided infective endocarditis present differently than those with left-sided infective endocarditis due to the differences in hemodynamic changes.

Left-Sided Infective Endocarditis

◆ Occurs when a valve on the left side of the heart is affected.

◆ More commonly occurs with previously damaged valves.

◆ May result in systemic embolization to the brain, spleen and kidneys.

◆ Usually results in a greater hemodynamic compromise.

Symptoms

The symptoms in subacute infective endocarditis develop slowly over time, while the symptoms associated with acute infective endocarditis are sudden onset and usually more severe. Patients with subacute infective endocarditis most frequently report symptoms of fever, malaise, fatigue, and weight loss. The fever of subacute infective endocarditis is usually low grade and persists over weeks. Night sweats and back pain may also accompany the "flu-like" symptoms.

Symptoms associated with acute infective endocarditis are more severe with rapid onset. A high-grade fever with chills and the rapid onset of symptoms of congestive heart failure are reported. Congestive heart failure with prosthetic valve infective endocarditis occurs earlier and is often more severe than with native valve infective endocarditis. Often the sudden onset of symptoms is the result of either an embolic event or acute valve dysfunction. The symptoms of heart failure are dependent on the affected valve. Right-sided symptoms, as with tricuspid valve disease, include peripheral edema, jugular venous distention, hepatomegaly, and ascites. Symptoms that occur with an affected valve on the left side of the heart are usually related to decreased cardiac output and fluid overload. These patients present with symptoms of shortness of breath and fatigue.

Other symptoms are related to the effects of embolization of the vegetations located on the valves. The rate of embolization is related to the organism, the size of the vegetation, and the rate of growth. Mitral valve vegetation has a higher rate of embolization than vegetation of other valves. IE of the right side usually involves the tricuspid valve and results in embolization to the lungs with symptoms related to pulmonary emboli. The most common areas of embolization from the left side of the heart include the brain, spleen and kidneys; however, embolization to the retina, spinal cord, coronary artery, or bowel may also occur. For many patients, presenting with symptoms of cerebral emboli may lead to a diagnosis of infective endocarditis.

Physical Examination

◆ Fever

❖ Low-grade fever in subacute infective endocarditis.

❖ High-grade fever in acute infective endocarditis.

◆ Murmurs

❖ Regurgitant murmurs occur with a high frequency in subacute infective endocarditis.

❖ A new murmur in the presence of a fever is highly suspicious of infective endocarditis.

❖ If no murmur is noted, the diagnosis of infective endocarditis becomes less feasible and other options should be evaluated, keeping in mind there are some patients with infective endocarditis who do not present with a murmur.

❖ Some patients with involvement of the tricuspid valve may not have an audible murmur due to the low-pressure gradients on the right side of the heart. If there is no murmur present with a high suspicion of tricuspid involvement, as with intravenous drug abusers, further investigation is warranted.

527

Chapter 12

♦ Peripheral signs of infective endocarditis have been reported in as few as 20% and as many as 75% of patients with infective endocarditis. Their presence supports a diagnosis of infective endocarditis but their absence does not rule out the diagnosis of infective endocarditis. These signs are usually the result of emboli or an allergic vasculitis.

❖ Petechiae are the most frequently noted peripheral signs and may be present on the top of the hands and feet as well as the neck, anterior chest, the abdominal wall and the mucosa of the mouth.

❖ Splinter hemorrhages are dark red linear streaks on the distal tips of the nail beds.

❖ Osler's Nodes are small, tender, red-purple raised nodules most commonly found on the pads of the fingers and toes. They may also be present in the palms of the hands and the soles of the feet.

❖ Janeway Lesions are non-tender red-purple macules, 1-5mm in size, that are usually found on the palms of the hands and the soles of the feet.

❖ Roth's Spots (retinal hemorrhages) are small (3-10mm) white spots on the retina.

❖ Blue toe syndrome is embolization of vegetation debris to distal extremities causing ischemia, cyanosis and ultimately necrosis (gangrene).

♦ Clinical findings associated with heart failure (right- or left-sided) may be present.

♦ Clinical findings associated with embolic events may be present.

❖ Cerebral emboli and infarct (signs associated with a stroke).

❖ Splenic emboli and infarct (left upper quadrant abdominal pain radiating to the shoulder, signs of pleural effusions, splenomegaly).

❖ Renal emboli and infarct (hematuria, oliguria, flank or back pain, hypertension).

❖ Coronary artery emboli and infarct.

❖ Pulmonary emboli and infarct (dyspnea, blood tinged sputum, pleuritic chest pain, tachycardia, anxiety).

♦ Additional clinical findings would include normal findings associated with acute and chronic valvular heart disease.

Diagnosis

A complete patient history that focuses on a recent history of invasive procedures, surgery, or dental work assists in the diagnostic process. The Duke Criteria, published by Durak et al in 1994, is utilized as a basis for diagnosis of infective endocarditis (Table 12.3). In 2000, modifications for the Duke Criteria were recommended by Li et al. (2000) (Table 12.4). The increased utilization of transesophogeal echocardiography was one of the primary reasons for the recommended changes. Blood cultures and echocardiography are the cornerstones for the diagnosis of infective endocarditis.

Blood Cultures

♦ Positive blood cultures with typical organisms from two separate blood draws are diagnostic for infective endocarditis. Those typical organisms include:

❖ Streptococcus (alpha-hemolytic and *S. Viridans*).

❖ Staphylococci (*S. Aureus, S. Epidermis*).

❖ Pseudomonas aeruginosa .

❖ Enterococci.

❖ HACEK gram-negative organisms:

★ *Haemophilus aphrophilus.*

★ *Actinobacillus actinomycetemcomitans.*

Inflammatory Cardiovascular Diseases: Diseases Involving the Pericardium, Myocardium and Endocardium

- ☆ *Cardiobacterium hominis*
- ☆ *Eikenella corrodens*
- ☆ *Kingella kingae*

◆ If cultures are not positive with the typical organisms, then persistent bacteremia with any other organism is also a major criterion for IE. Persistent is defined by the Duke criteria as a) two positive cultures greater than 12 hours apart, or b) three positive cultures, or c) a majority of 4 or more cultures greater than one hour apart (Durack et al., 1994).

◆ About 5% of the patients with IE have negative cultures (Einhorn, Adair, Voorhees, 2001). The most common cause for culture-negative IE is inadequate treatment of a prior incidence of IE. Patients may also present with negative cultures if they have been very recently treated with antibiotics for some other suspected infective process.

Echocardiogram

◆ Echocardiography provides valuable information about the condition of the valves and the progression of vegetation. Positive blood cultures with echocardiographic findings consistent with IE confirm the diagnosis of IE.

◆ Transthoracic echocardiogram (TTE) provides the diagnostic evidence of IE 50-70% of the time, whereas a transesophageal echocardiogram (TEE) is 95% sensitive for detecting vegetation (Einhorn, Adair, & Voorhees, 2001).

◆ A TTE may be acceptable for initial diagnostic testing. A negative TTE does not necessarily rule out IE. If the patient history, symptoms and blood cultures are highly suggestive of IE and the TTE is negative, then a TEE should be done.

◆ TEE is indicated as the first line diagnostic test over TTE in patients with prosthetic valves, suspected right-sided IE vegetation, or suspected myocardial abscess.

Other Tests

◆ Abnormal lab work, while not diagnostic, may point towards IE.
- ❖ Elevated white blood cell count.
- ❖ Elevated erythrocyte sedimentation rate.
- ❖ Proteinuria.
- ❖ Hematuria.
- ❖ Elevated BUN and creatinine.
- ❖ Anemia in subacute IE.
  - ☆ Normocytic anemia.
- ❖ Positive serum rheumatoid factor in subacute IE.

Chapter 12

Table 12.3 Duke Criteria for Diagnosis of Infective Endocarditis

Clinical criteria for infective endocarditis requires:
    Two major criteria, OR
    One major and three minor criteria, OR
    Five minor criteria.

Major Criteria   1. Positive blood culture for Infective Endocarditis as defined below:
         a. Typical microorganism consistent with IE from 2 separate blood cultures:
            - viridans streptococci, *Streptococcus bovis*, or HACEK organisms.
         OR
            - community-acquired *Staphylococcus aureus* or enterococci, in the absence of a primary focus.
         b. Persistently positive blood cultures (any organism) defined as:
            - 2 positive cultures of blood samples drawn >12 hours apart.
         OR
            - 3 positive cultures.
         OR
            - a majority of 4 separate cultures of blood (with first and last sample drawn > 1 hour apart).
    2. Evidence of infective endocarditis as defined below:
         a. Oscillating intracardiac mass on valve or supporting structures, in the path of regurgitant jets, or on implanted material in the absence of an alternative anatomic explanation, abscess or new partial dehiscence of prosthetic valve.
         OR
         b. New valvular regurgitation (worsening or changing of pre-existing murmur not sufficient).

Minor Criteria   1. Predisposition: predisposing heart condition or intravenous drug use.
    2. Fever: Temperature > 38.0° C (100.4° F).
    3. Vascular phenomena: major arterial emboli, septic pulmonary infarcts, mycotic aneurysm, intracranial hemorrhage, conjunctival hemorrhages, and Janeway lesions.
    4. Immunologic phenomena: glomerulonephritis, Osler's nodes, Roth spots, and rheumatoid factor.
    5. Microbiological evidence: Positive blood culture without meeting major criterion as noted above, or serological evidence of active infection with organism consistent with infective endocarditis. (Excludes single positive cultures for coagulase-negative staphylococci, diphtheroids, and organisms that do not commonly cause endocarditis).
    6. Echocardiographic findings: Consistent with infective endocarditis without meeting a major criterion.

Adapted from Durack, D.T., Lukes, A.S., Bright, D.K., 1994.

Inflammatory Cardiovascular Diseases: Diseases Involving the Pericardium, Myocardium and Endocardium

---

Table 12.4
Proposed Modifications to the Duke Criteria for Diagnosing Infective Endocarditis

1. Criteria for "possible infective endocarditis" should be defined as:

   a. At least 1 major and 1 minor criteria

   OR

   b. 3 minor criteria.

2. Eliminate: Minor criterion of echocardiographic findings consistent with endocarditis without meeting a major criterion, due to the global use of transesophogeal echocardiography to accurately diagnose infective endocarditis.

3. Bacteremia with *S. aureus* should be considered a major criterion regardless if nosocomial in nature or if a primary focus is present.

4. Positive fever should be considered a major criterion.

Adapted from Li, J.S, Sexton, D.J., Mick, N., Nettles, R., Fowler, V.G., Jr., & Ryan, T., et al., 2000.

Treatment

The goals of treatment include early recognition, elimination of the infection, timely surgical intervention and treatment of complications.

Antibiotic Therapy

◆ Intravenous antibiotics are the key therapeutic intervention and are usually given for 4-6 weeks, sometimes longer, based on the response to treatment. Once patients are stable and responding to therapy, they are discharged on home intravenous antibiotic therapy.

◆ The fever usually returns to normal after 3 days of antibiotic therapy.

◆ If the fever persists, there may be a secondary infection or a resistance to the antibiotic.

Surgical Intervention

◆ Valve replacement may be necessary for some patients. Indications for surgical intervention include:

   ❖ IE with heart failure that is not responsive to medical treatment (NYHA Class III or IV).

   ❖ Recurrent or persistent infection.

   ❖ Large or hypermobile vegetation.

   ❖ Acute valvular dysfunction.

   ❖ A major embolic event or signs and symptoms of small frequent emboli.

   ❖ New onset conduction abnormalities (bundle branch blocks, AV blocks).

   ❖ Myocardial abscess or fistulas (ventricular septal defects, atrial septal defects).

   ❖ Urgent surgery for severe heart failure with significant aortic regurgitation.

   ❖ Any infected prosthetic valve that should be replaced.

◆ In acutely ill patients, surgical intervention improved long-term outcomes over medical therapy alone; therefore, acute infection should not be considered a contraindication to surgery.

◆ The development of heart failure with an abnormal valve is an indication for surgical intervention. Nurses should be cognizant of the indications for surgery so they can properly recognize when a change in patient condition could result in a change in the treatment plan from a medical plan to a surgical plan.

Chapter 12

◆ Fungal infections do not often respond to medical therapy and require surgical intervention.

◆ If the IE is the result of an infected permanent pacemaker with vegetation evident on the pacemaker wires, the entire pacemaker system must be removed after antibiotics are initiated. Patients who are pacemaker-dependent require a period of time with a temporary transvenous pacemaker in place while the antibiotics work to sterilize the blood before a new permanent pacemaker system is placed (Ellenbogen & Wood, M.A., 2002).

Anticoagulants

◆ Anticoagulation is not indicated; there is no evidence supporting the initiation of anticoagulation therapy for the prevention of emboli related to the IE.

◆ Patients previously on warfarin (coumadin) therapy for other reasons, such as a mechanical valve implant or a history of atrial fibrillation, should continue with this treatment regime; however, there is an increased risk for cerebral hemorrhage, so lowering the dose of the anticoagulant during the acute phase should be considered (Keys, 2004).

Other Treatment Considerations

◆ Other therapy is dependent on the patient's signs and symptoms, such as treatment for heart failure.

◆ Patients should be monitored for signs of embolization.

◆ Strict sterile technique should be utilized for any test or procedure that is invasive, including insertion of intravenous catheters.

◆ Care of indwelling catheters requires meticulous attention.

◆ Assure good oral hygiene.

◆ Bed rest is usually necessary early in the process, as the infection places a large metabolic demand on the body. Meticulous skin care should be carried out to maintain the integrity of the skin and prevent skin breakdown.

◆ Careful monitoring of the patient's temperature is important to recognize the response to antibiotic therapy.

◆ Monitoring of the patient for signs of heart failure may indicate progression of valvular disease and the need for surgical intervention.

◆ Intravenous drug abusers require support, as they experience drug withdrawal.

◆ Emotional support for patients and families is an important aspect of treatment. IE often requires a long hospitalization, with further antibiotic requirements after discharge.

Complications

◆ The most common complications in IE include:
  ❖ Valve dysfunction
  ❖ Congestive heart failure
  ❖ Myocardial (valvular) or septal abscesses
  ❖ Metastatic infection
  ❖ Embolic events
  ❖ Organ dysfunction from embolic events
  ❖ Pericarditis
  ❖ Myocarditis
  ❖ Glomerulonephritis and acute renal failure
  ❖ Mycotic aneurysm is the result of embolization of infected thrombotic material from an infected cardiac valve or other source. The thrombotic material most commonly travels to the branches

Inflammatory Cardiovascular Diseases: Diseases Involving the Pericardium, Myocardium and Endocardium

of the middle cerebral artery. Bacterial embolization causes inflammation and diminishes the integrity of the arterial wall resulting in rupture and intracerebral or subarachnoid hemorrhage.

Follow-Up Care

◆ Blood cultures are repeated 3-4 days after the initiation of antibiotics to assure that antibiotic treatment is effective.

◆ Education about reoccurrence should occur prior to discharge from the hospital. Compliance with the post hospital antibiotic regime should be stressed. The patient must be aware of the signs to watch for, indicating a reoccurrence of infection, including fever, anorexia, or any other symptoms that the patient experienced prior to treatment. The patient should be particularly alert for these symptoms within the first two weeks after antibiotic treatment was completed. Make sure the patient notifies the physician if any signs of reinfection occur. Meticulous dental hygiene should be stressed to prevent dental caries and the development of periodontal disease.

◆ Antibiotic prophylaxis prior to procedures that are likely to cause bacteremia is required for patients with a history of IE. Procedures that most frequently result in bacteremia include dental procedures, gastrointestinal procedures, genitourinary procedures, or gynecological procedures.

Outcomes

Left untreated, IE is fatal. With the development of antibiotics and more aggressive surgical intervention, the mortality rate from IE has decreased significantly. Outcomes vary depending on the invading organism, the affected valve, and the patient. Mortality rates are higher in acute cases of IE than in subacute cases. There is an increased mortality rate in cases with heart failure and renal failure, as well as culture-negative cases, gram-negative invasions or fungal infections. Cases with multiple valve or prosthetic valve involvement have less favorable outcomes. Cases with left-sided involvement have a poorer prognosis than those with right-sided involvement. Involvement of the aortic valve is associated with higher mortality rates than involvement of the mitral valve. The development of cardiac abscesses worsens the prognosis, as does systemic embolization. Those with late prosthetic valve infective endocarditis usually have better outcomes than those with early prosthetic valve infective endocarditis.

Situations that support improved outcomes are early diagnosis, young age, penicillin-sensitive streptococcal infections, and young intravenous drug users with *S. aureus* infection of the tricuspid valve (Einhorn, Adair, & Voorhees, 2001). Intravenous drug abusers can experience a 90% cure rate; however, they have a high rate of reoccurrence. Native valve streptococcal infections treated early have the best outcomes.

Special Note Regarding Antibiotic Prophylaxis

In April 2007 the American Heart Association published new guidelines for the prevention of endocarditis. These guidelines significantly alter the past practices related to antibiotic administration prior to specific procedures in patients who were felt to be at high risk for the developed infective endocarditis. Within the new guidelines the committee noted that it is no longer reasonable to believe that antimicrobial prophylaxis is effective in the prevention of infective endocarditis associated with dental, GI or GU procedures (Wilson, Taubert, Gewitz, Lockhart, Baddour, and Levison et al, 2007). The guidelines provide the following as rationale for the changes to the guidelines:

1. Infective endocarditis is much more likely to result from frequent exposure to random bacteremias associated with daily activities than from bacteremia caused by a dental, GI tract, or GU tract procedure.

2. Prophylaxis may prevent an exceedingly small number of cases of infective endocarditis, if any, in individuals who undergo dental, GI tract, or GU tract procedures.

533

Chapter 12

3. The risk of antibiotic associated adverse events exceeds the benefit, if any of prophylactic therapy.

4. Maintenance of optimal oral health and hygiene may reduce the incidence of bacteremia from daily activities and is more important than prophylactic antibiotics for dental procedure to reduce the risk of infective endocarditis. (Wilson, Taubert, Gewitz, Lockhart, Baddour, and Levison et al, 2007).

The new guidelines recommend prophylaxis for only those with the highest risk for the development of infective endocarditis. The American Heart Association panel identified the following population as those at the highest risk for the development of infective endocarditis:

1. Prosthetic cardiac valve

2. Previous infective endocarditis

3. Congenital heart disease

4. Cardiac transplant recipients who develop cardiac valvulopathy (Wilson et al., 2007).

Linking Knowledge to Practice

✔ *A new murmur in the presence of a high fever is a strong predictor of infective endocarditis.*

✔ *While sterile and clean techniques should be carefully adhered to with all patients, they should be of particular importance in those with prosthetic or abnormal native valves.*

✔ *Meticulous oral hygiene should be encouraged in patients with a prosthetic or abnormal native valve to prevent dental caries or periodontal disease.*

✔ *Patients with infective endocarditis should be carefully monitored for signs of embolization.*

✔ *Patients with infective endocarditis and their families require strong emotional support for this disease process that necessitates a prolonged treatment plan.*

✔ *Acute infective endocarditis places a great metabolic demand on the body with increased energy utilization. Bedrest may be necessary during the first several days of treatment.*

TEST YOUR KNOWLEDGE

1. The following is true regarding the fibrous pericardium:
    a. It normally holds up to 20 ml of serous fluid.
    b. It is contiguous with the epithelial layer of the heart.
    c. It is also known as the visceral layer of the pericardium.
    d. It helps to maintain the shape and size of the heart, especially in fluid overload situations.

2. Symptoms of pericarditis include all of the following, except:
    a. Sharp stabbing chest pain.
    b. Pain that eases when lying in the left lateral position.
    c. Pain that increases with deep inspiration, movement or cough.
    d. Shallow respiratory pattern.

Inflammatory Cardiovascular Diseases: Diseases Involving the Pericardium, Myocardium and Endocardium

3. Nursing interventions in the patient with pericarditis include all of the following, except:

    a. Provide comfort by administering pain medications and proper positioning.

    b. Auscultate heart sounds to assess for muffled heart sounds.

    c. Administer anticoagulants to prevent thrombus in the pericardium.

    d. Monitor for JVD and hypotension.

4. When differentiating the ST-segment changes of pericarditis from the ST-segment changes of acute myocardial infarction, the nurse knows the ST-segment elevation of pericarditis typically has the following pattern:

    a. Diffuse ST elevation with concave upward ST-segments.

    b. Diffuse ST elevation with convex upward ST-segments.

    c. ST elevation with concave upward ST-segment in aVR and V_1 only.

    d. ST elevation with convex upward ST-segments in aVR and V_1 only.

5. Pericardial effusion occurs when there is an abnormal accumulation of which of the following in the pericardial space?

    a. Blood

    b. Pus

    c. Fluid

    d. a and c

    e. All of the above.

6. Patients with pericardial effusions should be assessed for the development of the following complication of effusion:

    a. Thrombocytopenia

    b. Tamponade

    c. AV fistula

    d. Endocarditis

7. Following pericardiocentesis, the nurse should monitor the patient for

    a. development of pneumothorax.

    b. bleeding from groin site.

    c. pupil responsiveness.

    d. sudden increase in urine output.

Chapter 12

8. Which of the following readings represents an abnormal pulsus paradoxus?

   a. Systolic BP during expiration only, 120 mm Hg, with systolic BP during expiration and inspiration 110 mm Hg

   b. Systolic BP during inspiration only, 120 mm Hg, with systolic BP during inspiration and expiration 110 mm Hg

   c. Systolic BP during expiration only, 120 mm Hg, with systolic BP during expiration and inspiration 106 mm Hg

   d. Systolic BP during inspiration only, 120 mm Hg, with systolic BP during inspiration and expiration 106 mm Hg

9. Beck's classic triad of symptoms for cardiac tamponade include:

   a. Hypotension, muffled heart sounds, jugular venous distension

   b. Hypertension, muffled heart sound, jugular venous distension

   c. Hypotension, muffled heart sounds, pulmonary edema

   d. Hypertension, muffled heart sound, pulmonary edema

10. Treatment strategies that may be helpful in stabilizing the patient in acute cardiac tamponade may include:

    a. Increase preload, increase afterload, increase contractility.

    b. Increase preload, increase afterload, decrease contractility.

    c. Increase preload, decrease afterload, increase contractility.

    d. Decrease preload, decrease afterload, increase contractility.

11. The patient with constrictive pericarditis is at particular risk for a decrease in cardiac output in which of the following situations?

    a. Atrial fibrillation

    b. Dehydration

    c. VVI Pacing

    d. All of the above.

12. Patients presenting with acute myocarditis will most likely have which of the following hemodynamic profiles?

    a. Decreased preload, decreased afterload, decreased contractility

    b. Decreased preload, increased afterload, increased contractility

    c. Increased preload, increased afterload, decreased contractility

    d. Increased preload, decreased afterload, decreased contractility

Inflammatory Cardiovascular Diseases: Diseases Involving the Pericardium, Myocardium and Endocardium

13. Patients with infective endocarditis should be monitored for signs of

    a. embolization.

    b. hypertension.

    c. pleural effusion.

    d. cardiac tamponade.

14. Treatment strategies for infective endocarditis include which of the following?

    a. Anticoagulation

    b. Antibiotics

    c. Beta blockers

    d. Valuloplasty

15. Patient education for the patient with a prosthetic valve or abnormal valve should include

    a. meticulous oral hygiene.

    b. antibiotic therapy prior to oral, gastrointestinal, genitourinary or gynecological procedures.

    c. signs and symptoms of infective endocarditis.

    d. All of the above.

ANSWERS

1.	D	9.	A
2.	B	10.	C
3.	C	11.	D
4.	A	12.	C
5.	E	13.	A
6.	B	14.	B
7.	A	15.	D
8.	C		

Chapter 12

REFERENCES

Alspach, J.G. (2006). *Core curriculum for critical care nursing* (6th ed.). St. Louis: Saunders.

Antman, E.M., Anbe, D.T., Armstrong, P.W., Bates, E.R., Green, L.A., Hand, M., Hochman, J.S., Krumholz, H.M., Kushner, F.G., Lamas, G.A., Mullany, C.J., Ornato, J.P., Pearle, D.L., Sloan, M.A., & Smith, S.C. Jr. (2004). ACC / AHA guidelines the management of patients with ST-elevation myocardial infarction: executive summary: A report of the ACC / AHA task force on practice guidelines (Committee to Revise the 1999 Guidelines on the Management of Patients with Acute Myocardial Infarction). *Journal of the American College of Cardiology, 44,* 671-719

Apple, M.S. (2005). Common cardiovascular disorders. In P.G. Morton, D.K. Fontaine, C.M. Hudak, & B.M. Gallo (Eds.), *Critical care nursing: A holistic approach* (8th ed., pp. 378-392). Philadelphia: Lippincott, Williams and Wilkins.

Atar, S., Darovic, G.O., & Siegel, R.J. (2002). Cardiomyopathies and pericardial disease. In G.O. Darovic (Ed.), *Hemodynamic monitoring: Invasive and noninvasive clinical application* (3rd ed., pp 601-636). Philadelphia: Saunders.

Attman, W.G. & Tahon, S.E. (1999). Minimally invasive closed mitral commissurotomy. *Texas Heart Institute Journal:* 26(4), 269-274.

Baddour, L.M., Wilson, W.R., Bayer, A.S., Fowler, V.G., Bolger, A.F., Levison, M.E., Ferrieri, P., Gerber, M.A., Tani, L.Y., Gewitz, M.H, Tong, D.C., Steckelberg, J.M., Baltimore, R.S.,. Shulman, S.T., Burns, J.C., Falace, D.A., Newburger, J.W., Pallasch, T.J., Takahashi, M., &Taubert, K.A. Infective endocarditis: Diagnosis, antimicrobial therapy, and management of complications: A statement for healthcare professionals from the Committee on Rheumatic Fever, Endocarditis, and Kawasaki Disease, Council on Cardiovascular Disease in the Young, and the Councils on Clinical Cardiology, Stroke, and Cardiovascular Surgery and Anesthesia, American Heart Association: Endorsed by the Infectious Diseases Society of America. *Circulation, Jun 2005*; 111: e394-e434.

Bloomquist, J. & Love, M.M. (2000). Cardiovascular assessment and diagnostic procedures. In L.D. Urden, & K.M. Stacy (Eds.), *Priorities in critical care nursing* (pp. 99-145). St Louis: Mosby.

Bojar, R.M.(2005). Manual of perioperative care in adult cardiac surgery (4th ed.). Malden, Massachusetts: Blackwell Publishing.

Bond, E.F. (2005). Cardiac anatomy and physiology. In S.L.Woods, E.S. Froelicher, S.U. Motzer, & E.J. Bridges (Eds.), *Cardiac nursing* (5th ed., pp. 3-48). Philadelphia: Lippincott, Williams and Wilkins.

Brusch, J. (2005). Infective endocarditis. Emedicine. Retrieved March 23, 2006, from http://www.emedicine.com/MED/topic671.htm

Carabello, B.A. & Ganzes, P.C. (2001). *Cardiology pearls* (2nd ed.). Philadelphia: Hanley and Belfus.

Conover, M.B. (2003). *Understanding electrocardiography* (8th ed.). St. Louis: Mosby.

Crawford, M.H. (2004) *Essentials of diagnosis and treatment in cardiology*. New York: McGraw-Hill.

Critical care challenges: disorders, treatments and procedures. (2003). Philadelphia: Lippincott, Williams and Wilkins.

Dauber, I.M. (2003). Endocarditits. In P.E. Parsons & J.P. Wiener-Kronish (Eds.), *Critical care secrets* (3rd ed., pp 185-190). Philadelphia: Hanley & Belfus, Inc.

De Castro, M.A. & Schwartz, D.E. (2003). Pericardial disease (pericarditis and pericardial tamponade). In P.E. Parsons & J.P. Wiener-Kronish (Eds.), *Critical care secrets* (3rd ed., pp. 163-171). Philadelphia: Hanley & Belfus, Inc.

Dennison, R.D. (2000). *Pass ccrn* (2nd ed.). St.Louis: Mosby.

Dirks, J. (2000). Cardiovascular therapeutic management. In L.D. Urden & K.M. Stacy (Eds.), *Priorities in critical care nursing* (pp. 183-209). St Louis: Mosby.

Durack, D.T., Lukes, A.S., & Bright, D.K. (1994). New criteria for diagnosis of infective endocarditis: utilization of specific echocardiographic findings. *American Journal of Medicine, 96*(3): 200-209.

Einhorn, A., Adair, O.V., & Voorhees, D.P. Endocarditis. In A. V. Adair (Ed.), *Cardiology secrets* (2nd ed., pp.129-135). Philadelphia: Hanley and Belfus, Inc.

Ellenbogen, K.A. & Wood, M.A. (2002). *Cardiac pacing and ICDs* (3rd ed.). Malden, Massachusetts: Blackwell Science, Inc.

Goyle, K. & Walling, A.D. (2002). Diagnosing pericarditis. *American Family Physician, 66* (9). Retrieved August 3, 2006, from http://www.aafp.org/afp/20021101/1695.html

Hambach, C. (1998). Opening a window ion pericardial effusion. *Nursing,* August 1998. Retrieved March 23, 2006, from http://findarticles.com/p/articles/mi_qa3689/is_199808/ai_n8824630

Howes, D.S. (2005). Myocarditis. Emedicine. Retrieved July 14, 2006, from http://www.emedicine.com/EMERG/topic326.htm

Keys, T. (2004). Infective endocarditis. Cleveland Clinic Medical Education. Retrieved August 17, 2006, from http://www.clevelandclinicmeded.com/diseasemanagement/infectiousdisease/infectendo/infectendo.htm

Khasnin, A. & Lokhandwala, Y. (2002). Clinical signs in medicine: Pulusus paradoxus. *Journal of Postgraduate Medicine, 48*(1) pp. 46-49.

Kowalak, J. P., Welsh, W. & Mills, E.J. (Eds.). (2003). *Critical care challenges: Disorders, treatments, and procedures.* Philadelphia: Lippincott, Williams and Wilkins.

Kumar, V., Abbas. A.K., & Fausto, N. (2005). *Pathologic basis of disease* (7th ed.). Philadelphia: Elsevier Saunders.

Lewis, S.M., Heitkemper, M.M. & Dirksen, S.T. (2004). *Medical surgical nursing: Assessment and management of clinical problems* (6th ed.). St. Louis: Mosby.

Li, J.S, Sexton, D.J., Mick, N., Nettles, R., Fowler, V.G., Jr., Ryan, T., Bashore, T., & Corey, G.R. (2000). Proposed modification to the Duke criteria for the diagnosis of infective endocarditis. *Clinical Infectious Disease, 30*(4): 633-638.

Marill, K. (2006). Endocarditis. Emedicine. Retrieved July 14, 2006 from http://www.emedicine.com/emerg/topic164.htm

Marinella, M.A. (1998). Electrocardiographic manifestations and differential diagnosis of acute pericarditis. *American Family Physician, 57*(4). Retrieved August 3, 2006, from http://www.aafp.org/afp/980215ap/marinell.html

Chapter 12

Marini, J.J. & Wheeler A.P. (2006). *Critical care medicine the essentials* (3rd ed.). Philadelphia: Lippincott, Williams and Wilkins.

Marriott, H.J.L. (1999). *Board review manual of electrocardiography* (2nd ed.). Riverview, FL: Marriott Foundation/ACCN.

Marriott, H.J.L. (1997). *Emergency electrocardiography*. Naples, FL: Trinity Press.

Massie, B.M. & Amiodon, T.M. (2004). Heart. In L.M. Tierney, Jr., S.J. McPhee, & M.A. Papadakis, *Current medical diagnosis and treatment* (43rd ed., pp. 315-400). New York: McGraw-Hill.

McNeil, M. (2005). Pericardial, myocardial and endocardial disease. In Woods, S.L., Froelicher, E.S., Motzer, S.U., & Bridges, E.J. (Eds.), *Cardiac nursing* (5th ed., pp. 776-793). Philadelphia: Lippincott, Williams and Wilkins.

Mendoza, R. & Trujillo, N. (2001). Complication and care following myocardial infarction. In A.V. Adair (Ed.), *Cardiology secrets* (2nd ed., pp. 113-117). Philadelphia: Hanley and Belfus, Inc.

Meyerson, S. & D'Amico, T.A. (2006). Pericardial procedures. ACS Surgery Online. Retrieved March 23, 2006, from http://www.medscape.com/viewarticle/535596

O'Brien, T. (2005). Pericarditis, constrictive. Emedicine. Retrieved March 23, 2006, from http://www.emedicine.com/med/topic1782.htm

O'Donnell, M. & Dirks, J. (2000). Cardiovascular disorders. In L.D. Urden & K.M. Stacy (Eds.), *Priorities in critical care nursing* (pp. 146-182). St Louis: Mosby.

Opie, L.H. (2004). *Heart physiology from cell to circulation* (4th ed.). Philadelphia: Lippincott, Williams and Wilkins.

Perea, M.A. & Sherry, P.D. (2001). Pericardial disease. In A.V. Adair (Ed.), *Cardiology secrets* (2nd ed., pp. 139-142). Philadelphia: Hanley and Belfus, Inc.

Porth, C.M. (Ed.). (2004). *Essentials of pathophysiology: concepts of altered health states*. Philadelphia: Lippincott, Williams and Wilkins.

Shabeti, R. (1998). Pericardial disease. In D.L. Brown (Ed.), *Cardiac intensive care* (pp. 469-475). Philadelphia: W.B. Saunders.

Smith, S.W., Zvosec, D.L., Sharkey, S.W., & Henry, T.D. (Eds.) (2002). *The ECG in acute MI*. Philadelphia: Lippincott, Williams and Wilkins.

Spodick, D.H. (2004). Decreased recognition of the post-myocardial infarction (dressler) syndrome in the postinfarct setting. *Chest, 126*:1410-1411. Retrieved August 3, 2006, from http://www.chestjournal.org/cgi/content/full/126/5/1410

Stein, R.A. & Gonzalez, J. M. Myocarditis. In A.V. Adair (Ed.), *Cardiology secrets* (2nd ed., pp.152-155). Philadelphia: Hanley and Belfus, Inc.

Strimel, W. (2005). Pericardial effusion. Emedicine. Retrieved March 23, 2006, from http://www.emedicine.com/MED/topic1786.htm

Tang, W.H.W. & Young, J.B. (2005). Myocarditis. Emedicine. Retrieved March 3, 2006, from http://www.emedicine.com/med/topic1569.htm

Valley, V.T. (2005). Pericarditis and cardiac tamponade. Emedicine. Retrieved March 3, 2006, from http://www.emedicine.com/EMERG/topic412.htm

White, M.J. (2001). Anticoagulants and antiplatelet drugs. In A.V. Adair (Ed.), *Cardiology secrets* (2nd ed., pp. 113-117). Philadelphia: Hanley and Belfus, Inc.

Wilson, W., Taubert, K., Gewitz, M., Lockhart, P., Baddour, L., Levison, M., Bolger, A., Cabell, C., Takahashi, M., Baltimore, R., Newburger, J., Strom, B., Tani, L., Gerber, M., Bonow, R., Pallasch, T., Shulman, S., Rowley, A., Burns, J., Ferrieri, P., Gardner, T., Goff, D., & Durack, D. (2007). Prevention of endocarditis guidelines from the American Heart Association: A guideline from the American Heart Association rheumatic fever, endocarditis, and Kawasaki disease committee, council on cardiovascular disease in the young, and the council on clinical cardiology, council on cardiovascular surgery and anesthesia, and the quality of care and outcomes research interdisciplinary working group. Retrieved June 3, 2007 from www.circ.ahajournals.org

Yariagadda, C. (2002). Cardiac tamponade. Emedicine. Retrieved March 23, 2006, from http://www.emedicine.com/MED/topic283.htm

CHAPTER 13:
PERIPHERAL ARTERIAL DISEASE AND ISCHEMIC STROKE

PERIPHERAL ARTERIAL DISEASE OVERVIEW

Peripheral arterial disease (PAD) as defined in the ACC/AHA Guidelines for the Management of Patients of Peripheral Arterial Disease includes: stenotic, occlusive, and aneurysmal diseases of the aorta and its branch arteries, including the abdominal aorta, renal and mesenteric arteries, and lower extremity arteries.

PAD includes vascular diseases caused by atherosclerotic, thromboembolic, degenerative, inflammatory, or traumatic pathology. The most common cause of PAD is atherosclerosis.

Patients with PAD are likely to have co-existing cardiovascular and cerebral vascular disease and are at an increased risk for ischemic events. Coronary artery disease exists in > 60% of those people with lower extremity PAD (Hirsch et al., 2005). Ischemic events associated with coronary and carotid disease are more common and more life threatening than ischemic events of the lower extremities.

PAD is a prevalent but under-recognized condition. Early detection and management of PAD can improve quality of life and lower the rate of ischemic events in this patient population.

LOWER EXTREMITY PAD

Prevalence

Lower extremity PAD is a common syndrome affecting a large portion of the adult population. Patients with lower extremity PAD have a 3 to 5 times overall greater risk of cardiovascular mortality. Of the patients who have symptoms, 30% have stenosis of the aorta or iliac arteries, 80% have stenosis of the femoral or popliteal arteries, and 40% have stenosis of the tibial and peroneal arteries (Creager, 2002). The high number of patients with multiple areas of stenosis accounts for the overlapping percentages.

Atherosclerotic Risk Factors for Lower Extremity PAD

- Cigarette smoking: Smoking is 2-3 times more likely to cause lower extremity PAD than coronary artery disease. Additionally > 80% of patients with lower extremity PAD are current or former smokers (Hirsch et al., 2006). The risk associated with smoking increases as the number of packs per day and number of years the patient has smoked increases.
- Diabetes: Diabetes is present in 12 to 20% of patients with lower extremity PAD (Hirsch et al., 2006). Diabetic patients with lower extremity PAD are also more likely to require an amputation than non-diabetic patients with lower extremity PAD.
- Dyslipidemia.
- Hypertension.
- Hyperhomocysteinemia: 30 to 40% of patients with lower extremity PAD have elevated levels of homocysteine.
- Increased levels of C reactive protein.
- Age > 70 years.
- Age 50-69 with history of smoking or diabetes.
- Age < 50 with diabetes and one or more additional atherosclerotic risk factors.

Chapter 13

Medical Conditions with High Risk for Lower Extremity PAD
- Coronary artery disease.
- Carotid/cerebral vascular disease.
- Renal artery stenosis.

Clinical Signs and Symptoms Indicating High Risk for Lower Extremity PAD
- Leg pain (claudication or rest pain).
- Abnormal lower extremity pulses.

Assessment Questions for Lower Extremity PAD
- Walking impairment?
  - Fatigue?
  - Aching?
  - Numbness?
  - Pain (buttock, thigh, calf, foot)?
- Classic claudication symptoms?
- Rest pain localized to the lower extremities (associated with upright or recumbent position)?
- Poor healing of lower extremity wounds?
- Abdominal pain after eating associated with weight loss?
- Family history of first degree relative with abdominal aortic aneurysm?

Physical Assessment in PAD
- Bilateral arm blood pressure: assessing for variation in readings.
- Assessment of carotid pulses (carotid upstroke).
- Palpation of abdomen (presence of aortic pulsation and maximal diameter).
- Auscultation for carotid, abdominal, and femoral artery bruits.
- Peripheral pulse assessment and scoring on 0-3 scale (0 = absent, 3 = bounding).
  - Brachial
  - Radial
  - Ulnar
  - Femoral
  - Popliteal
  - Dorsalis pedis
  - Posterior tibial.
- Inspection and palpation of feet for color, temperature and lesions.
- Inspection of additional finding, such as distal hair loss and hypertrophic nails.

544

Non-Invasive Diagnostic Studies for Peripheral Arterial Disease

Ankle Brachial Index (ABI)
- The ABI is ankle systolic BP divided by brachial systolic BP.
- The ABI – can be used in asymptomatic lower extremity disease or in patients with claudication. The ABI is the most cost effective diagnostic tool and provides an accurate and objective assessment of lower extremity PAD. ABI is used not only as a diagnostic tool, but also as a tool for monitoring effectiveness of treatment.
- The ABI does not correlate strongly with walking ability because an ABI does not assess the supply and demand relationship. Patients can have an abnormal ABI without symptoms of claudication.
- Patients with lower extremity PAD may have normal resting ABI if collaterals are present.
- Some patients have calcified vessels that are not very compressible (systolic BP cannot be abolished by inflation of the cuff). These patients may have high ankle pressures resulting in a high ABI measurement. Patients at risk for these calcified vessels are those with chronic renal failure or a long history of diabetes, or the elderly.

ABI Measurement (Figure 13.1)
- Systolic BP is recorded in both brachial arteries. There should be < 12 mm Hg difference between arms.
- If arm pressures are not equal, axillary or subclavian stenosis is presumed and the higher pressure is used in calculating the ratios. (Note: Subclavian and axillary occlusive disease exists more frequently in patients with lower extremity arterial disease.)
- Systolic BP is taken in both posterior tibial and dorsalis pedis arteries after patient has been in supine resting position for 10 minutes.
- BP cuffs are sized to the lower calf right above the ankle, and systolic pressures are recorded using a hand-held Doppler.
- In healthy individuals the ankle pressure is 10 to 15 mm Hg higher than the brachial systolic pressure, resulting in a normal ratio of > 1.0.
- ABI measurements are recorded to 2 decimal places.
- ABI is performed in both legs to establish a baseline.

    ABI Values
    Above 0.90   Normal
    0.71-0.90   Mild Obstruction
    0.41-0.70   Moderate Obstruction
    < 0.40   Severe Obstruction

- Patients with ABI values > .5 are not likely to progress to critical limb ischemia.
- A normal or high ABI cannot exclude lower extremity PAD when symptoms are strongly suggestive. Alternative diagnostic tests should be done.
- A toe brachial index of < 0.7 is considered diagnostic for lower extremity PAD (Hirsch et al., 2006).

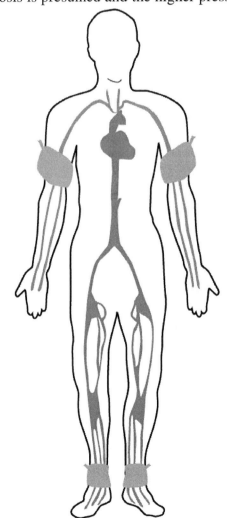

Figure 13.1: Arm and ankle blood pressure cuffs used to obtain ABI measurement.

Chapter 13

Indications for a Resting ABI
◆ Exertional leg symptoms.
◆ Non healing wounds.
◆ $\geq$ 70 years of age.
◆ $\geq$ 50 years of age with a history of smoking or diabetes.

Toe Brachial Index
Toe brachial index can be used in patients with non-compressible ankle arteries (most common in diabetic patients, elderly patients, or patients with end stage kidney disease) or for those with an ABI > 1.30. Obtaining toe pressures can measure digital perfusion when small-vessel arterial disease is present. Pulse volume recordings and Doppler waveform measurements can also be used in this group of patients.

Exercise Ankle Brachial Index
Exercise test with ankle brachial index is used to assess functional capacity and to diagnose patients with a normal resting ABI. Exercise treadmill tests are used to provide objective evidence of functional impairment. A specific exercise protocol (flat or graded exercise) is used to measure maximal walking distance and pain free walking distance. A 6-minute walk test can also be used in patients not able to tolerate exercise treadmill testing. The post exercise ABI is based on the principle that walking induces profound vasodilation. In patients with lower extremity PAD, the post exercise ankle pressure will fall resulting in a decreased ABI.

Continuous Wave Doppler Ultrasound
Continuous wave Doppler ultrasound is used as a non-invasive diagnostic tool to provide accurate assessment of lower extremity peripheral arterial disease. This diagnostic test will determine both location and severity of disease in addition to monitoring disease progression and quantitative improvement after revascularization. Continuous wave Doppler ultrasound obtains velocity waveforms and measures systolic blood pressure at sequential segments of lower extremity arteries.

Duplex Ultrasound
Lower extremity duplex ultrasound is used to diagnose both the location and degree of stenosis in lower extremity PAD. The most important diagnostic information in duplex ultrasound comes of analysis of the velocity of blood flow. Peak systolic velocity ratios are obtained within or beyond the site of stenosis and compared to the adjacent upstream segment. Duplex ultrasound is used for decision-making purposes prior to both interventional and surgical procedures. In addition, it is used as a component of routine follow up after surgical revascularization.

Other indications for duplex ultrasound include evaluation of aortic aneurysms, arterial dissections, and soft tissue masses.

Other Imaging Modalities
◆ Abdominal ultrasound, CT, or MRA for suspected aortic or abdominal aortic aneurysm.
◆ MRA or CTA can also be used to diagnose the anatomical location and degree of stenosis in lower extremity PAD. May be used as a guide in selecting endovascular and surgical procedures.

Invasive Diagnostic Procedures
◆ Contrast angiography is used when patient is being considered for revascularization. Contrast angiography has been the gold standard imaging modality in the diagnosis of peripheral arterial disease. Digital subtraction technology eliminates artifact caused by bony structure and dense body tissue.

Peripheral Arterial Disease and Ischemic Stroke

◆ Non-invasive imaging may be preferential to contrast angiography in certain situations such as in patients with critical limb ischemia or in patients with lesions in vessels below the knees. MRA and CTA offer a 3-dimensional view. Non-invasive imaging may be used for diagnosis or to aide in guiding invasive therapeutic procedures.

Contrast Induced Nephropathy

◆ Risk factors for contrast induced nephropathy include:
  ❖ Diabetes.
  ❖ Dehydration.
  ❖ Low cardiac output state.
  ❖ Baseline renal insufficiency.

◆ Contrast induced nephropathy is a potential complication of angiography. Interventions to limit contrast induced nephropathy include:
  ❖ Aggressive pre-procedure hydration with 0.9NS or sodium bicarbonate drip.
  ❖ N-acetylcysteine can also be given as pre-treatment for patients with creatinine > 2.0 mg /dL.
  ❖ Use of low osmolar contrast agents as well as minimizing quantity of contrast.
  ❖ Pre-procedure hemofiltration may play a role in prevention.

◆ Post-procedure renal function should be assessed within 2 weeks of the procedure.

Asymptomatic Lower Extremity PAD

Asymptomatic disease refers to the absence of classic claudication symptoms. Asymptomatic disease, however, can be associated with forms of leg dysfunction other than classic claudication. Other types of leg dysfunction found in patients without claudication include: 1) slower walking speed, 2) less distance walked per week, 3) slower time to rise from seated position, and 4) poor standing balance. Asymptomatic, therefore, does not mean that limb function is normal.

Asymptomatic patients also have an increased cardiovascular risk and, therefore, are treated with antiplatelet therapy.

Symptomatic Lower Extremity PAD: Claudication

◆ Definition: Ischemic pain or discomfort occurring in specific leg muscle groups during periods of exercise. Symptoms are relieved with 2 to 3 minutes of rest. Symptoms are reproducible to distance, severity, and location on leg. Claudication symptoms are typically stable and do not worsen or improve at rapid rates.

◆ Most common symptom in patients with lower extremity PAD; however, only a fraction of the patients with lower extremity PAD have intermittent claudication. Symptoms are present in only about 20% of patients with lower extremity PAD (Hirsch et al., 2005).

◆ Ischemia to the gastrocnemius (calf) muscle frequently causes claudication because the gastrocnemius muscle has a higher level of oxygen consumption than other muscle groups during walking.

◆ The pathophysiology of symptomatic lower extremity PAD is complex involving metabolic neurological, and inflammatory responses, in addition to the lack of blood flow from occlusive disease.

◆ The location of claudication symptoms is related to the location of the occlusive disease:
  ❖ Occlusive disease of the iliac arteries can produce pain in the hip, buttock, thigh or calf.
  ❖ Occlusive disease proximal to the origin of internal iliac arteries or bilateral iliac disease can also include erectile dysfunction in men.
  ❖ Occlusive disease of the femoral or popliteal artery typically produces calf pain.
  ❖ Occlusive disease of tibial arteries can produce calf pain, ankle or foot pain.

Chapter 13

- ◆ Other causes of leg pain to consider when making a differential diagnosis:
  - ❖ Lumbar disk disease (sciatica).
  - ❖ Spinal stenosis.
  - ❖ Osteoarthritis.
  - ❖ Muscle pain.
  - ❖ Neuropathy.
  - ❖ Chronic compartment syndrome.
  - ❖ Venous obstructive disease.

Critical Limb Ischemia

Critical limb ischemia (CLI) occurs when distal arteriole pressure is so low that there is no longer an adequate pressure gradient across the capillary bed to provide tissue perfusion to meet metabolic demands. The majority of patients with lower extremity PAD do not progress to CLI.

Only 2-4% of patients with claudication develop CLI (Creager, 2002).

Risk Factors for Development of CLI
- ◆ Non-diabetic patients with a decreased ABI < 0.4.
- ◆ Diabetic patients.
  - ❖ Neuropathy can mask pain of CLI.
  - ❖ CLI can also cause neuropathy.
- ◆ Patients with chronic renal failure.
- ◆ Low cardiac output states.
- ◆ Infection, injury or skin breakdown of affected extremity.

Signs and Symptoms
- ◆ Limb pain occurring at night or at rest (particularly in forefoot or toes) or pain requiring narcotics for relief.
- ◆ Ulcers or gangrene from arterial disease (likely to occur in forefoot or toes).
  - ❖ Arterial ulcers are painful and tender to touch.
  - ❖ Open ulcers are associated with infection and cellulitis.
  - ❖ Diabetic patients and immuno-compromised patients require systemic antibiotics.
  - ❖ Specialized wound care is needed in patients with open skin.
- ◆ Impending limb loss due to compromised blood flow.

Some patients have subclinical CLI; they deny rest pain and have no signs of gangrene or arterial ulcers. These patients need close observation because they are at risk for tissue loss with any trauma to the feet.

Other Signs of Chronic Ischemia
- ◆ Dependent redness.
- ◆ Pallor on elevation of extremity.
- ◆ Reduced capillary refill.
- ◆ Shiny / scaly skin due to subcutaneous tissue loss.
- ◆ Trophic skin changes.
- ◆ Loss of hair over dorsum of foot.
- ◆ Calf atrophy.
- ◆ Potential tissue loss.

Peripheral Arterial Disease and Ischemic Stroke

Patients with arterial occlusive disease who develop CLI most often have diffuse multi-vessel disease. The prognosis for the limb is very poor once critical limb ischemia develops unless adequate blood flow can be restored. The one-year survival rate for patients with CLI is approximately 25% due to their high risk of cardiovascular ischemic events (Creager, 2002).

CLI is considered chronic in nature and differs from acute limb ischemia. Acute onset of CLI in high-risk patients is suspicious for thromboembolism as the cause. Patients with suspicion for atheroembolization as the cause of CLI should be evaluated for the presence of arterial aneurysms. Inflammatory arteritis can also cause an acute onset of CLI.

Signs of CLI from Atherosclerotic Emboli

◆ Onset after recent endovascular procedures.

◆ Associated with systemic fatigue or systemic muscle discomfort.

◆ Increased creatinine levels.

◆ Bilateral limb symptoms.

◆ Skin discoloration with red non-blanched network pattern.

Acute Limb Ischemia

Acute limb ischemia is defined as a sudden decrease in limb perfusion that threatens the viability of the limb.

Causes

Acute limb ischemia is often caused by thrombosis associated with plaque rupture, thrombosis of a lower extremity bypass graft, or thromboemobolization from an aneurysm. The severity of the ischemia depends on the location and degree of obstruction, as well as the presence of collateral circulation and adequacy of cardiac output.

Collateral circulation is usually not well developed when the acute limb ischemia is caused by embolization. Arterial embolization is suspected when the onset is sudden and there is a suspected embolic source. The absence of preexisting lower extremity PAD and the presence of normal pulses in the unaffected leg are other signs that the cause of acute limb ischemia is embolic in origin. Emboli typically lodge at branch points in vessels.

Acute limb ischemia can be caused by factors other than atherosclerotic disease. Other causes include:

◆ Arterial trauma or arterial dissection.

◆ Arteritis or vasospasm.

◆ Compartment syndrome or external arterial compression.

◆ Hypercoagulable state.

◆ Atrial fibrillation.

Patients with existing lower extremity arterial occlusive disease who experience a low cardiac output state can have signs mimicking acute arterial occlusion. Other mimics of acute arterial occlusion include acute deep vein thrombosis (DVT) and acute nerve compression. Clues for differential diagnosis include edema associated with DVT and normal or above normal skin temperature associated with nerve compression.

Signs and Symptoms

The hallmark signs and symptoms of acute limb ischemia are described in Box 13.1.

549

Chapter 13

Box 13.1
Six Ps of Acute Limb Ischemia

- Pain
  - ❖ Not impacted by dependency
  - ❖ May be decreased if collaterals are present
- Paralysis
- Parathesias
- Pulselessness (pulses may be present if there is microembolization)
- Pallor (pallor early - followed by cyanosis if left untreated)
- Polar (cold) - unilateral.

Sensory deficits are subtle in the early phase. Numbness and weakness are associated with persistent acute ischemia. Diabetic patients can have pre-existing sensory deficits. Patients with persistent pain, sensory loss and toe muscle weakness are at risk for loss of limb.

Intervention

Patients with acute limb ischemia and a viable extremity should have an emergent evaluation for endovascular or surgical revascularization.

Treatment Goals in Lower Extremity PAD

- Reduce risk of ischemic events (MI and stroke).
- Relieve symptoms of claudication and increase functional capacity and quality of life.
- Salvage limb and reduce mortality if CLI is present.
- Reduce risk, identify, and treat all other forms of vascular disease.

Treatment (All Patients: High Risk, Asymptomatic Disease, and Symptomatic Disease)

Aggressive Risk Factor Modification

- Smoking cessation: The goal is complete cessation through behavior modification, nicotine replacement therapy, bupropion (Zyban, Wellbutrin) or varenicline (Chantix) therapy. Physician advice is critical to smoking cessation efforts. Physician advice results in a 1-year smoking cessation rate of approximately 5%. The addition of pharmacotherapy with nicotine replacement or bupropion results in 1-year smoking cessation rates of 16 and 30% (Hirsch et al., 2005).

- Lipid management: Statins are used to achieve LDL-C < 100 in all patients with lower extremity PAD. LDL-C < 70 mg /dL is an alternative goal for patients at high risk for ischemic events. Fibric acid derivatives can be used for patients with normal LDL-C but low HDL-C and high triglycerides.

- Blood pressure control: Goal is <140/90 mm Hg for all patients without diabetes and chronic renal disease and <130/80 mm Hg in patients with diabetes and chronic renal disease.
  - ❖ Beta blockers are not contraindicated in lower extremity PAD and do not adversely affect walking capacity.
  - ❖ ACE inhibitors may also be used in patients with asymptomatic lower extremity PAD for cardiovascular risk reduction.
  - ❖ Any antihypertensive therapy may decrease the limb perfusion pressure and potentially exacerbate symptoms of claudication or critical limb ischemia. Most patients, however, can tolerate antihypertensive therapy without adverse symptoms.

Peripheral Arterial Disease and Ischemic Stroke

◆ Blood sugar control: The goal is a glycosylated hemoglobin (Hgb A1C) < 7% in all diabetic patients to reduce microvascular complications, such as nephropathy and retinopathy. The Hgb A1C measures the amount of sugar carried by hemoglobin. Because sugar is attached to hemoglobin for the life of the cell (approximately four months) this measurement represents glucose levels over this extended period of time. A normal Hgb A1C is < 6%.

Diabetic Foot Care
◆ Proper foot wear.
◆ Routine care from podiatrist.
◆ Daily foot inspection.
◆ Skin cleansing and topical moisturizers to prevent dryness and fissures.
◆ Skin lesions addressed urgently.

Treatment (Asymptomatic and Symptomatic Lower Extremity PAD)
Antiplatelet Therapy
Antiplatelet therapy with aspirin or clopidogrel should be ongoing in all patients with PAD. Aspirin 75 mg to 325 mg should be used in all patients with lower extremity peripheral arterial disease to reduce the risk of MI, stroke and death. Clopidogrel can be used as an alternative to aspirin in patients with asymptomatic disease. Clopidogrel appears to be more effective than aspirin in preventing ischemic events in patients with symptomatic disease.

Warfarin is not indicated in the treatment of asymptomatic or symptomatic lower extremity PAD.

Treatment for Claudication
Supervised Exercise
Supervised exercise is recommended as initial treatment in all patients with intermittent claudication. Supervised exercise can also be used as an adjunctive treatment in patients being treated with pharmacotherapy or for patients undergoing revascularization.

The improved outcomes associated with supervised exercise training include:
◆ Increased speed, distance and duration of walking.
◆ Decreased claudication per each distance.
◆ 100-200% improvement in walking is expected over 3 to 6 months.
◆ Increase in routine activities of daily living.
◆ Increase in quality of life
◆ Improvements with supervised exercise exceed the improvements with medication therapy.
(Hirsch et al., 2005)

The benefits of supervised exercise begin to show at 4 to 8 weeks and increase progressively over 3 to 6 months. The maximal benefit occurs when exercise sessions last > 30 minutes and when sessions take place at least 3 times weekly and when the program lasts 6 months or longer. Walking to near maximal pain is the most effective form of exercise because this level of exercise results in the benefits discussed below.

Several factors may contribute to the improvements seen with supervised exercise at this level, including changes in skeletal muscle metabolism, muscle hypertrophy, change in gait pattern, and improvements in endothelial function.

Patients participating in supervised exercise should be evaluated for their cardiovascular risk. However, stress imaging studies are not routinely indicated prior to participation in supervised exercise. Treadmill testing can be used to assess for adverse response to exercise and to guide exercise prescription.

Chapter 13

Supervised exercise in a formal program with ECG, blood pressure and blood glucose monitoring is recommended. Patient monitoring during initial sessions of exercise can help determine the ongoing need for monitoring.

Components of Supervised Exercise Program
◆ Treadmill (most effective) or track walking minimum of 3 times per week.
◆ Minimum of 12 weeks duration of program.
◆ Each session 45 to 60 minutes.
◆ Workload is set to induce claudication within 3 to 5 minutes of walking.
◆ Patients walk until pain of a moderate severity and then rest for a brief period of time.
◆ Periods of exercise and rest are repeated throughout the session.
◆ Total exercise usually begins at 35 minutes and should be increased in 5-minute increments until the patient is able to exercise for 50 minutes a session.
◆ Resistance training to improve muscle strength can be used to complement walking, but not in place of walking. Resistance training itself does not improve walking ability.
◆ Arm ergometer training can be used to improve cardiovascular endurance in poorly conditioned patients or in patients who have undergone amputation and cannot participate in a walking program.

Pharmacological Treatment
Cilostazol (Pletal) (100 mg PO BID)
Cilostazol is a platelet aggregation inhibitor and has vasodilator properties. In addition, cilostazol modestly improves dyslipidemia by raising high-density lipoprotein cholesterol (HDL-C) and lowering triglyceride levels.

Cilostazol is recommended in all patients with lifestyle limitations who do not have heart failure. Improvement in walking distance of approximately 40-60% is seen after 12 to 24 weeks of therapy.

Cilostazol is a PDE III inhibitor. Other drugs in this class, such as milrinone, have been studied for their effectiveness as inotropic agents in severe heart failure and have shown increased mortality in the presence of systolic dysfunction. For this reason, cilostazol should not be used in patients with systolic heart failure.

Pentoxifylline (Trental) (400 mg TID)
Pentoxifylline is a second line alternative to cilostazol. The effectiveness of this medication has not been well documented.

Therapeutic actions include decreasing blood and plasma viscosity, increasing red and white blood cell deformability, inhibiting neutrophil adhesion and activation, and decreasing plasma fibrinogen concentrations. Pentoxifylline results in an approximate 20-25% improvement in maximal walking distance.

Other Agents
The effectiveness of L-arginine, propionyl-L-carnitine, and ginkgo biloba has not been well established.

L-arginine is a precursor to nitric oxide, which inhibits platelet aggregation and induces vasodilation. L-arginine has been shown to improve endothelial related vasodilation in patients with elevated cholesterol levels.

Cartinine is a co-factor for skeletal muscle metabolism. Propionyl -L-carnitine shows promise, but is not yet approved for this indication.

Ginkgo biloba decreases red blood cell aggregation, decreases blood viscosity, and inhibits platelet activating factor. Ginkgo biloba may be considered as an alternative therapy.

Therapies that are not recommended include:
◆ Oral vasodilator prostaglandins (beraprost and iloprost).

♦ Vitamin E
♦ Chelation: leaches calcium out of plaque and may have serious harmful effect of hypocalcemia.
Angiogenic growth factors to promote collateral vessels are being evaluated.

Revascularization

Revascularization (surgical or endovascular) is not indicated in asymptomatic patients as a prophylactic therapy or to prevent the progression of the disease to critical limb ischemia. The goal for revascularization is to improve quality of life.

Revascularization is indicated in people with lifestyle or job limiting disability due to claudication who are likely to have symptomatic improvement after the procedure. Patients should have a very favorable risk benefit ratio and should have failed pharmacological and exercise therapy. Approximately 5% of patients with intermittent claudication require revascularization procedures for lifestyle or vocational limiting symptoms (Hirsch et al., 2005).

Superficial femoral artery and proximal popliteal artery (Figure 13.2) stenosis are the most common lesions associated with intermittent claudication. Superficial femoral artery stenosis rarely leads to advanced ischemia because the deep femoral artery provides collateral to the popliteal artery. Popliteal and tibial artery occlusions are more likely to cause limb threatening ischemia because of the small number of distal collaterals. Revascularization is performed for hemodynamically significant lesions (presence of pressure gradient across the stenosis) that are producing symptoms.

Peripheral arterial lesions are classified into 3 categories: inflow disease, outflow disease, and run off disease. Table 13.1 describes each category.

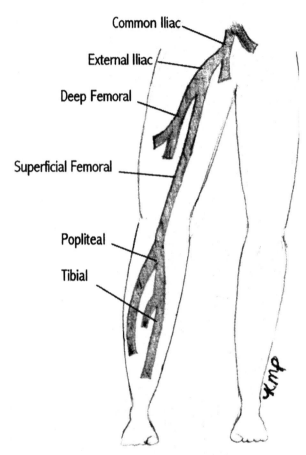

Figure 13.2: Lower extremity arterial anatomy.

Table 13.1 Classification of Lesions		
Inflow Disease	**Outflow Disease**	**Runoff Disease**
Stenosis in suprainguinal vessels that limit blood flow to common femoral artery. ♦ Infrarenal aorta. ♦ Iliac arteries.	Stenosis in lower extremity arterial tree below the inguinal ligament, from the common femoral artery to the level of the infrapopliteal trifurcation.	Stenosis in trifurcation vessels (anterior tibial, posterior tibial, peroneal) to the pedal arteries that cross the ankle.

Endovascular Treatment for Intermittent Claudication
Endovascular treatment is the preferred method of revascularization for a single stenosis in iliac lesions (common iliac and external iliac) and femoropopliteal lesions (superficial femoral and popliteal). The more severe the pre-procedure symptoms, the more likely the procedure is to be effective.

Stents can be used as primary therapy or salvage therapy after angioplasty in the iliac arteries. Most iliac lesions are treated with primary stenting. Stenting can be used as a salvage treatment for failed angioplasty in other vessels, but is not indicated for primary therapy in the femoral, popliteal, and tibial arteries (Hirsch et al., 2005).

Long-term patency for peripheral angioplasty is greatest for the common iliac artery. Duration of patency decreases as the lesion becomes more distal. The effectiveness of angioplasty also decreases with multiple lesions and in lesions with increased length. Patients who smoke and have diabetes have less durable results with angioplasty, as well.

Surgical Treatment for Intermittent Claudication
Surgery is recommended when longer and more diffuse lesions are present or endovascular treatment has failed. A preoperative cardiovascular evaluation is required prior to surgical intervention. CAD is the leading cause of early and late postoperative mortality in patients having surgery for peripheral vascular disease (Eagle et al., 2004). There is a benefit to having CABG prior to surgery for peripheral vascular disease if there is surgically correctable CAD.

During surgical revascularization in patients with both inflow and outflow lesions, inflow lesions are corrected first. After correction of inflow lesions, exercise and medication therapy may be effective in treating claudication. If outflow lesions do require grafting, there is improved flow and reduced chance of graft thrombosis when inflow lesions are corrected first.

Patients under the age of 50 who require surgery have a higher rate of graft failure compared with older patients, due to the aggressive nature of their atherosclerotic disease. Surgery is therefore avoided in younger patients if at all possible.

<u>Surgical Inflow Procedures</u>
Many patients have diffuse disease of the infrarenal aorta and iliac arteries with hemodynamically significant lesions in the iliac arteries. The most common surgical inflow procedure for this type of disease is the aortobifemoral bypass (Figure 13.3). In this procedure, a bifurcated synthetic graft is sewn to the aorta immediately below the origin of the renal arteries and distally to the common femoral arteries or deep femoral arteries.

Other less invasive procedures can be done including aortoiliac endarterectomy, or aortoiliac bypass or iliofemoral bypass (for unilateral disease). These procedures can be done with small flank incisions into the retroperitoneum. Combination endovascular and surgical procedures can also be done.

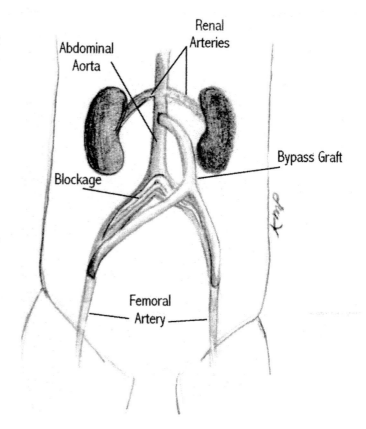

Figure 13.3: Aortobifemoral bypass.

For patients who cannot tolerate an open aortobifemoral bypass due to cardiovascular or surgical risk, an axillofemoral-femoral bypass can be performed. In this procedure a synthetic graft is tunneled from the axillary artery to one of the femoral arteries. A second femoral to femoral bypass is then constructed. This procedure is rarely performed.

Surgical Outflow Procedures

The most common surgical bypass for outflow lesions is the femoral-popliteal bypass (Figure 13.4). This procedure can be performed under general or regional anesthesia.

The two primary factors affecting the results of surgical outflow procedures are 1) the type of graft material and 2) the site of distal anastomoses. Vein grafts are superior to synthetic grafts in outflow procedures. If a vein is not available for a femoral-popliteal bypass, then synthetic graft material can be used.

There is accelerated failure of synthetic grafts with more distal anastomoses. Femoral-tibial bypassing with a vein is rarely done because of the increased risk for amputation with graft failure (Hirsch et al., 2006). Synthetic graft material is not used to bypass to tibial arteries because of the very high risk of graft failure and amputation (Hirsch et al., 2006).

Follow Up After Surgical Intervention

After lower extremity PAD vein graft surgery, the ACC/AHA Guidelines recommend an ongoing monitoring program for at least 2 years to assess for reoccurrence of the disease or development of new disease. Components of a follow-up program include:

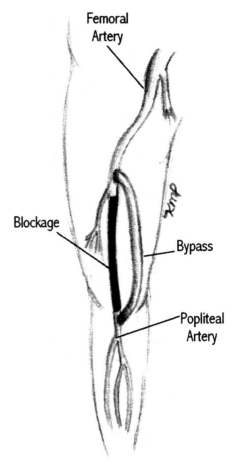

Figure 13.4: Femoral-popliteal bypass.

- History to assess for new symptoms.
- Physical exam to include palpation pulses: proximal, graft, and outflow vessels.
- Periodic resting and post-exercise ABIs.
- Duplex scanning of entire vein graft with peak systolic velocities and velocity ratios across all lesions. The benefit of duplex scanning in synthetic vein grafts is less well established.

Treatment for Critical Limb Ischemia (CLI)

The goal in treating critical limb ischemia is to reduce the risk for amputation. About 1/2 of patients with CLI require revascularization to salvage the limb. Patients who were ambulatory immediately prior to the development of CLI, and who have a life expectancy of greater than 1 year, should be evaluated for revascularization. After revascularization for CLI, patients remain on indefinite antiplatelet therapy.

Cardiovascular risk is higher if an open surgical procedure is required, so endovascular treatment is used as the first-line strategy. Patients who cannot undergo revascularization have a high risk for requiring major amputation within 6 months.

Patients with CLI frequently have 2 or more levels of arterial disease. Pressure gradients across stenotic lesions are taken to help determine the hemodynamic significance of each lesion. Inflow lesions are treated first. Treatment of inflow lesions often resolves resting pain. An outflow procedure is required if pain, infection, or ABI < 0.8 remain after inflow lesions are treated. An adequate blood flow to the foot is necessary to heal ischemic ulcers or gangrene.

Chapter 13

Special Considerations for Surgical Treatment

The same inflow procedures are used as with treatment of claudication. During outflow procedures, the most distal artery (with continuous flow from above the stenosis) should be used as the site of origin for the distal bypass graft. The tibial or pedal artery that is able to provide the best outflow to the foot is used for the site of distal anastomoses. Bypasses done for CLI are longer with more distal outflow anastomoses. The creation of an *in situ* or reversed saphenous vein graft bypass to a tibial vessel is a common revascularization procedure for CLI, and can be done with general or regional anesthesia. The most important goal in surgical revascularization for CLI is to achieve uninterrupted blood flow to the foot.

Amputation

Contributing factors for amputation:

◆ Significant necrosis of the weight bearing portion of foot.

◆ Uncorrectable flexion contracture.

◆ Paresis of the extremity.

◆ Refractory rest pain from ischemia.

◆ Sepsis.

◆ Very limited life expectancy.

Major amputation is associated with an increased risk for mortality and morbidity. Amputation also results in a significant impact on quality of life and often independence, especially in the elderly and other patients when there is a barrier to prosthesis use and rehabilitation. Prevention of amputation with timely revascularization is always the goal.

When revascularization is not an option, various medical treatments can be utilized, although none has been proven in clinical trials to be effective (Hirsch et al., 2006).

◆ Antiplatelet and anticoagulation therapy

◆ Intravenous (or intraarterial) prostanoids (vasodilator and platelet aggregation inhibitors) may be effective in a small number of patients to reduce ischemic pain and promote wound healing.

  ❖ Prostaglandin E1 (PGE1).

  ❖ Prostacyclin (PGI2) (Iloprost) Note: Oral Iloprost is not effective in reducing the risk of amputation or death.

◆ Parenteral pentoxifylline treatment is not useful for CLI.

◆ Maintenance of limb in dependent position.

◆ Treatment of infection to reduce demand.

CLI may improve with time if collateral vessels develop. Angiogenic therapies (administration of a gene or a protein) are being studied to promote the development of collateral vessels.

Treatment for Acute Limb Ischemia

Thrombosis is treated with systemic anticoagulation. Thrombosis resulting in acute limb ischemia may occur in native vessels or in failing bypass grafts.

Catheter-based thrombolysis is effective in patients with acute limb ischemia < 14 days in duration. Catheter-based thrombolysis involves the intra-arterial delivery of a thrombolytic (fibrinolytic) agent to site of thrombosis. Mechanical thrombectomy devices may be helpful to break up and remove clot. Thrombectomy can also be used in patients who are high-risk surgical candidates and who have contraindications to thrombolytic therapy. Both therapies may also be considered for patients with acute limb ischemia > 14 days.

556

Thrombolysis outcomes are better in more proximal or iliofemoral arteries than in infra-inguinal or more distal arteries. Urokinase has been the most studied lytic drug. Other drugs that have been studied include alteplase, reteplase, tenectaplase and streptokinase. Urokinase has better results and less bleeding than streptokinase. Otherwise, no single lytic agent has shown superiority over the others.

RENAL ARTERY DISEASE

Although most hypertension is essential, renal artery stenosis (RAS) is one of the more common causes of secondary hypertension and a common and progressive condition in patients with advanced age and atherosclerotic disease.

Complete renal artery occlusion occurs more frequently in diabetics, and in those with severe hypertension with severely stenotic lesions. The impact of RAS is determined by the degree of blood flow impairment, and ranges as listed below:

◆ Asymptomatic RAS
◆ Renovascular hypertension
◆ Ischemic nephropathy and atrophy
◆ End stage renal disease.

Higher levels of renal impairment result in higher mortality rates for those with RAS.

Diagnosis

Indications for Diagnostic Workup
There are several indications for a diagnostic workup to identify renal artery stenosis. These include:

◆ Hypertension onset before the age of 30 years.
◆ Onset of severe hypertension after the age of 55.
◆ Accelerated hypertension: sudden and persistent worsening of previously controlled hypertension.
◆ Resistant hypertension: Hypertension resistant to full dose, appropriate 3 drug therapy in which one of the drugs is a diuretic.
◆ Malignant hypertension: Hypertension with evidence of end organ damage.
◆ New azotemia or worsening renal function after the start of an ACE inhibitor or renin angiotensin receptor blocker.
◆ Variation in size between two kidneys (>1.5cm), or an atrophic kidney.
◆ Sudden unexplained pulmonary edema.
◆ Unexplained renal failure.

Other indications may include:
◆ Multi-vessel CAD or lower extremity PAD.
◆ Unexplained heart failure or refractory angina.

Note: Most hypertension is essential hypertension and is therefore not a result of RAS. A routine evaluation for RAS is not indicated in patients with hypertension.

Diagnostic Studies
◆ Duplex ultrasound sonography as a screening test
  ❖ Excellent test to monitor patency after surgical or endovascular revascularization (ultrasound is able to transmit through a stent).
  ❖ Limited ability to visualize accessory arteries.
  ❖ Imaging limitations with obese patients.

- ❖ Can measure renal artery resistive index to detect abnormalities in small vessels.
- ❖ Patient needs to be NPO for 8 to 12 hours prior to procedure.
- ❖ Requires skilled sonographer and should be performed in accredited ultrasound laboratory.
◆ MRI as a screening test
- ❖ Gandolinium used as contrast (less nephrotoxic than iodinated agent).
- ❖ Cannot image inside a stent to detect instent restenosis.
◆ CTA as a screening test in patients with normal renal function.
- ❖ Excellent 3 D images of aorta, renal, and visceral arteries.
- ❖ Requires iodinated contrast.
- ❖ Able to image metal stents.
◆ Catheter-based angiography
- ❖ When high clinical suspicion and noninvasive testing is inconclusive.
- ❖ When clinical suspicion exists and patient is undergoing angiography for coronary or lower extremity peripheral arterial disease.
- ❖ Historic gold standard; replaced by noninvasive modalities as first-line diagnostic tool.

The following diagnostic studies are **not** recommended:
◆ Captopril renal scintigraphy.
◆ Selective renal vein renin measurements.
◆ Plasma renin activity (with or without captopril administration).

RAS is best diagnosed with an imaging modality. The goal is to image both the main and accessory renal arteries and to evaluate the hemodynamic significance of any lesions. Evaluating for renal or adrenal masses and abdominal aortic aneurysms is also included in the diagnostic evaluation.

Pathophysiology

Approximately 90% of all RAS is due to atherosclerosis, which is part of a systemic process. Atherosclerotic RAS usually involves the proximal 1 cm of the main renal artery with the renal plaque extending into the aorta (Figure 13.5). Patients at high risk for significant RAS include those with: diabetes, advanced age, CAD, lower extremity PAD, heart failure, and female gender. Extensive CAD is strongest predictor of co-existing atherosclerotic RAS. The finding of atherosclerotic RAS also predicts co-existing CAD, when the RAS is diagnosed first.

Fibromuscular dysplasia is the second most common cause of RAS, and is most commonly seen in women with hypertension ages 25 to 50 years. Fibromuscular dysplasia usually involves the middle and distal 2/3 of both renal arteries and may also involve renal artery branches. The majority of fibromuscular dysplasia involves the medial layer of the artery.

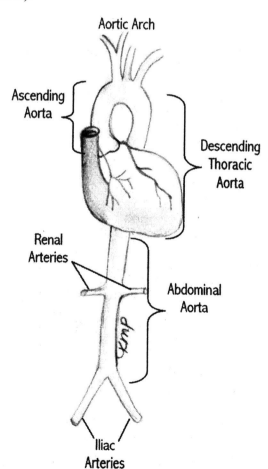

Figure 13.5: Location of renal arteries off abdominal aorta.

Peripheral Arterial Disease and Ischemic Stroke

Renovascular hypertension may also be caused by renal artery aneurysms. These aneurysms may require surgical or endovascular repair. Aneurysm rupture is of greatest concern in non calcified aneurysms > 2 cm in diameters. There is an increased risk for aneurysm rupture during pregnancy.

Acute unilateral RAS causes renin-mediated vasoconstrictive hypertension. This increases left ventricular afterload, which can result in adverse outcomes for patients with heart disease. Hypertensive effects of bilateral RAS or RAS to a solitary kidney are also impacted by an increase in extracellular circulating volume because the kidney(s) affected by RAS become ischemic, and cannot handle the extra volume that results from activation of the renin angiotensin aldosterone system. Mortality rates are increased in patients with severe RAS, and patients with bilateral RAS have a higher mortality rate than those with unilateral RAS.

Impact of Renin Angiotensin Aldosterone Blocking Medications with RAS

Angiotensin II produces many effects including the regulation of glomerular filtration rate in response to renal perfusion. During renal hypoperfusion, angiotensin II causes efferent arteriole vasoconstriction and helps preserve renal blood flow and glomerular filtration. Although ACE inhibitors and angiotensin II receptor blockers are considered renal protective, the introduction of these agents in patients with bilateral renal artery stenosis or in renal artery stenosis to a single kidney causes a decrease in glomerular filtration and can cause acute renal failure. Patients with bilateral renal artery stenosis or renal artery stenosis to a single kidney are dependent on efferent arteriole vasoconstriction to maintain adequate glomerular filtration.

Treatment

Goals of Treatment

◆ Achieve normal blood pressure.

◆ Preserve renal function.

◆ Reduce overall cardiovascular risk.

Medical Management

Multiple anti-hypertensive agents can be used to achieve hypertension treatment goals in the presence of renal artery stenosis. These agents include ACE inhibitors, angiotensin II receptor blockers, calcium channel blockers, beta blockers, hydrochlorothiazide, and hydralazine. In addition to controlling blood pressure, a decrease in the progression of renal dysfunction has been associated with the use of ACE inhibitors and calcium channel blockers (Hirsch et al., 2005). The progression of RAS itself, though, is unaffected by medical therapy.

Percutaneous Revascularization

Potential benefits of revascularization include reperfusion of the ischemic kidney(s), resulting in a decrease in the activation of the renin-angiotensin-aldosterone system. Increased renal perfusion promotes glomerular filtration and natriuresis. After revascularization (especially for bilateral RAS or RAS to a solitary kidney), patients may be able to tolerate long term ACE inhibitor or ARB therapy. This improves ability to manage patients with cardiovascular disease. ACE inhibitors and angiotensin II receptor blockers are renal protective in patients with proteinuria or microalbuminuria because they reduce intraglomerular pressure.

Percutaneous techniques are much more common than surgical techniques in treating atherosclerotic RAS. Stents are superior to balloon angioplasty alone in the treatment of atherosclerotic RAS because the plaque commonly extends into the aorta and is subject to recoil. Stents result in a higher procedural

Chapter 13

success rate as well as a decrease in restenosis rate. Most restenosis occurs within the first year. Balloon angioplasty with bail out stenting is the preferred treatment method for fibromuscular dysplasia lesions.

Patients with severe RAS who have hypertension that is accelerated, resistant, or malignant, usually benefit from revascularization, with an improved control in blood pressure and possible reduction in number of required medications for control. Patients with atherosclerotic RAS who have only focal RAS with secondary hypertension are more likely to receive clinical benefit than those who have clinical manifestations of more systemic atherosclerosis. A complete cure of renovascular hypertension with revascularization is rare. Patients with atherosclerotic RAS are older and are more likely to have co-existing essential hypertension.

Revascularization is also effective in stabilizing or improving renal function in patients with symptomatic atherosclerotic RAS. Improved renal function with revascularization is most likely to occur in patients with atherosclerotic RAS who exhibited a more sudden onset of renal impairment.

Indications

◆ Asymptomatic but hemodynamically significant bilateral renal artery stenosis (or in the presence of one solitary kidney).

  ❖ Absence of end organ dysfunction.

  ❖ ≥ 50 -70% stenosis with peak gradient across the lesion ≥ 20 mm Hg, or a mean gradient ≥ 10 mm Hg, or any stenosis ≥ 70%.

  ❖ Endovascular procedures in asymptomatic patients is controversial.

◆ Hemodynamically significant stenosis in presence of accelerated, resistant, or malignant hypertension; hypertension with unexplained unilateral small kidney; or hypertension where patient is unable to tolerate medications.

  ❖ Renal artery stenosis in presence of progressing chronic renal insufficiency or disease.

  ❖ Chronic kidney disease is defined as estimated decreased in glomerular filtration rate to less than 60 ml/min per 1.73 m^2 that lasts for at least 3 months (Hirsch et al., 2005).

◆ Patients with end stage renal disease are not ideal candidates because of existing intrinsic renal disease.

◆ Hemodynamically significant stenosis in the presence of heart failure, pulmonary edema, or unstable angina.

  ❖ RAS causes peripheral arterial vasoconstriction and volume overload. In addition, angiotensin II has direct effects on myocardial function. These factors may exacerbate cardiac conditions, such as ischemia or congestive heart failure.

  ❖ Cardiac conditions may also be aggravated by the inability to administer secondary prevention medications, such as ACE inhibitors and angiotensin II receptor blockers in the presence of RAS.

(Hirsch et al., 2006)

Surgical Revascularization

Indications

◆ Complex disease, such as disease in multiple small vessels or the co-existing presence of renal anuerysmal disease.

◆ Atherosclerotic RAS when the patient needs additional treatment for abdominal aortic aneurysms or severe aortoiliac peripheral arterial occlusive disease.

Patients with RAS caused by fibromuscular dysplasia are more likely to benefit from surgical revascularization than those with atherosclerotic RAS. Surgical risk for renal revascularization increases when patients require additional aortic reconstructive procedures, or when the patient has existing renal insufficiency.

Aortorenal bypass is the most common surgical procedure used to treat atherosclerotic RAS. It is usually used for single renal artery disease. Reversed saphenous vein grafts can be used for single or multiple vessel bypassing. Synthetic graft material can be used if there are no acceptable veins, if the renal artery is large, or if the graft starts from a synthetic aortic prosthesis. Aortorenal bypass requires clamping of the aorta. If clamping of the aorta is contraindicated, a non-anatomic bypass can be done: hepatorenal, splenorenal, or iliorenal. Aortorenal endarterectomy is another surgical option and often performed if there is bilateral disease or multiple renal arteries involved.

A secondary surgical nephrectomy may be needed when surgical revascularization fails to result in control of blood pressure. This is only done when a reoperation to salvage the kidney is not an option. A primary nephrectomy may be indicated in certain situations in which it is not likely that revascularization will help with blood pressure control or will have any benefit on improved renal function. In certain situations, ischemia to the kidney has caused atrophy that cannot be repaired.

Indications that a kidney will not benefit from revascularization include:
- A kidney that contributes to < 10% of combined renal function.
- Small kidney < 5 cm long.
- Extensive cortical infarction.

Potential Complications of Angiography and Percutaneous Treatment of Peripheral and Renal Artery Disease

- Contrast Induced Renal Failure
    - Increased risk in diabetes and chronic kidney disease.
    - Risk < 3% in patients with no diabetes or kidney disease; 5-10% in patients with diabetes; 10-20% in patients with chronic kidney disease; and 25-50% when both diabetes and chronic kidney disease are present (Hirsch et al., 2005).
    - Risk reduction strategies:
        - Adequate pre-procedure hydration with 0.9NS or sodium bicarbonate drip.
        - Use of alternatives to iodinated contrast (carbon dioxide, gandolinium, iso-osmolar noninionic).
        - Oral acetylcysteine in high-risk patients.
        - Hemofiltration before and after procedure in high risk patients.
- Contrast Allergic Reaction.
- Distal embolization.
- Access site complications.
    - Hematoma
    - Pseudoaneurysm
    - Arteriovenous fistula
    - Bleeding.

DISEASES OF THE AORTA: ANEURYSMS

Abdominal Aortic Aneurysms

An abdominal aortic aneurysm (AAA) (Figure 13.6) is considered present when the anteroposterior diameter of the aorta reaches 3 cm. Gender is taken into account because women have slightly smaller normal aortic diameters. The most common abdominal aortic aneurysms extend below the renal arteries and involve the entire infrarenal aorta; they often extend to involve the common iliac arteries.

Risk Factors for AAA

- Male Gender
- Family History
  - Familial aneurysms may develop at an earlier age.
- Advanced Age
  - Degenerative changes occur in the aorta as part of the normal aging process.
  - Can accelerate in patients with bicuspid aortic valves and during pregnancy.
- Cigarette Smoking
  - Tobacco smoke causes degradation of elastin.
  - Medication use (inhalers and steroids) used to treat COPD may also influence the development and expansion of AAAs.
- Polycystic kidney disease and other renal disease
- Cardiovascular, cerebral vascular or lower extremity peripheral arterial disease
- Known popliteal aneurysms
- Marfan Syndrome
  - Frequently associated with cystic medial necrosis of the aorta.
  - 11% of patients with Marfan's syndrome will have an aortic dissection (Hirsch et al., 2005).

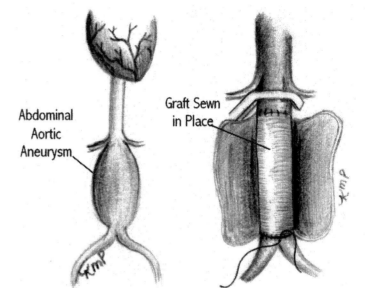

Figure 13.6: Abdominal aortic aneurysm and graft repair.

Screening (physical exam and ultrasound screening) for AAA

- Men ≥ 60 years of age with family history (sibling/parent).
- Men 65 to 75 years of age who have smoked.

Pathophysiology

Most aortic and peripheral aneurysms represent degeneration of the medial layer of the aorta. There is also a destruction of the structural matrix proteins, such as elastin and collagen. The inflammatory process may also contribute to the pathophysiology of AAAs. Localized aneurysms differ from systemic arteriomegaly in which there is a generalized dilatation and elongation of arteries.

Inflammatory aneurysms, a special subset of aneurysms, are seen most commonly in smokers. These aneurysms have a distinct appearance of a very thickened aneurysmal wall, with white shiny fibrotic material around the aneurysm. The aneurysm adheres to adjacent abdominal structures. Patients with inflammatory aneurysms are more likely to have symptoms and a higher operative mortality (Hirsch et al., 2005).

Peripheral Arterial Disease and Ischemic Stroke

Another subset of aneurysms is infectious aneurysms. Secondary infection of the aorta can arise from an existing aneurysm. Primary infection of the aorta is not common. The most common pathogens associated with infectious aneurysms are staphylococcus and salmonella. *C. pneumoniae* may be associated with atherosclerotic aortic aneurysms (Hirsch et al., 2005).

Diagnostic Studies

◆ Most aneurysms are asymptomatic and are discovered during a diagnostic work up (CT, MRI, ultrasound, nuclear scan, plain film radiograph) for another medical condition.

◆ Arteriography is not the preferred diagnostic exam to determine true diameter of aneurysms.

◆ Ultrasound (B mode or real time) is an excellent diagnostic tool.

  ❖ Accurate for measuring infrarenal (below renal arteries) aneurysms.

  ❖ More limitations with aneurysms close to or above the renal arteries.

  ❖ Used for initial screening and for follow-up monitoring.

  ❖ Measurement of aneurysm diameter done after overnight fasting to aid in visualization.

◆ CTA or MRA are commonly used for mapping before surgical intervention and for postoperative evaluation.

◆ Patients with small atherosclerotic abdominal aneurysms commonly have co-existing coronary artery disease. Any patient with a discovered abdominal aortic aneurysm should also be evaluated for the presence of additional aneurysms.

Physical Exam

◆ Palpation of abdominal and lower extremity pulses to detect presence of widened pulses.

◆ Palpation for actual aneurysm.

  ❖ Difficult in obese patient or with small aneurysms.

  ❖ Palpation does not cause rupture.

Classification of Aneurysms

Abdominal aortic aneurysms are classified according to their relationship to the renal arteries (Table 13.2).

Table 13.2 Classification of Abdominal Aortic Aneurysms	
Infrarenal	Below the renal arteries
Juxtarenal	Just below the renal arteries
Pararenal	Involving the origin of one or both renal arteries
Suprarenal	Involving the aortic segment containing the visceral arteries
Type IV thoracoabdominal	Suprarenal aneurysms that extend to the level of the diaphragm

Complications of Aneurysms

◆ Dissection resulting in rupture or occlusion

  ❖ Rupture most common complication.

  ❖ Mortality associated with rupture is as high as 90% (Hirsch et al., 2005).

  ❖ Associated with aneurysms of abdominal aorta, common iliac, and visceral arteries.

  ❖ Aneurysm size most important predictor for rupture.

  ❖ Other factors increasing risk for rupture include: hypertension, COPD, tobacco use, family history and female gender.

Chapter 13

- ◆ Thromoembolic ischemic events.
- ◆ Compression and resulting damage to nearby anatomical structures
  - ❖ Very large or inflammatory aneurysms can compress the duodenum.
  - ❖ Popliteal aneurysms can compress the popliteal veins and cause venous insufficiency.
  - ❖ Very uncommon but devastating complications are aortoenteric fistula, causing GI bleed or aortocaval fistula causing acute congestive heart failure.

Treatment for Asymptomatic Aneurysms
Most important treatment goal is to prevent fatal rupture.

When To Repair To Prevent Rupture?
- ◆ Infrarenal or juxtarenal aneurysms 5.5 cm or >.
- ◆ Suprarenal > 5.5 to 6.0 cm.
  - ❖ Aneurysms above the renal arteries have a higher postoperative mortality and higher risk for renal insufficiency and other complications. This is the reason for the larger diameter size required for elective repair.
- ◆ Aneurysms that have demonstrated a growth spurt.

When To Monitor?
- ◆ Infrarenal aneurysms 4.0 to 5.4 cm (annually).
- ◆ Asymptomatic (infrarenal) < 5.0 in men; < 4.5 in women.
- ◆ < 4.0 cm infrarenal (every 2 to 3 years).
- ◆ Iliac aneurysms < 3.0 cm.
- ◆ Note: Larger aneurysms tend to expand more rapidly than smaller aneurysms and need to be monitored more closely.

Other Treatment Considerations
- ◆ Hypertension and smoking accelerate the rate of aneurysm growth; therefore, smoking cessation and tight blood pressure control are important aspects of patient management.
- ◆ Beta blockers may be used in appropriate patients to decrease rate of aneurysm expansion

Treatment for Symptomatic Aneurysms (Aortic or Iliac)
Symptomatic aneurysms are surgically treated regardless of size. An evaluation for urgent surgery is done with the following presentation:
- ◆ Back pain or abdominal pain
  - ❖ Pain is most common symptom.
  - ❖ Pain is a long lasting steady pain, not generally affected by movement, but some relief may be obtained with knees in a bent position.
  - ❖ Abrupt, severe, worsening pain, or pain radiating toward lower extremities is sign of impending rupture.
- ◆ Hypotension
  - ❖ Hemorrhagic shock develops rapidly.
- ◆ Pulsatile abdominal mass
  - ❖ Mass is not pulsatile with significant hypotension.

Elective Repair of AAA

Preoperative Assessment
- Anterior / posterior diameter of aneurysm.
- Relationship of aneurysm to renal arteries.
- Identification of other aneurysms or co-existing occlusive disease in the renal or iliac arteries.
- Both CTA and MRA can be used. Both technologies are rapidly developing.

Perioperative Management
Beta blockers are given during the perioperative period to reduce mortality and cardiovascular morbidity. Patients with symptomatic coronary artery disease have a high rate of surgical mortality.

Surgical Considerations
- Mid-line transabdominal approach or extraperitoneal left flank incision.
- Pararenal, suprarenal and type IV aneurysms require aortic cross-clamping above the renal arteries.
- Thoracoretroperitoneal approach necessary for type IV aneurysms.
  - Infrarenal aneurysm repair has the lowest operative mortality and type IV aneurysms have the highest operative mortality (Hirsch et al., 2005).
- Endovascular repair (Figure 13.7) with stent grafts using a transfemoral approach is an option to open surgical repair.
  - Done with regional or local anesthetic.
  - Advantage for patients with severe cardiopulmonary operative risk factors.
  - Long term results of endovascular treatment compared to open surgical treatment in low risk patients are still the subject of current research.
  - Endografts are modular; metallic skeleton is secured to fabric of the graft.

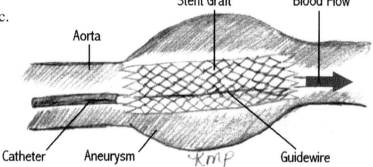

Figure 13.7: Stent graft used in endovascular repair of abdominal aortic aneurysm.

  - There are anatomical limitations to aortic graft repair. Must have adequate length of normal aorta below the renal arteries for proximal graft attachment or use of newer device with hooks long enough to secure the graft to the visceral segment of the aorta above the renal arteries. The proximal seal of the graft has to be below the renal arteries because the fabric portion of the graft cannot overlap the renal arteries.
  - Endograft leaks are a common complication of endovascular repair and result in continued blood flow into the aneurismal sac. Follow-up imaging to detect graft leaks is required every 6 to 12 months after surgery. Endoleaks typically occur within 1 year after surgery and are the most common reason for repeat intervention after endovascular aneurysm repair.
    - Type I Endograft Leak: Caused by problem with proximal or distal graft attachment sites. This type of leak can cause high pressures to build inside the aneurismal sac and can lead to rupture. These types of leaks must be repaired.
    - Type II Endograft Leak: These leaks are caused by retrograde flow from branch vessels. This is a very common type of endograft leak. It can be corrected by arterial cannulation and purposeful embolization; however, the majority of these leaks seal spontaneously. This type of leak has less risk for rupture than Type I leaks and is considered the most benign of the 4 types of leaks.

Chapter 13

      ☆ Type III Endograft Leak: Type III leaks are caused by a defect in the actual graft, such as disruption of modular connection or tear in the graft fabric. These types of leaks require prompt surgical repair.

      ☆ Type IV Endograft Leak: Type IV leaks are diffuse leaks throughout the graft and rarely occur.

◆ Endotension is another complication in which there is no leak, but excluded aneurismal sac continues to enlarge and remain under high pressure.

◆ Endografts may also migrate if the proximal aorta expands. Graft diameters are oversized to accommodate the future expansion of the aorta. Graft migration can occur as a late complication and require repeat surgical intervention.

◆ Limb ischemia can also occur as a complication within months after endovascular repair.

◆ Graft occlusion is now a less frequent complication due to improvements in graft design, including more stable metallic skeletons.

Postoperative Complications

◆ Postoperative renal insufficiency is the most common complication in patients requiring aortic cross-clamping above the renal arteries.

◆ Surgery for Type IV aneurysm repair also has a small risk for spinal cord ischemia.

◆ Late graft complications after open surgical repair are uncommon.

◆ Endovascular treatment of larger aneurysms has a higher complication rate than for smaller aneurysms.

Emergent Repair

Non-elective surgeries have a higher mortality rate than elective aneurysm repairs.

Surgical repair for ruptured aortic aneurysm carries an operative mortality rate ranging from 40-70% (Hirsch et al., 2005).

Lower Extremity Aneurysms

The diameter of lower extremity arteries increases in size by 25% over the course of adulthood. Patients with lower extremity arterial aneurysms have a high rate of co-existing abdominal aortic aneurysms. However, only a small percentage of patients with AAA have co-existing lower extremity arterial aneurysms.

Lower extremity arterial aneurysms differ from abdominal aortic aneurysms, frequently resulting in thrombosis and thromboembolism.

Lower extremity arterial aneurysms include femoral and popliteal aneurysms, with popliteal being the more common. Popliteal aneurysms occur more commonly in men, often bilaterally. Ultrasound can be used to assess for lower extremity arterial aneurysms; popliteal aneurysms can often be palpated.

Thromboembolic complications of popliteal aneurysms can result in limb loss. To avoid the complications of thrombosis and thromboembolic events to the calf and foot, all popliteal aneurysms ≥ 2 cm in diameter should be repaired (Hirsch et al., 2005). Popliteal aneurysms < 2 cm may be observed if they contain no thrombus.

Thromboembolic complications of popliteal aneurysm resulting in acute limb ischemia can be treated with catheter-directed thrombolysis or mechanical thrombectomy. Antiplatelet therapy may be used to prevent and treat thromboembolic complications of lower extremity arterial aneurysms.

Femoral aneurysms are more likely than popliteal aneurysms to rupture. In addition to thrombosis and thromboembolic complications, femoral aneurysms can cause compression of the femoral nerve or venous system if 3 cm in diameter or larger. All symptomatic femoral aneurysms should be repaired. Asymptomatic aneurysms < 3 cm can be monitored.

Peripheral Arterial Disease and Ischemic Stroke

Femoral Artery Pseudoaneurysm

In addition to true femoral artery aneurysms from arterial degeneration, there are also false or pseudoaneurysms related to arterial injury. A pseudoaneurysm is a pulsatile hematoma that is contained by partial elements of the arterial wall and is surrounded by subcutaneous fibrous tissue. The hematoma communicates with the artery through a defect in the arterial wall.

Pseudoaneurysm can occur as a late complication of aortofemoral bypass surgery using a synthetic graft. Pseudoaneurysm also occurs in 3.5 to 5.5% of patients following interventional cardiology procedures (Hirsch et al., 2005). The risk of pseudoaneurysm increases with longer procedure time, larger-sized sheath, use of systemic anti-coagulation, and difficulty with arterial access.

Suspected pseudoaneurysms are evaluated by duplex ultrasound. Treatment includes ultrasound-guided compression or ultrasound-guided thrombin injection. Thrombin injection is generally preferred over compression therapy. A risk of thrombin injection is distal arterial embolization. Small pseudoaneurysms < 2 cm can spontaneously heal. Surgical repair may be needed for pseudoaneurysms ≥ 2 cm or for those that persist after ultrasound guided therapy. Any femoral aneurysm (true or false) that erodes into adjacent soft tissue requires surgical repair. Large pseudoaneurysms can rupture into the peritoneal space.

Linking Knowledge to Practice

✔ *Large hematomas should be auscultated for the presence of a bruit to aid in the differentiation between a hematoma and a pseudoaneurysm.*

Thoracic Aortic Aneurysms (Ascending and Descending)

Thoracic aortic aneurysms typically develop in elderly patients with hypertension, lung disease and diffuse atherosclerosis. The exception is in ascending aortic aneurysms, which are typically a result of degenerative changes in the medial layer of the artery, as seen in patients with connective tissue disorders such as Marfan Syndrome. Thoracic aneurysms that arise in the distal aorta, the thoracic aorta, and the thoraco-abdominal aorta are usually atherosclerotic in nature. Aneurysms may develop as a result of the expansion of a chronic dissection.

Ascending Aortic and Aortic Arch Aneurysms
Indications for Surgical Repair

◆ Symptomatic aneurysms.
◆ Expanding aneurysms.
◆ Aneurysms > 5 cm (with Marfan Syndrome) or > 5.5 cm (without Marfan Syndrome).
◆ Aneurysms between 4.5 and 5.0 cm if aortic valve surgery is indicated.
◆ Any acute Type A dissection, as described below.
◆ Mycotic (infected) aneurysms.

(Bojar, 2005)

Surgical Considerations

Coronary angiography is done preoperatively in patients requiring surgical repair of ascending aorta or aortic arch aneurysms to determine the need for CABG. If CABG is needed, it is done at the same time as the aneurysm resection and repair.

Cardiopulmonary bypass is required for repair of ascending aortic aneurysms. Depending on the location of the aneurysm, either aortic cross clamping or a period of deep hypothermic circulatory arrest is used. During deep hypothermic circulatory arrest, the core body temperature is lowered to 18° C. At this

Chapter 13

temperature there is presumed electroencephalographic inactivity. Safe arrest can be maintained for 45 to 60 minutes with minimal risk of neurological complication (Bojar, 2005). Multiple strategies are used to improve cerebral protection during this period of circulatory arrest. Deep hypothermia and subsequent rewarming produce coagulopathies as a complication.

Repair of distal aortic arch aneurysms can be performed via left thoracotomy without cardiopulmonary bypass.

Descending Thoracic and Thoracoabdominal Aneurysms
Surgical Indications
- Symptomatic aneurysms.
- Aneurysms > 6.5 cm.
- Complicated acute Type B dissections, as described below. Uncomplicated acute Type B dissection if low risk patient.

Surgical Considerations and Potential Complications
An evaluation for the presence of CAD is done prior to elective surgery. If CAD is present, intervention or CABG may need to be performed preoperatively to reduce the surgical risk associated with aneurysm repair.

Repair of descending thoracic and thoracic abdominal aneurysms involves a thoracotomy incision and possible involvement of the diaphragm. There is a large incision and extensive pain.

Creatinine should return to baseline after angiography or intervention to reduce the risk of postoperative renal dysfunction from cross clamping of the aorta during surgery. Renal perfusion is optimized with loop or osmotic diuretics. Many patients have co-existing COPD, so there is a high potential for pulmonary complications, and > 10% require tracheostomy and extended ventilator support (Bojar, 2005).

A thorough preoperative neurological exam is important prior to surgery. There is an increased risk for stroke and seizures if deep hypothermic circulatory arrest is used and there is a risk of paraplegia if aortic cross clamping is used. Medications, cerebral spinal fluid drainage, and shunting of blood (draining blood proximal to aorta cross clamp and returning it distal to cross clamp) are used to prevent spinal cord injury during aortic cross clamping. Paraplegia may be reversed if promptly recognized and treated. Treatment includes:
- Increase systemic BP.
- High dose steroids.
- CSF drainage.

DISEASES OF THE AORTA: DISSECTIONS

Pathophysiology

Aortic dissection (Figure 13.8) involves an intimal tear that allows the pressurized blood to enter into the media and create a false channel. The outer medial and adventitial layers of the aorta contain the blood. The outer wall containing the blood is thinner than the original media and has a higher risk of rupture. The dissection resulting in a hematoma can extend with each force of ventricular contraction. This can occlude arterial branches of the aorta.

The majority of aortic dissections involve the ascending aorta. A smaller percentage involves the aortic arch and descending thoracic aorta. Dissections of the abdominal aorta are rare.

Dissections typically extend antegrade (travel distally) down the aorta. Dissections can also travel retrograde and involve the coronary arteries, most commonly the right coronary artery. A retrograde dissec-

568

tion can also involve the aortic valve and result in loss of commissural support for the aortic valve cusps, resulting in aortic insufficiency.

Risk Factors and Predisposing Conditions

- Hypertension is present in most patients with dissections.
- Congenital disorders affecting connective tissue, such as Marfan Syndrome or Ehlers-Danlos syndrome; also presence of bicuspid aortic valve.
- 3rd trimester of pregnancy.
- After procedures where aorta or the aortic branches have been cannulated.

Classification

Dissections diagnosed within 2 weeks of onset are considered acute. Those diagnosed outside the two-week window are considered chronic.

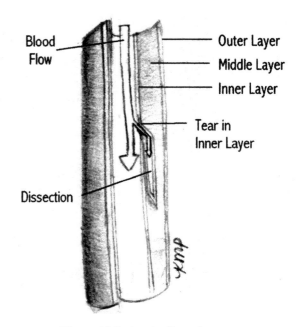

Figure 13.8: Aortic dissection.

The most current classification system is the Stanford system involving Type A and Type B dissections (Figure 13.9).

- Type A Dissections: Dissections involving the ascending aorta.
- Type B Dissections: Dissections involving the descending thoracic aorta. These dissections begin distal to the left subclavian artery.

Complications

- Aortic regurgitation from retrograde dissection involving aortic valve or from aortic dilatation.
- MI from retrograde coronary artery dissection.
- Cardiac tamponade from ascending aorta or aortic arch rupture. (Parietal pericardium is attached to ascending aorta.)
- Intraplerual rupture from descending aortic dissection that ruptures into the intrapleural space – most commonly left-sided.
- Retroperitoneal bleed from rupture of abdominal aorta dissection.
- Stroke from brachial artery compromise.
- Paraplegia; reduced blood flow to kidneys, bowels, and lower extremities from compromise of arterial branches.

There is a very high mortality rate (90% at 3 months) for untreated dissections (White & Schwartz, 2001). Cardiac tamponade is the most common cause of mortality (Bojar, 2005).

Signs and Symptoms and Diagnosis

Chest or back pain with variation in upper extremity blood pressure is a key assessment finding in aortic dissection. Recurrent chest or back pain can indicate extension or rupture. The presence of aortic regurgitation in the setting of chest pain is also suspicious for aortic dissection.

Diagnosis can be made with:
- Chest x-ray. An abnormality of the aorta can usually be seen as a widening of the aorta and mediastinum. Calcium present in the intima is separated from the outer border of the false channel.

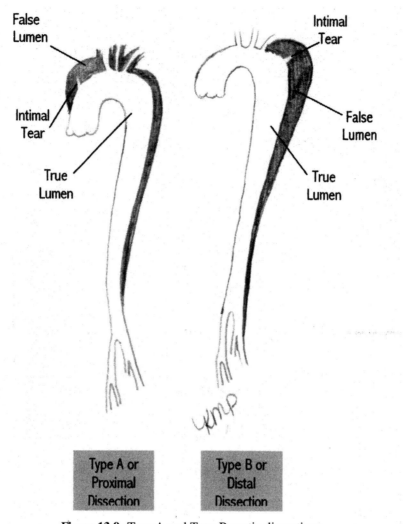

Figure 13.9: Type A and Type B aortic dissections.

- Transthoracic echocardiography and transesophageal echocardiography. A visible intimal flap separates the true and false lumens. Echocardiography is most helpful with type A dissections. Transesophageal echocardiography is very valuable and can be performed at the bedside.
- CT is particularly helpful in evaluating dissections of the thoracic aorta.
- MRI is an excellent diagnostic tool but has limitation because it cannot be used emergently or in critically ill patients.
- Angiography is a definitive diagnostic tool required for patients having elective repair of the thoracic aorta.

Treatment

The overall treatment goal is to stop the dissection. Control of hypertension is an important strategy. The systolic blood pressure is maintained in the range of 100 to 120 mm Hg, with a mean arterial pressure between 60 - 65 mm Hg. The goal is to achieve the lowest possible pressure without compromising perfusion to vital organs. The velocity of left ventricular ejection, in addition to the rate of rise of aortic pressure, is as important as systolic blood pressure in controlling dissection. A beta blocker, such as esmolol, in combination with sodium nitroprusside is used to manage hypertension and decrease left ventricular velocity and the rate of rise of aortic pressure.

Trimethaphan, a ganglionic blocking agent, can be used as an alternative to sodium nitroprusside. A beta blocker is not needed if trimethaphan is used (White & Schwartz, 2003).

Labetolol can also be used instead of sodium nitroprusside and a beta blocker (Gill, 2001).

Pain control, along with decreasing environmental and emotional stressors, is also an important feature of initial treatment.

Type A Dissections

Dissections (acute or chronic) involving the ascending aorta (Stanford Type A dissection) require surgical repair. Type A dissections require deep hypothermic circulatory arrest for construction of the distal anastomoses. The portion of the aorta containing the proximal intimal tear is resected and the entrance to the false channel is obliterated. However, the distal false channel is not completely eliminated; therefore, the patient remains at risk for future aneurysms.

The resected ends of the aorta are typically reapproximated using a Dacron graft. There is a risk for bleeding, and aprotinin and BioGlue can be used to help control bleeding. A simultaneous replacement of the aortic valve may be done for those with aortic regurgitation. Reimplantation of the coronary arteries may also be necessary when retrograde dissection has occurred.

Hypertension management (as discussed above) is critical in the preoperative and early postoperative period to prevent rupture.

Surgical considerations are similar to those for ascending aortic aneurysms, as discussed above. Surgical mortality for Type A dissections is approximately 15-20% and therefore aggressive surgical treatment in the elderly is controversial (White & Schwartz, 2003).

Type B Dissections

Stanford Type B dissections are usually treated medically. Patients with these types of dissections tend to be higher surgical risk candidates due to advanced age, extensive atherosclerotic disease, and existing co-morbidities. Surgery is limited to complicated dissections, which include:

◆ Persistent pain.

◆ Uncontrolled hypertension.

◆ Evidence of expansion or rupture.

◆ Circulatory compromise to visceral, renal, or lower extremity vessels and resultant organ ischemia.

◆ 6 to 6.5 cm diameter in chronic dissections.

(Bojar, 2005)

Surgical considerations and potential complications are similar to those for descending thoracic aneurysms, as described above.

Chapter 13

CAROTID DISEASE AND ISCHEMIC STROKE

Stroke Prevention

There are more than 700,000 strokes per year, resulting in more than 160,000 deaths. Stroke is the 3rd leading cause of death and number one cause of disability. Twenty percent of stroke survivors require institutional care 3 months after the stroke and between 15 - 30% of stroke survivors are left with a permanent disability. Greater than 70% of all strokes are first time events. There was a 60% decline in stroke mortality in the 30 years from 1969 to 1999; however, the mortality rate has currently leveled off in many regions (Goldstein et al., 2006).

Ischemic Stroke Risk Factors

Many risk factors for ischemic stroke overlap with those for coronary artery disease. However, there are some important risk factor considerations specific to stroke. Specific information regarding the reduction of common risk factors is covered in Chapter 7.

Non-Modifiable Risk Factors

◆ Age: Stroke risk doubles with each decade after the age of 55.

◆ Gender: Stroke more common in men, except between ages 35-44, and after the age of 85. However, 1 in 6 women die of stroke compared to 1 in 25 who die of breast cancer.

◆ Ethnicity: African Americans and some Hispanics have higher stroke incidence and mortality compared to European Americans.

◆ Family history: The exact relationship between genetic factors and environmental factors is not yet fully understood.

Modifiable Risk Factors and Medical Conditions Increasing Risk for Stroke

◆ Previous transient ischemic attack (TIA).

◆ Vascular disease in another bed: Antiplatelet therapy (aspirin/clopidogrel) can reduce the risk.

◆ Hypertension: Increases both the risk of ischemic and hemorrhagic stroke. Effective antihypertensive treatment is associated with a 35-44% reduction in incidence of stroke. Reduction of blood pressure is more important in reducing risk than the specific agent used (Goldstein et al., 2006).

◆ Smoking: Approximately doubles the risk for ischemic stroke. Also increases the risk for hemorrhagic stroke 2 to 4 fold. Smoking also increases the stroke risk associated with oral contraceptive use.

◆ Diabetes: Independent risk factor for ischemic stroke. Tight blood pressure control (< 130/80) with an ACE inhibitor or angiotensin II receptor blocker reduces the risk of stroke in diabetics. Statins in diabetics also reduces the risk of first time stroke (Goldstein et al., 2006).

◆ Cholesterol: There is an association between increased total cholesterol and ischemic stroke. Statins are approved for the prevention of ischemic stroke in patients with CAD. There is also a positive relationship between homocysteine levels and stroke risk.

◆ Sedentary lifestyle is associated with an increased risk for stroke.

◆ Increased body weight and abdominal fat are directly associated with an increase stroke risk.

◆ Alcohol use: Excessive intake increases risk for hemorrhagic stroke. Light to moderate intake of wine is associated with a decreased risk of stroke. One serving of wine is 4 to 5 ounces.

◆ Oral contraceptives: The overall stroke risk with the use of oral contraceptives is low. Women with other risk factors for stroke are encouraged not to use oral contraceptives.

◆ Migraine headache is associated with stroke in younger women. There are no specific recommended treatment approaches to reduce stroke risk in younger women with migraines.

Peripheral Arterial Disease and Ischemic Stroke

◆ Sleep apnea may be an independent risk factor for stroke. In addition, successful treatment of sleep apnea reduces blood pressure.

◆ Hypercoagulability: Most hypercoagulable states are associated with venous thrombosis rather than arterial thrombosis. The presence of antiphospholipid antibodies increases risk for arterial thrombosis. High levels of antiphospholipids are often found in young women with stroke (Goldstein et al., 2006).

◆ Atrial fibrillation: Patients with paroxysmal or persistent atrial fibrillation and valvular heart disease are at the highest risk for embolic events. Atrial fibrillation results in a 3 to 4 fold increased risk of stroke. Strokes associated with atrial fibrillation are typically large and result in disability. Stroke risk is reduced by 60% with warfarin and by 20% with aspirin (AHA). Direct thrombin inhibitors are not approved at this time for stroke prevention. Anticoagulation is underutilized in the elderly. Warfarin is indicated in the elderly if the benefit of stroke prevention outweighs the risk of bleeding. A target INR in non-valvular atrial fibrillation is generally 2 to 3. Some practitioners use a target INR of 2 in the elderly. Blood pressure control for those on warfarin is very important, not only to reduce ischemic stroke risk, but also to reduce the risk of intracerebral hemorrhage. Aspirin can be used for those who are at low risk for stroke.

◆ Other cardiac conditions: Dilated cardiomyopathy, ST-elevation MI with extensive regional wall motion abnormality, valvular heart disease (including endocarditis), and congenital defects increases ischemic stroke risk due to embolization. The incidence of stroke is inversely proportional to the ejection fraction. The use of warfarin in patients with idiopathic cardiomyopathy and low ejection fraction is controversial. Warfarin can be prescribed post ST-elevation MI when there is significant left ventricular dysfunction or left ventricular aneurysm creating high risk for mural thrombi.

◆ Cardiac surgical procedures, particularly open heart surgery.

◆ Sickle cell disease is an autosomal dominant genetic disorder in which patients suffer from severe hemolytic anemia with episodes of vaso occlusive crises. Stroke risk is significant for those with homozygous sickle cell disease. At least 11% of these patients have a stroke by the age of 20 (AHA). In this subset of patients, transcranial Doppler is used to screen for children who would benefit from transfusion therapy to prevent stroke. Adults with sickle cell disease are managed according to the general stroke prevention guidelines.

Additional Considerations for Stroke Prevention

Patients with asymptomatic carotid stenosis should be screened for all modifiable risk factors and treatable conditions that increase the risk for stroke. Aggressive measures should be put in place to reduce stroke risk. Aspirin therapy is recommended in these patients unless contraindicated (AHA). Patients with asymptomatic carotid bruits and asymptomatic carotid artery stenosis have a high likelihood of having co-existing coronary artery disease.

Aspirin is also recommended for prevention of cardiovascular complications in patients who are at high risk, and where the benefit of aspirin therapy outweighs any risk.

Carotid endarterectomy as a prevention strategy may be indicated in select patients with high-grade asymptomatic carotid artery stenosis. Carotid angioplasty with stenting may be considered in these select patients who are at high risk for a surgical procedure. The evidence is less strong regarding the benefit of prophylactic procedures in patients with high-grade stenosis who are asymptomatic. Carotid endarterectomy and carotid stenting are discussed below.

Hormone replacement therapy with estrogen, and with or without progestin, is not indicated for primary stroke prevention. Other forms of hormone replacement therapy are the subject of current research.

Although bacterial agents have been found in carotid (as well as coronary atherosclerotic plaque) treatment with antibiotics has not been proven to lower the risk of stroke and there are currently no recommendations for the use of antibiotics in stroke prevention.

Neuro Anatomy and Physiology

Major components of the brain include (Figure 13.10):
- Cerebral hemispheres (discussed below)
- Diencephalon
    - Thalamus
        - Central command for incoming sensory impulses.
        - Gross awareness of pain.
        - Involved in recticular activating system.
    - Hypothalamus
        - Controls visceral, endocrine, and emotional function.
        - Coordinates autonomic responses.
        - Controls hormonal secretion of pituitary gland.
        - Regulation of temperature, appetite, water balance, and sleep.
    - Limbic System
        - Self preservation.
        - Basic drives.
        - Emotional affect.
        - Some memory function.
- Brainstem: Origin of all cranial nerves except I and II, relay station between brain and lower level nervous system
    - Midbrain:
        - Origin of reticular activating system responsible for wakefulness and attention span.
        - Cranial nerves III and IV.
        - Responsible for pupillary response to light.
    - Pons
        - Contains respiratory centers.
        - Cranial nerves V, VI, VII, and VIII.
    - Medulla
        - Contains cardiac, vasomotor and respiratory centers.
        - Vomiting, gagging, coughing, and sneezing reflexes.
        - Cranial nerves IX, X, XI, and XII.
- Cerebellum
    - Coordinates smooth muscle movement with sensory input.
    - Balance and posture.

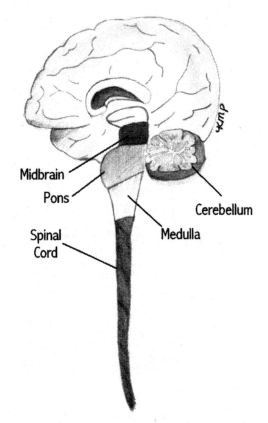

Figure 13.10: Central nervous system anatomy.

There are two cerebral hemispheres connected by the corpus callosum. The corpus callosum allows fibers to travel between the two hemispheres. The outer layer of cerebrum is the cerebral cortex containing both gray matter and white matter. Each cerebral hemisphere receives sensory input from the opposite side of the body and also has control of skeletal muscle function on the opposite side of the body. Each hemisphere has four lobes named for the underlying skull bones (Figure 13.11).

Cerebral Hemisphere Key Functions
- Left: Analysis, problem solving, language, mathematics, abstract reasoning.
- Right: Spatial relationships, non-verbal communication, music, artistic ability.

Cerebral Lobe Key Functions
- Frontal Lobe: Voluntary motor function, intellectual function, personality.
- Temporal: Memory function and emotion.
- Parietal: Sensory function, object recognition and position sense, body awareness and image.
- Occipital: Visual reception.

Cerebral Circulation (Figure 13.12)
- Four cerebral vessels carry oxygenated blood to the brain.
  - Two internal common carotid arteries anteriorly.
    - Internal carotid arteries supply the major blood supply to the brain.
    - Internal carotids arise from the common carotids.
    - Left common carotid is branch of left subclavian artery.
    - Right common carotid arises from right brachiocephalic trunk.
    - Common carotid bifurcates at angle of jaw into internal and external carotids.
    - Internal carotids supply optic nerves, retina, and the majority of the cerebral hemispheres.
    - Divides into:
      - Anterior cerebral artery.
      - Middle cerebral artery.
  - Two vertebral arteries posteriorly
    - Arise from right and left subclavian arteries.
    - Enter posterior fossa through foramen magnum.
    - Vertebral arteries merge to form basilar artery; basilar artery divides into two posterior cerebral arteries.

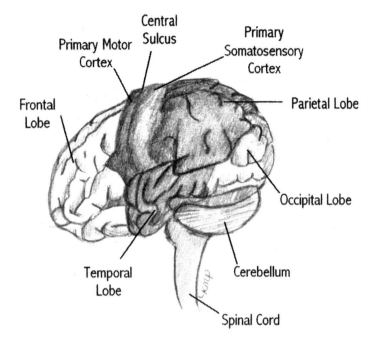

Figure 13.11: Lobes of cerebral hemispheres.

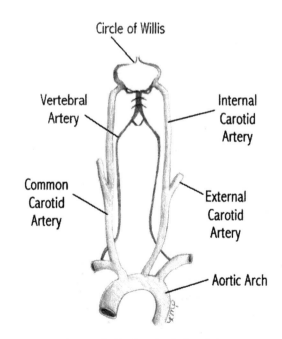

Figure 13.12: Cerebral circulation.

★ Vertebrobasilar system, including the posterior cerebral arteries, supplies the cervical cord, brainstem (hindbrain, pons, midbrain), medulla, cerebellum, caudal part of diencephalons, medial and posterior temporal lobes, and the occipital lobes.
- Circle of Willis (Figure 13.13): an anatomical ring of vessels joining the carotid artery system and the vertebrobasilar system. The four arteries of the Circle of Willis are:
  - Posterior communicating artery.
  - Posterior cerebral artery.
  - Anterior communicating artery.
  - Anterior cerebral artery.

Cerebral Blood Flow

- Normal: 750 ml/min or 6-15% of the cardiac output.
- Brain takes up 2% of total body weight; but uses 20% of body's oxygen consumption.
- Autoregulation.
  - Capacity to maintain constant cerebral blood flow despite systemic blood pressure. Autoregulation also allows adjustments for local metabolic needs of brain tissue.
  - Autoregulation is most efficient with MAP between 60 and 140 mm Hg.
  - MAP < 50 or > 150 mm Hg = failure of autoregulation.
  - The autoregulation range shifts higher in patients with hypertension.
  - Autoregulation is altered in an injured brain. There is oligemia (reduced blood flow) in the first 24 hours after injury.
  - When autoregulation fails, cerebral blood flow alters with changes in systemic pressure. Hypotension = hypoperfusion and ischemia.

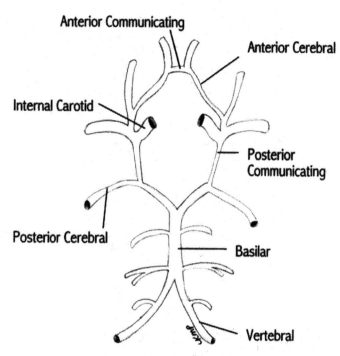

Figure 13.13: Circle of Willis.

- Metabolic factors increasing regional cerebral blood flow:
  - Acidosis (↑ $PaCO_2$).
  - Increased metabolic rate.
  - Decreased oxygen.
- Metabolic factors decreasing regional cerebral blood flow:
  - Alkalosis (↓ $PaCO_2$).
  - Decreased metabolic rate.
  - Increased oxygen.

Peripheral Arterial Disease and Ischemic Stroke

Cerebral Perfusion Pressure (CPP)

- Pressure at which the brain is perfused.
- Cerebral blood flow is impacted by CPP.
- CPP = MAP – ICP.
- Normal: 80-100 mm Hg.
- Acceptable: 60-150 mm Hg.
- Injured brain needs a CPP > 70 mm Hg.

Linking Knowledge to Practice

✔ *It is important to maintain an adequate MAP in an injured brain in order to maintain an adequate cerebral perfusion pressure.*

Definitions

- Ischemic Stroke: Sudden, severe disruption of the cerebral circulation with a subsequent loss of neurologic function caused by thrombus or embolism.
- TIA – Transient Ischemic Attack
  - ❖ Episode of neurologic impairment.
  - ❖ Focal cerebral ischemia.
  - ❖ Resolves within 24 hours.
  - ❖ Places patient at high risk for future stroke.
- RIND – Reversible Ischemic Neurologic Deficit
  - ❖ Focal cerebral ischemia.
  - ❖ Lasts longer than 24 hours.
  - ❖ Usually resolves 1-3 days; may take 3-4 weeks.

Pathophysiology of Ischemic Stroke

Ischemic strokes account for 75% of all strokes. Ischemic strokes can be caused by thrombosis or by embolism.

Subsets of Ischemic Stroke

- Large artery atherosclerotic disease involving either thrombosis or embolic plaque often affects the cortex of the brain. Cerebral atherosclerotic plaques are commonly found at vessel bifurcations. Thrombotic strokes are more common in older persons with extensive atherosclerotic disease. Thrombotic strokes can be progressive, exhibiting worsening symptoms over minutes, hours, or days. Thrombosis is often associated with a nighttime stroke due to more sluggish blood flow at night.

- Small or penetrating vessel occlusive disease causes lacunar strokes, affecting the deeper non-cortical areas of the brain. Other causes of lacunar strokes have been proposed, including embolism, hypertension, vasospasm, small intracerebral hemorrhage, and hematologic disorders.
  Infarcted brain tissue leaves small cavities referred to as lacunes. Multiple lacunes can impair intellectual capacity, and dementia can be a complication. Lacunar strokes do not typically cause cortical deficits such as aphasia or apraxia. Typical lacunar symptoms include pure motor or pure sensory hemiplegia and dysarthria with clumsy hand syndrome. CT scan is not sensitive enough to detect lacunar strokes.

- ◆ Cardiogenic embolic stroke from cardiac sources such as atrial fibrillation, ventricular aneurysm, or bacterial endocarditis. These strokes usually affect large proximal cerebral vessels and frequently lodge at bifurcations. The middle cerebral artery is a common location for these strokes, and they have a sudden onset with maximum deficit occurring immediately.
- ◆ Cryptogenic strokes are of unknown cause. Some experts believe cardiogenic emboli are likely the source in many of these strokes, although the exact etiology is not discovered.
- ◆ Unusual causes include carotid dissections, migraines, and coagulapathies.
- ◆ Watershed or border zone infarct is an area of focal ischemia from decreased perfusion pressure, and typically occurs bilaterally in boundary zones between major vessels. Bilateral watershed infarcts are usually caused by systemic hypotension.

An ischemic cascade begins with the onset of an ischemic stroke.

- ◆ Primary cell death occurs within 4 to 5 minutes. This is the core central area of irreversible damage. Dying cells in this core area release toxins that can damage nearby cells.
- ◆ Secondary cell death can occur in compromised cells surrounding the core area of injury. The penumbra (Figure 13.14) is the area surrounding the core and contains cells with potential for recovery. These cells receive low levels of blood flow, resulting in the potential to preserve neurological function. Reperfusion must occur early (within 3 hours) to salvage the penumbra. Other factors that can impair the salvage of the penumbra include toxins released from dying cells, development of cerebral edema, and loss of auto regulation.
- ◆ The inflammatory and immune responses occur in response to the initial injury. The chemical mediators of these responses impair the ability of the body to dissolve existing clot. In addition, the inflammatory response results in cerebral edema. The presence of cerebral edema after an ischemic stroke increases the chance of intracerebral hemorrhage as a complication of ischemic stroke. Large ischemic strokes are at particularly high risk for developing a hemorrhagic complication.

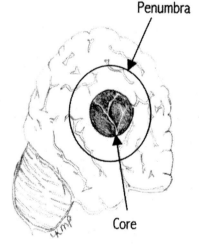

Figure 13.14: Areas of injury in an ischemic stroke.

Key Signs and Symptoms of Stroke

- ◆ Numbness – especially on one side of the body.
- ◆ Confusion – sudden onset.
- ◆ Difficulty speaking or slurred speech.
- ◆ Sudden visual problems in one or both eyes.
- ◆ Loss of balance or coordination.
- ◆ Severe dizziness.
- ◆ Sudden severe headache with no explanation.

The presentation of the patient depends on location and size of the stroke. Stroke symptoms are typically sudden in onset and focal in presentation. Infarcts involving the carotid artery usually involve unilateral symptoms. Infarcts involving the vertebrobasilar system may involve bilateral symptoms.

Diagnosing Ischemic Stroke

- ◆ CT
  - ❖ Most widely used diagnostic tool.
  - ❖ Identifies presence or absence of a mass or hemorrhage.

Peripheral Arterial Disease and Ischemic Stroke

- ❖ May show distortion or shift of ventricle.
- ❖ Insensitive to recent ischemic strokes (within 24 hours) and insensitive to brain stem and small infarcts.
- ◆ MRI
  - ❖ Sensitive and accurate for ischemic stroke.
  - ❖ May replace CT as initial diagnostic tool to rule out hemorrhagic stroke.
- ◆ Transcranial Doppler (TCD)
  - ❖ Differentiate thrombotic or hemorrhagic stroke *(not time effective)*.
- ◆ Cerebral Angiogram
  - ❖ Identifies occlusion, stenosis, aneurysm, hemorrhage in arterial system.

Treating Ischemic Stroke

A primary goal in the treatment of acute ischemic stroke is to maintain cerebral perfusion. It is important to avoid hypotension and maintain an adequate mean arterial pressure. Most patients with ischemic stroke present with hypertension. These patients may require a higher mean arterial pressure to achieve an optimum cerebral perfusion pressure. An optimum cerebral perfusion pressure is necessary to support perfusion to ischemic areas of the brain via collateral circulation. Hypotension can extend the stroke.

Intravenous fibrinolytics are a treatment option in patients who meet criteria, do not have contraindications, and who can receive therapy within three hours of symptom onset. The three-hour time frame begins with last known time of normal assessment. Current guidelines require fibrinolytics to be given within the window of three hours from symptom onset; however, current research is evaluating the extension of the window for administration. The baseline CT scan must exclude hemorrhage or a territory larger than 1/3 the middle cerebral artery territory (very large ischemic strokes are at high risk for hemorrhage). The patient must also score > 4 on the National Institutes of Health Stroke Scale Score. Components of the stroke scale include: LOC, visual, facial palsy, motor arm, motor leg, limb ataxia, sensory, language, and dysarthria. The higher the score on the scale, the more severe the stroke. At least two of the points of the score must come from a motor deficit. Table 13.3 outlines specifics of fibrinolytic therapy.

Table 13.3 Fibrinolytic Therapy		
Agents	**Time Frames**	**Contraindications**

◆ Activase (alteplase)
  ❖ Total dose = .9 mg/kg
  ❖ 10% of dose over first minute; 90% over next 60 minutes
◆ Other potential agents
  ❖ desmotoplase
  ❖ reteplase
  ❖ tenecteplase
	◆ Door to doctor: 10 minutes
	◆ Door to CT:15 minutes
	◆ CT to Read: 45 minutes
	◆ Door to Drug: 90 minutes
		◆ Rapid improving deficit
		◆ BP > 185/ 110
		◆ Recent surgery
		◆ Bleeding disorder/anticoagulants (Patients with INR ≤ 1.7 can receive therapy)
		◆ Seizure at stroke onset
		◆ Stroke or head trauma within 3 months
		◆ Recent non-compressible arterial puncture
		◆ Glucose < 50 mg/dL or > 400 mg/dL

Chapter 13

Complications of Fibrinolytic Therapy

The development of cerebral hemorrhage as a complication of an ischemic stroke is the primary and most important complication associated with fibrinolytic therapy. Careful patient selection can help minimize risk.

Patients with acute ischemic stroke are treated with platelet aggregation inhibitors. Most patients should receive aspirin within the first 48 hours of a stroke. Aspirin is not a replacement for fibrinolytic therapy (Adams et al., 2005). Anticoagulants may or may not be used, depending on the clinical situation. Patients with progressive thrombotic stroke may benefit from anticoagulation; however, in patients with a large completed thrombotic stroke, anticoagulants may increase the risk of post stroke intracerebral hemorrhage.

Current recommendations for the use of antithrombotics after fibrinolytic therapy include holding antithrombotic therapy for the first 24 hours after administration. Studies are currently evaluating the use of anticoagulants and antiplatelets immediately after fibrinolytic therapy administration to reduce the risk of reocclusion.

Sedation is avoided, if possible, in acute stroke to optimize the neurological exam.

Additional Treatment Options
◆ Intra-arterial thrombolysis
  ❖ Delivers directly to lesion; can be used for middle cerebral artery occlusion.
  ❖ Can extend window of opportunity in some patients up to 6 hours.
  ❖ Favorable outcomes have been demonstrated.
  ❖ No evidence of superiority over intravenous delivery, and therefore, intravenous delivery should not be delayed to wait for intra-arterial administration.
  ❖ Combination intravenous and intra-arterial delivery is being investigated.

Treatment Options Under Investigation
◆ Mechanical thrombolysis
  ❖ Angioplasty
  ❖ Laser
  ❖ Snare
  ❖ Intra-arterial suction devices/clot retrieval devices
  ❖ Therapeutic ultrasonography.
◆ Hypothermia
  ❖ Extends window.
  ❖ Improves penumbral survival.
  ❖ Techniques
    ★ Surface
    ★ Intravenous
    ★ Radiant catheter.
◆ Volume expansion and drug induced hypertension
  ❖ Goal is to improve cerebral perfusion.
  ❖ Potential complications: brain edema and hemorrhage.

Peripheral Arterial Disease and Ischemic Stroke

Long Term Treatment

Rehabilitation to prevent complications and maximize functional capacity and secondary prevention are the hallmarks of long-term stroke treatment. Range of motion exercises and physical therapy are key for improving physical functional capacity and preventing complications of immobility. Special emphasis is given to adequate nutrition and aspiration prevention due to frequent swallowing abnormalities.

Complications of Stroke

- Death.
- Recurrent stroke.
- Myocardial infarction.
- Deficit-related complications (falls, aspiration, DVT, UTI, constipation).
- Disability.
- Depression.

Common Deficits That Occur With Stroke

- Pain or numbness.
- Hemi-neglect syndrome: Ignoring affected side and environmental factors on that side.
- Visual field problems.
- Bowel/bladder problems.
- Fatigue.
- Sensory deprivation.
- Rapid mood changes.
- Depression.
    - ❖ Nearly universal with stroke survivors.
    - ❖ Impacts physical recovery.
- Reflex crying.
    - ❖ Crying when some emotion triggers the reflex, which would normally not cause crying.
    - ❖ The cortex of the brain (highest level) inhibits reflexes controlled by spinal cord. Crying is a reflex that is easily released when the cortex is damaged.
- There are additional deficits based on the involved hemisphere (Table 13.4).

Table 13.4 Changes with Right and Left Brain Strokes	
Changes Specific to Right Brain Strokes	**Changes Specific to Left Brain Strokes**
◆ Left-sided paralysis. ◆ Impulsiveness: often act as if unaware of deficits and try to do things beyond their ability. ◆ Spatial deficit. Example: missing the table with coffee cup while reading.	◆ Right sided paralysis. ◆ Hesitancy: tend to be slow, cautious and disorganized. ◆ Aphasia: in right-handed people the language center is generally on the left side of the brain.

Surgical and Interventional Treatment Options for Prevention of Ischemic Stroke

Carotid Endarterectomy

A carotid endarterectomy involves the surgical removal of plaque for the prevention of ischemic events. A high percentage of ischemic strokes is a result of atherosclerotic lesions of the carotid artery, frequently in the location of the carotid bifurcation.

Indications

Carotid endarterectomy (Figure 13.15) has been shown to reduce the risk of ischemic stroke in a select groups of patients with carotid artery stenosis.

- Symptomatic disease with hemodynamically significant carotid stenosis.
- Asymptomatic disease with critical carotid stenosis.

Surgical Considerations

- Aspirin is continued up to and including the day of surgery to reduce risk of thromboembolic complications (Moore, 2002).
- Cervical portion of carotid can be done with general anesthesia or cervical block anesthesia
- Clamping of carotid interrupts blood flow
    - Clamping of carotid may be tolerated if open collaterals from contra lateral carotid artery and from the vertebral arteries are present.
    - Lack of adequate collaterals requires an internal shunt to maintain cerebral circulation.
    - Several surgical techniques can be used, based on plaque location and anatomical features. The basic surgical procedure involves an arteriotomy. The artery may be sutured or a prosthetic graft or saphenous vein graft may used to patch the artery.
    - Post-surgical imaging (angiography or direct duplex scanning) is done while the patient is still on the table to assure optimal technical results.

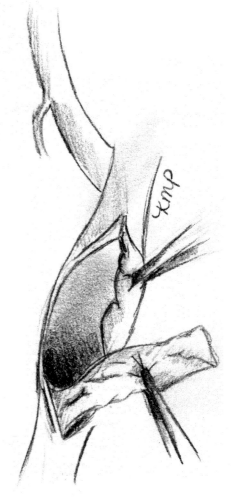

Figure 13.15: Carotid endarterectomy.

Post Operative Care

- Assessment of neurological status
    - Vagus nerve and hypoglossal nerve function are tested after patient is fully awake.
    - Cranial nerve damage is potential complication.
- Management of blood pressure
    - Avoid both hypertension and hypotension.
    - Temporary auto regulation can be lost on operative side.
- Assessment of wound
    - Assess for hematoma.
    - Maintain adequate airway if hematoma present.
    - Surgical evacuation required for hematoma.

Follow-Up

Follow-up includes ongoing assessment of carotid bruits and bilateral duplex scanning. Assessment for both restenosis and development of disease on contralateral side is important.

Carotid Artery Stenting

Carotid endarterectomy has been the gold standard of treatment for stroke prevention in patients with significant carotid artery stenosis. Carotid artery stenting is now a treatment option in patients at high risk for surgical revascularization.

Procedural Considerations

◆ Potential advantages include:

  ❖ Avoidance of surgical incision, as well as potential complications of cranial nerve damage and hematoma development at surgical site.

  ❖ Avoidance of anesthesia.

◆ Potential disadvantage is the production of emboli, causing upstream complications; most procedures are done with distal protection devices.

◆ Clopidogrel and aspirin are used for 48 hours pre-procedure and for 4 weeks post-procedure.

◆ Aspirin is continued indefinitely.

(Kirshner, Biller & Callhan, 2005)

Linking Knowledge to Practice

✔ *Age > 70 years, smoking and diabetes are the 3 most significant risk factors for lower extremity peripheral arterial disease (PAD). These patients need careful assessment for presence of lower extremity PAD.*

✔ *When assessing for walking impairment, it is important to assess the amount of walking done by the patient. Many patients with lower extremity PAD reduce their activity to minimize symptoms.*

✔ *Many patients with lower extremity PAD have coexisting CAD, and special instruction is needed regarding activity and response to symptoms. Patients with lower extremity PAD are instructed to walk to near maximal claudication pain, rest briefly, and resume walking. Patients need to understand that the response to chest discomfort with activity is much different.*

✔ *Caution and careful assessment must be used in initiating ACE inhibitors in patients with cardiovascular disease due to the chance of undiagnosed RAS predisposing to the development of acute renal failure.*

✔ *It is important to control force of left ventricular ejection and the rate of rise in aortic pressure, while also controlling systolic blood pressure when treating symptomatic aortic aneurysms and dissections. For this reason, beta blockers are used in conjunction with sodium nitroprusside.*

✔ *Because the window of opportunity for fibrinolytic administration is so small, it is important for nurses to actively educate patients and the community regarding the early recognition of stroke symptoms and the need for immediate response.*

✔ *If blood pressure must be reduced to meet criteria for fibrinolytic therapy, it is important to use caution to avoid hypotension, or a significant decrease in blood pressure that will adversely affect cerebral perfusion pressure. Patients with acute stroke lose auto regulation abilities and are dependent on higher pressures to maintain adequate cerebral perfusion.*

✔ *It is important to rule out hypo or hyperglycemia as a cause of change in neurological condition prior to the administration of fibrinolytics for presumed acute stroke.*

Chapter 13

✔ *It is important for all stroke patients to be assessed for depression and adequate treatment of depression prior to discharge.*

✔ *Patients who develop a surgical site hematoma after carotid endarterectomy need careful assessment and potential management to maintain adequate airway.*

TEST YOUR KNOWLEDGE

1. The majority of patients with lower extremity peripheral arterial disease present with claudication symptoms.
   a. True.
   b. False.

2. A normal ankle brachial index is
   a. < 0.9.
   b. < 0.1.
   c. > 0.9.
   d. > 0.1.

3. Supervised walking programs are more effective than medications in treating lower extremity PAD with claudication.
   a. True.
   b. False.

4. The following are indications that a patient with lower extremity PAD has critical limb ischemia:
   a. Pain with walking
   b. Pain at rest or pain at night
   c. Ischemic ulcers on the toes
   d. Skin ulcers on the buttocks from sitting
   e. b and c.

5. Revascularization for lower extremity PAD is indicated for the following reasons:
   a. To improve symptoms and quality of life in patients with lifestyle or occupational limiting claudication.
   b. To prevent progression of disease to CLI in patients who are asymptomatic.
   c. To restore blood flow in CLI to avoid amputation.
   d. All of the above.
   e. a and c.

584

Peripheral Arterial Disease and Ischemic Stroke

6. Which of the following is not a sign of acute limb ischemia?

   a. Pain

   b. Paralysis

   c. Pulselessness

   d. Petechiae

7. During revascularization procedures for PAD, inflow lesions (vessels limiting flow to the common femoral artery) are corrected first.

   a. True.

   b. False.

8. The following patients warrant evaluation for renal artery stenosis, except

   a. a patient who develops hypertension before the age of 30 years.

   b. a patient who has resistant hypertension on 3 anti-hypertensives, including a diuretic.

   c. a patient who develops renal failure after the start of an ACE inhibitor.

   d. a patient who has a rise in creatinine after receiving contrast for an invasive procedure.

9. A patient presents to the emergency department with sudden and severe continuous abdominal pain. The patient complains of abdominal fullness and is profoundly hypotensive. What diagnosis do you anticipate being confirmed?

   a. Ruptured abdominal aortic aneurysm

   b. Cardiac perforation

   c. Systemic septic myocarditis

   d. Hemothorax with referred pain

10. Aortic dissections are most common in the abdominal aorta.

    a. True.

    b. False.

11. Type B aortic dissections have a very low surgical risk, and therefore are treated aggressively with surgery as the initial intervention.

    a. True.

    b. False.

12. Postoperative care of the patient with carotid endarterectomy involves:

    a. Maintenance of blood pressure between 80 and 90 mm Hg systolic to avoid injury to the involved artery

    b. Trendelenburg position to improve cerebral perfusion

    c. Assessment of intact cranial nerves

    d. Application of manual pressure to surgical site to prevent hematoma

585

Chapter 13

13. Changes common with a right-sided stroke include
    a. aphasia.
    b. hesitancy.
    c. right-sided weakness.
    d. impulsiveness.

14. The following patient is a possible candidate for fibrinolytic therapy for acute stroke:
    a. Went to bed normal at 10:00 pm; awakened by wife at 6:00 am, with noted deficits
    b. Patient with known valvular disease on warfarin with an INR of 2.3
    c. Patient with a stroke score on the NIH scale of 6
    d. Patient with positive CT scan for hemorrhagic stroke

15. A contraindication for fibrinolytic therapy in an acute stroke is
    a. Blood pressure 160/90
    b. Blood glucose of 35 mg/dL
    c. Cardiac catheterization one week ago
    d. INR of 1.7

ANSWERS
1. B
2. C
3. A
4. E
5. E
6. D
7. A
8. D
9. A
10. B
11. B
12. C
13. D
14. C
15. B

REFERENCES

Adams, H., Adams, R., Del Zoppo, G., & Goldstein, L.B. (2005). Guidelines for the Early Management of Patients With Ischemic Stroke: 2005 Guidelines Update A Scientific Statement From the Stroke Council of the American Heart Association/American Stroke Association *Stroke, Apr 2005; 36*:916-923.

Alspach, J.G. (2006). *Core curriculum for critical care nursing* (6th ed.). St. Louis: Saunders.

Ayerdi, J., Edwards, M.S., & Hansen, K.J. (2002). Endovascular procedures for renovascular disease: Introduction. *ACS Surgery Online*. Retrieved from http://www.medscape.com/viewarticle/535538_print

Bloch, M.J. & Basile, J. (2003). The diagnosis and management of renovascular disease: A primary care perspective. *Journal of Clinical Hypertension, 5*(3), 210-218.

Bojar, R.M. (2005). *Manual of perioperative care in adult cardiac surgery* (4th ed.). Malden, MA: Blackwell Publishing.

Creager, M.A. (2002). Peripheral arterial disease: Peripheral atherosclerosis. *ACP Online*. Retrieved from http://www.medscape.com/viewarticle/535394_print

Critical care challenges: disorders, treatments and procedures. (2003). Philadelphia: Lippincott, Williams and Wilkins.

Dennison, R.D. (2000). *Pass ccrn* (2nd ed.). St.Louis: Mosby.

Eskandari, M.K. (2002). Aortoiliac reconstruction: Introduction. *ACS Surgery Online*. Retrieved from http://www.medscape.com/viewarticle/535535_print

Gill, E.A. (2001). Aortic dissections and diseases of the aorta. In A.V. Adair (Ed.), *Cardiology secrets* (pp. 136-138). Philadelphia: Hanley and Belfus, Inc.

Goldstein, L.B., Adams, R., Alberts, M.J., Appel, L.J., Brass, L.M., Bushnell, C.D., et al. (2006). Primary Prevention of Ischemic Stroke: A Guideline From the American Heart Association/American Stroke Association Stroke Council: Cosponsored by the Atherosclerotic Peripheral Vascular Disease Interdisciplinary Working Group; Cardiovascular Nursing Council; Clinical Cardiology Council; Nutrition, Physical Activity, and Metabolism Council; and the Quality of Care and Outcomes Research Interdisciplinary Working Group: The American Academy of Neurology affirms the value of this guideline. *Stroke, Jun 2006; 37*:1583-1633.

Hirsch, A.T., Haskal, Z.J., Hertzer, N.R., Bakal, C.W., Creager, M.A., Halperin, J.L., et al. (2006). ACC/AHA Guidelines for the Management of Patients with Peripheral Arterial Disease (Lower Extremity, Renal, Mesenteric, and Abdominal Aortic): A Collaborative Report from the American Association for Vascular Surgery/Society for Vascular Surgery, Society for Cardiovascular Angiography and Interventions, Society of Interventional Radiology, Society for Vascular Medicine and Biology, and the American College of Cardiology/American Heart Association Task Force on Practice Guidelines (Writing Committee to Develop Guidelines for the Management of Patients With Peripheral Arterial Disease). American College of Cardiology WebSite. Available at: http://www.acc.org/clinical/guidelines/pad/index.pdf

Kastrup, A. & Gröschel, K. (2005). Treatment of symptomatic and asymptomatic internal carotid artery stenosis in older adults. *Geriatrics Aging, 8*(5), 23-26.

Kirshner, H.S., Biller, J., & Callahan, A. (2005). Long-term therapy to prevent stoke. *The Journal of the American Board of Family Practice, 18*(6), 528-450.

Marini, J.J. & Wheeler A.P. (2006). *Critical care medicine the essentials* (3rd ed.). Philadelphia: Lippincott, Williams and Wilkins.

McIntyre, K.E. (2005). *Aortoiliac occlusive disease.* Retrieved from http://www.e-medicine.com/med/topic2759.htm

Moore, W.S. (2002). Carotid arterial procedures: Introduction. *ACS Surgery Online.* Retrieved from http://www.medscape.com/viewarticle/535532_print

Morton, P.G., Fontaine, D., Hudak, C.M., & Gallo, B.M. (Eds.). (2005) *Critical care nursing – a holistic approach* (8th ed.). Philadelphia: Lippincott, Williams and Wilkins.

Porth, C.M. (Ed.). (2004). *Essentials of pathophysiology: concepts of altered health states.* Philadelphia: Lippincott, Williams and Wilkins.

Rosner, M.H. (2001). Renovascular hypertension: Can we identify a population at high risk? *Southern Medical Association Journal, 94*(11), 1058-1064.

Wargo, K.A., Chong, K., & Chan, E.C.Y. (2003). Acute renal failure secondary to angiotensin II receptor blockade in a patient with bilateral renal artery stenosis. *Pharmacotherapy, 23*(9), 1199-1204.

White, T.R. & Schwartz, D.E. (2003). Aortic Dissection. In P.E. Parsons & J.P. Wiener-Kronish (Ed.) *Critical Care Secrets* (3rd ed.) (pp. 145-152). Philadelphia: Hanley and Belfus, Inc.

CHAPTER 14:
CARDIOVASCULAR DRUGS

There are many types of drugs used to treat cardiovascular diseases and manage hemodynamics, including the following:

ACE inhibitors (ACEI)	Calcium channel blockers
Aldosterone blockers	Diuretics
Angiotensin receptor blockers (ARB)	Inotropes
Antiarrhythmics	Nitrates
Anticoagulants	Platelet inhibitors
Antihypertensives	Fibrinolytics
Anti-lipid agents	Vasodilators
Beta blockers	Vasoconstrictors

A major goal of this chapter is to provide an understanding of the "why" of drug therapy, not just facts about drugs. Facts can be obtained from drug reference books, but an understanding of the physiology underlying drug actions provides a basis for understanding drug therapy and facilitates patient teaching related to cardiovascular drugs.

Information about specific drugs in this chapter comes from the references listed at the end of the chapter. Refer to the individual drug insert and to drug reference books, such as the Physician Desk Reference or pharmacology text books for more detailed information and dosing of specific drugs.

PHYSIOLOGIC BASIS OF CARDIOVASCULAR DRUG THERAPY

The job of the cardiovascular (CV) system is to provide oxygen and nutrients to every cell in the body so that each cell and organ system can perform its own individual function. In order for the CV system to do its job, the following four things have to work optimally:

HEART: the pump.

ARTERIES: carry oxygenated blood to all cells in the body.

VEINS: return blood to the heart.

BLOOD VOLUME: must be adequate for the size of the vascular space.

Problems with any of the above components can lead to hemodynamic instability and failure of the CV system to perform its function. It is these components that we can evaluate with physical assessment or invasive hemodynamic monitoring, and it is these same components that we can treat with drug therapy in order to reestablish hemodynamic stability. The sympathetic nervous system, the endocrine system, and various substances produced by the body that constrict or dilate blood vessels or alter contractile function of the heart affect how the CV system does its job.

Chapter 14

The following physiological concepts are reviewed in this section and provide a basis for understanding drug therapy for cardiovascular diseases:

Determinants of cardiac output

Myocardial O_2 supply and demand

Sympathetic nervous system

Renin-angiotensin-aldosterone system.

Determinants of Cardiac Output

Cardiac output (CO) is the amount of blood pumped by the heart each minute, normally 4-8 liters per minute in a normal-sized person. Cardiac output is a product of heart rate (HR) times stroke volume (SV). Stroke volume is the amount of blood ejected with each heart beat and varies widely among individuals, normally around 60-100 ml per beat. The formula for CO is:

$$CO = HR \times SV$$

Understanding this formula is key to understanding drug therapy aimed at optimizing CO. The two sides of the equation must balance each other. Therefore, if the CO is low, look at the other side of the equation to determine why: it must be either low HR or low SV (or both). Conversely, if you want to increase CO, you must go to the other side of the equation to do it: increase either HR or SV.

Stroke volume has three major determinants:

◆ **Preload** is ventricular fiber length prior to contraction. Starling's Law of the Heart says that up to a certain point the longer the fibers, the better they contract. In the ventricles, blood volume is what stretches the fibers, so we think of preload as volume. Up to a point, the more volume in the ventricles, the better they contract. However, if the fibers get too long or "overstretched," their performance declines and stroke volume is reduced. Each ventricle has a preload: right atrial pressure (RAP) or CVP is used as the clinical indicator of right ventricular (RV) preload; pulmonary artery occlusive pressure (PAOP) is used as the clinical indicator of left ventricular (LV) preload. Preload is dependent on the following:

❖ Blood volume – hypovolemia reduces preload, hypervolemia increases preload.

❖ Distribution of blood volume. Blood has to be able to fill the ventricles in order to stretch the fibers; therefore, anything that prevents blood from entering the ventricles reduces preload and therefore stroke volume. The following factors determine whether blood returns to the ventricles or is distributed away from them:

☆ Venous tone – venous dilation causes volume to stay in the dilated venous system rather than being returned to the heart. Venous dilation is one of the main ways we can reduce preload in heart failure – nitrates (nitroglycerin and its relatives) are primarily venous dilators.

☆ Body position. Sitting upright with feet on the floor is the best position for a patient in pulmonary edema because it uses gravity to help distribute blood away from the heart into the dependent extremities. Conversely, lying flat with legs elevated is a body position used in hypotension to help redistribute blood from the peripheral circulation back up to the heart.

☆ Intrathoracic pressure. The heart sits in the thorax and is affected by intrathoracic pressure. Normal intrathoracic pressure does not interfere with ventricular filling, but if intrathoracic pressure rises, that pressure is transmitted to the heart and pushes on the heart from the outside, thus limiting the ability of the ventricles to expand and fill. Examples of high intrathoracic pressure that can lead to preload reduction include pneumothorax and the addition of positive end-expiratory pressure (PEEP) to a ventilator.

590

☆ Intrapericardial pressure. The heart is surrounded by a non-distensible fibrous pericardial sac that normally contains between 10-30 ml of fluid to lubricate the heart as it moves during contraction and relaxation. If excess fluid accumulates in the pericardial sac, it limits ventricular filling in the same way that a pneumothorax does, by constricting the ventricles and limiting their ability to fill.

❖ Atrial kick - refers to atrial contribution to ventricular filling. Normally in sinus rhythm, the atria contract before the ventricles and contribute 20-30% more volume into the ventricles just before ventricular contraction, thus increasing preload by stretching ventricular fibers a little more, just prior to contraction. Any rhythm that causes a loss of atrial kick, such as atrial fibrillation, atrial flutter, or any rhythm that results in AV dissociation, can reduce preload.

❖ Left ventricular function - refers to how well the ventricles handle the volume they are being asked to handle. A normally functioning LV is able to handle additional volume by increasing its rate and force of contraction. With LV dysfunction, however, the ventricle is unable to compensate for increased volume and, therefore, ventricular pressures rise, resulting in pulmonary congestion and heart failure.

Figure 14.1 summarizes the determinants of preload.

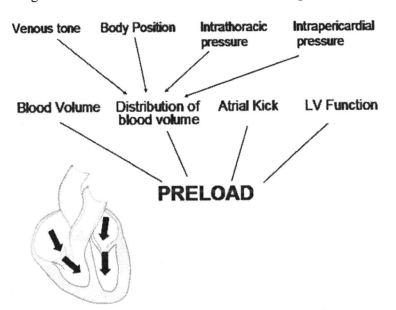

Figure 14.1: Preload.

Conditions that Alter Preload:
Hypovolemia
    Hemorrhage
    Dehydration
    Burns
    Overdiuresis
    Third Spacing

Hypervolemia
    Overhydration
    HF
    Renal disease

Altered Size of Vascular Space
    Sepsis
    Spinal or epidural anesthesia
    Anaphylaxis
    Venous dilating drugs

The way we increase preload is to administer volume, either crystalloid, colloid, or blood products. Reestablishing and maintaining sinus rhythm in atrial fibrillation or flutter with antiarrhythmic drugs also increases preload.

The two main ways to decrease preload are diuretics and venous dilators.

◆ **Afterload** is the amount of work a ventricle has to do in order to eject its volume. Clinically we think of resistance to ejection as afterload. Afterload is determined by the following:

❖ Vascular resistance is determined by the amount of arteriolar vasoconstriction, which, in turn, is determined by sympathetic nervous system activity and by circulating vasoconstrictors such as endothelin and angiotensin II. The RV must eject its volume into the pulmonary system; therefore, pulmonary vascular resistance (PVR) is the clinical indicator of RV afterload. The LV ejects into the systemic circulation, so systemic vascular resistance (SVR) is the clinical indicator of LV afterload.

- ❖ Vascular compliance refers to the "elasticity" or ability of blood vessels to stretch to accommodate blood volume. A stiff, noncompliant aorta increases LV afterload, and a stiff pulmonary artery increases RV afterload.
- ❖ Valve stenosis also contributes to the work of ventricular ejection. Pulmonic and aortic stenosis increase afterload for the RV and LV, respectively.
- ❖ Outflow tract obstruction – hypertrophic obstructive cardiomyopathy (HOCM) is obstruction of the left ventricular outflow tract due to septal and LV free wall hypertrophy. This contributes to increased afterload for the LV in the same way as aortic stenosis.

Figure 14.2 illustrates determinants of LV afterload:

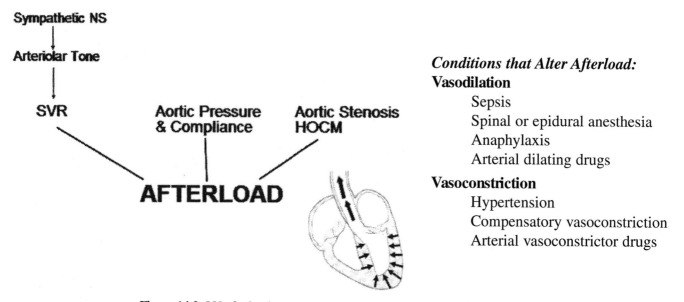

Figure 14.2: LV afterload.

Drugs that cause pulmonary or peripheral arterial vasodilation are used to decrease afterload, commonly referred to as "afterload reduction therapy." Arterial dilators include: nitroprusside (Nipride), milrinone (Primacor), hydralazine (Apresoline), labetalol (Trandate, Normodyne), nesiritide (Natrecor), ACE inhibitors, angiotensin receptor blockers, Ca^{++} channel blockers, and other antihypertensive agents.

Drugs that cause vasoconstriction increase afterload and thus increase the work load on the heart. Vasoconstrictor drugs include norepinephrine, epinephrine, high-dose dopamine, neosynephrine, and vasopressin.

- ◆ **Contractility** refers to the ability of cardiac fibers to develop tension and shorten. Shortening of cardiac fibers causes ejection of blood from the chamber. The term "inotropic" refers to the contractile state of the heart. Substances or drugs that increase contractility are positive inotropes, while drugs that decrease contractility are negative inotropes. Ventricular contractility is affected by the following:
  - ❖ Ventricular muscle mass – refers to the number of alive and functioning fibers in the ventricle. Myocardial infarction kills muscle fibers and reduces the number of fibers available to eject blood.
  - ❖ Catecholamines – circulating substances released by the sympathetic nervous system (SNS) and the adrenal glands that increase contractility of muscle fibers. Norepinephrine is released by the SNS and epinephrine is released by the adrenal glands; both are positive inotropes.

❖ The metabolic state of blood perfusing cardiac fibers is a very important determinant of contractility. Too many H⁺ ions (acidosis), too much CO_2, and reduced delivery of O_2 to the myocardium (either hypoxemia or ischemia) all decrease contractility.

Figure 14.3 illustrates determinants of contractility:

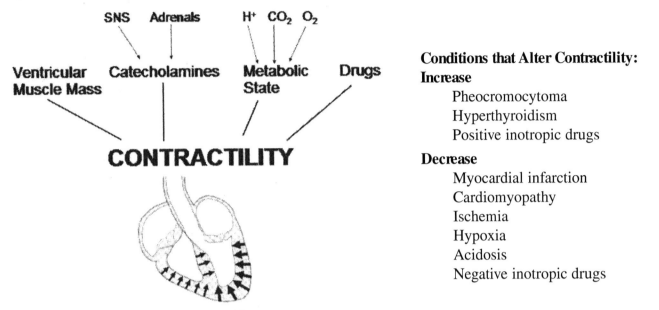

Figure 14.3: Contractility.

Positive inotropic drugs include: dopamine, dobutamine, milrinone, epinephrine, norepinephrine (Levophed), and digoxin.

Negative inotropic drugs include beta blockers, calcium channel blockers, most antiarrhythmics, many sedatives, anesthetics, and some chemotherapy agents.

Heart rate is the other major determinant of CO. Unless the HR is very slow or extremely fast, it is unlikely to be the cause of a low CO. Tachycardia can decrease CO in three ways:

1. Fast HR increases the amount of time the heart is in systole and reduces the amount of diastolic time. Since the ventricles fill with blood during diastole, rapid HR decreases preload and SV by reducing diastolic filling time.

2. The coronary arteries perfuse the myocardium during diastole; therefore, a rapid HR reduces coronary perfusion time.

3. The faster the heart goes the more O_2 it requires; therefore, rapid HR increases myocardial O_2 consumption (MVO_2) and can contribute to angina and heart failure.

Chapter 14

PHARMACOLOGIC MANIPULATION OF CARDIAC OUTPUT

Increase heart rate:
Atropine
Epinephrine
(Other drugs that also increase
HR but are used for other
reasons: dopamine, dobutamine,
norepinephrine)

Decrease heart rate:
Beta blockers
Ca^{++} blockers
Digoxin
Adenosine
Antiarrhythmics

$$CO \quad = \quad HR \quad X \quad SV$$

Preload   Afterload   Contractility

Increase:
Fluids
   Colloids
   Crystalloids
Blood products

Decrease:
Arterial dilators:
   ACEI
   Antihypertensives
   ARBs
   Ca^{++} blockers
   Milrinone
   Nesiritide
   Nipride

Increase:
Digoxin
Dobutamine
Dopamine
Milrinone

Decrease:
Diuretics
Aldosterone blockers
Venous Dilators:
   ACEI
   ARBs
   Morphine
   Nesiritide
   NTG, oral nitrates

Increase:
Vasopressors:
   Dopamine (high dose)
   Epinephrine
   Neo-synephrine
   Norepinephrine (Levophed)
   Vasopressin

Decrease:
Beta blockers
Ca^{++} blockers
Others:
   Anesthetics
   Antiarrhythmics
   Chemotherapy
   Propofol

Cardiovascular Drugs

Myocardial O₂ Supply and Demand

Angina is a result of a mismatch between myocardial O₂ supply and the demand of the heart for O₂. Chest pain can occur with reduced O₂ delivery to the myocardium or when the heart's demand for O₂ increases above the available O₂ supply. O₂ supply is dependant on open coronary arteries, adequate cardiac output, adequate O₂ content in the blood, and adequate number of red blood cells and Hb to carry the O₂. The heart's demand for O₂ is determined by heart rate, preload, afterload, and contractility.

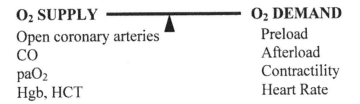

PHARMACOLOGIC MANIPULATION OF O₂ SUPPLY AND DEMAND

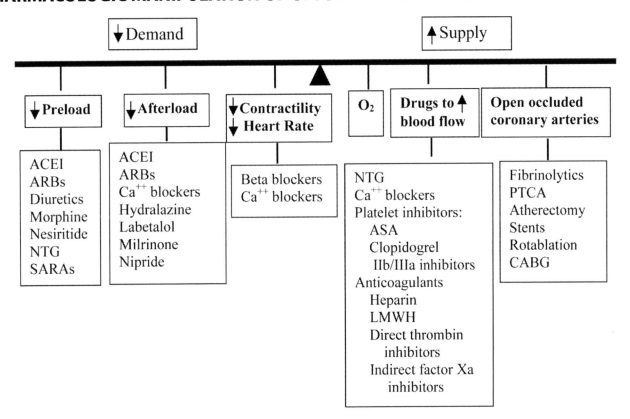

Sympathetic Nervous System (SNS)

The SNS plays an important role in the cardiovascular system in both the heart and blood vessels. The SNS works by stimulating either alpha or beta receptors. In terms of the CV system, alpha-1 receptors are located in arteries and veins, and when stimulated, they cause vasoconstriction. There are two types of beta receptors, ß₁ and ß₂. The heart is heavily populated with beta-1 receptors, and when they are stimulated, the result is an increase in heart rate, contractility, automaticity, and conduction velocity through the AV node. In the kidney, ß₁ stimulation results in renin release, which is discussed in more detail later. ß₂ stimulation in the blood vessels causes vasodilation, and in the lungs it causes bronchodilation. These effects are summarized in Figure 14.4.

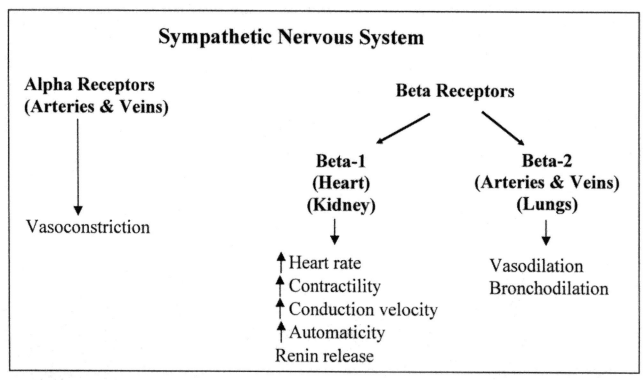

Figure 14.4: Sympathetic nervous system.

Drugs that stimulate alpha and/or beta receptors are called "sympathomimetic" agents because they cause the same effects as SNS stimulation. Drugs that block alpha and/or beta receptors cause the opposite effects. Alpha and beta stimulating and blocking drugs are used to help regulate cardiovascular function and are discussed later.

Renin-Angiotensin-Aldosterone System (RAAS)

The RAAS plays an important role in cardiovascular pathology, especially in hypertension and heart failure. The main function of the RAAS is renal protection in the presence of hypotension or decreased renal blood flow, but there are negative cardiovascular effects when this system is activated.

Renin is released from the juxtaglomerular cells in the kidney in response to decreased renal blood flow (e.g. hypotension, hypovolemia, sodium depletion), and increased Beta-1 stimulation. Renin causes the conversion of angiotensinogen (an inactive protein) to angiotensin I. Angiotensin I is converted to angiotensin II by an angiotensin converting enzyme (ACE), found primarily in pulmonary vascular endothelium, but also in other vascular beds. Angiotensin II causes two major effects: peripheral vasoconstriction (arterial and venous) and aldosterone release by the adrenal cortex. Aldosterone causes the renal tubules to reabsorb sodium and water, thus increasing circulating blood volume. The combined effects of peripheral vasoconstriction and increased blood volume lead to an increase in BP and increased renal perfusion, which is the main goal of the RAAS. However, when the decrease in renal perfusion is due to a failing LV, the effects of vasoconstriction (higher afterload) and increased blood volume (higher preload) are deleterious to cardiac function and can worsen heart failure and lead to hypertension.

Figure 14.5 illustrates the RAAS:

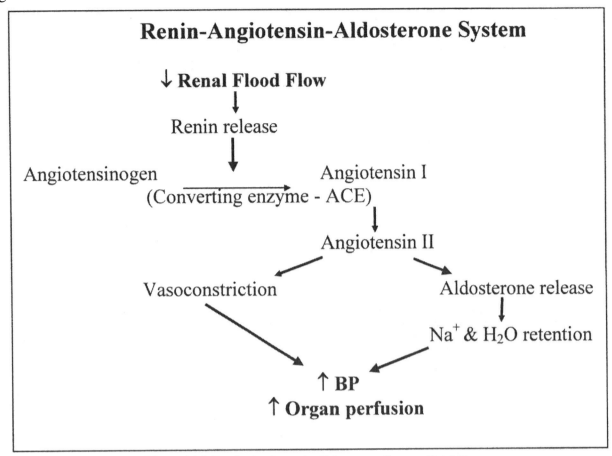

Figure 14.5: Renin-Angiotensin-Aldosterone System (RAAS).

Angiotensin II can also be formed in tissues via non ACE pathways, including in the ventricles. Whether angiotensin II is formed via ACE or non ACE pathways, it stimulates angiotensin receptors to exert its effects on the heart and blood vessels.

Four types of drugs can be used to block the RAAS to treat hypertension and heart failure, and for myocardial protection following myocardial infarction (MI). These drugs are:

- Beta blockers – block renin release by juxtaglomerular cells in the kidney.
- Angiotensin converting enzyme inhibitors (ACEI) – block the enzyme responsible for converting angiotensin I to angiotensin II (only work on ACE pathways).
- Angiotensin receptor blockers (ARB) – block angiotensin II at its receptor sites, regardless of the pathway used for angiotensin II formation.
- Aldosterone blockers (also called aldosterone receptor antagonists) – block aldosterone at its receptor sites.

Chapter 14

ACE INHIBITORS

Mechanism of Action

ACE inhibitors block the conversion of angiotensin I to angiotensin II, resulting in arterial and venous vasodilation and reduced Na^+ and H_2O reabsorption by the kidney. They also block the breakdown of bradykinin, increasing bradykinin levels. Bradykinin is a vasodilator itself, but it also causes the release of two vasodilator substances in vascular endothelium: nitric oxide and vasodilatory prostaglandins. The actions of bradykinin are thought to potentiate the beneficial effects of ACEI.

The net effects of ACEI include:

◆ Preload reduction due to decreased Na^+ and H_2O reabsorption and venous dilation.

◆ Afterload reduction due to arterial dilation.

◆ Increased levels of bradykinin due to inhibition of the enzyme that breaks down bradykinin, resulting in vasodilation.

◆ Increased prostaglandin and nitric oxide production in vascular endothelium, causing vasodilation and endothelial protection.

◆ Decreased ventricular remodeling by decreasing filling pressures in the ventricles (preload), which results in less thinning and dilation of ventricular myocardium.

Indications for ACE Inhibitors

◆ Heart failure – preload and afterload reduction.

◆ Hypertension– preload and afterload reduction.

◆ Acute MI – acute stage and as follow-up therapy to reduce mortality, decrease ventricular remodeling and prevent reinfarction.

◆ Nephropathy – renoprotective in Type I and Type II diabetic and nondiabetic nephropathy.

Recent studies have suggested that ACE inhibitors and angiotensin receptor blockers may significantly reduce the incidence of new onset type 2 diabetes in patients with or without hypertension (Jandeleit-Dahm, Tikellis, Reid, Johnston, & Cooper, 2005).

Side Effects of ACE Inhibitors

◆ Cough – most common side effect, probably due to increased bradykinin and prostaglandin levels.

◆ Hypotension – especially in patients with low Na^+ levels (<130 mEq/L), diuretic therapy, volume depletion, or with severe HF. Because of the risk of hypotension, a test dose is recommended when initiating therapy.

◆ Hyperkalemia – lower aldosterone levels cause K^+ retention by renal tubules especially if given with K^+ sparing diuretics, aldosterone blockers, or in patients with acute kidney injury.

◆ Renal failure – can be precipitated by excessive hypotension, severe HF, renal artery stenosis (bilateral renal artery stenosis is a contraindication to ACE inhibitors).

◆ Angioedema (swelling of face, tongue, larynx) – rare but very dangerous. Probably related to increased bradykinin levels.

◆ Rash – most common with captopril.

◆ Neutropenia and agranulocytosis – occur most often with high dose captopril and may occur with others.

598

Cardiovascular Drugs

Contraindications for ACE Inhibitors

- Bilateral renal artery stenosis.
- Renal artery stenosis of a single kidney.
- Immune based renal disease (especially collagen vascular disease).
- Severe renal failure.
- Preexisting hyperkalemia.
- History of angioedema.
- Pregnancy.

Combination Therapy and Drug Interactions

- Diuretics – thiazides and lasix enhance hypotensive effects. Risk of hyperkalemia with K^+ sparing diuretics (aldosterone blocking agents). Diuretic dose should be decreased or discontinued on initiation of ACE inhibitor therapy and reinstituted, as needed for BP or volume control in HF.
- Digoxin – used as combination therapy for HF. Captopril increases digoxin levels.
- Beta blockers – additive effects (both classes of drug decrease renin effects).
- Ca^{++} blockers – good combination for hypertension, additive effects on BP; both cause arterial dilation and may cause excessive hypotension.
- Nitrates – additive effects on preload reduction, so may cause excessive hypotension.
- NSAIDS – decrease cough side effect, but also decrease effects of ACE inhibitors by blocking prostaglandins. They also cause vasoconstriction, which increases afterload and can lead to worsening HF; therefore, non-aspirin NSAIDS should be generally avoided in patients with preexisting HF.

Types of ACE Inhibitors

Class I: Captopril – active as it is (does not need to be metabolized in order to exert its effects), but has active metabolites.

Class II: Prodrugs – parent drug is inactive until converted to active form by hepatic metabolism. This class includes most ACEI. The active form of the drug is the name of the parent drug with "at" on the end (i.e. enalapril is the parent drug; enalaprilat is the active form of the drug).

Class III: Water soluble and not metabolized. Lisinopril is the ACEI in this class.

Linking Knowledge to Practice

- ✔ *The initial dose of an ACEI should be low (e.g. 15-25% of the maximal recommended dose) and slowly increased to attain treatment goals. Once the response is known (i.e. BP, creatinine, and K+ level) the dose can be increased if the drug is tolerated.*

Chapter 14

<table>
<tr><td colspan="5" align="center">Table 14.1
ACE Inhibitors</td></tr>
<tr><td>DRUG</td><td>PEAK RESPONSE</td><td>DURATION</td><td>DOSE: TEST/ MAINTENANCE</td><td>PRECAUTIONS NURSING IMPLICATIONS</td></tr>
<tr><td>Benazapril (Lotensin) [Benazaprilat]</td><td>2-4 hr</td><td>24 hrs</td><td>10 mg/
20-40 mg qd
One or two doses</td><td>No effects from food.
Monitor labs: Na$^+$, K$^+$, creatinine, BUN.
Initial dose 5 mg/day if renal impairment.</td></tr>
<tr><td>Captopril (Capoten)</td><td>1-1.5 hrs</td><td>6-12 hrs</td><td>6.25 mg/
25-50 mg bid or tid</td><td>Take one hour before meals.
Take 2 hours apart from antacids.
Sulfhydryl group may cause bad taste, neutropenia, rash, renal disease (immune based side effects). Neutropenia more common in patients with collagen vascular disease and renal failure.
Monitor BP response carefully.
Monitor labs: Na$^+$, K$^+$, BUN, creat, WBC.
Elevates digoxin levels.</td></tr>
<tr><td>Enalapril (Vasotec) [Enalaprilat]

Enalaprilat IV</td><td>4-6 hrs</td><td>24 hrs</td><td>2.5 mg/
5-40 mg qd PO

1.25 mg IV q 6 h</td><td>Less risk of immune-based side effects (no sulfhydryl group).
Food does not affect absorption.
Monitor BP response.
Monitor labs: Na$^+$, K$^+$, creat, BUN.
If taking diuretic or has renal failure, initial dose 2.5 mg, adjust slowly for BP control.</td></tr>
<tr><td>Fosinopril (Monopril) [Fosinoprilat]</td><td>3 hrs</td><td>24 hrs</td><td>10 mg/
20-40 mg qd
Max 80 mg/day</td><td>Take antacids 2 hrs apart from drug.
No effects from food.
Monitor WBC, Na^{++}, K$^+$, creat, BUN.
Can cause pancreatitis, hepatitis, bronchospasm.</td></tr>
<tr><td>Lisinopril (Zestril, Prinivil)</td><td>7 hrs</td><td>24 hrs</td><td>2.5 mg/
20-40 mg qd
Once a day dosing</td><td>Less risk of immune-based side effects (no sulfhydryl group).
Not metabolized by liver.
Monitor labs: Na^{++}, K$^+$, creat, BUN.</td></tr>
<tr><td>Moexipril (Univasc)</td><td>1.5 hr</td><td>24 hrs</td><td>3.75mg/
7.5-30 mg qd
One or two doses</td><td>Take 1 hour before meals.
If renal impairment, 3.75 mg/day, adjust to maximum of 15 mg/day.
Monitor labs: Na$^+$, K$^+$, creat, BUN.</td></tr>
<tr><td>Perindopril (Aceon)</td><td>1 hr</td><td>Unknown</td><td>4 mg/
4-8 mg qd
Max 16 mg/day</td><td>If renal impairment, 2 mg/day, maximum 8 mg/day. If patient taking diuretic, 2-4 mg/day and watch BP closely for several hours. Monitor labs: Na$^+$, K$^+$, creat, BUN.</td></tr>
<tr><td>Quinapril (Accupril) [Quinaprilat]</td><td>2-6 hrs</td><td>24 hrs</td><td>10 mg/
20-80 qd</td><td>Take on empty stomach.
Monitor labs: Na$^+$, K$^+$, creat, BUN.
If taking diuretic, start with 5 mg bid; if renal impairment, 2.5-5 mg/day.</td></tr>
<tr><td>Ramipril (Altace) [Ramiprilat]</td><td>1-3 hrs</td><td>24 hrs</td><td>2.5 mg/
2.5-20 mg qd
Once a day dosing</td><td>Monitor labs: Na$^+$, K$^+$, creat, BUN.
If renal impairment, 1.25 mg/day, max 5mg/day. Risk of hypoglycemia with insulin or oral diabetic agents.</td></tr>
<tr><td>Trandolapril (Mavik)</td><td>1-10 hrs</td><td>24 hrs</td><td>1 mg/
2-4 mg/day
One or two doses</td><td>If hepatic or renal disease, initial dose is 0.5 mg daily.
Monitor labs: Na$^+$, K$^+$, creat, BUN.
Can cause first-degree block, bradycardia, pancreatitis, neutropenia, leukopenia.</td></tr>
</table>

Cardiovascular Drugs

ANGIOTENSIN RECEPTOR BLOCKERS (ARB)

Mechanism of Action

ARBs block the effects of angiotensin II at receptor sites, regardless of the pathway by which angiotensin II was formed. This results in vasodilation and decreased volume retention, just like ACEI, but ARBs have no effect on bradykinin, which decreases the side effects of cough and angioedema.

Indications for ARBs

◆ Heart failure – preload and afterload reduction.

◆ Hypertension – preload and afterload reduction.

◆ Acute MI – acute stage and as follow-up therapy to reduce mortality, decrease ventricular remodeling and prevent reinfarction in ACEI intolerant patients.

◆ Nephropathy – renoprotective in Type II diabetes.

Side Effects of ARBs

◆ Hypotension.

◆ Hyperkalemia.

◆ Much less likely to cause a cough than ACEI.

Contraindications for ARBs

◆ Pregnancy.

◆ Bilateral renal artery stenosis.

DRUG	PEAK RESPONSE	DOSE RANGE	RECOMMENDED INITIAL DOSE	PRECAUTIONS NURSING IMPLICATIONS
Table 14.2				
Angiotensin II Receptor Blockers (ARBs)				
Candesartan (Atacand)	3-4 hrs	8-32 mg/day Once or twice daily	16 mg/day	Fatigue, peripheral edema, back pain, headache, dizziness, upper respiratory symptoms, N&V, abdominal pain, small ↑ in creat, BUN, K⁺, liver enzymes, bilirubin. May take with food. May take with diuretics or other antihypertensives.
Eprosartan (Teveten)	1-3 hrs	400-800 mg/day	600 mg/day	May take with food. Same as candesartan.
Irbesartan (Avapro)	1.5-2 hrs	75-300 mg/day	150 mg /day	May take with food. Same as candesartan.
Losartan (Cozaar)	1-4 hrs	25-100 mg/day	25-50 mg/day	May take with food. Same as candesartan.
Olmesartan (Benicar)	1-2 hrs	20-40 mg/day	20 mg/day	May take with food. Same as candesartan.
Telmisartan (Micardis)	0.5-1 hr	20-80 mg/day	40 mg / day	May take with food. Don't open blister pack until ready to take, discard unused scored tablets. Same as candesartan.
Valsartan (Diovan)	2-4 hours	80-320 mg/day	80 mg/day	May take with food. Same as candesartan.

Chapter 14

ALDOSTERONE BLOCKERS

Aldosterone has several negative effects in heart failure, including: retention of Na+ and H2O (increased preload), loss of Mg++ and K+ (which can cause arrhythmias), activation of the SNS (increased preload and cardiotoxic effects), myocardial and vascular fibrosis (contributes to ventricular remodeling and inhibits ability of blood vessels to dilate), endothelial dysfunction (increases formation of endothelin which is a potent vasoconstrictor). Blocking the effects of aldosterone is a beneficial effect in treating heart failure and hypertension.

A nonselective aldosterone blocker, spironolactone (Aldactone), has been used as a K⁺ sparing diuretic for many years. It effectively blocks the effects of aldosterone and has beneficial effects in treating heart failure and hypertension, but it also blocks androgen receptors and stimulates progesterone receptors, which causes undesirable side effects such as gynecomastia, menstrual problems, and sexual dysfunction, thus decreasing patient compliance with therapy.

Selective aldosterone receptor antagonists (SARAs) are being developed to block aldosterone but not affect the other receptors that cause undesirable side effects. One such agent is available at this time: eplerenone (Inspra). This drug is indicated for treatment of heart failure and hypertension, but it does not cause the same undesirable effects as spironolactone. Other drugs in this class are under development.

Linking Knowledge to Practice

✔ *Patients receiving ACEI or ARBs are usually also on diuretics and may be taking a beta blocker or a Ca⁺⁺ channel blocker as well. All of these drugs can cause hypotension, especially when used together. Follow these precautions when caring for patients on these drugs:*

  ❖ *Check postural pressures the first time a patient gets out of bed to make sure there is no significant orthostatic drop. If a significant drop occurs, check postural pressures each time up.*

  ❖ *Teach patients to get out of bed slowly, sitting on side of bed and moving their feet for a minute before standing. This should also be included in the discharge instructions.*

✔ *Hyperkalemia is a risk in patients on ACEI and ARBs. Check K⁺ levels on initiation of therapy and whenever the dose is altered, and follow closely during hospitalization.*

✔ *Patients on ACEI and ARB therapy probably do not need K⁺ supplements because these drugs cause K⁺ reabsorption. Hold K⁺ supplements on initiation of therapy and check with physician about discontinuing supplements if K⁺ level rises on drug therapy. Instruct patients to avoid potassium-containing salt substitutes.*

✔ *The goal of drug therapy with ACEI and ARBs in heart failure is to make it easier for the heart to work by both preload and afterload reduction. Blood pressure is expected to be lower than what we as nurses are used to tolerating in our patients. Pressures in the 80s are not uncommon and, in fact, are desirable in many patients. DO NOT automatically hold these medications because of low BP unless the patient is symptomatic. Verify with the physician what BP parameters are desired for each individual patient.*

✔ *Cough is a common side effect of ACEI, but it can also be a sign of worsening heart failure. Perform a good physical assessment to rule out worsening HF before assuming the cough is a side effect of ACEI therapy.*

✔ *African Americans are less responsive to ACEI and ARB therapy than Caucasians. A combination of hydralazine (an arterial dilator) and isosorbide dinitrate (a venous dilator) is recommended as part of standard therapy in addition to beta blockers and ACE-inhibitors for African Americans with LV systolic dysfunction.*

Cardiovascular Drugs

BETA BLOCKERS

The SNS exerts its cardiovascular effects by stimulating alpha and beta receptors in the heart and/or blood vessels. Refer to the discussion under sympathetic nervous system above for a summary of the effects of alpha and beta stimulation.

Mechanism of Action

Beta blockade results in the following effects:

Heart: ↓ heart rate (sinus bradycardia).
  ↓ contractility (↓ LV function, HF).
  ↓ AV conduction (AV block).

Blood Vessels: Prevents vasodilatation in arterioles and veins so allows alpha receptors to work unopposed, resulting in vasoconstriction. Can worsen angina that is due to coronary vasospasm and cause claudication in peripheral vascular disease.

Lungs: Prevents bronchodilation and can cause bronchospasm. Non cardioselective beta blockers are contraindicated in patients with reactive airway disease.

Kidney: Decreases renin secretion.

Types of Beta Blockers

Nonselective: block both β_1 and β_2 receptors, so effects include undesired bronchoconstriction and peripheral vascular constriction (because blockade of β_2 receptors in peripheral vessels leaves the alpha vasoconstrictor receptors unopposed).

Cardioselective: block only the β_1 receptors so avoid the undesired pulmonary and peripheral vascular effects. Cardioselectivity occurs with lower doses of these drugs; at high doses the β_2 receptors are also blocked.

Vasodilating beta blockers: combined alpha and beta blockade results in peripheral vasodilation. Another vasodilatory mechanism is called ISA (intrinsic sympathomimetic activity) in which β_2 receptors are stimulated to result in vasodilation. Drugs with ISA are not used as often as other beta blockers.

Indications for Beta Blocker Therapy

Table 14.3 illustrates the cardiovascular indications for beta blocker therapy and the mechanism of action for each indication.

Table 14.3 Indications for Beta Blocker Therapy	
USE	**MECHANISM OF ACTION**
Hypertension	↓ heart rate = ↓ CO = ↓ BP. BP = CO X SVR. ↓ contractility = ↓ CO = ↓ BP. ↓ renin release in kidney causes less angiotensin I to angiotensin II.
Classic Angina (due to atherosclerotic obstruction of coronary arteries)	↓ O_2 demand by ↓ HR, ↓ contractility, ↓ BP. ↑ O_2 supply by ↓ HR which increases diastolic filling and coronary perfusion time.

603

Chapter 14

<table>
<tr><td colspan="2" align="center">**Table 14.3 (continued)**
Indications for Beta Blocker Therapy</td></tr>
<tr><td>**USE**</td><td>**MECHANISM OF ACTION**</td></tr>
<tr><td>**Acute MI and**
MI follow-up</td><td>↓ automaticity in ventricle so ↓ risk of VF early in MI.
Preserves ischemic myocardium by ↓ O₂ demands (↓ HR, ↓ contractility, ↓ BP.</td></tr>
<tr><td>**Arrhythmias**
(atrial fibrillation, atrial flutter, SVT, some VT, congenital long QT)</td><td>↓ automaticity so ↓ VT, VF.
↓ AV conduction so can slow ventricular response to atrial fibrillation, atrial flutter, and may terminate PSVT.
Blunt adrenergic surge that causes torsades de pointes in long QT syndrome.</td></tr>
<tr><td>**Heart Failure** (low dose beta blockade to block neurohormonal SNS response)</td><td>↓ HR = longer diastolic filling time, ↑ coronary perfusion time, ↓ myocardial O₂ demands.
Protect heart from cardiotoxic effects of high norepinephrine levels that occur in HF; cause upregulation of beta receptors.
↓ renin release so ↓ angiotensin II levels.</td></tr>
<tr><td>**Obstructive Cardiomyopathy**</td><td>↓ contractility so reduces outflow track obstruction
↓ HR allows longer diastolic filling time so more blood in ventricle to keep outflow tract open.</td></tr>
<tr><td>**Migraine Headaches**</td><td>Inhibits β mediated vasodilatation in cerebral vessels.</td></tr>
</table>

Contraindications to Beta Blocker Therapy

- Hypotension (systolic BP less than 90 mm Hg)
- Severe bradycardia, sick sinus syndrome.
- Heart block – first, second, or third degree block.
- Cardiogenic shock.
- Acute decompensated heart failure.
- Angina due to coronary vasospasm.
- Severe asthma or bronchospasm.
- Peripheral arterial disease with ischemic pain at rest.

Side Effects of Beta Blockers

Cardiac:

- Bradycardia – depressed sinus node automaticity.
- AV block – decreased conduction through AV node.
- HF – decreased contractility with higher doses.
- Hypotension – decreased contractility lowers BP.

Pulmonary:

- Bronchoconstriction (with non-selective agents or high doses of cardioselective agents) – due to ß₂ blockade, which prevents bronchodilation.
- Pulmonary edema – due to decreased contractility in the setting of depressed LV function.

Cardiovascular Drugs

Peripheral Vascular:

◆ Worsening of peripheral arterial disease due to ß2 blockade, which leaves alpha receptors unopposed and causes vasoconstriction.

Metabolic:

◆ Masks signs of hypoglycemia (tachycardia, sweating, etc.) in diabetics.

◆ Non selective agents decrease formation of glucose in liver and can augment the hypoglycemic action of insulin.

◆ Increase serum triglycerides

Central Nervous System:

◆ Fatigue.

◆ Sleep disturbances: insomnia, nightmares.

◆ Depression, sexual dysfunction.

Combination Therapy and Drug Interactions

ß blockers can be used with all other classes of cardiovascular drugs. Additive effects can occur between ß blockers and other drugs that slow heart rate, decrease AV conduction, and depress contractility, especially calcium channel blockers.

Table 14.4 Beta Blockers				
Drug Name (Trade Name)	**Half-life**	**Dose for Angina**	**Dose for Hypertension**	**IV dose**
Non-cardioselective Agents				
Propranolol (Inderal)	1-6 hours	80 mg bid. (may give 160 mg bid). 80-320 mg qd.	10-40 mg bid. Mean dose 160-320 mg/day. (1 or 2 doses) 80-320 mg qd.	1-6 mg.
(Inderal LA)	8-11 hours			
Carteolol [ISA] (Cartrol)	5-6 hours		2.5-10 mg qd.	
Nadolol (Corgard)	20-24 hours	40-80 mg qd up to 240 mg.	40-80 mg qd up to 240 mg.	
Penbutalol [ISA] (Levatol)	20-25 hours		10-20 mg qd.	
Sotalol (Betapace) (for arrhythmias)	7-18 hours (mean 12)	80-240 mg bid for ventricular arrhythmias. 160 mg bid for atrial fib, flutter.	80-320 mg/day.	
Timolol (Blocadren)	4-5 hours	Post MI: 10 mg bid.	10-20 mg bid.	

605

Chapter 14

			Table 14.4 (continued) Beta Blockers		
Drug Name (Trade Name)	**Half-life**	**Dose for Angina**	**Dose for Hypertension**	**IV dose**
Cardioselective Agents				
Acebutolol [ISA] (Sectral)	8-13 hours		400-1200 mg/day	
Atenolol (Tenormin)	6-7 hours	50-200 mg qd	50-100 mg qd	5mg over 5 minutes, repeat in 5 minutes
Betaxolol (Kerlone)	14-22 hours		10-20 mg qd	
Bisoprolol (Zebeta)	9-12 hours	10 mg qd	2.5-40 mg qd *For heart failure:* First dose: 1.25 mg, Week 3: 3.75 mg, Week 5-6: 5 mg, Final dose: 10 mg	
Metoprolol (Lopressor) **Metoprolol SR**	3-7 hours	50-200 mg bid	50-400 mg qd (I or 2 doses) *For heart failure:* First dose: 12.5-25 mg, Week 3: 50 mg, Week 5-6: 100 mg, Final dose: 200 mg	5 mg three times q 2 minutes to total of 15 mg
Vasodilatory Beta Blockers, non-cardioselective				
Carvedilol (Coreg) Alpha & beta blocker **Coreg CR**	6 hours	*For heart failure:* First dose: 3.125 mg bid, Week 3: 6.25 mg bid, Week 5-6: 12.5 mg bid, Final dose: 25 mg bid 10 mg qd (equivalent to 3.125 bid of Coreg) 20 mg qd (equivalent to 6.25 mg bid of Coreg) 40 mg qd (equivalent to 12.5 mg bid of Coreg) 80 mg qd (equivalent to 25 mg bid of Coreg)	12.5-25 mg bid	
Labetalol (Trandate, Normodyne) Alpha & beta blocker	6-8 hours	300-600 mg qd in three doses; max dose 2400 mg/day	300-600 mg qd in three doses; max dose 2400 mg/day	IV infusion 2.5-30 mcg/kg/min
Pindolol [ISA] (Visken)	4 hours		5-30 mg/day in 2 doses	

CALCIUM CHANNEL BLOCKERS

Mechanism of Action

Ca^{++} plays a major role in depolarization of the sinus node and the AV node. Ca^{++} binds to actin and myosin proteins in cardiac and smooth muscle fibers to facilitate contraction of the heart and of the smooth muscle layer in peripheral blood vessels. Ca^{++} blockers inhibit inward flow of Ca^{++} ions through the L-type calcium channel in smooth muscle and myocardium.

Effects of Ca^{++} Channel Blockers:

Heart: ↓ heart rate (verapamil and diltiazem).
     ↓ conduction velocity through AV node (verapamil and diltiazem).
     ↓ contractility (especially verapamil).

Blood Vessels: prevents contraction of muscle layer in blood vessels.
     Coronary – vasodilation (prevents coronary vasospasm).
     Peripheral – vasodilation (afterload reduction).

Types of Ca^{++} Channel Blockers

Dihydropyridines (DHP)

DHP type calcium channel blockers have more effect on peripheral blood vessels than on the heart, but there is still the potential for cardiac depression with these drugs. Because of their relative vascular selectivity, DHPs are used to treat effort angina and hypertension. Nifedipine is the prototype of this group of Ca^{++} channel blockers, and other drugs whose generic name ends in "pine" are also DHPs. Newer generation DHPs, like felodipine and amlodipine, have very little cardiac depressant activity and are better tolerated in patients with HF.

Nondihydropyridines

These drugs have more cardiac effects than peripheral effects and are considered to be heart rate lowering (HRL) drugs. Verapamil and diltiazem are the two agents in this class of Ca^{++} blockers; they both decrease HR and AV conduction and are used primarily to treat supraventricular arrhythmias. Both drugs also have some peripheral vasodilating effects; diltiazem is often used to prevent spasm in radial artery grafts used in cardiac bypass surgery.

Chapter 14

Indications for Ca^{++} Channel Blockers

Table 14.5 outlines the clinical uses and mechanism of action for Ca^{++} blockers.

Table 14.5 Indications for Calcium Channel Blockers	
USE	**MECHANISM OF ACTION**
Angina:	
Coronary Spasm	Prevent vasoconstriction by ↓ amount of Ca^{++} available for contraction = coronary vasodilation.
Classic Angina (All agents)	Coronary vasodilation = ↑ collateral blood flow to ischemic areas. ↓ MVO2 by ↓ heart rate, ↓ contractility, and ↓ afterload.
Hypertension (All agents)	**BP = CO x SVR** ↓ CO by ↓ contractility, ↓ SVR by vasodilation.
Arrhythmias: SVT (Verapamil & Diltiazem)	Slow AV conduction so ↓ ventricular response to atrial fib & flutter. Can terminate AV nodal active arrhythmias (AVNRT, accessory pathway tachycardias).
Hypertrophic Cardiomyopathy (Verapamil & Diltiazem)	↓ contractility lessens outflow tract obstruction. ↓ HR allows longer diastolic filling time so more blood in ventricle ↓ outflow tract obstruction. DHPs contraindicated due to more profound ↓SVR, which increases pressure gradient between LV and aorta.

Side Effects of Ca^{++} Channel Blockers

◆ Bradycardia – due to ↓ sinus rate (verapamil, diltiazem).
◆ AV block – due to ↓ AV node conduction (verapamil, diltiazem).
◆ Hypotension – due to vasodilation, especially with DHPs.
◆ HF – due to ↓ contractility, especially verapamil.
◆ Flushing, headaches, peripheral edema, constipation.
◆ Short acting nifedipine causes a precipitous drop in BP and should not be used to treat acute coronary ischemia. NEVER put the contents of a nifedipine gel capsule under the tongue to treat angina. Long acting Procardia XL can be used safely to treat effort angina, vasospastic angina, and hypertension.
◆ DHPs can cause reflex tachycardia if they cause the BP to drop significantly.

Contraindications for Ca^{++} Channel Blockers

◆ Dihydropyridines: severe aortic stenosis, obstructive cardiomyopathy, heart failure, unstable angina (impending infarction), preexisting hypotension.
◆ Verapamil and diltiazem: bradycardia, heart block, heart failure, hypotension, WPW syndrome.

Combination Therapy and Drug Interactions

◆ Additive effects with β blockers and digoxin on ↓ HR and ↓ AV conduction (verapamil & diltiazem).
◆ Additive effects with other vasodilators (ACE inhibitors, ARBs, nitrates, antihypertensives) on BP.
◆ Verapamil can ↑ digoxin levels and statin levels.

Cardiovascular Drugs

Table 14.6 Calcium Channel Blockers			
DRUG	**DOSE**	**MAJOR EFFECTS/CLINICAL USES**	**PRECAUTIONS**
Verapamil (Calan, Isoptin)	80-120 mg tid po 2.5-10 mg IV	Most potent first generation Ca^{++} blocker on slowing AV conduction. Used for atrial fibrillation or flutter to decrease ventricular rate and to terminate SVT. ↓ contractility and arterial vasodilation. Used for angina, hypertension. Can be used for obstructive cardiomyopathy. Short duration (half-life 3-7 hrs).	Negative inotropic effect = hypotension and HF. Potential for severe AV node block when given IV with ß blockers. DO NOT use with wide complex tachycardias or in WPW complicated by atrial fibrillation.
Diltiazem (Cardizem)	120-360 mg in divided doses 3-4 times/day po IV: 0.25 mg/Kg over 2 min. May repeat with 0.35 mg/Kg. Infusion: 5-15 mg/hr for up to 24 hrs.	Most potent first generation Ca^{++} channel blocker on slowing sinus rate. Short duration (half-life 4-7 hrs). Used for angina, hypertension, ventricular rate control in atrial fibrillation or flutter, and to terminate SVT.	Same as for verapamil with possibly less negative inotropic effect.
Nifedipine (Procardia) (Procardia XL)	10-30 mg tid to qid po 10 mg sublingual 30-90 mg once daily	Most potent first generation Ca^{++} channel blocker on arterial vasodilation and least effect on AV node conduction. Short duration (half-life 3 hrs). Used for hypertension and angina. Safest Ca^{++} blocker to combine with ß blockers due to less HR effect.	Contraindicated in obstructive cardiomyopathy and aortic stenosis due to peripheral dilation and ↑ pressure gradient; and in unstable angina. Negative inotropic effect can cause HF. Hypotension, tachycardia, and headache, flushing, dizziness due to vasodilation.
Amlodipine (Norvasc)	2.5-10 mg daily	Major advantage is slower onset and longer duration of action (elimination half-life is 35-48 hours) so can be dosed once a day. Used for hypertension and angina. No reflex tachycardia.	Same general side effects and precautions as nifedipine. Has less negative inotropic effect than nifedipine.
Felodipine (Plendil)	2.5-10 mg bid	More vascular effects and fewer cardiodepressant effects than nifedipine. Medium duration of action (half-life 8 hrs). Used for hypertension and angina.	Same as nifedipine with less negative inotropic effect and less incidence of HF.
Nicardipine (Cardene)	20-40 mg tid po IV infusion: 5 mg/hr to start. ↑ by 2.5 mg/hr q 15 min to max. of 15 mg/hr if nec.	More vascular specific and less cardio-depression than nifedipine. Short duration (half-life 4 hrs). Used for hypertension and angina. Can be used IV for acute BP control.	Same as nifedipine.
Isradipine DynaCirc) (2nd generation)	5-10 mg bid or tid	Vascular selective, less cardio-depression. Used for hypertension and angina. Medium duration (half-life 8 hrs).	Same as nifedipine.

609

Chapter 14

Linking Knowledge to Practice

✔ *Beta blockers and the heart rate lowering (HRL) calcium blockers (Verapamil and Diltiazem) have the same effects on the heart: they both decrease HR and contractility. Both types of drugs are used to treat angina and hypertension; therefore, many patients are on both a beta blocker and a HRL calcium channel blocker and may experience additive effects of these drugs. Watch for bradycardia, AV block, and hypotension in patients taking both a beta blocker and a HRL calcium channel blocker. If combination therapy is not tolerated, the calcium channel blocker is usually discontinued and the beta blocker is continued due to the positive mortality benefits of beta blockers. Drug induced bradycardia can be an indication for pacing.*

✔ *Some classes of drugs can be recognized by the suffix in their generic name. For example:*

❖ *Beta blockers all end in "olol:" metoprolol, atenolol, propranolol, etc.*

❖ *ACEI all end in "pril:" captopril, lisinopril, fosinopril, etc.*

❖ *ARBs all end in "sartan:" losartan, candesartan, valsartan, etc.*

❖ *Ca++ channel blockers that are dihydropyridines and cause peripheral vasodilation end in "pine": nifedipine, nicardipine, amlodipine, etc.*

DIURETICS

Diuretics alter renal function to cause increased loss of water and electrolytes in urine, thus reducing intravascular volume and decreasing preload in the heart. Volume reduction also lowers the blood pressure; therefore, diuretics are used to treat heart failure and hypertension. Three types of diuretics are available: thiazides, loop diuretics, and potassium sparing diuretics.

Mechanism of Action

◆ Loop diuretics:

❖ Work in the ascending limb of the Loop of Henle and cause loss of Na^+, K^+, Cl^-, H^+, and H_2O.

❖ Cause relatively more loss of H_2O and less loss of Na^+ and K^+ than thiazides.

❖ Cause venous dilation which reduces preload even before diuresis begins.

❖ Rapid onset but short duration of action.

❖ Can be effective in the presence of renal dysfunction.

❖ "High ceiling" diuretics – increasing diuresis with increasing doses. Potent diuretics.

◆ Thiazide diuretics:

❖ Inhibit reabsorption of Na^+ and Cl^- in the distal tubule.

❖ Delayed onset but longer duration of action than loops.

❖ "Low ceiling" diuretics - maximal response is reached at relatively low doses.

❖ Less potent diuretics than loops.

❖ Diminished effectiveness in presence of renal failure.

◆ Potassium sparing diuretics:

❖ Work in distal tubule and collecting ducts to cause loss of Na^+ and reabsorption of K^+.

❖ Weak diuretic activity, usually given with thiazides.

Indications for Diuretics

◆ Heart failure – chronic and acute decompensation.

◆ Hypertension.

Cardiovascular Drugs

	Table 14.7 Diuretics	
DRUG	**DOSE**	**SIDE EFFECTS**
Thiazide Diuretics		
Bendrofluazide (Naturetin)	1.25-2.5 mg for BP 10 mg for HF	General side effects of thiazide diuretics: Blood Chemistry changes: Hypokalemia ($\downarrow$ K$^+$) Hyperglycemia ($\uparrow$ blood sugar) Hyperuricemia ($\uparrow$ uric acid) Hypercalcemia ($\uparrow$ Ca^{++}) Decreased glomerular filtration in kidneys ($\uparrow$ BUN, creatinine) $\uparrow$ cholesterol $\uparrow$ triglycerides $\downarrow$ HDL cholesterol Other side effects: Impaired glucose tolerance Gout Impotence Ventricular arrhythmias ($\downarrow$ K$^+$) Nausea, dizziness, headache
Benthiazide (Aquatag, Exna)	50-200 mg	
Chlorothiazide (Diuril)	250-1000 mg	
Chlorthalidone (Hygroton)	12.5-50 mg	
Cyclothiazide (Anhydron)	1-2 mg	
Hydrochlorothiazide (HCTZ) (HydroDiuril, Esidrix)	12.5-25 mg for BP 25-100 mg for HF	
Hydroflumethazide (Saluron, Diucardin)	12.5-25 mg for BP 25-200 mg for HF	
Indapamide (Lozol)	1.25-2.5 mg for BP 2.5-5 mg for HF	
Metolazone (Zaroxolyn)	2.5-5 mg for BP 5-20 mg for HF	
Polythiazide (Renese)	1-2 mg	
Trichlormethiazide (Metahydrin, Naqua)	1-4 mg	
Loop Diuretics		
Bumetanide (Bumex)	0.5-2 mg PO 1-2 times daily for HF; 5 mg PO or IV for oliguria	General side effects of loop diuretics: Blood Chemistry changes (less severe than with thiazides): Hypokalemia ($\downarrow$ K$^+$) Hyperglycemia ($\uparrow$ blood sugar) Hyperuricemia ($\uparrow$ uric acid) $\uparrow$ cholesterol $\uparrow$ triglycerides $\downarrow$ HDL cholesterol Other side effects: Gout Impaired glucose tolerance Ototoxicity (deafness, reversible)
Furosemide (Lasix)	10-40 mg bid for BP; 20-80 mg 2-3 times daily for HF; up to 250-2000 mg PO or IV	
Torsemide (Demadex)	5-10 mg PO qd for BP; 10-20 mg PO or IV qd for HF	
K$^+$ Sparing Diuretics		
Amiloride (Midamor)	2.5-20 mg	Risk of hyperkalemia with all K$^+$ sparing diuretics. Acidosis can occur (rare)
Eplerenone (Inspra) [Aldosterone blocker]	50-100 mg	
Spironolactone (Aldactone) [Aldosterone blocker]	25-200 mg	Gynecomastia, sexual dysfunction, menstrual problems
Triamterene (Dyrenium)	25-200 mg	

Table 14.7 (continued) Diuretics		
DRUG	**DOSE**	**SIDE EFFECTS**
Combination Diuretics (Thiazide + K⁺ Sparing Diuretic)		
Aldactazide (Spironolactone + HCTZ)	25/25 25 mg of each drug.	
Dyazide (HCTZ + triamterene)	25/50 (25 mg HCTZ + 50 mg triamterene).	
Maxzide (HCTZ + triamterene)	50/75 (50 mg HCTZ + 75 mg triamterene).	
Maxzide-25 (HCTZ + triamterene)	25/37.5 (25 mg HCTZ) + 37.5 mg triamterene).	
Moduretic (HCTZ + amiloride)	50/5 (50 mg HCTZ + 5 mg amiloride).	

SYMPATHOMIMETIC DRUGS

Drugs that work by stimulating alpha or beta receptors are called sympathomimetics because they mimic the actions of the SNS to cause either increased contractility (inotropic effect), or to constrict or dilate blood vessels. Sympathomimetic drugs include phenylephrine (Neosynephrine), isoproterenol, dobutamine, dopamine, epinephrine, and norepinephrine. Figure 14.6 illustrates the sites of action of these drugs. Individual drugs are discussed below.

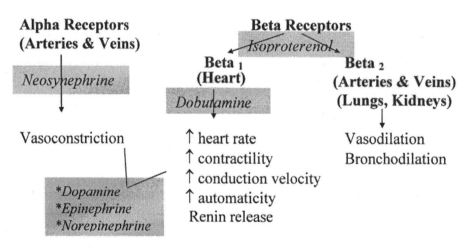

Figure 14.6: Sites of sympathomimetic drugs.

INOTROPES

Inotropes increase myocardial contractility by a variety of mechanisms. Sympathomimetic drugs mimic the inotropic actions of the SNS; milrinone is a phosphodiesterase inhibitor that results in increased contractility. Digoxin is also a positive inotropic drug, but it is no longer used in acute situations and is not discussed here. Several drugs have more than one effect on the cardiovascular system: dopamine, epinephrine, and norepinephrine increase contractility, heart rate, and cause vasoconstriction; isoproterenol and milrinone increase contractility and cause vasodilation. They are all discussed in this section as inotropes.

Cardiovascular Drugs

Dobutamine (primarily ß₁ Stimulation)

Dobutamine (Dobutrex) is a synthetic analog of dopamine that primarily stimulates ß₁ receptors. There is mild ß₂ stimulation, which may lead to hypotension, but ß₁ stimulation is the major effect.

Actions

◆ Increased cardiac contractility.

◆ Mild ß₂ stimulation.

◆ Reflex fall in SVR may occur due to increased cardiac output.

Indications

◆ Used as positive inotrope to increase cardiac output in acute LV failure.

◆ Cardiogenic shock.

◆ Excess beta blockade.

Dose

◆ Available IV only, used as continuous infusion.

◆ 2-20 mcg/kg/min is usual dose for heart failure; 40mcg/kg/min is maximum dose.

◆ Dose related increase in CO (the more drug given, the more the increase in CO).

Side effects

◆ Tachycardia (sinus, increased ventricular rate in atrial fibrillation or flutter).

◆ Reflex fall in SVR may cause hypotension.

◆ Headaches, tremors, anxiety.

◆ Tolerance can develop after prolonged infusion.

◆ Can cause myocardial ischemia due to increased contractility and HR.

◆ May cause ventricular arrhythmias.

◆ Can cause hypokalemia - monitor K^+ levels.

Special Considerations

◆ Half life = 2 minutes.

◆ Maximal effect 10-20 minutes after starting or changing infusion rate (must give drug time to work before evaluating its effects or changing infusion rate).

◆ Central line preferred.

◆ Must be titrated down before discontinuing if prolonged infusions are used.

Dopamine (Alpha & Beta Stimulation)

Dopamine is a precursor of norepinephrine and causes release of norepinephrine from cardiac nerve endings. It stimulates dopaminergic receptors at low doses, beta receptors at moderate doses, and alpha receptors at high doses.

Actions

◆ At lower doses (0.5-3 mcg/kg/min) dopamine dilates both afferent and efferent arterioles in the nephrons of the kidney. This results in an increase in renal blood flow and urine output, but there is little evidence that this has a renal protective effect. The previous notion that "renal dose" dopamine could prevent or treat renal failure is now outdated, although clinically, low dose dopamine is still sometimes used for renal perfusion.

613

Chapter 14

◆ At moderate doses (3-10 mcg/kg/min), dopamine stimulates β_1 receptors and primarily results in increased cardiac output.

◆ At higher doses, starting at about 10 mcg/kg/min, alpha effects predominate and dopamine causes peripheral vasoconstriction, but maintains its positive inotropic action on contractility.

◆ The maximum effective dose is 20 mcg/kg/min. There is no additional effect at doses higher than this, so if hypotension is still present at this dose, it is time to add or switch to another drug.

Indications

◆ Heart failure (low or moderate doses).

◆ Shock states.

◆ Keep dose as low as possible to prevent peripheral and renal vasoconstriction.

Dose

◆ Available IV only.

◆ Start at 0.5-1 mcg/kg/min and titrate up until desired effects achieved.

◆ Keep dose as low as possible for renal blood flow.

◆ Is a vasoconstrictor starting at about 10 mcg/kg/min.

Side Effects

◆ Nausea.

◆ Tachycardia, ventricular arrhythmias.

◆ Hypertension.

◆ Angina, myocardial ischemia due to increased HR and contractility.

◆ Can increase ventricular rate in atrial fibrillation or flutter.

◆ May depress ventilation and increase pulmonary shunting in hypoxic patients.

Special Considerations

◆ Half life = 2 minutes.

◆ Tissue necrosis can occur with extravasation; central line preferred.
  ❖ Phentolamine (Regitine) can be used to treat local extravasation. Dilute 5-10 mg of Regitine in 10 ml of NS and infiltrate area subcutaneously with approximately 1 ml of solution within 12 hours of extravasation. Do not exceed 0.1-0.2 mg/kg or 5 mg total. If dose is effective, normal skin color should return to the blanched area within 1 hour.

◆ Must be titrated down before being discontinued if higher doses are used.

Epinephrine (Alpha & Beta Stimulation)

Epinephrine (Adrenalin) stimulates both alpha and beta receptors and is a "selective" vasoconstrictor (it causes vasoconstriction in all vascular beds except heart, brain and skeletal muscle – the "fight or flight" response). At lower doses it is an inotrope and a vasodilator, and at higher doses it is a vasoconstrictor. It is also used in acute allergic reactions and anaphylactic shock, but only its use as a cardiovascular agent is discussed here.

Actions

◆ Beta stimulation = increased myocardial contractility.

◆ Alpha stimulation = selective vasoconstriction (everywhere except heart, brain, skeletal muscle).

Indications

◆ Blood pressure support and inotropic support in hypotension, often used following cardiac surgery.

◆ As a vasopressor in cardiac arrest.

Dose

◆ Can be used IV, SQ, IM intratracheal.

◆ IV infusion: 1-10 mcg/min (occasionally higher in severe cardiac dysfunction).

◆ At 20 mcg/min, it is pure alpha stimulator and causes peripheral vasoconstriction.

◆ 1 mg IV q 3-5 min in cardiac arrest.

◆ Intratracheal in intubated patients: use 2-2.5 mg via ET tube.

Side Effects

◆ Tachycardia.

◆ Hypertension.

◆ Headache.

◆ Can increase myocardial ischemia due to increased HR and contractility.

◆ Arrhythmias.

◆ Can increase ventricular rate in atrial fibrillation or flutter.

◆ Pulmonary edema.

Special Considerations

◆ Half life = 2 minutes.

◆ Tissue necrosis can occur with infiltration, central line preferred.

  ❖ Phentolamine (Regitine) can be used to treat local extravasation. Dilute 5-10 mg of Regitine in 10 ml of NS and infiltrate area subcutaneously with approximately 1 ml of solution within 12 hours of extravasation. Do not exceed 0.1-0.2 mg/kg or 5 mg total. If dose is effective, normal skin color should return to the blanched area within 1 hour.

Norepinephrine (Levophed) (Alpha & Beta Stimulation)

Levophed is very similar to epinephrine with equal beta stimulating effects, but it is a "nonselective" vasoconstrictor and results in constriction of most vascular beds. It is used most often in vasodilatory shock states to cause vasoconstriction and support the BP.

Actions

◆ Beta = increases contractility.

◆ Alpha = widespread vasoconstriction.

Indications

◆ BP support in vasodilated shock states (sepsis, neurogenic shock).

◆ BP support for severe hypotension.

Dose

◆ Available IV only, used as infusion.

◆ Infusion 8-12 mcg/min.

Chapter 14

Side Effects

◆ Tachycardia.

◆ Hypertension.

◆ Can increase myocardial ischemia due to increased HR and afterload.

◆ Can increase ventricular rate in atrial fibrillation or flutter.

Special Considerations

◆ Half life = 3 minutes.

◆ Tissue necrosis can occur with infiltration, central line preferred.

  ❖ Phentolamine (Regitine) can be used to treat local extravasation. Dilute 5-10 mg of Regitine in 10 ml of NS and infiltrate area subcutaneously with approximately 1 ml of solution within 12 hours of extravasation. Do not exceed 0.1-0.2 mg/kg or 5 mg total. If dose is effective, normal skin color should return to the blanched area within 1 hour.

Isoproterenol (Isuprel) (ß₁ and ß₂ Stimulation)

Isuprel stimulates both ß₁ and ß₂ receptors and has no alpha effect. It is used mostly in cardiac transplant patients because it has direct myocardial stimulation in the denervated heart. Its use outside of heart transplantation has dropped due to its side effects, primarily ventricular arrhythmias and hypotension.

Actions

◆ Stimulates ß₁ receptors in heart to increase contractility

◆ Stimulates ß₂ receptors in blood vessels to cause vasodilation.

Indications

◆ As an inotrope and to support HR and increase contractility following cardiac transplant.

◆ Sometimes used to support HR in patients with high grade or complete heart block until pacing can be instituted.

Dose

◆ Infusion at 0.5-10 mcg/min.

Side Effects

◆ Tachycardia.

◆ Hypotension.

◆ Arrhythmias, especially ventricular.

◆ Can cause myocardial ischemia due to increased HR.

◆ Headache, tremor, sweating.

Milrinone (Primacor)

Milrinone is a phosphodiesterase inhibitor that increases contractility and causes peripheral vasodilation by a different mechanism than sympathomimetic drugs. It offers inotropic support that is not mediated by beta receptors, so may be effective in patients on beta blockers or whose beta receptors are downregulated in chronic heart failure. Its vasodilation properties result in both preload and afterload reduction.

Cardiovascular Drugs

Actions

◆ Moderate inotrope.

◆ Potent vasodilator (arterial and venous).

Indications

◆ Acute heart failure.

◆ Inotropic support following cardiac surgery.

Dose

◆ Loading dose: IV dose of 50 mcg/kg over 10 minutes.

◆ Maintenance Infusion
   ❖ Minimum dose = .375 mcg/kg/min.
   ❖ Standard dose = .5 mcg/kg/min.
   ❖ Maximum dose = .75 mcg/kg/min.
   ❖ No need to titrate for effect.
   ❖ Reduce dose in renal failure.

Side Effects

◆ Hypotension.

◆ Ventricular arrhythmias.

◆ Headaches.

◆ Can increase ventricular rate in atrial fibrillation or flutter.

Contraindications

◆ Acute MI.

◆ Severe aortic stenosis.

◆ Hypertrophic obstructive cardiomyopathy.

Special Considerations

◆ Half life = 2.5 hours.

◆ Do not give lasix in same line – precipitate forms.

VASOPRESSORS

Vasopressors cause constriction of peripheral arteries and increase SVR and afterload. Levophed, epinephrine, and dopamine (high dose) are vasopressors, as well as positive inotropes, and are discussed above.

Phenylephrine (Neosynephrine) (Pure Alpha Stimulation)

Neosynephrine stimulates alpha receptors and has no beta effects. It causes peripheral vasoconstriction, which increases SVR and BP.

Actions

◆ Peripheral vasoconstriction.

◆ No direct cardiac effects, but indirectly increases afterload by causing increased SVR.

Chapter 14

Indications

◆ Used to support BP in vasodilated shock states (i.e. sepsis, neurogenic shock, anesthesia induced hypotension).

◆ Occasionally used to terminate SVT in patients who are very hypotensive. Its mechanism of action in this situation is to cause peripheral vasoconstriction and elevate BP, which stimulates baroreceptors and initiates a reflex stimulation of the vagus nerve to slow AV conduction.

Dose

◆ Can be used as bolus or IV infusion.

◆ Bolus dose for acute hypotension: 0.1-0.5 mg IV every 10-15 minutes as needed.

◆ Bolus dose for terminating SVT: 0.25-0.5 mg IV over 20-30 seconds.

◆ Infusion: start at 100-180 mcg/min to increase pressure.

◆ Maintenance infusion at 40-60 mcg/min.

◆ Drug is usually run for effect, so higher doses may be needed.

Side Effects

◆ Hypertension.

◆ Reflex bradycardia.

◆ Headache, anxiety, restlessness.

Special Considerations

◆ Tissue necrosis can occur with infiltration, central line preferred.

❖ Phentolamine (Regitine) can be used to treat local extravasation. Dilute 5-10 mg of Regitine in 10 ml of NS and infiltrate area subcutaneously with approximately 1 ml of solution within 12 hours of extravasation. Do not exceed 0.1-0.2 mg/kg or 5 mg total. If dose is effective, normal skin color should return to the blanched area within 1 hour.

Vasopressin (Antidiuretic Hormone - Pitressin)

Antidiuretic hormone is released from the posterior pituitary in response to hypovolemia, hypotension, high osmolality in the blood, and angiotensin II. The major action of ADH is to conserve body water by causing the renal tubules to reabsorb water. It also causes peripheral vasoconstriction, thus elevating BP and increasing afterload.

Actions

◆ Blood vessels = direct peripheral vasoconstriction.

◆ Kidneys = increased water reabsorption.

◆ No beta effects so no increase in myocardial O_2 consumption.

Clinical Uses

◆ Diabetes insipidus.

◆ GI bleeding.

◆ Cardiac arrest (VF/pulseless VT, asystole, PEA). May be used as alternative to first or second dose of epinephrine.

◆ Distributive shock states (i.e. sepsis).

◆ Any hypotensive or shock state not responsive to catecholamines.

Cardiovascular Drugs

Dose

◆ 40 units IV in cardiac arrest.

◆ Vasodilatory shock/septic shock: I.V infusion at 0.01-0.04 units/minute.

Side Effects

◆ Myocardial ischemia (high doses).

◆ Abdominal cramps, diarrhea, flatulence.

◆ Pale skin, perioral blanching.

◆ Toxicity = water intoxication (confusion, drowsiness, headache, weight gain, difficulty urinating, seizures, coma.

Linking Knowledge to Practice:

✔ *Patients who are taking beta blockers may not get an adequate response from drugs like dopamine, dobutamine, levophed, or epinephrine because the beta blocker interferes with the beta stimulating effects of those drugs. In such patients, a better response may be obtained by using a drug that is not a sympathomimetic agent, such as milrinone, for inotropic support.*

VASODILATORS

Drugs that dilate blood vessels, either veins, arteries, or both, are called vasodilators. Venous dilation reduces preload; arterial dilation reduces afterload. There are several mechanisms by which drugs can cause vasodilation:

1. ACE inhibitors and ARBs are vasodilators that reduce both preload and afterload by inhibition of the RAAS. (Used to treat heart failure and hypertension.)

2. Ca^{++} channel blockers (especially the dihydropyridines) inhibit Ca^{++} entry into the muscle layer of arterial blood vessels and result in arterial dilation and afterload reduction. (Used to treat hypertension and prevent spasm.)

3. Drugs that block post-synaptic alpha-1 receptors in peripheral arteries result in arterial dilation. Examples: prazosin (Minipres), terazosin (Hytrin), and doxazosin (Cardura). (Used to treat hypertension.)

4. Drugs that stimulate central or pre-synaptic alpha receptors cause peripheral dilation. Examples: clonidine (Catapres), guanfacine (Tenex), methyldopa (Aldomet). (Used to treat hypertension)

5. Drugs that directly dilate peripheral arteries (the mechanism of this action is not well understood) include hydralazine (Apresoline) and minoxidil (Loniten). (Used to treat hypertension.)

6. Phosphodiesterase inhibitors cause peripheral arterial and venous dilation as well as increased myocardial contractility. Example: milrinone (Primacor). (Used to treat heart failure, hypertension, and hypertensive emergencies.)

7. Drugs that increase nitric oxide in vascular tissue cause vasodilation. Examples: nitrates, which are primarily venous dilators; nitroprusside (Nipride) is a more balanced dilator with slightly more arterial than venous effect. (Used to treat heart failure and hypertension. Nipride is also used for hypertensive emergencies.)

Chapter 14

8. Nesiritide (Natrecor) is a recombinant preparation that is identical to the hormone BNP (B-type natriuretic peptide) that is produced by the ventricles in response to volume overload. Nesiritide causes both arterial and venous dilation and is used to treat acute decompensated heart failure.

Nitrates

Nitrates cause dilation of coronary arteries and peripheral arteries and veins, with relatively more venous dilation than arterial dilation. Their major benefit in treating angina is preload reduction, which reduces myocardial O_2 demand, and redistribution of coronary blood flow to collateral vessels in the heart to relieve ischemia. They can also relieve coronary artery spasm which can cause angina.

Indications

◆ Angina – acute treatment and prophylaxis, unstable angina.

◆ Heart failure – preload reduction in acute and chronic heart failure.

◆ Acute pulmonary edema.

Types of Nitrates

◆ Nitroglycerin: available in many forms, including sublingual, oral, spray, patch, ointment, IV.

◆ Isosorbide dinitrate (Isordil) – available in many forms, including sublingual, oral, spray, chewable tablet, IV. Longer acting than nitroglycerin and comes in a slow release form for angina prophylaxis.

Usual IV Dosage

◆ IV nitroglycerin: start at 5-10 mcg/min, increase by 5-10 mcg every 5-10 minutes to desired effect or maximal dose of 200 mcg/min (larger doses are sometimes used if tolerated).

◆ IV nitroglycerin is primarily a venous dilator at doses < 100 mcg/min. At higher doses there is arterial dilation as well.

◆ IV Isordil: 1.25-5 mg/hour.

Side Effects

◆ Hypotension.
◆ Headache.
◆ Syncope.
◆ Tachycardia (and sometimes bradycardia).
◆ Tolerance develops unless there is a nitrate-free period. Transdermal forms (patches, ointment) should be removed for 8-12 hours, usually at night. Long acting oral forms should be dosed eccentrically (i.e. at 8 AM and 3 PM, instead of evenly spaced every 12 hours) so that there is a nitrate-free period at night.

Contraindications

◆ Right ventricular infarction - preload reduction is contraindicated because the right ventricle needs adequate preload in order to send enough blood forward to left ventricle.

◆ Hypotension – systolic BP less than 90 mm Hg.

◆ Recent ingestion (24-48 hours) of drugs used to treat erectile dysfunction.

◆ Use with caution in obstructive cardiomyopathy – decreased LV volume can contribute to outflow tract obstruction.

Drug Interactions

◆ Drugs used for erectile dysfunction in combination with nitrates can precipitate profound hypotension. Male patients presenting with chest pain must be asked about the use of these drugs before administration of nitrates. It is recommended that nitrates not be used for 24 hours after taking sildenafil (Viagra) or vardenafil (Levitra), and 48 hours after taking tadalafil (Cialis).

◆ Heparin – high dose IV nitroglycerin can cause heparin resistance, requiring higher doses of heparin to maintain PTT at desired levels.

◆ Additive effects with other drugs that dilate blood vessels and can cause significant hypotension (Ca^{++} blockers, ACEI, ARBs, antihypertensives).

Nesiritide (Natrecor)

Nesiritide represents a new class of drug used to treat acute decompensated heart failure. It is a recombinant form of B-type natriuretic peptide (BNP), which is produced in the ventricles in response to stretch and volume overload.

Actions

◆ Arterial and venous dilation, resulting in preload reduction and afterload reduction.

◆ Causes diuresis (loss of H_2O) and natriuresis (loss of Na^+).

◆ No increase in HR, BP or myocardial O_2 demands.

◆ No inotropic effect and not arrhythmogenic.

◆ Symptomatic relief of dyspnea.

Indications

◆ Acute decompensated heart failure in patients with dyspnea at rest or with minimal activity (NYHA class III, IV).

Dosage and Administration

◆ IV bolus of 2 mcg/kg given over 1 minute, followed by infusion at 0.01 mcg/kg/min. Give in a dedicated line due to incompatibilities.

◆ **Initiation:** Mix one vial (1.5 mg) in 250 ml D_5W. Bolus dose is 2 mcg/kg removed from bag (NEVER directly from vial), using a weight-based dosing chart that comes with drug.

◆ **Continuous infusion:** 0.01 mcg/kg/min using dosing chart that comes with drug. Can increase up to 0.03 mcg/kg/min if tolerated.

Side Effects

◆ Hypotension.

◆ VT.

◆ Headache.

◆ Abdominal pain, nausea.

◆ When compared to IV NTG, the incidence of hypotension was about the same, but the duration was longer with Natrecor (about 2 hours) than with NTG.

◆ Recent concern has been raised about the effects of Nesiritide on increased risk of worsening renal failure and death after treatment of acutely decompensated heart failure (Sackner-Bernstein, Kowalski, Fox, & Aaronson, 2005; Sackner-Bernstein, Skopicki, & Aaronson, 2005).

Chapter 14

Contraindications

◆ SBP < 90 mm Hg.
◆ Cardiogenic shock.
◆ Hypovolemia.

Nitroprusside (Nipride)

Nipride is a rapid acting vasodilator that affects both arteries and veins to cause afterload and preload reduction, but its predominant effect is arterial dilation. It has a 1-3 minute duration of effect which makes it easy to titrate because changes in BP occur quickly, and effects disappear quickly when the drug is discontinued. It is very potent and some patients are very sensitive to it, which requires starting at a very low dose and titrating up, as tolerated.

Actions

◆ Arterial dilation (↓ afterload).
◆ Venous dilation (↓ preload).

Indications

◆ Severe LV failure.
◆ Mitral and aortic regurgitation – afterload reduction allows more blood to be ejected into the aorta and less back into the atrium in mitral regurgitation or back into the LV in aortic regurgitation.
◆ Dissecting aneurysm.
◆ Hypertensive emergencies.
◆ After cardiac surgery to treat hypertension.

Dosage and Administration

◆ Start slow – 0.25-2.5 mcg/kg/min.
◆ Increase as tolerated every 5-10 minutes until BP reaches desired level or until maximum dose is reached.
◆ Maximum dose is 10 mcg/kg/min. If BP is not controlled within 10 minutes at maximum dose, stop drug.

Side Effects

◆ Hypotension.
◆ Fatigue, nausea, vomiting.
◆ Cyanide toxicity (confusion, weakness, hyperreflexia, convulsions, disorientation, acidosis). Cyanide is a byproduct of Nipride metabolism and can accumulate to lethal levels with high doses or prolonged infusions, or with renal or liver failure.
◆ Hypoxia (due to ventilation-perfusion mismatch with pulmonary vasodilation).

Special Considerations

◆ Shield from light, change every 24 hours.
◆ Wean slowly to avoid withdrawal in heart failure.
◆ Monitor BP continuously during infusion.
◆ Do not administer at maximum dose (10 mcg/kg/min) for more than 10 minutes.

622

Cardiovascular Drugs

Linking Knowledge to Practice

✔ *The half life of a drug is the amount of time that it takes for the plasma concentration of the drug to fall to half its original level. Drugs with a long half life stay in the body longer than those with a short half life. It takes about 5 half lives for 95% of a drug to be eliminated, and about 7 half lives for 99% of a drug to be eliminated. Clinically, most drugs are considered to be "gone" in about 5 half lives. For example, amiodarone has a very long half life (average of 53 days) so it takes approximately 265 days for 95% of the drug to disappear; while adenosine has a half life of 9 seconds, so 95% of it is gone in 45 seconds.*

✔ *Most IV drugs that have cardiac and vascular effects need to be titrated down prior to discontinuation rather than terminated abruptly. Drugs with a short half life need to be titrated more slowly than drugs with a longer half life. Many vasoactive drugs like dopamine, dobutamine, and nitroprusside have a half life of about 2 minutes and should be weaned over a period of 2-3 hours while monitoring the patient's response as the infusion rate is decreased. Drugs like lidocaine and milrinone, with a half life of about 2 hours, can be discontinued and the body will "wean" the drug over the next few hours. If hypotension or other adverse effects occur when a drug is initiated, it can be discontinued immediately.*

✔ *Older patients have reduced drug clearance due to decreased renal or hepatic function and need to be monitored for signs of drug accumulation and toxicity.*

ANTITHROMBOTIC DRUGS

Thrombus formation in a coronary artery is the most common cause of acute myocardial infarction. Thrombus formation begins with injury to vascular endothelium that activates platelet activity and triggers the clotting cascade to cause a blood clot that can occlude the vessel. This process can be interrupted at several stages of thrombus formation, including inhibition of platelet activity, inhibition of the clotting cascade, and breakdown of the thrombus once it is formed. Three types of antithrombotic drugs are discussed here: antiplatelet drugs, anticoagulants, and fibrinolytics.

Information on the coagulation cascade and drugs that inhibit it comes from the following sources listed in the references: (Abrams, 2005; Brunton, Lazo, & Parker, 2006; Guyton & Hall, 2000; Leung, 2004).

The Role of Platelets in Acute Coronary Syndrome

Rupture of atherosclerotic plaque is a trigger for thrombus formation in an artery. Plaque rupture can occur spontaneously or can be caused by interventional procedures such as angioplasty, atherectomy, or stent deployment in the artery. Platelets respond to rupture by first adhering to the ruptured area (platelet adhesion) by binding to von Willebrand factor, after which they are activated by collagen that is exposed at the site of rupture and by tissue factor released from the ruptured plaque. Activated platelets change their shape and express GP IIb/IIIa receptor sites that bind to circulating fibrinogen; the fibrinogen then binds to a receptor site on another activated platelet, allowing the platelets to stick together (platelet aggregation). Activated platelets also secrete substances, such as thromboxane A2 and adenosine diphosphate (ADP), which stimulate further platelet activation and perpetuate the formation of the platelet plug ("white clot"), as well as substances that activate the clotting cascade and contribute to thrombus formation.

Figure 14.7 illustrates a plaque rupturing in a coronary artery and platelets coming in contact with substances released by the plaque. Platelets change shape as the GP IIb/IIIa receptors are formed, and fibrinogen is able to bind one platelet's receptor to another platelet's receptor, resulting in platelet aggregation.

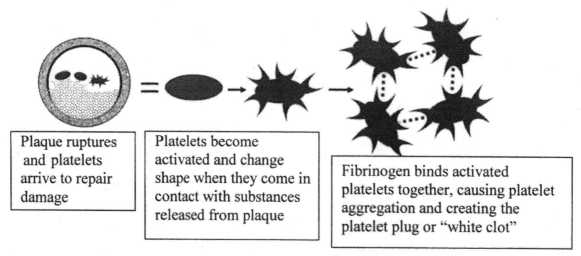

Figure 14.7: Plaque rupture in coronary artery.

Figure 14.8 (A) illustrates several pathways by which platelets can become activated. The final common pathway is formation of the GP IIb/IIIa receptor sites which allow fibrinogen to bind platelets together (platelet aggregation). (B) shows the site of action of GP IIb/IIIa platelet inhibitors: abciximab (Reopro), eptifibatide (Integrilin), and tirofiban (Aggrastat).

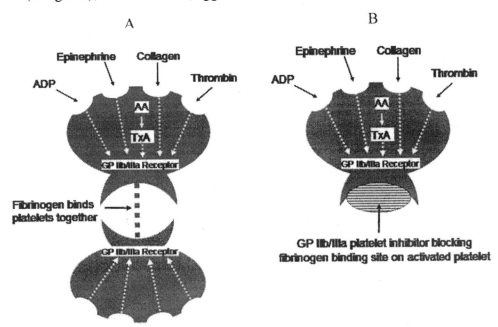

Figure 14.8: Pathways for platelet activation.

The Role of the Coagulation Cascade in Clot Formation

Blood clot formation is a complicated process involving a cascade of chemical reactions in the blood that results in the formation of fibrin fibers that trap red blood cells, platelets, and plasma to form a clot. Traditionally this process is described in terms of an intrinsic and an extrinsic pathway by which the coagulation cascade becomes activated. It is now thought that the primary physiologic event that initiates clotting is stimulation of the extrinsic pathway by tissue damage, and that the intrinsic pathway plays a less important role (Leung, 2004; Opie & Gersh, 2005). Vessel wall damage or ruptured plaque initiates clot formation via the extrinsic pathway in ACS, so this review is limited to the role of the extrinsic pathway in blood clot formation.

Plaque rupture or damage to the vascular endothelium initiates platelet adhesion, activation, and aggregation, as described above. In addition, tissue factor (TF) is released from the damaged tissue and triggers the initiation of clotting in the following way:

◆ Tissue factor binds with blood coagulation factor VII to create the activated form of factor VII, called VIIa.

◆ Factor VIIa causes coagulation factor X to convert to its active form, Xa.

◆ Factor Xa combines with TF, factor V, and substances released from activated platelets to form a complex called prothrombin activator.

◆ Prothrombin activator, in the presence of Ca^{++}, causes the conversion of prothrombin (which is formed in the liver) to thrombin.

- Thrombin causes conversion of fibrinogen (also formed in the liver) to fibrin strands; and fibrin strands create the meshwork that traps red blood cells, more platelets, and plasma to form the clot.
    - Thrombin is also a powerful stimulant for platelet activation, which causes further aggregation of platelets at the site of injury; it accelerates the actions of clotting factors VIII, IX, X, XI to perpetuate clot formation (Guyton & Hall, 2000; Opie & Gersh, 2005).

Figure 14.9 illustrates the extrinsic pathway and the sites of action of heparin and warfarin.

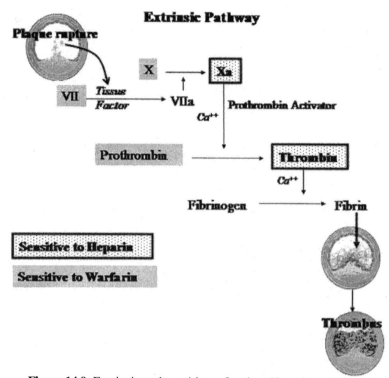

Figure 14.9: Extrinsic pathway/sites of action. Heparin and Warfarin.

Fibrinolysis – The Breakdown of Blood Clots

If allowed to proceed unchecked, the clotting cascade would lead to extensive clot formation in the vascular system and result in tissue damage. The process of blood clot formation is balanced by several control mechanisms that turn off the clotting cascade. One of the most important inhibitors of coagulation is antithrombin, which is a circulating substance that inactivates thrombin and several clotting factors to prevent further clot formation after the initial bleeding at the site of injury has been controlled.

Once blood clots have been formed, they can be broken down and removed from the blood vessel by a process called fibrinolysis (or thrombolysis). The removal of small blood clots by this system restores patency of blood vessels and allows blood to continue to circulate.

- During clot formation, plasminogen is trapped in the clot, along with other plasma proteins and clotting factors.
    - When activated, plasminogen converts to plasmin, which is the substance that dissolves clots by breaking down the fibrin strands, as well as by digesting many of the clotting factors involved in clot formation.

◆ Tissue plasminogen activator (t-PA) is released slowly by the injured tissue and vascular endothelium about a day after the clot has stopped the bleeding, causing plasminogen to convert to plasmin, which then dissolves the blood clot and re-establishes flow through the vessel.

❖ During ACS, drugs that stimulate the fibrinolytic system (e.g. tPA and its derivatives) can be given to dissolve the clot and restore vessel patency.

The Role of Antithrombotic Drugs

Antithrombotic drugs interrupt the clotting process by interfering with platelet activation, platelet aggregation, or the clotting cascade itself, or by breaking down the clot once it has formed.

◆ Drugs that interfere with platelet activation include:
  ❖ Aspirin (ASA).
  ❖ Clopidogrel (Plavix).
  ❖ Heparin.
◆ Drugs that interfere with platelet aggregation are the glycoprotein IIb/IIIa inhibitors:
  ❖ Abciximab (Reopro).
  ❖ Eptifibatide (Integrilin).
  ❖ Tirofiban (Aggrastat).
◆ Drugs that interfere with the clotting cascade include:
  ❖ Heparin – inhibits thrombin.
  ❖ Warfarin (Coumadin) – interferes with prothrombin formation in the liver.
  ❖ Direct thrombin inhibitors (argatroban, bivalirudin, lepirudin).
  ❖ Indirect Factor Xa inhibitors (fondaparinux).
◆ Drugs that break down clots are called fibrinolytic (or thrombolytic) agents. They include:
  ❖ Tissue plasminogen activator (tPA).
    ☆ Alteplase (tPA).
    ☆ Tenecteplase (TNK-tPA).
    ☆ Reteplase (R-tPA).
  ❖ Streptokinase.
  ❖ APSAC (anisoylated plasminogen streptokinase activator complex).
  ❖ Urokinase (used primarily for acute peripheral arterial occlusion).

Antiplatelet Drugs

Aspirin (ASA)

Actions

Aspirin interferes with the formation of thromboxane A_2 inside the platelet by inhibiting cyclooxygenase (COX-1), an effect that lasts for the lifespan of the platelet. Since thromboxane A_2 is one of the pathways of platelet activation, ASA inhibition of this pathway ultimately inhibits platelet aggregation. Aspirin also has anti-inflammatory effects that may contribute to its cardiovascular protection.

Indications

◆ Acute coronary syndrome – including unstable angina, the acute phase of MI, and as follow-up therapy after AMI.
  ❖ Aspirin should be administered as soon as possible after presentation and continued indefinitely (Antman et al., 2004; Braunwald et al., 2002).
◆ Secondary prevention in patients with prior MI and stable angina.

Chapter 14

◆ After ischemic stroke.

◆ After coronary artery bypass surgery.

◆ After percutaneous interventional cardiology (PCI) procedures.

◆ Atrial fibrillation for stroke prevention when warfarin cannot be taken, or in patients at low risk for stroke.

◆ Artificial heart valves to prevent embolization.

Dose

◆ In acute MI: initial dose of 162-325 mg chewed as soon after symptom onset as possible.
   ❖ Maintenance dose: 75-162 mg PO daily.

◆ After CABG surgery: 75-325 mg PO daily, starting within 24 hours after surgery when possible.

◆ After PCI with stent placement: 325 mg daily for 1 month with bare metal stent, 3 months with sirolimus stent, and 6 months with paclitaxel stent. Continue 75-162 mg daily indefinitely.

◆ For secondary prevention in ischemic stroke: 75-162 mg daily indefinitely.

Side Effects

◆ Bleeding – especially GI and GU.

◆ GI symptoms – nausea, dyspepsia, vomiting.

◆ Impaired renal function – especially in elderly.

◆ Decreased excretion of uric acid – especially in elderly.

Contraindications

◆ Inherited or acquired bleeding disorders.

◆ History of GI bleeding.

◆ Peptic ulcer disease.

◆ Asthma.

◆ Aspirin intolerance.

◆ Pregnancy (especially 3rd trimester).

◆ Thrombocytopenia.

Drug Interactions

◆ Ibuprofen interferes with cardioprotective effects of ASA by competing for a common binding site on COX-1. This effect may be mitigated by taking ibuprofen at least two hours after ASA.

◆ ACE inhibitors promote formation of vasodilatory prostaglandins, while ASA inhibits their formation, so ASA may reduce the effects of ACE inhibitors. This interaction does not contraindicate the use of these two types of drugs together in heart failure or hypertension.

◆ Alcohol, steroids, and other non-steroidal anti-inflammatory drugs may increase the potential for GI bleeding.

◆ Thiazide diuretic and ASA combination may increase the risk of gout.

Clopidogrel (Plavix)

Actions

Plavix irreversibly inhibits the ADP pathway of platelet activation, which ultimately prevents formation of the GP IIb/IIIa receptor on the platelet, therefore preventing platelet aggregation.

Indications

◆ In acute coronary syndrome –with or without PCI or CABG (Antman et al., 2004; Braunwald et al., 2002).

Cardiovascular Drugs

❖ In patients who are unable to take ASA because of hypersensitivity or GI intolerance.

❖ In patients for whom an early non-interventional approach is planned and in those for whom PCI is planned and are not at high risk for bleeding, added as soon as possible and continued for at least one month up to 9 months.

❖ If elective CABG is planned, the drug should be stopped for 5-7 days prior to surgery.

◆ Reduction of atherosclerotic events (MI, stroke, vascular death) in patients with atherosclerosis documented by recent MI, recent stroke, or established peripheral arterial disease (PAD).

◆ Investigational use - prevention of CABG saphenous vein graft closure.

Dose

◆ Loading dose: 300-600 mg PO in patients with non-ST-elevation MI (NSTEMI) and in patients having PCI, unless urgent CABG is planned.

❖ 600 mg dose has maximal platelet inhibition at 2 hours.

❖ 300 mg dose has maximal platelet inhibition in 24-48 hours.

❖ For prevention of saphenous vein bypass graft closure – 300 mg 6 hours after procedure.

◆ Maintenance dose: 75 mg PO daily.

❖ Continue for a minimum of one month, ideally up to one year after bare metal stent.

❖ Continue for at least 12 months after a drug eluting stent.

Side Effects

◆ Bleeding – increased risk when used with ASA or other antiplatelet drugs.

◆ GI problems – abdominal pain, dyspepsia, gastritis, constipation.

Contraindications

◆ Active bleeding.

◆ Coagulation disorders.

Abciximab (Reopro)

Actions

Reopro is a GP IIb/IIIa receptor inhibitor that blocks the final common pathway to platelet aggregation by preventing fibrinogen from binding with the GP IIb/IIIa receptors on the platelet membrane.

Indications

◆ PCI – to inhibit platelet aggregation during the procedure and up to 12 hours following.

❖ A platelet GP IIb/IIIa inhibitor should be administered, in addition to ASA and heparin, to patients in whom PCI is planned (can be given just prior to PCI) (Braunwald et al., 2002; Popma et al., 2004).

❖ It is reasonable to start treatment with abciximab as early as possible before primary PCI, with or without stenting, in patients with ST elevation myocardial infarction (STEMI) (Antman et al., 2004).

◆ Unstable angina not responding to medical therapy, with PCI planned within 24 hours (Opie & Gersh, 2005; Popma et al., 2004).

Dose

◆ For PCI: 0.25 mg/kg bolus 10-60 minutes prior to PCI, then 0.125 mcg/kg/min (maximum of 10 mcg/kg/min) for 12 hours.

◆ For ACS: same bolus dose and infusion rate up to 24 hours. Stop 1 hour after PCI.

629

Chapter 14

Side Effects

◆ Bleeding - drug is administered with heparin and with ASA, which compounds bleeding risk.

◆ Thrombocytopenia - rare but serious side effect, especially when used with heparin.

Contraindications

◆ Active internal bleeding or recent GI or GU bleeding within 6 weeks.

◆ History of CVA within 2 years.

◆ Thrombocytopenia.

◆ Major surgery or trauma within 6 weeks.

◆ Intracranial tumor, AV malformation or cerebral aneurysm.

◆ Severe uncontrolled hypertension.

◆ Not to be given with other GP IIb/IIIa agents.

Special Considerations

◆ Draw bolus through filter and administer infusion with filtered IV set.

◆ Monitor platelet counts: before starting drug, 2-4 hours after bolus, at 24 hours or before discharge.

Eptifibatide (Integrilin)

Actions

Integrilin is a GP IIb/IIIa receptor inhibitor that blocks the final common pathway to platelet aggregation by preventing fibrinogen from binding with the GP IIb/IIIa receptors on the platelet membrane. It has lower affinity for these receptors than the other GP IIb/IIIa agents, so doses are higher.

Indications

◆ Acute coronary syndromes – unstable angina, NSTEMI, with or without PCI (Braunwald et al., 2002).

❖ Eptifibatide or tirofiban should be administered to patients with continuing ischemia, an elevated troponin, or other high-risk features in whom an invasive strategy is not planned.

◆ PCI – to inhibit platelet aggregation during and after procedure up to 24 hours or hospital discharge, whichever comes first (Antman et al., 2004; Braunwald et al., 2002; Popma et al., 2004).

❖ A platelet GP IIb/IIIa inhibitor should be administered, in addition to ASA and heparin, to patients in whom PCI is planned (can be given just prior to PCI).

❖ Treatment with tirofiban or eptifibatide may be considered before primary PCI, with or without stenting, in patients with STEMI.

Dose

◆ For ACS: bolus of 180 mcg/kg (maximum 22.6 mg) over 1-2 minutes, then infusion at 2 mcg/kg/min (maximum 15 mg/hr) up to 72 hours.

❖ If PCI done, continue infusion 18-24 hours after PCI.

◆ For PCI: 180 mcg/kg bolus (maximum 22.6 mg) just before PCI, infusion at 2 mcg/kg/min, repeat bolus in 10 minutes, continue infusion for 12-24 hours.

◆ Reduce infusion to 1 mcg/kg/min in renal disease.

Side Effects

◆ Bleeding - drug is administered with heparin and with ASA, which compounds bleeding risk.

◆ Thrombocytopenia - rare but serious side effect, especially when used with heparin.

Cardiovascular Drugs

Contraindications

◆ Active bleeding or history of bleeding diathesis within 30 days.

◆ History of CVA within 30 days, history of hemorrhagic stroke.

◆ Severe uncontrolled hypertension.

◆ Major surgery within 6 weeks.

◆ Do not give with other GP IIb/IIIa inhibitors.

Special Considerations

◆ Monitor platelet counts: before starting drug, 2-4 hours after bolus, at 24 hours or before discharge.

Tirofiban (Aggrastat)

Action

Aggrastat is a GP IIb/IIIa receptor inhibitor that blocks the final common pathway to platelet aggregation by preventing fibrinogen from binding with the GP IIb/IIIa receptors on the platelet membrane.

Indications

◆ Acute coronary syndrome – with or without PCI (Antman et al., 2004; Braunwald et al., 2002).

  ❖ Eptifibatide or tirofiban should be administered to patients with continuing ischemia, an elevated troponin, or other high-risk features in whom an invasive strategy is not planned.

  ❖ A platelet GP IIb/IIIa inhibitor should be administered, in addition to ASA and heparin, to patients in whom PCI is planned (can be given just prior to PCI).

  ❖ Treatment with tirofiban or eptifibatide may be considered before primary PCI, with or without stenting, in patients with STEMI.

Dose

◆ Infusion of 0.4 mcg/kg/min for 30 minutes, then 0.1 mcg/kg/min for 12-24 hours after PCI.

◆ Reduce dose if renal disease.

Side Effects

◆ Bleeding – drug is administered with heparin and with ASA, which compounds bleeding risk.

◆ Thrombocytopenia – rare but serious side effect, especially when used with heparin.

Contraindications

◆ Active bleeding or history of bleeding diathesis within 30 days.

◆ History intracranial neoplasm, AV malformation, cerebral aneurysm.

◆ History of CVA within 30 days or any history of hemorrhagic stroke.

◆ Severe uncontrolled hypertension.

◆ Major surgery or trauma within 4 weeks.

◆ Do not give with other GP IIb/IIIa inhibitors.

Special Considerations

◆ Monitor platelet counts: before starting drug, 2-4 hours after bolus, at 24 hours or before discharge.

Anticoagulant Drugs

Heparin

Actions

Heparin has both anticoagulant and antiplatelet effects. As an anticoagulant, heparin binds to antithrombin and accelerates its ability to inactivate circulating thrombin and other clotting factors in the coagulation cascade. Since thrombin is a strong platelet activator, its inhibition by heparin also blocks a major

Chapter 14

pathway of platelet activation. Heparin also binds to and inhibits von Willebrand factor to prevent platelet adhesion and activation. Heparin has no effect on thrombin that is bound to fibrin in the clot, and is susceptible to inactivation by circulating inhibitors released from activated platelets. Its ability to bind to platelet factor 4 (PF4) can cause heparin induced thrombocytopenia (HIT), discussed in the section on side effects below.

Types of Heparin
◆ Unfractionated heparin (UFH)
  ❖ Long chains that are capable of binding with antithrombin to inhibit thrombin as well as inhibiting the actions of other clotting factors (especially Xa).
  ❖ Obtained from bovine lung or porcine intestinal mucosa.
  ❖ UFH also binds to several other proteins and has highly variable dose-effect relationship from person to person, requiring frequent laboratory monitoring of its anticoagulant effects.
  ❖ Activity is monitored by activated partial thromboplastin time (aPTT) and by anti-factor Xa activity (HEPACT). Platelet counts should be monitored.
  ❖ Must be given IV or SQ.
◆ Low molecular weight heparin (LMWH)
  ❖ Derived from cleavage of UFH into shorter chains, most of which are not long enough to bind with antithrombin but do inhibit factor Xa.
  ❖ Activity cannot be monitored by aPTT because of limited antithrombin activity, but can be monitored by anti-factor Xa activity (HEPACT).
  ❖ Has a more consistent anticoagulant effect than UFH because of reduced binding to other proteins, longer duration of anticoagulant effect, good correlation between anticoagulant response and body weight.
  ❖ Given SQ once daily or every 12 hours.
  ❖ Laboratory monitoring not necessary due to consistent anticoagulant effect.
  ❖ Considered equivalent to or preferable to UFH for most indications.
  ❖ Two most commonly used: enoxaparin (Lovenox), dalteparin (Fragmin). They are not interchangeable.

Indications
◆ Acute coronary syndrome
  ❖ Unstable angina and NSTEMI- with ASA to help prevent MI (Braunwald et al., 2002).
    ✰ Subcutaneous LMWH or IV UFH should be added to antiplatelet therapy with ASA and/or Clopidogrel.
    ✰ Enoxaparin is preferable to UFH in patients with UA/NSTEMI in the absence of renal failure and unless CABG is planned within 24 hours.
  ❖ Acute MI - in addition to thrombolysis or PCI (Antman et al., 2004).
    ✰ UFH in patients undergoing reperfusion therapy with alteplase, reteplase, or tenecteplase.
    ✰ UFH given IV to patients treated with nonselective fibrinolytic agents (streptokinase, anistreplase) who are at high risk for systemic emboli (large or anterior MI, atrial fibrillation, previous embolus, known LV thrombus).
    ✰ LMWH can be an alternative to UFH in patients less than 75 years old receiving fibrinolytic therapy, if significant renal dysfunction not present.

632

Cardiovascular Drugs

- PCI
    - As an adjunct to prevent acute closure due to clot formation at the site of intervention.
- Prevention and treatment of deep vein thrombosis (DVT).
- Treatment of pulmonary embolism.

Dose
- UFH
    - When used with fibrinolytic therapy: bolus of 60 Units/kg IV (maximum 4000 Units), followed by infusion of 12 Units/kg/hr (maximum 1000 Units/hr), adjusted to keep aPTT at 1.5 to 2.0 times control (approximately 50-60 seconds) (Antman et al., 2004).
    - When used without fibrinolytics: bolus of 60-70 Units/kg IV, followed by infusion at 12-15 Units/kg/hr to keep aPTT 1.5-2.0 times control (Antman et al., 2004).
    - With PCI: keep activated clotting time (ACT) 250-350 seconds if no GP IIb/IIIa platelet inhibitor used; 200-250 seconds if GP IIb/IIIa used (Popma et al., 2004).
- LMWH
    - Enoxaparin (Lovenox) – 1 mg/kg SQ every 12 hours.
    - Dalteparin (Fragmin) – 120 IU/kg (max: 10,000 IU) SC every 12 hours for 5-8 days, beginning within 72 hours of the onset of symptoms.

Side Effects
- Bleeding
    - Increased risk in patients with peptic ulcers, liver disease, hematological disorders, subacute bacterial endocarditis, severe uncontrolled hypertension, thrombocytopenia, age greater than 65 in women.
    - UFH can be reversed with protamine (1 mg/100 units of heparin).
    - LMWH is only partially reversed with protamine.
- Osteoporosis – if UFH given for more than 6 months.
- Heparin induced thrombocytopenia (HIT) (Coutre, 2005; Warkentin, 2004).
    - Type I – nonimmune drop in platelet count that occurs within 2 days after heparin initiation and returns to normal with no clinical consequences.
    - Type II – dangerous immune-mediated disorder that occurs usually 4-10 days after heparin is started and involves formation of antibodies against the heparin-platelet factor 4 (PF4) complex. This heparin-PF4-antibody complex binds to platelets, causing further platelet activation and thrombin generation that results in intravascular thrombosis. The activated platelets aggregate and are removed from the circulation, leading to thrombocytopenia. HIT is considered to be an acquired hypercoagulability syndrome and occurs more often with UFH than with LMWH.
        - Occurs in 0.3-3% of patients who receive heparin for more than 4 days. Rapid-onset HIT (large platelet count reduction within 24 hours of starting heparin) may occur in patients who have circulating antibodies due to previous exposure to heparin within the last 100 days (especially within the last month).
        - Platelet count usually falls by 50% or more from baseline - this is the initial sign of HIT.
        - HIT results in both arterial and venous thrombosis that can result in DVT, pulmonary embolism, limb gangrene, stroke, MI, and other organ infarction.
        - Treatment of HIT includes discontinuing all heparin products (including heparin coated catheters and heparin flushes), and use of direct thrombin inhibitors, such as lepirudin (Refludan) or argatroban (Novastan) to manage intravascular clotting.

Chapter 14

Contraindications
◆ Active bleeding.
◆ Severe thrombocytopenia.
◆ Suspected intracranial hemorrhage.
◆ Hypersensitivity to heparin or any components.

Special Considerations
◆ Monitor platelet counts, Hb, Hct.
◆ Adjust dose based on aPTT, HEPACT, or ACT.

Direct Thrombin Inhibitors
Actions
Direct thrombin inhibitors (DTI) are highly specific for both soluble and clot-bound thrombin, binding directly to thrombin rather than depending on antithrombin as heparin does. Because they do not bind to PF4, they do not cause HIT.

Types and Indications
◆ Argatroban (Novastat)
  ❖ Prophylaxis or treatment of thrombosis in adults with HIT.
  ❖ Adjunct to PCI in patients who have or are at risk of thrombosis associated with HIT.
◆ Bivalirudin (Angiomax)
  ❖ Approved as an alternative to heparin in patients with STEMI and NSTEMI/ UA who undergo PCI.
  ❖ Can consider as an alternative to UFH in patients who are treated with streptokinase and who have known HIT.
◆ Lepirudin (Refludan)
  ❖ Anticoagulation in patients with HIT and associated thromboembolic disease in order to prevent further thromboembolic complications.

Dose
◆ Argatroban
  ❖ Prophylaxis of thrombosis in HIT
    ☆ Initial dose: IV infusion at 2 mcg/kg/minute.
    ☆ Maintenance dose: adjusted according to aPTT or HEPACT. See drug insert for specific dosing information.
  ❖ PCI
    ☆ Bolus dose of 350 mcg/kg (over 3-5 minutes) and IV infusion of 25 mcg/kg/minute. ACT should be checked 5-10 minutes after bolus infusion; proceed with procedure if ACT >300 seconds.
    ☆ Maintenance dose: adjusted according to aPTT or HEPACT. See drug insert for specific dosing information.
◆ Bivalirudin
  ❖ During PCI
    ☆ Initial bolus of 0.75 mg/kg.
    ☆ IV infusion of 1.75 mg/kg/hour for the duration of procedure up to 4 hours post-procedure.
    ☆ Infusion may be continued beyond initial 4 hours at 0.2 mg/kg/hour for up to 20 hours, if needed.

❖ See drug insert for more specific dosing information.

◆ Lepirudin (Refludan)
  ❖ Use in HIT.
    ★ Bolus dose: 0.4 mg/kg IV (over 15-20 seconds).
    ★ Continuous infusion at 0.15 mg/kg/hour.
  ❖ Use in PCI.
    ★ Bolus dose: 0.2 mg/kg IVP (over 15-20 seconds).
    ★ Continuous infusion at 0.1 mg/kg/hour.
  ❖ See drug insert for more specific dosing information.

Side Effects
◆ Bleeding.

Contraindications
◆ Active bleeding.
◆ Sensitivity to drug or any component.

Warfarin (Coumadin)

Action
Coumadin inactivates vitamin K in the liver and interferes with the production of prothrombin and several other clotting factors (factors II, VII, IX, and X). The anticoagulant effect of coumadin is delayed until the normal clotting factors are cleared from the circulation, and the components of the intrinsic coagulation pathway are also reduced. Because of the long half-life of prothrombin, the onset of action of coumadin can be delayed for 2-7 days. Heparin and coumadin treatment should overlap by four to five days, when warfarin is initiated in patients with thrombotic disease, to allow time for the vitamin K dependent coagulation factors to be inactivated. Coumadin is the most commonly used oral anticoagulant, with excellent absorption and a consistent half-life of about 37 hours (Opie & Gersh, 2005). Effectiveness is monitored by the international normalized ratio (INR), discussed below.

Indications
◆ MI
  ❖ For 3-6 months after MI in patients at high risk for systemic embolization due to atrial fibrillation, heart failure, low ejection fraction, large anterior wall MI, or prior venous thromboembolism.
◆ DVT or pulmonary embolism (PE)
  ❖ For 3-6 months or longer after initial occurrence to prevent recurrent thrombosis.
  ❖ For prevention of DVT after orthopedic or gynecologic surgery.
◆ Atrial fibrillation
  ❖ In patients with atrial fibrillation of > 48 hours or unknown duration, anticoagulation with coumadin for 3 weeks prior to chemical or electrical cardioversion; continued for at least 4 more weeks.
  ❖ Chronic therapy in patients with chronic atrial fibrillation.
◆ Prosthetic heart valves (Bonow et al., 2006)
  ❖ Chronic therapy in patients with mechanical prosthetic valves.

Chapter 14

- ❖ For the first 3 months after biologic prosthetic valves, then either ASA or coumadin, depending on location of valve and associated risk factors (atrial fibrillation, LV dysfunction, previous thromboembolism, hypercoagulable condition):
  - ☆ For bioprosthesis in mitral or aortic position and no risk factors = ASA.
  - ☆ For bioprosthesis in aortic position and risk factors = coumadin, INR 2-3.
  - ☆ For bioprosthesis in mitral position and risk factors = coumadin, INR 2.5-3.5.

Dose

- ◆ The usual adult dose of coumadin is 5 mg per day for 5 days, followed by 2 to 10 mg per day, as indicated by measurements of the INR (see special considerations below).
- ◆ Lower starting doses may be required for patients with hepatic impairment, poor nutrition, HF, elderly, or a high risk of bleeding.
- ◆ Higher starting doses (10 - 15 mg daily) can be used if an urgent effect is needed, but it is preferable to avoid large initial doses.
- ◆ Coumadin must be started at least 4 days before heparin is discontinued to allow time for inactivation of vitamin K-dependent coagulation factors.

Side Effects

- ◆ Bleeding – risk increases with intensity (dose) and duration of therapy.
- ◆ Skin necrosis
  - ❖ Rare complication involving appearance of skin lesions 3-10 days after coumadin started.
  - ❖ Due to widespread thrombosis of microvasculature, can spread and become necrotic.
- ◆ Birth defects can occur if given during pregnancy.
- ◆ There are many drug interactions with coumadin.

Contraindications

- ◆ Bleeding.
- ◆ Uncontrolled hypertension.
- ◆ Recent stroke.
- ◆ Hepatic cirrhosis.
- ◆ Potential GI or GU bleeding (peptic ulcers, gastritis, cyctitis, colitis, proctitis).

Special Considerations

- ◆ INR is used to monitor effectiveness.
  - ❖ INR is based on the patient's PT drawn 8-14 hours after the last dose of coumadin. The PT is compared to a World Health Organization Standard.
  - ❖ The target INR depends on the condition being treated; in general, it is between 2 and 3 for DVT or PE.
  - ❖ In high risk situations (like prosthetic valves), the INR range is 2.5-3.5, sometimes up to 4.5.
  - ❖ In low risk patients (like nonvalvular atrial fibrillation), it can be 1.5.
- ◆ Bleeding precautions:
  - ❖ Watch for bleeding from puncture sites, gums, nose.
  - ❖ Check urine and stools for blood.
  - ❖ Monitor for mental status changes.
  - ❖ Avoid unnecessary venous punctures (use heparin lock for blood draws); hold puncture sites or bleeding areas for at least 10 minutes.

◆ Be aware of multiple drug interactions and disease processes that can either potentiate or block the effects of coumadin.

◆ Dietary considerations:

❖ Foods high in vitamin K (eg, beef liver, pork liver, green tea and leafy green vegetables) inhibit anticoagulant effect.

❖ Avoid large amounts of alfalfa, asparagus, broccoli, Brussels sprouts, cabbage, cauliflower, green teas, kale, lettuce, spinach, turnip greens, watercress.

❖ Do not change dietary habits once stabilized on warfarin therapy.

❖ It is recommended that the diet contain a consistent vitamin K content of 70-140 mcg/day.

◆ Management of overdose and bleeding (Opie & Gersh, 2005):

❖ Minor bleeding: reduce dose or discontinue temporarily until INR is down to 2.0-3.0.

❖ Significant bleeding or INR > 9.0: give 3-5 mg of oral vitamin K to reduce INR within 24-48 hours.

❖ In emergency: 5-10 mg vitamin K IV over 30 minutes. Fresh frozen plasma can be used if immediate reversal is needed.

❖ Vitamin K should be avoided in patients with prosthetic valves unless there is life-threatening intracranial bleed.

Fibrinolytics (Thrombolytics)

Fibrinolytic therapy is used clinically to treat arterial and venous thromboembolic disorders, including MI, stroke, and pulmonary embolism. The goal in AMI is early reperfusion of the occluded artery to reestablish blood flow to the myocardium, which has been shown to limit infarct size, preserve left ventricular function, and reduce mortality. Fibrinolytic agents accomplish this by dissolving the thrombus that is responsible for the occlusion.

Actions

Fibrinolytic agents accelerate the conversion of plasminogen, an inactive precursor, to plasmin, an enzyme that breaks up fibrin strands and dissolves the clot.

Types of Fibrinolytics (See Table 14.8)

◆ Tissue plasminogen activators

❖ **Alteplase** (recombinant tissue-type plasminogen activator, tPA) – naturally occurring enzyme produced by several tissues, including endothelial cells. It binds directly to fibrin in the clot and converts entrapped plasminogen to plasmin, which breaks down fibrin strands and dissolves the clot. Non-fibrin-bound tPA in the systemic circulation does not extensively activate plasminogen.

❖ **Reteplase** (recombinant plasminogen activator, rPA) – less fibrin selective and has a longer half-life than alteplase.

❖ **Tenecteplase** (TNK-tPA) – genetically engineered mutant of tPA with a longer plasma half-life and is more fibrin specific than alteplase.

◆ Streptokinase is a single chain polypeptide derived from beta-hemolytic streptococcus cultures. It binds to plasminogen to form a complex that becomes an enzyme that converts plasminogen to plasmin. High doses are necessary to counteract antistreptococcal antibodies in the blood. Streptokinase is antigenic and can cause allergic reactions, particularly with repeat administration.

◆ Urokinase is a nonselective plasminogen activator that activates fibrin-bound and circulating plasminogen. Urokinase is used primarily in the management of pulmonary embolism, but can also be used to treat DVT and occluded IV catheters.

Chapter 14

Indications

◆ Patients with chest pain suggestive of an acute MI presenting up to 12 (and possibly up to 24) hours after symptom onset and having ECG evidence of an acute MI manifested by ST elevations >1 mm in two contiguous leads (after nitroglycerin to rule out coronary vasospasm) that are considered to represent ischemia (Antman et al., 2004).

◆ Patients with typical and persistent symptoms in the presence of a new or presumably new left bundle branch block or a true posterior MI are also considered eligible.

◆ Administration of alteplase is indicated for patients with acute ischemic stroke, provided that treatment is initiated within three hours of clearly defined symptom onset.

Table 14.8 **Fibrinolytics**		
DRUG	**DOSE**	**COMMENTS**
Alteplase	**Accelerated dose in AMI** Dose for weight > 67 kg: • 15 mg IV bolus over 1-2 minutes, then • 50 mg over 30 minutes, then • 35 mg over next 60 minutes. Dose for weight < 67 kg: • 15 mg IV bolus over 1-2 minutes, then • 0.75 mg/kg over 30 minutes, then • 0.5 mg/kg over 60 minutes. **For acute ischemic stroke:** Recommended total dose: 0.9 mg/kg (maximum dose should not exceed 90 mg) infused over 60 minutes. • Load with 0.09 mg/kg as an I.V. bolus over 1 minute, followed by • 0.81 mg/kg as a continuous infusion over 60 minutes.	Better outcomes than streptokinase. More expensive. Short half-life. Concurrently, begin heparin 60 units/kg bolus (maximum: 4000 units) followed by continuous infusion of 12 U/kg/hour (maximum: 1000 units/hour), and adjust to aPTT to 1.5-2 times the upper limit of control. Heparin should not be started for 24 hours or more after starting alteplase for stroke.
Reteplase	10 Units over 2 minutes. Repeat 10 Unit bolus in 30 minutes.	Withhold second dose if serious bleeding or anaphylaxis occurs. Concurrently, begin heparin 60 units/kg bolus (maximum: 4000 units) followed by continuous infusion of 12 U/kg/hour (maximum: 1000 units/hour), and adjust to aPTT to 1.5-2 times the upper limit of control.

Cardiovascular Drugs

<table>
<tr><td colspan="3" align="center">Table 14.8 (continued)
Fibrinolytics</td></tr>
<tr><td>DRUG</td><td>DOSE</td><td>COMMENTS</td></tr>
<tr>
<td>Tenecteplase</td>
<td>The recommended total dose should not exceed 50 mg and is based on weight. Administer as a bolus over 5 seconds:
• < 60 kg: 30 mg dose
• 60 to 69 kg: 35 mg
• 70 to 79 kg: 40 mg
• 80 to 89 kg: 45 mg
• > 90 kg: 50 mg.</td>
<td>Concurrently, begin heparin 60 units/kg bolus (maximum: 4000 units) followed by continuous infusion of 12 U/kg/hour (maximum: 1000 units/hour), and adjust to aPTT to 1.5-2 times the upper limit of control.

Easiest to administer.</td>
</tr>
<tr>
<td>Streptokinase</td>
<td>1.5 million units over 30-60 minutes.</td>
<td>Much less expensive.
Worse outcomes than with tPA.
Not used much in US.
Heparin is recommended if patient at high risk for thrombo-embolism: large anterior MI, atrial fibrillation, previous embolus, known LV thrombus.</td>
</tr>
</table>

Side Effects
◆ Bleeding is the primary complication of all fibrinolytic agents, and hemorrhagic stroke is the greatest concern.

◆ Allergic reactions can occur with streptokinase, especially on repeat administration.

Contraindications
◆ Absolute contraindications:
  ❖ Previous intracranial hemorrhage.
  ❖ Known structural cerebral vascular lesion.
  ❖ Known malignant intracranial neoplasm.
  ❖ Ischemic stroke within three months, except acute ischemic stroke within 3 hours.
  ❖ Suspected aortic dissection.
  ❖ Active bleeding or bleeding diathesis.
  ❖ Significant closed-head or facial trauma within 3 months.
◆ Relative contraindications:
  ❖ History of chronic severe, poorly controlled hypertension
  ❖ Severe uncontrolled hypertension on presentation (SBP > 180 mm Hg or DBP > 110 mm Hg).
  ❖ Ischemic stroke more than three months previously.
  ❖ Dementia or other intracranial pathology.
  ❖ Traumatic or prolonged cardiopulmonary resuscitation (>10 minutes) or major surgery (within 3 weeks).
  ❖ Recent internal bleeding(within 2 to 4 weeks).
  ❖ Noncompressible vascular puncture.
  ❖ For streptokinase: prior exposure (more than five days previously) or prior allergic reaction to this agent.

Chapter 14

❖ Pregnancy.
❖ Active peptic ulcer.
❖ Current use of anticoagulants: the higher the INR, the higher the risk of bleeding.

Linking Knowledge to Practice:

✔ *All types of drugs that interfere with clot formation can cause bleeding as a side effect. Monitor all patients receiving any of these antithrombotic agents for bleeding:*

✔ *Bleeding precautions:*

❖ *Watch for bleeding from puncture sites, gums, nose.*
❖ *Check urine and stools for blood.*
❖ *Monitor for mental status changes.*
❖ *Avoid unnecessary venous punctures (use PRN adapter for blood draws); hold puncture sites or bleeding areas for at least 10 minutes.*
❖ *Monitor groin access site for oozing, hematoma.*
❖ *Do not remove arterial sheath until aPTT is less than 50 seconds (or HEPACT is less than 0.4 U/ml) or ACT less than 175 seconds; hold pressure for minimum of 15-20 minutes.*

ANTIARRHYTHMIC DRUGS

Antiarrhythmic drugs are currently grouped into four classes based on the major ion channels that the drug affects. Many of these drugs affect more than one ion channel, giving them multiple actions that vary with heart rate, disease states, electrolyte concentrations, and other factors. The major effects of each class of drugs are listed in Table 14.9.

Cardiovascular Drugs

<table>
<tr><td colspan="2" align="center">**Table 14.9**
Classification of Antiarrhythmic Drugs</td></tr>
<tr><td>**Drug Class**</td><td>**Effects on Action Potential & ECG**</td></tr>
<tr><td>**Class I: Na⁺ channel blockers**</td><td></td></tr>
<tr><td>**Class IA:**
Quinidine
Procainamide (Pronestyl)
Disopyramide (Norpace)</td><td>Depress phase 0 depolarization.
Slow conduction through heart - widen QRS.
Prolong repolarization time slightly – prolong QT.
Proarrhythmic.</td></tr>
<tr><td>**Class IB:**
Lidocaine
Tocainide
Mexilitine</td><td>Block Na⁺ channels and depress phase 0 in depolarized tissue.
Slow conduction through ischemic tissue.
Shorten repolarization time.
↓ automaticity (slows Phase 4 depolarization).
No effect on PR, QRS, QT intervals.</td></tr>
<tr><td>**Class IC: "super slowers"**
Flecainide (Tambocor)
Propafenone (Rhythmol)</td><td>Markedly depress phase 0 depolarization.
Marked slowing of conduction – widen QRS.
Prolong repolarization time – prolong QT.
Highly proarrhythmic.</td></tr>
<tr><td>**Class II: Beta Blockers**
The "olols":
Atenolol (Tenormin)
Metoprolol (Lopressor)</td><td>Depress spontaneous phase 4 depolarization.
Slow conduction through AV node – prolong PR.
Slow heart rate.
Block sympathetic activity.
Antihypertensive and anti-ischemic effects.</td></tr>
<tr><td>**Class III: Repolarization inhibitors**
(K⁺ channel blockers)
Amiodarone (Cordarone)
Sotalol (Betapace)
Ibutilide (Corvert)
Dofetilide (Tikosyn)</td><td>Markedly prolong phase 3 repolarization time.
Prolong refractory period – prolong QT.
Ibutilide and dofetilide are pure class III agents with
 no other effects.
Amiodarone and sotalol are "mixed" agents with other
 actions that can slow conduction.
Proarrhythmic (amiodarone less than others).</td></tr>
<tr><td>**Class IV: Calcium Channel Blockers**
Verapamil (Calan)
Diltiazem (Cardizem)</td><td>Inhibitory effects on calcium dependent cells in SA and AV
 node.
Slow conduction through AV node – prolong PR.
Increases AV node refractory period.
Slow heart rate.</td></tr>
</table>

Each class of drug works on a different part of the cardiac action potential (refer to Chapter 1 for explanation of the cardiac action potential). Figure 14.10 illustrates the site of action of antiarrhythmic drugs on the action potential (AP).

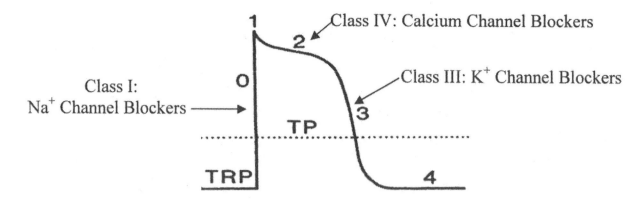

Figure 14.10: Site of action: antiarrhythmic drugs.

Figure 14.11 shows the major effects of Class I and Class III agents on conduction time (Phase 0) and repolarization (Phase III) of the AP. The solid line represents the normal AP, and the dotted lines show drug effects.

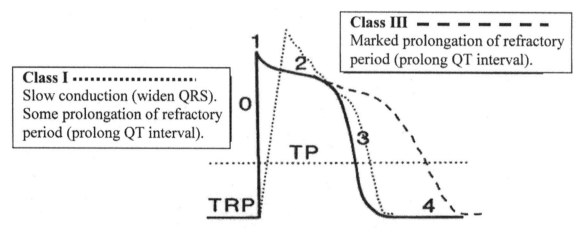

Figure 14.11: Major effects of Class I and Class III agents.

In addition to drugs that are classified as antiarrhythmics according to the above classification system, there are many other drugs used for heart rate and rhythm control that are not classified as "antiarrhythmics." Drugs such as atropine, adenosine, digitalis, epinephrine, and magnesium are used to treat arrhythmias but are not "antiarrhythmics," according to the current classification system.

Figure 14.12 illustrates drugs that can be used to increase or decrease sinus node rate, increase or decrease AV conduction, suppress atrial or ventricular arrhythmias, and slow conduction through an accessory pathway. There are other drugs that have some of these effects, but are not specifically used for this purpose (e.g. dopamine and dobutamine can also increase heart rate and speed AV conduction but they are not used for that purpose).

DRUGS USED FOR HEART RATE AND RHYTHM CONTROL

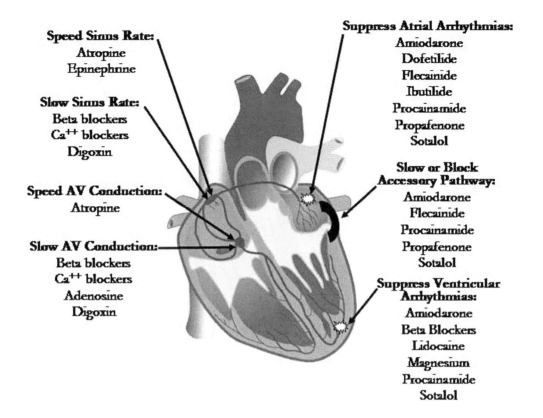

Figure 14.12: Heart rate and rhythm control drugs.

Specific information about drugs used for heart rate and rhythm control can be found in Table 14.10.

Table 14.10
Drugs Used for Heart Rate and Rhythm Control

DRUG (CLASS)	INDICATIONS	DOSE/ADMINISTRATION Therapeutic Level Half-Life	SIDE EFFECTS	COMMENTS
Adenosine (unclassified) (Adenocard)	First line therapy to terminate AV nodal active SVTs: (AV Nodal Re-entry or Circus Movement Tachycardia using an accessory pathway). Can be diagnostic in AV nodal passive rhythms by causing AV block and revealing underlying atrial mechanism, and in wide complex tachycardias of uncertain origin. VT arising in the right ventricular outflow tract that is due to afterde-polarizations may respond to adenosine.	6 mg given very rapidly IV followed by rapid saline flush. May follow with 12 mg if needed and repeat 12 mg if no effect. Half-life = 9 seconds.	Acute onset of AV block usually lasting a few seconds. May result in brief period of asystole or bradycardia, which is not responsive to atropine. Torsades can occur in patients who are susceptible to bradycar-dia-dependent arrhythmias. Flushing, hot flash, acute dyspnea, chest pressure. Side effects last only a few seconds due to short half life of drug. Can precipitate bronchoconstric-tion in asthmatic patients.	Very short half-life so side effects are transient. Warn patients about side effects before giving drug – especially dyspnea. It may be helpful to have patient take a deep breath while injecting drug to ↓ sensation of dyspnea. Should not be used when arrhyth-mia is known to be atrial fib or flutter. Monitor ECG during administra-tion and be prepared for car-dioversion. May accelerate accessory pathway conduction and should not be used when antegrade conduction is occurring over accessory pathway. May rarely accelerate ventricular rate in atrial flutter. **Drug interactions:** Theophylline (and related drugs) and caffeine antagonize effects of adenosine and make it ineffective. Dipyridamole and carbamazepine potentiate effects of adenosine.

Table 14.10 (continued)
Drugs Used for Heart Rate and Rhythm Control

Cardiovascular Drugs

DRUG (CLASS)	INDICATIONS	DOSE/ADMINISTRATION Therapeutic Level Half-Life	SIDE EFFECTS	COMMENTS
Amiodarone (III) (Cordarone)	Life-threatening ventricular arrhythmias: recurrent VF, recurrent hemodynamically unstable VT. Also used for: Conversion of atrial fibrillation to sinus rhythm and maintenance of NSR. Treatment of atrial tachycardia, CMT. Slows conduction through accessory pathways in atrial fibrillation or CMT. Prophylaxis 5-7 days prior to cardiac surgery to prevent atrial fibrillation.	PO: 800-1600 mg qd in divided doses for 1-2 weeks, then 400-800 mg qd for 1-3 weeks. Maintenance: 100-400 mg/day. IV for VT: 1000 mg over first 24 hours given as follows: First rapid infusion: 150 mg over first 10 min (15 mg/min). [Add 3ml (150mg) to 100ml D5W]. Infuse 100ml over 10minutes. Followed by slow infusion: 360 mg over next 6 hours (1 mg/min). [Add 18ml (900mg) to 500ml D5W]. Infuse at 33.6ml/hr. Maintenance infusion: 540 mg over next 18 hours (0.5 mg/min). [Decrease rate of slow loading infusion to 0.5 mg/min] Infuse at 16.8ml/hr May continue with 0.5 mg/min for 2-3 weeks if needed. Central line recommended for long term infusions. If breakthrough VT occurs, may give supplemental doses of 150 mg over 10 min. [150 mg added to 100 ml D5W]. For shock-resistant cardiac arrest: IV bolus of 5 mg/kg, may repeat with 2.5 mg/kg if needed. IV for atrial fibrillation: 5mg/kg over 20 minutes, then 500-1000 mg over 24 hours, then 0.5 mg/min. Start oral during loading if possible. Therapeutic level = 1-2.5 mcg/ml. Very long half-life (26-107 days, average 53 days).	Bradycardia, heart block. Torsades de pointes is rare unless other risk factors are present. Hypotension with IV form. Pulmonary fibrosis, corneal microdeposits, photosensitivity, blue skin, thyroid dysfunction (hypo and hyper), liver dysfunction. Tremor, malaise, fatigue, GI upsets, dizziness, poor coordination, peripheral neuropathy, involuntary movements. Liver enzyme elevations are common but occur in patients with MI, HF, shock, multiple defibrillations, etc. It is unknown if elevations in liver enzymes are due to amiodarone or to associated conditions commonly present in these patients. Hepatocellular necrosis has occurred in patients who received IV amiodarone at rates higher than recommended.	Give with meals to ↓ GI intolerance. Baseline chest x-ray, renal, liver, thyroid function tests. Takes several weeks to achieve therapeutic blood levels and for effects to decrease after stopping drug. Is not dialyzable. Monitor K+ and Mg++ levels. Monitor QTc interval . **Drug interactions:** Additive proarrhythmic effects with many drugs (1A antiarrhythmics, phenothiazines, tricyclic antidepressants, thiazide diuretics, sotalol). ↑ protime with coumadin, may cause bleeding. ↑ serum levels of digoxin, quinidine, procainamide, cyclosporine. May double flecainide level. Cimetidine ↑ serum amiodarone levels. Cholestyramine and phenytoin (Dilantin) ↓ serum amiodarone levels. Additive effects on ↓ HR and ↓ AV conduction with beta blockers and Ca++ blockers. Special precautions with IV form: Physically incompatible with aminophylline, heparin, cefamandole, cefazolin, mezlocillin, sodium bicarb. Must be delivered using a volumetric pump (not drop counter) because drop size is altered by drug.

Chapter 14

Table 14.10 (continued)
Drugs Used for Heart Rate and Rhythm Control

DRUG (CLASS)	INDICATIONS	DOSE/ADMINISTRATION Therapeutic Level Half-Life	SIDE EFFECTS	COMMENTS
Atenolol (beta blocker) (Tenormin)	Ventricular rate control in atrial fibrillation/flutter. Slow conduction through AV node in AVNRT and CMT.	Initial dose: 12.5 - 25 mg PO qd Maintenance dose: 50-100 mg PO qd. IV: 5 mg over 5 minutes, may repeat in 5 minutes. Beta blocking plasma concentration = 0.2-5 mcg/ml Half-life = 6-7 hours.	Hypotension, bradycardia, AV block. Diarrhea, wheezing, HF.	Cardioselective beta blocker used primarily for hypertension and angina. **Drug interactions:** Additive effects on HR, AV conduction, BP, and ↑ potential for HF when given with negative inotropic drugs, Ca⁺⁺ blockers, digoxin.
Atropine (Anticholinergic, parasympatholytic)	Treatment of symptomatic bradycardia (sinus, junctional, AV block) and asystole.	Symptomatic bradycardia: 0.5-1 mg IV. May repeat q 3-5 minutes to total of 3 mg. Asystole: 1 mg IV, repeat q 3-5 minutes to total vagolytic dose of 0.04 mg/kg. May be given down ET tube during cardiac arrest if no IV available: use 2 to 2.5 mg. Half-life = 2-5 hours.	CV: tachycardia, chest pain, ventricular tachycardia/fibrillation (rare). CNS: drowsiness, confusion, dizziness, insomnia, nervousness. GI: dry mouth, ↓ GI motility, constipation, nausea. Other: urinary retention, hot flushed skin, rash.	Doses < 0.5 mg may cause paradoxical bradycardia. Causes pupils to dilate (significant when checking pupils during cardiac arrest situation). **Drug interactions:** Incompatible with aminophylline, metaraminol, norepinephrine, pentobarbitol, sodium bicarbonate.
Digoxin (unclassified)	Ventricular rate control in atrial fibrillation/flutter. Also used as an inotropic agent in HF.	PO loading dose: 0.5-1 mg divided into 3 or 4 doses at 6-8 hour intervals. PO maintenance dose: 0.125-0.5 mg qd. IV loading dose: 0.5-1 mg divided into 3 or 4 doses given at 4-8 hour intervals. Therapeutic level = 0.8-2 ng/ml. Half-life = 36-48 hours.	CV: bradycardia, AV block Digoxin Toxicity: sinus exit block, AV block, atrial tachycardia with block, bidirectional tachycardia, fascicular tachycardia, accelerated junctional rhythm, regularization the ventricular response to atrial fibrillation. Visual disturbances (halo vision), anorexia, nausea, vomiting, malaise, headache, weakness, disorientation, seizures.	Contraindicated in patients with WPW. Digoxin toxicity is more common in the presence of hypokalemia, renal failure, pulmonary or thyroid disease and in older people. **Drug interactions:** The following drugs ↓ digoxin levels: cholestyramine, antacids, kaopectate, neomycin, sulfasalazine, PAS. The following drugs ↑ digoxin levels: Erythromycin, tetracycline, quinidine, amiodarone, verapamil, spironolactone, nicardipine, indomethacin.

646

Cardiovascular Drugs

Table 14.10 (continued)
Drugs Used for Heart Rate and Rhythm Control

DRUG (CLASS)	INDICATIONS	DOSE/ADMINISTRATION Therapeutic Level Half-Life	SIDE EFFECTS	COMMENTS
Diltiazem (**Ca⁺⁺ blocker**) (**Cardizem**)	Ventricular rate control in atrial fibrillation/flutter. Slow conduction through AV node in AVNRT and CMT.	120-360 mg/day in divided doses. IV: 0.25 mg/kg bolus over 2 min. If needed, repeat with 0.35 mg/kg after 15 minutes. IV infusion: 5-15 mg/hr Therapeutic level = 50-200 ng/ml Half-life = 3-5 hours.	Bradycardia, heart block, sinus node dysfunction, HF, hypotension, flushing, angina, syncope, insomnia, ringing ears, edema, headache, nausea. Less depression of contractility than with verapamil, but watch for HF.	Contraindicated in patients with wide QRS tachycardia, sick sinus syndrome, heart block. **Drug interactions:** Additive effects on HR, AV conduction with amiodarone, beta blockers, digoxin. Decreased BP, and ↑ potential for HF when given with negative inotropic drugs, beta blockers.
Disopyramide (**IA**) (**Norpace**)	Effective in treating PVCs but not recommended due to proarrhythmic effects. Suppresses sustained VT. Effective in preventing atrial fibrillation and flutter. Slows conduction through accessory pathways.	Total daily dose = 400-800 mg in divided doses, usually 150mg q6h. SR form = 300mg q12h. Therapeutic level = 3-6 mcg/ml. Half-life = 4-10 hours.	Anticholinergic effects: dry mouth, urinary retention, constipation, precipitation or exacerbation of glaucoma, increased conduction through AV node. CV: marked negative inotropic effects, HF, prolongs QT interval, proarrhythmic (less than quinidine or procainamide), hypotension.	Monitor QT interval. **Drug Interactions:** May potentiate effect of coumadin. Additive negative inotropic effects with beta blockers or Ca⁺⁺ blockers. Phenobarbitol, dilantin, rifampin ↓ disopyramide levels. Quinidine ↑ disopyramide level.
Dofetilide (**III**) (**Tikosyn**)	Conversion of atrial fibrillation or flutter to NSR and maintenance of NSR after conversion.	Dose based on creatinine clearance: if normal renal function, 500 mcg bid. If abnormal renal function, 250 mcg bid. Do not give if creatinine clearance < 20 ml/min. Half-life = 9.5 hours.	Torsade de pointes (1.3 - 4% incidence), usually occurs within 3 days after initiating therapy. Has no negative inotropic effects and does not lower BP.	Patient must be on telemetry during initiation of therapy or with increase in dosage (recommendation is for 3 days monitoring). Monitor QT interval every 2-3 hours: if QTc increases > 15% or if QTc is > 500 ms, reduce dose. If QTc after second dose is > 500 ms, drug should be discontinued. **Drug Interactions:** Drugs that increase dofetilide levels include verapamil, ketoconazole, cimetidine, macrolide antibiotics, ritonavir, prochlorperazine, magesterol. Maintain normal K⁺ and Mg⁺⁺ levels.

Table 14.10 (continued)
Drugs Used for Heart Rate and Rhythm Control

DRUG (CLASS)	INDICATIONS	DOSE/ADMINISTRATION Therapeutic Level Half-Life	SIDE EFFECTS	COMMENTS
Epinephrine **(Adrenalin)**	Treatment of any cardiac arrest situation requiring CPR: VF, pulseless VT, asystole, PEA.	1 mg IV bolus every 3-5 minutes during resuscitation efforts. May be given via ET tube if IV access not available: use 2 to 2.5 mg. May be infused at 2-10 mcg/min to maintain BP during symptomatic bradycardia.	CV: tachycardia, hypertension, arrhythmias, angina CNS: restlessness, headache, tremor, stroke. Other: nausea, ↓ urine output, transient tachypnea.	**Drug Interactions:** Has potential to cause arrhythmias when given with bretylium, digoxin, other sympathomimetic agents. Physically incompatible with aminophylline, ampicillin, cephapirin, sodium bicarbonate and other alkaline solutions.
Esmolol **(beta blocker)** **(Brevebloc)**	Rapid control of ventricular rate in atrial fibrillation/flutter.	Loading infusion: 500 mcg/Kg/min for 1 min. Maintenance infusion: Use steps of 50, 100, 150, 200 mcg/kg/min over 4 minutes each - stop at desired effect. Use dosing chart that comes with drug. Beta blocking plasma concentration = 0.15 - 1 mcg/ml Half life of 9 minutes	Hypotension, peripheral ischemia, confusion, thrombophlebitis, skin necrosis from infiltration. bradycardia, bronchospasm. Contraindicated in bradycardia, heart block, cardiogenic shock, heart failure.	Cardioselective beta blocker. Short half life so effects reversed within 10-20 minutes after stopping drug. **Drug interactions:** May increase digoxin level. Additive effects on HR, AV conduction, BP, and ↓ potential for HF when given with negative inotropic drugs, Ca⁺⁺ blockers, digoxin. Incompatible with sodium bicarbonate, lasix, valium, thiopental.

Cardiovascular Drugs

Table 14.10 (continued)
Drugs Used for Heart Rate and Rhythm Control

DRUG (CLASS)	INDICATIONS	DOSE/ADMINISTRATION Therapeutic Level Half-Life	SIDE EFFECTS	COMMENTS
Flecainide (IC) (Tambocor)	In absence of structural heart disease: Conversion of atrial fibrillation to sinus and maintenance of NSR. Treatment of SVTs: AVNRT, CMT. Slow conduction through accessory pathways in atrial fibrillation or CMT. Life-threatening ventricular arrhythmias (sustained VT).	100-400 mg PO q 12 h. Therapeutic level = 0.2-1 mcg/ml (Plasma levels do not correlate with efficacy but incidence of CV toxicity greater when levels > 1mcg/ml). Half-life = 13-19 hours.	CV: Marked proarrhythmia, marked negative inotropic effects (HF), bradycardia, heart block CNS: Blurred vision, dizziness, flushing, ringing ears, drowsiness, headache. Other: bad taste, constipation, edema, abdominal pain	Higher mortality rate in post MI patients when studied in CAST. Safest in patients with normal LV function. Should not be used in patients with recent MI. Prolongs QT interval, potential for proarrhythmia (torsades de pointes). Monitor for HF. Full therapeutic effect may take up to 5 days. **Drug Interactions:** ↑ digoxin levels. Cimetidine, amiodarone, propranolol increase flecainide levels. Additive negative inotropic effects with beta blockers, Ca⁺⁺ blockers, disopyramide.
Ibutilide (III) (Corvert)	Conversion of atrial fibrillation or flutter to sinus.	IV infusion of 1 mg over 10 minutes. May repeat same dose in 10 minutes if needed. In patients < 60 Kg: 0.01 mg/kg. Half-life = 6 hours (2-12 hours).	Hypotension, VT, bundle branch block, AV block, torsades, nausea, headache.	Prolongs QT interval and may be proarrhythmic. Proarrhythmia usually occurs within 40 minutes. Monitor ECG continuously during administration and at least 4 hours after. Conversion to NSR usually occurs within 20-40 minutes of infusion. Correct hypokalemia and hypomagnesemia. **Drug interactions:** Do not give other Class I or Class III agents within 4 hours.

649

Table 14.10 (continued)
Drugs Used for Heart Rate and Rhythm Control

DRUG (CLASS)	INDICATIONS	DOSE/ADMINISTRATION Therapeutic Level Half-Life	SIDE EFFECTS	COMMENTS
Lidocaine (IB)	Treatment of ventricular arrhythmias: VT, VF Effective for PVC suppression, but PVC suppression not usually recommended.	For VT: 1 mg/kg IV bolus over 3 minutes followed by infusion at 2-4 mg/min. Repeat bolus of 0.5 mg/kg in 10 minutes to maintain therapeutic level. May repeat to total of 3 mg/kg. For VF or pulseless VT: 1.5 mg/kg IV bolus. May repeat with same amount and follow with infusion at 2-4 mg/min. May be given down ET tube during cardiac arrest if no IV available. Therapeutic level = 1.4-5 mcg/ml. Half-life of bolus = 10 minutes. Half-life once therapeutic level reached = 1.5-2 hours.	Side effects relatively rare. CNS: lightheadedness, dizziness, tremor, agitation, tinnitus, blurred vision, convulsions, respiratory depression and arrest. CV: bradycardia, asystole, hypotension, shock.	↓ dose to half if liver disease or low liver blood flow (shock, HF). **Drug Interactions:** Beta blockers and cimetidine increase lidocaine levels. Glucagon and isoproterenol may increase liver blood flow and ↓ lidocaine levels.
Magnesium	May be useful for treatment or prevention of both supraventricular and ventricular arrhythmias following MI or cardiac surgery. Treatment of choice for torsades de pointes and VF or pulseless VT refractory to other drugs.	1-2 gm diluted in 10 ml D5W over 1-2 minutes. May be given IV push for VF or torsades. Infusion of 0.5 - 1 gm/hr for up to 24 hours.	CV: hypotension, bradycardia, heart block, cardiac arrest. CNS: Weakness, drowsiness, peripheral neuromuscular blockade, absent deep tendon reflexes. Other: ↓ respiratory rate, respiratory paralysis.	**Drug Interactions:** CNS depression when used with general anesthetics, barbiturates, opiate analgesics. Additive effects with neuromuscular blocking agents. Incompatible with calcium, sodium bicarbonate, ciprofloxacin.
Metoprolol (beta blocker) (Lopressor)	Ventricular rate control in atrial fibrillation/flutter. Slow conduction through AV node in AVNRT and CMT. May be used to treat some ventricular arrhythmias.	PO: 50-200 mg qd. IV: 2.5-5 mg q 5 minutes up to 15 mg. Beta blocking plasma concentration = 50-100 ng/ml. Half-life = 3-7 hours.	Hypotension, bradycardia, AV block	Cardioselective beta blocker. **Drug interactions:** Additive effects on HR, AV conduction, BP, and ↑ potential for HF when given with negative inotropic drugs, Ca⁺ blockers, digoxin.

Cardiovascular Drugs

Table 14.10 (continued)
Drugs Used for Heart Rate and Rhythm Control

DRUG (CLASS)	INDICATIONS	DOSE/ADMINISTRATION Therapeutic Level Half-Life	SIDE EFFECTS	COMMENTS
Mexiletine (IB) (**Mexitil**)	Acute and chronic treatment of symptomatic VT.	PO loading dose = 400 mg. Maintenance dose = 200-400 mg q8h. Therapeutic level = 1 - 2 mcg/ml. Half-life = 10-17 hours.	GI: nausea, vomiting, heartburn, anorexia, diarrhea. CNS: tremor, dizziness, ataxia, slurred speech, paresthesias, seizures, hallucinations, emotional instability, insomnia, memory impairment. CV: bradycardia, hypotension, HF, proarrhythmia (rare). Other: thrombocytopenia, fever, rash, positive ANA.	Often given in combination with other antiarrhythmics with increased effectiveness (quinidine, disopyramide, propafenone, amio-darone). Drug interactions: Phenobarbitol, dilantin, rifampin ↓ mexiletine levels. Cimetidine ↑ mexiletine levels. Mexiletine ↑ theophylline levels.
Procainamide (IA) (**Pronestyl**)	Conversion of atrial fibrillation to sinus & maintenance of NSR. Suppresses PACs, atrial tachycardia, atrial flutter and fib. Slows conduction through accessory pathways. Effective in terminating and preventing VT. Effective in treating PVCs but not recommended due to proarrhythmic effects.	PO dose 3-7.5 gm qd in divided doses 3-4 times a day (never more than 6 hr between doses). SR forms q 6 h. IV loading dose: 17 mg/kg at 25 mg/min. If rapid loading is needed, give 100mg doses over 5 minutes to total of 1gm in first hour. IV drip 2-4 mg/min. Therapeutic level = 4-10 mcg/ml. Half-life = 3.5 hours. Active metabolite is NAPA: therapeutic level = 9-12 mg/L.	GI: nausea, vomiting, anorexia CV: bradycardia, heart block, proarrhythmia (less than with quinidine). Prolongs QT interval. Hypotension with IV use. CNS: headache, insomnia, dizziness, psychosis, hallucinations, depression. Lupus-like syndrome with long-term use (15-25% of patients who take drug > 1 year). Other: rash, fever, swollen joints, agranulocytosis, pancytopenia.	Monitor QT interval, QRS width, PR. Monitor NAPA level (active metabolite). Watch for hypotension with IV use. **Drug Interactions:** Amiodarone, cimetadine, raniti-dine increase procainamide levels. Alcohol ↓ procainamide levels. Additive effects on conduction system disease when given with other class IA, class IC, tricyclic antidepressants, or Ca⁺⁺ blockers.
Propafenone (IC) (**Rhythmol**) Also has beta blocker effects.	Conversion of atrial fibrillation to sinus & maintenance of NSR. Slow conduction through accessory pathways. Life-threatening ventricular arrhythmias (sustained VT).	150-300 mg tid. Therapeutic level = 0.2-3 mcg/ml. Half-life = 2-10 hours in normal metabolizers, up to 32 hours in slow metabolizers.	GI: nausea, anorexia, constipation, metallic taste CNS: dizziness, headache, blurred vision CV: HF, bradycardia, AV block, bundle branch block, proarrhythmia	Was not included in CAST, but is same class as drugs shown to cause higher mortality post MI. Watch for proarrhythmia. **Drug interactions:** ↑ digoxin levels. Potentiates coumadin. Has mild beta blocker and Ca⁺⁺ blocker effects. ↑ cyclosporin levels. Quinidine and cimetidine increase propafenone levels.

Chapter 14

Table 14.10 (continued)
Drugs Used for Heart Rate and Rhythm Control

DRUG (CLASS)	INDICATIONS	DOSE/ADMINISTRATION Therapeutic Level Half-Life	SIDE EFFECTS	COMMENTS
Propranolol (beta blocker) (Inderal)	Ventricular rate control in atrial fibrillation/flutter. Treatment of SVTs (slow AV node conduction): AVNRT, CMT Effective in some types of VT: exercise induced, digitalis induced. Effective in reducing incidence of VF and sudden death post MI.	PO: 40-240 mg qd in divided doses. IV: 1-6 mg (0.15 mg/kg) at rate of 1 mg/min. Beta blocking plasma concentration = 50-100 ng/ml. Half-life = 1-6 hours.	CV: bradycardia, heart block, hypotension, HF GI: Nausea, vomiting, stomach discomfort, constipation, diarrhea CNS: dreams, hallucinations, insomnia, depression Other: bronchospasm, exacerbation of peripheral vascular disease, fatigue, hypoglycemia, impotence	Non-cardioselective beta blocker. **Drug interactions:** Additive effects on HR, AV conduction, BP, and ↑ potential for HF when given with negative inotropic drugs, Ca⁺⁺ blockers, digoxin.
Quinidine (IA)	Rarely used Conversion of atrial fibrillation to sinus & maintenance of NSR. May be used for other SVTs: atrial tachycardia, AVNRT, accessory pathways. Effective in treating PVCs and VT but not recommended due to proarrhythmic effects.	Sulfate: 200-400 mg q 6-8 h Gluconate: 324 mg SR tabs, 1-2 q 8-12 h. Therapeutic level = 2-5 mcg/ml. Half-life = 7-9 hours.	GI: nausea, diarrhea, abdominal pain. CV: hypotension, bradycardia, tachycardias, torsades de pointes, HF. Prolongs QTc interval, proarrhythmia. CNS: cinchonism (tinnitus, hearing loss, confusion, delirium, visual disturbances, psychosis). Other: fever, headache, rashes, leukopenia, thrombocytopenia.	Give with food. Monitor QT interval, QRS width, PR. Watch for proarrhythmia (torsades). IV use rare (hypotension). **Drug Interactions:** ↑ Digoxin levels. Increased bleeding when used with coumadin. Dilantin, phenobarb, rifampin, nifedipine, sodium bicarb, thiazide diuretics all ↓ Quinidine levels. Cimetidine, amiodarone, verapamil – all increase Quinidine levels.
Sotalol (III) (Betapace) Has beta blocker effects.	Conversion of atrial fibrillation to sinus & maintenance of NSR. Treatment of SVT. Slow conduction through accessory pathways. Life-threatening VT, VF.	80 mg bid X 3 days, then 160 mg bid for 3 days. 160-480 mg daily in two divided doses. Therapeutic level = 1-4 mcg/ml (not clinically useful). Half-life = 12 hours.	CV: Bradycardia, heart block, HF, proarrhythmia. Other: Bronchospasm, fatigue, weakness, GI symptoms, dizziness, dyspnea, hypotension.	Prolongs QT interval, potential for proarrhythmia with IA agents or diuretics. Watch for bradycardia, AV block and new or worsening HF.
Verapamil (Ca⁺⁺ blocker) (Calan)	Ventricular rate control in atrial fibrillation/flutter. Slow conduction through AV node in AVNRT and CMT.	PO: 120-360 mg qd in 2-3 doses. IV: 2.5-5 mg over 2 min. May repeat with 5-10 mg if needed. Therapeutic level = 80-400 ng/ml. Half-life = 3-7 hours.	Bradycardia, heart block, HF, hypotension, fatigue, headache, edema, constipation.	Contraindicated in patients with wide QRS tachycardias, bradycardia, AV block, sick sinus syndrome. **Drug interactions:** increases digoxin levels. Additive effects on HR, AV conduction with beta blockers, digoxin. Hypotension, and ↑ potential for HF when given with other negative inotropic drugs.

Cardiovascular Drugs

Abbreviations used in Table 14.10:

ACLS = Advanced Cardiac Life Support; AVNRT = atrioventricular nodal re-entrant tachycardia; BP = blood pressure; CAST = Cardiac Arrhythmia Suppression Trial; CMT = circus movement tachycardia; CNS = central nervous system; CV = cardiovascular; HF = heart failure; HR = heart rate; PR = PR interval; QT = QT interval; SVT = supraventricular tachycardia; VF = ventricular fibrillation; VT = ventricular tachycardia

ANTI-LIPID DRUGS

Several types of drugs can be used to treat dyslipidemias: statins, fibric acid derivatives, bile acid sequestrates, nicotinic acid, and cholesterol absorption blockers. Table 14.11 includes detailed information about specific types of anti-lipid drugs.

Statins are the most effective and best tolerated of these drugs, and are the first choice in treating hypercholesterolemia. In addition to lowering LDL-C, which is their major effect, statins may also have the following cardioprotective effects:

◆ Improved endothelial function by enhancing endothelial production of nitric oxide.

◆ Enhance plaque stability in arteries.

◆ Antiinflammatory effects.

◆ Antioxidant effects.

◆ Reduce platelet aggregation.

Lipid lowering is beneficial for both primary and secondary prevention of coronary disease in patients with dyslipidemias. Several statins (atorvastatin, lovastatin, pravastatin, simvastatin) have been shown to be effective in reducing coronary events, strokes, and overall mortality. Some studies have suggested that statins may also have beneficial effects in preventing diabetes, increasing bone formation and thus possibly protecting against osteoporosis, lowering blood pressure, decreasing the risk of or progression of dementia, and preserving renal function. More studies are needed to prove or refute these possible additional effects of statins.

In general, the most effective drugs for effecting specific lipids are:

◆ Lower LDL-C – statins.

◆ Increase HDL-C – nicotinic acid.

◆ Decrease triglycerides – fibric acid derivatives.

653

Chapter 14

<table>
<tr><td colspan="5" align="center">Table 14.11
Anti-Lipid Drugs</td></tr>
<tr><td>DRUG</td><td align="center">MECHANISM
OF ACTION</td><td align="center">EFFECT ON LIPIDS</td><td align="center">DOSE</td><td align="center">PRECAUTIONS
COMMENTS</td></tr>
<tr>
<td>Bile Acid Sequestrants
(Resins)

Cholestyramine
(Questran)

Colestepol
(Colestid)

Colesevelam
(Welchol)</td>
<td>Bind bile acids in intestine and excretes them in feces. This causes increased synthesis of hepatic bile acids, which decreases the amount of cholesterol in liver. ↓ cholesterol in liver causes a compensatory ↑ in LDL-C receptors on hepatic cells, which increases clearance of LDL-C and lowers blood LDL-C and total cholesterol levels.</td>
<td>↓ LDL-C by 10-15% at low doses; up to 25% at maximum doses.

Little effect on HDL-C (↑ 4-5%).

May ↑ TG levels slightly, then usually return to baseline.</td>
<td>Cholestyramine:
8-16 Gm/day, increase slowly q 2-4 weeks to max. of 24 Gm/day in 2-4 divided doses
(Powder or candy bar)

Colestipol:
10-30 Gm/day in 2-4 divided doses.
(Powder)

Colesevelam:
3.75 – 4.375 g/day</td>
<td>Side Effects: Mainly GI: nausea, constipation, flatulence, cramps.

Other drugs should be taken 1 hr before or 4 hrs after these drugs (resins interfere with absorption by binding with digoxin, thyroxine, thiazides, furosemide, propranolol, warfarin).</td>
</tr>
<tr>
<td>Nicotinic Acid

Niacin
Niacor
Niaspan</td>
<td>Blocks release of free fatty acids from adipose tissue, resulting in less hepatic conversion of FFA into triglycerides. Results in ↓ production of LDL-C.</td>
<td>↓ LDL-C by 10-25%.

↓ TG by 35-50%.

↑ HDL-C by 15-35%.</td>
<td>Initial: 100 mg 2-3 times/day
Increase to 1.5-2 g/ day

Niaspan = start with 500 mg nightly and titrate up to 1-2 g at bedtime</td>
<td>Side Effects: Vasodilation resulting in flushing, hypotension, dizziness, tachycardia.
Brown skin discoloration, itching. GI symptoms, hyperglycemia, liver toxicity, ↑uric acid levels (gout), ↑ homocysteine levels.

Taking ASA 30 minutes prior can ↓ flushing.
Best taken with food to ↓ GI effects.</td>
</tr>
<tr>
<td>HMG-CoA reductase inhibitors:

Atorvastatin (Lipitor)

Fluvastatin (Lescol)

Lovastatin
(Mevacor)

Pravastatin
(Pravachol)

Rosuvastatin
(Crestor)

Simvastatin
(Zocor)</td>
<td>Reduces synthesis of cholesterol in liver by inhibiting the enzyme, HMG-CoA reductase, that is the rate-limiting step in cholesterol biosynthesis.

Decreased cholesterol synthesis in the liver results in increased LDL-C receptors on the surface of hepatic cells, which increases removal of LDL-C from the blood and lowers LDL-C levels.</td>
<td>↓ LDL-C by 20-60% depending on specific drug (effect is dose dependent).

↓ triglycerides by 20-40%, depending on specific drug (effect is dose dependent).

↑ HDL-C by 5-10%.</td>
<td>Take at bedtime (atorvastatin and rosuvastatin can be taken any time of day).

Atorvastatin: 10-80 mg/day.

Fluvastatin: 20-80 mg.

Lovastatin: 20-80 mg /day.

Pravastatin: 10-80 mg/day.

Rosuvastatin: 5-40 mg/day.

Simvastatin: 20-80 mg/day.</td>
<td>Side Effects:
Generally well tolerated.

Liver enzyme elevation (0.5-3%): usually in first 3 months and is dose dependent.

Myopathy (muscle injury) ranging from muscle weakness and pain to rhabdomyolysis and renal failure. Incidence of rhabdomyolysis is about 0.01%, but risk increases with increased dose and when statins are used with the following drugs: fibrates, cyclosporine, digoxin warfarin, macrolide antibiotics, mibefradil, niacin, amiodarone, nefazodone.</td>
</tr>
</table>

Cardiovascular Drugs

		Table 14.11 (continued) Anti-Lipid Drugs			
DRUG	**MECHANISM OF ACTION**	**EFFECT ON LIPIDS**	**DOSE**	**PRECAUTIONS COMMENTS**	
Fibric Acid Derivatives (Fibrates): Gemfibrozil (Lopid) Fenofibrate (Tricor, Lipantil)	Stimulate synthesis of enzymes that increase fatty acid oxidation, which enhances clearance of triglyceride-rich lipoproteins and VLDL-C.	↓ TG by 35-50% (major indication). ↑ HDL-C 15-30%. Lower LDL-C 5-20% if TG normal, but may ↑ LDL-C if TG high.	Gemfibrozil: 600 mg bid (30 minutes before AM and PM meal). Fenofibrate: 54-150 mg/day with food.	*Side Effects:* Liver enzyme elevations. Myositis (increased risk when combined with a statin) = myoglobinuria and renal failure. Possible ↑ risk of gall-stones. Interfere with warfarin metabolism – reduce dose of warfarin.	
Cholesterol Absorption Blockers: Ezetimibe (Zetia) Ezetimibe/simvastatin combination (Vytorin)	Decrease absorption of dietary cholesterol from small intestine.	↓ total cholesterol by 12%. ↓ LDL-C by 18%. Vytorin = ↓ LDL-C by 60%.	10 mg daily with or with-out food.	No known adverse effects.	

Abbreviations used in Table 14.11:

HDL-C = high density lipoprotein cholesterol; LDL-C = low density lipoprotein cholesterol; TG = triglycerides; VLDL=C = very low density lipoprotein cholesterol.

TEST YOUR KNOWLEDGE

There may be more than one correct answer for many of these questions.

1. Ca^{++} channel blockers cause which of the following effects?

   a. Increased blood pressure

   b. Decreased contractility

   c. Decreased heart rate

   d. Peripheral vasodilation

   e. Coronary vasospasm

2. Drugs that can decrease preload in a patient with heart failure include

   a. nitroglycerin.

   b. high dose dopamine.

   c. amiodarone.

   d. diuretics.

   e. ACE inhibitors.

Chapter 14

3. Dobutamine is used for which of the following?

   a. Angina

   b. Hypertension

   c. To increase cardiac output in left ventricular failure

   d. To increase preload in HF

4. All of the following are true of beta blockers except

   a. they decrease heart rate.

   b. they increase contractility.

   c. they can cause AV block.

   d. they can be used for supraventricular and ventricular arrhythmias.

5. ACE inhibitors are indicated for treatment of

   a. hypertension and heart failure.

   b. supraventricular arrhythmias.

   c. acute renal failure.

   d. angina.

6. Which of the following drugs is a pure beta stimulant and is used primarily to increase cardiac contractility?

   a. Digitalis

   b. Epinephrine

   c. Levophed

   d. Dobutamine

7. Epinephrine is indicated as the first line drug for any pulseless condition because it has the following actions:

   a. Is an inotrope and selectively shunts blood to the heart and brain.

   b. Converts VF to sinus rhythm.

   c. Slows the heart rate and improves contractility.

   d. Causes decreased contractility.

8. The following drugs are indicated for the treatment of ventricular arrhythmias:

   a. Levophed and dobutamine

   b. Captopril and inderal

   c. Lidocaine and amiodarone

   d. Isuprel and esmolol.

Cardiovascular Drugs

9. Supraventricular arrhythmias may be successfully treated with all of the following drugs except:
   a. Diltiazem
   b. Metoprolol
   c. Captopril
   d. Adenosine

10. All of the following drugs are indicated for the treatment of hypertension except:
    a. Beta blockers
    b. Lipitor
    c. ACE inhibitors
    d. Ca^{++} channel blockers

11. Atrial fibrillation may be successfully treated by all of the following drugs except:
    a. Ibutilide
    b. Adenosine
    c. Digitalis
    d. Ca^{++} channel blockers
    e. Procainamide
    f. Beta blockers

12. Which of the following is indicated for treatment of acute coronary ischemia?
    a. Captopril
    b. Atropine
    c. Nitroglycerin
    d. Adenosine
    e. Sublingual nifedipine

13. A patient with angina and hypertension may be treated with which of the following drugs to decrease myocardial oxygen demand?
    a. Dobutamine
    b. Diuretics
    c. Dopamine
    d. ACE inhibitor
    e. Angiotensin receptor blocker

Chapter 14

14. A patient is admitted to the telemetry unit following a syncopal episode at home. Her rhythm is sinus bradycardia at a rate of 32 beats per minute. She is on multiple medications for treatment of angina and hypertension. Which of the following medications might be contributing to her bradycardia and syncope?

   a. Lipitor

   b. Atenolol

   c. Lisinopril

   d. ASA

   e. Diltiazem

15. For the patient in question #14, which of the following therapies might be effective in managing her symptomatic bradycardia?

   a. Amiodarone

   b. Metoprolol

   c. Atropine

   d. Temporary transvenous pacing

16. You are caring for a patient following stent placement in the left anterior descending coronary artery as treatment for an acute anterior MI. He has a history of hypertension and is in chronic atrial fibrillation. He is receiving multiple medications listed below. Which of the following drugs are used to prevent stent thrombosis following his procedure?

   a. Metoprolol (Lopressor)

   b. Eptifibatide (Integrilin)

   c. ASA

   d. Simvastatin (Zocor)

   e. Clopidogrel (Plavix)

   f. Lisinopril (Zestril)

   g. Coumadin

17. For the patient in question #16, which drugs can be used to treat his hypertension?

18. For the patient in question #16, which drugs are indicated for management of his chronic atrial fibrillation?

19. For the patient in question #16, which drugs might contribute to an increased risk of bleeding?

Cardiovascular Drugs

20. A patient arrives in the ED with an ECG showing ST elevation MI. This facility does not have a cardiac cath lab and the transport time to the nearest cath facility is about 2 hours. Which of the following drugs are indicated in the acute treatment of this patient in the absence of contraindications?

    a. Ca^{++} blocker

    b. ASA

    c. tPA

    d. Beta blocker

    e. Diuretics

    f. Amiodarone

21. The above patient is successfully treated for his AMI. A cardiac echo shows an ejection fraction of 35%, but he has no overt signs of heart failure. Which of the following types of drugs should the patient be discharged with (in the absence of contraindications)?

    a. Diuretics

    b. Beta blocker

    c. Ca^{++} blocker

    d. Ace inhibitor

    e. Anticoagulant

    f. ASA

    g. Statin

22. Which of the following drugs reduce left ventricular afterload?

    a. Nitroprusside

    b. Dopamine

    c. Dobutamine

    d. Milrinone

    e. Hydralazine

23. Which of the following drugs are positive inotropic agents?

    a. Nitroprusside

    b. Dobutamine

    c. Amiodarone

    d. Atenolol

    e. Dopamine

    f. Digoxin

Chapter 14

24. Which of the following drugs inhibit platelet activation or aggregation?

  a. ASA

  b. tPA

  c. Plavix

  d. Coumadin

  e. Reopro

  f. Integrilin

ANSWERS

1.	B, C, D	13.	B, D, E
2.	A, D, E	14.	B, E
3.	C	15.	C, D
4.	B	16.	B, C, E
5.	A	17.	A, F
6.	D	18.	A, G
7.	A	19.	B, C, E, G
8.	C	20.	B, C, D
9.	C	21.	B, D, F, G
10.	B	22.	A, D, E
11.	B	23.	B, E, F
12.	C	24.	A, C, E, F

REFERENCES

2005 American Heart Association Guidelines for Cardiopulmonary Resuscitation and Emergency Cardiovascular Care, Part 4: Adult Basic Life Support. (2005). *Circulation, 112*(suppl IV), IV-1-IV-211.

Amiodarone: drug information. (2006). Retrieved April 15, 2006, from www.uptodate.com

Atorvastatin: drug information. (2006). *Lexi-Comp, Inc.* Retrieved April 18, 2006, from www.uptodate.com

Ezetimibe: drug information. (2006). *Lexi-Comp, Inc.* Retrieved Aprill 18, 2006, from www.uptodate.com

Fluvastatin: drug information. (2006). *Lexi-Comp, Inc.* Retrieved April 18, 2006, from www.uptodate.com

Lovastatin: drug information. (2006). *Lexi-Comp, Inc.* Retrieved April 18, 2006, from www.uptodate.com

Pravastatin: drug information. (2006). *Lexi-Comp, Inc.* Retrieved April 18, 2006, from www.uptodate.com

Simvastatin: drug information. (2006). *Lexi-Comp, Inc.* Retrieved April 18, 2006, from www.uptodate.com

Abrams, C.S. (2005). Platelet biology. Retrieved January 25, 2006, from www.uptodate.com

Antman, E.M., Anbe, D.T., Armstrong, P.W., Bates, E.R., Green, L.A., Hand, M., et al. (2004). ACC/AHA Guidelines for the management of patients with ST-elevation myocardial infarction: executive summary: A report of the ACC/AHA Task Force on Practice Guidelines (Committee to Revise the 1999 Guidelines on the Management of Patients with Acute Myocardial Infarction). *Journal of the American College of Cardiology, 44,* 671-719.

Bonow, R.O., Carabello, B., Chatterjee, K., de Leon, A.C., Faxton, D.P., Freed, M.D., et al. (2006). ACC/AHA 2006 guidelines for the management of patients with valvular heart disease: a report of the American College of Cardiology/American Heart Association Task Force on Practice Guidelines (Writing Committee to Develop Guidelines for the Management of Patients with Valvular Heart Disease). [Electronic Version] from http://www.americanheart.org

Braunwald, E., Antman, E.M., Beasley, J.W., Califf, R.M., Cheitlin, M.D., Hochman, J.S., et al. (2002). ACC/AHA 2002 guideline update for the management of patients with unstable angina and non-ST-segment elevation myocardial infarction: summary article: a report of the American College of Cardiology/American Heart Association Task Force on Practice Guidelines (Committee on the Management of Patients with Unstable Angina). *Circulation, 106,* 1893-1900.

Brunton, L.L., Lazo, J.S., & Parker, K.L. (Eds.). (2006). *Goodman & Gilman's Pharmacological Basis of Therapeutics* (11th ed.). New York: McGraw-Hill.

Coutre, S. (2005). Heparin-induced thrombocytopenia. *UpToDate.* Retrieved June 20, 2006, from www.uptodate.com

Guyton, A.C., & Hall, J.E. (2000). *Textbook of Medical Physiology.* Philadelphia: Saunders.

Jandeleit-Dahm, K.A., Tikellis, C., Reid, C.M., Johnston, C.I., & Cooper, M.E. (2005). Why blockade of the renin-angiotensin system reduces the incidence of new-onset diabetes. *Journal of Hypertension, 23,* 463-473.

Leung, L.L.K. (2004). Overview of hemostasis. Retrieved January 25, 2006, from www.uptodate.com

Opie, L.H. & Gersh, B.J. (2005). *Drugs for the Heart* (6th ed.). Philadelphia: Elsevier.

Popma, J.J., Berger, P., Ohman, E.M., Harrington, R.A., Grines, C., & Weitz, J.I. (2004). Antithrombotic Therapy During Percutaneous Coronary Intervention: The Seventh ACCP Conference on Antithrombotic and Thrombolytic Therapy. *Chest, 126,* 576S-599S.

Sackner-Bernstein, J.D., Kowalski, M., Fox, M., & Aaronson, K.D. (2005). Short-term risk of death after treatment with nesiritide for decompensated heart failure: a pooled analysis of randomized controlled trials. *JAMA, 293,* 1900-1905.

Sackner-Bernstein, J.D., Skopicki, H.A., & Aaronson, K.D. (2005). Risk of worsening renal function with nesiritide in patients with acutely decompensated heart failure. *Circulation, 111*(12), 1487-1491.

Chapter 14

Warkentin, T.E. (2004). Heparin-induced thrombocytopenia: recognition, treatment, and prevention. The Seventh ACCP Conference on Antithrombotic and Thrombolytic Therapy. *Chest, 126*(3), 311S-332S.

CHAPTER 15:
CARDIAC CATHETERIZATION & INTERVENTIONAL CARDIOLOGY

Cardiac catheterization is done to confirm and define the extent of coronary artery disease; to evaluate cardiac function in other types of heart disease (e.g. valvular disease, heart failure, congenital heart disease); and to perform catheter-based interventional procedures to treat coronary artery disease and other cardiac disorders. This chapter provides an overview of diagnostic cardiac catheterization and percutaneous coronary interventional procedures. For more detailed information on these topics, refer to references at the end of the chapter. It is beyond the scope of this chapter to discuss other interventional procedures that are done to treat valve disease, close patent foramen ovale, and occlusion of the left atrial appendage for stroke prevention in chronic atrial fibrillation.

DIAGNOSTIC CARDIAC CATHETERIZATION

Right Heart Catheterization

Right heart catheterization is done for the following reasons:

◆ to measure right atrial and right ventricular pressures.

◆ to measure pulmonary artery pressure.

◆ to measure O_2 content of right heart chambers and pulmonary artery.

◆ to detect left to right intracardiac shunt.

◆ to determine cardiac output.

◆ to evaluate tricuspid and pulmonic valves.

◆ to evaluate mitral valve function via the transseptal approach.

◆ to perform certain interventional procedures (e.g. closure of patent foramen ovale).

◆ to perform electrophysiology studies (see Chapter 17).

Right heart catheterization is usually done via femoral venous access but alternate venous access sites can be used, including the internal jugular veins, subclavian vein, or brachial veins. Once the superior or inferior vena cava is reached, the catheter is advanced through the right atrium, right ventricle, and into the pulmonary artery. Pressures are recorded and O_2 saturations are obtained when indicated. Contrast dye can be injected for imaging of the right atrium, right ventricle, or pulmonary artery. Cardiac output is determined using the thermodilution technique (see Chapter 4). In some procedures, such as catheter-based mitral valve repair or closure of patent foramen ovale, the left atrium is accessed via transseptal puncture through the atrial septum.

Left Heart Catheterization

Left heart catheterization is done for the following reasons:

◆ to evaluate coronary artery anatomy.

◆ to determine location and significance of coronary artery lesions.

◆ to measure left ventricular and aortic pressures.

◆ to evaluate mitral and aortic valve function.

◆ to evaluate left ventricular function.

- to perform interventional procedures on coronary arteries.
- to perform catheter-based valve procedures or closure of patent foramen ovale.

Left heart catheterization is usually performed percutaneously using the right femoral artery to gain access to the arterial circulation, and advancing the catheter up the aorta to the aortic root. Alternative arterial access sites include the brachial and radial arteries. An introducer sheath is inserted into the artery and guide wires and catheters are inserted and exchanged through the sheath. Once the catheter is in the aortic root, it can be placed into the ostium of the right coronary artery or the left main coronary artery, or advanced retrograde through the aortic valve into the left ventricle. Figure 15.1 illustrates femoral access sites for right and left heart catheterization. Figure 15.2 illustrates intracardiac catheter placement.

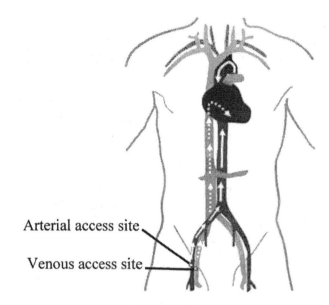

Figure 15.1: Femoral access sites.

Left heart catheterization = solid arrows

Right heart catheterization = dotted arrows

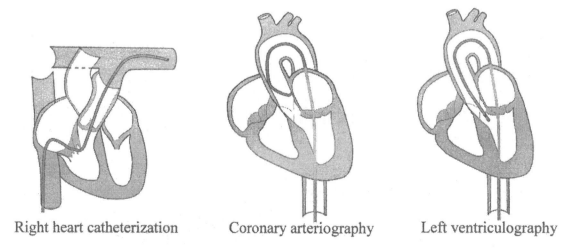

Figure 15.2: Intracardiac catheter placement.

Coronary Arteriography

Preformed catheters are used to access the ostia of the right coronary artery (RCA) and the left main coronary artery. Contrast material is injected through the catheter into the artery, and radiographic pictures of the coronary anatomy are obtained. A suspended C-arm rotates around the patient and can be placed at various angles to acquire different views of coronary anatomy. Figure 15.3 illustrates angiographic views of the right and left coronary arteries (note significant narrowing of circumflex at arrow).

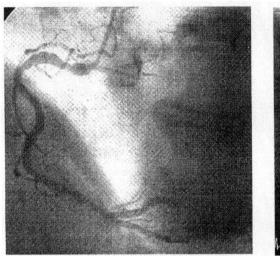
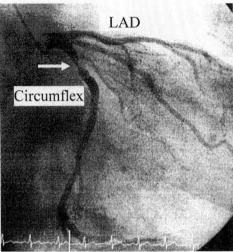

Right Coronary Artery   Left Coronary Arteries

Figure 15.3: Angiographic views of coronary arteries.

Ventriculography

Ventriculography is done by advancing a specialized catheter with multiple side holes retrograde across the aortic valve into the left ventricular cavity, and injecting contrast material into the left ventricle (see Figure 15.2). Ventricular wall motion can be filmed in single or biplane views to show wall motion abnormalities. Valve structure and function can be evaluated, and ejection fraction can be determined. Figure 15.4 shows a left ventriculogram in diastole and systole.

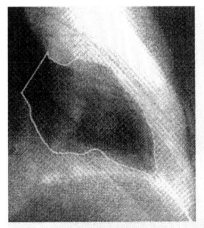
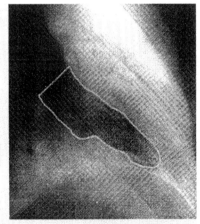

Diastole   Systole

Figure 15.4: Left ventriculogram.

Chapter 15

Contrast Agents

The "dye" used in coronary arteriography and ventriculography contains iodine that absorbs x-rays, and thus provides the images displayed on film or acquired digitally. The agents used are either ionic or non-ionic, and have variable osmolality. Ionic agents (e.g. Hypaque) dissociate into ions when dissolved in water and have a higher osmolality than blood. Nonionic agents (e.g. Omnipaque) do not dissociate into separate particles when dissolved in water; therefore, they have lower osmolality than ionic agents. First generation agents have an osmolality about 6 times higher than plasma. Low-osmolal agents have an osmolality about 3 times higher than plasma. The newest agent available, Visipaque, is iso-osmolal. The relatively high osmolality of contrast agents causes water to move from the extravascular space into the intravascular space and acts as an osmotic diuretic. Nonionic low-osmolal and iso-osmolal agents are associated with a lower incidence of contrast-induced renal failure and are the preferred agents, especially in patients with underlying renal insufficiency, diabetic nephropathy, or advanced heart failure (Rudnick & Tumlin, 2006).

Measures to prevent contrast induced nephropathy include using as low a dose of contrast as possible; hydration with IV normal saline or isotonic sodium bicarbonate before and after the procedure; and administration of acetylcysteine (Mucomist), which has antioxidant and vasodilatory effects, on the day before and the day of the procedure (Rudnick & Tumlin, 2006). Nephrotoxic drugs (e.g. some antibiotics, cyclosporine, non-steroidal anti-inflammatory drugs) and metformin should be withheld 24 hours prior to the procedure and 48 hours afterwards. The use of nonionic contrast agents and administration of corticosteroids and an antihistamine (diphenhydramine [Benadryl]) and H2 blocker (cimetadine or ranitidine) prior to the procedure can decrease the incidence of allergic reactions to contrast agents that occur in about 1% of patients (Carroza, 2006).

Post Procedure Care

At the end of a diagnostic procedure, catheters and sheaths are usually removed in the cath lab and manual pressure is applied to the access site for 20-30 minutes until bleeding is controlled. Mechanical compression devices, such as the C-clamp or Femostop, are sometimes used instead of manual pressure, but a staff member still needs to observe the patient and the site to make sure the device remains positioned correctly and that bleeding does not occur. Sometimes arterial puncture closure devices (APCD) are used to seal the arterial puncture site. APCDs are either absorbable collagen devices, such as Angioseal or Vasoseal; suture mediated devices, such as Perclose or ProStar; or staples or clip devices, such as Starclose. The use of such devices reduces bedrest time for the patient and eliminates the need for prolonged arterial compression, but may increase the risk for bleeding and pseudoaneurysm formation (Nikolsky et al., 2004), and the risk of local infection or endarteritis (Geary, Landers, Fiore, & Riggs, 2002).

Nursing care following a diagnostic catheterization includes vital signs, observation of the access site for bleeding or hematoma formation, distal pulse checks (i.e. pedal pulses for femoral access, radial pulses for radial or brachial access), and observation of the extremity below the access site for color, temperature, movement, and sensation. These observations are usually documented every 15 minutes for the first hour, every 30 minutes for the second hour, then hourly until patient is fully ambulatory or discharged. Continuous ECG monitoring is not routinely done for diagnostic procedures. The patient remains on bedrest with the affected leg straight for 2-4 hours, depending on the size of the sheath used and hospital protocol. If a closure device was used, bedrest times can be as short as 1 hour.

Cardiac Catheterization & Interventional Cardiology

Complications

The risk of major complications during diagnostic cardiac catheterization is less than 1%. Major complications include:

◆ Death – 0.08% to 0.14% incidence. Higher risk patients include those over 60 years of age, women, NYHA class IV heart failure, valvular heart disease, renal insufficiency, insulin-dependent diabetes, peripheral or cerebrovascular disease, pulmonary insufficiency.

◆ Myocardial infarction – < 1% incidence. Patients at higher risk are those with left main disease, recent unstable angina or non-ST elevation MI, and insulin-dependent diabetes.

◆ CVA – 0.07%-0.1% incidence. Risk factors include severity of coronary artery disease, length of fluoroscopy time, and aortic stenosis with retrograde catheterization across the aortic valve.

The most common complications of cardiac catheterization are local vascular problems at the insertion site.

◆ Hematoma formation is a common occurrence and results from bleeding into the soft tissues of the thigh. It appears as a swelling or hard knot at the access site under the skin and is often associated with discoloration resembling bruising due to accumulation of blood under the skin. It is usually self limited and resolves over several days. An enlarging hematoma should be treated with manual pressure for 15-30 minutes until bleeding is controlled. Occasionally surgery is necessary to repair a tear in the artery.

◆ Retroperitoneal bleeding occurs when a hematoma dissects into the retroperitoneal space. Symptoms can include hypotension, severe back or lower quadrant abdominal pain, a drop in hematocrit, bradycardia or tachycardia. A CT scan or ultrasound can be diagnostic. Treatment includes bedrest, fluid resuscitation or transfusion to maintain blood pressure, reversal of anticoagulation, and occasionally surgery to repair the artery.

◆ Pseudoaneurysm is a hematoma that remains in communication with the lumen of the artery, allowing blood to flow in and out of the hematoma cavity during systole and diastole. It usually presents as a pulsatile mass with a systolic bruit over the insertion site. Major risk factors for development of a pseudoaneurysm are inadequate manual compression, puncture of the superficial femoral artery, large sheath size, and post procedure anticoagulation. Pseudoaneurysm can be diagnosed by ultrasound and color flow mapping. Management may include ultrasound guided compression, ultrasound guided injection of thrombin into the aneurysm cavity, or surgical repair.

◆ Arteriovenous fistula is a communication between the femoral artery and vein, usually the result of puncture below the common femoral artery. This may present as a pulsatile mass with a continuous bruit at the insertion site. Surgical repair is usually necessary.

◆ Thrombosis at the arterial insertion site can reduce or completely occlude blood flow distal to the clot. Signs and symptoms include pain or paresthesia in the involved leg, loss of color in the leg, and reduced or absent distal pulses. The six P's indicate obstructed blood flow: Pallor, Polar, Pain, Pulseless, Paresthesia, Paralysis. These symptoms should be reported immediately, as surgery may be necessary to preserve the limb.

◆ Distal embolization of a clot into the extremity can present with the same six P's mentioned above, but appear lower in the leg or foot.

Other complications can occur during or after cardiac cath:

◆ Arrhythmias can occur during the procedure due to catheter manipulation in the heart and injection of contrast into coronary arteries. PVCs are common during catheter introduction into either ventricle. Ventricular tachycardia and fibrillation can occur with catheter manipulation or injection of contrast into the RCA and less often into the left system. Bradycardia commonly occurs during coro-

Chapter 15

nary injections (especially RCA) or due to vagal reactions. Having the patient cough after the injection helps to clear the contrast and restore normal rhythm. Atropine may be needed if a vagal reaction occurs. Third degree block or asystole are rare, but can occur especially with RCA interventions. A temporary pacemaker can be introduced through the venous sheath if needed for treatment of severe bradycardia or asystole. Atrial fibrillation or flutter can occur with catheter introduction into the right atrium.

◆ Allergic reactions to lidocaine used as a local anesthetic or to contrast agents can occur. Bupivicaine or mepivicaine can be used as alternative local anesthetics. See section above on contrast agents for information related to contrast allergies. Severe allergic reactions are usually treated with IV or IM epinephrine, according to the institution's protocol.

◆ Renal dysfunction following cardiac cath can be due to contrast agents or to atheroembolism from debris scraped from the aortic wall during catheter advancement. Contrast-induced nephropathy occurs in at least 5% of patients (with reported incidence ranging from 0 to 50%) (Carroza, 2006; Rudnick & Tumlin, 2006). The risk is greatest in patients with renal insufficiency and diabetes or heart failure. In most patients, renal failure is apparent within 24-48 hours after the procedure, diagnosed by a rise in creatinine, and resolves within 3-5 days. Renal failure due to atheroembolism is often delayed for days to weeks after the procedure, is accompanied by signs of embolism elsewhere (i.e. purple toes, a blue-reddish skin discoloration), and lasts much longer, frequently with little or no recovery of renal function (Rudnick & Tumlin, 2006). See the section above on contrast agents for recommendations to reduce contrast-mediated nephropathy.

◆ Infection is rare following cardiac cath procedures and occurs more often with the brachial approach than with the femoral approach.

◆ Radiation exposure can result in skin burns that may not develop for 2 weeks after the procedure if fluoroscopy times are longer than 60 minutes.
(Carroza, 2006; Smith et al., 2005)

PERCUTANEOUS CORONARY INTERVENTIONAL PROCEDURES

Percutaneous coronary intervention (PCI) is treatment of coronary artery disease via catheter-based procedures and includes percutaneous transluminal coronary angioplasty (PTCA), stents, directional atherectomy, rotational atherectomy (rotablation), and transluminal extraction atherectomy. PCI is performed via left heart catheterization, as described in the section above.

Table 15.1 lists Class I and Class IIa indications for PCI, according to AHA/ACC Guidelines ((Smith et al., 2005), and defines the angina grading scale used in the indications. In addition to these indications, PCI can also be used to reopen coronary arteries after failed fibrinolytic therapy or when ischemia occurs following CABG surgery. Refer to the guidelines for specific information on all indications for PCI.

Cardiac Catheterization & Interventional Cardiology

Table 15.1 (1 of 3) **Indications for Percutaneous Coronary Intervention**	
Class I: Conditions for which there is evidence for and/or general agreement that a procedure or treatment is beneficial, useful and effective.	**Patients with UA/NSTEMI** who have no serious comorbidity and coronary lesions amenable to PCI, and who have any of the following high-risk features: - recurrent ischemia despite intensive anti-ischemic therapy. - elevated troponin level. - new ST-segment depression. - HF symptoms or new or worsening MR. - depressed LV systolic function. - hemodynamic instability. - sustained VT. - PCI within 6 months. - prior CABG. **Primary PCI should be performed:** - in patients with STEMI (including true posterior MI) or new or presumably new LBBB who can undergo PCI of the infarct artery within 12 hours of symptom onset, if performed in a timely fashion (balloon inflation within 90 minutes of presentation) by persons skilled in the procedure (perform more than 75 PCI procedures per year, ideally at least 11 PCIs per year for STEMI). The procedure should be supported by experienced personnel in an appropriate laboratory environment (one that performs > 200 PCI procedures per year, of which at least 36 are primary PCI for STEMI, and that has cardiac surgery capability). The goal is a medical contact-to-balloon or door-to-balloon time within 90 minutes. - in patients < 75 years old who develop shock within 36 hours of MI and are suitable for revascularization that can be performed within 18 hours of shock (unless further support is futile because of patient's wishes or contraindications). - in patients with severe CHF and/or pulmonary edema and onset of symptoms within 12 hours. **Fibrinolytic-ineligible patients** who present with STEMI within 12 hours of symptom onset.
Class IIa: Conditions for which the weight of evidence/opinion is in favor of usefulness/efficacy.	**Patients with asymptomatic ischemia or CCS Class I or II angina:** - with 1 or more significant lesions in 1 or 2 coronary arteries. - with recurrent stenosis after PCI with a large area of viable myocardium or high-risk criteria on noninvasive testing. - with significant left main CAD (> 50% diameter stenosis) who are candidates for revascularization but are not eligible for CABG. *Continued on next page.*

Chapter 15

	Table 15.1 (2 of 3) **Indications for Percutaneous Coronary Intervention**
Class IIa (continued)	**Patients with CCS Class III angina:** - with single or multi-vessel CAD who are undergoing medical therapy and who have 1 or more significant lesions in 1 or more coronary arteries. - with single or multi-vessel CAD who are undergoing medical therapy with focal saphenous vein graft lesions or multiple stenosis who are poor candidates for reoperative surgery. - with significant left main CAD who are candidates for revascularization, but are not eligible for CABG. **Patients with UA/NSTEMI** who have no serious comorbidity and coronary lesions amenable to PCI: - with single or multi-vessel CAD who are undergoing medical therapy with focal saphenous vein graft lesions or multiple stenosis and are poor candidates for reoperative surgery. - with amenable lesions and no contraindication for PCI in the absence of high-risk features associated with UA/NSTEMI. - with significant left main CAD who are candidates for revascularization but are not eligible for CABG. **Patients with STEMI:** - selected patients 75 years or older who develop shock within 36 hours of MI, and are suitable for revascularization that can be performed within 18 hours of shock. - in patients with onset of symptoms within the prior 12 to 24 hours and 1 or more of the following: severe CHF, hemodynamic or electrical instability, evidence of persistent ischemia. Fibrinolytic-ineligible patients with onset of symptoms within the prior 12 to 24 hours, and 1 or more of the following: - severe CHF. - hemodynamic or electrical instability. - evidence of persistent ischemia.
	Angina grading scale used in above indications from Canadian Cardiovascular Society:
Class I	Ordinary physical activity does not cause angina, such as walking or climbing stairs. Angina occurs with strenuous, rapid or prolonged exertion at work or recreation.
Class II	Slight limitation of ordinary activity. Angina occurs on walking or climbing stairs rapidly; walking uphill; walking or stair climbing after meals; in cold, in wind or under emotional stress; or only during the few hours after awaking. Angina occurs after walking more than 2 blocks on the level and climbing more than one flight of ordinary stairs at a normal pace and under normal conditions.

Continued on next page.

Cardiac Catheterization & Interventional Cardiology

	Table 15.1 (3 of 3) **Indications for Percutaneous Coronary Intervention**	
Class III	Marked limitations of ordinary physical activity. Angina occurs on walking 1-2 blocks on the level and climbing one flight of stairs under normal conditions and at a normal pace.
Class IV	Inability to carry on any physical activity without discomfort – anginal symptoms may be present at rest.

Source: Smith, S. C., Hirshfeld, J. W., Jacobs, A. K., Kern, M. J., King, S. B., Morrison, D. A., et al. (2005). ACC/AHA/SCAI 2005 Guideline Update for Percutaneous Coronary Intervention: a report of the American College of Cardiology/American Heart Association Task Force on Practice Guidelines (ACC/AHA/SCAI Writing Committee to Update the 2001 Guidelines for Percutaneous Coronary Intervention). [Electronic Version] from www.americanheart.org/presenter.jhtml?identifier=3035436.

Abbreviations used in the table:
CABG = coronary artery bypass graft.
CAD = coronary artery disease.
CCS = Canadian Cardiovascular Society.
CHF = congestive heart failure.
HF = heart failure.
LBBB = left bundle branch block.
LV = left ventricular.
MR = mitral regurgitation.
NSTEMI = non ST elevation myocardial infarction.
STEMI = ST elevation myocardial infarction.
UA = unstable angina.
VT = ventricular tachycardia.

Percutaneous Transluminal Coronary Angioplasty (PTCA)

PTCA is a procedure that involves placement of a balloon across a stenotic lesion in a coronary artery, dilation of the balloon to compress the plaque and dilate the artery, and deflation and withdrawal of the balloon, leaving a larger luminal diameter at the lesion site (see Figure 15.5). PTCA causes the plaque to crack and creates injury that activates a platelet response and the coagulation cascade, resulting in acute thrombosis. To prevent this complication, anticoagulation is used during the procedure and antiplatelet drugs are administered following the procedure. The other major complication of PTCA is restenosis of the diseased segment, with rates ranging from 30-50% at 6 months (Cutlip & Baim, 2006b; Mann & Davies, 2002; O'Murchu & Myler, 2002). With advances in technology and the use of intracoronary stents and other interventional devices, plain balloon angioplasty is rarely used as a stand-alone procedure any longer, but is commonly used as an adjunct to other PCI procedures.

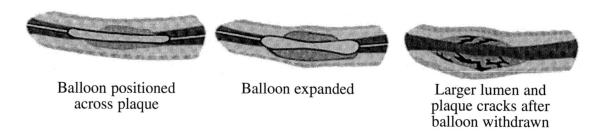

Balloon positioned across plaque

Balloon expanded

Larger lumen and plaque cracks after balloon withdrawn

Figure 15.5: Balloon positioned across plaque.

Cutting Balloon Angioplasty

The cutting balloon (Figure 15.6) has 3 or 4 longitudinal blades mounted on the surface of the balloon that are protected before inflation by the folds of the balloon. These blades are 3 to 5 times sharper than conventional surgical blades, and when the balloon is expanded they create controlled cuts in the plaque that widen as the balloon is inflated, thus allowing lower balloon inflation pressures and reducing the cracking and tissue damage caused by traditional balloon inflation (Bertrand, Meerkin, & Bonan, 2002; Cutlip & Baim, 2005). Cutting balloon angioplasty may be superior to traditional PTCA in treating ostial lesions and for in-stent restenosis (Cutlip & Baim, 2005).

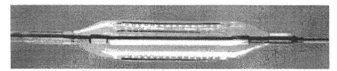

Figure 15.6: Cutting balloon.
Photo courtesy of Boston Scientific, 2006.

Intracoronary Stents

A stent is a metal scaffolding inserted into a coronary artery at the lesion site to hold the artery open. With improvements in stent design and stent delivery systems, the complications of acute vessel closure and restenosis that were common with PTCA have been dramatically reduced, thus intracoronary stenting is now done in almost all PCI procedures.

Stents (Figure 15.7) are most often made of stainless steel, although other metals such as nitinol, tantalum, and platinum/iridium are used in some models (Almond, 2002; Cutlip, Levin, & Baim, 2005). Bare metal stents are still used in some cases today, but the most commonly used stents are drug eluting stents discussed below. Stents differ in strut design, flexibility, length, diameter, and delivery method. Self-expanding stents are constrained on a delivery catheter by a membrane sheath that is retracted to allow the stent to expand to its preformed diameter once it is positioned at the lesion site. Balloon-expandable stents are mounted on a balloon and are expanded by inflation of the balloon once the stent is positioned at the lesion site. Typically, PTCA is performed before the stent is delivered, although direct stenting without predilation is being done in certain situations.

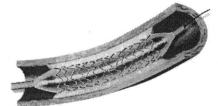

Figure 15.7: Balloon-mounted stent deployment in a coronary artery.
Photo courtesy of Boston Scientific, 2006.

Cardiac Catheterization & Interventional Cardiology

The healing process after stent implantation involves growth of the intima around the struts of the stent (endothelialization) to form a smooth lining that covers the metal struts and provides a smooth surface for blood to flow through. One of the complications of bare metal stents is intimal hyperplasia, which is overgrowth of smooth muscle cells and other cell types that eventually reocclude the artery, a process referred to as in-stent restenosis. Also contributing to restenosis is local vessel injury that occurs with balloon expansion and stent deployment. Bare metal stents reduced the 6 month restenosis rate from approximately 40% with PTCA alone to 20-30% with stenting. In an effort to further decrease the rate of restenosis, drug eluting stents were developed and have become the most commonly used stents in most centers.

Drug Eluting Stents

Drug eluting stents (DES) are metal stents coated with a polymer covering that contains an anti-restenotic drug that is released over a period of 14 to 30 days (Cutlip & Baim, 2006b). Drugs currently used in DES are sirolimus and paclitaxel (Taxol), both of which have immunosuppressive and antiproliferative properties that prevent the overgrowth of cells responsible for in-stent restenosis. Sirolimus is released over a period of 4-6 weeks, while paclitaxel is released within 2 weeks. Large clinical trials done so far have shown significant reductions of in-stent restenosis with DES, compared to bare metal stents: 3% versus 35% with sirolimus (Moses et al., 2003) and 8% versus 27% with paclitaxel (Stone et al., 2004). These benefits occurred in all subgroups of patient (e.g. diabetics, small vessels, long lesions), and are maintained for at least 2 years (Aoki et al., 2005), and up to 4 years in some follow-up studies (Sousa et al., 2005). In head-to-head comparison trials, sirolimus appears to be slightly superior to paclitaxel (Kastrati et al., 2005; Roiron, Sanchez, Bouzmondo, Lechat, & Montalescot, 2006).

Recent evidence indicates that there is a risk of late stent thrombosis (acute thrombus within a stent >30 days old) and hypersensitivity reactions associated with DES ("FDA Statement on Coronary Drug-Eluting Stents", 2006; Joner et al., 2006; Pfisterer et al., 2006). The antiproliferative effects of DES may delay or prevent endothelialization of the stent, allowing the metal struts to remain exposed to the blood. Platelets can then become activated and aggregate, leading to thrombus formation in the stent and resulting in myocardial infarction and death. In addition, hypersensitivity reactions have been reported and may also contribute to late stent thrombosis by stimulating an inflammatory response to the metal, the polymer or the drug on the stent (Virmani et al., 2004). The risk of late stent thrombosis appears to be highest in patients who discontinue taking ASA and Plavix, even for short periods of time. There has been no long term survival benefit shown with DES, and they are very expensive compared to bare metal stents.

Linking Knowledge to Practice

✔ *Nurses should be aware of the importance of continued ASA and Plavix therapy in patients following DES implantation and stress the importance of taking these drugs when doing patient teaching. Patients should be told to consult with their cardiologist before discontinuing ASA or Plavix for diagnostic or surgical procedures, such as colonoscopy, orthopedic procedures, etc.*

Atherectomy

Atherectomy devices remove plaque from the artery by either cutting it out (directional atherectomy) or "sanding" it out (rotational atherectomy). While these devices may improve acute procedural success, they have not resulted in improved survival and have been associated with increased rates of MI and other adverse cardiac events when compared with PTCA (Cutlip & Baim, 2005). While atherectomy (and use of other specialized devices like laser angioplasty) are used in less than 3% of PCI procedures,

673

they are effective in special types of lesions. Rotational atherectomy is more effective than other procedures in calcified lesions, and directional atherectomy is effective in large bifurcation lesions (Casterella & Teirstein, 2002; Ramsdale & Grech, 2002).

Directional Coronary Atherectomy (DCA)

Directional atherectomy removes plaque by cutting it away from the artery wall using a device that consists of a circular cutting blade housed inside a window with a balloon opposite the window (Ramsdale & Grech, 2002) (see Figure 15.8). When the device is positioned at the plaque area, the balloon is inflated to push the window against the plaque, forcing the plaque into the window, then the cutter is advanced down the window and shaves the plaque off into a distal nosecone. The device can then be turned to remove plaque in other areas of the lesion. PTCA is usually done following the procedure, and a stent can be inserted if DCA fails to open the artery satisfactorily. DCA is sometimes used to remove heavy plaque prior to stenting.

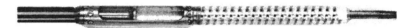

Image courtesy of Abbott Vascular. © 2006 Abbott Laboratories. All rights reserved.

Figure 15.8: Directional atherectomy device.

Rotational Coronary Atherectomy (Rotablation)

Rotational atherectomy (RA) removes calcified plaque by grinding it into micro-particles that are small enough to flow downstream in the coronary circulation. The device consists of an elliptical shaped burr that is coated on the leading half with diamond microchips that act like sandpaper (see Figure 15.9). The burr is welded to a flexible drive shaft connected to a turbine that rotates the burr at speeds of up to 200,000 revolutions per minute when activated by a foot pedal (Casterella & Teirstein, 2002). Progressively larger burrs are used to obtain the final desired lumen diameter. RA is especially useful in heavily calcified lesions that cannot be cut or dilated with a balloon; however, it is associated with a high rate of restenosis and MI. It may be used prior to stenting when heavy plaque is present that could interfere with stent expansion.

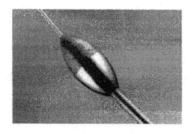
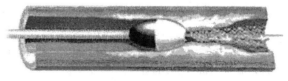

Figure 15.9: Rotational atherectomy device.
Photos courtesy of Boston Scientific, 2006.

Cardiac Catheterization & Interventional Cardiology

Transluminal Extraction Atherectomy

The transluminal extraction catheter (TEC) is a device that extracts plaque and thrombus from both native coronary arteries and saphenous vein grafts. The TEC device consists of an atherectomy catheter with a central lumen, a cutting head with two rotating blades, a drive unit that rotates the cutting blades at about 750 revolutions per minute, and a vacuum bottle at the proximal end of the system that collects excised atheroma and thrombus extracted from the artery (Mehta, Margolis, & Hidalgo, 2002). A guidewire is placed as distally as possible in the involved artery and the cutting head is positioned at the proximal end of the lesion. The drive unit is activated by hand and the cutting head is advanced slowly across the lesion, while saline is flushed through the guiding catheter. Excised plaque, thrombus, and saline are vacuumed through the central lumen of the TEC catheter into the collection bottle. Typically, one to three passes across the artery are made, and progressively larger cutting heads can be used to obtain optimal lumen diameter. Figure 15.10 illustrates a TEC device.

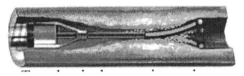

Figure 15.10: Transluminal extraction catheter.

Intravascular Ultrasound (IVUS)

Intravascular ultrasound (IVUS), or intracoronary ultrasound (ICUS), allows visualization of the anatomy of the coronary artery wall by using a miniature transducer at the end of a flexible catheter. The IVUS catheter is inserted into a coronary artery (or peripheral vessel) and transmits ultrasound from the transducer through the wall of the vessel. The ultrasound is reflected back to the transducer when it encounters structures of different acoustic impedance, creating a high resolution cross-sectional grayscale image of the vessel lumen, vascular wall components, and atherosclerotic plaque (Bose, von Birgelen, & Erbel, 2007; Gulel, Sipahi, & Tuzcu, 2007; Weissman, 2006). The ultrasound image from a normal coronary artery produces a bright echo from the intima, or inner lining of the blood vessel at the lumen-intima border; and a darker area from the media, or muscle layer of the vessel at the external elastic membrane border (Gulel, Sipahi, & Tuzcu, 2007; Weissman, 2006). Figure 15.11 shows an IVUS image of a coronary artery with plaque narrowing the lumen of the vessel.

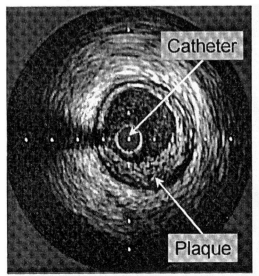
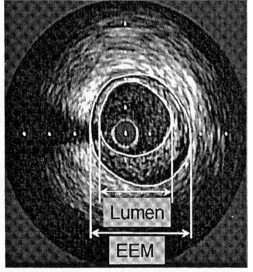

Figure 15.11: IVUS image of a coronary artery with plaque. EEM = external elastic membrane.

From Schoenhagen et al., (2001), Arterial remodeling and coronary artery disease: The concept of "dilated" versus "obstructive" coronary atherosclerosis. *JACC, 38,* 297-306. With permission from Elsevier.

Chapter 15

IVUS has some advantages over angiography. Angiography via dye injection into an artery shows a silhouette of the coronary anatomy but does not visualize the wall of the artery. Angiography demonstrates lumen narrowing once plaque has accumulated in sufficient quantity to protrude into the lumen and restrict blood flow. However, plaque growth is initially accommodated by vessel remodeling, which means that the blood vessel expands in size to accommodate the plaque in the early stages of atherosclerosis in an effort to maintain normal lumen size (Schoenhagen, Ziada, Vince, Nissen, & Tuzcu, 2001). In this early stage, angiography cannot detect the presence of atherosclerotic disease, but IVUS can demonstrate the presence of plaque within the arterial wall well before it becomes large enough to create luminal narrowing.

Uses of IVUS (Bose, von Birgelen, & Erbel, 2007; Gulel, Sipahi, & Tuzcu, 2007)
◆ Determine vessel and lumen size.
◆ Evaluate type and extent of vessel remodeling.
◆ Determine extent, morphology, and distribution of plaque within an artery.
◆ Provide information about plaque composition (e.g. lipid, fibrous tissue, calcium)
   ❖ Helps guide type of PCI procedure, e.g. rotablation is better for highly calcified lesions.
   ❖ May also be useful in identifying vulnerable plaque that is more prone to rupture.
◆ Assess stent deployment and stent strut apposition to arterial wall during PCI.
◆ Detect residual plaque burden following atherectomy (may demonstrate need for more aggressive plaque removal during procedure).
◆ Detect artery dissection and intramural hematoma.
◆ Assessment of in-stent restenosis
   ❖ Differentiate intimal hyperplasia (most common mechanism of restenosis) from other causes (e.g. stent underexpansion, dissection, thrombus).
◆ Differentiate between true and pseudoaneurysm in the vessel.
◆ Identification of transplant vasculopathy following cardiac transplant.
◆ Follow progression or regression of atherosclerosis to evaluate drug effects and other therapies for cardiovascular disease.

New technology that analyzes the radiofrequency data from the ultrasound signal obtained by IVUS is being developed to provide more accurate information about tissue properties and plaque composition (Mehta, McCrary, Frutkin, Dolla, & Marso, 2007). These new techniques are better able to differentiate distinct components of plaque (fibrous tissue, lipid, calcium) and display them in color images that provide "virtual histology" of the arterial wall. Research is ongoing in developing this technology and determining its application in assessment and management of atherosclerotic disease.

Outcomes of PCI Procedures

The success of PCI procedures is defined by angiographic, procedural and clinical criteria. The AHA/ACC Guidelines define PCI outcomes as follows:
◆ Angiographic success – minimum stenosis diameter reduction to < 20%.
   ❖ Reported rates range between 82% and 98% depending on device used and types of lesions attempted.
   ❖ Success rate for opening a total occlusion associated with STEMI is > 90%.
◆ Procedural success – achievement of angiographic success without major clinical complications (e.g. MI, death, emergency CABG) during hospitalization.
   ❖ Success rate is 90%-95% with currently used devices and adjunctive drug therapy.

Cardiac Catheterization & Interventional Cardiology

◆ Clinical success.
  ❖ Short term – anatomic and procedural success with relief of signs and symptoms of myocardial ischemia after the patient recovers from the procedure.
  ❖ Long term – anatomic and procedural success remains durable, and there is persistent relief of signs and symptoms of myocardial ischemia for more than 6 months after the procedure.

Adjunctive Drug Therapy and PCI

All PCI procedures cause vascular injury that is a trigger for thrombus formation, and stents are foreign substances that are thrombogenic. In addition, many patients receiving PCI procedures present with acute coronary syndromes in which thrombus is in various stages of formation in the coronary artery. The use of antithrombotic drugs during and after the procedure is mandatory to prevent acute and late thrombosis at the interventional site. Recommendations from the American Heart Association/American College of Cardiology/ Society for Cardiovascular Angiography and Interventions (Smith et al., 2005) and the American College of Chest Physicians for use of antithrombotic therapy during PCI are presented here (Popma et al., 2004). Refer to Chapter 14 for specific information about these drugs.

Antiplatelet Therapy

Aspirin
◆ Patients already taking daily chronic ASA therapy should take 75-325 mg before the procedure.
◆ Patients not on chronic ASA therapy should take 300-325 mg at least two hours and preferably 24 hours prior to the procedure.
◆ For long-term treatment after PCI in patients without contraindications, patient should take 162-325 mg daily for at least one month after bare metal stent, at least three months after sirolimus stent, at least 6 months after paclitaxel stent, after which a daily dose of 75-162 mg should be continued indefinitely.

Clopidogrel (Plavix)
◆ Clopidogrel is favored over ticlopidine (Ticlid).
◆ Loading dose of 600 mg before or when the PCI is performed. If PCI is within 12-24 hours of fibrinolytic therapy then the loading dose of clopidogrel is 300 mg.
◆ In aspirin intolerant patients: clopidogrel 300 mg at least 24 hours prior to planned PCI.
◆ After stent placement: clopidogrel 75 mg daily for at least 12 months after a drug eluting stent if not at high risk of bleeding; and at least one month (ideally up to 12 months) after a bare metal stent (unless patient is at high risk of bleeding, then at least two weeks).
◆ Following stent placement, combination of aspirin and clopidogrel is favored over systemic anticoagulation therapy.

GP IIb/IIIa Inhibitors
◆ All patients undergoing PCI, especially those with primary PCI or refractory UA or other high-risk features, should receive either abciximab (Reopro) or eptifibatide (Integrilin). In patients with STEMI undergoing PCI, abciximab is preferred over eptifibatide. Whenever possible, abciximab should be started prior to balloon inflation.
◆ Recommended administration of abciximab: 0.25 mg/kg bolus, followed by a 12-hour infusion at 10 mcg/min.
◆ Recommended administration of eptifibatide: double bolus of 180 mcg/kg, each given 10 minutes apart, followed by an 18 hour infusion at 2 mcg/kg/min (1 mcg/kg/min in patients with renal disease).
◆ For patients with NSTEMI/UA, who are designated moderate-to-high risk, either abciximab or eptifibatide should be started as soon as possible prior to PCI.

Chapter 15

◆ In patients with NSTEMI/UA and elevated troponin, abciximab should be started within 24 hours of planned PCI.

Antithrombin Therapy
Unfractionated Heparin
◆ Should be administered to all patients undergoing PCI.
◆ In patients with heparin induced thrombocytopenia (HIT), bivalirudin or argatroban should be used.
◆ In patients receiving a GP IIb/IIIa inhibitor, heparin bolus of 50-70 IU/kg to achieve target ACT > 200 sec.
◆ In patients not receiving GP IIb/IIIa inhibitor, heparin bolus of 60-100 IU/kg to achieve ACT of 250-350 sec.
◆ Post procedure heparin is not recommended after uncomplicated PCI.

Low Molecular Weight Heparin (LMWH)
◆ LMWH is a reasonable alternative to unfractionated heparin in patients with UA/NSTEMI.
◆ In patients who have received LMWH prior to PCI, additional anticoagulation is dependent on the timing of the last dose of LMWH:
  ❖ If last dose of enoxaparin (Lovenox) was < 8 hours prior to PCI: no additional anticoagulation.
  ❖ If last dose of enoxaparin was between 8 and 12 hours prior to PCI: 0.3 mg/kg IV bolus of enoxaparin at time of PCI.
  ❖ If last dose of enoxaparin was > 12 hours prior to PCI: conventional anticoagulation therapy during PCI.

Direct Thrombin Inhibitors (bivalirudin [Angiomax])
◆ For patients undergoing PCI who are not treated with a GP IIb/IIIa inhibitor: bivalirudin 0.75 mg/kg IV bolus followed by infusion of 1.75 mg/kg/h for duration of PCI procedure (recommended over use of heparin during PCI).
◆ In patients at low risk for complications: bivalirudin can be used as an alternative to heparin as an adjunct to GP IIb/IIIa inhibitors.
◆ In patients at high risk for bleeding: bivalirudin recommended over heparin as adjunct to GP IIb/IIIa inhibitors.

Warfarin
◆ Not recommended post PCI unless other indications for systemic anticoagulation therapy (i.e. atrial fibrillation).

Complications of PCI

In addition to all of the potential complications discussed under Diagnostic Cardiac Catheterization, the complications discussed here are specific to interventional procedures. More than 90% of PCI procedures involve stent implantation, so most of these complications are stent-related. However, all PCI procedures disrupt the integrity of the vessel lumen and predispose to thrombus formation, and all have the potential to cause coronary artery dissection or perforation, and to dislodge atheromatous material that can embolize downstream. Aggressive use of antiplatelet and antithrombotic drugs has reduced the incidence of acute and late thrombosis; use of drug-eluting stents has significantly decreased the incidence of restenosis.

Cardiac Catheterization & Interventional Cardiology

Stent Thrombosis

Acute stent thrombosis occurs within 24-48 hours, while subacute thrombosis usually occurs within the first week (rarely 3-4 weeks) after stent placement. The reported incidence is about 0.5% with both bare metal and drug eluting stents in patients treated with aspirin and clopidogrel (Cutlip & Baim, 2006a). Late stent thrombosis occurring as long as a year after stent implantation is rare and usually associated with cessation of antiplatelet therapy. Stent thrombosis usually presents clinically as profound ischemia or infarction, and is usually treated with emergency PCI to reopen the vessel.

Coronary Artery Dissection

Dissection of the coronary artery occurs when the intimal layer is separated from the medial layer of the blood vessel, and can be caused by passage of guidewires or other PCI devices, or by inflation of the balloon in the artery. Larger dissections can result in abrupt closure of the vessel and MI. Dissection has become less common since PTCA is rarely done without stent implantation, and stenting is the treatment for most dissections.

Coronary Artery Perforation

Perforation of a coronary artery is potentially catastrophic and can result in cardiac tamponade, emergency CABG, MI, and death. Perforation occurs in about 0.2-0.6% of patients undergoing PTCA (Carroza & Baim, 2006), and more often with use of atherectomy devices or intravascular ultrasound (Levin, Cutlip, & Baim, 2006). Nonsurgical management includes inflation of a balloon at the perforation site to control bleeding and possibly seal a small tear, insertion of a covered stent (specialized fabric-like material covers the stent and acts like a graft) at the perforation site, and pericardiocentesis to remove large accumulations of blood from the pericardial space and relieve tamponade. Emergency CABG is indicated if bleeding cannot be controlled any other way.

Coronary Ischemia

Chest pain within 48 hours after PCI can result from subacute vessel closure due to thrombosis at the site, transient coronary spasm, side branch occlusion by a stent, or distal embolization of debris from the lesion site (Carroza & Baim, 2006; Levin, Cutlip, & Baim, 2006). If ECG changes occur with chest pain, there is a significantly increased incidence of MI, repeat procedure, and death. Elevated cardiac enzymes (CK-MB and troponin) occur in up to 30% of patients, indicating a periprocedural MI. Elevated enzymes are thought to be the result of distal embolization of plaque constituents (especially with rotational atherectomy) and occlusion of side branches of coronary circulation. Nonischemic chest pain after PCI usually occurs without ECG changes or enzyme elevations and is atypical of the patient's anginal pain. The proposed cause of most nonischemic chest pain is overexpansion of the stent (Levin, Cutlip, & Baim, 2006).

Post-procedure Care

In addition to routine post-catheterization management (see section on Diagnostic Cardiac Catheterization), nurses must be attentive to the following issues:

Monitoring for Ischemia

Interventional patients must be monitored for myocardial ischemia that can be due to acute vessel occlusion following the procedure. Patients need to be taught to report chest pain immediately, and if pain occurs, an ECG should be obtained as soon as possible. If ST segment monitoring is available in the bedside monitoring equipment, it should be utilized to detect both overt and silent myocardial ischemia.

Chapter 15

Continuous 12 lead ECG monitoring is preferred if available (Drew, Adams, Pelter, & Wung, 1996; Drew et al., 1998). If two leads can be monitored, it is recommended that lead V1 be used for arrhythmia monitoring, and the second lead should be chosen to monitor for ST segment deviation based on the interventional artery (Jacobson, 2006). Since most bedside monitors allow use of only one V lead, the second lead has to be a limb lead. If the interventional artery is the RCA, limb leads II, III, or a VF are appropriate choices for ST monitoring. If the interventional artery is the circumflex, limb leads I or a VL are appropriate. If the LAD is the interventional artery, the best lead is V3, but limb leads III or a VF are appropriate choices to show reciprocal ST depression due to reocclusion of the LAD.

Linking Knowledge to Practice

✔ *If you work in a cardiac catheterization lab and have the capability of monitoring multiple leads during the procedure, document which leads showed ST elevation or depression during balloon inflation. This is useful information to include in report to nurses receiving the patient following the procedure.*

✔ *If you are receiving a patient following a PCI procedure, ask which leads showed ST elevation or depression during balloon inflation and then choose an appropriate lead for bedside monitoring.*

Anticoagulation Issues

Most interventional patients are on an intravenous GP IIb/IIIa agent (usually abciximab or eptifibatide) for several hours following the procedure. The nurse must assure that the infusion rate is accurate and that the infusion is discontinued at the appropriate time. Patients should be taught to report blood in urine or stool, and gum bleeding with tooth brushing. The patient must be monitored for signs of intracranial or GI bleeding, and lab draw sites and other puncture sites should be held for longer periods of time to control bleeding. Hct, Hb, and platelet count should be monitored following the procedure to detect occult bleeding. Any signs of bleeding should be reported to the physician so a decision can be made about the need to discontinue antiplatelet drugs.

Linking Knowledge to Practice

✔ *If an anticoagulant is ordered for every 12 hour administration, such as low molecular weight heparin, start the drug when the patient arrives from the procedure rather than waiting for the usual scheduled time if waiting would leave the patient unprotected for several hours. For example, every 12 hour dosing is usually 9 AM and 9 PM, but if the patient arrives from the procedure at noon, give the first dose soon after arrival rather than waiting until the 9 PM dose.*

Access Site Management

Access site management is more complicated following PCI because sheaths are often left in place after the procedure, and patients are on antiplatelet infusions and sometimes anticoagulants as well. If sheaths are left in place, they are not removed until the ACT is between 150-180 seconds, depending on protocol. Oozing around the sheaths is common following PCI because of heparin given during the procedure and continued infusion of GP IIb/IIIa inhibitors. If oozing becomes severe, the physician should be notified and a decision made about early removal of the sheath. The use of sandbags over the insertion site is discouraged because they dissipate pressure over too large an area to be effective in controlling oozing, and they obstruct visual inspection of the site.

The patient remains on bedrest with the affected leg straight while sheaths are in place and for 4-6 hours following sheath removal, depending on the hospital's protocol. Nurses should instruct the patient to keep the affected leg straight and to avoid raising his or her head, coughing, or straining, as these activities can increase the risk of access site bleeding. The head of the bed can be elevated to about 30 degrees for patient comfort. The patient can be turned to the affected side as long as the affected groin does not flex. Back pain is the most common complaint during the bedrest period; pain medication, sedation, and back rubs can be used for patient comfort during this time. Patients are cautioned that if bleeding does occur, the bedrest period starts over. If an arterial closure device is used, the length of bedrest can be as short as an hour, depending on the device used and hospital protocol.

Sheath removal must be done carefully with special attention paid to properly placed and prolonged pressure at the insertion site (see Figure 15.12). Typically, manual pressure is held or a compression device (e.g. C-clamp or Femostop) is left in place for a minimum of 20-30 minutes following sheath removal. The use of arterial closure devices is common after PCI procedures, but the site must still be carefully monitored for hematoma formation. If bleeding occurs around a closure device, manual pressure or a compression device is applied for a minimum of 20-30 minutes, and the patient remains on bedrest as described above.

Many patients experience a vagal reaction during or after sheath removal. This occurs more commonly in men, and can occur during the procedure or hours later. Symptoms of a vagal reaction include bradycardia, hypotension, sweating, yawning, diaphoresis, and anxiety. Vagal reactions can often be prevented by the use of sedation (e.g. Versed) and analgesia (e.g. morphine) as well as local infiltration of the access site area with lidocaine to reduce pain during pressure application. Atropine 0.5 mg IV can be used prophylactically prior to sheath removal or can be given if a vagal reaction occurs. Normal saline should be given to treat hypotension. Vagal reactions are usually of short duration and are easily managed with Atropine and fluid administration.

Figure 15.12

The skin insertion site is slightly distal to the actual artery puncture site. The white arrow indicates the direction of blood flow in the artery. Pressure needs to be applied proximal to the arterial access site in order to occlude blood flowing towards the access site. To remove an arterial sheath, place three fingers just proximal to the skin insertion site so that the arterial puncture site and the artery proximal to it are occluded by pressure. This allows the skin insertion site to remain visible so bleeding can be easily seen.

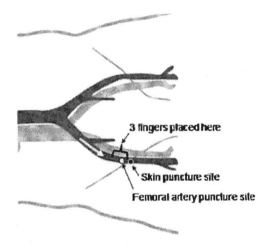

Figure 15.12: Comparison of skin and femoral artery puncture sites

Linking Knowledge to Practice

✔ *Be proactive related to the potential for a vagal reaction during sheath removal. Make sure there is a functioning IV in place and have normal saline running at a TKO rate. Have atropine at the bedside and use adequate sedation and pain medication prior to the procedure. At the first sign of a vagal reaction (yawning, bradycardia, hypotension, change in level of consciousness) open the IV up and*

Chapter 15

give atropine 0.5 mg IV. When atropine is administered watch for tachycardia. Some patients may become ischemic and develop chest pain if their heart rate increases too much with atropine, requiring treatment with NTG.

◆ *Patient teaching goes a long way in terms of patient compliance with bedrest restrictions and the need to keep the affected leg straight for a few hours. If patients know that "the clock starts all over again" if they re-bleed, they are more likely to be compliant with restrictions. A draw sheet across the knee on the affected leg serves as a reminder to keep the leg straight and is less restraining than tying the foot down.*

◆ *Back pain is a problem for many patients during the bedrest period following sheath removal. Sometimes placing a pillow under the unaffected knee or allowing the patient to lie on their side with the affected leg kept straight helps relieve back pain.*

Follow-up Care

Following PCI, patients should be taught about their disease process and given information about their specific risk factors for coronary disease. Depending on the patient's risk factors, teaching and written information should be provided on blood pressure control, diet, weight reduction, smoking cessation, lipid control, management of diabetes, and the benefits of regular exercise. The importance of taking prescribed medications should be emphasized, especially antiplatelet therapy (e.g. ASA, Plavix), beta blockers, statins, and ACE inhibitors. Patients should be referred to a cardiac rehabilitation program for help with an exercise program and risk factor modification. Patients should also be encouraged to keep follow-up visits with the primary care provider to monitor compliance with prescribed therapy and progress toward risk factor modification. Discharge teaching should also include information on access site monitoring, return to normal activities, and when and how to seek emergency help if symptoms should reoccur.

TEST YOUR KNOWLEDGE

There may be more than one correct answer.

1. Right heart catheterization can be accomplished by which of the following vascular access sites?

    a. Femoral vein

    b. Radial artery

    c. Femoral artery

    d. Subclavian vein

2. Left heart catheterization can be accomplished by which of the following vascular access sites?

    a. Femoral vein

    b. Radial artery

    c. Femoral artery

    d. Subclavian vein

Cardiac Catheterization & Interventional Cardiology

3. Left heart catheterization can provide information about which of the following?

    a. Coronary artery anatomy

    b. Pulmonary artery pressures

    c. Right ventricular function

    d. Left ventricular function

    e. Mitral valve function

4. Contrast agents used during coronary arteriography can cause which of the following complications?

    a. Myocardial infarction

    b. Pulmonary embolism

    c. Renal failure

    d. Stroke

5. Percutaneous interventional procedures (PCI) include which of the following?

    a. Stent placement

    b. Cardiac output determination

    c. Rotational atherectomy

    d. Pulmonary artery catheterization

    e. PTCA

6. PCI procedures create injury to the intima at the site of the procedure. Which of the following complications is a direct result of this local injury?

    a. Stroke

    b. Renal failure

    c. Acute thrombosis

    d. Cardiac tamponade

7. Drug eluting stents were developed to reduce which of the following complications?

    a. In-stent restenosis

    b. Acute thrombosis

    c. Coronary artery dissection

    d. Stroke

683

Chapter 15

8. Questions 8-12 refer to this patient:

    You are caring for a patient who had three stents placed in his RCA. The procedure was long and complicated, and he had rotational atherectomy to remove heavily calcified plaque prior to stenting. What drugs do you expect to administer to prevent thrombosis in the interventional artery?

    a. Beta blockers
    b. ASA
    c. Ca^{++} blockers
    d. Plavix
    e. Integrilin

9. The patient is at risk for which of the following complications due to the drugs he is on following the procedure?

    a. Ischemic stroke
    b. MI
    c. Renal failure
    d. Bleeding

10. The patient should be monitored in which of the following ECG leads to detect reocclusion of his RCA?

    a. V_1
    b. Lead III
    c. Lead I
    d. V_6

11. Your initial assessment of this patient reveals a BP of 130/76, NSR in the 70s, clear lungs, no JVD, skin is warm and dry. He is receiving NS at 100ml/hr, which is to be discontinued when the liter finishes. He has no pain but is sleepy from sedation used during the procedure. A right femoral artery sheath is still in place with slight oozing around the insertion site. What routine monitoring is indicated in this patient following the procedure?

    a. Continuous ECG monitoring
    b. Groin access site checks every 15 minutes
    c. Pedal pulse checks every 15 minutes
    d. BP every 15 minutes
    e. Vital signs and groin checks every 4 hours

Cardiac Catheterization & Interventional Cardiology

12. Forty-five minutes after returning to your unit, this patient's pressure drops to the 80s, HR is 116, and he complains of chest pain. His neck veins are elevated, his skin is cool and pale, and he feels SOB, but his lung sounds are clear. His pressure is continuing to fall and he is very anxious. You obtain a stat 12 lead ECG, which is unchanged from the ECG obtained immediately after the procedure. His femoral access site is unchanged. Which of the following is the most likely cause of these symptoms?

    a. Reocclusion of the RCA

    b. Cardiac tamponade

    c. Retroperitoneal bleeding

    d. Acute renal failure

13. When removing the arterial sheath, which of the following are true statements?

    a. Sheath can be safely removed any time following the procedure.

    b. Manual pressure or a mechanical pressure device can be used.

    c. ACT should be < 180 sec.

    d. Pressure should be applied just distal to the skin insertion site.

    e. Pressure should be maintained for at least 20-30 minutes.

    f. Atropine and fluid should be available at the bedside in case a vagal reaction occurs.

14. Following sheath removal, which of the following are true statements?

    a. The site no longer needs to be monitored once the sheath is out.

    b. Hematoma can still occur once the sheath is out.

    c. Bleeding is no longer a potential complication once the sheath is out.

    d. Access site monitoring should continue every 15 minutes for about an hour to monitor for complications.

    e. A vagal reaction can occur even after the sheath is removed.

ANSWERS

1.	A, D	8.	B, D, E
2.	B, C	9.	D
3.	A, D, E	10.	B
4.	C	11.	A, B, C, D
5.	A, C, E	12.	B
6.	C	13.	B, C, E, F
7.	A	14.	B, D, E

Chapter 15

REFERENCES

Almond, D. (2002). Coronary stenting I: intracoronary stents - form, function and future. In E. Grech & D. R. Ramsdale (Eds.), *Practical Interventional Cardiology* (2nd ed., pp. 63-76). London: Martin Dunitz.

Aoki, J., Colombo, A., Dudek, D., Banning, A.P., Drzewiecke, J., Zmudka, K., et al. (2005). Persistent remodeling and neointimal suppression 2 years after polymer-based, paclitaxel-eluting stent implantation: insights from serial intravascular ultrasound analysis in the TAXUX II study. *Circulation, 112*(25), 3876-3883.

Bertrand, O.F., Meerkin, D., & Bonan, R. (2002). Cutting balloon angioplasty. In E. Grech & D.R. Ramsdale (Eds.), *Practical Interventional Cardiology* (2nd ed., pp. 55-61). London: Martin Dunitz.

Bose, D., von Birgelen, C., & Erbel, R. (2007). Intravascular ultrasound for the evaluation of therapies targeting coronary atherosclerosis. *Journal of the American College of Cardiology, 49*(9), 925-932.

Carroza, J.P. (2006, September 15, 2006). Complications of Diagnostic Cardiac Catheterization. *UptoDate* Retrieved December 5, 2006

Carroza, J.P., & Baim, D.S. (2006). Periprocedural complications of percutaneous transluminal coronary angioplasty. *UpToDate* Retrieved June 20, 2006, from www.uptodate.com

Casterella, P.J., & Teirstein, P.S. (2002). Rotational Coronary Atherectomy. In E. Grech & D.R. Ramsdale (Eds.), *Practical Interventional Cardiology* (2nd ed., pp. 127-141). London: Martin Dunitz.

Cutlip, D., & Baim, D.S. (2005). Specialized revascularization devices in the management of coronary heart disease. Retrieved December 12, 2005, from www.uptodate.com

Cutlip, D., & Baim, D.S. (2006a). Coronary artery stent thrombosis. *UptoDate* Retrieved June 8, 2006, from www.uptodate.com

Cutlip, D., & Baim, D.S. (2006b). Drug-eluting intracoronary stents to prevent restenosis. *UptoDate* Retrieved December 1, 2006, from www.uptodate.com

Cutlip, D., Levin, T.N., & Baim, D.S. (2005). General principles of the use of intracoronary stents. *UptoDate* Retrieved June 8, 2006, from www.uptodate.com

Drew, B.J., Adams, M.G., Pelter, M.M., & Wung, S.F. (1996). ST-segment monitoring with a derived 12-lead electrocardiogram is superior to routine CCU monitoring. *American Journal of Critical Care, 5*, 198-206.

Drew, B.J., Pelter, M.M., Adams, M.G., Wung, S.F., Chou, T.M., & Wolfe, C.L. (1998). 12-lead ST-segment monitoring vs single-lead maximum ST-segment monitoring for detecting ongoing ischemia in patients with unstable coronary syndromes. *American Journal of Critical Care, 7*, 355-363.

FDA Statement on Coronary Drug-Eluting Stents. (2006, September 2006). from www.fda.gov/cdrh/news/091406.html

Geary, K., Landers, J.T., Fiore, W., & Riggs, P. (2002). Management of infected femoral closure devices. *Cardiovascular Surgery, 10*(2), 161-163.

Gulel, O., Sipahi, I., & Tuzcu, E.M. (2007). Intravascular untrasound: Questions and answers. *The Anatolian Journal of Cardiology, 7*, 169-178.

Jacobson, C. (2006). Bedside cardiac monitoring. In S. Burns (Ed.), *AACN Protocols for Practice: Noninvasive Monitoring* (2nd ed., pp. 3-30). Boston: Jones and Bartlett Publishers.

Joner, M., Finn, A.V., Farb, A., Mont, E.K., Kolodgie, F.D., Ladich, E., et al. (2006). Pathology of Drug-Eluting Stents in Humans: Delayed Healing and Late Thrombotic Risk *J Am Coll Cardiol, 48*(1), 193-202.

Kastrati, A., Dibra, A., Eberle, S., Mehilli, J., Suarez de Lezo, J., Goy, J.J., et al. (2005). Sirolimus-eluting stents vs paclitaxel-eluting stents in patients with coronary artery disease: meta-analysis of randomized trials. *Journal of the American Medical Association, 294*(7), 819-825.

King, S.B., Smith, S.C., Hirshfeld, J.W., Jacobs, A.K., Morrison, D.A., & Williams, D.O. (2008). 2007 Focused Update of the ACC/AHA/SCAI 2005 Guideline Update for Percutaneous Coronary Intervention: A Report of the American College of Cardiology/American Heart Association: Task Force on Practice Guidelines: 2007 Writing Group to Review New Evidence and Update the ACC/AHA/SCAI 2005 Guideline Update For Percutaneous Coronary Intervention. *Journal of the American College of Cardiology, 51,* 172-209.

Levin, T.N., Cutlip, D., & Baim, D.S. (2006). Early complications of intracoronary stents. *UptoDate* Retrieved June 8, 2006, from www.uptodate.com

Mann, J.M., & Davies, M.J. (2002). Epidemiology and pathophysiology of coronary artery disease. In E. Grech & D. R. Ramsdale (Eds.), *Practical Interventional Cardiology* (2nd ed., pp. 1-8). London: Martin Dunitz.

Mehta, S., Margolis, J., & Hidalgo, A. (2002). Transluminal Extraction Catheter Atherectomy. In E. Grech & D. R. Ramsdale (Eds.), *Practical Interventional Cardiology* (2nd ed., pp. 155-164). London: Martin Dunitz.

Mehta, S.K., McCrary, J.R., Frutkin, A.D., Dolla, W.J.S., & Marso, S.P. (2007). Intravascular ultrasound radiofrequency analysis of coronary atherosclerosis: an emerging technology for the assessment of vulnerable plaque. *European Heart Journal, 28,* 1283-1288.

Moses, J.W., Leon, M.B., Popma, J.J., Fitzgerald, P.J., Holmes, D.R., O'Shaughnessy, C., et al. (2003). Sirolimus-eluting stents versus standard stents in patients with stenosis in a native coronary artery. *New England Journal of Medicine, 349*(14), 1315-1323.

Nikolsky, E., Mehran, R., Halkin, A., Aymong, E.D., Mintz, G.S., Lasic, Z., et al. (2004). Vascular complications associated with arteriotomy closure devices in patients undergoing percutaneous coronary procedures: a meta-analysis. *J Am Coll Cardiol 44*(6), 1200-1209.

O'Murchu, B., & Myler, R. (2002). Percutaneous transluminal coronary angioplasty: history, techniques, indications and complications. In E. Grech & D.R. Ramsdale (Eds.), *Practical Interventional Cardiology* (2nd ed., pp. 25-34). London: Martin Dunitz.

Pfisterer, M., Brunner-La Rocca, H., Buser, P.T., Rickenbacher, P., Hunziker, P., Mueller, C., et al. (2006). Late Clinical Events After Clopidogrel Discontinuation May Limit the Benefit of Drug-Eluting Stents. *J Am Coll Cardiol, 48,* 2584-2591.

Popma, J.J., Berger, P., Ohman, E.M., Harrington, R.A., Grines, C., & Weitz, J.I. (2004). Antithrombotic Therapy During Percutaneous Coronary Intervention: The Seventh ACCP Conference on Antithrombotic and Thrombolytic Therapy. *Chest, 126,* 576S-599S.

Ramsdale, D.R., & Grech, E. (2002). Directional Coronary Atherectomy. In E. Grech & D.R. Ramsdale (Eds.), *Practical Interventional Cardiology* (2nd ed., pp. 103-125). London: Martin Dunitz.

Roiron, C., Sanchez, P., Bouzmondo, A., Lechat, P., & Montalescot, G. (2006). Drug eluting stents: an updated meta-analysis of randomised controlled trials. *Heart, 92*, 641-649.

Rudnick, M.R., & Tumlin, J.A. (2006, September 15, 2006). Radiocontrast media-induced acute renal failure. *UptoDate* Retrieved December 5, 2006, from www.uptodate.com

Schoenhagen, P., Ziada, K.M., Vince, D.G., Nissen, S.E., & Tuzcu, E.M. (2001). Arterial remodeling and coronary artery disease: The concept of "dilated" versus "obstructive" coronary atherosclerosis. *Journal of the American College of Cardiology, 38*, 297-306.

Smith, S.C., Hirshfeld, J. W., Jacobs, A. K., Kern, M. J., King, S. B., Morrison, D.A., et al. (2005). ACC/AHA/SCAI 2005 Guideline Update for Percutaneous Coronary Intervention: a report of the American College of Cardiology/American Heart Association Task Force on Practice Guidelinnes (ACC/AHA/SCAI Writing Committee to Update the 2001 Guidelines for Percutaneous Coronary Intervention). [Electronic Version] from www.americanheart.org/presenter.jhtml?identifier=3035436

Sousa, J.E., Costa, M.A., Abizaid, A., Feres, F., Seixas, A.C., Tanajura, L.F., et al. (2005). Four-year angiographic and intravascular ultrasound follow-up of patients treated with sirolimus-eluting stents. *Circulation, 111*(18), 2326-2329.

Stone, G.W., Ellis, S.G., Cox, D.A., Hermiller, J., O'Shaughnessy, C., Mann, J.T., et al. (2004). A polymer-based, paclitaxel-eluting stent in patients with coronary artery disease. *New England Journal of Medicine, 350*(3), 221-231.

Virmani, R., Guagliumi, G., Farb, A., Musumeci, G., Grieco, N., Motta, T., et al. (2004). Localized Hypersensitivity and Late Coronary Thrombosis Secondary to a Sirolimus-Eluting Stent. *Circulation, 109*, 701-705.

Weissman, N.J. (2006). Technique and interpretation of intravascular (intracoronary) ultrasonography. *Uptodate* Retrieved May 20, 2007.

CHAPTER 16:
OPEN HEART SURGERY AND CORONARY ARTERY BYPASS GRAFTING (CABG)

OVERVIEW

Surgical revascularization performed by coronary artery bypass grafting (CABG) was first introduced in 1967.

Goals of Revascularization

◆ Improve Survival. In asymptomatic patients, revascularization is only performed if there is an expected survival advantage.

◆ Minimize Complications of Ischemia.

◆ Relieve Ischemic Symptoms.

◆ Improve Functional Capacity

(Eagle et al., 2004).

Indications for CABG

◆ Left main disease or multi-vessel disease with impaired LV function (proven survival benefit) (Antman et al., 2004; Braunwald et al., 2002; Eagle et al., 2004; Gibbons et al., 2002).

◆ Left main equivalent disease: significant left anterior descending (LAD) and left circumflex blockage.

◆ Proximal LAD disease with > than 75% occlusion, plus another vessel, plus a very positive stress test and an abnormal ECG.

◆ Survivors of sudden death with CAD.

◆ Multi-vessel disease in diabetes

(Eagle et al., 2004).

Contraindications to CABG

◆ Lack of adequate conduit.

◆ Small (< 1-1.5 mm) coronary arteries distal to stenosis.

◆ Severe atherosclerosis of the aorta (places patient at very high risk for neurological complications).

◆ Severe left ventricular failure and coexisting peripheral vascular, renal and pulmonary disease.

◆ Other limiting conditions:

❖ Advanced or metastatic cancer with a life expectancy of less than 1 year.

❖ End-stage cirrhosis with severe portal hypertension.

❖ Intracranial disorders that limit the ability to anticoagulate or substantially limit cognitive function (Braunwald et al., 2002).

Chapter 16

Survival Benefit

◆ CABG increases the chance of survival in patients with reduced left ventricular function, severe ischemia, or potential for severe ischemia (Braunwald et al., 2002).

◆ The worse the left ventricular function, the greater the potential mortality benefit with CABG (Eagle et al., 2004). *Note:* Reduced left ventricular function can be a result of chronic hypoperfusion as well as a past myocardial infarction (MI). Areas with chronic hypoperfusion can be assessed for viability using noninvasive cardiac testing.

◆ CABG has the greatest survival benefit for patients who are at greatest risk of death without surgery (Gibbons et al., 2002).

◆ Compared to high-risk patients, lower-risk patients receive only a modest survival benefit with CABG. Low-risk patients are generally only considered for CABG when their symptoms have been unresponsive to medical treatment and are limiting their quality of life or functional capacity.

Symptom Benefit

◆ Angina is initially relieved in more than 90% of patients who undergo CABG (LeDoux & Luikart, 2005).

◆ Approximately 80% of patients remain free from angina at 5 years (Gibbons et al., 2002). These results are superior to medical treatment alone. Return of angina can indicate graft stenosis or progression of the patient's underlying CAD.

Patient Characteristics

There has been a change in patient population receiving CABG surgery over time. Today the CABG population profile includes the following characteristics:

◆ An older population.

◆ More women than previously.

◆ More patients with recent MI.

◆ More patients with left ventricular dysfunction.

◆ Increased number of patients with three-vessel disease.

◆ Increased patients with complicated co-morbidities.
   ❖ Diabetes mellitus.
   ❖ Lower extremity peripheral arterial disease.
   ❖ Renal insufficiency.
   ❖ Anemia.
   ❖ Chronic obstructive pulmonary disease.
   ❖ Valvular heart disease

(LeDoux & Luikart, 2005).

PREOPERATIVE CARE
Routine Preoperative Screening

◆ Thorough history and physical and detailed nursing assessment
   ❖ Coagulation abnormalities / previous problems with bleeding.
   ❖ Previous vein stripping / varicose veins.
   ❖ Skin lesions or rash (especially near planned incisions).
   ❖ Recent or current infection.
   ❖ Recent or current anticoagulant or antiplatelet use (particularly clopidogrel).

Open Heart Surgery and Coronary Artery Bypass Grafting

❖ Bilateral arm blood pressure assessment.

❖ History of alcohol use.

❖ Baseline neurological and functional status for postoperative comparison.

❖ Psychosocial, cultural, and educational needs.

◆ Chest x-ray.

◆ ECG.

◆ Complete blood count, complete chemistry panel, urinalysis, coagulation panel, and type and screen/crossmatch.

Preoperative Medications

◆ All antianginal, antihypertensive, and heart failure medications should be continued right up until the time of surgery, including the morning of surgery. Patients admitted the morning of surgery should take these medications prior to coming to the hospital. This is important to avoid any preoperative myocardial ischemia.

◆ Possible exceptions are ACE inhibitors (ACEI) and angiotensin II receptor blockers, which may be held 24 hours prior to surgery. These medications reduce systemic vascular resistance during surgery, and may contribute to postoperative renal insufficiency in high-risk patients. The use of ACE inhibitors in conjunction with Aprotinin (an antifibrinolytic, sometimes used to reduce the risk of bleeding in high risk patients) results in a higher risk for perioperative renal failure (Kincaid et al., 2005).

◆ In addition, non-steroidal anti-inflammatory medications (NSAIDs) are commonly held preoperatively in patients with or at risk for renal impairment, and in those with a high risk for bleeding.

◆ Insulin and oral hypoglycemic agents are held or given in reduced dose the morning of surgery.

◆ Routine preoperative mupirocin administration is recommended for all patients. Mupirocin is a patient administered topical antibiotic that eliminates nasal *S aureus*. Preoperative administration should begin at least one day before surgery (Engelman et al., 2007).

◆ Preoperative intravenous prophylactic antibiotics are not given until the patient is in the operating suite so the administration can be timed to be 30 to 60 minutes prior to the initial incision.

Preoperative Anticoagulants and Antiplatelet Medications

◆ When unfractionated heparin is indicated, it should be continued up until the time of surgery to avoid preoperative ischemia. Central lines can be placed with the patient on heparin. Any patient on unfractionated heparin should have his or her platelet count checked prior to surgery to assess for the development of heparin-induced thrombocytopenia.

◆ Low molecular weight heparin must be stopped at least 12 hours (preferably 24 hours) prior to surgery. The use of low molecular weight heparin can be replaced with unfractionated heparin.

◆ Short acting direct thrombin inhibitors can be continued until immediately before surgery. Bilvarudin has the shortest half life of all the direct thrombin inhibitors. All direct thrombin inhibitors lack reversibility (Ferraris & Ferraris et al., 2007).

◆ GP IIb/IIIa inhibitors tirofiban and eptifibatide should be stopped 4 to 6 hours prior to surgery. Abciximab should be stopped 12 to 24 hours prior to surgery. In patients who proceed to CABG after receiving abciximab, platelet aggregation does not return to normal for 48 hours. These patients receive special precautions during CABG to minimize the risk of bleeding.

◆ Aspirin is held for 2-3 days prior to elective surgery only. Aspirin should not be discontinued preoperatively in patients with acute coronary syndrome.

Chapter 16

◆ Clopidogrel should be stopped for 5 to 7 days prior to elective surgery. In patients with drug eluting stents, clopidogrel should be discontinued with great caution due to the concern regarding instent thrombosis. Other alternatives in these patients include hospitalization to convert clopidogrel therapy to a short acting glycoprotein IIb/IIIa inhibitor or a direct thrombin inhibitor.

◆ Warfarin is stopped 4 days prior to surgery. If surgery is urgent, vitamin K can be given. If surgery is emergent, fresh frozen plasma (FFP) is given.

◆ Most high intensity antiplatelet and anticoagulation medications are associated with an increased risk of bleeding. The timing of the discontinuation of these medications depends on both the half-life of the medication as well as the ability to reverse the effects of the medication.

◆ The goals of managing antiplatelet and anticoagulant medications during the preoperative period include preventing ischemic cardiac events while reducing the risk of surgical bleeding.

Table 16.1 summarizes the time frames for preoperative discontinuation of medications affecting platelets and coagulation.

Table 16.1 Preoperative Discontinuation Time Frames for Drugs Impacting Coagulation	
Aspirin	2-3 days (only in elective patients, not discontinued in acute coronary syndrome)
Clopidogrel	5 to 7 days (caution in withdrawal with drug eluting stents)
Tirofiban and Eptifibatide	4 to 6 hours
Abciximab	12 to 24 hours
Warfarin	4 days
Unfractionated Heparin	Continued up to time of surgery
Low Molecular Weight Heparin	12 to 24 hours
Direct Thrombin Inhibitors	Continued up to time of surgery

(Ferraris & Ferraris et al., 2007)

Preoperative Angina and Ischemia

◆ Patients who are unstable with active ischemia should be aggressively managed during the preoperative period. Medications may include IV nitrates and beta blockers, unfractionated heparin, antiplatelet therapy, and sedation.

◆ An IABP should be placed for refractory ischemia to reduce afterload and increase coronary perfusion.

◆ Factors that increase myocardial oxygen demand should be avoided during the preoperative period.

Preoperative Interventions to Decrease Transfusions

◆ Identifying patients at high risk for bleeding is a key preoperative intervention. It is important that perioperative strategies to decrease bleeding be applied to this high-risk group of patients. Risk factors for bleeding include:

❖ Advanced age.

❖ Preoperative anemia.

❖ Small body size.

❖ Acquired or congenital coagulation abnormalities.

❖ Preoperative antiplatelet or antithrombotic medications.

692

Open Heart Surgery and Coronary Artery Bypass Grafting

- ❖ Multiple comorbidities.
- ❖ Combined valve and CABG surgery.
- ❖ Urgent or emergent surgery.
- ❖ Reoperation.

◆ Limiting antiplatelet and antithrombotic drugs according to guidelines is another preoperative intervention to decrease perioperative bleeding and the need for transfusion.

◆ Recombinant human erythropoietin (EPO) can be used to restore red blood cell volume in patients undergoing preoperative autologous transfusion. EPO is also an alternative in low risk elective patients who are anemic (hemoglobin < 13 g/dL). In elective patients, EPO is started several days to a few weeks before surgery and is given in conjunction with iron therapy.

- ❖ EPO is an endogenous glycoprotein hormone that stimulates red blood cell production in response to hypoxia and anemia.
- ❖ EPO is produced by the kidney and is significantly decreased in patients with renal dysfunction. Beta blockers suppress endogenous EPO production. Cytokines released during the systemic inflammatory response also limit the production of EPO.
- ❖ The primary side effect of recombinant EPO is hypertension.
- ❖ The onset of action in recombinant EPO is 4 to 6 days.
- ❖ EPO is not typically used in patients with angina due to lack of safety data.

Preoperative Interventions to Decrease Postoperative Risk of Pulmonary Complications

◆ Most common preoperative pulmonary dysfunction is COPD. Most common parameter to assess pulmonary function is forced expiratory volume in one second. Patients with moderate to severe COPD have results < 50%-70% of predicted value, or less than 1.5 L. The diagnosis of clinical COPD is based on the following:

- ❖ Age.
- ❖ Smoking history.
- ❖ Preoperative arrhythmias.
- ❖ Previous hospitalizations for shortness of breath.
- ❖ COPD on chest radiograph (Eagle, et al. 2004).

◆ Pulmonary function studies and ABGs will be ordered for patients with COPD to assess preoperative pulmonary status.

◆ Smoking cessation is an important intervention to decrease the risk of pulmonary complications in patients electively undergoing CABG. Ideally patients should be smoke free for one month prior to surgery.

◆ Before surgery, it is important for patients to receive incentive spirometry and to perform deep breathing exercises. This preoperative treatment also provides instruction for postoperative exercises. It is important to accomplish preoperative respiratory teaching (incentive spirometry and deep breathing), even in patients without pre-existing lung disease, because postoperative sedation and pain interfere with the patient's ability to learn during the early postoperative period.

◆ All pulmonary infectious processes should be resolved prior to surgery.

◆ Bronchodilator therapy may be indicated preoperatively.

◆ Any evidence of congestive heart failure or fluid overload should be aggressively treated to achieve optimal fluid status preoperatively.

◆ If possible, weight loss should be achieved in obese patients electively undergoing CABG to decrease the risk of pulmonary and other complications.

Chapter 16

Preoperative Carotid Evaluation

◆ Carotid duplex scanning is often done routinely before surgery. Patients with symptomatic carotid bruits always need carotid duplex scanning prior to surgery.

◆ Patients who also have symptomatic or severe carotid stenosis should be treated with carotid endarterectomy prior to CABG.

◆ Carotid endarterectomy is generally not performed in asymptomatic carotid disease unless stenosis is 80% or greater (Eagle et al., 2004).

TRADITIONAL CABG

Transesophageal Echocardiography (TEE) and Epiaortic Imaging

◆ TEE probe is placed after patient is anesthetized and before patient is given heparin.

◆ TEE is used to determine global left and right ventricular function, ischemia, and valvular function.

◆ TEE is the most sensitive means for detecting myocardial ischemia via regional wall motion abnormality.

◆ Epiaortic imaging is typically used instead of TEE to assess the aortic arch and ascending aorta for atherosclerotic plaque.

◆ TEE is used to detect any intracardiac air (important in mitral valve surgery or when left side of heart has been entered), and valvular leaks, check competence of a repaired valve, and assess for global and regional ventricular function.

❖ Technical problems with blood flow through grafts can cause regional blood flow abnormalities.

❖ Intracardiac air can pass into the right coronary artery and cause RV dysfunction. Return to cardiopulmonary bypass (CPB) is necessary to de-air the aorta and bypass grafts.

◆ TEE is also used during weaning from CPB. TEE can be helpful in determining how to treat hypotension. PA catheter readings to determine volume status are not accurate because the pressure volume curve is affected due to the decreased compliance of the ventricle from cardioplegia. TEE, along with cardiac output measurements, can be used to assess ventricular filling pressures.

Anesthesia

◆ Narcotic based anesthesia is usually used to minimize myocardial depression.

◆ Narcotic induced hypotension is counteracted with fluids and vasopressors. Hypotension should be treated aggressively since it places the patient at risk for myocardial ischemia.

◆ A combination of agents are used, including:

❖ Induction agents.

❖ Anxiolytics.

❖ Amnetics.

❖ Analgesics.

❖ Muscle relaxants.

❖ Inhalation anesthetics.

◆ Use of low dose fentanyl or sufentanil, inhalation anesthetics, midazolam, and propofol allow for early postoperative extubation. Dexmedetomidine, a sedative/anesthetic, is another option because it also has analgesic and anxiolytic properties.

◆ Most common induction involves thiopental, narcotic, neuromuscular blocker (to prevent chest wall rigidity associated with high dose narcotic inductions.)

- ◆ Muscle relaxants are also given throughout the operation to minimize patient movement and suppress shivering during hypothermia.
- ◆ If a patient continues to be paralyzed in the ICU postoperatively, it is important that adequate sedation is maintained.
- ◆ Bispectral (BIS) EEG monitoring can be used to minimize the amount of medication needed.

Median Sternotomy

An incision is made in the center of the sternum from the top to bottom. This incision allows for access to the heart and thoracic vessels throughout surgery.

Cardiopulmonary Bypass (CPB) or Heart/Lung Machine (Figure 16.1)

Cardiopulmonary bypass allows for surgery to be performed on a still and bloodless heart while at the same time providing perfusion to other organs of the body.

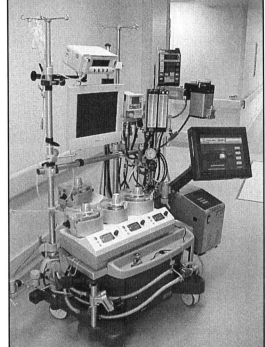

Figure 16.1: Cardiopulmonary bypass or heart/lung machine.
Courtesy of Chuck Vansickle and Aultman Heart Center, Aultman Hospital, Canton, Ohio.

- ◆ Perfusionists are responsible for the management of the heart lung machine (Figure 16.1).
- ◆ Blood is drained (usually by gravity) from the right atrium into a venous reservoir. Perfusionists can administer a wide variety of medications via a line within the venous reservoir.
- ◆ From there blood is oxygenated, cooled or warmed, and returned to the patient through an arterial cannula usually placed in the ascending aorta.
- ◆ The circuit also contains a vent to the left ventricle to prevent distention of the left ventricle when the aorta is cross-clamped (Ledoux & Luikart, 2005).
- ◆ The circuit has a direct connection to a cell saving device and may have the capability of several types of in-line monitoring such as temperature, blood gases, electrolytes and hematocrit. There are also recirculation lines to allow for venting of air and to prevent the stagnation of blood.
- ◆ Suction lines are used to aspirate blood from the surgical field. This blood is returned to the cardiotomy reservoir. This helps maintain pump volume. Blood removed from the surgical field contains fat, procoagulant factors, and proinflammatory factors. The return of this blood into the circuit typically causes systemic hypotension. Cell saver devices are used to aspirate, then wash shed blood. This process eliminates fat and many of the procoagulant and proinflammatory factors. Coagulation factors and platelets are eliminated during centrifugation but red blood cells are preserved.
- ◆ The circuit contains an arterial line filter to remove microemboli before returning blood to the patient. Microemboli can consist of air, blood, fat, and platelet microaggregates.
- ◆ The circuit also has hemoconcentrators to remove excess volume. This feature can hemoconcentrate the pump contents at the end of the case for retransfusion through the venous cannula.
- ◆ Pump prime volume is typically 1.2 to 2 L. There is normovolemic hemodilution from the pump prime. Hemodilution reduces blood viscosity and improves microcirculatory blood flow (Bojar, 2005; LeDoux & Luikart, 2005). However, excessive hemodilution reduces oncotic flow and increases the need for fluid.

Chapter 16

- The pump is primed with a balanced electrolyte solution. A colloid such as albumin may be added to the pump prime to increase oncotic pressure and decrease fluid requirements. Albumin may also delay fibrinogen absorption and delay platelet activation (Bojar, 2005). Retrograde autologous priming can also be used to reduce hemodilutional effects of the prime solution. The crystalloid prime is drained back into the circuit and aspirated into the cell saver.
- Systemic temperature is typically maintained with some degree of hypothermia to provide end organ protection. There is no conclusive evidence about the benefits of specific temperature management (Bojar, 2005).

Pump

- Systemic circulation is provided by a nonpulsatile flow. A roller pump or centrifugal pump can be used to provide nonpulsatile flow.
- Both types of pumps have similar effects on bleeding and the systemic inflammatory response.
- Roller pumps are not sensitive to pressure and can pressurize the arterial line, even with increased outflow resistance. Centrifugal pumps, however, are sensitive to pressure.
- High arterial line pressure may cause line disconnection if roller pumps are used.

Oxygenator (Figure 16.2)

- Lungs are not typically ventilated during CPB. Oxygenation occurs within the oxygenator. CO_2 is also eliminated through the oxygenator. Arterial blood gases are monitored every 30 minutes during surgery to assure adequate oxygenation and CO_2 removal.
- The ventilation of lungs during CPB has been suggested as a strategy to improve postoperative lung function. However, research results have not shown proven benefit, and this strategy is not routinely recommended (Vohra, Levine, & Dunning, 2005).
- The oxygenator maintains adequate O_2 concentration via an adjustable FIO_2. PaO_2 is maintained above 250 mm Hg to assure adequate oxygenation in case of temporary flow reduction through the CPB circuit.
- The oxygenator also has a sweep rate that determines gas flow and elimination of CO_2. CO_2 production decreases and pH rises with hypothermia. The $PaCO_2$ and pH are maintained at close to normal by adjusting the sweep rate.

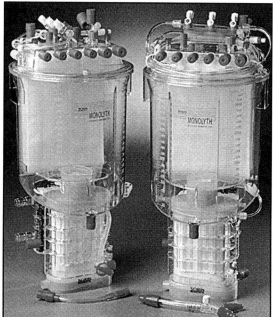

Figure 16.2: Oxygenator.

- The oxygenator can be coated with heparin or silicone to improve the biocompatibility.
- The modern membrane oxygenator contains the venous reservoir and heat exchanger. The heat exchanger is usually located proximal to the oxygenator. Water and blood pass countercurrently over a stainless steel interface. Heat is transferred by conduction.
- The oxygenator mimics the natural alveolar membrane by placing a thin membrane between the gas and the blood. The oxygenator is positioned after the roller or centrifugal pump to mimic the right ventricle pumping blood to the lung.
- Arterialized (oxygenated) blood then leaves the oxygenator prepared to enter the systemic circulation.

Cannulation

- Figure 16.3 displays the CPB circuit in relation to the patient.
- Venous drainage is typically done via a single cannula (Figure 16.4B). The cannula is placed through the right atrial appendage or through the right atrial free wall with the distal end in the inferior vena cava. Blood drains from the inferior vena cava and from the right atrium via side holes. This is the most common cannulation technique when surgery does not need to be done on the right side of the heart.
- Cannulation of the superior and inferior vena cavae (bicaval cannulation) is required for surgery involving the tricuspid valve and is often used for surgery involving the mitral valve (Figure 16.4A).
- Femerol venous cannulation may be used in emergent situations.
- Venous drainage is important because inadequate drainage distends the heart and stretches myocardial fibers. This overstretch may result in myocardial injury.
- There is a potential for entry of air into the venous lines at the point of cannulation. This is prevented with good suture technique around the cannula.
- Arterial cannulation involves placement of a cannula in the ascending aorta just proximal to the innominate artery. This is the most common arterial cannulation site (Figure 16.5). Alternate cannulation may be needed in patients having re-operation or in those patients with calcified or atherosclerotic aortas. The femoral artery may be used as an alternate cannulation site (Figure 16.5), however, there is a risk of retrograde dissection or retrograde cerebral embolism with femoral artery cannulation (Bojar, 2005).
- The size of the cannula is based on flow rate, which is determined by the patient's body surface area. Some cannulas have a distal net designed to trap embolic material.
- Epiaortic imaging is the gold standard for identifying atherosclerotic plaque in the aorta. Transesophageal echocardiography may also be used. In patients with severe ascending aortic atherosclerosis, it has been suggested that the tip of the cannula be placed beyond the left subclavain artery to avoid cerebral emboli. Off pump surgery is another option, which is discussed later.
- Cannulas can be placed percutaneously or via a surgical cut down.

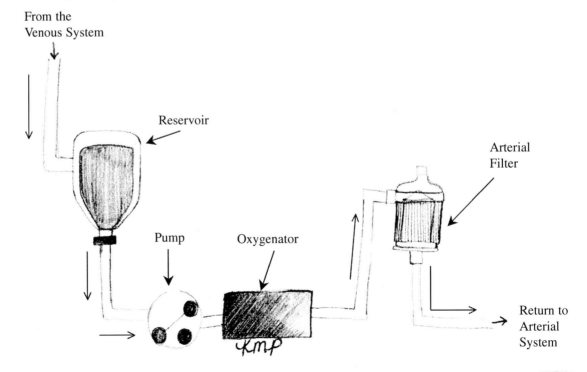

Figure 16.3: Cardiopulmonary bypass circuit.

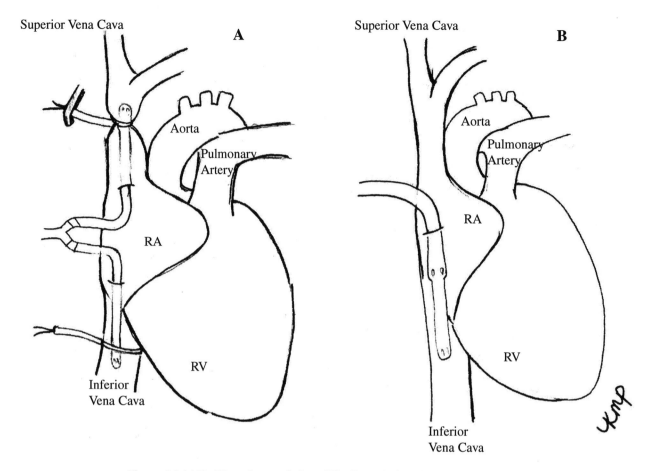

Figure 16.4 (A): Bicaval cannulation; **(B):** Cannulation via single cannula.

Myocardial Protection/Cardioplegia

◆ The combination of extracorpeal circulation, aortic cross-clamping, and cardioplegic arrest allows the surgeon to operate on a bloodless still-operating field. The heart is arrested with cardioplegia solution after the aorta is cross-clamped and coronary circulation is interrupted.

◆ Administration of cardioplegia is required when the aorta is clamped to prevent myocardial ischemia and injury. Cardioplegia solutions can extend the period of ischemic arrest to over 3 hours (Bojar, 2005). Without cardioplegia solution, ischemic arrest from aortic cross-clamping would be limited to 15 to 20 minutes in order to prevent significant myocardial injury (Bojar, 2005; LeDoux & Luikart, 2005).

◆ There is a separate heat exchanger in the bypass circuit to allow for the warm or cold delivery of cardioplegia solution.

  ❖ Myocardial oxygen demand is reduced by 90% by arresting the heart at normothermia. This is significantly more reduction in myocardial oxygen demand than can be achieved by hypothermia alone.

  ❖ Systemic hypothermia with additional topical cooling of the left ventricle is routinely used in patients receiving cold cardioplegia. The phrenic nerve must be protected from cold injury.

  ❖ Warm cardioplegia can also be used. The potential advantages of warm cardioplegia are that cellular repair is improved at normothermia and there is improved metabolic recovery. The potential disadvantage of warm cardioplegia is that the heart can resume electrical activity at normothermia so cardioplegia can only be briefly interrupted.

Open Heart Surgery and Coronary Artery Bypass Grafting

- ❖ Warm cardioplegia can also be used in conjunction with cold cardioplegia at the beginning and ending of aortic cross clamping.
- ◆ Cardioplegia solution contains a combination of potassium and other additives such as magnesium and procainamide to produce immediate cardiac arrest. The solution contains 20 to 25 mEq/L of KCl. Potassium levels are monitored frequently. An increase in potassium may require a change in the cardioplegia solution. Diuretics or insulin may also need to be given to control potassium.
- ◆ Cardioplegia solutions contain additional substances to aid in myocardial protection:
  - ❖ Glucose, glutamate, or aspartate as an energy source.
  - ❖ Bicarbonate or phosphate to buffer acidosis.
  - ❖ Calcium, steroids, or procaine to stabilize cardiac membranes.
  - ❖ Solution is made to be hyperosmolar to prevent myocardial edema
  (LeDoux & Luikart, 2005).
- ◆ Cardioplegia solution can be crystalloid or a crystalloid and blood mixture.
  - ❖ Crystalloid solutions are used to arrest the heart at cold temperatures. The use of standard crystalloid solutions can result in a depletion of adenosine triphosphate stores (LeDoux & Luikart, 2005). Ventricular fibrillation occurs when the heart is maintained at a cold temperature during cardioplegia arrest and usually requires defibrillation (Bojar, 2005).
  - ❖ Solutions involving the use of blood are commonly used because of the increased oxygen carrying capacity and to maintain oncotic pressure and reduce myocardial edema. Another benefit of blood cardioplegia is the ability of blood proteins to act as scavengers for oxygen free radicals (LeDoux & Luikart, 2005). Solutions containing blood are recommended in emergent and urgent cases as well as in patients with depressed left ventricular function (Bojar, 2005).
- ◆ Cardioplegia can be infused either antegrade through the coronary arteries or retrograde through the coronary veins.
  - ❖ Cardioplegia is initially administered antegrade via the aortic root and then can be administered retrograde via the coronary sinus.
  - ❖ The potential advantage for retrograde infusion is better distribution to the myocardium by avoiding blockages in the coronary arteries. Infusion pressure must be monitored particularly during retrograde infusion. Infusion pressure should not exceed 40 mm Hg to prevent rupture of the coronary sinus.
  - ❖ A combination of antegrade and retrograde infusion can be used to provide optimal myocardial protection.
  - ❖ In high risk patients a combination of antegrade and retrograde blood cardioplegia is used.

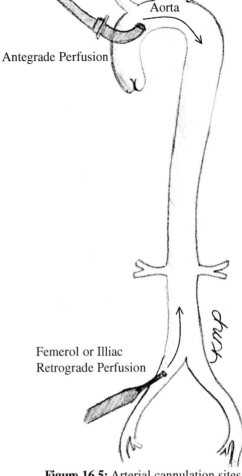

Figure 16.5: Arterial cannulation sites.

Chapter 16

◆ Maintenance of arrest is accomplished by the readministration of cardioplegia solution with a lower KCl concentration every 15 to 20 minutes. Cold blood alone can also be used as an alternative to additional cardioplegia doses as long as this is sufficient to keep the heart arrested. The cold blood is given retrograde via the coronary sinus. Using cold blood instead of additional cardioplegia helps eliminate high KCl levels. A modified cardioplegia solution is given prior to the release of the cross clamp to provide additional myocardial protection.

◆ Intermittent ischemic arrest can also be used with multiple short periods of cross-clamping.

◆ The optimal type and delivery of cardioplegia remains the subject of current research. Most methods have similar results in low risk patients. All methods have the potential to provide suboptimal protection to the right ventricle, especially in patients with RCA disease. The RCA can be grafted first during surgery and additional cardioplegia can be administered via the graft.

◆ Surgery may also be performed on a hypothermic fibrillating heart where the aorta is not clamped. This method is called deep hypothermic circulatory arrest. However, this method may not provide adequate myocardial protection. Today there are improved stabilizing devices, and patients who need to avoid cross clamping of the aorta usually have surgery done on a beating heart.

◆ Beating heart surgery can also be performed while on CPB. In this type of surgery there is no cross-clamping of the aorta. There is less myocardial oxygen demand on an empty beating heart.

Table 16.2 summarizes variables involved in cardioplegia administration.

Table 16.2 Summary of Cardioplegia Administration	
Solution:	Crystalloid Crystalloid and Blood Mixture
Delivery:	Antegrade Retrograde Combined antegrade or retrograde
Temperature:	Cold Tepid Warm
Timing:	Continuous Intermittent

Additional Myocardial Protection

Prophylactic use of an intra-aortic balloon pump two or more hours before cardiopulmonary bypass can increase myocardial protection in high-risk patients. Intra-aortic balloon counterpulsation involves the placement of a balloon catheter in the descending aorta. The balloon is inflated during diastole and deflated during systole, delivering counterpulsation therapy. With balloon inflation during diastole, myocardial perfusion is increased. Perfusion to other organs is also increased. However, the myocardium receives the most benefit due to the proximity of the balloon. With balloon deflation just before systole, a vacuum is created in the aorta to reduce afterload, thereby reducing the work of the left ventricle. Intra-aortic balloon pumping is discussed in detail in Chapter 4.

Open Heart Surgery and Coronary Artery Bypass Grafting

INTRAOPERATIVE PATIENT MANAGEMENT ISSUES

Blood Pressure During CPB

◆ Blood pressure initially decreases from hemodilution and a decrease in blood viscosity.

◆ Optimal mean blood pressure during CPB remains controversial. It has been suggested that a higher mean BP may be associated with decreased neurological complications.

◆ Mean blood pressure is typically kept around 60 to 65 mm Hg (between 50 and 70 mm Hg) during bypass (Bojar, 2005; LeDoux & Luikart, 2005). Diabetic patients, hypertensive patients, those with untreated carotid disease, and patients with renal insufficiency (creatinine > 1.5 mg/dl) need a higher MAP and shorter pump times to protect renal function. These patients may also be considered for off pump surgery.

◆ Hypotension during CPB can be related to several factors:
  ❖ Administration of preoperative vasodilators.
  ❖ Autonomic dysfunction.
  ❖ Aortic insufficiency.
  ❖ Inadequate systemic flow rates on CPB.
  ❖ Impairment of venous drainage on CPB.
  ❖ Return of large amounts of cardiotomy suctioned blood back into circulation.
  ❖ Administration of cardioplegia containing KCl.
  ❖ Vasodilation that occurs during rewarming.

◆ Vasoplegia caused by autonomic dysfunction and resulting in profound hypotension occurs in rare occasions. It also occurs more frequently in patients on multiple preoperative antihypertensives, and those on preoperative ACE inhibitors, calcium channel blockers, and amiodarone. Vasoplegia typically responds to vasopressin, which helps in restoring catecholamine sensitivity. Methylene blue is another alternative treatment for vasoplegia.

◆ Hypertension during CPB can be caused by:
  ❖ Vasoconstriction from hypothermia.
  ❖ Elevated endogenous levels of catecholamines.
  ❖ Alterations in acid base balance.
  ❖ Dilution of narcotics from pump prime.

Systemic Flow During CPB

◆ Systemic flow rate is set based on the patient's body surface area and adjusted based on degree of hypothermia. The flow rate is typically 2.2 L/min/mm^2 at normothermia (LeDoux & Luikart, 2005). Flow rate is decreased to 1.5 to 1.7 L/min/mm^2 at 30 degrees C (Bojar, 2005).

◆ Blood is cooled during CPB to decrease metabolic demands.

◆ Adequate flow rates must be maintained because the use of alpha agents to maintain blood pressure shunts blood away from the muscles and splanchnic circulation.

◆ The proposed benefits of low flow bypass during moderate hypothermia are:
  ❖ Myocardial protection.
  ❖ Reduced hemolysis.
  ❖ Reduced fluid requirements.

◆ Due to concerns about keeping MAP above the autoregulation threshold, there are some proponents of high flow (2-2.4 L/min/mm^2) rather than low flow during hypothermia.

Chapter 16

- Venous oxygen saturation (SVO_2) is measured to assure adequate systemic flow. A $SVO_2 > 65\%$ is associated with adequate systemic flow.
  - Venous oxygen saturation will increase with systemic hypothermia due to decreased oxygen extraction.
  - SVO_2 decreases during rewarming, requiring an increase in flow rate.
  - SVO_2 assesses global oxygenation, but does not assess the adequacy of regional blood flow. The brain and kidneys autoregulate to maintain flow, but skeletal and splanchnic flow are not under autoregulation.
  - Renal autoregulation is impaired during hypothermia.

Cerebral Blood Flow During CPB

- Cerebral blood flow is determined by blood pressure and blood flow, but may be more dependent on blood pressure than blood flow.
- Cerebral blood flow is maintained by autoregulation until the cerebral pressure falls below 40 mm Hg. Higher pressures are needed in diabetic hypertensive patients. Blood pressure must be maintained regardless of flow rate, and vasopressors are used if necessary. Vasopressors may improve cerebral oxygenation but reduce flow to other regions of the body such as kidneys.
- Measurement of cerebral oxygenation can be accomplished by fiberoptic jugular bulb oximetry or cerebral oximetry, using bifrontal sensors with near infrared spectroscopy.
- Cerebral perfusion ($ScO2$) should be kept > 40 mm Hg to reduce neurological complications. $ScO2$ can be reduced even when the SVO_2 is normal. $ScO2$ is at risk for falling with the initiation of CPB and during rewarming.

Oxygen Delivery During CPB

- Oxygen delivery is determined by the hematocrit and the systemic flow rate.
- Hemodilution from the pump prime can reduce oxygen delivery by 25%. The lower limit of hematocrit is considered to be 18%; however, there is some evidence that outcomes are superior with a hematocrit of $\geq 22\%$.

Blood Sugar Control During CPB

- Blood sugar increases and, resistance to insulin increases with the hormonal stress response to surgery and CPB.
- Reducing blood sugar may be important to decrease neurological complications. Blood sugars should be maintained at a level below 180 mg/dL. Many glycemic protocols use < 150 mg/dL as the target glucose.

Anticoagulation During CPB

- Anticoagulation is needed during CPB to prevent production of thrombin and fibrin monomers caused by the interaction between the blood and the synthetic interlining of the CPB circuit.
- 3 mg/kg of heparin is typically given before cannulation (LeDoux & Luikart, 2005). ACT should ideally be 480 seconds or greater.
- Heparin coated circuits have reduced, but not eliminated, the need for anticoagulation.
  - ACTs are kept at > 250 seconds in low risk cases.
  - ACTs are kept at > 400 seconds in high risk cases (reoperations and valve surgery).

702

Open Heart Surgery and Coronary Artery Bypass Grafting

◆ Activated clotting time (ACT) is monitored every 15 to 30 minutes during CABG (Bojar, 2005; LeDoux & Luikart, 2005). Circulating levels of heparin can also be monitored to guide heparin and protamine administration. Ecarin clotting times (ECT) can be used to measure the effectiveness of direct thrombin inhibitors in patients with heparin induced thrombocytopenia (Koster et al., 2003).

◆ Heparin resistance is present when 5mg/kg of heparin fails to raise the ACT to an adequate level. Heparin resistance is usually related to an antithrombin III deficiency (heparin binds to antithrombin III). Heparin resistance is seen more frequently in patients who receive heparin, IV nitroglycerin, or an intra aortic balloon pump preoperatively, as well as in those with infective endocarditis.

  ❖ Antithrombin III may need to be given either in fresh frozen plasma or in a commercially available product.

Anticoagulation with Heparin Induced Thrombocytopenia (HIT)

◆ Heparin administration should be delayed for 3 months in patients with HIT documented by thrombocytopenia and serologic tests.

◆ Antibodies usually disappear within this time and a heparin challenge is considered safe.

◆ Readministration of heparin with confirmed HIT (antibodies and thrombocytopenia) can produce profound thrombocytopenia and widespread thrombosis.

◆ The presence of the antibody for HIT alone, without thrombocytopenia, is not a contraindication for receiving heparin during surgery.

◆ If HIT is present, pretreatment or simultaneous treatment with antiplatelet medications (aspirin, GP IIb/IIIa inhibitors, prostaglandin analogs) is necessary to permit the use of heparin, or an alternative method of anticoagulation must be selected.

  ❖ Bivalrudin – a direct thrombin inhibitor; is a synthetic hirudin analog.

  ❖ R – hirudin (lepirudin) – a direct thrombin inhibitor.

  ❖ Argatroban – a direct thrombin inhibitor – primarily metabolized in the liver so is preferred option with renal dysfunction.

  ❖ Danaparoid sodium – is a heparinoid that inhibits factor Xa and therefore inhibits thrombin formation; there is a 10% cross-reactivity with antiheparin antibodies; half life is 20 hours so it is not reversible; has been associated with significant bleeding with CPB.

Antifibrinolytic Drugs to Decrease Bleeding

◆ Antifibrinolytic drugs to reduce blood loss are given to patients at highest risk for bleeding:

◆ Aprotinin (Trasylol), a serine protease inhibitor is both an antifibrinolytic and an antiinflammatory. The use of aprotinin became controversial with a February 2006 public health advisory warning of the possible increase risk of MI, stroke, and renal dysfunction with the use of aprotinin.

  ❖ High dose aprotinin is indicted to reduce blood loss and limit transfusions in high risk patients. The benefits of aprotinin must be weighed against the risk of renal dysfunction (Ferraris & Ferraris et al., 2007).

  ❖ Low dose aprotinin is also indicated to decrease blood loss and number of transfusions in patients having cardiac surgery (Ferraris & Ferraris et al., 2007).

◆ e–aminocaproic acid (Amicar) is often used during first time and uncomplicated cases. It has antifibrinolytic properties and may also preserve platelet function by inhibiting the conversion of plasminogen to plasmin. Unlike aprotinin, there is no effect on ACT (Bojar, 2005). Tranexamic acid (Cyclokapron) has similar properties to e-aminocaproic acid, but it is more potent. It can be used to reduce blood loss during on pump and off pump surgeries. It has been shown in some studies to be

703

Chapter 16

as effective as aprotinin (Bojar, 2005), and has no effect on the ACT. Both e-aminocaproic acid and tranexamic acid are slightly less potent than aprotinin in their blood sparing effect (Ferraris & Ferraris et al., 2007).

Heparin Reversal

◆ After successful weaning from CPB protamine is given to counteract the effect of heparin. Protamine is given at a 1:1 mg/mg ratio to return the ACT to baseline. Protamine itself is an anticoagulant and may contribute to mediastinal bleeding when given in a ratio > 1.5/1.

◆ Infusion of blood that is spun down in cell saving devices contains some heparin. Approximately 10% of heparin is retained.

◆ The ACT can remain elevated in patients with significant thrombocytopenia (ACT not affected by mild thrombocytopenia), or in patients with other coagulopathies. Platelets are dysfunctional after CPB, and the ACT will remain elevated with moderate thrombocytopenia.

◆ Heparin rebound may occur when heparin reappears after protamine neutralization (half-life of protamine is only about 5 minutes). Heparin rebound is more common with large doses of heparin and in obese patients.

◆ Intravenous protamine may cause a histamine release from the lungs and a resultant drop in SVR and blood pressures. This effect is not seen with intra-arterial administration of protamine.

◆ Protamine reactions are not common but are more frequently seen in patients who are taking NPH insulin, or who have medication or fish allergies, history of vasectomy, or previous protamine exposure (Bojar, 2005; LeDoux & Luikart, 2005). Protamine is administered slowly to allow for assessment of a response (LeDoux & Luikart, 2005). A quick response to a reaction is necessary because there is an increase in perioperative mortality associated with a reaction.

❖ Type I
 ★ Caused by rapid administration producing a histamine induced drop in SVR and BP.
 ★ Prevented by infusing protamine over 10 to 15 minutes.
 ★ Reversed by treating with alpha agents.

❖ Type II (Types IIA, IIB, and IIC)
 ★ Caused by anaphylactic or anaphylactoid reaction.
 ★ Results in hypotension, tachycardia, bronchopasm, flushing and pulmonary edema.

❖ Type III
 ★ Produces catastrophic pulmonary vasoconstriction - elevated PA pressures and dilated right ventricle.
 ★ Decreased left atrial pressure.
 ★ Systemic hypotension from peripheral vasodilation and decreased LV cardiac output.
 ★ Myocardial depression.

◆ Hemodynamic support is required to treat protamine reactions.

❖ Calcium chloride to improve SVR and provide inotropic support.

❖ Alpha agents to support SVR.

❖ Beta agents for inotropic support and to reduce pulmonary resistance. (Low dose epinephrine and dobutamine.)

❖ Drugs to decrease preload (venous vasodilators) and to decrease pulmonary pressures (NTG, Nitric Oxide, and Prostaglandin E1).

Open Heart Surgery and Coronary Artery Bypass Grafting

❖ Aminophylline for wheezing.

❖ Heparin can also be given to reverse the effects of a protamine reaction.

◆ Other options to stop bleeding without the use of protamine:

❖ Heparinase - I.

❖ Recombinant platelet factor 4.

❖ Heparin removal device.

❖ Low molecular weight protamine (investigational) (Bojar, 2005).

Weaning Off CPB

◆ Patient is rewarmed toward normothermia beginning 30 minutes before terminating CPB (LeDoux & Luikart, 2005). Even in normothermic CPB, active warming is required to keep temperatures > 35° C (Bojar, 2005). Aggressive over warming can contribute to adverse neurological outcomes. An inflow temperature > 38° C is avoided to minimize protein denaturation and potential cerebral damage.

◆ When the cross clamp is removed, lidocaine and magnesium may be given to suppress arrhythmias. Ventricular fibrillation may occur requiring internal defibrillation.

◆ If the left atrium, left ventricle, or aorta have been entered, then air must be removed before the cross clamp is removed in order to prevent air embolism (LeDoux & Luikart, 2005).

◆ When the bypass surgery has been completed:

❖ The lungs are ventilated.

❖ Pacing is initiated if needed.

❖ 1 gram of calcium chloride may be given to increase SVR and provide inotropic support.

◆ CPB is weaned by gradually reducing venous return, administering increased volume, and decreasing arterial flow rate. When adequate blood pressure and cardiac index are achieved, the heparin can be reversed and cannulae removed.

◆ Hypotension may need to be treated with:

❖ Volume (if LV function is adequate).

☆ Volume from the pump can be transfused after protamine is administered and the blood is processed through the cell saver.

☆ Colloids can also be used. Albumin is preferred to hetastarch, which can increase bleeding.

❖ Inotropic agents.

❖ Vasopressors.

◆ Inotropic support may be needed prior to terminating CPB in the following situations:

❖ Pre-existing LV dysfunction.

❖ LV hypertrophy.

❖ Preoperative ischemia.

❖ Recent MI.

❖ Incomplete revascularization.

❖ Long cross clamp periods.

◆ If alpha agents were needed on pump for blood pressure support, then they will most likely be needed in the immediate post CPB period.

◆ When myocardial performance is not adequate for weaning, the following are options:

❖ Resume CPB to re-perfuse the heart at a low workload.

❖ Insert intra-aortic balloon pump (IABP).

❖ Possible use of assist device if above measures fail.

(Bojar, 2005 and LeDoux & Luikart, 2005).

Chapter 16

◆ Hypothermia can occur post-pump when the chest is still open and hemostasis is being achieved. This is called afterdrop and occurs because there is a difference between temperature of the core, and the periphery and heat is re-distributed to the periphery, causing a decrease in core temperature. Heat loss is also exacerbated by additional factors.

❖ Strategies to prevent afterdrop:

★ Increase warming phase on CPB.

★ Warm the periphery.

★ Pharmcological vasodilation with nitroprusside.

COMPLICATIONS OF CARDIOPULMONARY BYPASS

Systemic Inflammatory Response During CPB

◆ Several responses are initiated due to the contact of blood with non-endothelial surfaces within the circuit:

❖ Kallikrein response.

❖ Coagulation system – the bypass circuit itself is an activator of the coagulation system, causing generation of factor Xa and thrombin that contribute to the inflammatory response.

❖ Complement system.

❖ Proinflammatory cytokines contribute to neutrophil adhesion.

❖ Systemic inflammatory response.

❖ Neutrophil – endothelial cell adhesion (endothelial activation and dysfunction). This neutrophil adhesion is thought to contribute to transient left ventricular dysfunction postoperatively (LeDoux & Luikart, 2005).

The inflammatory state caused by CPB may cause low flow within the coronary circulation. In addition, the initiation of the systemic inflammatory response alters both the coagulation and immune systems (LeDoux & Luikart, 2005). The longer the patient is on CPB, the greater the systemic effect.

◆ Hemodilution causing an increased need for fluid, which can increase the systemic inflammatory response, capillary leak, and tissue edema.

◆ Endothelial dysfunction, which has been associated with myocardial reperfusion damage, pulmonary dysfunction, renal dysfunction, neurological changes, and generalized capillary damage and leaking. No significant clinical effects are seen in most patients. However, in patients with hemodynamic instability or in patients with long pump times, there can be clinically significant effects from the systemic inflammatory response.

◆ Many strategies are used during CPB to decrease the associated inflammatory response:

❖ Membrane oxygenators

❖ Heparin coated circuits that improve biocompatibility and reduce complement, neutrophril and platelet activation. They also decrease the release of proinflammatory mediators.

❖ Centrifugal pumps.

❖ Leukocyte filters: The administration of leukocyte-poor blood and leukocyte depletion via filtration during the perioperative period has been shown to be beneficial in improving myocardial performance during acute or chronic ischemia (Eagle et al., 2004). Patients undergoing CABG today are older and have more co-morbidities than patients of the past. However, advances in CABG continue to occur to allow for improved outcomes, even for higher risk patients.

❖ Mannitol.

Open Heart Surgery and Coronary Artery Bypass Grafting

❖ Steroids: Preoperative corticosteroids block complement activation and reduce the levels of pro-inflammatory cytokines. (Steroids may not be indicated in diabetic patients.)

❖ High dose aprotinin: Aprotinin, a serine protease inhibitor and hemostatic agent used in high-risk patients to prevent bleeding, also has a role as an antiinflammatory agent because it blocks complement activation and cytokine release. Aprotinin is an expensive medication and is not widely used for this purpose.

Coagulopathy with CPB

◆ Coagulopathy is present to some degree with all CPB. A coagulopathy can develop from activation of platelets and the fibrinolytic system. In addition, there is a dilution of clotting factors and platelets during CPB.

◆ Increased coagulopathies associated with longer pump times and increased number of required transfusions while on pump.

◆ Autologous blood withdrawal before the induction of bypass protects platelets from the damaging effects of CPB.

  ❖ This procedure can reduce transfusion requirements.

  ❖ Can be used in patients whose hematocrit on pump remains adequate after the withdrawal of 1 to 2 units of blood, followed by replacement with fluid.

◆ Cell saver blood that is shed and washed in the operating room contains no clotting factors or platelets. This blood retains some amount of heparin, and if large quantities are transfused, additional protamine may be needed. Hemofilters, as opposed to cell savers, preserve the platelets and clotting factors.

◆ Point of care testing can be used to assess PT, PTT, platelet count and platelet function to guide therapy.

◆ General treatment guidelines:

  ❖ Platelet transfusions for:

    ☆ Preoperative aspirin or clopidogrel.

    ☆ Patients with uremia.

  ❖ Fresh frozen plasma transfusions for:

    ☆ Preoperative warfarin.

    ☆ Hepatic dysfunction.

    ☆ Multiple transfusions while on pump.

Additional Potential Problems During CPB

◆ Systemic air embolism requires cessation of CPB, venting of air from the aorta and removal of air from the CPB circuit. Ventilation with 100% oxygen, trendelenburg position, and retrograde perfusion via the SVC are used to eliminate air from the cerebral circulation. Steroids, barbiturates, and deep hypothermia may be used to minimize cerebral injury. TEE is the best method for detecting returned air. There is also risk of air embolism when air gets trapped in the left side of the heart. The most common site for systemic air embolism during valve surgery is the right coronary artery. This can result in temporary right ventricular dysfunction.

◆ Cold reactive autoimmune disease (caused by an IgM autoimmune antibody) can cause red blood cell agglutination and hemolysis on CPB at cold temperatures. This results in microvascular thrombosis and potential end organ damage. Less than 1% of patients have cold agglutinins, so preoperative screening is not routinely done. In addition, there is rarely a problem during CPB since hemodi-

Chapter 16

lution lowers antibody titers. When high titers are present, systemic hypotension and cold blood cardioplegia must be avoided; off-pump CABG (OPCAB) may even be considered. If the problem is not discovered until the patient is on CPB, normothermia is restored and crystalloid cardioplegia is given to flush out the coronary arteries.

ALTERNATIVES TO TRADITIONAL CABG

Off-pump CABG (OPCAB)

Off-pump CABG is an alternative method to performing CABG. This surgery is done without CPB but involves a median sternotomy. A full sternotomy offers better access to bypass the vessels that supply the lateral and posterior walls. Both pleural spaces are entered during OPCAB. Intraoperative techniques are used to stabilize the coronary arteries and to clear the operative field of blood, allowing the surgeon to operate on a beating heart.

The avoidance of CPB eliminates the need to clamp the aorta in patients with high-risk aortic atherosclerosis and may be the most beneficial in patients with severe aortic atherosclerosis. Other potential advantages include:

1) A decreased need for blood transfusions.

2) Less myocardial enzyme release.

3) Less renal dysfunction.

4) Less early neurological dysfunction

(Selke et al., 2005).

A potential disadvantage with OPCAB is decreased graft patency from difficulty with constructing anastomoses on a beating heart.

Technicalities of OPCAB

- The patient is positioned in trendelenburg with the table rotated to the right. Pericardial sutures are used to retract the heart and apical suction catheters are used to rotate the heart up and to the right.

- In trendelenburg position, filling pressures are elevated. There is also an increased risk for the development of cerebral edema.

- Blood pressure is kept at approximately 120 to 140 systolic (Bojar, 2005) to assure optimal coronary blood flow, especially through collateral vessels. Alpha agents are used to maintain blood pressure if needed.

- If inotropic support is needed, low dose epinephrine is usually the first line agent. Prophylactic IABP may also be used in high risk patients. Patients who have persistant instability should be converted to on-pump surgery. Patients requiring return to on-pump surgery have a higher risk of mortality and other complications compared to completed OPCAB or traditional CABG with CPB (Selke et al., 2005).

- Stabilizers using pressure or suction can be used to stabilize the field at the site of anastomosis.

- There is an increased risk for ischemia to the region being supplied by the vessel being anastomosed. Intra-coronary or aortocoronary shunting can be used to provide distal blood flow during anastomosis. Ischemic pre-conditioning can also be used during OPCAB. Ischemic pre-conditioning is accomplished by transient reduction in blood flow to the myocardium, preparing it to tolerate future longer periods of ischemia.

- Distal perfusion is at risk during the sewing of the graft to the aorta until the clamp is removed. The lower blood pressure maintained during clamping also increases the risk of renal hypoperfusion.

Open Heart Surgery and Coronary Artery Bypass Grafting

Even during OPCAB, if a saphenous vein is used, the ascending aorta is usually partially clamped while the anastomoses is made. Newer technology such as the aortic connector system, has been developed to avoid clamping, but this technology has not yet been proven (Nishizaki & Seki, 2005).

◆ Magnesium may be given intraoperatively while completing the anastomoses to reduce the threshold for arrhythmias.

◆ Ischemia detection via ST segment monitoring is impaired due to the manipulation of the heart. SVO₂ monitoring is used as an indirect measurement of ischemia significant enough to result in a decrease in cardiac output.

◆ During OPCAB, hemodynamics are controlled by the patient's heart, not by the CPB system. Myocardial performance is affected by positioning of the heart, myocardial ischemia, ventricular arrhythmias, bleeding, and valvular regurgitation. More intense monitoring is required for off pump surgery.

◆ During OPCAB the patient temperature is kept as close to normothermic as possible to prevent arrhythmia, bleeding and postoperative shivering.

  ❖ Room temperature is kept at a higher temperature (mid-70s).

  ❖ Some type of warming device or temperature control system is used.

  ❖ Fluids are warmed.

  ❖ Heated humidifier is used in the ventilatory circuit

  (Bojar, 2005).

◆ Heparinization is required during off-pump surgery because coagulation is activated by release of tissue factor and activation of extrinsic factor. Surgery itself causes activation of platelets and fibrinogen. ACTs ≥ 300 seconds protect from any clinical problems related to this procoagulant effect. In addition there can be prothrombotic effects with OPCAB because of the absence of effects associated with CPB (hemodilution, platelet dysfunction, and fibrinolysis) (Bojar, 2005).

◆ Antifibrinolytic therapy may have some benefit in decreasing bleeding in OPCAB. Although blood does not come into contact with the tubing from the CPB circuit, heparinization itself does induce some fibrinolysis.

◆ There is no hemodilution associated with CPB; however, large amounts of fluid may be given to maintain an adequate blood pressure due to the positioning of the heart during surgery. Diuresis is usually required during the postoperative period.

In the state of New York, 27% of CABG procedures in the year 2000 were done off pump (Racz et al., 2004). However, many surgeons reserve OPCAB for patients with limited disease due to the potential problems with graft patency. Additional research is needed to more fully evaluate the potential benefits of OPCAB. Based on research to date, length of stay, mortality, long term neurological function, and cardiac outcomes appear to be similar between OPCAB and traditional CABG with CPB (Selke et al., 2005). The greatest benefit may be for the patients at risk for neurological deficit due to clamping of an atherosclerotic aorta. At the present time the skill and experience of the surgeon plays an important role in the outcomes associated with OPCAB (Selke et al., 2005).

Minimally Invasive CABG (MIDCAB)

Minimally invasive CABG is performed on a beating heart without CPB and without the use of a median sternotomy to gain access. Due to limited access through an anterolateral thoracotomy, this procedure is typically done to the easily accessible proximal LAD. This approach is cosmetically appealing for patients because the incision from a small thoracotomy is less noticeable than an incision from a median sternotomy. However, this procedure is technically challenging because visibility is not the same as with

Chapter 16

a sternotomy. In addition, the intercostal nerves can be irritated, producing increased postoperative pain (Niinami, Ogasawara, Suda, & Takeuchi, 2005).

Another approach being used for MIDCAB is the ministernotomy. In this approach, the LAD and right coronary artery (RCA) can be bypassed using the same incision (Niinami, Ogasawara, Suda, & Takeuchi, 2005). Internal mammary artery grafts can be used during MIDCAB with both approaches; however, access to the internal mammary arteries is improved with the ministernotomy approach. To allow for suturing on a beating heart, medications such as beta blockers or adenosine, can be given to slow or temporarily stop the heart. Mechanical stabilizers are now predominantly used to hold the coronary artery still while suturing occurs. The advantages of MIDCAB are associated with its avoidance of the sternotomy and CPB. Some patients experience less pain with no sternotomy and require fewer blood transfusions by avoiding CPB. Both of these factors can lead to shorter hospital stays. However, with improved interventional cardiology techniques and the ability to do off-pump CABG with a full sternotomy, most surgeons no longer use the MIDCAB technique.

One lung anesthesia is used during MIDCAB. During one lung anesthesia, a pneumothorax is induced to collapse the left lung to facilitate the dissection of the internal mammary artery. The right lung is ventilated. There are potential hemodynamic and pulmonary complications of one lung ventilation (Murkin, 2001).

There is significant chest wall pain from the thoracotomy and rib retraction, and epidural anesthesia or intercostal bupivacaine can be used to reduce splinting (Bojar, 2005). No pacing wires are placed during MIDCAB.

Other Techniques

Other advances in cardiac surgery include port access and video-assisted CABG with a closed chest. During this procedure, the aorta can be occluded and cardioplegia delivered via endovascular techniques. Cardiopulmonary bypass is used during this procedure, and access occurs through the femoral artery and vein. One advantage of this technique is the avoidance of a median sternotomy. However, this procedure has not yet been evaluated through large controlled trials (Eagle et al., 2004). Additional techniques for CABG using robotics are also being investigated.

Computer assisted robotic surgeries for CABG are being tested in many centers. Many techniques are being developed to allow for port access CABG for multiple vessels to be performed on a beating heart (Ledoux & Luikart, 2005).

Transmyocardial Laser Revascularization

Transmyocardial laser revascularization (TMLR) is limited to patients who have angina refractory to maximal medical treatment, and who are not candidates for other forms of revascularization. These patients usually have very diffuse small vessel disease or no available conduit for revascularization. Patients must have reversible ischemia of the left ventricular free wall and coronary artery disease corresponding to the ischemia.

During this procedure, a series of transmural endomyocardial channels is created with lasers to improve myocardial blood supply. These channels are created on the epicardial surface and go through to the endocardium. The typical number of channels ranges from 20 to 40, with the size of the channels approximately 1mm wide. The physiology behind the treatment is more complex than simply creating channels for oxygenated blood to flow from the endocardium up through the myocardium to the epicardium. Two theories are proposed regarding the mechanism of action: 1) The laser treatment causes an inflammatory process and stimulates angiogenesis, which, in turn, improves the regional blood flow to the ischemic area of myocardium, and 2) The laser treatment creates denervation of the myocardium and an improvement of symptoms (Bridges et al., 2004). TMLR has been effective in improving anginal symptoms, functional capacity, and quality of life. This procedure is typically done in the cardiac surgery suite as a standalone surgery, or it can be done with CABG when not all ischemic areas can be reached by grafting. Percutaneous options are currently being investigated.

GRAFT MATERIAL IN CABG

Saphenous Vein Graft

- The most common vein graft material is taken from the greater saphenous vein of the leg.
- Vein grafts can be harvested using standard incisions or endoscopically.
    - Endoscopic harvest has become the primary practice in many centers, leaving standard incisions for emergent cases or cases where the vein is too deep for an endoscopic approach.
    - Endoscopic vein harvesting requires a puncture to hook the vein. Assessing for ecchymosis at the puncture site, usually in the thigh, is very important. Bleeding increases the risk for both compression and infection.
    - Laser is used to dissect/cauterize the vein.
    - Endoscopic harvesting minimizes patient discomfort and edema, promotes early ambulation, and improves cosmetic appearance. In addition, there is an improvement in wound healing, which decreases risk for infection.
- The vein graft is a free graft, is attached at one end to the ascending aorta and at the other end to the coronary artery distal to the blockage (Figure 16.6).
- Flow through vein grafts depends on pressure, and patients with hypotension or poor left ventricular function are at increased risk for acute vein graft closure.
- Failure of saphenous vein grafts has been a limiting factor in CABG and is often the cause of recurrent angina post CABG.
- Vein grafts can develop intimal fibroplasia and vein graft atherosclerosis.
- Up to one half of all vein grafts close within 10 years after surgery (Eagle et al., 2004).
- Antiplatelet therapy with aspirin reduces short-term vein graft occlusion.
- Lipid-lowering therapy with statins reduces long-term occlusion.

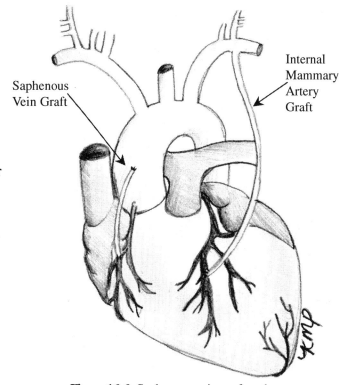

Figure 16.6: Saphenous vein graft and Internal mammary artery graft.

Arterial Grafts

Internal Mammary (Thoracic) Arteries

- A very important surgical advancement is the success of internal mammary artery grafts with a major improvement in late patency rates and more than 90% patency at 10 years (Eagle et al., 2004).
- Internal mammary artery grafts have improved long-term survival rates and reduced postoperative mortality (Eagle et al., 2004).

Chapter 16

- The left internal mammary artery (LIMA) is most commonly used to bypass the LAD, improving the long-term outcomes in this group of patients (Antman et al., 2004; Eagle et al., 2004).

- When used as a pedicle graft (a graft left attached to the original site), the proximal end of the internal mammary artery is left intact and the distal end is sutured beyond the site of stenosis (Figure 16.6).

- Both internal mammary arteries can be used. Due to the decrease in sternal blood flow, there is an increased risk for sternal wound infection when both internal mammary arteries are used. This is of particular concern in diabetic patients.

- Most CABG surgeries involve a combination of a left internal mammary artery graft and saphenous vein grafts.

Radial Artery

- The radial artery can be used as conduit; however, it is prone to spasm because of its thick muscular nature.

- The risk of spasm can be decreased with the use of nitrates and calcium channel blockers, both intraoperatively and postoperatively. Intravenous diltiazem 0.1 mg/kg/hr (5-10 mg/hr) or intravenous nitroglycerin 5-20 μg/kg/min are common dosages. IV vasodilators are started in OR and are continued for 18 to 24 hours postoperatively. IV medications are converted to oral long acting diltiazem or imdur and are continued for 6 months (Bohar, 2005).

- The advantage of the radial artery is its length, which enables it to be used to reach most distal targets.

- The radial artery is not used unless the patient has adequate patency of the ulnar artery.

- The radial artery is most often harvested from the patient's non-dominant hand.

Right Gastroepiploic Artery

- The right gastroepiploic artery supplies blood to the greater curvature of the stomach.

- When this artery is used as graft material in CABG, a more extensive surgery results because abdominal entry is also required.

- This artery can be used as a pedicle graft or a free graft.

Alternative Graft Material

- When patients have no available arterial or venous conduit, homologous cryopreserved saphenous vein grafts or umbilical vein grafts that have been treated with glutaraldehyde can be used.

- Unfortunately, these grafts have poor long-term patency, so they are used only when no other options are available.

- Other non-homologous grafts have been used, but also have had poor patency. These grafts include bovine internal mammary arteries and synthetic grafts (Eagle et al., 2004).

In some young patients, revascularization with all-arterial grafts may be considered, with the hope of achieving longer-term patency and avoiding the need for re-operation. The need for one or more re-operations is a concern in younger patients because re-operation carries a higher risk. Lack of an acceptable conduit is also a concern if re-operation must be performed more than once.

Open Heart Surgery and Coronary Artery Bypass Grafting

POSTOPERATIVE CARE

◆ Priority assessment parameters during and immediately after transport from the operating room to the ICU are ventilatory status, rhythm, and blood pressure.

◆ A chest x-ray may be done immediately in the postoperative period to reassess endotracheal tube placement and to confirm the absence of a pneumothorax. A chest x-ray should always be done with any change in respiratory status or with any concern for an air leak.

◆ A 12-lead ECG is also completed to assess for ischemia.

◆ An arterial line and pulmonary artery (PA) catheter are frequently used to monitor systemic and intracardiac pressures, cardiac output, and central venous oxygen saturation. There is a trend toward less PA catheter use and more use of less invasive strategies to obtain needed hemodynamic data.

◆ Cardiac rhythm and ST-segment monitoring and pulse oximetry are also used.

◆ Foley catheter may contain a temperature probe. Catheter is usually removed by 2nd postoperative day.

◆ NG tube to low intermittent suction may be used while patient is intubated.

Blood Pressure Management

◆ Systolic blood pressure should be kept between 90 mm Hg and 140 mm Hg. Hypotension or hypertension can result in additional complications in the postoperative period. The goal is typically to achieve a MAP of at least 65-70 mm Hg.

◆ Hypotension in the immediate postoperative period is usually caused by low circulating volume and responds to treatment with volume. If there is no immediate response to volume administration, 500 mg of IV calcium chloride is often given. Existing vasopressors, such as norepinephrine, can also be adjusted.

◆ Chest tubes should always be assessed for evidence of hemorrhage when there is a low blood pressure.

◆ Hypotension frequently occurs in the early postoperative period as the patient warms up. Vasodilation occurs for several other reasons during the early postoperative period.

   ❖ Analgesics and anxiolytics are vasodilators.

   ❖ NTG, if needed for ischemia, produces predominant venous vasodilation and decreases preload. Unless there is ischemia, NTG should be avoided during the rewarming phase.

   ❖ Resolution of hypothermia leads to peripheral vasodilation.

   ❖ Improvement in cardiac output also results in a resolution of vasoconstriction.

◆ Alpha agents norepinephrine (α and ß) and phenylephrine (pure α) are used to keep systolic blood pressure > 100 mm Hg when filling pressures are adequate.

◆ Failure of fluid challenges to raise preload may indicate the presence of capillary leak and fluid shifting into the interstitial space. Patients with longer CPB times are at greater risk for capillary leak. In patients with capillary leak, a large amount of fluid is required to maintain adequate circulating volume. Administration of large amounts of volume also increases the interstitial volume. Inotropes and vasopressors may also be needed for hemodynamic support in the patient with capillary leak.

◆ When preload rises in response to volume but cardiac output does not improve, there may be excessive ventricular distention. Inotropes are indicated in this situation.

◆ When α agents are not able to maintain adequate blood pressure in the presence of adequate filling pressures, then vasoplegia may be present.

◆ Vasoplegia is the failure to respond to catecholamines. There are several theories behind the cause of vasoplegia, including leukocyte activation and the release of pro-inflammatory mediators during CPB. Vasoplegia, however, can also be seen after OPCAB.

713

Chapter 16

❖ Nitroglycerin or nitroprusside are used to keep systolic blood pressure < 130 mm Hg. Nitroprusside is preferred in the treatment of hypertension because it has less effect on preload and helps minimize the amount of needed fluid. However, nitroglycerin is indicated in the presence of any ischemia.

❖ Hypertension in the presence of tachycardia may be treated with beta blockers.

❖ Control of hypertension is important during the postoperative period to reduce the risk of bleeding. Arterial lines are removed when blood pressure management no longer requires intravenous pharmacological support, and when post-extubation ABGs are satisfactory. Arterial lines left in place > 3 days are associated with vessel thrombosis and line sepsis.

Fluid Management

◆ Total body fluid is increased postoperatively due to third spacing from increased vascular permeability (capillary leak) and decreased oncotic pressure from hemodilution. Fluid administration may be necessary to maintain circulating volume. If capillary leak is the basic reason for low circulating volume, colloids should be avoided.

◆ Vasoconstriction from hypothermia can mask intravascular hypovolemia.

◆ If the basic reason for low circulating volume is vasodilation of peripheral and splanchnic beds, then colloids can expand intravascular volume better than crystalloids.

❖ Packed red blood cells can be used for volume replacement if the hematocrit is low.

◆ If the PAOP is not elevated, the patient should tolerate either crystalloids or colloids without an increase in interstitial lung volume.

◆ Fluid resuscitation is also necessary during rewarming.

❖ Typically, A 500 cc bolus of crystalloid (lactated ringers) is given initially.

❖ If there is no impact on filling pressure, 5% albumin or hetastarch is used.

❖ Hetastarch increases intravascular volume more effectively than crystalloid and is effective longer than albumin. If using hetastarch, the total infusion volume should not exceed 20 ml/kg in 24 hours to minimize adverse effects on coagulation. Hetastarch is also avoided in patients with significant mediastinal bleeding.

◆ Excessive fluid administration > 2 L within 6 hours may cause interstitial edema and delay extubation. Excessive fluid administration causes hemodilution and also reduces clotting factors.

◆ Response to fluid depends on:

❖ Compliance of left side of heart.

❖ Amount of capillary leak.

❖ Intensity of vasoconstriction – when fluid challenges raise cardiac output, constricted vessels relax.

◆ When there is excessive urine output, the blood sugar should be assessed to assure there is no hyperglycemia causing osmotic diuresis. If blood sugar is normal and no diuretics have been given, then a large urine output in the immediate postoperative period is most likely reflective of a good cardiac output. Postoperatively, patients have an increased amount of total body fluid, and in the presence of good left ventricular function, the excess fluid mobilizes to produce large amounts of urine. Fluids are given to keep fluid balance only slightly negative.

◆ After capillary leak has ended the patient may be aggressively diuresed to mobilize fluids and eliminate excessive salt and water. The goal is return to preoperative weight. Use of acetazolamide (Diamox) in conjunction with other diuretics can help correct primary metabolic alkalosis caused by diuresis. Diuresis may begin on post op day 1, especially in patients demonstrating signs of congestive heart failure or hypoxemia.

Open Heart Surgery and Coronary Artery Bypass Grafting

- Patients who need more intravascular volume frequently have diuresis held until postop day 2. Patients who are hypotensive in the early postoperative period are usually hypovolemic and need volume. Also, patients with left ventricular dysfunction may require higher filling pressures in order to maintain adequate cardiac output. The ventricle can be noncompliant in the postoperative period. A noncompliant ventricle will cause a rise in pulmonary artery diastolic and pulmonary artery occlusive pressures in the absence of volume overload.

Management of Hypothermia

- CPB is often accompanied by systemic hypothermia of 32° to 34° C, and the patient is rewarmed to a core temperature of at least 36°. This rewarming typically occurs prior to the patient returning to the ICU.
- OPCAB patients are usually around 35° on arrival to ICU.
- Patients are prone to a drop in temperature after the rewarming that occurs in CPB. This phenomenon is called afterdrop.
- Postoperative hypothermia in the ICU is associated with adverse outcomes:
  - ❖ Predisposes to atrial and ventricular arrhythmias and lower fibrillation threshold.
  - ❖ Increases SVR and systemic hypertension.
    - ☆ Vasoconstriction may mask hypovolemia.
    - ☆ Hypertension can increase mediastinal bleeding.
    - ☆ Increased afterload can impair LV function.
  - ❖ Can induce shivering which increases peripheral O_2 consumption and CO_2 production. Shivering also causes patient discomfort.
  - ❖ Causes platelet dysfunction and impairs aspects of the coagulation cascade. Can increase mediastinal bleeding.
  - ❖ Prolongs time to extubation and impairs speed of recovery.
- Patients are peripherally vasoconstricted to assist in providing core warming.
  - ❖ Vasodilation with nitroprusside or propofol can redistribute heat to the periphery and improve tissue perfusion. However, there is a potential to delay core warming because peripheral vasodilation also augments heat loss.
  - ❖ Use of warming blankets or other devices can minimize peripheral heat loss.
  - ❖ Other methods to prevent heat loss include warming IV fluids and the humidifiers in the ventilator circuit. Although these methods help prevent heat loss and worsening hypothermia, they do not significantly contribute to core rewarming.
- Shivering can be treated with:
  - ❖ Meperidine.
  - ❖ Dexmedetomidine.
  - ❖ Clonidine.
  - ❖ Ketanserin.
  - ❖ Doxapram.
  - ❖ Propofol – reduces total body oxygen consumption and may also reduce shivering.
    - ☆ Uncontrolled shivering may need to be treated with pharmacological paralysis. Sedation must always be used in conjunction with paralysis.
- As the patient warms, there is peripheral vasodilation and decreased filling pressure; hypotension can develop if the patient is hypovolemic.

Chapter 16

❖ Crystalloids and colloids can be given to keep the pulmonary artery occlusive pressure (PAOP) between approximately 18 to 20 mm Hg. Patients with abnormal ventricular compliance may require higher pressures for optimal cardiac output.

❖ If PAOP goal is achieved, then an alpha agent can be added to support blood pressure if the cardiac index is > 2.2 L/min/mm.²

❖ If cardiac index is low, then an agent(s) that provides both alpha and beta (inotropic) support is indicated.

PA Catheter and Left Atrial Line

◆ In low risk, non-complicated patients, a CVP line rather than a PA catheter may be used to guide therapy.

◆ PA catheters in surgery are more commonly placed through the internal jugular rather than the subclavian vein. The internal jugular has a higher risk of arterial puncture but has less risk of catheter malposition and pneumothroax.

◆ PA catheter is removed when vasoactive drugs are no longer needed.

◆ A left atrial line may be placed in patients with severe left ventricular dysfunction or in those with pulmonary hypertension secondary to mitral valve disease. This line allows for a more accurate assessment of left-sided filling pressure. The line is placed via the right superior pulmonary vein. There is a risk of an air embolism with a left atrial line, so it is always aspirated before being flushed. The line is connected to a constant infusion containing an air filter. The left atrial line is removed with chest tubes still in place in case there is any intrapericardial bleeding from the insertion site.

◆ Additional information regarding PA catheters is discussed in Chapter 4.

Cardiac Output and Delivery of Oxygen

◆ The goal is a cardiac index > 2.2 L/min/mm.²

◆ Inotropic support may be required for several hours into the postoperative period while the heart recovers from the operative ischemia and reperfusion associated with cardioplegic arrest.

◆ The decision to use inotropes in based on blood pressure response to volume, urine output and venous oxygen saturation.

◆ The sympathomimetics epinephrine, dobutamine, or dopamine may be used for inoptropic support. Epinephrine is the preferred first line agent. Phosphodiesterase inhibitors (e.g. milrinone) are another option for inotropic support if the patient has an adequate SVR. If the SVR is not adequate, then milrinone may be given in combination with an alpha-stimulating agent such as norepinephrine.

◆ Increased SVR from hypothermia can adversely affect myocardial performance and may require vasodilator therapy to optimize cardiac output.

◆ Intra aortic balloon pump therapy may be required when cardiac output does not improve in response to inotropic support and reduction in afterload.

◆ Venous oxygen saturation level provides the best global assessment of tissue oxygen.

◆ Some patients with normal contractility can have poor cardiac output postoperatively, due to diastolic dysfunction, which can become worse due to the ischemic and reperfusion injury associated with CPB. TEE can be used to diagnose diastolic dysfunction during surgery. Patients with diastolic dysfunction require a higher filling pressure. Drugs that have a lusitropic effect (ability to help heart relax and fill) can be given; these include phosodiesterase inhibitors and nesiritide. Low doses of calcium channel blockers and beta blockers can also be given to aid in diastolic relaxation.

716

Open Heart Surgery and Coronary Artery Bypass Grafting

◆ Right ventricular dysfunction is an additional problem, and can be due to right ventricular infarction or can occur as a result of elevated pulmonary pressures. In addition, the right ventricle is often not adequately protected during CPB. Right ventricular dysfunction is treated with fluids and inotropic support. Vasodilators to dilate the pulmonary bed can also be used. In severe cases, circulatory assist may be needed.

Ventilation and Oxygenation

◆ In some situations, based on type of anesthetic, there is the potential for extubation in the operating room. However, narcotic based anesthesia leaves patients sedated and most patients return to the ICU intubated with mechanical ventilation for a minimum of 2 to 4 hours. Most patients are able to be extubated within 12 hours of admission to the ICU.

◆ Approximately 5% of patients require mechanical ventilation > 48 hours and approximately 1% of patients suffer from acute respiratory insufficiency while on the ventilator (Bojar, 2005). Postoperative pulmonary dysfunction can persist for several months after surgery. Table 16.3 describes intra operative factors that impact postoperative pulmonary function.

◆ FIO_2 starts at 1.0 and is weaned to 0.4 if SaO_2 remains > 95%. Low levels of PEEP (5 cm H₂0) are routinely added to prevent atelectasis. This substitutes for loss of physiologic PEEP, but does not recruit unopened alveoli.

◆ Initial blood gases are drawn 15 to 20 minutes after arrival to ICU. Extubation should occur as soon as patient is able to protect his airway and maintain adequate ventilation and oxygenation. Some degree of suboptimal oxygenation is expected after surgery; however, extubation should be achieved within 12 hours in most patients.

Table 16.3
Intra-operative Factors Impacting Postoperative Pulmonary Function

◆ Anesthesia (decreases respiratory drive and respiratory muscle function).

◆ Median sternotomy (causes pain and splinting).

◆ Use of internal mammary artery (pleural entry decreases chest wall compliance and increases risk of pleural effusion and phrenic nerve injury).

◆ Fluid administration and hemodilution during CPB (can cause pulmonary edema).

◆ SIRS from CPB (can decrease lung surfactant and contribute to atelectasis).

  ❖ Due to capillary leak from the systemic inflammatory response associated with CPB, there is an increased amount of interstitial lung water in the early postoperative period. Minimizing the positive fluid balance associated with surgery is an important factor in the ability to achieve early extubation.

◆ Transfusion (may increase PVR and PA pressures).

◆ Oxygenation is assessed by the PaO_2 / FIO_2 ratio, the alveolar – arterial oxygen gradient, and the oxygen saturation level. A lower PaO_2 / FIO_2 ratio is typically seen in smokers or in patients with preoperative pulmonary dysfunction.

◆ Mild respiratory alkalosis (low $PaCO_2$) is acceptable in the early postoperative period when patient is hypothermic. This mild respiratory alkalosis:

  ❖ Decreases the patient's respiratory drive.

  ❖ Allows for increased CO_2 production associated with shivering and rewarming.

  ❖ Compensates for mild metabolic acidosis from hypoperfusion associated with the vasoconstriction of hypothermia.

Chapter 16

◆ Significant respiratory alkalosis needs to be treated by lowering the respiratory rate or by increasing the dead space via an increase in tubing length. Lowering the rate as opposed to lowering the tidal volume is preferred because adequate tidal volume helps prevent postoperative atelectasis. Significant respiratory alkalosis has detrimental effects:

 ❖ Hypokalemia – predisposing to ventricular arrhythmias.
 ❖ Shifting of oxyhemoglobin curve to the left and interfering with release of oxygen to the tissues.

◆ Rate and tidal volume are also adjusted for increased CO_2 production associated with warming and shivering. A slightly elevated $PaCO_2$ is accepted during the weaning process if the patient is still slightly sedated. $PaCO_2$ levels may also be elevated to compensate for metabolic alkalosis caused by aggressive diuresis in the early postoperative period.

◆ Note: A lower tidal volume may be needed in some patients to decrease tension on a short internal mammary artery pedicle graft. If so, CO_2 levels will need to be adjusted using respiratory rate and ventilator circuit dead space.

Table 16.4 defines postoperative strategies to minimize pulmonary complications. Table 16.5 lists benefits and potential disadvantages associated with early extubation. Table 16.6 defines patients who are excluded from early extubation.

Table 16.4   **Postoperative Strategies for Improving Pulmonary Function**
◆ Aggressive treatment of bleeding to minimize use of blood products.   ◆ Aggressive diuresis after hemodynamic stability.   ◆ Short acting sedatives.   ◆ Adequate analgesia to avoid splinting but also avoiding respiratory depression.

Table 16.5   **Benefits of Early Extubation in Appropriate Patients**
1. Improved hemodynamics.   2. Fewer pulmonary complications.   3. Less postoperative medication.   4. Earlier mobility.   5. Decreased length of stay and overall reduced hospital costs.
Potential Disadvantages of Early Extubation
1. Increased sympathetic tone that can cause myocardial ischemia and HTN. HTN can also increase the risk of bleeding.   2. Increased pain and splinting if less analgesia is used. Increased splinting can result in hypoventilation and atelectasis.

Open Heart Surgery and Coronary Artery Bypass Grafting

Table 16.6 Exclusion Criteria for Early Extubation	
Preoperative Conditions	◆ Intubation. ◆ Sepsis. ◆ Pulmonary edema. ◆ Cardiogenic shock .
Intra-operative Factors	◆ Deep hypothermic circulatory arrest. ◆ Coagulopathy. ◆ Severe left ventricular dysfunction. ◆ Excessive length of time on CPB (> 4-6 hours).
Postoperative Complications	◆ Mediastinal bleeding. ◆ Hemodynamic instability. ◆ Need for intra aortic balloon pump. ◆ Stroke. ◆ Acute renal failure. ◆ Respiratory failure.

◆ When weaning criteria are met (Table 16.7), the patient is weaned from propofol. Most patients awaken within 20 minutes. To achieve early extubation, patients must be weaned based on clinical condition, not based on time of day or on unit routines. Ventilator weaning is discussed in detail in Chapter 3. Extubation criteria are listed in Table 16.7. Signs of weaning failure are described in Table 16.8.

◆ Although there are multiple risk factors for prolonged intubation, patients should be extubated based on clinical condition, not pre-existing risk factors.

◆ Acute changes in pulmonary status (ventilation or oxygenation problem) can be caused by the following:

   ❖ Pneumothorax.

   ❖ Atelectasis or lobar collapse.

   ❖ Aspiration pneumonia.

   ❖ Pulmonary edema.

   ❖ Cardiac tamponade.

   ❖ Pulmonary embolus.

Chapter 16

Table 16.7
Weaning and Extubation Criteria

Initial Weaning Criteria	Extubation Criteria

◆ Awake with stimulation.
◆ Effective reversal of any neuromuscular blockade.
◆ Chest tube drainage < 50 ml/hour.
◆ Core temperature > 35.5° C.
◆ Hemodynamic Stability.
  ❖ CI > 2.2 L/min/m².
  ❖ Systolic BP 100-120 mm Hg, MAP > 65 mm Hg.
  ❖ Heart rate < 120 BPM.
  ❖ Stable cardiac rhythm.
◆ Satisfactory ABGs while on ventilator.
  ❖ PaO_2 / FIO_2 ratio > 150.
  ❖ $PaCO_2$ < 50 mm Hg.
  ❖ pH 7.30-7.50.
	◆ Awake without stimulation.
	◆ Negative inspiratory force > 25 cm H_2O.
	◆ TV > 5 ml/kg.
	◆ Vital capacity > 10-15 ml/kg.
	◆ Respiratory rate < 24.
	◆ ABGs on 5 cm or less of continuous positive airway pressure (CPAP) or pressure support ventilation (PSV).
	  ❖ PaO_2 / FIO_2 ratio > 150 and improving.
	  ❖ $PaCO_2$ < 48 mm Hg.
	  ❖ pH 7.32-7.48.

Table 16.8
Signs of Weaning Failure

◆ Somnolence.

◆ Agitation.

◆ Increase in systolic BP.

◆ Tachycardia.

◆ Increased respiratory rate.

◆ Diaphoresis.

◆ Need for vasoactive medications.

◆ PaO_2 / FIO_2 ratio < 150.

◆ SaO_2 < 90%.

◆ $PaCO_2$ > 50 mm Hg with respiratory acidosis.

◆ Post-Extubation Issues

  ❖ 40% to 70% humidified oxygen via mask may be needed for a few days if the patient has underlying pulmonary disorders.

  ❖ BiPAP can be used if needed to improve oxygenation and prevent reintubation. BiPAP prevents an increase in extravascular lung water associated with the weaning process.

  ❖ Oxygen via nasal cannula may be continued after the patient is discharged from the ICU.

  ❖ Incentive spirometry done correctly each hour while awake may help maintain functional residual capacity and prevent atelectasis.

  ❖ Deep breathing is important, and a pillow can be used during coughing to decrease pain and prevent splinting.

  ❖ Adequate analgesia is also important to improve respiratory effort.

Open Heart Surgery and Coronary Artery Bypass Grafting

❖ When patient has been diuresed to preoperative weight, room air should be sufficient to maintain an adequate oxygen saturation level.

◆ There are 3 primary reasons for unresolved pulmonary problems and prolonged ventilatory support.

❖ Ventilatory failure where patient is unable to perform or sustain the work of breathing. Problems with respiratory drive, respiratory muscle dysfunction, or disorders increasing CO_2 production can cause ventilatory failure.

❖ Persistent hypoxemia due to hemodynamic compromise and pulmonary edema or to pulmonary pathology, such as COPD or pneumonia.

❖ Development of ARDS.

Epicardial Temporary Pacing Wires

◆ The number and location of epicardial pacing wires vary with the surgeon. Patients may have one or two atrial wires, and/or one or two ventricular wires, and possibly a ground wire.

◆ Bradycardia can occur postoperatively, especially in patients who have undergone valve repair or replacement. The suture lines from valve surgery are close to the conduction system, and postoperative edema can cause temporary heart block.

◆ If AV conduction is intact, atrial pacing in the AAI mode can be used to increase heart rate (see Chapter 17 for more information on pacing modes). If both atrial and ventricular wires are present, dual chamber pacing in the DDD or DVI mode can be used.

◆ If there is AV block, or if only ventricular wires are present, ventricular pacing in the VVI mode must be used.

◆ If atrial fibrillation or flutter is present, atrial pacing cannot be used; ventricular pacing in VVI mode is necessary if pacing is required.

◆ A pacing rate of 90 to 100 may be required to achieve the desired cardiac index.

◆ If pacing wires are not being used, they should be placed in some type of insulating material (e.g. needle cap or finger from glove) to keep isolated from stray electrical current.

◆ Pacing wires are removed before chest tubes if possible to help identify the source of any bleeding complications. The patient should be assessed for tamponade after removal of pacing wires.

Chest Tubes

◆ Mediastinal chest tubes are placed when mediastinal incision is used, and pleural chest tubes are placed when the pleural spaces have been entered. Pleural and mediastinal chest tubes are connected to water-seal chambers and 20 cm of suction. Standard chest tubes are 32 F, but smaller silastic drains may also be used.

◆ Assessment of chest tube patency is a key nursing function. Chest tubes should be gently milked to prevent formation of clots. Stripping of chest tubes postoperatively should be avoided because of the risk of damaging bypass grafts. Aggressive stripping causes a negative 300 cm H_2O pressure in the mediastinum and may increase bleeding. This is also painful to the patient.

◆ Decreased breath sounds, increased inspiratory pressures on the ventilator, or widening of the mediastinum on chest radiograph warrant suspicion for undrained blood in the pleural space or in the mediastinum.

◆ The color of drainage should be assessed to determine if arterial or venous.

◆ Dumping of blood with a position change may indicate an acute onset of bleeding. However, if the blood is dark in color and there is minimal additional drainage, then an acute problem can be ruled out.

721

Chapter 16

◆ Postoperative bleeding should taper off within the first several hours after surgery. Average total blood loss is approximately 1 L (Ferraris et al., 2003). Approximately 1-3% of patients have excessive bleeding requiring re-expoloration.

◆ Chest tube drainage is recorded a minimum of every hour. During the first 2 hours of the immediate postoperative period, drainage is usually recorded every 15 minutes. If drainage is > 100 cc/hr a stat PT, PTT, and platelets should be drawn. Persistent bleeding depletes clotting factors and causes coagulopathy.

◆ Excessive mediastinal bleeding is an emergency situation. Uncontrolled bleeding accumulating around the heart can lead to cardiac tamponade. Signs of tamponade include:

  ❖ Rising filling pressures with a decreased cardiac output and hypotension. CVP, PAOP, and PAD pressures that are equal can indicate tamponade. Clot formation next to the right or left atria may cause pressure increases consistent with either right or left heart failure.

  ❖ Sudden drop/stop in previously significant mediastinal bleeding.

  ❖ Narrowing of pulse pressure.

  ❖ Classic pulsus paradoxus is not a sign of tamponade in the ventilated patient because positive pressure ventilation reverses the blood pressure response to respiration.

  ❖ Tachycardia, dysrhythmias, and decreased ECG voltage.

  ❖ Decrease in urine output from fall in cardiac output.

◆ Transthoracic or transesophageal echo are helpful in the diagnosis of tamponade.

Patients with the following chest tube drainage criteria require surgical re-exploration:
- > 400 ml for 1 hour.
- > 300 ml/hr for 2-3 hours.
- > 200 ml/hr for 4 hours.
- Drainage > 1000 ml within the first 3 to 4 hours.
- Acute onset of bleeding (> 300 ml/hr) after period of stable and minimal bleeding.

◆ There is an increase in mortality and morbidity associated with the need for re-exploration (Bojar, 2005).

◆ Chest tubes are removed when total drainage is < 100 ml for 8 hours.

◆ Chest tubes are clamped prior to removal.

◆ A chest x-ray is done after removal of pleural chest tubes to assess for pneumothorax if there is any change in respiratory status, any previous signs of air leak, or any new subcutaneous air.

Transfusion and Strategies for Managing Mediastinal Bleeding

◆ Management of Mediastinal Bleeding:

  ❖ Warming of patient and control of shivering.

  ❖ Control of hypertension.

  ❖ Control of agitation.

  ❖ Increased levels of PEEP to augment mediastinal pressure. PEEP exerts mechanical pressure on the myocardium and may limit microvascular bleeding. When PEEP is effective, the results are usually seen within 1 hour. There is limited research regarding the risk and benefits for the use of PEEP in this situation. Prophylactic increased levels of PEEP to reduce the risk of postoperative bleeding are not indicated (Ferraris & Ferraris et al., 2007).

  ❖ Platelets and or fresh frozen plasma based on coagulation study results. Aggressive treatment with blood components is used because persistent bleeding depletes clotting factors and contributes to ongoing coagulopathy.

Open Heart Surgery and Coronary Artery Bypass Grafting

- ❖ Colloids, especially hetastarch, are generally avoided because of the dilutional effects on clotting factors.
- ❖ Protamine 25 to 50 mg, given slowly (5mg/min) if PTT is elevated. Excessive protamine is avoided because of anticoagulation effect.
- ❖ Aprotinin 2 million units can be considered in the postoperative period, even if other antifibrinolytic drugs were given.
- ❖ Desmopressin (DDAVP) raises von Willebrand's factor by approximately 50%. Mediastinal bleeding can be due to an acquired deficiency of von Willebrand's factor. May also be effective when dysfunctional platelets are the cause of bleeding, such as with uremia or in patients who received preoperative antiplatelet therapy. Peripheral vasodilation and hypotension are side effects of the infusion.
- ◆ Transfusion Issues and Guidelines
  - ❖ Several factors increase the patient's risk of needing a blood transfusion during or after surgery, including:
    - ☆ Increased age.
    - ☆ Coagulation abnormalities.
    - ☆ Increased time on CPB.
    - ☆ Re-operation.
    - ☆ Emergent or urgent operation.
    - ☆ Combined valve and CABG surgery.
    - ☆ Low red blood cell volume preoperatively (preoperative anemia or small body size)
    - ☆ Fibrinolytics, anticoaugulants or antiplatelet therapy therapy (particularly clopidogrel) preoperatively.
  - ❖ The risk of complications from transfusion increases when the transfused blood is older than 1 month (Raghavan & Marik, 2005).
  - ❖ Transfusion is associated with several complications:
    - ☆ Introduction of vasoactive cytokines and activation of systemic inflammatory response.
    - ☆ Transfused hemoglobin less effective at oxygen transport.
    - ☆ Increased risk of infection due to immunosuppressive effect.
    - ☆ Increased risk of pulmonary and renal complications.
    - ☆ Risk of viral transmission, especially cytomegalovirus.
  - ❖ Leukodepletion reduces the risk of transmission of cytomegalovirus.
  - ❖ Actively bleeding patients require red blood cell transfusions in addition to clotting factors and platelets in order to maintain an adequate hematocrit.
  - ❖ Calcium chloride may be indicated if multiple units of citrate-preserved blood are administered within a short period of time because citrate binds calcium. However, hypocalcemia is not common because citrate is rapidly metabolized by the liver.
  - ❖ Platelets and FFP are often needed for patients with CPB times > 3 hours, or in patients who receive multiple transfusions of packed red blood cells.
    - ☆ Each unit of platelets increases platelet count by 7,000-10,000 per microliter. Platelet transfusion is given for platelet count < 100,000 per microliter or for presumed platelet dysfunction when patient has been on preoperative antiplatelet therapy.

723

Chapter 16

☆ FFP contains all clotting factors except for platelets. One unit is 250 cc of volume, and FFP is the colloid of choice in the bleeding patient. FFP must be transfused within 2 hours of thawing.

☆ Cryoprecipitate contains 40-50% of the plasma content of factor VIII and von Willebrand's factor, and is also a source of fibrinogen (factor I) and factor XIII. It must be administered within 6 hours of thawing.

❖ Recombinant factor VII (NovoSeven) can be given to control bleeding when a severe coagulopathy is present. It combines with tissue factor and activates the extrinsic coagulation system, resulting in thrombin formation at the site of tissue injury. Systemic thrombosis has not been observed.

❖ Postoperative mediastinal shed blood reinfusion using a washing or cell saving technique is an alternative strategy that can be considered. Washing of the shed blood decreases the lipid emboli and the concentration of inflammatory cytokines. Direct reinfusion of shed mediastinal blood from chest tube drainage systems is not recommended (Ferraris & Ferraris et al., 2007).

◆ Emergency resternotomy

❖ A small subxiphoid incision may relieve some the pressure around the heart; however, it may take less time to open the entire sternotomy incision. After the chest is opened, manual pressure can be used to stop visualized bleeding, and the chest is suctioned. Relief of tamponade should improve myocardial performance. Internal massage may be done if the chest is opened due to cardiac arrest or profound hypotension. The mediastinum is irrigated with normal saline or an antibiotic solution, and drains may be left in place for antibiotic irrigation.

Pain Control and Sedation

◆ Pain control initiatives begin immediately in the postoperative period.

◆ Low dose fentanyl or other short acting narcotics given by anesthesia allow patients to awaken more easily. Amnestic agents with long half-lives, such as midazolam, are only given in the pre-bypass period.

◆ Short acting agents are given in the ICU to allow for early extubation. Small dose narcotics and low dose propofol are frequently used.

◆ Elderly patients or those with hepatic disease may take longer to wake up after anesthesia. If a patient does not wake up in 24 to 36 hours, the differential diagnoses of stroke or encephalopathy must be considered.

◆ Nonsteroidal anti-inflammatory agent such as ketorolac (Toradol) are often given before propofol is discontinued to provide pain control. The use of ketorolac is limited to 72 hours and cannot be used in patients with renal dysfunction or with any bleeding concerns. In addition, there have been recent concerns regarding the risk of cardiovascular thrombotic events, including MI and stroke, associated with non-steroidal anti-inflammatory agents. Future guidelines may include the avoidance of non-steroidal anti-inflammatory agents after CABG.

◆ A continuous infusion of low dose morphine or morphine via PCA pump is also an option. Continuous infusions of low dose narcotics can help avoid the peaks and valleys of breakthrough pain and respiratory depression associated with bolus dosing.

◆ Breakthrough pain is treated with IV morphine or IV ketoralac.

◆ Longer acting agents can be used if early extubation is not planned.

Open Heart Surgery and Coronary Artery Bypass Grafting

Laboratory Testing

◆ Hemoglobin, hematocrit, and potassium levels are monitored every several hours during the immediate postoperative period.

◆ Potassium levels can be high from cardioplegia, but in the postoperative period, patients with normal renal function have excessive diuresis from hemodilution and are at risk for hypokalemia.

◆ Decrease in exchangeable potassium and magnesium invariably occurs when renal function is normal. Maintain serum potassium 4.5 ± 0.5 mEq/L and magnesium > 2.0 mEq/L to decrease incidence of cardiac arrhythmia.

◆ Mild to moderate degrees of ionized hypocalcemia are common following cardiac surgery and generally don't require treatment. Excess calcium administration may worsen ischemic reperfusion injury.

◆ New transfusion guidelines recommend transfusion at a Hgb < 6.0 g/dL as a life saving strategy. It is considered reasonable to transfuse most patients at a Hgb < 7.0 g/dL. It may also be reasonable to transfuse patients with higher hemoglobin levels who are exhibiting signs of organ ischemia (Ferraris & Ferraris et al., 2007).

◆ Coagulation study results should always be correlated to the amount of bleeding.

  ❖ Prothrombin time (PT) / INR – assesses extrinsic cascade. Abnormal INR is corrected with fresh frozen plasma (FFP). Cryoprecipitate may also be used.

  ❖ Partial thromboplastin time (PTT) – assesses intrinsic cascade. Can detect residual or rebound heparin effects. Protamine can be used to correct heparin effects.

  ❖ Platelet count – CPB reduces platelet count by 30-50% and also alters platelet function (Bojar, 2005). Assessment of fibrinolysis can be made by elevated D-dimer, fibrinogen (factor I) levels < 150 mg /dL, and decreased levels of factor VIII. An elevated D-dimer may also be seen after an autotransfusion of shed blood. If fibrinolysis is confirmed, aprotinin may be considered in the postoperative period. There is a risk of achieving a prothrombic state with the use of aprotinin.

◆ Glucose levels are closely monitored and protocols are used to keep the glucose level as close to normal as possible.

Antibiotics

◆ Postoperative antibiotics are given for 48 hours or less.

◆ A single dose prophylaxis may be used in select circumstances when the surgeon considers it optimal practice.

◆ Decisions regarding antibiotic prophylaxis are not guided by the presence of indwelling catheters. (Edwards, et al., 2006).

Stress Ulcer Prophylaxis

Debate remains regarding stress ulcer prophylaxis in the critical care setting. Although the rate of clinically important gastrointestinal bleeding is low, the consequences when it occurs are devastating. H_2 receptor blockers and proton pump inhibitors both work by raising gastric pH and blocking the secretion or production of gastric acid. Sucralfate contains aluminum and binds to the hydrochloric acid in the stomach, acting as a buffer. The potential advantage of sucralfate is a lower incidence of the development of pneumonia. However, there is inconsistent evidence regarding an increased risk for pneumonia with H_2 receptor blockers and proton pump inhibitors. Insitution specifc protocols are used to guide appropriate stress ulcer prophylaxis (Allen & Kopp, 2004).

Chapter 16

Deep Vein Thrombosis (DVT) Prophylaxis

◆ Early mobilization is the most effective intervention in preventing DVT.

◆ Graded compression stockings or intermittent pneumatic devices can be used after surgery. Intermittent pneumatic compression devices have a higher rate of compliance in the intensive care unit where there is increased monitoring. Graded compression stockings should be worn on both legs because DVT frequently occurs in the leg contra-lateral to the SVG harvest.

◆ In patients who are not mobile, unfractionated heparin 5,000 units SQ BID is the strategy least likely to cause excessive bleeding. Low molecular weight heparin causes an increased risk of bleeding in the postoperative period. In patients with an increased number of risk factors, strategies other than unfractionated heparin may be considered. Direct factor Xa inhibitors or oral direct thrombin inhibitors may play a future role in DVT prophylaxis (Goldhaber & Schoepf, 2004).

Arrhythmia Management

Ventricular Arrhythmias

◆ Lidocaine is often used when aortic cross-clamp is removed to suppress reperfusion arrhythmias. This may be continued into the immediate postoperative period.

◆ Patients with poor left ventricular function who have VT postoperatively may need placement of an implantable defibrillator.

◆ If left ventricular function is normal, ventricular arrhythmias are treated with beta blockers and amiodarone, if needed.

Atrial Arrhythmias

Atrial fibrillation occurs in anywhere from 10% to 50% of postoperative patients (Brantman & Howie, 2006), and is most commonly seen on the second to third hospital day (LeDoux & Luikart, 2005). Probable causes include cessation of preoperative beta blocker or the lack of myocardial protection to the atria during CPB.

◆ The standard therapy for the reduction of postoperative atrial fibrillation is the initiation of beta blockers preoperatively or very early postoperatively.

◆ Amiodarone can be used if beta-blockers are contraindicated. Amiodarone, a class III antiarrhythmic, has been shown to reduce the occurrence of postoperative atrial fibrillation by 50% in some studies (Brantman & Howie, 2006). Amiodarone is a predominant class III antiarrhythmic (potassium channel blocker) but also has actions of all the Vaughn-Williams antiarrhythmic classes. Amiodarone also has some alpha blocking activity. As a predominant class III antiarrhythmic, amiodarone delays repolarization and prolongs refractoriness. Common side effects of short term amiodarone include bradycardia and hypotension. Hypotension is most often seen during IV loading.

◆ Digoxin and calcium channel blockers can be used for ventricular rate control, but are not currently recommended for prophylaxis.

◆ Additional information on these pharmacological agents can be found in Chapter 14.

Postoperative Antiplatelet Therapy

◆ Early postoperative aspirin administration, initiated at least within the first 48 hours to prevent saphenous vein graft closure. Aspirin also reduces many other postoperative complications and decreases postoperative mortality (Eagle et al., 2004; Ferraris et al., 2003). Aspirin is usually given within 6 hours after surgery, or as soon as mediastinal bleeding has stopped. Aspirin therapy is continued indefinitely.

Open Heart Surgery and Coronary Artery Bypass Grafting

◆ Clopidogrel may also be prescribed for one year post CABG if the patient had a preoperative NSTE-MI. Clopidogrel does not inhibit platelet function for at least 5 days after surgery (Bojar, 2005).

◆ The platelet count should be assessed before the initiation of antiplatelet therapy.

Fast Tracking

Low-risk patients can be selected for fast tracking after CABG. These patients are targeted for early extubation, early ambulation, and early discharge. Special pathways are used to guide care in patients being fast tracked. Patients who are fast tracked are sedated postoperatively with short-acting agents, and receive lower doses of opioids to allow for earlier extubation. Patients can be extubated postoperatively when they are awake, respond appropriately, and are able to have pain controlled without using medications that interfere with extubation. Prior to extubation, patients must also have no serious postoperative bleeding and have stable vital signs.

Pharmacological strategies to prevent atrial fibrillation are also a key component of fast tracking. Early ambulation and phase I cardiac rehabilitation exercises are also a part of the fast track program. Patients who are fast tracked are generally discharged 3 to 5 days postoperatively. Older patients are commonly more difficult to fast track because of higher numbers of preoperative co-morbidities.

POSTOPERATIVE COMPLICATIONS

Summary of Potential Postoperative Complications

◆ Myocardial depression / low cardiac output state.
  ❖ Perioperative MI.
  ❖ Reversible conditions.
◆ Neurological complications
  ❖ Type I.
  ❖ Type II.
◆ Bleeding.
◆ Cardiac tamponade
◆ Ventricular arrhythmias.
◆ Atrial fibrillation.
◆ Pulmonary.
  ❖ Pulmonary edema.
  ❖ Atelectasis.
  ❖ Pneumothorax.
  ❖ Pleural effusion.
◆ Renal impairment.
◆ Gastrointestinal complications.
◆ Postpericardiotomy syndrome.
◆ Wound infection.
◆ Death.

Systemic Inflammatory Response Syndrome

The use of CPB causes a diffuse inflammatory response. This response results in transient multi-organ dysfunction and can also delay recovery after surgery.

Chapter 16

Low Cardiac Output State

◆ The most common cause of mortality after CABG is a low cardiac output state (Eagle et al., 2004).

◆ Perioperative MI is a cause of a low cardiac output state. Perioperative MI can occur due to graft spasm, embolization into the graft, or a complication of CPB if myocardial protection is not adequate. Incomplete revascularization, stenosis at the anastomosis site, or acute graft closure are other causes of perioperative MI.

◆ Patients with perioperative MI are at increased risk for adverse outcomes.

◆ Treatment of perioperative MI involves medical therapy, including antiplatelet agents, beta blockers, and angiotensin converting enzyme (ACE) inhibitors.

◆ Low cardiac output after CABG can be also caused by reversible conditions, including acidosis and hypoxemia.

◆ The ECG should be assessed for regional ischemic changes. Patients frequently have pericarditis postoperatively, which can mimic an acute MI. Generalized pericarditis can be differentiated from an acute MI based on the wide spread ST segment elevation seen with pericarditis. Regional changes confirmed by reciprocal changes are helpful in the accurate identification of a perioperative MI. Echocardiography can also be used to assess regional wall motion abnormalities.

◆ Because myocardial enzymes are elevated in nearly 90% of all CABG patients, the following guidelines are used in the diagnosis of perioperative MI.

  ❖ CKMB 10 times the upper limit of normal. CKMB greater than 5 times the upper limit of normal places the patient at higher risk for subsequent events (Eagle, et al., 2004).

  ❖ Troponin > 15-20 µg/dL.

◆ If graft closure is suspected as the cause of ischemia, then emergency angiography and PCI are indicated. Surgical re-exploration may also be indicated.

Neurological Complications

◆ The second most common cause of postoperative mortality is postoperative stroke (Eagle et al., 2004).

◆ Neurological complications can be caused by intraoperative or postoperative hypoxia, emboli from CPB, hemorrhage, or metabolic abnormalities (Eagle et al., 2004).

◆ Neurological complications after CABG are classified as Type I or Type II.

◆ Risk factors for Types I and II neurological complications are advanced age and hypertension. Increased time spent on CPB also increases the risk for neurovascular complications.

◆ Hyperglycemia can also worsen neurological impairment.

◆ Peripheral neurovascular complications, including brachial plexus injury and ulnar nerve injury, can also occur as complications of surgery.

Type I Neurological Complications

◆ Type I deficits include major focal deficits and coma.

◆ Additional risk factors for Type I complications include atherosclerosis of the proximal aorta, previous history of neurological disease, unstable angina or diabetes, and intraoperative use of an intra-aortic balloon pump.

◆ Other factors that contribute to postoperative stroke are recent anterior wall MI with left ventricular thrombus and recent stroke. Patients with recent stroke should not have CABG for at least 4 weeks. If CABG is done within 4 weeks of a stroke, then the patient is at high risk for hemorrhagic complications of stroke.

Open Heart Surgery and Coronary Artery Bypass Grafting

◆ Minimizing Type I complications is critical because stroke is the second leading cause of mortality. A Type I neurological injury can produce a 21% mortality rate (Eagle et al., 2004).

◆ The use of ultrasound via epiaortic imaging or transesophageal echocardiography to assess the aorta for the presence of atherosclerotic plaque is a technique to help minimize Type I complications. When atherosclerotic plaque is identified in the ascending aorta, the patient is at high risk for an adverse neurovascular outcome. Embolization of atherosclerotic plaque is the most common cause of perioperative strokes (LeDoux & Luikart, 2005). Atherosclerotic emboli can be dislodged from the aortic arch during cannulation for CPB or during clamping of the aorta. In very high-risk patients, a no-clamp strategy may be used (Eagle et al., 2004).

Type II Neurological Complications

◆ Type II deficits include various degrees of intellectual deterioration and memory loss.

◆ Additional risk factors for Type II complications include prior CABG, alcohol consumption, arrhythmias, heart failure, and history of peripheral vascular disease (Eagle et al., 2004).

◆ Type II complications may be related to the brain's own microcirculation in addition to microemboli during CPB. Sophisticated arterial line filters within the bypass circuit help protect against microemboli. Type II complications have been associated with periods of hypotension or hypoperfusion and may be reversible.

Atrial Fibrillation

Atrial fibrillation not only extends length of stay but also greatly increases the risk of postoperative stroke. If atrial fibrillation persists more than 24 hours, intravenous heparin and warfarin can be initiated to prevent clot formation and future stroke. The benefits of full anticoagulation must be balanced against the increased risk of postoperative bleeding. The decision to cardiovert is based on the individual patient situation. Cardioversion within 24 hours of onset is probably safe without anticoagulation (Eagle et al., 2004). Postoperative atrial fibrillation usually resolves on its own 6 to 8 weeks after surgery (Brantman & Howie, 2006).

Additional potential complications of postoperative atrial fibrillation:

◆ Ventricular arrhythmias.

◆ Myocardial ischemia.

◆ Hemodynamic alterations.

Chapter 16

> ### *Risk Factors for Development of Postoperative Atrial Fibrillation*
>
> **Preoperative**
> - Advanced age.
> - Male gender.
> - Peripheral arterial disease.
> - Valvular heart disease.
> - Chronic obstructive pulmonary disease (COPD) or proximal RCA disease (can cause right ventricular and right atrial enlargement).
> - Left atrial enlargement or atrial arrhythmias preoperatively.
> - Cessation of beta blockers prior to surgery.
> - Previous cardiac surgery
>
> (Eagle et al., 2004; Brantman & Howie, 2006).
>
> **Intraoperative**
> - Increased cross-clamp time, producing atrial ischemia.
> - Atrial incisions and surgical trauma to the atria.
> - Placement of venous cannulas
>
> (Eagle et al., 2004; Brantman & Howie, 2006).
>
> **Postoperative**
> - Increased circulating catecholamines (endogenous and exogenous).
> - Pneumonia and prolonged mechanical ventilation.
> - Volume overload.
> - Hypoxia.
> - Electrolyte disturbances
>
> (LeDoux & Luikart, 2005).

Of all the risk factors, advanced age is a consistent predictor of postoperative atrial fibrillation. With advanced age there are several degenerative changes that increase the risk of re-entry circuits within the atria, including atrial fibrosis, dilatation or atrophy of atria, and decreased tissue conductivity.

Wound Infection

Mediastinitis, or deep sternal wound infection, is a serious complication of CABG, resulting in a mortality rate as high as 25% (Eagle et al., 2004). Sternal wound infections typically manifest several days to 2 weeks after surgery (LeDoux & Luikart, 2005). Skin and nasopharyngeal gram-positive organisms are the leading cause of deep sternal wound infections postoperatively (Eagle et al., 2004).

Prevention

◆ Routine mupirocin administration is recommended for all patients. Mupirocin is a patient administered topical antibiotic that eliminates nasal *S aureus,* including methicillin-resistant strains of *Staphyloccocus.* The most common organism cultured in cardiac wounds is *Staphylococcus,* and colonization is considered the major factor in wound contamination ((Engelman et al., 2007).

◆ Properly timed preoperative antibiotic administration (within 30 minutes of incision time) is important to assure adequate tissue levels at the time of incision (Eagle et al., 2004). National core quality indicators require administration within 1 hour of incision.

◆ Additional antibiotic dosing may be required for longer surgeries.

◆ Postoperative intravenous (IV) antibiotics are continued for up to 48 hours (Edwards et al., 2006).

Open Heart Surgery and Coronary Artery Bypass Grafting

◆ A cephalosporin (typically cefazolin) is the antibiotic of choice (Engelman, et al., 2007).

◆ Vancomycin may be added to a cephalosporin in patients at high risk for a staphylococcal infection (Engelman, et al., 2007).

◆ Vancomycin is recommended (along with additional gram-negative coverage) in patients who are considered lactam or penicillin allergic and cannot receive a cephalosporin (Engelman et al., 2007).

◆ Meticulous aseptic technique during surgery: a) Double gloving of OR team; b) reduced OR traffic.

◆ Proper hand hygiene throughout perioperative period.

◆ Clipping rather than shaving of hair and avoidance of hair removal.

◆ Shorter CPB times.

◆ Avoidance of unnecessary electrocautery.

◆ Strict control of blood sugars during and after surgery.

◆ Protecting the sternum: a) Keeping patient arms and hands away from sternum; b) avoiding excess coughing; and c) minimizing the use of arms for weight bearing, pushing, and pulling.

Risk Factors for Development of Infection
- Obesity.
- Diabetes.
- End stage renal disease.
- Re-operation.
- Excessive use of electrocautery.
- Use of both internal mammary arteries (decreased blood flow to the sternum).

Treatment

◆ Superficial wounds are treated with antibiotics and drainage.

◆ Deep sternal wounds need surgical debridement and closure with a muscle flap (LeDoux & Luikart, 2005).

Renal Dysfunction

Renal dysfunction is another potential complication after CABG because CPB decreases glomerular filtration rate. Mortality is high for those who develop renal dysfunction perioperatively and is especially high for those who require dialysis. Early recognition of renal insufficiency and assurance of adequate volume administration are key nursing interventions to prevent postoperative renal failure. Adequate cardiac output at the end of CPB is important to prevent postoperative renal dysfunction.

Nephrotoxic medications, including nonsteroidal anti-inflammatory drugs and aminoglycoside antibiotics, should be avoided in high-risk patients. Patients with end-stage renal disease are at very high risk for mortality and morbidity if they undergo CABG. However, their risk for mortality may be even higher if they do not undergo revascularization; therefore, CABG may be considered for some of these patients. Patients with end-stage renal disease have a particularly high risk of developing postoperative infection and sepsis (Eagle et al., 2004).

731

Chapter 16

> **Risk Factors for Postoperative Renal Dysfunction following Cardiac Surgery**
> - Preoperative renal dysfunction.
> - Congestive heart failure.
> - Age (adults > 70 years).
> - Prolonged CPB time (> 4 h) or acute reduction in cardiac output.
> - Aminoglycoside antibiotics.
> - Non steroidal antinflammatory agents in high risk patients.
> - Preoperative ACE inhibitors in patients receiving aprotinin.
> - Preoperative contrast nephropathy.
> - Type I diabetes.
> - Prior CABG
>
> (Eagle et al., 2004).

Pulmonary Complications

Patients with postoperative pulmonary complications are at a higher risk for atrial and ventricular arrhythmias.

Mild pulmonary complications can occur simply as a result of CPB. Most patients also experience post-operative atelectasis. Postoperative thoracic and abdominal surgery patients are prone to hypoventilation due to postoperative pain. Postoperative pain control is an effective intervention to prevent atelectasis by promoting adequate ventilation. Chest tube removal, as soon as clinically indicated, will help with pain control and promotion of optimal ventilation.

> **Risk Factors for Development of Pulmonary Complications**
> The most common preoperative pulmonary problem is (COPD). Those with moderate to severe COPD, including those with elevated pCO_2 levels and those who use home oxygen, are at increased risk for postoperative complications. These patients are also at increased risk of ventricular arrhythmias postoperatively (Eagle et al., 2004).
> Additional risk factors for pulmonary complications include:
> - Increased age.
> - Smoking.
> - Depressed LV function.
> - Preoperative clinical HF.
> - Obesity.
> - Diabetes.

Acute respiratory distress syndrome (ARDS) is a serious potential complication. Patients undergoing re-operation, emergent operation, those requiring blood transfusions, and those with poor LV function or experiencing shock are at higher risk for developing ARDS. Preoperative pulmonary edema should be resolved prior to surgery because pulmonary edema increases with CPB. Patients who develop acute respiratory insufficiency and ARDS usually suffer a major perioperative insult, such as shock or sepsis, which is imposed on a pre-existing lung problem or significant risk factor.

Patients who are unable to be extubated in a prompt manner are at increased risk of developing nosocomial pneumonia and ARDS. These patients are usually ventilated using low tidal volume. The use of low tidal volume is one lung-protective strategy to limit damage to pulmonary tissue caused by mechanical

Open Heart Surgery and Coronary Artery Bypass Grafting

ventilation. Patients requiring prolonged ventilatory support > 5 days have an increased risk for multi-organ dysfunction.

Pneumothorax can also occur as a postoperative complication and can happen at the time of removal of pleural chest tubes.

The development of pleural effusion is not uncommon after CABG. Left pleural effusion is more common when the pleural cavity has been entered for LIMA takedown because both blood and serous fluid ooze from the chest wall. Right pleural effusion is more commonly from serous fluid as a result of fluid overload. Hemothorax may also result as a complication if blood spills over from the pericardial space in patients with large amounts of mediastinal bleeding (Bojar, 2005).

Most postoperative pleural effusions are asymptomatic and resolve either spontaneously over time or in response to diuretics. Patients who have moderate-sized pleural effusions or underlying lung disease may be symptomatic and require thoracentesis. Large pleural effusions may require chest tube insertion. A large pleural effusion can cause cardiac tamponade, even in the absence of pericardial effusion (Bojar, 2005).

Postoperative Bleeding

Contributing factors to mediastinal bleeding include:
- Residual effects of heparin.
- Thrombocytopenia or platelet dysfunction.
- Clotting factor depletion.
- Fibrinolysis.
- Hypothermia.
- Postoperative hypertension.
- Surgical technique.

Postoperative bleeding is usually venous and usually caused from bleeding at the site of sutures. Bleeding can also occur from pericardial adhesions during a re-operation.

Causes

◆ Surgical bleeding.
◆ Rebound or residual heparin effect.
◆ Thrombocytopenia or dysfunctional platelets.
  ❖ Hemodilution and CPB reduce platelet count by 30-50% (Bojar, 2005).
  ❖ Protamine transiently reduces platelets.
  ❖ Platelet function is also affected by: CPB, preoperative antiplatelets and herbals, uremia, and hypothermia post CPB.
◆ Clotting factor deficiency
  ❖ Hepatic dysfunction.
  ❖ Hemodilution.
  ❖ Intraoperative cell saving devices.
◆ Fibrinolysis
  ❖ Plasminogen is activated during CPB.
  ❖ Heparin also induces some fibrinolysis.

733

Chapter 16

Strategies to Reduce the Risk of Bleeding

◆ Heparin coated circuits for CPB to allow for reduction in heparin administration.

◆ Retrograde autologous priming of circuit involving withdrawal of cystalloid prime.

◆ Avoidance of cardiotomy suction. Blood aspirated from pericardial space has been in contact with tissue factor and has fibrinolytic properties.

◆ Limit hemodilution.

◆ Avoid surgery in anemic patients.

◆ Liberal use of antifibrinolytic drugs.

Postpericardiotomy Syndrome

Weeks to months after CABG, some patients experience an autoimmune response of the pericardial tissue. This response causes inflammation of the pericardium and is termed *post-pericardiotomy syndrome*. The pleural space can also be involved. Patients are treated with NSAIDs, and steroids can also be used, if needed. Cardiac tamponade can occur alone or as a complication of post-pericardiotomy syndrome. Late tamponade is most typically seen in patients on warfarin (LeDoux & Luikart, 2005).

Angina after CABG

Up to 20% of patients presenting with unstable angina have undergone CABG. These patients are at higher risk for mortality and morbidity than patients who have never received revascularization (Braunwald et al., 2002). Patients who present with ACS or other symptoms suggestive of ischemia after having CABG are generally candidates for cardiac catheterization because it is difficult to distinguish between graft closure and progression of native vessel disease using only noninvasive testing. Most patients who present with ischemia within 30 days of surgery have graft failure due to thrombosis. This acute graft closure can occur in vein grafts and arterial conduits. These patients are usually candidates for PCI to treat the focal stenosis. If multiple vein grafts are stenosed or if the stenotic graft is supplying the LAD, then repeat CABG is often indicated.

SPECIAL PATIENTS POPULATIONS

Emergency CABG Patients

Any emergent or urgent surgery carries an increased risk of mortality and morbidity. Whenever possible, PCI, an intra-aortic balloon pump, and medical treatment should be used to stabilize the patient prior to surgery. Failed PCI procedures in patients who are ischemic or who have hemodynamic instability may warrant emergency CABG. Emergency CABG may also be performed at the time of a repair of a mechanical complication of acute MI, such as septal or papillary muscle rupture. Emergency CABG is not performed in patients with only a small area of myocardium at risk, and who are hemodynamically stable (Antman et al., 2004).

Acute MI Patients

Patients who have had acute MIs have higher mortality with CABG for the first several days after the infarction. For patients with large MIs who are stabilized, surgery should be delayed to allow the myocardium to recover. However, some patients with acute MIs are unable to wait to have CABG, including those with left main or triple vessel disease and those with symptomatic valve disease. CABG mortality is elevated for the first 3 to 7 days after an MI (Antman et al., 2004).

Open Heart Surgery and Coronary Artery Bypass Grafting

Right Ventricular MI Patients

Patients with large right ventricular MIs are at particularly high risk and may need surgery delayed for up to 4 weeks to allow for recovery of the right ventricle. During surgery, the pericardium is no longer able to contain the acutely injured right ventricle, and it dilates. This dilatation may even prevent the chest from closing (Eagle et al., 2004).

Elderly Patients

The greatest increase in patients having CABG is among the over 85 age-group. The elderly have increased risk of mortality and morbidity; however, improvement in functional capacity and quality of life can be achieved in most patients in this age-group (Eagle et al., 2004). Patients ≥ age 85 years have:

◆ Higher incidence of left main and multivessel disease.
◆ More advanced left ventricular dysfunction.
◆ Co-existing valve disease.
◆ More non cardiac co-morbid conditions.

Women

Some studies have found differences in CABG mortality and morbidity rates when comparing women to men, with women having higher complication rates. However, the evidence is conflicting as to whether gender is the determining factor. General consensus is that risk factors and patient co-morbidities are more important than gender, and CABG should not be delayed as a treatment option for women (Eagle et al., 2004). Recent research indicates that women may have improved outcomes with OPCAB.

Diabetics

Patients with diabetes have an increased risk of mortality with CABG compared to nondiabetic patients, regardless of level of preoperative blood sugar control (Woods, Smith, Sohail, Sarah, & Eagle, 2004). However, CABG was shown in the Bypass Angioplasty Revascularization Investigation (BARI[3]) trial to provide a greater survival benefit to appropriate patients with diabetes when compared to PCI (Woods, Smith, Sohail, Sarah, & Engle, 2004). In addition to diabetes, any hyperglycemia during the perioperative period increases risk, especially for sternal wound infections. Hyperglycemia can occur in nondiabetic patients due to surgical stress, hypothermia, commonly used postoperative medications, and other complex metabolic changes that occur during CABG (Lorenz, Lorenz, & Codd, 2005). Tight glycemic control, with the use of intravenous insulin, is recommended in CABG patients (Lorenz, Lorenz, & Codd, 2005).

Patients with Peripheral Vascular Disease

Patients with peripheral vascular disease commonly have co-existing CAD, and those who undergo CABG have an increased short- and long-term risk for mortality.

Patients with Low Ejection Fractions

Patients with low ejection fractions or clinical heart failure also have an increased risk of operative mortality. However, this group of patients, when treated with CABG, also have the greatest survival benefit when compared to treatment with medical therapy. In addition, this population can benefit from symptom relief and improvement in functional capacity (Gibbons et al., 2002).

Chapter 16

Patients with Valve Disease

Patients with co-existing moderate to severe aortic stenosis commonly undergo aortic valve replacement at the time of CABG. In addition, patients who have clinically symptomatic mitral regurgitation with structural abnormalities undergo mitral valve repair at the time of CABG (Bonow et al., 1998; Eagle et al., 2004). If the mitral valve is structurally normal and regurgitation is not severe, the regurgitation may be caused by reversible ischemia that is corrected with the revascularization procedure. Combined procedures increase the operative risk of complications and mortality. When a valve procedure is added to CABG, the risk of stroke substantially increases (Bonow et al., 1998; Eagle et al., 2004).

Patients with End Stage Renal Disease

Cardiovascular disease is the number one cause of death in patients with end stage kidney disease. Revascularization provides improved survival options in some patients. Although revascularization is associated with a high risk of mortality and morbidity in these patients, there may be an even higher risk without revascularization. Although long term survival may be limited, patients may have symptom improvement and increased quality of life.

Patients for Re-operation

Mortality and morbidity risks are higher for patients who undergo repeat CABG. These patients may have limited available graft options and long-term results, including symptomatic relief, are not as successful with repeat operations as with initial operations. In addition, the surgery is longer and the risk of bleeding is higher due to the presence of scar tissue. Re-operation candidates may have many of the characteristics below, placing them at high risk:

◆ Advanced age.

◆ Advanced coronary and non coronary atherosclerotic disease.

◆ Diminished left ventricular function.

◆ Limited acceptable conduit.

POST-DISCHARGE CARE

Administration of postoperative aspirin is continued indefinitely. All patients also receive statin therapy to reduce the progression of vein graft disease. CABG patients are placed on a lifting restriction for 6 to 8 weeks after discharge. The restriction varies by surgeon, but is typically a 5 to 10 lb restriction. Bypass patients generally wait to drive, even after their restrictions are over, due to chest soreness and fear of injury. A formal cardiac rehabilitation program referral should be made for all patients prior to discharge. Patients usually begin participation in outpatient cardiac rehabilitation 3 to 8 weeks after surgery. In one long-term study of CABG patients who participated in cardiac rehabilitation, outcomes at 5 years included increased physical mobility, perception of better health, and perception of better overall life situation. Compared to those who do not participate in cardiac rehabilitation, a larger percentage of those who complete the program are working at 3 years (Eagle et al., 2004). Assessment of depression and presence of psychosocial support are important nursing interventions in the post-discharge period. Depression occurs in up to 33% of patients after CABG (Eagle et al., 2004). Psychosocial interventions for CABG patients are similar to those for patients with CAD. These interventions are discussed in detail in Chapter 8. Facilitating participation in cardiac rehabilitation is a key nursing intervention in the prevention and treatment of postoperative depression and social isolation.

Many patients and their caregivers experience major psychosocial adjustments after discharge. Adapting to postoperative pain, changes in body image, activity limitations, and financial burdens are a few of the areas for which nurses need to provide support during the discharge transition (Theobald & McMurray, 2004). Telephone follow-up programs are one method of providing postoperative support, especially to assure a smooth home transition in patients who are fast tracked.

Linking Knowledge to Practice

Key hemodynamic considerations in the postoperative period:

✔ *Optimize pre-load (PAOP 18-20 mm Hg) and HR (90-100 BPM) as first line strategies for maintaining adequate cardiac output.*

✔ *Use an inotrope if cardiac index is < 2.0 L/min/mm²*
   ❖ *Epineprhine.*
   ❖ *Dopamine if decreased SVR (beta 1 and alpha).*
   ❖ *Dobutamine if elevated SVR (beta 1 with modest beta 2; beta 2 stronger than alpha).*
   ❖ *Inamrinone / milrinone if elevated SVR (inotrope with venous and arterial vasodilation).*

✔ *Use an alpha agent if blood pressure and SVR is low*
   ❖ *Phenylephrine if cardiac index is satisfactory.*
   ❖ *Norepinephrine if cardiac index is marginal.*
   ❖ *Vasopressin or single dose methylene blue when blood pressure not responsive to norepinephrine.*

✔ *Use a vasodilator if SVR is elevated.*
   ❖ *Nitroprusside.*
   ❖ *Niroglycerin if evidence of ischemia.*

TEST YOUR KNOWLEDGE

1. The patient who would be a good candidate for coronary artery bypass graft surgery (CABG) is
    a. a patient with 90% left main occlusion.
    b. a patient with a 50% LAD occlusion and a 60% circumflex occlusion.
    c. a patient with a 95% RCA lesion with a significant amount of myocardium at risk.
    d. a patient with very diffuse and very small vessel disease.

2. Preoperative clopidogrel should be held for how many days preoperatively?
    a. 1-2 days
    b. No days
    c. 30 days
    d. 5-7 days

Chapter 16

3. The term OPCAB refers to
   a. the use of thoracotomy instead of sternotomy.
   b. patients who are fast tracked to be discharged in less than 5 days.
   c. CABG surgery without the use of CPB.
   d. combination open heart surgery and percutaneous procedure.

4. Neurological complications after CABG are most likely to occur in which of the following patients:
   a. A previously healthy 50-year-old woman undergoing CPB.
   b. A patient with an atherosclerotic aorta undergoing CPB.
   c. A patient undergoing OPCAB.
   d. A 67-year-old man having a MIDCAB to the LAD with no known history of hypertension.

5. A characteristic of a fast-track pathway after CABG would include
   a. extubation by the third post-op day.
   b. anticipated discharge between post-op days 7 and 8.
   c. liberal use of opioid medications to increase patient comfort during the ventilator weaning process.
   d. a defined medication strategy to prevent post-operative atrial fibrillation.

6. Medistinal drainage in the following amount meets criteria for re-exploration:
   a. > 400 ml for 1 hour
   b. > 300 ml/hr for 2-3 hours
   c. > 200 ml/hr for 4 hours
   d. All of the above.

7. Patients with prolonged CPB times are likely to experience
   a. a decrease in total body fluid due to dehydration.
   b. an increase in coagulopathies.
   c. a decrease in chest tube drainage.
   d. an increased likelihood of early extubation.

8. Sternal wound infections typically manifest by post-op day 1.
   a. True.
   b. False.

Open Heart Surgery and Coronary Artery Bypass Grafting

9. Hypothermia in the immediate postoperative period is associated with what physiological effects?

   a. Increase in SVR and systemic hypertension

   b. Decrease in SVR and hypotension

   c. Improved platelet function

   d. Protection provided from incisional pain via shivering

10. Acceptable postoperative extubation criteria include all of the following, except:

    a. Awake without stimulation

    b. Negative inspiratory force > 25 cm H_2O

    c. TV < 5 ml/kg

    d. Respiratory rate < 24

11. Aprotinin is a pharmacological agent used to decrease bleeding in the high risk patient. It works by coating and protecting the platelets during CPB.

    a. True.

    b. False.

12. To prevent postoperative infection, prophylactic antibiotic administration is

    a. not recommended.

    b. recommended in insulin dependent diabetic patients only.

    c. recommended for a minimum of 7 days for maximum effect.

    d. recommended for a maximum of 24 to 48 hours.

13. The <u>first line</u> strategy to maintain an adequate cardiac index postoperatively includes

    a. optimizing pre-load and heart rate.

    b. initiating an inotrope.

    c. initiating a vasopressor.

    d. None of the above.

14. Patients with right ventricular infarcts are at high risk and have improved outcomes if surgery is done immediately after the infarct.

    a. True.

    b. False.

15. Antianginal medications in a patient waiting for CABG surgery should be

    a. given up to the time of surgery.

    b. held, beginning at 12 midnight, before surgery.

    c. held as soon a surgery is scheduled to prepare the heart for cardioplegia.

    d. None of the above.

Chapter 16

16. Strategies to decrease sternal wound infections include all of the following, except
    a. strict glycemic control during the perioperative period.
    b. shorter CPB times.
    c. shaving of hair prior to surgery.
    d. administration of preoperative antibiotics within 30 minutes of incision.

17. Patients who develop atrial fibrillation post CABG are protected from stroke for several weeks due to the anticoagulation received during surgery.
    a. True.
    b. False.

18. The potential benefits of OPCAB are related to
    a. avoidance of cross-clamping of the aorta .
    b. avoidance of the systemic effects of CPB.
    c. avoidance of a sternotomy.
    d. a and b.

19. The following factors increase bleeding risk in patients undergoing CABG:
    a. Development of coagulopathies from CPB
    b. Administration of antiplatelet agents during the preoperative period
    c. Hypothermia
    d. All of the above.

20. During the immediate postoperative period, total body fluid may be increased while circulating volume is decreased.
    a. True.
    b. False.

Open Heart Surgery and Coronary Artery Bypass Grafting

ANSWERS

1.	A	11.	B
2.	D	12.	D
3.	C	13.	A
4.	B	14.	B
5.	D	15.	A
6.	D	16.	C
7.	B	17.	B
8.	B	18.	D
9.	A	19.	D
10.	C	20.	A

REFERENCES

Allen, M.E. & Kopp, B.J. (2004). Stress ulcer prophylaxis in the postoperative period. *American Journal of Health-System Pharmacy, 61*(6), 588-596.

Antman, E.M., Anbe, D.T., Armstrong, P.W., Bates, E.R., Green, L.A., Hand, M., Hochman, J.S., Krumholz, H.M., Kushner, F.G., Lamas, G.A., Mullany, C.J., Ornato, J.P., Pearle, D.L., Sloan, M.A., & Smith, S.C. Jr. (2004). ACC/AHA guidelines for the management of patients with ST-elevation myocardial infarction: executive summary: a report of the ACC / AHA task force on practice guidelines (Committee to Revise the 1999 Guidelines on the Management of Patients with Acute Myocardial Infarction). *Journal of the American College of Cardiology, 44,* 671-719.

Bojar, R.M. (2005). *Manual of perioperative care in adult cardiac surgery* (4th ed.). Malden, Massachusetts: Blackwell Publishing.

Braunwald, E., Antman, E.M., Beasley, J.W., Califf, R.M., Cheitlin, M.D., Hochman, J.S., Jones, R.H., Kereiakes, D., Kupersmith, J., Levin, T.N., Pepine, C.J., Schaeffer, J.W., Smith, E.E., III, Steward, D.E., & Thoroux, P. (2002). *ACC/AHA 2002 guideline update for the management of patients with unstable angina and non ST elevation myocardial infarction: A report of the American College of Cardiology / American Heart Association Task Force on Practice Guidelines* (Committee on the Management of Patients with Unstable Angina). Retrieved from: http://www.acc.org/clinical/guidelines/unstable/unstable.pdf

Bridges, C.R., Horvath, K.A., Nugent, W.C., Shahian, D.M., Haan, C.K., Shemin, R.J., Allen, K.B., & Edwards, F.H. (2003). The Society of Thoracic Surgeons practice guideline series: Transmyocardial laser revascularization [Electronic Version]. *Society of Thoracic Surgeons*. Retrieved on December 22, 2004 from http://www.sts.org

Eagle, K.A., Guyton, R.A., Davidoff, R., Edwards, F.H., Ewy, G.A., Gardner, T.J., Hart, J.C., Herrmann, H.C., Hillis, L.D., Hutter, A.M. Jr., Lytle, B.W., Marlow, R.A., Nugent, W.C., & Orszulak, T.A., (2004). *ACC/AHA 2004 guideline update for coronary artery bypass graft surgery: A report to the American College of Cardiology/American Heart Association Task Force on Practice Guidelines* (Committee to Update the 1999 Guidelines for Coronary Artery Bypass Graft Surgery). American College of Cardiology Web Site. Available at http://www.acc.org/clinical/guidelines/cabg/cabg.pdf

Edwards, F.H., Engelman, R.M., Houck, P., Shahian, D.M., & Bridges, C.R. (2006). The Society of Thoracic Surgeons practice guideline series: Antibiotic prophylaxis in cardiac surgery, part I: Duration. *Annals of Thoracic Surgery, 81,* 397-404.

Engelman, R., Shahian, D., Shemin, R., Guy, T.S., Bratzler, D., Edwards, F., Jacobs, M., Fernando, H., & Bridges, C. (2007). The Society of Thoracic Surgeons practice guideline series: Antibiotic prophylaxis in cardiac surgery, part II: Antibiotic choice. *Annals of Thoracic Surgery, 83,* 1569-1576.

Ferraris V.A., Ferraris, S.P., Moliterno, D.J., Camp, P., Walenga, J.M., Messmore, H.L., Jeske, W.P., Edwards, F.H., Royston, D., Shahian, D.M., Peterson, E., Bridges, C.R., & Despotis, G. (2003). The Society of Thoracic Surgeons practice guideline series: aspirin and other anti-platelet agents during operative coronary revascularization. *Society of Thoracic Surgeons.* Retrieved on December 22, 2004 from http://www.sts.org

Ferraris, V.A., Ferraris, S.P., Saha, S.P., Hessel E.A., Haan, C.K., Royston, B.D., Bridges, C.R., Higgins, R.S.D., Despotis, G., Brown, J.R., Spiess, B.D., Shore-Lesserson, L., Stafford-Smith, M., Mazer, C.D., Bennett-Guerrero, E., Hill, S.E., & Body, S. (2007). Perioperative blood transfusion and blood conservation in cardiac surgery: The Society of Thoracic Surgeons and The Society ofCardiovascular Anesthesiologists clinical practice guideline. *Annals of Thoracic Surgery, 83*, S27-86.

Goldhaber, S.Z. & Schoepf, U.J. (2004). Pulmonary embolism after coronary artery bypass grafting. *Circulation, 109*, 2712-2715.

Kincaid, E.H., Ashburn, D.A., Hoyle, J.R., Reichert, M.G., Hammon, J.W., & Kon, N.D. (2005). Does the combination of aprotinin and angiotensin-converting enzyme inhibitor cause renal failure after cardiac surgery? *Annals of Thoracic Surgery, 80*, 1388-1393.

Koster, A., Chew, D., Gründel, N., Bauer, M., Kuppe, H., Spiess, B. (2003). *Bivalirudin monitored with the ecarin clotting time for anticoagulation during cardiopulmonary bypass.* The International Anesthesia Research Society. Retrieved on March 31, 2007 from http://www.anesthesia-analgesia .org/cgi/reprint/96/2/383.pdf

LeDoux, D. & Luikart, H. (2005). Cardiac surgery. In S.L.Woods, E.S. Froelicher, S.U. Motzer, & E.J. Bridges (Eds.), *Cardiac nursing* (5th ed., pp. 628-658). Philadelphia: Lippincott, Williams and Wilkins.

Lorenz, R.A., Lorenz, R.M., & Codd, J.E. (2005). Perioperative blood glucose control during adult coronary artery bypass surgery [Electronic Version]. *Association of Operating Room Nurses AORN Journal, 81*(1), pp. 126-148.

Mangano, D.T., Miao, Y., Vuylsteke, A., Tudor, I.C., Juneja, R., Filipescu, D., et al., (2007). Mortality associated with aprotinin during 5 years following coronary artery bypass graft surgery. *JAMA,* (297), 5, 471-479.

Murkin, J. (2001). Anesthesia for robotic heart surgery: An overview. *The Heart Surgery Forum,* (4), 4, 311-314.

Niinami, H., Ogasawara, H., Suda, Y., & Takeuchi, Y. (2005). Single vessel revascularization with minimally invasive direct coronary artery bypass: minithoracotomy or ministernotomy? *Chest, 27*(1), 47-52.

Nishizaki, K., & Seki, T. (2005). Early results on aortic connector system for proximal anast-moses of the saphenous vein graft. *Annals Thoracic Cardiovascular Surgery,* (11), 2, 98-104.

Racz, M.J., Hannan, E.L., Isom, O.W., Subramanian, V.A., Jones, R.H., Gold, J.P., et al. (2004). A comparison of short- and long-term outcomes after off-pump and on-pump coronary artery bypass graft surgery with sternotomy. *Journal of American College of Cardiology, 434*, 557-564.

Raghavan, M. & Marik, P.E. (2005). Anemia, allogenic blood transfusion and immunomodulation in the critically ill [Electronic Version]. *Chest, 127*(1), 295-308.

Selke, F.W., DiMaio, J.M., Caplan, L.R., Ferguson, T.B., Gardner, T.J., Hiratzka, L.F., Isselbacher, E.M., Lytle, B.W., Mack ,M.J., Murkin, J.M., & Robbins, R.C. (2005). Comparing On-Pump and Off-Pump Coronary Artery Bypass Grafting: Numerous Studies but Few Conclusions: A Scientific Statement From the American Heart Association Council on Cardiovascular Surgery and Anesthesia in Collaboration With the Interdisciplinary Working Group on Quality of Care and Outcomes Research *Circulation, 111,* 2858 - 2864.

Smith, S.C. Jr., Dove, J.T., Jacobs, A.K., Kennedy, J.W., Kereiakes, D., Kern, M.J., Kuntz, R.E., Popma, J.J., Schaff, H.V., & Williams, D.O. (2001). ACC/AHA guidelines for percutaneous coronary intervention: executive summary and recommendations: a report of the American College of Cardiology / American Heart Association Task Force on Practice Guidelines (Committee to Revise the 1993 Guidelines for Percutaneous Transluminal Coronary Angioplasty). *Journal of the American College of Cardiology, 37*, 2215-2238.

Sundt, T.M. (2004). Adult cardiac surgery: Coronary artery bypass grafting surgery. *Society of Thoracic Surgeons.* Retrieved on December 22, 2004 from http://www.sts.org

Theobald, K. & McMurray, A. (2004). Coronary artery bypass graft surgery: Discharge planning for successful recovery [Electronic Version]. *Journal of Advanced Nursing, 47*, 483-491.

Vohra, H.A., Levine, A., & Dunning, J. (2005). Can ventilation while on cardiopulmonary bypass improve post-operative lung function for patients undergoing cardiac surgery? *Interactive CardioVascular and Thoracic Surgery, 4*, 442-446.

Woods, S.E., Smith, J.M., Sohail, S., Sarah, A., & Engle, A. (2004). The influence of type 2 diabetes mellitus in patients undergoing coronary artery bypass graft surgery: An 8-year prospective cohort study [Electronic Version]. *Chest, 126,* 1789-1793.

CHAPTER 17:
ELECTRICAL MANAGEMENT OF ARRHYTHMIAS:

DEFIBRILLATION, CARDIOVERSION, PACEMAKERS, IMPLANTABLE CARDIOVERTER DEFIBRILLATORS, ELECTROPHYSIOLOGY STUDIES, RADIOFREQUENCY ABLATION

This chapter focuses on the electrical management of cardiac arrhythmias, including defibrillation and cardioversion for terminating tachyarrhythmias; single and dual chamber pacemaker concepts; and implantable cardioverter defibrillators (ICD) in sudden cardiac death (SCD) survivors and patients at high risk for SCD. Pacemakers and ICDs have become very complicated, and it is increasingly difficult for nurses to keep up with new technology and feel comfortable dealing with these devices. This chapter focuses on basic concepts of single and dual chamber pacemakers and ICDs, but does not attempt to cover all technology associated with these devices.

DEFIBRILLATION

Defibrillation is the delivery of electrical energy to the myocardium to terminate ventricular fibrillation (VF) and pulseless ventricular tachycardia (pVT). The defibrillating shock depolarizes all cells in the heart simultaneously, stopping all electrical activity and allowing the sinus node to resume its function as the normal pacemaker of the heart. Early defibrillation is the only treatment for VF or pVT, and should not be delayed for any reason when a defibrillator is available. If a defibrillator is not immediately available, cardiopulmonary resuscitation (CPR) should be started until a defibrillator arrives.

Defibrillation is usually done transcutaneously, using two paddles applied to the skin in the anterolateral position (Figure 17.1). The procedure can also be done through hands-free adhesive pads in either the anterolateral or the anteroposterior position (Figure 17.2), but this method is usually only used in patients with frequent, recurrent VF requiring repeated shocks. Defibrillation can also be done via transvenous electrodes as part of an ICD system, which is covered later in this chapter.

Electrical output used for defibrillation (and for cardioversion) is quantified in joules (J) or watt-seconds. Traditional machines utilize a monophasic waveform that delivers energy in one direction through the myocardium. Newer machines utilize a biphasic waveform that delivers the initial energy in one direction and the last portion of energy in the opposite direction. Biphasic waveforms are more effective than monophasic waveforms in terminating arrhythmias. At this time there is no concensus on how biphasic waveform energy relates to monophasic waveform energy. The current Advanced Cardiac Life Support (ACLS) guidelines from the American Heart Association indicate that defibrillation with a 120j – 150j biphasic shock is at least as effective as higher energy monophasic shocks (Hamdan, Dorostkar, & Scheinman, 2000).

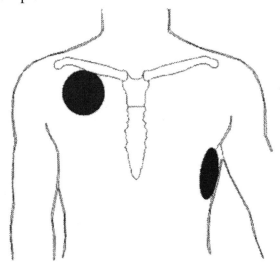

Figure 17.1: Anterolateral position for placing paddles or hands-free adhesive pads for defibrillation.

Chapter 17

New ACLS guidelines recommend an initial energy of 360 J with a monophasic defibrillator and the manufacturer's recommended energy level for biphasic defibrillators (*Advanced Cardiovascular Life Support Provider Manual,* 2006). Since there are two types of biphasic waveforms available, the manufacturer often designates on the machine what the initial energy should be. If this is not known, ACLS guidelines recommend using a 200 J shock. Since VF and pVT result in loss of consciousness, sedation is not necessary for defibrillation. Several factors should be considered for safety and increased efficacy when performing defibrillation.

◆ Use conductive gel pads on the patient's skin (or conductive gel or paste on paddles) to decrease transthoracic impedance and protect the skin from burns.

◆ Apply approximately 25 pounds of pressure to each paddle to reduce impedance when delivering the shock.

◆ Make sure no one is touching the patient, the bed, or anything attached to the patient when the shock is delivered (call "all clear" and visually verify before delivering shock).

◆ Make sure patient and operator are not in water during delivery of shock.

◆ Keep paddles on chest and re-verify rhythm before delivering subsequent shocks.

◆ Avoid placing paddles near medication patches. Remove medication patches if necessary.

◆ Do not place paddles over pacemaker or ICD pulse generators – stay 4-6 inches away. Use AP position whenever possible.

Procedure for Defibrillation

◆ Identify rhythm as VF or pVT. If rhythm appears to be asystole, check another lead to make sure it is not fine VF. Verify that patient has no pulse.

◆ Position patient supine and flat.

◆ Turn on defibrillator.

◆ Apply conductive gel pads to chest (or put conductive gel or paste on paddles).

◆ Place paddles over protective pads and apply 25 lbs of pressure.

◆ Charge machine to 360 J if using a monophasic defibrillator (this may take a few seconds). Most machines beep when charged. Charge to 200 J or manufacturer's recommended energy with biphasic defibrillators.

◆ Call "all clear" and look around to verify that no one (including you) is touching the patient or the bed.

◆ Depress both discharge buttons simultaneously to release the energy. The shock is delivered immediately when both buttons are pushed.

◆ Immediately resume CPR for 2 minutes before rhythm and pulse check (this may be modified in a monitored situation where ECG and hemodynamic monitoring is available).

CARDIOVERSION

Cardioversion is the delivery of electrical energy that is synchronized to the QRS complex so that the energy is delivered during systole in order to avoid the T wave and the vulnerable period of ventricular repolarization. The delivery of electrical energy near the T wave can lead to ventricular fibrillation. Synchronized cardioversion is used to terminate both supraventricular and ventricular tachycardias and is usually an elective procedure, although it should be performed urgently if the patient is hemodynamically unstable. Rhythms due to re-entry are suitable for cardioversion, while rhythms due to automaticity (i.e. sinus tachycardia, atrial tachycardia, junctional tachycardia) do not respond to cardioversion. Rhythms for which cardioversion is an appropriate therapy include:

Electrical Management of Arrhythmias

- Re-entrant SVTs – AV nodal re-entry tachycardia (AVNRT) and circus movement tachycardia (CMT) using an accessory pathway.
- Atrial flutter with rapid ventricular response and hemodynamic instability, or electively to terminate atrial flutter.
- Atrial fibrillation with rapid ventricular response and hemodynamic instability, or electively to terminate atrial fibrillation.
- Sustained monomorphic VT with a pulse and blood pressure present; if the patient is pulseless, defibrillation is required.

Cardioversion can be performed via anterolateral electrode placement or via anteroposterior (A-P) electrode placement (Figure 17.2). A-P placement is preferred because less energy is required and the success rate is higher when energy travels through the short axis of the chest. Electrodes can be either paddles or hands-free adhesive pads.

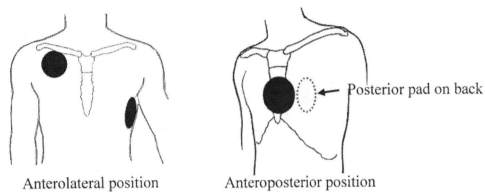

Figure 17.2: Cardioversion.

Initial energy level for cardioversion varies with different arrhythmias. If the first shock is unsuccessful, the energy level is increased for subsequent shocks. Table 17.1 shows recommended initial and subsequent monophasic energy levels for different arrhythmias. Biphasic equivalents have not yet been determined.

Table 17.1
Energy Levels for Cardioversion

Rhythm	Initial Energy Level (monophasic waveform)	Subsequent Energy Levels
Atrial flutter	50 J	100 J, 200 J, 300 J, 360 J
SVT	50 J	100 J, 200 J, 300 J, 360 J
Atrial fibrillation	100 J – 200 J	300 J, 360 J
Monomorphic VT	100 J	200 J, 300 J, 360 J

Source: Advanced Cardiovascular Life Support Provider Manual, American Heart Association, 2006

The same safety practices described above in the defibrillation section apply to cardioversion. A main difference is that the machine must be synchronized to the QRS complex for cardioversion. Most machines put a bright dot or similar marker on the QRS complex when in the "synch" mode. The machine will not discharge its energy until it sees the synch marker. Make sure to visually verify that the synch marker is actually on the QRS complex and not on a tall T wave. The machine synchronizes on the tallest complex it recognizes; if that happens to be the T wave, change leads until the machine is able to synch on the QRS. When delivering energy during cardioversion, push and hold both discharge buttons until the energy is delivered. Unlike defibrillation, when the energy is delivered as soon as the buttons are pushed, the synchronized machine will not discharge until it sees a QRS complex.

Another difference is that sedation is required for cardioversion since the patient is usually awake and alert and able to feel the pain caused by the procedure. Sedation can be accomplished with drugs like midazolam (Versed), methohexitol (Brevital), propofol (Diprovan), or others at the discretion of the physician, or an anesthesiologist may be used to administer deep sedation. Follow your institution's procedural sedation policy when monitoring patients during and after cardioversion. An emergency cart, emergency drugs (lidocaine, epinephrine, amiodarone, atropine), sedation reversal agent, O_2 delivery equipment, suction equipment, O_2 saturation monitor, and non-invasive BP monitoring equipment should be in the room.

Procedure for Cardioversion

- Verify the presence of the following items before doing cardioversion: a defibrillator that has been quality checked according to institutional policy, a functioning IV line for administration of fluids and sedation, O_2 and nasal cannula or mask, ambu bag, suction equipment, O_2 saturation monitor, non-invasive BP monitor, appropriate sedation and reversal agent, emergency cart and medications.
- Clip hair on chest and back in area where pads are to be placed. (Excess hair increases transthoracic impedance and makes application of adhesive pads difficult.)
- Place adhesive "hands-free" pads in the AP position whenever possible. (Or place protective gel pads in the anterolateral position if paddles are used.)
- Position patient supine and flat.
- Administer sedation as directed by physician, or assist anesthesiologist as needed.
- Turn on defibrillator.
- Press the Synch button and verify that the synchronization marker is on the QRS complex.
- Select desired energy level based on arrhythmia being treated (most machines power on at 200 J).
- If using paddles, place them over protective pads and apply 25 lbs of pressure.
- Charge machine. Most machines beep when charged.
- Call "all clear" and look around to verify that no one (including you) is touching the patient or the bed.
- Depress both discharge buttons simultaneously and hold until energy is discharged.
- Reassess rhythm; if necessary, increase energy and repeat procedure. Remember to push the Synch button prior to each subsequent shock.
- Follow your institution's procedural sedation policy regarding frequency of monitoring vital signs, rhythm, level of consciousness, etc. until patient is awake and able to maintain airway and handle secretions.

The following rhythm strip shows monomorphic VT with the synchronization marker on the QRS complex. The shock is delivered on a QRS complex, and sinus rhythm is restored.

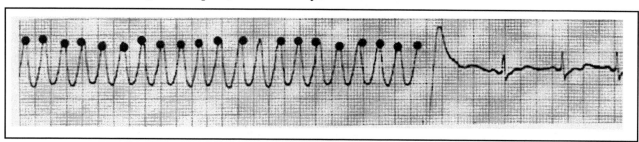

Electrical Management of Arrhythmias

PACEMAKERS

Indications for Pacing

Pacemakers were originally developed to treat symptomatic bradycardia, which can be due to sinus node dysfunction or to conduction failure in or below the atrioventricular (AV) node. Pacemaker therapy can have beneficial effects on hemodynamics and clinical status by providing rate response for patients with chronotropic incompetence, meaning that the sinus node is not capable of increasing its rate appropriately in response to the body's need for increased cardiac output. Dual-chamber pacemaker therapy can preserve stroke volume in patients with left ventricular dysfunction, hypertrophic cardiomyopathy, or dilated cardiomyopathy by ensuring AV synchrony and providing optimal AV intervals to enhance ventricular filling. Cardiac resynchronization therapy (CRT) with biventricular pacing improves septal wall motion, mitral valve function, and the dynamics of left ventricular contraction in patients with severe heart failure or dilated cardiomyopathy. Pacemaker therapy can also be used to terminate both supraventricular and ventricular tachyarrhythmias, usually in conjunction with implantable cardioverter defibrillators (ICDs).

The American College of Cardiology and American Heart Association have published guidelines for implantation of permanent pacemakers and antiarrhythmia devices. The following outline lists the class I indications for permanent pacing according to the guidelines (Gregoratos et al., 2002). Refer to the guidelines for class II indications.

Class I Indications for Permanent Pacing

◆ Acquired Atrioventricular Block
  ❖ Third-degree and advanced second-degree AV block at any anatomic level, associated with any one of the following conditions:
    ★ Bradycardia with symptoms (including heart failure) presumed to be due to AV block.
    ★ Arrhythmias and other medical conditions that require drugs that result in symptomatic bradycardia.
    ★ Documented periods of asystole greater than or equal to 3.0 seconds or any escape rate less than 40 bpm in awake, symptom-free patients.
    ★ After catheter ablation of the AV junction.
    ★ Postoperative AV block that is not expected to resolve after cardiac surgery.
    ★ Neuromuscular diseases with AV block, such as myotonic muscular dystrophy, Kearns-Sayre syndrome, Erb's dystrophy (limb-girdle), and peroneal muscular atrophy, with or without symptoms, because there may be unpredictable progression of AV conduction disease.
  ❖ Second-degree AV block regardless of type or site of block, with associated symptomatic bradycardia.
◆ Pacing for Chronic Bifascicular and Trifascicular Block
  ❖ Intermittent third-degree AV block
  ❖ Type II second-degree AV block
  ❖ Alternating bundle branch block.
◆ Pacing for Atrioventricular Block Associated with Acute Myocardial Infarction
  ❖ Persistent second-degree AV block in the His-Purkinje system with bilateral bundle branch block or third-degree AV block within or below the His-Purkinje system after AMI.
  ❖ Transient advanced (second or third-degree) infranodal AV block and associated bundle branch block. If the site of block is uncertain, an electrophysiologic study may be necessary.

749

Chapter 17

❖ Persistent and symptomatic second or third-degree AV block.
◆ Pacing in Sinus Node Dysfunction
❖ Sinus node dysfunction with documented symptomatic bradycardia, including frequent sinus pauses that produce symptoms. In some patients, bradycardia is iatrogenic and will occur as a consequence of essential long-term drug therapy of a type and dose for which there are no acceptable alternatives.
❖ Symptomatic chronotropic incompetence.
◆ Pacing to Prevent Tachycardia
❖ Sustained pause-dependent VT, with or without prolonged QT, in which the efficacy of pacing is thoroughly documented.
◆ Pacing in Hypersensitive Carotid Sinus Syndrome and Neurocardiogenic Syncope
❖ Recurrent syncope caused by carotid sinus stimulation; minimal carotid sinus pressure induces ventricular asystole of more than 3 seconds' duration in the absence of any medication that depresses the sinus node or AV conduction.
◆ Pacing for Hypertrophic Cardiomyopathy
❖ Class I indications for sinus node dysfunction or AV block, as described previously.
◆ Pacing for Dilated Cardiomyopathy
❖ Class I indications for sinus node dysfunction or AV block, as described previously.

Types of Pacing

Temporary Pacing

Temporary pacing is indicated to treat symptomatic bradycardia after acute myocardial infarction (AMI) or when associated with hyperkalemia or drug toxicity; bradycardia dependent VT; before permanent pacemaker implantation in symptomatic patients; and in reversible conditions that will not likely result in the need for permanent pacing, such as bacterial endocarditis, Lyme disease, or cardiac trauma. Inferior MI can cause intranodal block that is usually benign and temporary, and requires pacing only if it results in symptomatic bradycardia or bradycardia dependent VT.

Second or third-degree AV block associated with anterior MI and bundle-branch block often requires temporary pacing. Prophylactic temporary pacing is often done in the presence of new right bundle-branch block with either anterior or posterior hemiblock, in left bundle-branch block with first-degree AV block, and in alternating right and left bundle-branch block. Temporary pacing is often used after cardiac surgery to treat symptomatic bradycardia and is sometimes used prophylactically in high-risk patients during cardiac catheterization or with electrical or chemical cardioversion. Overdrive atrial pacing is sometimes used in an attempt to terminate atrial flutter or fibrillation after cardiac surgery when atrial epicardial leads are in place. Temporary pacing can be accomplished via transvenous, epicardial, or transcutaneous methods.

Single Chamber Pacing

Single chamber pacing means that only the atria or the ventricles, but not both, are paced. This requires only one pacing lead inserted into either the right atrium or the right ventricle. Single chamber ventricular pacing is the most frequently used temporary transvenous type of pacing and is also often used for permanent pacing. Single chamber atrial or ventricular pacing can also be done using epicardial pacing wires.

Electrical Management of Arrhythmias

Dual Chamber Pacing

Dual chamber pacing means that both the atria and the ventricles are paced and requires two pacing leads: one in the right atrium and one in the right ventricle. Dual chamber pacing is a frequently used method of permanent pacing and can also be used with epicardial pacing wires. Temporary transvenous dual chamber pacing can be done, but it is difficult to place temporary atrial wires and it is not as reliable as ventricular pacing.

Biventricular Pacing

Biventricular pacing means that both ventricles are paced simultaneously via a pacing lead in the right ventricular apex and another lead threaded through the coronary sinus and down a lateral vein in the left ventricle. Biventricular pacing is used to treat severe heart failure and cardiomyopathy, and usually incorporates an atrial lead for dual chamber pacing as well.

Rate Adaptive Pacing

Rate adaptive pacing is used when the heart is unable to increase its rate appropriately when the body's need for cardiac output increases (chronotropic incompetence). The pacing system contains a physiologic sensor that tells the pacemaker to pace faster in response to the sensed parameter. The most frequently used sensors at this time are motion sensors and minute ventilation sensors. Motion sensors are activated by increased body movement that occurs with exercise, and signal the pacemaker to pace faster. Minute ventilation sensors measure transthoracic impedance and increase the pacing rate when the respiratory rate is increased in response to exercise, fever, emotional states, etc.

Classification of Pacemakers

The nomenclature used to describe the expected function of a pacemaker was established by members of the North American Society of Pacing and Electrophysiology (NASPE) and the British Pacing and Electrophysiology Group (BPEG) and is designated the NBG code for pacing nomenclature. The code describes the expected function of the device according to the site of the pacing electrodes and the mode of pacing (Hayes, 2006).

◆ The first letter describes the chamber that is paced: A = atrium, V = ventricle, D = dual (both atrium and ventricle), O = none.

◆ The second letter describes the chamber where intrinsic electrical activity is sensed: A = atrium, V = ventricle, D = dual (both atrium and ventricle), O = none.

◆ The third letter describes the pacemaker's response to sensing of intrinsic electrical activity: I = inhibited, T = triggered, D = dual (inhibits or triggers), O = none.

◆ The fourth letter reflects rate modulation: R = rate modulation, using a sensor that controls pacing rate in response to the body's need for increased cardiac output, O = no rate response feature.

◆ The fifth letter specifies the location or absence of multi-site pacing (stimulation of both atria, both ventricles, or multiple pacing sites in a single chamber: A = multi-site pacing in the atria, V = multi-site pacing in the ventricles (i.e. biventricular pacing), D = multi-site pacing in both atria and ventricles, O = no multi-site pacing feature.

Table 17.2 illustrates the pacemaker code.

Chapter 17

Table 17.2
NBG Code for Pacing Nomenclature

First Letter: Chamber Paced	Second Letter: Chamber Sensed	Third Letter: Response to Sensing	Fourth Letter: Rate Modulation	Fifth Letter: Multi-site Pacing
O = None A = Atrium V = Ventricle D = Dual (A & V)	O = None A = Atrium V = Ventricle D = Dual (A & V)	O = None I = Inhibited T = Triggered D = Dual (I & T)	O = None R = Rate modulation	O = None A = Atrial V = Ventricular D = Dual

The most commonly used pacing modes are VVI and DDD (or VVIR and DDDR). The VVI mode means that the electrode is in the ventricle and paces the ventricle (first V), senses ventricular activity (second V), and inhibits its output when it senses intrinsic ventricular depolarization (I in third position). VVI is the most commonly used mode of pacing with temporary transvenous leads because it is the quickest and easiest method of pacing in an emergency, and it is difficult to get a temporary atrial lead to stay in place. VVI is often used with epicardial leads after cardiac surgery, especially if third-degree AV block is present, and this is the mode most often used for permanent pacing in patients with chronic atrial fibrillation. The DDD mode means that both atrial and ventricular pacing leads are present and both chambers are paced (first D), and sensed (second D), and the device either inhibits or triggers an output in response to sensed intrinsic activity. (D in third position means dual response to sensing.) DDD is the most frequently used permanent pacing mode, unless the patient has chronic atrial fibrillation or flutter.

Pacing Terminology

See the glossaries for single chamber and dual chamber pacing terminology at the end of this pacemaker section for definitions of terminology used in cardiac pacing.

Basics of Pacemaker Operation

Electrical current flows in a closed-loop circuit between two pieces of metal (poles). For current to flow, there must be conductive material (i.e., a lead, muscle, or conductive solution) between the two poles. In the heart the pacing lead, cardiac muscle, and body tissues serve as conducting material for the flow of electrical current in the pacing system. The pacing circuit consists of the pulse generator (the power source), the conducting lead (pacing lead), and the myocardium. The electrical stimulus travels from the pulse generator through the pacing lead to the myocardium, through the myocardium, and back to the pulse generator, thus completing the circuit (Figure 17.3).

Bipolar Pacing System

In any pacing system, there are two metal poles in the pacing circuit. The term bipolar means that both of these poles are in or on the heart. In a bipolar system, the pulse generator initiates the electrical impulse and delivers it out the negative terminal of the pacemaker to the pacing lead. The impulse travels down the lead to the distal electrode (negative pole or cathode) that is in contact with myocardium. As the impulse reaches the tip, it travels through the myocardium and returns to the positive pole (or anode) of the system, completing the circuit. In a bipolar system, the positive pole is the proximal ring located a few millimeters proximal to the distal tip of the pacing lead. The circuit over which the electrical impulse travels in a bipolar system is small because the two poles are located close together. This results in a small pacing spike on the electrocardiogram (ECG) as the pacing stimulus travels between the two poles.

Unipolar Pacing System

A unipolar system has only one of the two poles in or on the heart. In a permanent unipolar pacing system, the back of the pulse generator serves as the second pole. In a temporary epicardial pacing system, a ground lead placed in the subcutaneous tissue in the mediastinum serves as the second pole. Unipolar pacemakers work the same way as bipolar systems, but the circuit over which the impulse travels is much larger because of the distance between the two poles, resulting in a large pacing spike on the ECG.

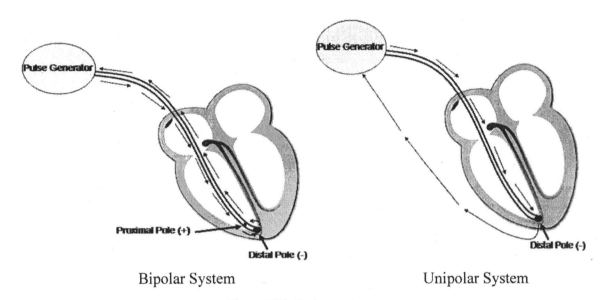

Bipolar System   Unipolar System

Figure 17.3: Pacing systems.

Asynchronous (Fixed Rate) Pacing Mode

A pacemaker programmed to an asynchronous mode paces at the programmed rate, regardless of intrinsic cardiac activity. This can result in competition between the pacemaker and the heart's own electrical activity. Asynchronous pacing in the ventricle is unsafe because of the potential for pacing stimuli to fall in the vulnerable period of repolarization and cause VF. Asynchronous pacing in the atria is less dangerous, but can cause atrial fibrillation.

Demand Mode

The term "demand" means that the pacemaker only paces when the heart fails to depolarize on its own, i.e. the pacemaker fires only "on demand." In the demand mode the pacemaker's sensing circuit is capable of sensing intrinsic cardiac activity and inhibiting pacer output when intrinsic activity is present. Sensing takes place between the two poles of the pacemaker. A bipolar system senses over a small area because the poles are close together, and this can result in "undersensing" of intrinsic signals. A unipolar system senses over a large area because the poles are far apart, and this can result in "oversensing." A unipolar system is more likely to sense myopotentials caused by muscle movement and inappropriately inhibit pacemaker output, potentially resulting in periods of asystole. The demand mode should always be used for ventricular pacing to avoid the possibility of VF.

Transvenous Pacing

Transvenous pacing is usually done by percutaneous puncture of the internal jugular, subclavian, antecubital, or femoral vein and threading a pacing wire into the apex of the right ventricle for ventricular pacing. The procedure can be done under fluoroscopy in a cardiac cath lab or without fluoroscopy at the bedside. Transvenous pacing is usually only necessary for a few days until the rhythm returns to normal or a permanent pacemaker is inserted. Temporary transvenous pacing wires are bipolar and have two tails, one marked positive or proximal and the other marked negative or distal, and are connected to the pulse generator via a bridging cable.

To initiate ventricular pacing using a transvenous wire (Figure 17.4):

1. Connect the negative terminal of the pulse generator to the negative tail of the bridging cable; connect the negative port of the bridging cable to the distal tail of the pacing wire.
2. Connect the positive terminal of the pulse generator to the positive tail of the bridging cable; connect the positive port of the bridging cable to the proximal tail of the pacing wire. (Remember: PP = "proximal is positive.")
3. Set the rate at 60-80 beats per minute, or as ordered by the physician.
4. Set the output at 5 mA, then determine stimulation threshold (as discussed later in this chapter) and set 2-3 times higher.
5. Set the sensitivity at 2 mV and adjust according to sensitivity threshold.

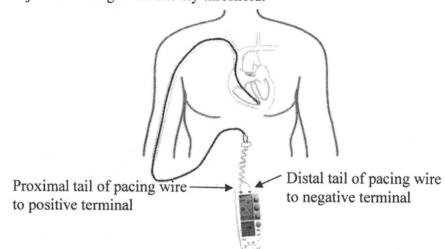

Figure 17.4: Ventricular pacing using transvenous wire.

Epicardial Pacing

Epicardial pacing is done through electrodes placed on the atria and/or ventricles during cardiac surgery. The pacing electrode end of the wire is looped through or loosely sutured to the epicardial surface of the atria and/or ventricles, and the other end is pulled through the chest wall, sutured to the skin, and attached to an external pulse generator. A ground wire is often placed subcutaneously in the chest wall and pulled through with the other wires. The number and placement of wires varies with the surgeon.

To initiate unipolar atrial or ventricular pacing:

1. Connect the negative terminal of the pulse generator to the wire on the chamber to be paced (atrial wire for atrial pacing, ventricular wire for ventricular pacing).
2. Connect the positive terminal of the pulse generator to the ground wire.
3. Set the rate at 60-80 beats per minute or as ordered by the physician.
4. Set the output at 10 mA for atrial pacing and 5 mA for ventricular pacing, then determine stimulation threshold and set 2-3 times higher.
5. Set the sensitivity at the lowest possible number for atrial pacing and at 2 mV for ventricular pacing.

Electrical Management of Arrhythmias

To initiate bipolar atrial or ventricular pacing:

1. Connect the negative terminal of the pulse generator to one of the wires on the chamber to be paced (atrial wire for atrial pacing, ventricular wire for ventricular pacing)
2. Connect the positive terminal of the pulse generator to the other wire on the chamber to be paced.
3. Set the rate at 70-80 beats per minute, or as ordered by the physician.
4. Set the output at 10 mA for atrial pacing and 5 mA for ventricular pacing, then determine stimulation threshold and set 2-3 times higher.
5. Set the sensitivity at the lowest possible number for atrial pacing and at 2 mV for ventricular pacing.

Figure 17.5 illustrates epicardial pacing.

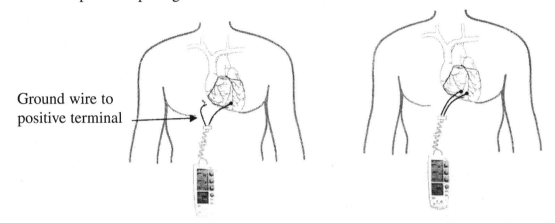

Figure 17.5: Epicardial pacing.

Linking Knowledge to Practice

✔ *Nurses need to know which epicardial wires are atrial and which are ventricular so that in an emergency, pacing can be initiated quickly. The number and placement of wires varies with the surgeon: some have atrial wires exiting to the right on the chest and ventricular wires exiting to the left, while others have atrial wires exiting above ventricular wires. In any case, nurses need to identify which wires are which and label them. One method of labeling wires that are not being used for pacing is to cut the fingers off of a glove and place the ends of the atrial wires in one finger, the ventricular wires in another, and the ground wire (if present) in a third finger. Coil the wires on the chest with their metal ends in the finger, place gauze on top of the coil and tape to the chest. Label the tape with "atrial," "ventricular," or "ground" for easy identification.*

✔ *If both atrial and ventricular wires are present, the nurse can choose to initiate either atrial or ventricular or dual chamber epicardial pacing. Remember that if AV block is present it does no good to pace the atria, so ventricular pacing is needed, either alone or with dual chamber pacing. Follow these guidelines when initiating temporary epicardial pacing:*

  ❖ *Sinus bradycardia with intact AV conduction = atrial pacing.*
  ❖ *Slow junctional rhythm = dual chamber pacing if possible to provide AV synchrony, or ventricular pacing.*
  ❖ *AV block = dual chamber pacing if possible to maintain AV synchrony, or ventricular pacing.*
  ❖ *Atrial fibrillation with slow ventricular rate = ventricular pacing*

✔ *Transvenous and epicardial pacing wires provide a direct route for stray electrical current to travel directly to the ventricles and initiate ventricular fibrillation. Some electrical safety precautions include:*

❖ *Wear gloves when handling pacing wires to protect wires from static electricity.*
❖ *Touch a metal surface (e.g. bedrail, IV pole) before touching the pacing system.*
❖ *Keep bare metal connections and wire ends wrapped in non-conductive material such as a glove.*
❖ *Do not wrap tape around the ends of pacing wires. Tape is not an insulator, and it may make the wire ends so sticky that they don't make good contact with the pacemaker when pacing is needed.*
❖ *Keep dressings over epicardial pacing sites dry (wet dressings conduct electricity).*
❖ *Make sure all electrical equipment in room is safe and checked as required by biomedical department.*

Transcutaneous Pacing (TCP)

Transcutaneous pacing is a noninvasive method of pacing used as a temporary measure in emergency situations for treatment of asystole, severe bradycardia, or overdrive pacing for tachyarrhythmias until a transvenous pacing wire can be inserted. Large surface adhesive electrodes are attached to the anterior and posterior chest wall and connected to an external pacemaker (Figure 17.6). The pacing current passes through skin and chest wall structures to reach the heart; therefore, large energies are required to achieve capture, and sedation is usually needed to minimize discomfort felt during pacing.

To initiate transcutaneous pacing:

1. Attach ECG leads from pacemaker to patient.
2. Connect pacing cable from pacemaker to pacing pads.
3. Place anterior pacing pad over lower sternum.
4. Place posterior pacing pad on back directly opposite anterior pad.
5. Turn transcutaneous pacemaker on and increase energy (mA) until capture occurs.
    a. The lowest amount of energy required to obtain 1:1 capture is the pacing threshold.
    b. Set current about 10 mA higher than threshold to assure a safety margin for capture.

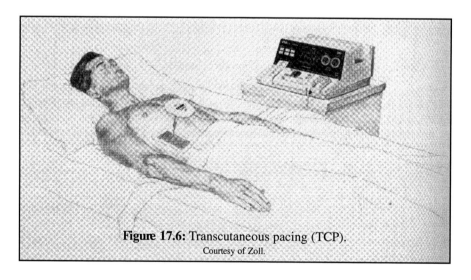

Figure 17.6: Transcutaneous pacing (TCP).
Courtesy of Zoll.

Electrical Management of Arrhythmias

Evaluating Pacemaker Function

Evaluation of pacemaker function requires knowledge of the mode of pacing expected (VVI, DDD, etc.); the minimum rate of the pacemaker, or pacing interval; and any other programmed parameters in the pacemaker. The basic functions of a pacemaker include stimulus release, capture, and sensing. *Stimulus release* refers to pacemaker output, or the ability of the pacemaker to generate and release a pacing impulse. *Capture* is the ability of the pacing stimulus to result in depolarization of the chamber being paced. *Sensing* is the ability of the pacemaker to recognize and respond to intrinsic electrical activity in the heart. Pacemaker operation is evaluated by assessing these three functions. Since ventricular pacing is the most common type of single chamber pacing, evaluation of VVI pacemakers is discussed here. The concepts presented for ventricular pacemaker evaluation can be applied to atrial pacemaker evaluation as well.

VVI Pacemaker Evaluation

A VVI pacemaker is expected to pace the ventricle at the set rate unless intrinsic ventricular activity occurs to inhibit pacing. The lower rate of the pacemaker, or pacing interval, is measured from one pacing stimulus to the next consecutive pacing stimulus with no intervening sensed beats between the two. In a normally functioning VVI pacemaker, pacing spikes occur at the preset pacing interval and each spike results in a ventricular depolarization (capture). If intrinsic ventricular activity occurs (either a normally conducted QRS or a PVC), that activity is sensed, the next pacing stimulus is inhibited, and the pacing interval timing cycle is reset. If no intrinsic ventricular activity occurs, a pacing stimulus is released at the end of the timing cycle.

Figure 17.7 illustrates normal VVI pacemaker function. The solid lines at the bottom of the strip represent the programmed lower rate of the pacemaker, or the pacing interval. The dotted lines represent resetting of the pacing interval and inhibition of the pacer spike by sensed beats (the 3rd beat is probably a normally conducted sinus beat, and the 5th beat is a PVC – both were sensed by the pacemaker).

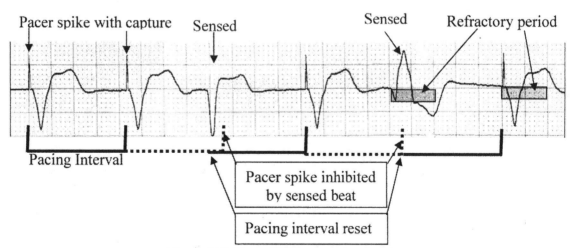

Figure 17.7: Normal VVI pacemaker function.

The pacemaker has a *refractory period,* which is a period of time following either pacing or sensing in the ventricle during which the pacemaker is unable to respond to intrinsic activity. During the refractory period, the pacemaker, in effect, has its eyes closed and is not able to see spontaneous activity. If an intrinsic QRS should occur during the pacemaker's refractory period, it will not be sensed because the pacemaker is "blind" at that time.

Stimulus Release

Stimulus release is verified on the ECG by the presence of a pacer spike. A pacer spike indicates that the pacemaker battery has enough power to initiate a stimulus and that the stimulus was delivered into the body. Identify the automatic interval by measuring two consecutive pacer spikes. Spikes should appear regularly at this interval unless the pacer is in the demand mode and sensing intrinsic ventricular activity.

Absence of stimulus release may be due to:

- Pacemaker is not turned on.
- Oversensing – pacemaker is set to be so sensitive that it is sensing external electrical signals, T wave potentials, or myopotentials from surrounding muscle. The pacemaker interprets these signals as QRS complexes so it doesn't pace. Common sources of external interference include electromagnetic or radiofrequency fields (cell phones) and electronic equipment in use near the pacemaker (radios, electric razors, cautery, etc.)
    - Try turning the sensitivity down – make the pacemaker less sensitive by increasing the sensitivity value (i.e. if sensitivity is set at 0.5 mV, change it to 0.8 mV).
    - Decrease mA if they are set very high, as this can produce an afterpotential that can be sensed by the pacemaker.
    - Put in asynchronous mode to verify that the pacemaker is capable of releasing stimuli.
- Loose or broken connections – can produce "false signals" from intermittent separation of a broken lead or intermittent contact of connections in the pacemaker.
    - Check and tighten all connections (pulse generator to cable and cable to pacing lead connections).
    - Chest x-ray to check for broken lead.
- Battery failure
    - Change battery.
- Rule out hysteresis: in some pacemakers the escape interval (interval from a sensed beat to the next paced beat) is longer than the automatic interval. The pause following a sensed beat is longer than the automatic interval and may appear to be failure of stimulus release.

The following strip illustrates a VVI pacemaker with appropriate stimulus release. Pacing spikes appear regularly at the lower rate. Capture is verified by the presence of a wide QRS immediately following the pacer spike.

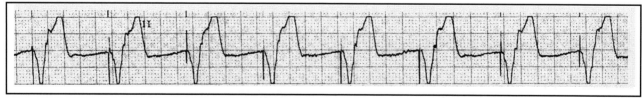

In the following example, the connections at the top of a temporary pacemaker were not tight, creating intermittent loss of contact with the bridging cable and the absence of pacer spikes where they would be expected. The solid lines represent the pacing interval based on the lower rate of the pacemaker. Pacer spikes should have appeared at arrows.

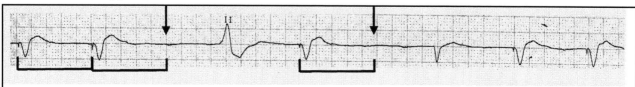

Capture

Capture is indicated by a wide QRS complex immediately following the pacemaker spike and represents the ability of the pacing stimulus to depolarize the ventricle. Loss of capture is recognized by the presence of pacer spikes that are not followed by paced ventricular complexes.

Loss of capture may be due to:

- Output too low. After 2-3 days, the output required to produce a response increases due to edema and fibrosis at the lead tip.
  - Turn up the mA.
  - Check capture threshold every shift and set output 2-3 times higher than threshold to avoid loss of capture.
- Pacing stimulus falls in the hearts refractory period. This is not a capture problem due to pacemaker malfunction – it is physiological failure to capture due to the heart's inability to respond to the stimulus. Pacer spikes should not fall in the refractory period if sensing is appropriate; therefore, it is most likely a sensing problem (discussed below).
- Catheter tip is no longer in contact with myocardium, or tip is lying in infarcted tissue.
  - Reposition patient to back, side, or whatever position re-establishes contact between the lead and the heart.
  - Monitor for pacer lead perforation.
    - Note direction of paced beats on monitor in lead V1 (pacing from the RV apex produces a LBBB pattern in Lead V1). A change in direction can indicate perforation of the lead into the left ventricle or migration of the tip into the RV outflow tract.
    - Watch for pacing of diaphragm or pectoral muscles indicted by hiccups or muscle twitching.
  - PA and lateral chest x-ray to verify lead position.
  - Pacing lead repositioning is done by a physician.
- Battery failure
  - Change battery.

Loss of capture in a totally pacemaker-dependent patient is an emergency because without an effective underlying rhythm, the patient may be asystolic or severely symptomatic due to a slow intrinsic rate. If loss of capture is intermittent, it may not result in symptoms but should be corrected as soon as possible. If the patient is asystolic or symptomatic with extreme bradycardia:

1. Begin CPR.
2. Initiate transcutaneous pacing ASAP.
3. Support with atropine or epinephrine until the problem is corrected.

The following strip illustrates loss of capture in a VVI pacemaker. Pacer spikes are present at the programmed pacing interval, but are not followed by QRS complexes. The underlying rhythm is atrial fibrillation with a slow ventricular response.

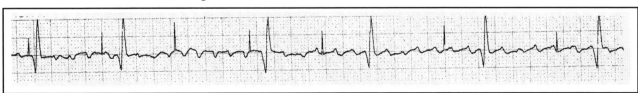

Chapter 17

In the following example, the first pacer spike (✱) fails to capture because it falls in the ventricle's refractory period when the ventricle is unable to respond. This represents a loss of sensing, not a loss of capture. Note that the 2nd and 3rd pacer spikes do capture, although the 2nd pacer spike should not have occurred so close to the previous QRS – this is another failure to sense.

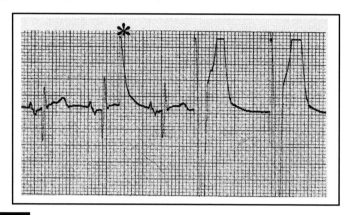

Linking Knowledge to Practice

✔ *New nurses often wonder what happens with the pacemaker when a patient dies. In the event of death, pacing spikes will be delivered to the heart at the basic pacing rate but no capture will occur because the heart is unable to respond to the electrical stimulus. If the patient is still connected to the bedside monitor, the monitor will show asystole with pacing spikes appearing at the basic pacing rate. There is no need to program the pacemaker off, and usual postmortem care can be provided.*

Sensing

Sensing of intrinsic ventricular electrical activity inhibits the next pacing stimulus and resets the pacing interval. Sensing cannot occur unless the pacemaker is given the opportunity to sense. It must be in the demand mode and there must be intrinsic ventricular activity present in order for the pacemaker to have an opportunity to sense.

The following strip illustrates appropriate sensing by a VVI pacemaker. The beats marked with ✱ are intrinsic beats that are sensed by the pacemaker and reset the pacing interval.

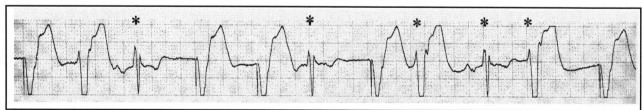

Undersensing means that the pacemaker fails to sense intrinsic activity that is present.

Undersensing may be due to:

◆ Asynchronous (fixed rate) mode of pacing.
  ❖ Turn to demand mode to activate the sensing circuit.
  ❖ Set sensitivity at 2 mV for ventricular sensing.
◆ Spontaneous ventricular activity falling in the pacemaker's refractory period. The pacemaker "closes its eyes" (refractory period) for a period of time after a paced or sensed ventricular beat. If another impulse comes along during that time, it cannot be sensed by the pacemaker because its "eyes are closed."

- ◆ Catheter out of position or lying in infarcted tissue.
  - ❖ Lead needs to be repositioned by a physician.
- ◆ Low QRS voltage reducing size of signal to sensing circuit. This can be due to drug therapy, electrolyte imbalances, or disease process.
  - ❖ Increase pacemaker's sensitivity (i.e. change from 0.8 to 0.5 mV).
  - ❖ Reposition patient.
  - ❖ PA and lateral chest x-ray to verify lead position.
  - ❖ Unipolarize the system to increase sensing signal.
    - ☆ Attach a monitoring electrode (one with a metal snap connector) on the chest near the ventricle.
    - ☆ Use an extra monitoring lead wire with a snap connection on one end to attach the chest electrode to the positive terminal of the pacemaker.
- ◆ Break in connections, faulty pulse generator, or battery failure.
  - ❖ Check and tighten all connections.
  - ❖ Replace battery.
  - ❖ Change pulse generator.
  - ❖ Take chest x-ray to check for lead fracture.

The following strip illustrates undersensing in a VVI pacemaker. The intrinsic beats marked with * are not sensed by the pacemaker and do not reset the pacing interval.

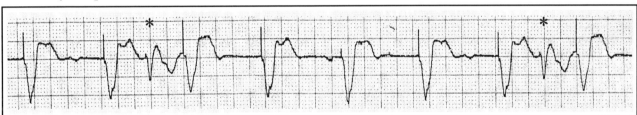

Oversensing means that the pacemaker is so sensitive that it inappropriately senses internal or external signals and inhibits its output. Common sources of external signals that can interfere with pacemaker function include electromagnetic or radio-frequency signals or electronic equipment in use near the pacemaker. Internal sources of interference can include large P waves, large T wave voltage, local myopotentials in the heart, or skeletal muscle potentials. Since a VVI pacemaker is programmed to inhibit its output when it senses, oversensing can be a dangerous situation in a pacemaker dependent patient, resulting in a dangerously slow rate or ventricular asystole.

Oversensing can be due to:

- ◆ Pacer sensitivity set too high (too sensitive), and pacemaker is sensing external stimuli or local potentials in the myocardium or surrounding muscle.
  - ❖ Decrease sensitivity of pacemaker (turn to a higher value, i.e. from 0.5 mV to 0.8 mV).
  - ❖ Decrease mA if they are very high, as this may produce an afterpotential that is sensed by the pacemaker.
  - ❖ Take chest x-ray to verify lead position. If pacer is sensing P waves, the lead may be in the right ventricular outflow tract or coronary sinus.

The following strip illustrates oversensing in a VVI pacemaker. In the middle of the strip, the pacing rate slows because the pacemaker senses something that resets the pacing interval.

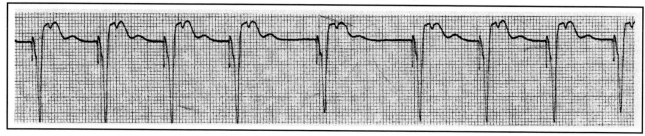

Stimulation Threshold Testing

The stimulation threshold is the minimum amount of voltage necessary to capture the heart consistently. It is recommended that stimulation threshold testing should be done every shift, since thresholds change over time. Once the threshold has been determined, set the output 2-3 times higher to ensure an adequate safety margin.

1. Verify that the patient is in a paced rhythm. Pacing rate may need to be temporarily increased to override an intrinsic rhythm.
2. Watch the monitor continuously while gradually decreasing output.
3. Note when the pacing stimulus no longer captures the heart (pacer spikes not followed by P wave (for atrial threshold) or QRS (for ventricular threshold).
4. Gradually turn output up until 1:1 capture resumes – this is the stimulation threshold.
5. Set output 2-3 times higher than threshold (i.e. if threshold is 2 mA, set output between 4 – 6 mA).

Sensitivity Threshold Testing

The sensitivity threshold is the minimum voltage of intrinsic cardiac activity that can be sensed by the pacemaker. The pacemaker becomes more sensitive (can see smaller signals) as the sensitivity dial is turned clockwise (or the sensitivity number gets smaller). It becomes less sensitive as the dial is turned counterclockwise (or the sensitivity number gets larger).

Sensitivity testing can only be done if the patient has a spontaneous rhythm at a rate capable of supporting hemodynamics while the test is being done. If the patient is completely pacer dependent or has a very slow intrinsic rate, do not do sensitivity testing. Otherwise, sensitivity threshold should be measured daily.

1. Verify that the patient is in a spontaneous rhythm. This may require temporarily turning the pacing rate down below the rate of spontaneous cardiac activity.
2. Slowly decrease sensitivity (make the pacemaker less sensitive) by turning the dial counterclockwise (or increasing the mV value) while watching the sense indicator light on the pulse generator. The sense indicator light will flash with each intrinsic P wave (for atrial pacing) or QRS (for ventricular pacing), as long as the pacemaker continues to sense.
3. Note when the sense indicator fails to flash with each spontaneous P wave or QRS. This is the sensitivity threshold.
4. Set the sensitivity at ½ the identified threshold (i.e. if threshold is 5 mV, set sensitivity at 2.5 mV).

Electrical Management of Arrhythmias

DUAL CHAMBER PACEMAKERS

Dual chamber pacemakers are complex and becoming even more challenging with advances in pacing technology. It is increasingly difficult for bedside nurses to keep up with new devices and all of their functions. This section presents the basics of dual chamber pacemaker timing cycles and basic information on evaluating atrial and ventricular capture and sensing. More detailed information on dual chamber pacemakers can be found in other references (see reference list at end of this chapter).

Dual Chamber Pacemaker Timing Cycles

Dual chamber pacemakers have a pacing lead in the atrium and one in the right ventricular apex. The pacemaker can function in several different pacing modes using combinations of atrial pacing, atrial sensing, ventricular pacing, and ventricular sensing. Common dual chamber pacing modes include: DDD, DVI, DDI, and VDD. The timing cycles used in DDD mode are presented here.

Lower Rate Interval (Base Pacing Rate) – minimum rate at which the pacemaker will pace if it does not sense any intrinsic activity. The pacing interval is measured between two consecutive ventricular pacing spikes without any intervening sensed beats in a ventricular-based pacing system or between two consecutive atrial pacing spikes in an atrial-based system.

AV Interval (or AV Delay) is the interval between an atrial pacing spike and a ventricular pacing spike (the electronic PR interval). In Figure 17.8, A = atrial pace, V = ventricular pace, R = intrinsic R wave, P = intrinsic P wave.

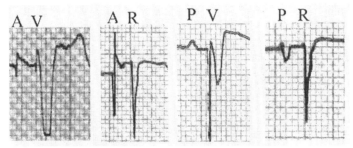

Figure 17.8: AV interval.

Atrial Escape Interval (AEI) or V-A Interval – interval from a sensed or paced ventricular event to the next atrial output spike. This is the amount of time that a dual chamber pacemaker will wait for atrial activity before pacing the atrium. This is not a programmable value but is derived by subtracting the AV delay from the basic pacing rate.

Figure 17.9 illustrates the above intervals:

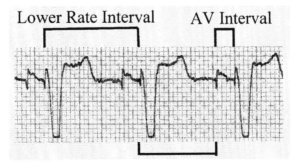

Figure 17.9: Atrial escape interval.

Total Atrial Refractory Period (TARP) is the period of time following a sensed or paced atrial event during which the atrial channel will not respond to sensed atrial activity. TARP consists of two parts: AVI and PVARP (Figure 17.10). The atrial channel is "asleep" during the AV interval and during PVARP.

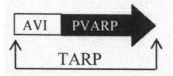

Figure 17.10: Total atrial refractory period (TARP).

Post Ventricular Atrial Refractory Period (PVARP) is the period of time following a ventricular paced or sensed event during which the atrial channel will not respond to sensed atrial activity. PVARP always follows the AV interval and always follows a sensed ventricular event (Figure 17.11 A).

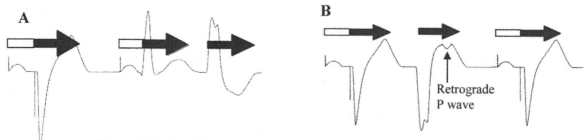

Figure 17.11 A and B: Post ventricular atrial refractory period (PVARP).

In Figure 17.11B, PVARP hides a retrograde P wave and prevents inappropriate ventricular pacing.

Ventricular Blanking Period (VBP) is a very short refractory period that occurs in the ventricular channel whenever an atrial output pulse is emitted. The ventricular channel "blinks" its eyes so it can't sense or see the atrial pacing output. Figure 17.12 shows the short VBP with each atrial output pulse.

Ventricular Refractory Period (VRP) is the period of time following a paced or sensed ventricular event during which the ventricular channel ignores intrinsic ventricular activity (arrows in Figure 17.12).

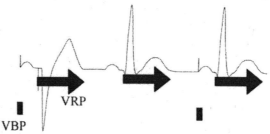

Figure 17.12: Ventricular blanking period (VBP).

Maximum Tracking Interval (MTI) or Upper Rate Limit is the maximum rate at which the ventricular channel will track atrial activity. This protects the ventricle from being paced too rapidly in response to rapid atrial rates. When the upper rate is reached, some type of blocking mechanism occurs to prevent rapid ventricular pacing rates.

In Figure 17.13, a PAC (3rd beat) results in a longer AV interval than on other beats because the MTI will not allow ventricular pacing to occur until its "arrow" times out.

Electrical Management of Arrhythmias

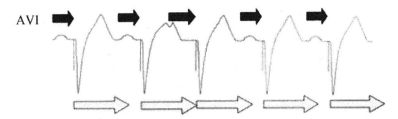

Figure 17.13: Maximum tracking interval (MTI).

Four States of Dual Chamber Pacing

♦ *Atrial and ventricular pacing (AV pacing state):* atrial spike followed by ventricular spike at the end of the programmed AV interval.

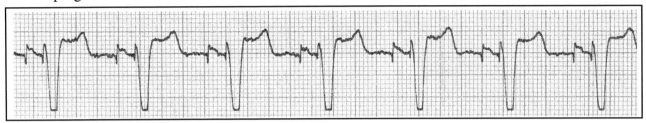

♦ *Atrial pacing with ventricular sensing (atrial pacing state):* atrial spike followed by an intrinsic conducted QRS within the programmed AV interval. Paces the atria and allows normal AV conduction to depolarize the ventricles.

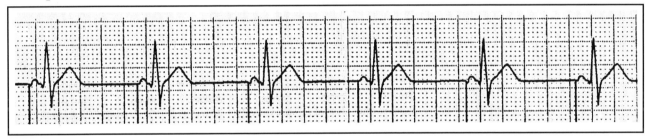

♦ *Atrial sensing, ventricular pacing (atrial tracking state):* intrinsic P wave followed by ventricular pacing at the end of the programmed AV interval. Normal atrial activity initiates the AV interval and paces the ventricle if no AV conduction occurs. This function is the reason for the upper rate limit – to prevent rapid atrial rates from causing rapid ventricular pacing.

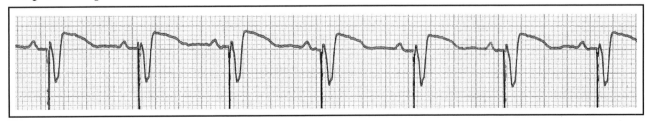

♦ *Atrial and ventricular sensing (inhibited state):* intrinsic atrial activity inhibits atrial pacing and conducts to the ventricle, inhibiting ventricular pacing.

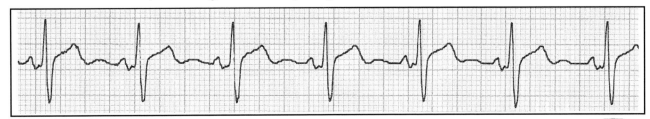

Evaluating Dual Chamber Pacemaker Function

In order to evaluate dual chamber pacemaker function, the following information must be known:
- Minimum rate
- Upper rate limit
- AV interval
- Atrial refractory period
- Ventricular refractory period
- Any special programmed parameters.

In reality, we often don't have access to all of this information, so we do the best we can using basic principles of capture and sensing. We can often figure out some of the parameters, like AV delay or minimum pacing rate, by measuring it when we see it on a strip. To evaluate basic DDD function, we assess atrial capture and sensing, and ventricular capture and sensing.

Atrial Capture

Atrial capture is present when an atrial spike is followed immediately and consistently by an obvious P wave or when an atrial spike is followed by a normal QRS within the programmed AV interval. Atrial capture is not as obvious as ventricular capture because the paced P wave is often very small and not easily visible. But if the atrial spike captures the atrium and that impulse conducts to the ventricle, the atrial spike will be followed by a normally conducted QRS complex before the AV interval times out. The following strips illustrate atrial capture. In A, each atrial spike is followed by an obvious P wave. In B, the second beat shows an atrial spike followed at the end of the AV interval by a normally conducted QRS complex.

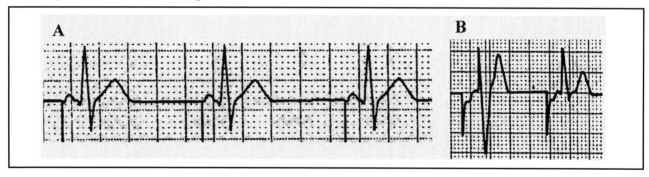

Atrial Sensing

Atrial sensing is present when an intrinsic P wave is followed by a paced QRS at the end of the programmed AV interval. If the P wave is sensed, it should start the AV interval and result in ventricular pacing at the end of the AV interval. The presence of a normal P wave followed by a normal QRS only proves that AV conduction is intact, not that atrial sensing has occurred. The two strips below illustrate atrial sensing.

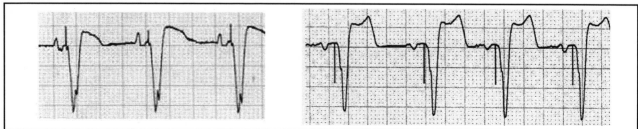

Electrical Management of Arrhythmias

Ventricular Capture

Ventricular capture is present when a ventricular pacing spike is followed by a wide QRS complex. In the following two strips, ventricular capture is present.

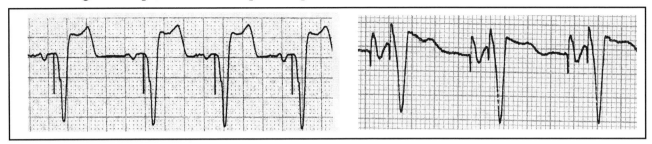

Ventricular Sensing

Ventricular sensing is present when an atrial spike is followed by a normal QRS within the programmed AV interval. Other proof of ventricular sensing includes resetting of the atrial escape interval by a PVC, and safety pacing (discussed later). In the following examples, A and B show atrial pacing spikes followed by normal QRS complexes, indicating that ventricular sensing is intact. In C, a sensed PVC (second beat) resets the atrial escape interval, proving intact ventricular sensing. In D, safety pacing occurs on the 3rd beat, indicated by the short AV interval, and proves that ventricular sensing is intact (see discussion later on safety pacing).

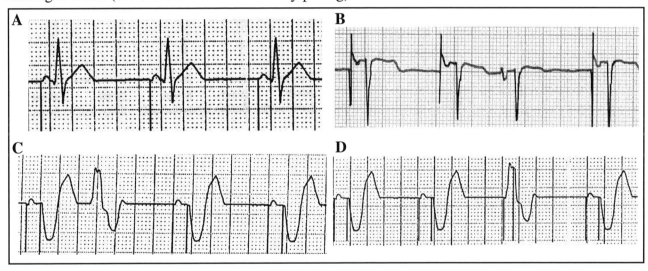

Dual Chamber Practice

Evaluate the following strips for atrial capture and sensing, ventricular capture and sensing:

1.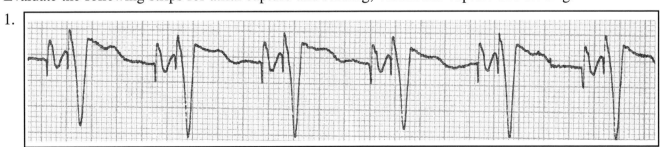

Atrial capture: Atrial sensing:

Ventricular capture: Ventricular sensing:

Chapter 17

2.
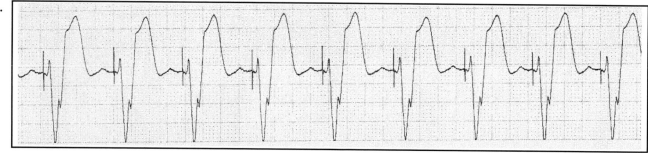

Atrial capture: Atrial sensing:

Ventricular capture: Ventricular sensing:

3.
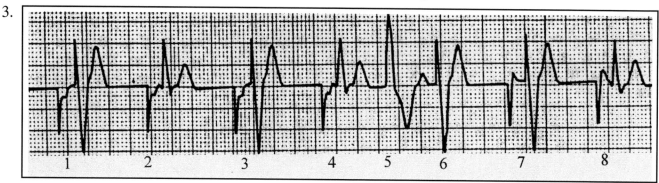

Atrial capture: Atrial sensing:

Ventricular capture: Ventricular sensing:

Dual Chamber Practice Answers

1. *Atrial capture*: probably good based on consistent deflection following atrial pacing spike.

   Atrial sensing: can't evaluate since there are no intrinsic P waves to be sensed.

   Ventricular capture: good. Each ventricular spike is followed by a wide QRS.

   Ventricular sensing: can't evaluate since there are no intrinsic QRS complexes to be sensed.

2. *Atrial capture*: can't evaluate since there is no atrial pacing.

   Atrial sensing: good. Each P wave is sensed and triggers a ventricular pace.

   Ventricular capture: good. Each ventricular spike is followed by a wide QRS.

   Ventricular sensing: can't evaluate since there are no intrinsic QRS complexes to be sensed.

3. *Atrial capture*: good. Beats 2, 4, and 8 show atrial spikes followed by intrinsic QRS complexes, indicating that conduction occurred from atrium to ventricle.

   Atrial sensing: good. Beat 6 shows an intrinsic P wave followed by a paced QRS complex

   Ventricular capture: good. Each ventricular spike is followed by a wide QRS.

   Ventricular sensing: good. Beats 2, 4, and 8 show atrial spikes followed by intrinsic QRS complexes that were sensed and inhibited ventricular pacing.

768

Electrical Management of Arrhythmias

Special Features of Dual Chamber Pacemakers

- *Differential AV Delay*
  - Shorter AV delay on sensed beats than on AV paced beats.

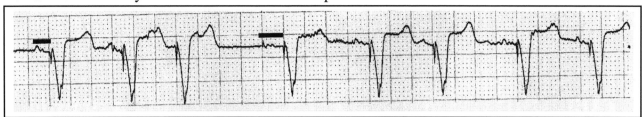

- *Rate Adaptive AV Delay*
  - AV delay shortens as pacing rate increases in response to activity.
  - Mimics the heart's normal physiologic response to exercise (i.e. shortens AV conduction time as heart rate increases).

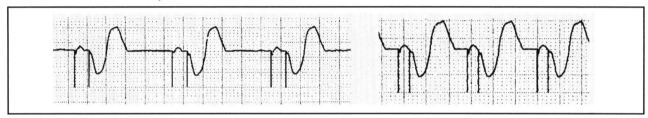

- *Mode Switching*
  - Switches to non-tracking mode (VVI or DDI) when atrial fib or flutter occurs.

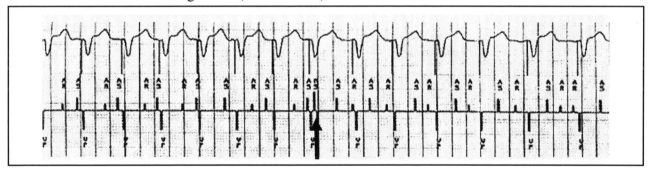

In the above strip, the atrial channel senses a rapid atrial rate and switches to a non-tracking mode at the arrow. Note slowing of the ventricular paced rate after mode switching as the ventricular channel stops trying to track the rapid atrial impulses.

- *Safety Pacing (also called non-physiological AV delay)*
  - Delivery of the ventricular pacing spike at a very short AV delay whenever the ventricular channel senses something early in the AV interval.
  - Used to prevent inappropriate inhibition of ventricular pacing by crosstalk.

The blanking period is supposed to prevent sensing of the atrial output pulse by the ventricular channel (crosstalk), but sometimes the ventricular channel still "sees" the atrial spike after the blanking period is over. If this occurs, the ventricular channel would normally inhibit ventricular pacing because it would think that the atrial spike was a QRS. In safety pacing, the ventricular channel delivers a pacing spike at a short AV delay whenever it senses something very early in the AV interval – that way it delivers a V spike if one is needed, but it delivers it at such a short AV delay that the V spike will avoid the T wave if a QRS is actually present.

769

See the following strips for explanation and illustration of safety pacing:

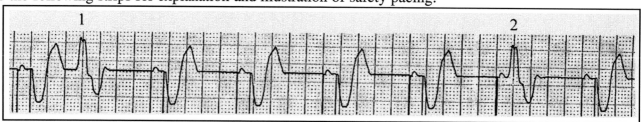

In the above strip, the first PVC occurs before the atrial pacing spike is due and appropriately inhibits the next atrial and ventricular outputs. The second PVC occurs during the AV interval after the atrial pacing spike has been delivered, is sensed by the ventricular channel, and appropriately inhibits the ventricular pacing spike.

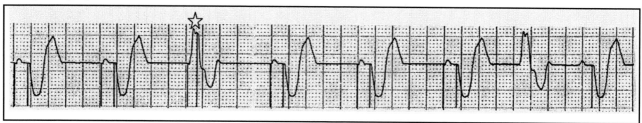

Safety pacing (☆) occurs on the first PVC in the above strip. The PVC occurs early in the AV interval right after the atrial pacing spike and right after the blanking period. When the ventricular channel "opens its eyes" at the end of the blanking period, it sees the PVC but it doesn't know whether it is seeing an atrial spike or a QRS, so it delivers a ventricular spike at a short AV interval (safety paces). This provides a ventricular pace but avoids the T wave of the PVC and prevents pacing into the vulnerable period of the ventricle.

In the following example, the programmed AV interval is evident on the first and fourth paced beats. On the second and third beats, the atrial output was sensed by the ventricular channel after the blanking period was over (crosstalk) and resulted in safety pacing at a short AV interval.

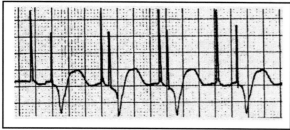

- ◆ *Upper Rate Responses*

    Since DDD pacemakers are capable of tracking P waves, there needs to be a way to limit the rate at which the ventricle will pace in response to sensed atrial activity. For example, if a patient develops an SVT at a rate of 180, it is not desirable to have the ventricle pace at that rate; therefore, the pacemaker can be programmed to pace at a rate no faster than 120. This is the upper rate limit of the pacemaker, is controlled by the maximum tracking interval (MTI), and is a programmable value. When the upper rate limit is reached or exceeded, the pacemaker limits the ventricular rate by going into its upper rate response. There are a variety of upper rate responses, but only two are illustrated here.

Wenckebach Upper Rate Response

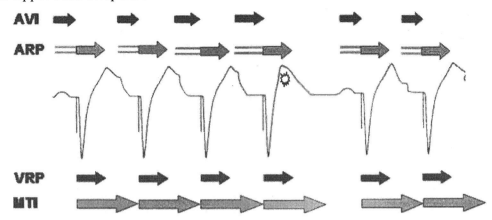

Figure 17.14: Wenkebach upper rate response.

In Figure 17.14, a sinus tachycardia is present at a rate faster than the upper rate limit (represented by the length of MTI arrow at bottom). Because the MTI will not allow ventricular pacing to occur until its arrow has timed out, the AV interval gradually increases with consecutive P waves (top arrows). This also gradually delays PVARP, which starts with each paced ventricular beat. The ventricular pace is gradually delayed due to the increasing AVI, causing PVARP to get closer and closer to the next P wave. Finally, one P wave falls in PVARP (✱) and is not sensed by the atrial channel, resulting in a pause which keeps the ventricular rate at or below the upper rate limit. A Wenckebach upper rate response can only occur if the MTI is longer than the total atrial refractory period (AVI + PVARP). The following strip illustrates sinus tachycardia at a rate of 115 with pacemaker Wenckebach upper rate response. The upper limit of the pacemaker is set at 110. Note the "group beating" that is typical of Wenckebach conduction. This is "pacemaker Wenckebach," not AV node Wenckebach. The Wenckebach upper rate response allows the ventricle to track more P waves and avoids a sudden reduction in paced ventricular rate during exercise.

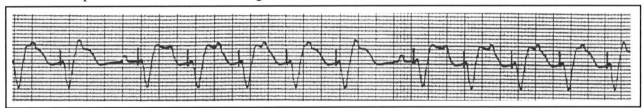

2:1 Block Upper Rate Response

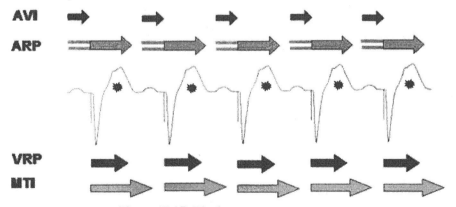

Figure 17.15: Block upper rate response.

In Figure 17.15, sinus tachycardia is present at a rate faster than the upper rate limit (length of MTI arrow at bottom). Alternate sinus beats are in the T wave. However, the total atrial refractory period (length of ARP arrows in second row) is longer than the MTI; therefore, every other P wave of the tachycardia falls into PVARP (*) and is not sensed. This reduces the ventricular rate to half of the atrial rate because only every other P wave is sensed by the atrial channel. To prevent a sudden decrease in ventricular rate with increasing sinus rates, PVARP needs to be programmed shorter so that the total atrial refractory period is shorter than the MTI; this would result in a Wenckebach response, as in Figure 17.14.

In the following strip, the upper rate limit of the pacemaker is 120 and the patient's sinus tachycardia gradually increases to a rate faster than the upper rate limit. At a critical atrial rate, alternate P waves fall in PVARP, resulting in 2:1 block. To prevent a sudden decrease in ventricular rate with increasing sinus rates, PVARP needs to be programmed shorter so that the total atrial refractory period is shorter than the MTI.

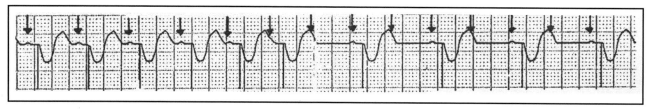

Pacemaker Mediated Tachycardia (PMT)

PMT is a re-entrant tachycardia that is sustained by continued participation of a dual chamber pacemaker as the antegrade limb of the circuit and retrograde conduction through the AV node, or an accessory pathway as the retrograde limb of the circuit. Another term for this tachycardia is "endless loop tachycardia." Anything that causes loss of AV synchrony in a dual chamber pacemaker can cause PMT if there is intact retrograde conduction through the AV node, including:

- PVC with retrograde conduction.
- PAC that prolongs the AV interval.
- Loss of atrial capture.
- Removal of a magnet after pacemaker testing.
- Myopotential tracking.

Figure 17.16 illustrates the mechanism of PMT. If a PVC occurs and conducts retrograde through the AV node, the atrial channel senses the retrograde P wave, initiates an AV interval, and causes a ventricular pace at the end of the AV interval. This paced ventricular beat then conducts retrograde into the atria and initiates another AV interval with another ventricular pace, and so on. PMT continues until either the AV node gets tired of conducting and blocks an impulse from reaching the atria, or a magnet is put on the pacemaker to disable atrial sensing.

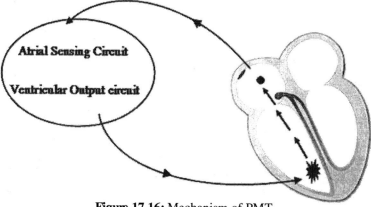

Figure 17.16: Mechanism of PMT.

Electrical Management of Arrhythmias

In the following strip, something triggered a V pace (possibly myopotential sensing), and retrograde conduction occurred to the atria. PVARP is shorter than the retrograde AV conduction time, allowing the atrial channel to sense the retrograde P wave (arrows), which sets up an AV interval and causes pacing in the ventricle at the end of the AV interval. As long as retrograde conduction continues, each sensed retrograde P wave sets up another AV interval and paces the ventricle.

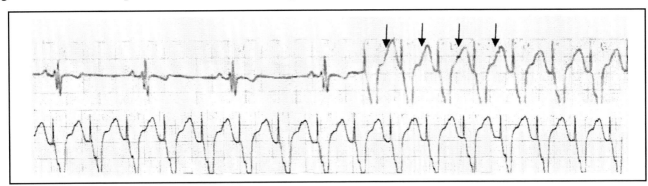

Most pacemakers have PMT termination algorithms that automatically terminate PMT after a programmable number of beats in tachycardia by either extending PVARP or omitting one ventricular paced beat.

Do the practice strips at the end of this chapter to apply the knowledge you have gained by reading this information!

Linking Knowledge to Practice

- ✔ *Placing a magnet over a permanent pulse generator turns off the sensing circuit and causes the pacemaker to pace in the asynchronous mode; it does not turn the pacemaker off. The danger posed by using the magnet is that an asynchronous pacemaker may pace on the T wave and cause ventricular tachycardia or fibrillation; therefore it should not be done indiscriminately.*
- ✔ *Some facilities have a written protocol that directs the staff to record an ECG with a magnet over the pulse generator when a patient with a pacemaker presents in a rhythm that is inhibiting the pacemaker. Otherwise, use of a magnet usually requires a physician's order.*
- ✔ *Appropriate use of a magnet includes:*
  - ❖ *Testing pacemaker function when the pacemaker is being inhibited by a faster intrinsic rhythm. It is appropriate to record an ECG with the magnet in place when a patient with a pacemaker presents with a faster intrinsic rhythm. The magnet will cause the pacemaker to pace asynchronously and allow the healthcare provider to determine if the pacemaker is capable of pacing and to evaluate capture when pacing stimuli are delivered at a time when the heart is able to respond to the stimulus.*
  - ❖ *Termination of PMT. Placing a magnet over a dual chamber pacemaker can terminate PMT because the atrial sensing circuit will be turned off, which will prevent sensing of the retrograde P wave and stop the PMT.*
- ✔ *When the magnet is removed the pacemaker returns to its programmed parameters and resumes normal function.*

BIVENTRICULAR PACING

Patients with chronic heart failure (HF) often have atrioventricular and intraventricular conduction delays that result in ventricular dyssynchrony, which impairs cardiac function. Up to 30% of patients with moderate to severe heart failure have a QRS duration greater than 120 msec, most often presenting as left bundle branch block (LBBB) (Abraham et al., 2002; Cazeau et al., 2001; Saxon & Ellenbogen, 2003). This intraventricular conduction delay causes electrical and mechanical abnormalities in ventricular function that interfere with ventricular filling, impair cardiac output, worsen mitral regurgitation, and contribute to mortality in patients with HF (Abraham et al., 2002; Littmann & Symanski, 2000). Although right bundle branch block (RBBB) is less common, it is associated with similar mechanical abnormalities and is a predictor of mortality in HF as much as LBBB (Fantoni et al., 2005).

Mechanisms of Dyssynchrony

Normally, when both bundle branches are functioning properly, both ventricles depolarize at the same time. The septum contracts and moves toward the left ventricle (LV), and participates in ejection of blood from the LV into the aorta. The papillary muscles in the LV contract slightly before the LV free wall, putting tension on the mitral valve leaflets and keeping them closed to prevent regurgitation of blood into the left atrium during ventricular systole. Figure 17.17 illustrates normal ventricular function when both bundle branches are working correctly. The small arrows represent the direction of ventricular wall and septal motion during systole, and the large arrow indicates blood flowing out of the LV into the aorta.

LBBB causes both electrical and mechanical abnormalities that result in ventricular dyssynchrony. Electrical abnormalities include:

- The right ventricle depolarizes normally
- The left ventricle depolarizes late and abnormally slowly via muscle cell-to-cell conduction (Figure 17.18A).
- The septum is activated from the right bundle branch and depolarizes before the left ventricle.

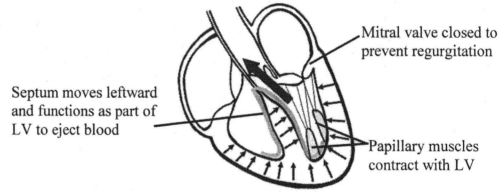

Figure 17.17: Normal ventricular function.

Mechanical abnormalities due to late LV activation and relaxation include (Figure 17.18B):

- LV activation is delayed but left atrial activation is not; therefore, the early passive LV filling phase and left atrial contraction occur simultaneously, which reduces LV filling and decreases LV preload.
- The septum finishes its contraction before the LV contracts.
- When the LV finally contracts, the septum bulges into the RV and contributes to reduced ejection of blood from the LV.
- The LV papillary muscles contract late, allowing the mitral valve to evert into the left atrium, causing mitral regurgitation.

- The combination of the above abnormalities reduces forward flow of blood through the aortic valve during LV systole, which decreases stroke volume.

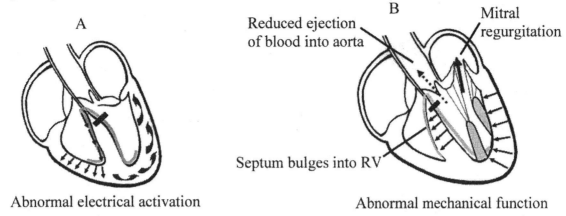

Figure 17.18 A and B: Electrical and mechanical abnormalities.

Cardiac Resynchronization Therapy (CRT)

Cardiac resynchronization therapy (CRT) is atrial-synchronized, biventricular pacing aimed at improving electromechanical activity in the failing heart. This therapy is meant to complement, not replace, optimum drug therapy for HF. The goals of CRT are to improve hemodynamics by restoring ventricular synchrony, and improve quality of life via symptom relief. CRT devices can be stand-alone pacemakers or combination ICD and biventricular pacemakers (CRT-D).

Candidates for CRT include patients with the following characteristics:

- Symptomatic heart failure (Class III or IV).
- Left ventricular ejection fraction ≤ 35%.
- Presence of significant intraventricular conduction delay (QRS duration ≥ 130 msec).
- Sinus rhythm.
- Symptomatic in spite of optimal drug therapy for heart failure.
- Most patients who meet these criteria are also candidates for ICD therapy and receive the combination device.

CRT is accomplished by placing standard pacing leads in the right atrium and into the right ventricular apex as is done for normal dual chamber pacing. A third lead is advanced through the coronary sinus and into a lateral or posterior left ventricular vein for pacing of the LV (Figure 17.19).

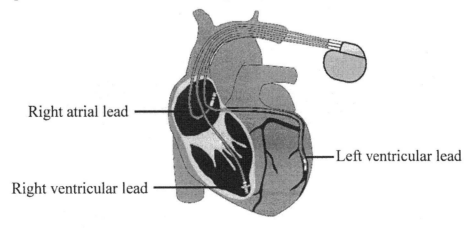

Figure 17.19: Cardiac resynchronization therapy (CRT).

Chapter 17

Mechanisms of Resynchronization

◆ Biventricular pacing allows the LV to complete contraction and begin relaxation earlier, which increases filling time and improves "atrial kick."

◆ Biventricular pacing causes the ventricles and septum to contract simultaneously; this forces the septum to contract with the LV and prevents it from bulging into the RV during systole.

◆ Atrial-biventricular pacing restores the normal timing between left atrial and left ventricular contraction, allowing the LV papillary muscles to contract earlier and put tension on the mitral valve leaflets to reduce or prevent mitral regurgitation.

Outcomes of CRT

Studies have indicated the following clinical benefits of CRT in patients with HF:

◆ Improved systolic and diastolic function (Abraham et al., 2004; Higgins et al., 2003; Linde et al., 2002; St. John Sutton et al., 2003).

◆ Decreased mitral regurgitation (Linde et al., 2002; St. John Sutton et al., 2003).

◆ Improved exercise capacity (Abraham et al., 2002; Auricchio et al., 2002; Cazeau et al., 2001; Linde et al., 2002; Young et al., 2003).

◆ Improved functional class (e.g. from Class III to Class II HF) (Abraham et al., 2002; Abraham et al., 2004; Higgins et al., 2003; Linde et al., 2002; Young et al., 2003).

◆ Improved quality of life (Abraham et al., 2002; Cazeau et al., 2001; Linde et al., 2002; Young et al., 2003).

◆ Decreased hospitalization for HF (Abraham et al., 2002; Bradley et al., 2003; Bristow et al., 2004; Cazeau et al., 2001; Leclercq et al., 2002).

◆ Reduced mortality (especially when combined with ICD) (Bradley et al., 2003; Bristow et al., 2004).

The ECG in Biventricular Pacing

This topic is extremely complex and beyond the scope of this chapter. However, some general observations can be made.

In single chamber RV pacing from the RV apex, the QRS produces a LBBB pattern, usually with a QRS width > .12 seconds. Lead V1 usually shows a wide negative QRS complex, as do leads II, III, and AVF. The QRS axis is usually directed leftward and superior as the ventricles depolarize from right to left.

Left ventricular pacing is more complicated due to the fact that the LV lead can be placed in either a lateral or posterior vein and can be located in an apical or a basal site within the vein. The resulting QRS varies in morphology, depending on the location of the LV lead, but, in general, LV pacing produces a RBBB pattern with a wide upright QRS complex in lead V1, and the QRS axis is often directed toward the right inferior quadrant and less often to the right superior quadrant (Barold, Herweg, & Giudici, 2005).

It makes logical sense that pacing both ventricles simultaneously would result in a narrow QRS complex preceded by a pacemaker spike, but this narrowing is not always obvious with biventricular pacing. Loss of capture in one or the other ventricle should cause a change in the morphology of the paced QRS that would indicate single chamber pacing from the ventricle that is still being captured. A shift in the frontal plane axis may also occur with loss of capture in one ventricle.

Some recommend recording four 12 lead ECGs at the time of implant: one during intrinsic conduction, one during RV pacing, one during LV pacing and one during biventricular pacing (Barold, Herweg, & Giudici, 2005). These ECGs should be examined to determine which lead best demonstrates an obvious difference between the four pacing states recorded, then the best lead should be used as the monitoring lead for pacemaker evaluation.

Electrical Management of Arrhythmias

SINGLE CHAMBER PACING TERMINOLOGY

Asynchronous (Fixed Rate) Pacing – the pacemaker releases a pacing stimulus at the programmed rate, regardless of the heart's intrinsic activity. No sensing occurs so the pacemaker fires in competition with the heart's natural rhythm. Examples of asynchronous modes are AOO, VOO, DOO.

Automatic Interval – the time period between two consecutive paced events without an intervening sensed event. Also known as the **lower rate interval** or **pacing interval.**

Base Rate – the rate at which the pacemaker paces when no intrinsic cardiac activity is present. Also called the **minimum rate** or **lower rate.**

Bipolar – having two poles. (1) A pacing lead with two electrical poles. The negative pole is the distal tip of the lead, and the positive pole is a metal ring located a few millimeters proximal to the distal tip. The stimulating pulse is delivered through the distal tip electrode. (2) A pacing system with both electrical poles in or on the heart.

Capture – ability of the pacing stimulus to depolarize the chamber being paced. Capture is recognized on the ECG whenever the pacing spike is followed immediately by the appropriate waveform: an atrial spike followed by a P wave or a ventricular spike followed by a wide QRS.

Demand Pacing – the pacemaker only paces when the heart's intrinsic rate is below the pacemaker's programmed rate (only when necessary or on demand). This mode means that the pacemaker senses intrinsic cardiac activity and inhibits its output when intrinsic activity is present.

Electrode – the exposed metal tip of a pacing lead that contacts myocardium and directly transmits the pacing stimulus to cardiac tissue.

Electromagnetic Interference – electrical signals from the environment (i.e. radio frequency waves), which can be sensed by the pacemaker and interfere with pacer function. Abbreviated **EMI.**

Escape Internal – the period of time between a sensed cardiac event and the next pacemaker output. The escape interval is usually equal to the basic pacing rate, but it can be programmed longer in some pacemakers (hysteresis).

Fusion Beat – a cardiac depolarization (either atrial or ventricular) that results from two foci, both contributing to depolarization of the chamber. In pacing, a fusion beat results when an intrinsic depolarization and a pacing stimulus occur simultaneously and both contribute to depolarization (usually seen in the ventricle).

Hysteresis – a programmable feature in most pacemakers that allows the escape interval to be programmed longer than the basic pacing interval (the pacing interval following a sensed beat is longer than the basic pacing interval). This allows more time for the heart's intrinsic activity to occur.

Inhibited Response – a type of response to sensing that inhibits pacemaker output when an intrinsic beat is sensed. This results in demand pacing, or pacing only when the heart's intrinsic activity is slower than the basic pacing rate.

Lead – the insulated wire and its electrode that transmits the pacing stimulus from the pulse generator to the heart and relays sensed intrinsic activity to the pulse generator. A single chamber pacemaker uses one lead, and a dual chamber pacemaker usually uses two leads, one in the atrium and one in the ventricle.

Magnet Mode – a term used for the pacemaker's response when a magnet is placed over the pulse generator. A magnet inactivates the sensing circuitry and causes a pacemaker to function asynchronously at a predetermined rate and in a preset manner. The magnet mode differs among manufacturers in pacing rate and number of impulses delivered with the magnet in place. A change in magnet-induced pacing rate is often an indicator of battery depletion and warrants pulse generator replacement.

777

Chapter 17

Myopotential – an electrical signal generated by muscle movement. Myopotentials are sometimes sensed by the pacemaker and cause inhibition of pacemaker output.

Output – the electrical stimulus delivered by the pulse generator, usually defined in terms of pulse amplitude (V = volts) and pulse width (milliseconds = ms).

Oversensing – detection of inappropriate electrical signals by the pacemaker's sensing circuit, resulting in inappropriate inhibition of pacer output. Sources of oversensing can include electromagnetic interference, myopotentials, T waves, or crosstalk between atrial and ventricular channels in dual chamber pacemakers.

Pacemaker Syndrome – adverse clinical signs and symptoms due to inadequate timing of atrial and ventricular contraction. The syndrome can be due to loss of AV synchrony in VVI pacing, inappropriate AV interval in dual chamber pacing, or inappropriate rate modulation. Symptoms include fatigue, confusion, unpleasant pulsations in neck or chest, limited exercise capacity, CHF, hypotension, syncope or near syncope.

Pacing Interval – the time between two consecutive paced events without an intervening sensed event. Measured in milliseconds (ms). AA interval = atrial pacing interval; VV interval = ventricular pacing interval.

Pacer Spike – term used to describe the small vertical "blip" recorded on the ECG with every pacemaker output pulse. The presence of a pacer spike indicates that a stimulus was released by the pacemaker.

Pseudofusion Beat – an electrocardiographic phenomenon resulting from delivery of a pacemaker spike into an intrinsic event. In the ventricle, it appears as a pacer spike in an intrinsic QRS complex, but since the ventricle is already depolarized, the spike is ineffective but may distort the QRS complex on the ECG.

Pulse Generator – the device that contains the power source (battery) and the electronic circuits that control pacemaker function. The term "pacemaker" is commonly used for the pulse generator.

Rate Modulation – the ability of a pacemaker to increase the pacing rate in response to physical activity or metabolic demand, also called **rate adaptation** or **rate response**. The pacemaker uses some type of physiologic sensor to determine the need for increased pacing rate. The most commonly used sensors at the present time are motion sensors and minute ventilation sensors.

Refractory Period – (1) In the heart, the period of time that the myocardium is incapable of responding to a stimulus. (2) In the pacemaker, an interval or timing cycle following a sensed or paced event during which the pacemaker will not respond to incoming signals. A single chamber pacemaker has one refractory period; a dual chamber pacemaker has an atrial refractory and a ventricular refractory period.

Sensing – the ability of the pacemaker to recognize and respond to intrinsic cardiac depolarization.

Sensing Threshold – the smallest intrinsic atrial or ventricular signal (measured in mV) that can be consistently sensed by the pacemaker.

Stimulation Threshold – the minimum amount of voltage necessary to capture the heart consistently. Also called **capture threshold** or **pacing threshold.**

Undersensing – failure of a pacemaker to sense intrinsic cardiac depolarizations. This can result in competition between the pacemaker and the intrinsic rhythm.

Unipolar – having one pole. (1) A unipolar lead has only one pole, located at the distal tip. (2) A pacing system with one pole in or on the heart and the second pole located remote from the heart to complete the circuit. Permanent unipolar systems utilize the back of the pulse generator as the second pole. Temporary epicardial pacing systems utilize a ground wire in subcutaneous tissue as the second pole.

Electrical Management of Arrhythmias

DUAL CHAMBER PACEMAKER TERMINOLOGY

Adaptive AV Delay (or Rate Adaptive AV Delay) – see AV Interval.

Alert Period – the portion of the pulse generator's timing cycle during which it can sense and respond to intrinsic cardiac activity. The alert period follows the refractory period.

Atrial Escape Interval – period of time from a sensed or paced ventricular event to the next paced atrial event. Also called the **V-A interval.**

Atrial Refractory Period – period of time during which the atrial channel is unable to respond to sensed signals. In dual chamber pacemakers, the total atrial refractory period is divided into two parts: the AV interval and the post ventricular atrial refractory period (PVARP).

Atrial Tracking – a state of pacing in which sensed atrial activity triggers a ventricular pacing output at the end of the programmed AV delay. Also known simply as tracking.

AV Interval (or AV Delay) – the "electronic PR interval," or the length of time between a sensed or paced atrial event and the delivery of the ventricular pacing output. The AV interval is programmable and is measured in milliseconds (e.g. an AV interval of 120 ms = a PR interval of .12 second). Many pacemakers have an **"adaptive AV delay,"** meaning that the AV delay can be programmed to shorten when the intrinsic atrial rate increases, thus mimicking the heart's own physiological increase in AV conduction as heart rate increases. Many devices also have a **"differential AV delay,"** meaning that the AV interval can be programmed to be longer on an atrial paced beat than on an atrial sensed beat (e.g. 200 ms when the atrium is paced, and 150 ms when P waves are sensed).

Blanking Period – a very short ventricular refractory period that occurs simultaneously with every atrial pacing output to prevent the ventricle from sensing the atrial stimulus. It is intended to prevent inhibition of ventricular output due to crosstalk (see definition below). Many pacemakers allow the blanking period to be programmed longer to prevent crosstalk.

Crosstalk – the sensing of a signal in one chamber by the sensing circuit in the other chamber, usually used in reference to the sensing of the atrial output pulse by the ventricular channel. Crosstalk due to sensing of atrial signals by the ventricular channel causes inhibition of ventricular pacing output because the ventricular channel thinks that the atrial output is a ventricular event.

Differential AV Delay – see AV Interval.

Endless Loop Tachycardia – see Pacemaker Mediated Tachycardia.

Maximum Tracking Rate (MTR) – the programmable upper rate limit of a dual chamber pacemaker that determines the fastest rate at which 1:1 tracking of atrial sensed events will occur. The MTR prevents the ventricular channel from pacing faster than the upper rate limit when the intrinsic atrial rate exceeds the programmed MTR. When the intrinsic atrial rate is faster than the upper rate limit, the pacemaker reverts to its "upper rate response" (see below) to prevent the ventricular rate from exceeding the MTR. MTR is also called the **ventricular tracking limit** or **upper rate limit.**

Pacemaker Mediated Tachycardia – a tachycardia induced by competition between the pacemaker and the intrinsic rhythm and sustained by the continued participation of the pacemaker. Most commonly used to describe the endless loop tachycardia that results when there is retrograde conduction from the ventricle to the atria, sensing of the retrograde P wave by the atrial channel, and pacing in the ventricle in response to the sensed P wave. This results in a re-entry tachycardia in which the pacemaker serves as the antegrade limb of the circuit and the intrinsic conduction system serves as the retrograde limb; also known as **endless loop tachycardia** or **pacemaker re-entry tachycardia.**

Chapter 17

Pseudopseudofusion Beat – an electrocardiographic phenomenon in which an atrial pacing spike is super-imposed on a native QRS complex. The atrial pacing spike cannot contribute to ventricular depolarization, but the presence of the spike can distort the native QRS complex on the ECG.

PVARP (Post Ventricular Atrial Refractory Period) – part of the total atrial refractory period that begins with a sensed or paced ventricular event. PVARP is a programmable parameter and is intended to prevent the atrial channel from sensing far-field ventricular signals, such as T waves or local myocardial potentials. PVARP can also be programmed to prevent the atrial channel from sensing retrograde P waves, thus preventing PMT.

Rate Response – ability of the pacemaker to increase its pacing rate in response to physical activity or increased metabolic demand. Rate responsive pacemakers have some type of sensor that detects physical activity or a physiological parameter that indicates the need for increased heart rate. Currently, the sensors most commonly used are vibration or motion sensors and minute ventilation sensors. Other sensors being evaluated include blood temperature, blood oxygen content, QT interval, and stroke volume. Rate response is also known as **rate modulation** or **rate adaptation.**

Rate Smoothing – a programmable function that prevents excessive cycle-to-cycle changes in pacing rate. Atrial tracking and rate response can occur, but no sudden acceleration or deceleration in pacing rate can occur.

Safety Pacing – the delivery of a ventricular output at a short AV interval whenever a signal is sensed early in the AV delay. The purpose of safety pacing is to prevent crosstalk inhibition of ventricular output, and is also called **non-physiological AV delay** or **ventricular safety standby.**

Total Atrial Refractory Period – the amount of time following a ventricular sensed or paced event during which the ventricular channel cannot respond to signals (in effect "has its eyes closed"). The purpose is to prevent the ventricular channel from seeing large repolarization signals (T waves) or other local myocardial signals.

IMPLANTABLE CARDIOVERTER DEFIBRILLATORS (ICD)

Sudden cardiac death (SCD) is defined as cardiac arrest with cessation of cardiac function and is most often due to VF or pulseless VT (pVT), although pulseless electrical activity (PEA), and asystole can also cause SCD. SCD occurs most often in patients with coronary artery disease, with cardiomyopathy being the second largest associated condition. Refer to the current guidelines from the American Heart Association for information on acute management of SCD and advanced cardiac life support. Patients who have survived a SCD episode are often treated with an ICD. This section describes ICD function and patient care issues related to ICDs.

Indications for ICD Implantation

The American College of Cardiology and American Heart Association have published guidelines for implantation of antiarrhythmia devices. The following outline lists the class I indications for antiarrhythmia devices according to the guidelines available at the time of this writing (Gregoratos et al., 2002).

Class I Indications for ICD Therapy

- Cardiac arrest due to VF or VT not due to transient or reversible cause.
- Spontaneous sustained VT in association with structural heart disease.
- Syncope of undetermined origin with sustained VT or VF induced at electrophysiology study (EPS) when drug therapy is ineffective, not tolerated, or not preferred.

- Nonsustained VT with coronary disease, prior MI, LV dysfunction, and inducible VF or sustained VT at EPS that is not suppressible by class I antiarrhythmic drugs.

Other Indications

- VT/VF while waiting for heart transplant.
- Familial or inherited conditions with high risk for life-threatening arrhythmias (long QT syndrome or hypertrophic cardiomyopathy).
- Brugada syndrome – syncope of unexplained etiology or family history of unexplained SCD associated with RBBB and ST segment elevation.
- Primary prevention of SCD in patients with documented MI and impaired left ventricular systolic function.
- Primary prevention in patients with cardiomyopathy and left ventricular ejection fraction $\leq 35\%$.

Overview of ICD Devices

An ICD system consists of a pulse generator and defibrillation lead capable of detecting ventricular arrhythmias and delivering therapy to terminate the arrhythmia. The pulse generator can be single or dual chamber with backup pacing capability (VVI/R or DDD/R), biventricular pacing capability, and antitachycardia therapies. The generator is implanted subcutaneously just like a permanent pacemaker, and the leads are most commonly placed transvenously like pacemaker leads. Arrhythmia detection and therapies are programmable functions and are discussed below.

Lead Systems

- Transvenous lead(s) placed in the right atrium and RV apex for dual chamber pacing.
- The RV lead is a coil that has pacing and sensing capabilities just like a pacemaker lead, but also has a large electrical surface area for defibrillation.
- Current devices have a "hot-can" where the case of the pulse generator serves as one pole for defibrillation and the RV lead is the second pole. The defibrillating current flows from the RV coil to the metal case of the generator, and frequently to a proximal coil placed in the superior vena cava. This type of defibrillation configuration lowers defibrillation thresholds.

Figure 17.20 illustrates ICD lead and generator placement.

ICD Function

ICDs must detect ventricular arrhythmias and then deliver therapy to terminate those arrhythmias. Because patients may have supraventricular arrhythmias as well, the device needs to be able to differentiate between supraventricular and ventricular rhythms and withhold therapy if the rhythm is not ventricular. In an effort to reduce inappropriate shocks, devices have several detection criteria that can be programmed

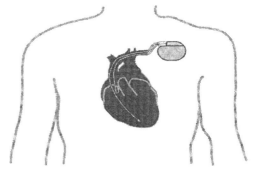

Figure 17.20: ICD generator and lead.

for each individual patient. Arrhythmia termination can be accomplished by antitachycardia pacing, cardioversion, or defibrillation therapies which can be programmed based on the patient's clinical tachycardias. Detection criteria and termination therapies are discussed below.

Arrhythmia Detection Criteria (vary among devices and are programmable options)

- **Heart rate** – the device continuously monitors ventricular rate and delivers therapy when the rate exceeds the programmed tachycardia detection rate.
  - Rate boundaries can be programmed to classify all possible rates into three zones: sinus, tachycardia, and fibrillation.
  - The tachycardia zone can be subdivided into one to three subcategories based on rate, depending on the patient's clinical tachycardias: tach 1, tach 2, tach 3. Figure 17.21 illustrates the different rate zones that can be programmed.

In Figure 17.21, the patient has three different VTs at three different rates. The sinus zone defines the sinus rhythm rate (e.g. up to 130 beats per minute). The tach 1 zone might include rates between 135 and 150 to capture the patient's slowest VT. The tach 2 zone might include rates between 151 and 180 to capture the patient's faster VT. The tach 3 zone might include rates between 181 and 250 to capture the patient's fastest VT. The V fib zone will capture VF rates. Termination therapies can be programmed differently for each tach zone (see below).

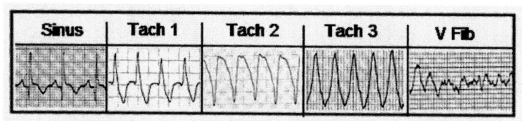

Figure 17.21: Tach zones.

- **Sudden onset** – detects sudden shortening of cycle length (sudden heart rate increase). Sinus tachycardia in response to exercise accelerates gradually, but VT occurs suddenly.
- **Interval stability (or rate stability)** – looks for variability in cycle lengths. VT usually has regular cycles while atrial fib has very irregular cycles.
- **Morphology** – measures width of the ventricular electrogram as seen by the ventricular lead and only treats if width is greater than a programmed value.

Combinations of the above detection criteria can be programmed to individualize detection for each patient, depending on the characteristics of the patient's arrhythmias.

Termination Therapies

Arrhythmia termination therapies include antitachycardia pacing (ATP), low energy cardioversion, and defibrillation. ATP therapy is usually painless and is used to terminate VTs that are in the slower rate ranges. Low energy cardioversion at energies of 2 joules or less are more comfortable than higher energy shocks. Defibrillation therapy is always delivered for VF.

- ATP (antitachycardia pacing) – one to several pacing therapies can be programmed for each tach zone.
  - *Burst* – delivery of a programmable number of pacing stimuli at a constant cycle length into the tachycardia (usually around 7-8 paced beats).
  - *Ramp* – a burst with progressively decreasing cycle length between paced beats.
  - *Decremental scanning* – allows successive bursts to be delivered at shorter cycle lengths (faster rates).
- Cardioversion shock – delivers shocks from 0.1 to 30 joules synchronized on the R wave of a VT.
- Defibrillating shock – delivers high energy (20 – 34 joules) unsynchronized shock for VF.

Example of Therapies Delivered by ICDs

◆ Antitachycardia Pacing (ATP)

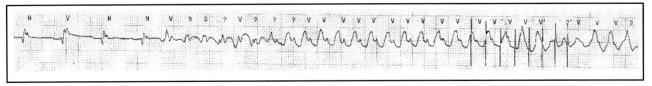

◆ Cardioversion

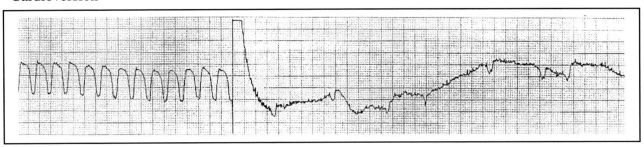

◆ Defibrillation

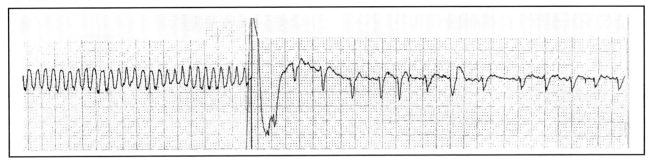

Other Device Features

- Bradycardia pacing capability – VVI, DDD, DDDR with mode switching.
- Atrial diagnostics – use of an atrial lead to monitor atrial activity and improve the device's ability to discriminate between SVT and VT.
- Stored electrograms – device is capable of storing arrhythmia events and displaying them in a variety of formats. Annotated atrial and ventricular electrograms can be displayed to show when sensing or pacing occurred, when detection criteria were met, and what therapies were delivered.
- Noninvasive EPS – device is capable of doing an EP study through implanted leads.

Implant Procedure

An ICD implant can be performed in the operating room, catheterization lab, or electrophysiology lab under local anesthesia with conscious sedation or general anesthesia. The procedure is almost identical to permanent pacemaker implantation, with a pocket made in the left pectoral area and leads introduced into subclavian or cephalic vein and threaded into the RV apex (and RA or coronary sinus for dual chamber or CRT devices). Stimulation and sensing thresholds are tested on the leads, then VF is induced and defibrillation thresholds (DFT) are done to determine the minimum amount of energy needed to reliably terminate VF. Defibrillation energy is set about 10 joules higher than DFT (usually between 20-34 joules). Leads are then connected to the generator, and VF is induced again to test the device's ability to detect and deliver therapy appropriately. The generator is implanted in the pocket after appropriate function is assured.

Chapter 17

Complications of Pacemaker/ICD Surgery and Therapy

Complications of Subclavian Vein Stick
◆ Pneumothorax.
◆ Hemothorax.
◆ Subclavian artery puncture.
◆ Air embolism.
◆ Bleeding.
◆ Hemoptysis (if lung punctured).
◆ Brachial plexus injury (pain or paresthesias in arm, hand, fingers).

Complications Related to Pulse Generator
◆ Pocket erosion.
◆ Pocket hematoma.
◆ Infection.
◆ Generator migration.
◆ Generator malfunction.
◆ Premature battery depletion.

Complications Related to Leads
◆ Perforation of RV, subclavian vein.
◆ Lead dislodgement.
◆ Insulation breaks, lead fracture.
◆ Diaphragmatic stimulation.
◆ Venous thrombosis.
◆ Pulmonary embolus.

Other Problems
◆ Shocks for non VT rhythms (e.g. atrial fib).
◆ Failure to deliver therapy when needed.
◆ Ineffective therapy.
◆ High DFTs (defibrillation thresholds).
◆ Device deactivation.

Postoperative Care

Routine Patient Care: Pacemaker or ICD implant
◆ Patient is usually placed in a monitored unit (telemetry) and usually discharged in 24 hours.
◆ Monitor rhythm continuously.
◆ Immobilize arm in sling.
◆ Monitor for signs of infection: redness, swelling at incision site, fever, elevated WBC.
◆ Monitor pulse generator pocket for bleeding and hematoma formation.
◆ Monitor for signs of tamponade: chest pain, SOB, hypotension, elevated neck veins, paradoxical pulse.

Status of ICD
◆ Place sign at head of bed, noting if device is on or off and the programmed rates.
◆ Know what therapies will be delivered for detected ventricular arrhythmias: pacing, cardioversion, or defibrillation. Make sure monitor technicians are aware that the patient has an ICD and what the programmed therapies are.

Emergency Care for VT/VF
◆ Device delivers therapy within 10-15 seconds and continues to deliver therapy as programmed if necessary.
◆ DO NOT WAIT for device to deliver all its therapies if patient is hemodynamically unstable or in VF.

Electrical Management of Arrhythmias

- ◆ Defibrillate with external paddles at maximum energy if necessary.
  - ❖ Avoid placing paddles directly over the pulse generator.
  - ❖ May need to alter paddle placement to anterior-posterior if first defibrillation is unsuccessful.
- ◆ Document rhythm strips in chart.
- ◆ Assess patient rhythm, vital signs, pain or other symptoms after device discharge.
  - ❖ Provide reassurance that device is doing what it is intended to do.
  - ❖ Note any symptoms patient may have experienced before device discharged.
- ◆ Notify physician of all appropriate and inappropriate discharges.

Linking Knowledge to Practice

✔ *There are reports of healthcare providers being shocked when doing CPR or intubating patients with an ICD that is delivering shocks to treat an arrhythmia. It is a good idea to wear gloves when providing emergency care, especially CPR and intubation, to patients with an ICD. It may be advisable to place a magnet over the ICD during intubation to suspend arrhythmia detection and delivery of shocks during the procedure.*

Inappropriate Firing of ICD

- ◆ Assess patient's rhythm and determine if ICD discharge is appropriate.
  - ❖ SVTs may occur at rates faster than the detection rate of ICD and the device may deliver therapy as programmed, even though the rhythm is not VT.
- ◆ If the device is firing inappropriately, notify physician and obtain an order to deactivate the device.
  - ❖ All ICDs can be turned off using a programmer.
  - ❖ If no programmer is available, placing a round magnet over the generator will deactivate arrhythmia detection and therapy.
  - ❖ Detection remains inhibited until the magnet is removed.

Patients going to surgery where cautery is to be used need to have their ICDs turned off or deactivated with a pacemaker magnet until after surgery.

- ◆ Notify surgery and anesthesia that patient has ICD.

Linking Knowledge to Practice

✔ *A pacemaker magnet works differently for ICDs than for pacemakers. Placing a magnet over an ICD deactivates arrhythmia detection and therefore prevents therapy from being delivered, but it does not affect the function of the pacemaker portion of the device; the pacemaker continues to operate as programmed even with the magnet in place. Once the magnet is removed, the ICD returns to programmed parameters and once again can detect and treat arrhythmias.*

Patient/Family Teaching

- ◆ Reason for ICD, how it works, and what to expect when it discharges.
- ◆ Signs of infection, erosion.
- ◆ Carry ID card at all times (may want to wear Medic Alert bracelet).
- ◆ Keep site dry for 4 days or as directed by physician.
- ◆ No lifting of arm on ICD side over the head; don't lift objects with that arm until physician approves.

Chapter 17

- ◆ What to do when device discharges:
  - ❖ If have warning symptoms (dizziness, palpitations), sit or lie down to prevent harm due to fall.
  - ❖ If receive only one shock and feel alright afterwards, notify physician.
  - ❖ If receive multiple shocks or feel very ill afterward, call 911 and get to hospital for evaluation.
  - ❖ Instruct family to call 911 any time patient is shocked and does not awaken immediately.
- ◆ When to notify physician:
  - ❖ After receiving shocks (unless instructed otherwise by physician or follow-up nurse).
  - ❖ If receive multiple shocks (two or more shocks in a row) or frequent shocks (i.e. several times a week or several in a day).
  - ❖ Any time patient feels terrible after a shock and doesn't recover as fast as usual.
  - ❖ Fever, redness, drainage from generator site, or other signs of infection.
- ◆ Family CPR.
- ◆ Importance of follow-up visits.
- ◆ What to avoid in environment that may interfere with device function:
  - ❖ Strong magnets
    - ★ Large stereo speakers (don't carry speaker close to device).
    - ★ Security search wands (if held over device for prolonged time or moved in repetitive fashion over device).
    - ★ Electronic article surveillance equipment (store security devices) – don't stand near them for prolonged periods or lean against them.
    - ★ Industrial magnets like those found in amusement rides.
  - ❖ Arc and resistance welders.
  - ❖ Large generators or power plants.
  - ❖ Large TV or radio transmitting towers (stay 25 feet away).
  - ❖ Industrial equipment, induction furnaces.
  - ❖ CB or ham radio antennas (avoid direct contact during transmission).
  - ❖ Electrocautery (i.e. at dentist office or in surgery).
  - ❖ Leaning over running motor of car or boat (turn engine off to repair).
  - ❖ MRI & diathermy (contraindicated).
  - ❖ CT scans (device should be turned off first).
  - ❖ Lithotripsy may damage ICD. Device should be turned off and beam should be directed away from the generator, and testing done after procedure to assess function of device.
- ◆ These things are safe for ICD patients to use:
  - ❖ Household appliances (toaster, blenders, can openers, etc.).
  - ❖ Hand held appliances (hair dryer, shaver, etc.).
  - ❖ Radios, TVs and VCR remote controls.
  - ❖ Lawnmowers, leaf blowers, etc.
  - ❖ Microwave ovens.
  - ❖ Garage door openers.
  - ❖ Light shop equipment (drills, table saws, etc.).
  - ❖ Electric blankets, heating pads.
  - ❖ Office equipment, computers, fax machines, etc.

Electrical Management of Arrhythmias

- ❖ Store and airport security systems (device may set off alarms but won't be harmed if you move through quickly).
- ❖ Diagnostic x-ray.
- ❖ Ultrasound.
- ❖ Lasers.
- ◆ Using cell phones
  - ❖ May be potential interaction between cell phones and ICDs: may either inhibit therapy or cause inappropriate therapy.
  - ❖ Keep phone at least 6 inches away from device – use on opposite ear.
  - ❖ Carry phone on opposite side of body and at least 6 inches away from ICD.
- ◆ Activities
  - ❖ No activity restriction due to ICD, except contact sports and driving.
  - ❖ Driving is usually restricted for 6 months to assess risk of shocks and how patient reacts when shocked. No commercial driving allowed.
  - ❖ May swim and boat, but not alone.
  - ❖ May perform all activities of daily living and exercise within tolerance.
- ◆ Support groups for patients with ICDs can be a source of information and emotional support for patients and their families.

Follow-up Care and Replacement

- ◆ Follow-up visits every 4-6 months with cardiologist.
  - ❖ Check battery status: when battery nears end of service, replacement can be scheduled.
  - ❖ Interrogate device and review stored electrograms to assess appropriate function and types of arrhythmias patient may have.
- ◆ Replacement surgery
  - ❖ Usually day surgery or overnight stay.
  - ❖ Remove and replace pulse generator only.

ELECTROPHYSIOLOGY STUDIES AND RADIOFREQUENCY CATHETER ABLATION FOR ARRHYTHMIAS

A cardiac electrophysiology study (EPS) is an invasive catheter based technique used for evaluation and treatment of cardiac arrhythmias. EPS can be used to evaluate the following:

- ◆ Sinus node function – when sinus node dysfunction is suspected as a cause of symptoms.
- ◆ AV node function – when AV block is suspected as a cause of symptoms.
- ◆ Narrow QRS tachycardias – to diagnose the mechanism of tachycardia (atrial tachycardia, AV nodal reentry tachycardia [AVNRT], or circus movement tachycardia [CMT] utilizing an accessory pathway); evaluate for ablation or surgical correction.
- ◆ Wide QRS tachycardias – to diagnose the mechanism of tachycardia (ventricular versus supraventricular); evaluate for ablation or surgical correction.
- ◆ Wolff-Parkinson-White (WPW) syndrome – locate accessory pathways and evaluate for ablation or surgical correction.
- ◆ Unexplained syncope – to determine if cardiac arrhythmia (bradycardia or tachycardia) is potential cause of symptoms.
- ◆ Survivors of cardiac arrest without evidence of acute MI as cause of arrest.

- Indications for device therapy – permanent pacemaker or ICD.
- Outcome of drug or device therapy (evaluate efficacy of drugs or devices in treating diagnosed arrhythmias).

EPS Procedure

EPS is usually done in a dedicated electrophysiology laboratory where several multipolar catheters are introduced percutaneously into the heart using fluoroscopy and positioned at specific sites for recording intracardiac signals and for pacing from specific locations in the heart. The procedure is usually done using intravenous sedation and local anesthesia at the catheter insertion sites, very similar to cardiac catheterization. The patient is connected to an external defibrillator (biphasic is preferred) via "hands-free" defibrillation pads, and the rhythm is continuously monitored via the ECG cable from the defibrillator as well as via the intracardiac signals obtained from the catheters. Blood pressure is monitored via non-invasive machine and sometimes via arterial line. In addition, O_2 saturation and often end-tidal CO_2 are monitored as part of the procedural sedation protocol.

Vascular access is usually via the femoral veins, where as many as three catheters can be placed in the right femoral vein, and often additional catheters are placed via the left femoral vein. Subclavian, internal jugular, or brachial access can also be used, usually for placement of a catheter in the coronary sinus. If ablation of a left-sided accessory pathway is planned, a right femoral arterial insertion site may also be used.

Catheter placement – flexible, multipolar catheters are placed in specific areas of the heart where intracardiac recordings are obtained and pacing can be done. Typical catheter placement for a SVT study includes: high right atrium, His bundle, right ventricular apex, and coronary sinus to record left atrial activation (see Figure 17.22). There are several specialized catheters of various shapes with as many as 30 or more poles that record from multiple sites within the atria or ventricles to locate arrhythmogenic foci or pathways in more advanced mapping studies.

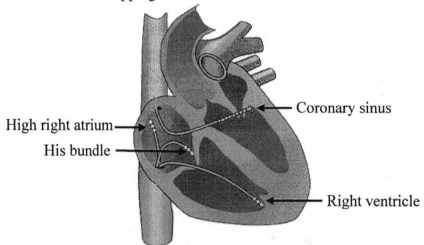

Figure 17.22: Catheter placement.

Intracardiac recordings are obtained from each of the catheters and displayed on a monitor along with three surface leads. As many as 120 electrograms can be displayed on more sophisticated monitoring equipment. (See Figure 17.23 for basic recordings).

In Figure 17.23, three surface leads are displayed: I, AVF, V1.

HRA = high right atrium.

HB = His bundle recordings (proximal, mid, and distal recordings displayed).

CS = coronary sinus recordings (proximal, mid, and distal recordings displayed).

RV = right ventricular recording.

Basic intervals are recorded and used to analyze baseline cardiac conduction, including:

- *AH interval* – measured from onset of atrial activation to the His bundle deflection and approximates AV node conduction time. In first degree AV block, the AH interval is prolonged.

- *HV interval* – measured from His deflection to onset of ventricular activation and reflects conduction time through the distal His-Purkinje system. In Type II AV block, the HV interval is prolonged.

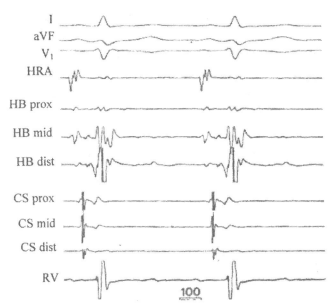

Figure 17.23: Intracardiac recordings.

Programmed Electrical Stimulation (PES) involves pacing according to pre-established protocols in the atria and ventricles, and sometimes from the His bundle or CS catheters as well. Pacing protocols are used to evaluate conduction system function; determine refractory period of the atria, AV node, and ventricle; and to induce supraventricular or ventricular arrhythmias.

Mapping refers to the precise placement and movement of a catheter around an area of the heart in an attempt to find a focus or electrical pathway responsible for an arrhythmia and locate the area where ablation might abolish the arrhythmia.

In most cases, once an arrhythmia has been induced and its focus located, an ablation is performed at the same time.

Radiofrequency Catheter Ablation

Radiofrequency (RF) energy is a form of electrical energy produced by high frequency alternating current. When this current is passed through a catheter tip to cardiac tissue, heat is created which causes thermal injury and local tissue destruction, resulting in a small fibrotic scar. RF energy directed at an arrhythmogenic focus or a re-entrant pathway in the myocardium destroys tissue that is responsible for many tachyarrhythmias and prevents their recurrence. Depending on the type and complexity of arrhythmia and the patient's cardiac anatomy, an ablation procedure can take several hours.

Indications for RF Ablation

Ablation can be done to treat a variety of supraventricular arrhythmias as well as ventricular tachycardia. The following section outlines indications for ablation and briefly describes the arrhythmias for which ablation can be effective treatment.

AV Nodal Re-entry Tachycardia (AVNRT)
- Responsible for about 60% of PSVT (paroxysmal supraventricular tachycardia), most commonly occurs in young to middle-aged adults and is more common in women.

- Usually not associated with structural heart disease.
- Symptoms include palpitations, dizziness, chest tightness, dyspnea, and occasionally syncope. This rhythm is usually fairly well tolerated.
- AVNRT is due to dual AV nodal pathways, one fast conducting with a long refractory period and one slow conducting with a short refractory period (Figure 17.24).
  - Usually initiated by a PAC that finds the fast pathway unable to conduct, so it travels down the slow pathway into ventricle (PAC has a long PR interval).
  - Impulse can then travel back up the fast pathway and re-enter the slow pathway, setting up a re-entry circuit within the AV node, resulting in tachycardia.
    - 90% of AVNRT are "slow/fast" – impulse travels anterograde through slow pathway and retrograde up fast pathway.
    - 10% are "fast/slow" – impulse travels anterograde through fast pathway and retrograde through slow pathway.
  - Presents as a narrow QRS tachycardia (unless bundle branch block is present) with no P waves visible; P waves are either hidden in the QRS or may peek out at the end of the QRS due to simultaneous atrial and ventricular depolarization.
- RF energy is usually directed at the slow pathway to destroy it and prevent its participation in the re-entry circuit, causing the tachycardia.
  - Success rate 90-100% (Arnsdorf, Morrissey, & Wilber, 2006).

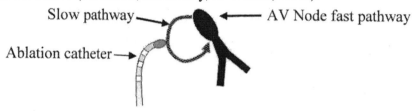

Figure 17.24: AV nodal re-entry tachycardia (AVNRT).

AVRT (AV re-entrant tachycardia) or CMT (circus movement tachycardia)
- Responsible for about 30% of PSVTs.
- CMT occurs in people who have accessory pathways (WPW syndrome) and involves both the AV node and the accessory pathway (AP) in the re-entry circuit. (See Figure 17.25.)
- Accessory pathways can be located anywhere around either the tricuspid or mitral valve ring.
  - 60% are left free wall.
  - 12% are right free wall.
  - Others are posteroseptal, anteroseptal, or midseptal.
- During sinus rhythm, if the AP is able to conduct in an antegrade direction (from atrium to ventricle) the impulse conducts through the AP faster than it does through the AV node, resulting in a short PR interval and an initial slurred portion of the QRS complex called a delta wave, which is due to premature stimulation of the ventricle via the AP.
- CMT usually presents as a narrow QRS tachycardia (unless BBB is present), and P waves may not be visible or may be seen in the ST segment or T wave. See Chapter 5 for more information on CMT.
- Symptoms during tachycardia may include palpitations, dizziness, chest tightness, dyspnea, and occasionally syncope.

- ◆ If atrial fibrillation occurs in the presence of an AP, ventricular rates can be extremely fast because the AP conducts the impulses without delay into the ventricle. This can result in VF.
- ◆ RF energy is directed at the accessory pathway to destroy it and prevent its participation in the re-entry circuit causing the tachycardia.
  - ❖ Success rate 90-95%, depending on number and location of APs (Knight, 2006).

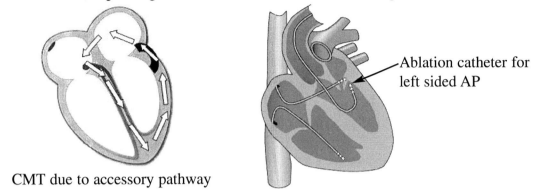

Figure 17.25: Circus movement tachycardia (CMT).

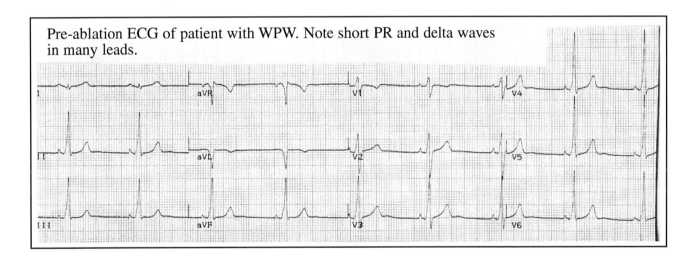

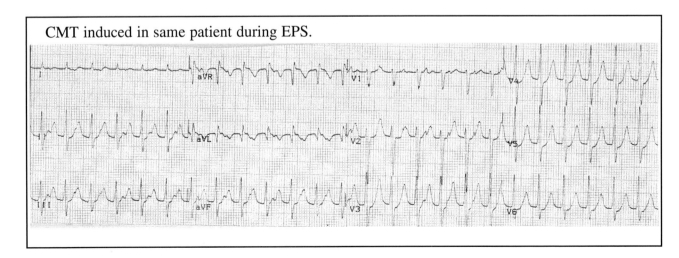

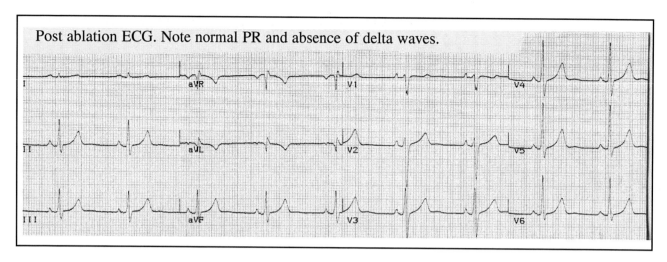

Post ablation ECG. Note normal PR and absence of delta waves.

AV Node Ablation
- RF energy is used to destroy the AV node in an effort to control ventricular rate in atrial fibrillation or flutter that is refractory to drug therapy.
- Destruction of AV node results in complete AV block and requires permanent pacing.

Atrial Flutter
- The most common type of atrial flutter involves a re-entry circuit in the right atrium that allows an electrical impulse to "chase its own tail" around in a circle at a rate of 250-350 times per minute – most common rate is 300.
- RF energy is directed at a portion of the re-entry circuit in the low right atrium with success rates around 95% (Cheng & Arnsdorf, 2006).

Atrial Tachycardia
- Incision lines, patch grafts, and scars in the atria from surgical correction of congenital problems can serve as a substrate for re-entry tachyarrhythmias.
  - Ablation is more difficult because re-entry pathways vary, depending on type of surgery and resulting changes in atrial anatomy.
- Focal atrial tachycardias can arise in the right atrium, near the ostia of the pulmonary veins in the left atrium, around the tricuspid valve, near the ostium of the coronary sinus, and other localized spots in either atrium.
  - These tachycardias are probably due to abnormal firing of foci in the atria rather than to reentry.
  - RF energy directed at the focus of the tachycardia can abolish it once mapping has identified the site.

Atrial Fibrillation
- AF often originates from ectopic sites within the atria, most commonly around the ostia of the pulmonary veins entering the left atrium; other sites around the superior vena cava and isolated sites within the atria are less common.
- Pulmonary vein isolation is complete electrical disconnection of the pulmonary veins from the left atrium by the use of RF ablation to create lesions around the ostia of the pulmonary veins. The goal is to prevent electrical impulses that originate in the pulmonary veins from crossing the lesions and entering the atria, triggering AF.
  - Segmental ostial isolation is performed by ablating specific sites of conduction between the ostia of the pulmonary veins and the left atrium without completely encircling the ostia.

Electrical Management of Arrhythmias

❖ Circumferential pulmonary vein ablation creates ablation lesions that completely encircle the ostia of the pulmonary veins. Additional ablation lines are sometimes made to anatomic landmarks like the mitral annulus.

◆ RF Maze procedure is the use of RF energy to create linear lesions within the atria to interrupt the reentrant pathways required for AF maintenance.

Ventricular Tachycardia

◆ Idiopathic VT occurs in people without structural heart disease and is amenable to ablation because it is focal in origin (70% of cases arise in RV outflow tract) (Arnsdorf & Ganz, 2006).

❖ Repetitive monomorphic VT usually occurs in young or middle-aged people and is often asymptomatic and associated with physical or emotional stress. It presents as repetitive runs of non-sustained VT with periods of sinus rhythm (frequent PVCs or couplets), usually has LBBB morphology with normal or rightward axis, and is usually not inducible during EPS.

❖ Paroxysmal sustained monomorphic VT presents with similar symptoms, but is often more symptomatic because VT is sustained for longer periods. It is more often inducible in EPS and may be terminated with adenosine, verapamil, Valsalva maneuver, carotid massage, or beta blockers.

❖ Idiopathic LV tachycardia usually occurs in young people and is often symptomatic and sustained. It usually has RBBB morphology with leftward axis, and commonly originates in the inferior left mid-septum or at the apex near the posterior fascicle. It is usually inducible at EPS and is unresponsive to beta blockers or adenosine, but may respond to verapamil.

❖ Ablation can be successful in all these types of VT.

❖ VT usually tolerated well enough for mapping to find focus.

☆ No scar or other myocardial abnormalities to interfere with delivery of RF energy to focus.

☆ Success rates around 75-100% depending on site of VT and experience of operator (Arnsdorf & Ganz, 2006).

◆ Bundle branch re-entry VT involves a macro-re-entry circuit in the ventricles – usually using the left bundle to conduct retrograde and the right bundle to conduct anterograde within the ventricles.

❖ Ablation of the right bundle or occasionally the left anterior or posterior fascicle can eliminate this type of VT.

❖ Ablation can eliminate bundle branch re-entry VT, but long term survival is limited by associated heart disease and underlying ventricular dysfunction.

The Ablation Procedure

After a diagnostic EPS, the arrhythmia focus or pathway is identified and an ablation catheter is placed at the target area. For right-sided ablations (e.g. atrial flutter, AV node, AVNRT, right-sided accessory pathways); the ablation catheter is inserted via the right femoral vein. For left-sided ablations, a femoral artery puncture is made and the ablation catheter is advanced up the aorta and retrograde across the aortic valve to reach the ablation site. Alternatively, a trans-septal puncture can be done and the catheter advanced from the right atrium into the left atrium through the puncture in the atrial septum. Heparin is given to prevent thrombus formation when left-sided ablations are done.

RF energy is delivered from the RF generator through the large tip of the ablation catheter to a grounding pad placed on the patient's back or hip. The RF energy heats up the tissue surrounding the electrode and results in thermal tissue necrosis in a small area of myocardium around the catheter tip, thus destroying the arrhythmogenic focus or part of the pathway required for a re-entry circuit. Energy is

793

Chapter 17

usually applied for 30-60 seconds (sometimes up to 2 minutes). Temperatures of 60-70 degrees centigrade at tip-tissue interface are optimal for adequate tissue heating. Temperatures of 90 degrees centigrade result in local coagulation at the catheter tip and interfere with the delivery of RF energy to the myocardium (Ganz, 2006). Newer ablation catheters are cooled by circulating saline within the catheter, which prevents temperatures high enough to create coagulation at the catheter tip. Numerous "burns" may be required to destroy the targeted tissue. Intracardiac signals are assessed for loss of conduction through involved tissue, and programmed stimulation is repeated to verify that the tachycardia is no longer inducible. The patient is usually monitored in the lab for 30-60 minutes after ablation to verify that conduction through targeted tissue does not resume.

Potential Complications (overall incidence < 4%)

◆ Cardiac perforation.
◆ Tamponade.
◆ Major venous thrombosis.
◆ Pulmonary embolism.
◆ Pneumothorax.
◆ Infection – sepsis.
◆ Bleeding.
◆ CVA.
◆ VT/VF.

Nursing Care of the EPS and Ablation Patient

Pre-procedure

◆ Patient/family education and support.
  ❖ Need for procedure.
    ☆ Explain patient's arrhythmia and how it relates to symptoms.
    ☆ Explain how procedure may affect arrhythmia and symptoms (expected outcome).
  ❖ What to expect during procedure
    ☆ Sedation, local anesthetic.
    ☆ Catheter insertion and sensation associated with this – usually not painful.
    ☆ Pacing and sensations associated with this – may feel heart beating rapidly.
    ☆ Induction of tachycardia is the objective and patient may feel same symptoms as with clinical tachycardia.
    ☆ Ablation and sensations associated with this (some people feel a burning sensation or pain).
    ☆ Need to be very still, especially during ablation.
    ☆ Importance of reporting any pain or other symptoms (SOB).
  ❖ Post procedure care.
  ❖ Expected discharge date/time.
◆ Consent forms for procedure.
◆ NPO for at least 6-8 hours prior to procedure.
◆ IV or Heparin lock.
◆ Labs: K+, PT or PTT, antiarrhythmic drug levels, if applicable.
◆ Foley catheter if long study anticipated.

Electrical Management of Arrhythmias

Post-procedure Care

◆ Bedrest for 4-6 hours with leg(s) straight.

◆ Head can elevate 20-30 degrees.

◆ VS, pedal pulse and groin checks q 15 min for 1 hour, then q 30 min for 1 hr, then q 4 hours, or according to hospital protocol.

◆ Observe all puncture sites for bleeding with VS checks. Be aware of all puncture sites used in procedure: femoral vein, femoral artery, subclavian, internal jugular, brachial.

◆ May eat usual diet and take usual meds.

◆ May have foley catheter if long SVT study – can be discontinued at end of bedrest period.

◆ Monitor rhythm continuously and notify EP physician if arrhythmia occurs.

◆ Monitor for signs of:

❖ Tamponade (hypotension, tachycardia, elevated neck veins, pulsus paradoxus).

❖ Cardiac perforation (hypotension, tachycardia, dyspnea, chest pain).

❖ Pneumothorax (dyspnea, unequal breath sounds).

❖ Pulmonary embolism (sudden dyspnea, chest pain, tachycardia, $\downarrow$ O$_2$ sat).

❖ Venous or arterial thrombosis ($\downarrow$ pedal pulses, cool extremities, numbness or tingling in legs, flushing or cyanotic extremities).

◆ Some ablation patients are outpatients and can go home after bedrest period.

◆ Discharge instructions per physician preference. These are common:

❖ Resume normal activities but avoid strenuous activity for a week.

❖ Avoid prolonged sitting.

❖ Watch puncture sites for bleeding or signs of infection (redness, swelling, exudate, warm).

❖ Report to physician or arrhythmia center nurse: dizziness, SOB, symptoms of tachycardias, signs of infection at puncture sites, fever or chilling.

❖ Inform patient that they may still feel "early beats," but these should no longer result in tachycardia.

❖ Teach about discharge medications.

Chapter 17

PRACTICE STRIPS

Pacemakers and ICDs

Strips 1-8 are VVI pacemakers.

1.
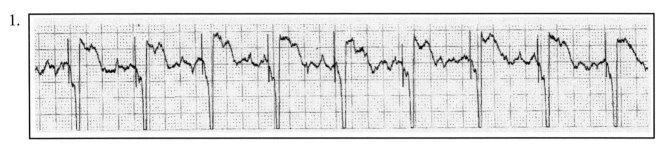

Capture:

Sensing:

2.
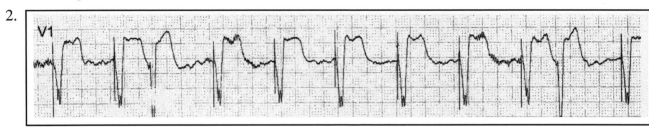

Capture:

Sensing:

3.
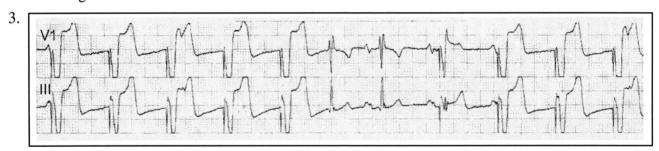

Capture:

Sensing:

4.
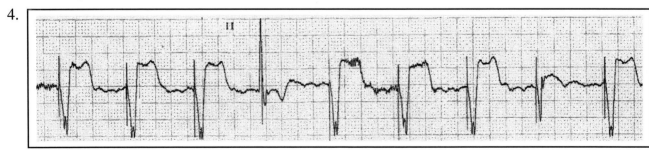

Capture:

Sensing:

5.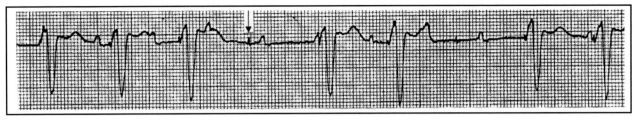

Capture:

Sensing:

6.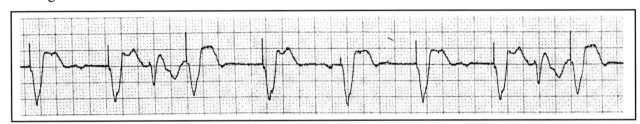

Capture:

Sensing:

7.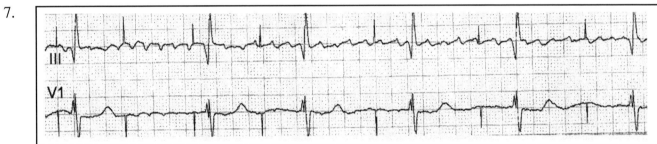

Capture:

Sensing:

8.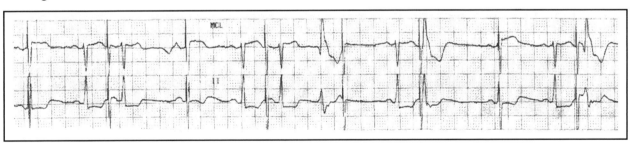

Capture:

Sensing:

Chapter 17

Strips 9-17 are DDD pacemakers.

9.
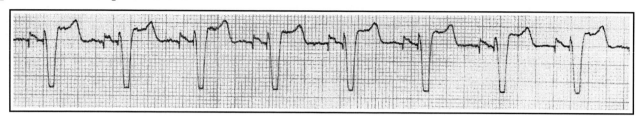
Atrial capture   Atrial sensing
Ventricular capture   Ventricular sensing

10.
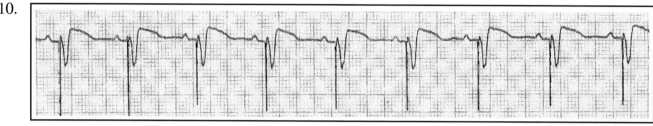
Atrial capture   Atrial sensing
Ventricular capture   Ventricular sensing

11.
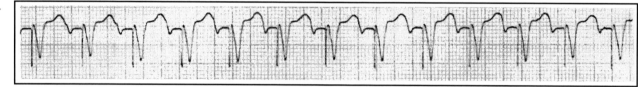
Atrial capture   Atrial sensing
Ventricular capture   Ventricular sensing

12.
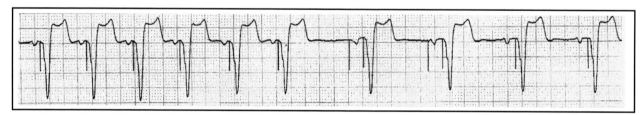
Atrial capture   Atrial sensing
Ventricular capture   Ventricular sensing

13.
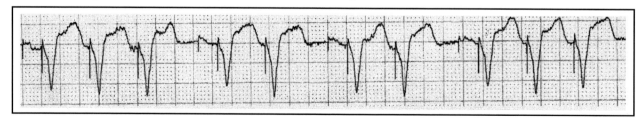
Atrial capture   Atrial sensing
Ventricular capture   Ventricular sensing

14.

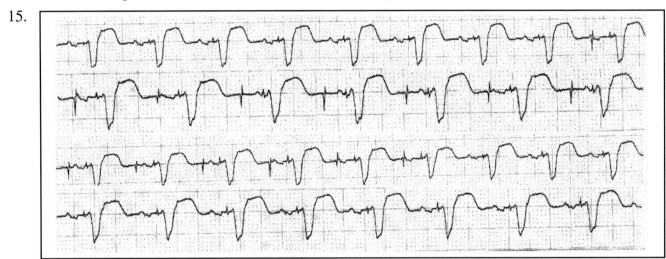

Atrial capture   Atrial sensing
Ventricular capture   Ventricular sensing

15.

Atrial capture   Atrial sensing
Ventricular capture   Ventricular sensing

16.

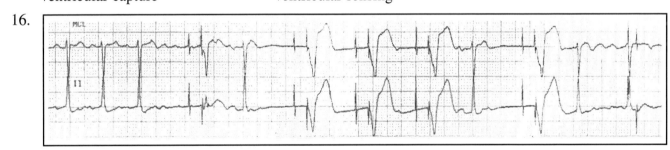

Atrial capture   Atrial sensing
Ventricular capture   Ventricular sensing

17.

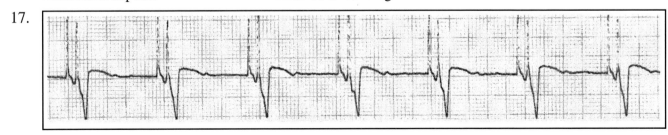

Atrial capture   Atrial sensing
Ventricular capture   Ventricular sensing

Chapter 17

Strips 18 – 20 are from patients with an ICD.

18. These two strips are the same episode in this patient:

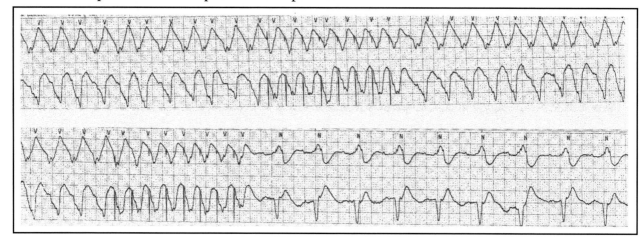

19.

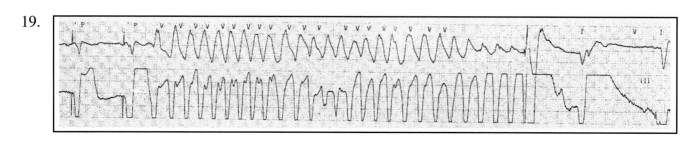

20.

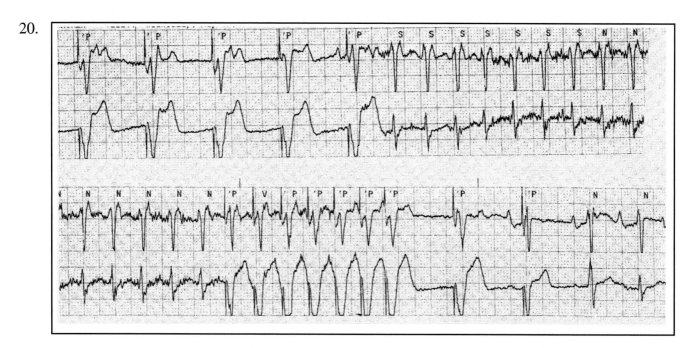

Electrical Management of Arrhythmias

Pacemaker and ICD Answers

1. Capture: normal.
    Sensing: can't tell. No opportunity for pacemaker to sense.
    Underlying rhythm is atrial fib. Normal VVI pacing.

2. Capture: normal.
    Sensing: normal. The 3rd and 10th intrinsic QRS complexes are sensed.
    Underlying rhythm is atrial fib. Normal VVI pacing and sensing.

3. Capture: normal.
    Sensing: normal. The 8th beat is a fusion beat between the pacemaker and the intrinsic QRS occurring at the same time.

4. Capture: normal.
    Sensing: probably normal. The 4th beat is a pseudofusion beat, and the 8th beat is a fusion beat. Both are just timing coincidences. Underlying rhythm is atrial fib.

5. Capture: intermittent loss.
    Sensing: can't tell. There are no intrinsic QRS complexes to be sensed.

6. Capture: normal.
    Sensing: loss of sensing. There are two intrinsic QRS complexes that should have been sensed and reset the pacing interval. Instead, pacing continues uninterrupted and in competition with the intrinsic beats.

7. Capture: total loss of capture.
    Sensing: sensing is normal in spite of the fact that pacer spikes #2 and #4 occur close to the preceding QRS complexes. QRS #1 and #2 fall in the pacemaker's refractory period, so the pacemaker has its eyes closed and can't "see" them. Therefore, the following spikes are delivered on time, which looks like failure to sense. Underlying rhythm is atrial fib with a VVI pacemaker at a rate of 60, with total loss of capture.

8. Capture: total loss of capture.
    Sensing: total loss of sensing.
    Pacemaker is set at a rate of 50. Underlying rhythm is sinus with PVCs.

9. Atrial capture: can't tell for sure but appears to have a "bump" after atrial spike.
    Atrial sensing: can't evaluate. No intrinsic atrial activity to sense.
    Ventricular capture: good.
    Ventricular sensing: can't evaluate. No intrinsic ventricular activity to sense.
    DDD pacemaker operating in AV sequential pacing state.

10. Atrial capture: can't evaluate. No atrial pacing is occurring.
    Atrial sensing: good. Every intrinsic P wave is followed by a paced QRS.
    Ventricular capture: good.
    Ventricular sensing: can't evaluate. No intrinsic ventricular activity to sense.
    DDD pacemaker operating in atrial tracking state.

11. Atrial capture: can't evaluate. No atrial pacing is occurring.
    Atrial sensing: good. Every intrinsic P wave is followed by a paced QRS.
    Ventricular capture: good.
    Ventricular sensing: can't tell. No intrinsic ventricular activity to sense.
    DDD pacemaker operating in atrial tracking state.

12. Atrial capture: difficult to be sure from this short strip. The two atrial pacing spikes do have a P

Chapter 17

wave after them, but they appear to alter their relationship to the spike.

Atrial sensing: good. Every intrinsic P wave is followed by a paced QRS.

Ventricular capture: good.

Ventricular sensing: can't evaluate. There is no intrinsic ventricular activity to sense.

DDD pacemaker operating in atrial tracking state. Underlying rhythm appears to be sinus arrhythmia or sick sinus syndrome.

13. Atrial capture: hard to tell. There is a P wave after the atrial pacing spikes, but the rhythm appears to be sinus tachycardia, and the P wave may be occurring at the same time as the atrial spike.

Atrial sensing: good. P waves are being sensed and triggering the ventricular paced beats.

Ventricular capture: good.

Ventricular sensing: can't evaluate. There is no ventricular activity to be sensed.

DDD pacemaker operating at upper rate limit in response to sinus tachycardia with a Wenckebach type response.

14. Atrial capture: Can't evaluate. The only atrial pacing spike (beat #7) occurs in an intrinsic P wave.

Atrial sensing: good. Sinus rhythm P waves are followed by paced QRS. There are 2 PACs (beats #2 and #9) that occur in PVARP so are not sensed, but do conduct to ventricles. Beat #6 is a PAC that occurs outside of PVARP, so is sensed and triggers a V pace, but at a longer than programmed AV interval due to upper rate limit.

Ventricular capture: good.

Ventricular sensing: good. The QRSs following the conducted PACs are sensed and inhibit pacing.

DDD pacemaker operating in atrial tracking state. Three PACs are present.

15. Atrial capture: complete loss of atrial capture. Note sinus rhythm P waves present within many of the AV intervals, but at varying relationships to the atrial pacing spikes. If the atrial spikes had captured the atrium, there could be no sinus rhythm P waves occurring in the AV interval.

Atrial sensing: good. Whenever the sinus P waves occur outside the atrial refractory period, they are sensed (i.e. first 8 beats in top strip).

Ventricular capture: good. All QRSs appear to be paced.

Ventricular sensing: can't evaluate. There is no intrinsic ventricular activity to sense.

DDD pacemaker with total loss of atrial capture. Sinus rhythm is present, and many sinus P waves are sensed and appropriately trigger a V pace. Other sinus P waves occur in the AV interval when the atrial channel is "asleep," so are not sensed.

16. Atrial capture: can't tell. There doesn't appear to be a P wave after atrial spikes or anywhere in the AV interval. There is no place where an atrial spike is followed by a normal QRS.

Atrial sensing: probably not good. The underlying atrial rhythm is intermittent atrial fib alternating with some sinus rhythm. Beat #4 shows an atrial spike during atrial fib, indicating that the pacemaker doesn't sense the atrial activity. Often atrial fib amplitude is too low to be sensed by the pacemaker.

Ventricular capture: good.

Ventricular sensing: good. All intrinsic QRSs appear to be sensed and inhibit pacing. The last beat is safety pacing due to an atrial pacing spike occurring at the same time an intrinsic QRS occurs. The ventricular channel blanks during the A spike, and when it "opens its eyes" at the end of the blanking period, it sees the intrinsic QRS, so it delivers a V pace at a shorter than programmed AV interval (safety pacing).

DDD pacemaker in a patient with intermittent atrial fib. This pacemaker does not appear to have a mode-switching option, which would cause it to switch to VVI or DDI pacing during atrial fib.

Electrical Management of Arrhythmias

17. Atrial capture: can't tell. There are no atrial spikes followed by normal QRSs.
    Atrial sensing: can't evaluate. There are no intrinsic P waves to be sensed.
    Ventricular capture: good.
    Ventricular sensing: good. This is safety pacing at a short AV interval due to crosstalk between the atrial pacing spike and the ventricular channel. The ventricular channel sees the atrial spike (which proves that ventricular sensing is OK) and paces at a short AV interval.

18. Top strip shows VT and ATP therapy with an 8 beat burst, which was not successful in terminating the VT. Second strip shows the next ATP therapy of 8 paced beats; this time it successfully converted the VT.

19. Onset of rapid VT with a cardioverting shock on the QRS complex that successfully converts the VT.

20. Ventricular paced rhythm with onset of VT in top strip. In second strip, ATP with a 7 beat burst terminates the VT.

REFERENCES

2005 American Heart Association Guidelines for Cardiopulmonary Resuscitation and Emergency Cardiovascular Care, Part 5: Electrical Therapies. *Circulation, 112(suppl IV)*, IV-1 – IV-211.

Advanced Cardiovascular Life Support Provider Manual. (2006). Dallas, TX: American Heart Association.

Arnsdorf, M.F. & Ganz, L.I. (2006). Catheter ablation for ventricular arrhythmias. *UptoDate.* Retrieved January 23, 2007, from www.uptodate.com

Arnsdorf, M.F., Morrissey, W., & Wilber, D. (2006). Catheter ablation for AV nodal reentrant tachycardia (junctional reciprocating tachycardia). *UptoDate.* Retrieved January 23, 2007, from www.uptodate.com

Arnsdorf, M.F. & Ganz, L.I. (2005). General principles of the implantable cardioverter-defibrillator. *UpToDate.* Retrieved December 14, 2005, from www.uptodate.com

Barold, S.S., Stroobandt, R.X., & Sinnaeve, A.F. (2004). *Cardiac pacemakers step by step.* Malden, MA: Blackwell Futura.

Blancher, S. (2005). Cardiac electrophysiology procedures. In S.L. Woods, E.S. Froelicher, S.U. Motzer, & E J. Bridges (Eds.), *Cardiac nursing* (5th ed.). Philadelphia: Lippincott.

Cheng, J. & Arnsdorf, M.F. (2006). Maintenance of sinus rhythm after cardioversion in atrial flutter. *UptoDate.* Retrieved Jamuary 23, 2007, from www.uptodate.com

Ganz, L.I. (2006). Catheter ablation of cardiac arrhythmias: Overview and technical aspects. *UptoDate.* Retrieved January 23, 2007, from www.uptodate.com

Gregoratos, G., Abrams, J., Epstein, A.E., Freedman, R.A., Hayes, D.L., Hlatky, M.A., et al. (2002). ACC/AHA/NASPE 2002 guideline update for implantation of cardiac pacemakers and antiarrhythmia devices: summary article. *Circulation, 106,* 2145-2161.

Hayes, D.L. (2006). Modes of cardiac pacing: Nomenclature and selection. *UptoDate.* Retrieved January 8, 2007, from www.uptodate.com

Chapter 17

Jacobson, C. & Gerity, D. (2005). Pacemakers and implantable defibrillators. In S.L. Woods, E.S. Froelicher, S.U. Motzer, & E.J. Bridges (Eds.), *Cardiac Nursing* (5th ed., pp. 709-755). Philadelphia: Lippincott Williams & Wilkins.

Jacobson, C. (2006). Advanced ECG concepts. In M. Chulay & S.M. Burns (Eds.), *AACN Essentials of critical care nursing* (pp. 391-430). New York: McGraw-Hill.

Kenny, T. (2005). *The nuts and bolts of cardiac pacing.* Malden, MA: Blackwell Futura.

Kenny, T. (2006). *The nuts and bolts of ICD therapy.* Malden, MA: Blackwell Futura.

Knight, B.P. (2006). Nonpharmacologic therapy of arrhythmias associated with the Wolff-Parkinson-White syndrome. *UptoDate.* Retrieved January 23, 2007, from www.uptodate.com

Levine, P.A. (2004). Dual chamber pacing system malfunction: evaluation and management. Retrieved 2005, from www.uptodate.com

Levine, P.A. (2004). Normal dual pacing system arrhythmias. Retrieved August 3, 2005, from www.uptodate.com

Podrid, P.J. (2005). Basic principles and technique of cardioversion and defibrillation. Retrieved August 11, 2005, from www.uptodate.com

Saxon, L.A., Kumar, U.N., & DeMarco, T. (2005). Cardiac resynchronization therapy (biventricular pacing) in heart failure. Retrieved August 3, 2005, from www.uptodate.com

Sljapic, T.N. & Bharucha, D.B. (2004). Driving restrictions in patients with an implantable cardioverter-defibrillator. *UpToDate.* Retrieved December 14, 2005, from www.uptodate.com

Strickberger, S.A., Conti, J., Daoud, E., Havranek, E., Mehra, M.R., Pina, I.L., et al. (2005). Patient selection for cardiac resynchronization therapy. *Circulation, 111,* 2146-2150.

Zipes, D.P., Camm, J.A., Borggrefe, M., Buxton, A.E., Chaitman, B., Fromer, M., et al. (2006). ACC/AHA/ESC 2006 guidelines for management of patients with ventricular arrhythmias and the prevention of sudden cardiac death – executive summary: a report of the American College of Cardiology/American Heart Association Task Force and the European Society of Cardiology Committee for Practice Guidelines. *Circulation, 114,* 1088-1132.

CHAPTER 18:
NON CARDIAC ISSUES IN THE CARDIAC PATIENT:
Pulmonary Pathophysiology, Electrolytes and Renal, Sepsis

PULMONARY PATHOPHYSIOLOGY
Acute Respiratory Failure

Acute respiratory failure is the failure of the respiratory system to provide for the exchange of oxygen and carbon dioxide between the environment and tissues in quantities sufficient to sustain life.

There are 2 types of acute respiratory failure: Oxygenation failure and ventilatory failure.

Type I Acute Respiratory Failure: Oxygenation Failure

◆ Hypoxemic but normocapnic
  ❖ Low PaO_2.
  ❖ Normal $PaCO_2$.
  ❖ Widened A-a gradient.
◆ Pathophysiology
  ❖ Significant diffusion defect.
  ❖ V/Q mismatching, resulting in intrapulmonary shunting.
  ❖ Untreated alveolar hypoventilation.
◆ Etiologies
  ❖ Pneumonia.
  ❖ Pulmonary edema.
  ❖ Pleural effusion.
  ❖ ARDS.
  ❖ High altitude.

Type II Acute Respiratory Failure: Ventilatory Failure

◆ Hypoxemic and Hypercapnic
  ❖ Low PaO_2.
  ❖ High $PaCO_2$.
  ❖ Normal A-a gradient.
◆ Pathophysiology
  ❖ Hypoventilation leading to hypercapnia.
  ❖ Hypercapnea results in acidemia.
◆ Etiologies
  ❖ CNS depressant drugs.
  ❖ Neuromuscular abnormalities.
  ❖ Spinal cord injury.
  ❖ Chest trauma.

Chapter 18

- ❖ Restrictive lung disease (decreased compliance).
- ❖ Acute exacerbation of obstructive lung disease (increased airway resistance).
- ❖ Increased dead space
  - ☆ Decreased cardiac output.
  - ☆ Pulmonary emboli.
  - ☆ High airway pressure (hyperinflated alveoli compress pulmonary capillaries).

Treatment

Treatment strategies include treating the underlying cause and providing support for ventilation and oxygenation. Patients with Type I respiratory failure may need to be intubated and placed on a ventilator in order to deliver PEEP and other treatments to support adequate oxygenation.

Indications for Ventilator Support

- ◆ Apnea.
- ◆ Acute Ventilatory Failure.
  - ❖ $PaCO_2 > 50$ and pH < 7.30.
- ◆ Impending Acute Ventilatory Failure.
- ◆ Severe Refractory Hypoxemia.
  - ❖ $PaO_2 < 60$ ($SaO_2 < 90\%$) with $FIO_2 > 60\%$.
- ◆ Clinical signs of increased work of breathing.

Criteria for Weaning from Ventilator

- ◆ Alert.
- ◆ Stable vital signs.
- ◆ Intact gag reflex.
- ◆ Arterial $PaO_2 > 60$ mm Hg on $FIO_2 < 0.50$ and PEEP of 0 to 5 cm of H_2O.
- ◆ Ventilation status.
  - ❖ Respiratory rate: < 30 per minute.
  - ❖ Tidal volume: > 5 ml/kg.
  - ❖ Rapid shallow breathing index (respiratory rate/tidal volume): < 100 breaths/min/L.
  - ❖ Vital capacity: > 10 ml/kg, ideally 15 ml/kg.
  - ❖ Minute ventilation: < 10 L.
  - ❖ Negative inspiratory force of at least -25 to -30 cm H_2O.

Spontaneous breathing trials are the most effective strategy for ventilator weaning. Chapter 3 discusses more detailed information about ventilator management.

Chronic Obstructive Pulmonary Disease (COPD)

- ◆ COPD includes the disorders of emphysema, chronic bronchitis, and small airway disease.
- ◆ Asthma also contains an obstructive component, but is no longer classified as COPD.
- ◆ Obstructive disease causes resistance to airflow and therefore alters effective ventilation. The work of breathing is increased.
- ◆ Decreased expiratory airflow is central to COPD pathophysiology and, as a result, residual volume, functional residual capacity, and total lung capacity can increase. Expiratory airflow (FEV) in one second (FEV_1) is measured by spirometry.

Non Cardiac Issues in the Cardiac Patient: Pulmonary Pathophysiology, Electrolytes and Renal, Sepsis

◆ COPD also involves chronic inflammation of all structures of the lungs including airways, lung parenchyma, and the pulmonary vasculature.

   ❖ White blood cells including neutrophils, macrophages, and T lymphocytes invade various parts of the lung. Inflammatory mediators are released from these cells.

   ❖ Inflammatory cells in the epithelium of the central airways cause edema, enlargement of mucous secreting glands, and an increased number of goblet cells (Fernandez, 2003). This results in excessive mucous secretion and ciliary dysfunction.

   ❖ Chronic inflammation in the peripheral airways leads to repeated damage and repair of the airways, resulting in destruction of the lung parenchyema, which then leads to pulmonary hyperinflation, and impaired gas exchange.

   ❖ Vascular changes lead to thickening of the vessel wall. Pulmonary hypertension and subsequent acute cor pulmonale can develop.

Emphysema

◆ Attacks alveolar walls and the elastic tissue support of small airways.

◆ The destruction of alveolar walls results in a decreased surface area for gas exchange.

◆ Inward elastic recoil is diminished, airway collapse and gas trapping occur.

◆ There is enlargement of air spaces distal to the terminal bronchioles. Elasticity and lung volumes are changed, and resistance of airways is increased.

◆ Air sacs are replaced by bullae.

◆ Resistance to blood flow is also increased because many alveolar walls have been destroyed with a subsequent loss of pulmonary capillaries.

◆ Alveolar hypoventilation: leads to hypercapnea, alveolar hypoxia and eventual arterial hypoxemia.

Chronic Bronchitis

◆ Mucous glands hypertrophy in response to tobacco smoke. There is excessive mucous production in the bronchial tree; excessive sputum production results. Tobacco smoke also damages cilia, and a cough is therefore necessary to clear excess sputum.

◆ Chronic inflammation causes swelling of the bronchial walls; excessive secretions can block airways.

◆ A diagnosis of chronic bronchitis is made when a patient has a chronic cough and sputum production on a daily basis for a minimum of three months a year, and not less than two consecutive years (Ellstrom, 2006).

Risk Factors and Exacerbations

Smoking is the primary risk factor for the development of COPD, although only a small percentage of smokers actually develop chronic bronchitis or emphysema as a result of smoking (Fernandez, 2003). Exacerbations of chronic bronchitis are usually related to an acute infection.

Clinical Presentation

◆ Cough and sputum production are the classic signs of chronic bronchitis.

◆ Dyspnea on exertion (progressing to dyspnea at rest) is the classic sign of emphysema. Patients with emphysema have an increased responsiveness to hypoxemia. Patients may be dyspneic with an adequate oxygen saturation.

807

Chapter 18

Clinical Implications

- Large lung volumes of COPD result in diminished breath sounds.
- COPD causes ventilation and perfusion mismatching.
- COPD results in hypoxemia and CO_2 retention.
- Chronic hypoxemia produces tissue hypoxia. In response, the kidneys release erythropoietin, which stimulates the bone marrow to produce more RBCs. Patients may have a dark red coloration of the skin from increased levels of hemoglobin.
- Patients may also have central cyanosis, which is a bluish coloring of conjunctivae of the eyes and the mucous membranes of the mouth. The skin will also be discolored in central cyanosis. (Note: In peripheral cyanosis, there is poor perfusion to the tissues. Oxygen saturation may be normal in peripheral cyanosis.) Central cyanosis is a result of arterial oxygen desaturation or as a result of the presence of an abnormal hemoglobin derivative. Central cyanosis results when there are 5 grams of desaturated hemoglobin per deciliter of blood. This is an absolute value; it is the amount of deoxygenated hemoglobin rather than the percentage. In the presence of anemia, the absolute amount of hemoglobin may be too low for central cyanosis to exist.
- COPD patients have more hypoxemia during sleep due to hypoventilation. Complications of nighttime hypoxemia include:
  - ❖ Increased pulmonary artery pressures.
  - ❖ Increased serum erythropoietin.
  - ❖ Increased ventricular arrhythmias.
  - ❖ Poor sleep quality.
  - ❖ Increased mortality when combined with CO_2 retention.
  - ❖ Right-sided heart failure is a result of COPD due to the increase in pulmonary vascular resistance.

Treatment

- Smoking cessation is the most important intervention.
- Pharmacology
  - ❖ Bronchodilators: Bronchodilators treat the reversible component of the airway obstruction in COPD. Bronchodilators decrease airway resistance, which decreases the work of breathing and improves ventilation. The effectiveness of bronchodilator therapy can be measured by spirometry, exercise tolerance, and quality of life.
    - ☆ Anticholinergics are the first-line medication in COPD maintenance therapy.
      - ✳ ipratropium (Atrovent).
    - ☆ Beta-agonists can be added if treatment with anticholinergics is not optimal.
      - ✳ Short acting
        - – racemic albuterol (Ventolin, Proventil, Accuneb).
        - – levalbuterol (Xopenex).
        - – metaproterenol (Alupent).
        - – pirbuterol (Exirel, Maxair).
      - ✳ Long acting
        - – salmeterol (Serevent).
        - – formoterol (Foradil, Oxeze).

Non Cardiac Issues in the Cardiac Patient: Pulmonary Pathophysiology, Electrolytes and Renal, Sepsis

☆ Theophylline is a long acting weak bronchodilator.
  ✱ Benefits
    – May have inotropic effect on diaphragm and decrease respiratory muscle fatigue.
    – Anti-inflammatory effect.
    – Increases mucocilliary clearance.
    – Increases central respiratory drive.
    – Improves exercise capacity (6-minute walk test).
    – Decreases night time declines in forced expiratory volume.
    – Decreases early morning respiratory symptoms.
  ✱ Cautions
    – Narrow therapeutic window.
    – Side effects can be serious: sleep disturbances, changes in mood, decrease in short term memory.
    (Fernandez, 2003)

❖ Antibiotics: Acute exacerbations of COPD can be caused by bacterial infections.

❖ Corticosteroids: Corticosteroids in the treatment of COPD remains controversial, but they are frequently used in treating exacerbations. Steroids are used as part of chronic treatment in some patients. Corticosteroids can also be combined with other medications.
  ☆ budesonide (Pulmicort)
  ☆ fluticasone and salmeterol (Advair)

❖ Expectorants/mucolytics.

◆ Oxygen: Arterial hypoxemia can exist in advanced COPD due to ventilation and perfusion mis-matching. Oxygen can improve survival in patients who are hypoxemic (Fernandez, 2003).

❖ Criteria for O_2 Administration
  ☆ Room air: PaO_2 < 55 mm Hg with saturation < 85%.
  ☆ PaO_2 56-59 and saturation 86-89%, with a qualifying secondary diagnosis.
    ✱ Pulmonary edema.
    ✱ Right-sided heart failure on ECG.
    ✱ Erythrocytosis with hematocrit > 56%.
    ✱ Drops in saturations during sleep or exercise.

❖ Goal of oxygen therapy is to obtain PaO_2 of 65-80 mm Hg while awake and at rest.

❖ Oxygen is typically delivered at 1-4 L/min via nasal cannula with an increase of 1 L during sleep and exercise.

❖ Oxygen should be given continuously at least 19 hours of each day.
(Fernandez, 2003)

◆ Pneumonia and influenza vaccines.

Treatment of Acute Exacerbation

◆ Conservative treatment is used whenever possible.

◆ Focus includes treating the underlying cause of exacerbation.

◆ Oxygen is used to treat hypoxemia. Hypercapnia is clinically better tolerated than hypoxemia.
  ❖ Oxygen is given to correct hypoxemia without interrupting hypoxic drive for ventilation (usually saturation between 90 and 92%).

Chapter 18

◆ Patient may require mechanical ventilation.
  ❖ Indications:
    ☆ Worsening of hypoxemia.
    ☆ Worsening of respiratory acidosis.
    ☆ Increased respiratory muscle fatigue.
    ☆ Decreased level of consciousness and non-arousable state.
  ❖ Avoid hyperventilation. Ventilate to a normal pH, but not to a normal CO_2 level. Many CO_2 retainers have developed renal compensation.

Obstructive Sleep Apnea

Obstructive sleep apnea can result in episodes of upper airway obstruction during sleep. Patients with obstructive sleep apnea also experience daytime drowsiness. The effect of obstructive sleep apnea is altered cardiopulmonary function. This altered cardiopulmonary function places patients at risk for:

◆ Diurnal hypertension.
◆ Nocturnal dysrhythmias.
◆ Pulmonary hypertension.
◆ Hypoxemia.
◆ Hypercapnia.
◆ Right- and left-ventricular failure.
◆ MI.
◆ Stroke.

Continuous positive airway pressure (CPAP) is the most common treatment for obstructive sleep apnea. Patients should also be counseled regarding needed lifestyle changes, including smoking cessation, limiting alcohol, and losing weight.

Pulmonary Embolism

Pulmonary embolism (PE) is the obstruction of blood flow to one or more arteries of the lung by a thrombus (or other emboli – fat, air, amniotic fluid) lodged in a pulmonary vessel. The lower lobes of the lung are frequently affected. The mortality associated with undiagnosed PE is 30% (Sharma, 2006; Feied & Handler, 2006).

Risk Factors

Virchow's triad describes the three primary risk factors for the development of venous thrombosis: venous stasis, hypercoagulability, and injury to the vascular endothelium. These same three risk factors are the primary risk factors for the development of PE.

◆ Stasis of blood
  ❖ Prolonged immobilization after surgical procedures.
  ❖ Plaster casts.
  ❖ Venous obstruction.
  ❖ Heart failure.
  ❖ Shock.
  ❖ Hypovolemia.
  ❖ Varicose veins.
  ❖ Obesity.

Non Cardiac Issues in the Cardiac Patient: Pulmonary Pathophysiology, Electrolytes and Renal, Sepsis

◆ Hypercoagulability
 ❖ Polycythemia vera.
 ❖ Sickle cell disease.
 ❖ Malignancy.
 ❖ Pregnancy.
 ❖ Recent trauma.
 ❖ Oral contraceptives
◆ Injury to the vascular endothelium
 ❖ Central venous and arterial catheters.
 ❖ Phlebitis.

Pathophysiology

Pulmonary vascular resistance increases when emboli block blood flow. However, this increase is not as great as expected due to a rise in pulmonary artery pressure. When pulmonary artery pressure rises, some capillaries not previously open will be recruited and therefore reduce overall resistance to flow. In response to higher pressure, capillaries also distend and change to a more circular shape. Distention also lowers pulmonary vascular resistance.

◆ > 90% of thrombi develop in deep veins of lower extremities (iliofemoral system) (Ellstrom, 2006).
◆ Thrombi can also originate in the right side of the heart, pelvic veins, and axillary or subclavian veins. Another source of thrombus is around indwelling catheters.
◆ Thrombus formation leads to platelet adhesiveness and release of serotonin (vasoconstrictor).
◆ Dislodgement of thrombus
 ❖ Intravascular pressure changes (standing, massaging legs, fluid challenge, valsalva maneuver).
 ❖ Natural clot dissolution (7-10 days after development).
◆ Clot lodges in pulmonary vessels.
◆ Lower lobes of lungs have greatest amount of perfusion and therefore are more frequently affected.
◆ Ventilation continues but perfusion decreases.
 ❖ Increase in alveolar dead space.
 ❖ Alveolar CO_2 decreases, which causes bronchoconstriction and alveolar shrinking. This allows for more inspired air into the perfused alveoli.
◆ Overperfusion of uninvolved lung results in a decreased V/Q ratio.
◆ Decreased blood flow damages type II pneumocytes, which results in a decrease in surfactant production. This leads to atelectasis.
◆ Pulmonary edema can develop secondary to the damage caused by the pulmonary embolus.
◆ Hypoxemia can occur due to ventilation perfusion mismatching.
◆ An increased PVR can lead to pulmonary hypertension and potential acute cor pulmonale.
◆ Cardiogenic shock can occur as the result of right-ventricular failure.
◆ Pulmonary infarction is infrequent, but may occur.
 ❖ Is not common due to bronchial arterial collateral circulation.
 ❖ More common when a large embolus is involved, or when the patient has pre-existing lung disease.
 ❖ Infarction results in alveolar filling with RBCs and inflammatory cells.
 ❖ Infarction complicated by infection leads to abscess.

Chapter 18

Signs and Symptoms

◆ Medium-sized emboli
  ❖ Dyspnea.
  ❖ Substernal chest discomfort/pleuritic chest pain.
  ❖ Many non-specific signs
    ★ Tachypnea.
    ★ Tachycarida.
    ★ Rales.
  ❖ Accentuated 2nd heart sound.
◆ Large to massive is when 50% of pulmonary artery bed is occluded. Massive PE is one of the most common causes of unexpected death and is often not diagnosed until autopsy (Feied & Handler, 2006). Patients who do survive a massive PE are at risk for recurrent PE and the development of pulmonary hypertension and cor pulmonale.
  ❖ Signs and symptoms as described under medium-sized emboli can be present.
  ❖ Impending doom.
  ❖ Hypoxemia.
  ❖ Syncope.
  ❖ Signs and symptoms of right heart strain or right-ventricular failure
    ★ Hypotension.
    ★ Engorged neck veins.
    ★ Signs of right-ventricular strain on ECG.
  ❖ Sudden shock.
  ❖ Pulseless electrical activity.
◆ Pulmonary infarction
  ❖ Pleuritic chest pain.
  ❖ Dyspnea.
  ❖ Hemoptysis.
  ❖ Cough.
  ❖ Pleural friction rub.

Linking Knowledge to Practice

✔ *Many patients with PE have no obvious initial signs or symptoms, or have atypical signs and symptoms, and the diagnosis of PE is frequently missed. PE should be considered in any high-risk patient.*

Treatment

◆ Prevent thrombus formation with aggressive DVT prophylaxis in immobile and other high risk patients.
  ❖ Compression stockings that provide a 30-40 mm Hg or higher gradient.
    ★ Used for prophylaxis.
    ★ Used to prevent progression of known thrombus.
  ❖ Low molecular weight heparin.
◆ Fibrinolytic therapy
  ❖ Indicated in patients with hypotension (even if resolved), hypoxemia, or evidence of right-ventricular strain (Feied & Handler, 2006).

Non Cardiac Issues in the Cardiac Patient: Pulmonary Pathophysiology, Electrolytes and Renal, Sepsis

❖ Troponin levels can also be used to guide decision-making in patients with sub-massive PE. Elevated troponin levels in PE indicate worse short-term and long-term prognosis (Horlander & Leeper, 2003).

❖ Pulmonary embolectomy is a surgical option when fibrinolytic therapy is contraindicated.

◆ Heparin is the treatment of choice for reducing mortality in PE.

❖ Heparin should be initiated prior to a confirmed diagnosis.

❖ Slows or prevents clot progression and decreases risk of further emboli.

☆ Ongoing embolization of new thrombi is a major contributor to mortality.
(Sharma, 2006; Feied & Handler, 2006).

◆ Oxygen is indicated, even in the absence of hypoxemia because it can reduce pulmonary vascular resistance.

◆ Pulmonary vasodilators to help reduce pulmonary vascular resistance.

◆ Treat right-ventricular failure with fluids and inotropes.

◆ Warfarin

❖ Warfarin is continued for 3 to 6 months if there is identifiable reversible risk factor.

❖ Warfarin is continued for a minimum of 6 six months if there is no identifiable risk factor.

❖ Long term warfarin is indicated in patients with recurrent PE or in patients with ongoing risk factors.
(Sharma, 2006)

◆ Surgical interruption of inferior vena cava with a filter, such as a Greenfield filter.

❖ Patients with contraindication to anticoagulants.

❖ Recurrent thromboembolism despite anticoagulant.

❖ Survivor of massive PE wherein another PE would likely be fatal.

Linking Knowledge to Practice

✔ *Cardiopulmonary resuscitation (CPR) and advanced cardiac life support are not effective in cardiopulmonary arrest produced by massive PE due to the obstruction of blood flow and inability to circulate oxygenated blood to the brain and other organs. Emergency cardiopulmonary bypass may be a life-saving option in this circumstance.*

Special Considerations With Fat Emboli

◆ Risk Factors

❖ Skeletal trauma: femur and pelvis.

❖ Major orthopedic surgery.

❖ 24 to 72 hours post insult.

◆ Signs and Symptoms

❖ Vague chest pain.

❖ Shortness of breath.

❖ Sudden restlessness – drowsiness.

❖ Fever.

❖ Petechiae (transient – axillary or subconjunctival).

◆ Release of free fatty acids causes endothelial injury and toxic vasculitis.

◆ Hemorrhage into lungs (decrease H&H and platelets).

◆ CXR pattern similar to ARDS.

◆ Steroids.

Chapter 18

Special Considerations With Air Emboli

◆ Large volume of air into venous system.
◆ Risk Factors
  ❖ Dialysis.
  ❖ Pulmonary artery catheters.
  ❖ Surgical procedures.
  ❖ CABG.
◆ Symptoms
  ❖ Dyspnea, chest pain, agitation, confusion, cough.
◆ Treatment
  ❖ 100% oxygen
  ❖ Left lateral/trendelenburg.
  ❖ Positive pressure ventilation.
  ❖ Aspiration of air.

Cor Pulmonale

Cor pulmonale is enlargement of right ventricle (either dilation or hypertrophy) as a result of pulmonary pathology, including diseases of the lungs (COPD) or the pulmonary circulation (thromboembolic disease or primary pulmonary hypertension).

Pathophysiology

The initial pathophysiology involves an increase in pulmonary vascular resistance. As resistance increases and the pulmonary artery pressure rises, the workload of the right ventricle increases.

Clinical Manifestations

◆ Accentuated A wave of jugular venous pulsation and prominent V wave on right atrial tracing from tricuspid regurgitation.
◆ Palpable left parasternal lift (Fernandez & Yanakakis, 2003).
◆ Accentuated pulmonic component of S2.
◆ Right-sided S4.
◆ Murmurs of tricuspid and pulmonic insufficiency.
◆ Right-sided abnormalities manifested by echocardiography, MRI, radionuclide studies, or right-sided cardiac catheterization.
◆ ECG criteria for right-ventricular hypertrophy.
  ❖ Right axis deviation or rightward axis shift
  ❖ Right atrial enlargement (tall P waves in lead II or dominant first 1/2 of P wave in V$_1$).
  ❖ RBBB.
  ❖ Right precordial T wave inversion.
  ❖ Delayed intrinsicoid deflection (measured from beginning of QRS complex to peak of R wave) in right precordial leads.
◆ Signs of right-sided heart failure.
  ❖ Jugular venous distention.
  ❖ Hepatomegaly.
  ❖ Peripheral edema.

Non Cardiac Issues in the Cardiac Patient: Pulmonary Pathophysiology, Electrolytes and Renal, Sepsis

Treatment

◆ Oxygen (pulmonary vasodilator) to decrease pulmonary vascular resistance and improve right-ventricular stroke volume.

◆ Diuretics if congested.

◆ Vasodilators can improve cardiac output but can also have adverse effects.
   ❖ Systemic hypotension (compromising coronary perfusion pressure).
   ❖ Blunting of hypoxic pulmonary vasoconstriction.

◆ Pulmonary specific vasodilators.
   ❖ IV
      ☆ Nitroglycerin.
      ☆ Sodium nitroprusside (Nipride).
      ☆ Prostaglandins (PGE1, PGI2).
      ☆ PDE1 (phosphodiesterase enzyme).
   ❖ Inhaled
      ☆ Any of the above IV medications.
      ☆ Nitric oxide.
      ☆ Prostacyclin (PGI2, Epoprostenol, Flolan) or derivative Iloprost.

◆ Inotropes may also be used with vasodilators.

◆ Phlebotomy may be used if polycythemia is present (hematocrit > 60%).

Pulmonary Edema

Pulmonary edema is the presence of extravascular accumulation of fluid in the lungs.

Pathophysiology

The lymphatic system can adjust to remove up to ten times the normal amount of fluid during pathological conditions. When the level of fluid exceeds this amount and cannot be removed by lymph drainage, then pulmonary edema occurs.

Fluid accumulates first in the interstitium, then in the alveoli because the capillary endothelium is more permeable to water and solute than the alveolar endothelium. Fluid in the interstitium is removed by the lymphatic system.

Pulmonary edema can be classified as cardiogenic or non cardiogenic. Cardiogenic pulmonary edema is accompanied by an elevated pulmonary artery occlusive pressure (PAOP). Non cardiogenic pulmonary edema is diagnosed when pulmonary edema exists in the presence of a normal PAOP. Non cardiogenic pulmonary edema is seen with acute lung injury and acute respiratory distress syndrome and is discussed later in this chapter.

Risk Factors

◆ Increase in pulmonary capillary hydrostatic pressure (cardiogenic pulmonary edema).
   ❖ Left ventricular failure.
   ❖ Increased fluid administration.
   ❖ Loss of atrial kick.
   ❖ Occlusion of pulmonary veins.

Chapter 18

- ◆ Loss of the integrity of the capillary endothelium and altered permeability.
  - ❖ Infections.
  - ❖ Circulating or inhaled toxins.
  - ❖ Oxygen toxicity.
- ◆ Additional Factors
  - ❖ Decrease in plasma colloidal osmotic pressure (hypoproteinemia, over administration of hypotonic solutions).
  - ❖ Blockage of lymphatic drainage system (tumor).
  - ❖ Post pneumonectomy (same amount of blood from right ventricle but less pulmonary vasculature).

Linking Knowledge to Practice

✔ *Pulmonary edema results in impaired diffusion of oxygen, which can lead to hypoxemia. Pulmonary edema also decreases lung compliance and can impair ventilation.*

Treatment

The pharmacological treatment of cardiogenic pulmonary edema is discussed in Chapter 9 in the section on acute decompensated heart failure and also in Chapter 4 in the section on cardiogenic shock. The treatment of non-cardiogenic pulmonary edema is discussed below in the section on acute respiratory distress syndrome.

Pneumonia

Pneumonia is inflammation caused by an acute infection of the lung parenchyma, including alveolar spaces and interstitial space.

Causes

- ◆ Bacteria (bacteria are different for community-acquired versus hospital-acquired).
- ◆ Virus.
- ◆ Fungi.
- ◆ Parasites.
- ◆ Mycoplasma.

Many normal protective mechanisms are in place in the pulmonary system and the general immune system to prevent the acquisition of pneumonia. A breakdown of these protective mechanisms or exposure to a very virulent agent, even with normal protective mechanisms, can lead to pneumonia.

Risk Factors for Acute Bacterial Pneumonia

- ◆ Previous viral respiratory infection.
- ◆ Gastro esophageal reflux disease (GERD).
- ◆ Chronic alcohol abuse.
- ◆ Cigarette smoking.
- ◆ Decreased level of consciousness.
- ◆ Anesthesia.
- ◆ Intubation.
- ◆ Lung disease.

Non Cardiac Issues in the Cardiac Patient: Pulmonary Pathophysiology, Electrolytes and Renal, Sepsis

◆ Diabetes mellitus.
◆ Use of corticorsteroids.
◆ Elderly.
(Schwarz, 2003)

Linking Knowledge to Practice

✔ *The use of deep breathing, incentive spirometry, and early ambulation is key to the prevention of pneumonia in postoperative patients.*

Pathophysiology

◆ Causative agent is inhaled or enters pharynx via direct contact.
◆ Alveoli become inflamed.
◆ Alveolar spaces fill with exudate and consolidate.
◆ Diffusion of O_2 obstructed ➤ hypoxemia.
◆ Goblet cells are stimulated to increase mucous ➤ increased airway resistance and work of breathing (ventilation problem).

Causative Agents

Common agents in community-acquired pneumonia in the generally younger and healthier population include:
◆ Streptococcus pneumoniae (most common agent in community acquired pneumonia).
◆ Mycoplasma pneumoniae.
◆ Chlamydia pneumoniae.
◆ Viral.

Haemophilus influenza is a common cause among smokers and *Klebsiella pneumoniae* may be a cause of community-acquired pneumonia in patients with chronic alcoholism.

Agents causing community-acquired pneumonia in the older population with more co-morbidities commonly include gram negative bacilli such as:
◆ *Moraxella catarrhalis* (particularly common in patients with chronic bronchitis).
◆ *Staphylococcus aureus* (in the setting of post viral influenza).
(Schwarz, 2003; Cunha, 2007)

Methicillin-resistant *Staphylococcus aureus* (MRSA) has also emerged in recent years as a cause of community-acquired pneumonia.

Clinical Presentation

◆ Flu-like symptoms.
◆ Pleuritic chest pain.
◆ Confusion in elderly.
◆ Tachycardia, tachypnea, fever.
◆ Crackles and wheezes.
◆ Productive cough.
◆ Clinical signs of dehydration.

The clinical presentation in the elderly may be more subtle including confusion, dehydration, and fever. This subtle presentation in the elderly makes diagnosis more difficult. Mortality rates for pneumonia in the elderly are higher, so accurate diagnosis and treatment are essential to preventing adverse outcomes.

Diagnosis

- The sputum gram stain is an important diagnostic tool. The results of the sputum gram stain guide the decision for initial antibiotic therapy.
- Sputum culture can be falsely positive due to oral pharyngeal contamination.
- Blood cultures are used to diagnose coexisting bacteremia. (Co-existing bacteremia is not present in the majority of patients with pneumonia.)
- Leukocytosis.
- Shift to left of WBCs.
- Blood gases/oxygen saturation show problems with arterial oxygen saturation. PCO_2 may also be elevated due to increased airway resistance from secretions.
- Chest x-ray – produces variable results but infiltrates are frequently seen on a chest x-ray (Figure 18.1). A chest CT may also be used to aid in the diagnosis of pneumonia.

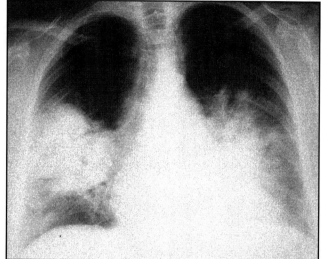

Figure 18.1: Infiltrates on chest x-ray.

Leukocytosis and a left shift of the white blood cell count is expected in the presence of bacterial pneumonia. Failure of the white blood cell count to rise in the presence of a bacterial infection is associated with an increased mortality rate (Schwarz, 2003). The failure of the white blood cell count to rise is seen more commonly in the immuno-suppressed, elderly, and alcoholics.

Complications

- Abscesses may form and rupture into pleural space leading to pneumothorax and/or empyema.
  - Video assisted thoracoscopy with debridement is a treatment option for empyema in the early organizing phase.
  - Full thoracotomy with decortication may be necessary in later organizing phases.
- Pleural Effusion.
- Acute respiratory failure.
- ARDS.
- Sepsis.

Mortality rates for nosocomial or hospital-acquired pneumonia are higher than those for community-acquired pneumonia.

Nosocomial (Hospital-Acquired) Pneumonia

Nosocomial pneumonia is typically caused by bacterial agents that are more resistant to antibiotic therapy.

Causative agents associated with nosocomial pneumonia:

- Aerobic gram negative rods
  - Klebsiella sp.
  - Psuedomonas sp.
  - Enterobacter sp.
  - Escherichia coli.
  - Proteus sp.

❖ Serratia sp.

❖ Enterococci.

◆ *Staphylococcus aureus* (including methicillin-resistant Staphylococcus aureus [MRSA]).

◆ Group B streptococci.

Sources

◆ Contamination of pharynx and perhaps stomach with bacteria (an increase in the pH of the stomach allows for bacterial overgrowth).

❖ Repeated small aspirations of oral pharyngeal secretions.

❖ Retrograde contamination from GI tract.

High Risk Patient Characteristics

◆ Intubation or ICU admission.

◆ Previous antibiotic use.

◆ Post operative condition.

◆ Chronic lung disease.

◆ Renal insufficiency.

◆ Elderly.

(Schwarz, 2003)

Strategies to Prevent Ventilator-Acquired Pneumonia

◆ Hand hygiene.

◆ Oral care (teeth brushing with tooth brush; use of chlorhexidine oral rinse in high risk patients).

◆ HOB elevated 30 to 40 degrees.

◆ Suction only when necessary (not routine).

◆ Routine installation of NS not recommended.

◆ Cover yankauer catheters when not in use.

◆ Ventilator circuit changes only when soiled or every week.

◆ Adequate endotracheal tube cuff pressure.

◆ Subglottic suctioning prior to repositioning or deflating cuff.

◆ Hold tube feeding for residuals > 150 cc.

◆ Discontinue nasogastric tubes as soon as possible.

◆ Extubate as soon as possible.

◆ Avoid nasal intubation.

◆ Stress ulcer prophylaxis with sucralfate (rather than with agents that increase gastric pH) may decrease risk of pneumonia.

◆ Avoid overuse of antibiotics.

Treatment

◆ Prevent nosocomial infections.

◆ Timely antibiotics.

◆ Hydration (monitor electrolytes).

◆ Deep breathing/incentive spirometry.

◆ Bronchodilators, expectorants, mucolytics.

◆ Avoid sedatives and antitussives.

◆ Early activity and mobility.

Chapter 18

Aspiration

Aspiration can result from vomiting or regurgitation. Vomiting is an active process, but regurgitation is a passive process that can occur even in the presence of paralyzed muscles. Laryngeal and cough reflexes protect from aspiration into the tracheobronchial tree. Patients with impaired reflexes, particularly the elderly and the critically ill, are at risk for aspiration.

Swallowing impairment is common in the elderly and in those who have had a prolonged illness. Silent aspiration may occur and go unrecognized until the later development of aspiration pneumonia. A swallowing evaluation can be used to determine the risk for aspiration. There is limited research regarding strategies to prevent aspiration in those at high risk and some strategies may be more effective with particular types of dysphagia. A few selected strategies that may be beneficial include:

◆ Avoiding sedation.
◆ Resting prior to meal time.
◆ Eating slowly.
◆ Flexing the head slightly to the "chin down" position.
◆ Determining food viscosity best tolerated (thickening liquids will improve swallowing in some patients).

Aspiration of a liquid has different results, depending on the pH of the liquid. Large volumes of acidic liquid – or any volume of very acidic liquid – will result in acute lung injury. The acid results in a chemical burn and type II surfactant-producing alveolar cells are destroyed. This results in an increase in pulmonary capillary permeability and an accumulation of blood and fluid in the alveolar space. When fluid is in the alveolar space, there is less room for air, resulting in a decreased V/Q ratio. Lung compliance is also decreased. More severe chemical burns can result in pulmonary hemorrhage or necrosis. Acidic fluid may also result in bronchospasm. Non-acidic aspirations are more transient and reversible compared to acidic aspirations.

The aspiration of a large particle will result in airway obstruction. The aspiration of smaller particles results in a sub acute inflammatory process and hemorrhage. Patients can have extensive hemorrhagic pneumonia within 6 hours of aspiration. Aspiration of material significantly contaminated with bacteria can be fatal (Ellstrom, 2006).

Acute Respiratory Distress Syndrome (ARDS)

Definition: A syndrome of acute respiratory failure characterized by non-cardiac pulmonary edema and manifested by refractory hypoxemia. ARDS does not include mild or early acute lung injury, but rather involves severe and diffused lung injury.

Risk Factors

◆ Sepsis (most common).
◆ Transfusion.
◆ Aspiration.
◆ Trauma.
◆ Massive transfusion.
◆ Pancreatitis.
(Turki & Parsons, 2003)

Pathophysiology

◆ Predisposing insult to lungs, resulting in acute lung injury.
  ❖ Direct lung injury
    ☆ Chest trauma.
    ☆ Near drowning.
    ☆ Smoke inhalation.
    ☆ Pneumonia.
    ☆ Pulmonary embolism.
  ❖ Indirect lung injury
    ☆ Sepsis.
    ☆ Shock.
    ☆ Multi-system trauma.
    ☆ Burns.
    ☆ CABG.
    ☆ Head injury.
◆ Acute lung injury causes stimulation of inflammatory and immune systems.
◆ Cells release toxic substances, causing micro vascular injury.
◆ Pulmonary capillary membranes (microvascular endothelium and alveolar type I epithelial cells) are damaged, resulting in an increase in capillary permeability.
◆ Protein containing fluid, inflammatory cells, and inflammatory cytokines leak into interstitium and alveolar spaces, causing pulmonary edema and rapidly progressive hypoxemia.
◆ Impaired production and dysfunction of surfactant.
◆ Alveolar collapse and massive atelectasis.
◆ Blood passes past atelectatic and fluid-filled lung units that are unable to participate in gas exchange, which results in poorly oxygenated blood returning to the left side of the heart. This is called intrapulmonary shunting.
◆ Pulmonary capillaries constrict to redirect blood away from poorly ventilated alveoli. This increases pulmonary vascular resistance.
◆ Fluid-filled and collapsed alveoli decrease the compliance of lung tissue and require high-peak inspiratory pressures to ventilate the lungs.
◆ Potential development of pulmonary fibrosis in chronic phase.
  ❖ Endothelium and epithelium expand.
  ❖ Interstitial space expands due to edema.
  ❖ Protein exudate inside the alveoli produces a hyaline membrane. This destroys the normal structure of the alveoli.

ARDS develops within 24 to 72 hours of initial predisposing insult.

Diagnostic Criteria

◆ Predisposing condition.
◆ PaO_2/FIO_2 ratio < 200.
◆ Chest x-ray: Diffuse bilateral infiltrates.
  (Chest CT may also be used.)

Chapter 18

◆ Decreased static compliance of lungs.

◆ PAOP < 18 mm Hg or no evidence of increased left-atrial pressure.

◆ No evidence of COPD.

◆ No other explanation for above.

Treatment

◆ It is important to avoid over-hydration in patients with ARDS because pulmonary edema is present. However, the appropriate fluid management strategy in ARDS is complex. The reason for the complexity is because of the co-existing right-ventricular effects in the presence of ARDS. The right ventricle often requires more fluid to provide the left ventricle with adequate preload. Inadequate fluid can result in a low left-ventricular preload and a decrease in tissue oxygen delivery. A conservative approach must be balanced with the need to protect end-organ perfusion. The ARDS Network Fluid Management Trial showed that a conservative fluid management strategy improved lung function and decreased the number of mechanical ventilator days (MacIntyre, 2006). Current practice in the management of ARDS often reflects a more liberal fluid management strategy. A more conservative fluid strategy reduces lung edema and improves the rate of lung recovery (MacIntyre, 2006). A pulmonary artery catheter may be of benefit when fluid balance is unclear or the patient has complicating factors, such as hypotension or low urine output. End-organ perfusion must always be the highest priority. More aggressive fluid management may be needed in the initial stages of the systemic inflammatory response system due to the systemic vasodilation.

◆ There is no evidence that the use of steroids reduces mortality in ARDS, and therefore the routine use of corticosteroids is not indicated in the treatment of ARDS. In addition, starting steroids longer than 2 weeks after the onset of ARDS may actually worsen outcomes (Steinberg, et al., 2006).

Mechanical Ventilator Management Strategies

There are several goals for mechanical ventilator therapy in ARDS.

◆ Prevent further injury to lung tissue.

◆ Prevent collapse or derecruitment of alveoli.

◆ Open (or recruit) fluid-filled collapsed alveoli.

Repetitive decruitment of alveoli with the need to re-open results in ventilator induced lung injury. When utilizing lung recruitment strategies it is important to understand the changes in lung tissue in ARDS. Different regions of the lung have different critical opening pressures in ARDS. Positive airway pressure must rise above the critical opening pressure before any air can enter the alveoli. Critical opening pressures are influenced by surface tension. Surface tension is adversely affected by a decrease in surfactant.

For these reasons, an airway pressure may be insufficient to overcome the critical opening pressure in one region, but may be an excessive amount of pressure in another healthier region. The over distention of healthy lung tissue can also cause ventilator-induced lung injury. An overall ventilator strategy includes limiting over distention of healthy lung units and preventing repetitive collapse and re-expansion of unhealthy lung units.

It is often difficult to fully recruit unhealthy lung units without over distending healthy lung units. Patients with ARDS may need a less than optimal PaO_2 ratio in order to protect healthy lung units.

◆ Lower tidal volume ventilation ($\leq$ 6ml/kg) as a lung protective strategy.

❖ Prevent over distention of healthy lung tissue.

❖ May require permissive hypercapnia due to lower tidal volume ventilation.

Non Cardiac Issues in the Cardiac Patient: Pulmonary Pathophysiology, Electrolytes and Renal, Sepsis

❖ Limit ventilatory support to prevent over distention of lung.

❖ Lower tidal volume ventilation was associated with decreased mortality in ARDS Network's study (Burns, 2005).

◆ Maintaining plateau pressure at < 30 cm H_2O as a lung protective strategy.

◆ PEEP to prevent decruitment of alveoli by maintaining end expiratory pressure and avoiding end expiratory alveolar collapse. Determining the appropriate level of PEEP to prevent derecruitment is a clinical challenge. Generally, the optimal level of PEEP is considered the PEEP that provides optimal oxygenation without compromising cardiac output.

◆ Higher levels of PEEP can also be used for lung recruitment. Other recruitment strategies can also be considered, such as a high level of CPAP for a short period of time. In this recruitment strategy, 30 to 40 cm H_2O CPAP is applied for up to 1 to 2 minutes. Increased sedation may be required for patients to tolerate recruitment maneuvers. Recruitment measures always carry the potential risk of over distending healthy lung tissue.

◆ Inverse I:E pressure control ventilation, airway pressure release ventilation (APRV), and high frequency oscillation are modes of mechanical ventilation focused on recruitment. These modes are referred to as open lung strategies and focus on the mean airway pressure.

◆ Independent lung ventilation may be required when there are vast differences between the lung tissue compliance of each lung.

◆ Extracorporeal membrane oxygenation (ECMO).

Positioning

◆ Proning while on mechanical ventilation has physiological benefit. Research continues to be conducted to validate improved outcomes.

❖ In the supine position in ARDS, higher critical pressures are required to open alveoli in the dependent areas of the lung. These higher pressures may over distend the alveoli in the upper areas of the lung. In addition, perfusion is greatest in the dependent areas of the lung. If alveoli are not open in the dependent areas of the lung, then V/Q mismatching occurs.

❖ The most important benefit is improved ventilation and perfusion matching by reducing the gradient between gravity dependent and non-dependent areas of the lung by moving the heart and abdominal structures away from the spine.

❖ Proning stiffens the chest wall and helps limit regional over distention.

❖ Proning may also improve the use of the muscles of the diaphragm by promoting a more natural curvature of the diaphragm.

❖ Suctioning may be required immediately after proning due to the mobilization of secretions.

❖ Preventing pressure injury to facial structures is a key nursing consideration in proning.

❖ The duration of proning remains controversial, but most protocols provide for at least 12 of 24 hours in the prone position.

❖ Proning has been shown to improve oxygenation, but further research is needed to confirm the benefit in terms of mortality reduction.

(MacIntyre, 2004).

The use of protocols to guide the weaning process results in improved clinical outcomes in ARDS patients (Burns, 2005).

Chapter 18

Clinical Implications/Complications

Many deaths in ARDS are a result of the initial insult causing lung injury. The focus of prevention lies in preventing the initial insult. Many deaths that occur after the development of ARDS are due to infection. The diagnosis of pneumonia in patients with ARDS is often difficult. Patients with ARDS without pneumonia may have fever, leukocytosis and purulent sputum. The overall mortality with ARDS can be as high as 40% (Turki & Parsons, 2003). Survivors of ARDS are left with a wide range of pulmonary dysfunction, ranging from none to severe. Most survivors are left with mild to moderate pulmonary dysfunction (Turki & Parsons, 2003).

Pneumothorax

A pneumothorax occurs when intrapleural space loses its negative pressure (by exposure to atmospheric pressure), and the lung collapses.

Closed (Simple) Pneumothorax (Figure 18.2)

- Air enters the intrapleural space through the lung, causing partial or total collapse of the lung.
- Possible etiology
    - Blunt trauma (lung laceration by rib fracture).
    - Positive pressure ventilation.
    - Tracheostomy.
    - Transthoracic needle aspiration procedures.
    - Subclavian needle sticks.
    - Thoracentesis.
    - Pleural or lung biopsies.
    - Post operative complication of lung resection/pneumonectomy (contralateral pneumothorax).
    - Cardiopulmonary resuscitation.
    - Spontaneous pneumothorax may occur in younger adults, typically under the age of 40 years.
        - ☆ Smoking increases the risk for spontaneous pneumothorax.
- Pathophysiology
    - Disruption of normal negative intrapleural pressure.
    - Lung collapse.
    - Decreased surface area for gas exchange.
    - Acute respiratory failure.
- Signs and Symptoms
    - Chest pain.
    - Dyspnea.
    - Asymmetrical chest excursion.
    - Diminished to absent breath sounds on affected side.
    - Dramatic increases in peak inspiratory pressures on a mechanical ventilator.
- Treatment
    - Oxygen.
    - Position.

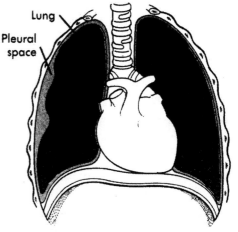

Figure 18.2: Closed (simple) pneumothorax.
From *Pass CCRN* (2nd ed.), by R.D. Dennison, 2000, St. Louis: Mosby. Reprinted with permission from Elsevier.

- ❖ Analgesics.
- ❖ Chest tube is required for pneumonthorax ≥ approximately 15%, or if the patient is symptomatic.

Tension Pneumothorax (Figure 18.3)

- ◆ Accumulation of air into the pleural space without a means of escape causes complete lung collapse and potential mediastinal shift.
- ◆ Potential etiology
  - ❖ Blunt trauma.
  - ❖ Positive pressure mechanical ventilation.
  - ❖ Clamped or clotted water seal drainage system.
  - ❖ Airtight dressing on open pneumothorax.
- ◆ Pathophysiology
  - ❖ Air rushes in – cannot escape pleural space.
  - ❖ Creates positive pressure in pleural space.
  - ❖ Ipsalateral lung collapse.
  - ❖ Mediastinal shift ⇨ contralateral lung compression ⇨ potential tearing of thoracic aorta.
  - ❖ Can also compress heart ⇨ decrease RV filling ⇨ shock.
- ◆ Treatment
  - ❖ Similar to closed pneumothorax.
  - ❖ If mediastinal shift may need to treat shock.
  - ❖ Oxygen (100%).
  - ❖ Emergency decompression.
  - ❖ Chest tube.
- ◆ Other as with closed pneumothorax.

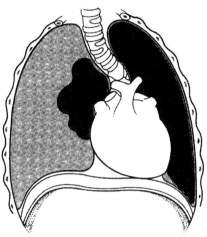

Figure 18.3: Tension pneumothorax.
From *Pass CCRN* (2nd ed.), by R.D. Dennison, 2000, St. Louis: Mosby. Reprinted with permission from Elsevier.

Open Pneumothorax (Figure 18.4)

- ◆ Air enters the pleural space through the chest wall.
- ◆ Etiology.
  - ❖ Penetrating trauma.
- ◆ Pathophysiology and Signs and Symptoms.
  - ❖ Equilibrium between intra thoracic and atmospheric pressures.
  - ❖ Patient condition depends on size of opening compared to trachea.
  - ❖ The affected lung collapses during inspiration.
  - ❖ May cause a tension pneumothorax.
  - ❖ Subcutaneous emphysema usually presents.
- ◆ Treatment
  - ❖ Similar to closed pneumothorax.
  - ❖ Closure of open wound with petroleum jelly gauze.
    - ☆ End expiration.
    - ☆ Modification for tension pneumothorax.
  - ❖ Chest tube and water seal drainage.

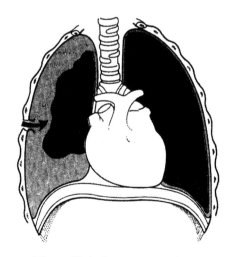

Figure 18.4: Open pneumothorax.
From *Pass CCRN* (2nd ed.), by R.D. Dennison, 2000, St. Louis: Mosby. Reprinted with permission from Elsevier.

Chapter 18

Chest Tubes

Chest tubes are used to evacuate fluid and or air from the pleural space. They also re-establish normal negative intrapleural pressure and allow the lung to re-expand. Small catheters can be used to evacuate air, while larger size tubing is needed for fluid drainage, such as required in treating hemothorax. A commonly used thoracostomy tube is 28 F and this can be used to drain both fluid and air (Halow & Bower, 2003). Mediastinal chest tubes can also be placed and are commonly used in cardiac surgical procedures.

There are 3 compartments in a sealed chest tube drainage system:

◆ The first compartment is connected to the chest tube and allows for collection of fluid from the pleural space.

◆ The 2nd compartment is connected to the 1st and creates a water seal. A small amount of sterile water (per manufacturer directions) is injected into the water seal chamber before the drainage system is connected to the patient. The main purpose of the water seal is to allow air to exit from the pleural space on exhalation and prevent air from entering the pleural cavity or mediastinum on inhalation.

◆ The 3rd compartment is connected to the 1st 2 sections and provides suction. Traditional units regulate the amount of suction by the height of a column of water in the suction chamber. Adjusting a system valve controls the amount of suction. -20 cm H_2O of suction is the typical amount applied to the system. Lower levels may be indicated for patients with friable lung tissue. The goal is to have an adequate amount of suction to keep open the pleural space, but not an excessive amount that will cause damage to the lung tissue. No more than -40 cm H_2O should be applied to a chest tube drainage system (Halow & Bowyer, 2003).

Chest tube complications can include infection and bleeding. There can also be equipment and technical-related problems. Strict sterile technique should be used during insertion of chest tubes. Prophylactic antibiotics are not indicated for chest tube insertion for a simple pneumothorax (Halow & Bowyer, 2003).

A rare but serious complication is the development of unilateral pulmonary edema in response to rapid re-expansion or rapid evacuation of pleural fluid. The impact of rapid treatment can cause an increase in capillary permeability, resulting in pulmonary edema. Avoiding suction with the initial drainage of a large pleural effusion or the expansion of a large pneumothorax and also clamping after the 2 liters of initial drainage are strategies for minimizing the risk of unilateral pulmonary edema (Halow & Bowyer, 2003).

Nursing Interventions with Chest Tubes

◆ Assure that the amount of sterile fluid in the water seal and suction chambers is at the manufacturer recommended levels.

❖ The column of fluid limits the amount of suction. Adjust the source suction to produce only gentle bubbling in the suction control chamber. Excessive external suction causes loud bubbling and also increases the evaporation of water from the suction control chamber. A lower level of water results in a lower amount of suction applied to the patient.

❖ To maintain an adequate water seal it is important to monitor the level of water in the water seal chamber and to keep the chest drainage unit upright at all times.

◆ Assess for air leak by checking water seal chamber for bubbles during inspiration. The water seal chamber may bubble gently with insertion, during expiration and with a cough. Continuous bubbling represents an air leak.

❖ Check for system leaks by clamping before each connection (system may need to be replaced).

❖ Check for leak where tube enters chest.

❖ Check chest x-ray to assure last hole of chest tube is inside chest.

Non Cardiac Issues in the Cardiac Patient: Pulmonary Pathophysiology, Electrolytes and Renal, Sepsis

◆ Assess the water seal chamber for slight fluctuation. Slight fluctuation (tidaling) in the water seal level (rising during spontaneous inspiration and falling during expiration) is normal. Lack of fluctuation with respiration may indicate kinking or other problems interfering with drainage. Lack of fluctuation may also be a good sign indicating lung re-expansion.

◆ Assess for excessive bleeding requiring surgical intervention.
   ❖ Drainage > 1500 ml in a short period of time represents approximately 40% of the circulating volume (Halow & Bowyer, 2003).
   ❖ General guidelines for surgical re-exploration after a surgical procedure are listed below. More specific guidelines may exist for specific types of surgery.
      ☆ 400 to 800 ml x 1 hour.
      ☆ 400 ml/hr x 2 hours.
      ☆ 200 ml/hr x 4 hours.
      ☆ A total of 800 ml in 8 hours.
   (Halow & Bowyer, 2003)

◆ Assess the insertion site for subcutaneous emphysema.
◆ Keep the collection unit below the level of the patient's chest.
◆ Do not clamp chest tube for transport (can cause tension pneumothorax with pleural chest tubes or tamponade with mediastinal chest tubes). Use portable suction if available or transport on gravity drainage with tubing from suction chamber open to air. Leaving the tubing open to air allows a vent for the escape of air.
◆ Avoid dependent loops in the drainage tubing.
◆ No routine stripping.

Criteria for Chest Tube Removal
◆ No air leak on water seal for 24 hours (absence of continuous bubbling in the water-seal chamber).
◆ Absence of fluctuations in the water-seal chamber of the collection device. Lack of fluctuation in the water seal can indicate that the lung has reexpanded and there is no further air leaking into the pleural space.
◆ Drainage < 50-100 ml for 24 hours.
   ❖ Post cardiac surgery chest tubes may be removed when drainage is < 100 ml in 8 hours.
◆ Complete expansion of lung confirmed by chest x-ray.
◆ Improvement in respiratory status.

A chest tube is typically removed by using a gauze pad and asking the patient to take a deep breath and hold (performing the valslava maneuver). This creates a positive pressure in the pleural space and prevents the development of a pneumothorax during removal. The use of an occlusive dressing (petrolatum gauze) with pleural chest tube removal prevents the entry of air into the pleural space. Although the traditional method of removal involves removing at the end of inspiration, some research has raised the question of whether or not this technique actually reduces the risk of development of pneumothorax (Halow & Bowyer, 2003). A chest x-ray is also typically done several hours after chest tube removal.

ELECTROLYTE ABNORMALITIES

Treatment of electrolyte abnormalities requires focus on the underlying cause in addition to the immediate abnormality. Electrolyte abnormalities often occur in groups rather than as isolated abnormalities. For this reason the clinical manifestations may be related to multiple abnormalities.

Chapter 18

Electrolyte imbalances should be suspected in patients with renal or endocrine diseases. An acute change in mental status or the development of ventricular arrhythmias warrants an electrolyte assessment.

Sodium

Sodium is a dominant extracellular cation. It is the primary determinant of serum osmolality and plays an important role in regulating extracellular volume. Because sodium is closely related to water, several factors must be considered when assessing sodium abnormalities:

◆ Serum and urine osmolality.
◆ Intravascular volume status/presence of edema.
◆ Serum albumin, lipids, and glucose.
◆ Medications (particularly diuretics) and IV fluids.
◆ Renal function.

Abnormalities in serum sodium impact neuronal and neuromuscular functioning.

Hyponatremia

Definition: Sodium less than 135 mEq/L.

Hyponatremic symptoms are related to the severity of the disorder and the rapidity at which it developed. In addition to symptoms related to low sodium, patients can have symptoms related to fluid balance abnormalities. The primary effects of hyponatremia are CNS-related, regardless of cause. At sodium levels < 125 mEq/L, there are changes in cognitive and motor function. Mortality approaches 50% when sodium is < 105 mEq/L (Marini & Wheeler, 2006).

Signs and Symptoms
◆ Muscle cramps.
◆ Twitching/tremors.
◆ Muscle weakness.
◆ Nausea and vomiting.
◆ Abdominal cramps.
◆ Irritability.
◆ Headache.
◆ Personality changes.
◆ Confusion.
◆ Lethargy progressing to coma.
◆ Seizures.

Permanent neurological changes occur at sodium levels < 110 mEq/L (Stark, 2006).

Hyponatremia can occur in isotonic, hypertonic, and hypotonic states. Hypotonic hyponatremia is the most common form of hyponatremia. Hypotonic hyponatremia results in an intracellular hypoosmolar state. This intracellular state is responsible for the signs and symptoms.

Isotonic hyponatremia occurs when a large amount of non-salt (glucose, mannitol) containing isotonic fluids are given.

Hypertonic hyponatremia occurs in the presence of non-sodium osmotically active substances. This occurs, for example, in hyperglycemia in which the extra-cellular fluid is hypertonic and the sodium level is low.

Non Cardiac Issues in the Cardiac Patient: Pulmonary Pathophysiology, Electrolytes and Renal, Sepsis

Hypotonic (Hyposmolar) Hyponatremia

Hypotonic hyponatremia occurs as a result of excess free water in relation to sodium. Patients with hypotonic hyponatremia can be hypovolemic, isovolemic, or hypervolemic (Table 18.1). Isovolemic hypotonic hyponatremia is the most common form of hypotonic hyponatremia and is typically caused by an inappropriate increased secretion of antidiuretic hormone (SIADH).

Table 18.1
Types of Hypotonic Hyponatremia

	Hypovolemic	Isovolemic	Hypervolemic
Pathophysiology	◆ Volume depletion with replacement fluids more hypotonic than plasma. ◆ Decreased free water clearance in volume depleted states (body protects volume at the expense of normal tonicity with continued release of vasopressin).	◆ Actual slight excess of total body fluid but considered isovolemic.	◆ Inadequate excretion of sodium and water. ◆ Water is retained in excess of sodium. ◆ 12 to 15 L of excess total body water before sufficient interstitial fluid accumulates and causes edema.
Specific Signs and Symptoms	◆ Thirst. ◆ Postural hypotension.	◆ Inappropriate concentrated urine (urine osmolality > serum osmolality).	◆ Edema is primary indicator.
Causes	◆ Bleeding. ◆ Diarrhea, vomiting. ◆ Third space loss. ◆ Diuretics. ◆ Osmotic diuresis. ◆ Adrenal insufficiency (aldosternone deficiency). ◆ Salt wasting nephropathy.	◆ Inappropriate secretion of ADH (SIADH). ◆ Water intoxication (psychogenic polydipsia).	◆ Renal dysfunction from most any type of acute or chronic renal failure. ◆ Congestive heart failure. ◆ Hypoproteinemia from hepatic failure or nephrotic syndrome.
Specific Treatment Based on Volume Status	◆ Isotonic saline to restore lost circulating volume.	◆ Free water restriction and treat underlying cause. ◆ Free water clearance with loop diuretic and replace volume with 0.9NS.	◆ Restrict fluid. ◆ Diuretics. ◆ Dialysis if needed.

(Marini & Wheeler, 2006; Society of Critical Care Medicine, 2001)

Treatment for Severe Hyponatremia

Sodium should be corrected to an initial level of 120 to 130 mEq/L over 12 to 24 hours. It is generally recommended to increase the serum sodium level not more than 8 to 12 mEq/L over 24 hours unless life-threatening symptoms are present (Society of Critical Care Medicine, 2001). In general, the rate of

Chapter 18

correction should be proportional to speed at which the hyponatremia developed. Accelerated correction is used in patients with life threatening symptoms, and slower rates of correction are used in patients who have chronic hyponatremia. When sodium is > 125 to 130 mEq/L, restriction of free water alone will allow a slow return to normal sodium levels.

Too rapid of a correction can lead to osmotic demyelinating syndrome and cause central nervous system injury (Society of Critical Care Medicine, 2001).

Hypernatremia

Definition: Sodium greater than 145 mEq/L with a serum osmolality > 295 mOsml/kg. Most cases of hypernatremia involve intracellular volume depletion from a loss of free water in excess of sodium. This produces a hyperosmolar state.

Hypernatremia rarely occurs in patients with normal ADH secretion, thirst mechanism, and ability to consume free water. Hypernatremia almost always causes cellular dehydration.

Causes
◆ Conditions in which patient is unable to consume free water (ICU setting).
◆ Hypertonic tube feedings without free water replacement.
◆ Increased sodium intake (sodium bicarbonate, hypertonic saline).
◆ Dehydration (burns, tachypnea, hyperthermia, diarrhea, vomiting).
◆ Osmotic diuretics with excessive free water clearance.
◆ Diabetes mellitus.
◆ Diabetes insipidus.

Signs and Symptoms
◆ Thirst (early symptom).
◆ Dry mouth and skin.
◆ Increased body temperature.
◆ Nausea and vomiting.
◆ Muscle weakness.
◆ Irritability and agitation.
◆ Lethargy.
◆ Seizures.
◆ Coma.

Treatment
Treatment is aimed at correcting the underlying cause and replacing free water. The goal is to decrease sodium levels 0.5 to 1 mEq/L per hour (Society of Critical Care Medicine, 2001). Too rapid of a correction can result in cerebral edema.
◆ Replacement of free water with D_5W, $D_50.2$ NS or 0.45 NS.
◆ 0.9NS may be used when patient is hemodynamically unstable and adequate circulating intravascular volume is the priority.
◆ Loop diuretics or dialysis are rarely needed to remove excess sodium.

Potassium

Approximately 95% of body potassium is intracellular. Much of the body's potassium is contained in muscle, and total body potassium declines with age based on the decrease in muscle mass. Although small in quantity, extracellular potassium is important because the ratio of extracellular to intracellular potassium

Non Cardiac Issues in the Cardiac Patient: Pulmonary Pathophysiology, Electrolytes and Renal, Sepsis

plays an important role in the maintenance of electrical membrane potentials. It is important to remember, however, that extracellular potassium does not adequately estimate total body potassium. The major body systems affected by potassium abnormalities are the gastrointestinal, neuromuscular, and cardiac systems. Dietary intake is the major source of potassium, and the kidneys are responsible for excretion.

Hypokalemia

Definition: K^+ less than 3.5 mEq/L.

Hypokalemia represents an approximate total body potassium deficit of approximately 5-10% (Marini & Wheeler, 2006).

Causes

Assessing urinary potassium levels, systemic acid base balance, and other electrolytes is important in evaluating the cause of hypokalemia.

◆ Poor K^+ intake.
   ❖ Elderly, alcoholics, anorexia.
   ❖ Urinary potassium levels will be low.
   ❖ Healthy kidneys can usually adjust potassium excretion to be less than dietary intake.
◆ Increased extra renal loss (GI loss): Urinary potassium levels will be low.
   ❖ Vomiting, diarrhea, nasogastric suctioning, laxative abuse.
   ❖ GI losses typically do not cause symptomatic hypokalemia; however, GI losses may lead to intravascular fluid volume deficit, which can lead to renal potassium wasting.
◆ Increased renal loss: Hypokalemia from renal loss represents a decrease in total body potassium. Urinary potassium will be high.
   ❖ Renal tubular acidosis or diabetic ketoacidosis (accompanied by systemic acidosis).
   ❖ Diuretics: Very common cause of hypokalemia (accompanied by systemic alkalosis).
      ✰ Increased distal tubular flow promotes exchange of sodium for potassium
         ✳ Loop diuretics.
         ✳ Thiazide diuretics.
         ✳ Acetazolamide (Diamox) (a carbonic anhydrase inhibitor).
   ❖ Excess mineral or glucocorticoid (accompanied by systemic alkolosis)
      ✰ Hyperaldosteronism.
      ✰ Cushing's syndrome.
      ✰ Cirrhosis.
      ✰ Volume depletions.
   ❖ Magnesium deficiency
      ✰ Caused by diuretics or excessive alcohol use.
   ❖ Certain antibiotics, such as amphotericin B, aminoglycosides, penicillin and penicillin analogs (Linas, 2003).
◆ Extracellular to intracellular shifts.
   ❖ Alkalosis
      ✰ Causes potassium to shift into the cell in exchange for hydrogen ions.
      ✰ Potassium levels decrease 0.1 to 0.4 mEq/L for each 0.1 unit increase in pH (Linas, 2003).
   ❖ Insulin (treatment of DKA or HHNK).

831

Chapter 18

- ❖ Catecholamines (beta adrenergic agonists).
- ❖ Note: This type of hypokalemia does not reflect total body potassium and treatment should be administered cautiously.

Signs and Symptoms

Effects of hypokalemia are related to altered membrane potentials and impaired muscle contractility. Low potassium levels cause an increase in the resting membrane potential of neural and muscular cells, therefore reducing the excitability of these cells. Symptoms typically occur when potassium is less than 3.0 mEq/L. Severity of effects of hypokalemia depends on calcium levels, systemic pH, and the rapidness of onset.

- ◆ GI: Nausea and vomiting, constipation, abdominal distention, cramping, and paralytic ileus.
- ◆ Orthostatic hypotension (vascular smooth muscle has an altered response to catecholamines).
- ◆ Parasthesias, weakness, fatigue and muscle cramps (2.5-3.0 mEq/L).
  - ❖ Muscles of the lower extremities are typically impacted first.
- ◆ Respiratory muscle weakness, dyspnea, paralysis and arrest (< 2.5 mEq/L).
- ◆ Enhanced digitalis effect (a variety of arrhythmias and conduction defects related to digitalis effect).
- ◆ Severe hypokalemia can result in rhabdomyolysis.
- ◆ ECG / cardiac rhythm changes.
  - ❖ Mild hypokalemia: delays ventricular repolarization.
    - ☆ ST depression, inverted T waves.
    - ☆ Heightened U waves, prolonged QT interval.
  - ❖ Lowered threshold for ventricular fibrillation; promotes re-entrant tachycardias, especially in the presence of acute myocardial ischemia.
  - ❖ Any arrhythmia – atrial or ventricular (especially in the presence of digoxin).
  - ❖ Severe hypokalemia.
    - ☆ Increased P wave amplitude.
    - ☆ Increased PR interval.
    - ☆ Increased QRS interval.

(Marini & Wheeler, 2006)

Treatment

- ◆ Treat cause.
- ◆ Correct alkalosis.
- ◆ Correct hypomagnesemia .
- ◆ Increase potassium intake (dietary or supplement) if potassium $\geq$ 3.0 mEq/L.
  - ❖ Foods high in potassium include: Orange juice, bananas, raisins, milk, green vegetables.
  - ❖ Oral supplements up to 40 mEq can be used safely several times per day.
  - ❖ Potassium chloride solutions placed in small bowel can cause irritation.
- ◆ Add potassium to maintenance IV fluid.
- ◆ IV potassium bolus for severe deficiency (less than 3.0 mEq/L if on digoxin, symptoms related to hypokalemia, or less than 2.5 mEq/L without symptoms).
  - ❖ Potassium should be diluted in a non-glucose solution. Glucose stimulates the release of insulin and causes the movement of potassium into cells.
  - ❖ Concentration should not generally exceed 10 mEq per 100 ml via peripheral line, or 20 mEq per 100 ml if central line.

Non Cardiac Issues in the Cardiac Patient: Pulmonary Pathophysiology, Electrolytes and Renal, Sepsis

☆ High concentrations can cause chemical phlebitis.

☆ Infiltration can cause necrosis.

❖ Safe dosage: 10 mEq/100 cc over an hour.

❖ May give 20 mEq over 1 hour if K^+ is < 3.5 mEq/L.

❖ If life threatening arrhythmias or paralysis 30-40 mEq over an hour may be given via central line (Marini & Wheeler, 2006).

❖ Potassium levels should be monitored every 1 to 2 hours during the acute replacement period.

❖ Continuous cardiac monitoring should be in place when doses > 10 mEq/hr are being used.

◆ Potassium is usually replaced with potassium chloride. If a phosphate deficiency is also present, potassium phosphate may be used. In the unusual circumstance where acidosis is present, potassium bicarbonate may be used.

Linking Knowledge to Practice

✔ *Potassium levels should be monitored closely during diuresis. Hypokalemia is a side effect of both loop and thiazide diuretics.*

✔ *Assess potassium level before the administration of digoxin. Hypokalemia enhances digitalis effect and places patient at risk for digitalis toxicity.*

✔ *Correct a low magnesium level prior to replacing potassium in a patient with hypokalemia.*

✔ *Potassium replacement should be done with caution in patients with an impaired ability to excrete potassium, including those with*

❖ *Renal disease.*

❖ *Diabetes.*

❖ *Medications.*

☆ *Aldosterone antagonists.*

☆ *ACE inhibitors or angiotensin II receptor blockers.*

☆ *Non-steroidal anti-inflammatory agents.*

✔ *Although unusual, hypokalemia in the presence of acidosis results in a more significant reduction in total body potassium (greater than 5-10%). This is because during acidosis, potassium shifts out of the cell into the extracellular space, typically causing hyperkalemia. Therefore, the presence of hypokalemia in acidosis represents a serious reduction in total body potassium. In addition, the correction of acidosis results in a worsening of hypokalemia.*

Hyperkalemia

Definition: K^+ greater than 5.0 mEq/L.

Causes

Hyperkalemia is a rare disorder in healthy persons because the kidneys are able to excrete excess potassium to maintain normal extracellular levels. The effective management of potassium is impaired in patients with diabetes and those with renal disease.

◆ Decreased potassium excretion.

❖ Renal disease.

☆ Inability of kidneys to excrete potassium due to distal tubular damage.

☆ Renal disease is the most common cause of hyperkalemia.

☆ When glomerular filtration falls to about 75% of normal, hyperkalemia can be seen in the

833

Chapter 18

presence of chronic renal failure. This loss of renal function is associated with a creatinine of > 4.0 mg/dL. The glomerular filtration rate typically falls to ≤ 10 ml/minute before chronic renal failure is the sole cause of hyperkalemia (Linas, 2003).

☆ In acute renal failure, the potassium may rise before the BUN and creatinine rise. However, in renal failure, the potassium typically does not rise faster than 0.5 mEq/L per day under normal circumstances (Marini & Wheeler, 2006).

☆ Acidosis as a result of renal failure further impairs the ability of the kidneys to excrete potassium.

❖ Decreased renal perfusion (pre-renal) also causes a decrease in potassium excretion due to a decrease in the availability of sodium for exchange with potassium.

❖ Decreased aldosterone: Addison's disease (adrenal insufficiency).

❖ Decreased aldosterone: Diabetes (hyporeninemic hypoaldosteronism due to impaired renin production).

❖ Sickle cell disease (renal distal tubule dysfunction).

❖ Antibiotics pentamidine and trimethoprim promote potassium retention (Stark, 2006).

❖ Drugs that inhibit aldosterone production or effects.

☆ Aldactone, eplerenone, and other aldosterone inhibitors (potassium sparing diuretics).

☆ ACE Inhibitors or angiotensin II receptor blockers.

☆ Non-steroidal anti-inflammatory medications.

☆ Heparin (suppresses aldosterone synthesis and secretion).

◆ Increased potassium intake (usually only causes hyperkalemia in patients with co-existing impaired excretory ability).

❖ Excessive use of salt substitutes containing potassium chloride.

❖ Transfusion of banked blood: The longer the storage, the higher the extracellular content.

❖ Potassium supplements.

❖ Lactated ringers solutions.

❖ High doses of penicillin preparations containing potassium.

◆ Intracellular to extracellular shift.

❖ Metabolic acidosis.

☆ Potassium is more sensitive to changes in sodium bicarbonate rather than blood pH, so respiratory acidosis does not significantly impact potassium movement.

☆ There is a rise in potassium of 0.6 mEq/L for every drop in pH of 0.1 units (Linas, 2003).

❖ Hypertonic glucose with insulin deficiency.

❖ Hyperosmolality.

❖ Digitalis toxicity.

☆ The sodium/potassium pump is damaged.

❖ Depolarizing neuromuscular blocking agents.

☆ Can cause an increase in serum potassium, especially in patients with neuromuscular disease.

❖ Beta blockers

☆ Block the cellular uptake of potassium, which is mediated by adrenergic receptors

◆ Cellular disruption with leak of intracellular K^+.

❖ Crush injuries.

❖ Rhabdomyolysis.

Non Cardiac Issues in the Cardiac Patient: Pulmonary Pathophysiology, Electrolytes and Renal, Sepsis

- ❖ Hemolysis (blood transfusion reaction).
- ❖ Early burns.
- ❖ Trauma.
- ❖ Large hematoma.
- ❖ Severe catabolic states.
- ❖ Lysis of tumor cells (chemotherapy).

Pseudohyperkalemia can occur with leukocytosis (WBC > 100,000/mm³ or with thrombocytosis platelets > 600,000/mm³). Both white blood cells and platelets can release potassium. Hemolysis secondary to phlebotomy is another potential cause of pseudohyperkalemia. Prolonged tourniquet application can cause hemolysis.

Signs and Symptoms

Symptoms don't typically develop until potassium level is > 6 mEq/L. Clinical effects are predominantly related to muscle and cardiac function. The neuromuscular effects of hyperkalemia can be complicated by acidosis and co-existing electrolyte abnormalities. Skeletal muscle effects are usually not seen until the potassium level reaches 7.0 mEq or higher.

- ◆ Parathesia: usually first symptom.
- ◆ Proximal lower extremity weakness: Most common symptom (Marini & Wheeler, 2006).
- ◆ Muscle irritability, numbness, or paralysis.
- ◆ Respiratory muscle weakness usually spared in hyperkalemia (Marini & Wheeler, 2006).
- ◆ Cardiac effects are the most significant.
    - ❖ Refractory hypotension.
    - ❖ ECG changes.
        - ☆ Tall narrow peaked T waves.
        - ☆ Widening QRS.
        - ☆ Decreasing amplitude of R waves.
        - ☆ Prolonged PR and flattened to absent P wave.
        - ☆ Dysrhythmias.
            - ✶ Bradycardia/Heart block.
            - ✶ Sine wave pattern (blending of QRS and T wave).
            - ✶ Asystolic cardiac arrest.
- ◆ Low sodium, low calcium, and high magnesium can magnify the neuromuscular effects of high potassium so these electrolytes should also be assessed and treated (Marini & Wheeler, 2006).

Treatment

Any potassium level > 6.0 mEq/L should be treated. The urgency of treatment depends on the clinical manifestations. Cardiac manifestations, as indicated by ECG changes, as well as any severe muscle weakness, warrant immediate treatment.

- ◆ Limit K⁺ intake.
- ◆ Volume expansion in dehydrated patients.
- ◆ K⁺ > 6.5, ECG changes or dysrhythmias, or severe muscle weakness.
    - ❖ Stabilize cardiac membrane.
        - ☆ Administering calcium IV if there are ECG changes due to hyperkalemia.
            - ✶ Usually 5-10 ml of 10% solution of calcium chloride to stabilize cell membrane and reduce myocardial irritability.

835

Chapter 18

* Give over 5-10 minutes. Effect is immediate, but lasts only 30-60 minutes (Society of Critical Care Medicine, 2001).
* Calcium given in the presence of digitalis toxicity will worsen the effects of toxicity. More calcium is able to enter the cell due to the damaged sodium/calcium exchange system.

❖ Shift potassium into the cell.
   ☆ 10 units regular insulin to shift potassium into the cell.
      * Give IV over 5-10 minutes; begins to work within minutes.
      * 50% dextrose IV given to prevent hypoglycemia (unless hyperglycemia is present).
      * Moves K^+ into cell.
      * Effects lasts a few hours.
   ☆ High dose inhaled beta agonists (albuterol 10-20 mg).
      * Acts synergistically with insulin to move potassium into the cell.
      * Not first line agent for shifting potassium into the cell.
   ☆ Administer sodium bicarbonate to correct acidosis.
      * 1 mEq/kg IV over 5-10 minutes.
      * Effects last 1-2 hours.
      * Potential for sodium overload.

❖ Eliminate total body potassium
   ☆ Sodium polystyrene (Kayexalate) is an exchange resin used to lower total body potassium.
      * Exchange sodium for potassium and moves potassium out via the gastrointestinal tract.
      * More sodium is gained than potassium lost, so there is potential for increased sodium and net fluid gain. This can cause fluid overload state in patients with renal disease or heart failure.
      * Can be given orally or as retention enema.
      * Oral dose is administered in sorbital.
         – Sorbital orally acts as osmotic laxative.
         – Sorbital can cause intestinal necrosis when given by enema.
      * Retention enema is administered in dextrose.
   ☆ Loop diuretics can help remove total body potassium in a person with functioning kidneys.
   ☆ Dialysis may be needed to remove total body potassium in patients with renal dysfunction. Hemodialysis can remove potassium more rapidly than peritoneal dialysis.

Linking Knowledge to Practice

✔ *Patients with heart failure are often on an ACE inhibitor or angiotensin receptor blocker and also on an aldosterone antagonist. These medications place the patient at risk for hyperkalemia. Nurses should always know the patient's potassium level prior to administering an ACE inhibitor, angiotensin receptor blocker, or aldosterone antagonist.*

✔ *In addition, patients with heart failure are instructed to eat a low sodium diet. The use of salt substitutes containing potassium chloride may further increase the risk for the development of hyperkalemia. Patient education and frequent monitoring of electrolytes are important aspects of long-term heart failure management.*

✔ *The ECG is important in determining the urgency of treatment in hyperkalemia so it should be performed immediately when a high potassium lab value is discovered. Follow up ECGs are also used to assess the effectiveness of treatment in stabilizing the cardiac membrane.*

Calcium

Calcium is a cation which is primarily located in the bone. The calcium located in the bone can be exchanged to maintain extracellular calcium as needed. One percent of calcium is located in the cells, and only 0.1-0.2% is in the extracellular fluid (Porth, 2004). There is a normal inverse relationship between serum calcium and serum phosphate.

Calcium is involved is several key physiological processes:

◆ Muscle contraction.
◆ Transmission of nervous system impulses.
◆ Hormone secretion.
◆ Blood clotting and wound healing.
◆ Cellular function.

Calcium is absorbed in the intestine with the aid of vitamin D. Less than 50% of dietary calcium is absorbed (Porth, 2004). The kidneys excrete calcium. Serum calcium is regulated by parathyroid levels, and vitamin D and is also influenced by serum phosphate levels. There are 3 types of serum calcium:

◆ > 40% of calcium is protein bound (mostly to albumin).
◆ Approximately 10% is chelated (non-ionized) with substances such as citrate or phosphate.
◆ Approximately 50% is ionized, meaning it is free to leave the extracellular fluid and participate in intracellular function.

Ionized calcium is the best measurement to assess the adequacy of calcium levels.

Hypocalcemia

Definition: Calcium < 8.8 mg/dL or ionized calcium < 4.65 mg/dL (Fischbach, 2004).

Hypocalcemia is a common disorder in critically ill patients. However, hypocalcemia is generally asymptomatic if the disorder develops slowly or if the levels of ionized calcium remain in the normal range.

Causes
Calcium levels can be decreased for multiple reasons (Table 18.2).

◆ Decreased calcium intake or absorption.
◆ Increased calcium excretion.
◆ Impaired ability to mobilize calcium from bone.
◆ Increased calcium binding.
   ❖ Calcium is removed from circulation by binding to drugs and chemicals, such as chelating agents or citrate anticoagulation used in banked blood.
   ❖ Calcium may also bind to abdominal fat during pancreatitis.
◆ Low protein (albumin) levels.
   ❖ A decrease in albumin of 1 gm/dL will result in a decrease in serum calcium by 0.8 mg/dL (Marini & Wheeler, 2006).

Chapter 18

<table>
<tr><td colspan="4" align="center">Table 18.2
Causes of Hypocalcemia</td></tr>
<tr><th>Decreased calcium intake or absorption</th><th>Increased calcium excretion</th><th>Impaired ability to mobilize calcium from bone</th><th>Increased calcium binding (Decreased ionized calcium)</th></tr>
<tr><td>Low dietary intake
Hypomagnesemia
Renal failure
Vitamin D deficiency
Liver disease
Steroid therapy
Cushing's disease
Gastrectomy or small bowel disorder.</td><td>Loop diuretics
Chronic diarrhea
Hyperphosphatemia.
(Phosphate elimination is impaired in renal failure.)</td><td>Inadequate levels of parathyroid hormone.
(Decreased magnesium inhibits parathyroid release.)</td><td>Alkalosis
Acute pancreatitis
Massive transfusion
Drugs
    Cimetidine
    Heparin
    Theophylline
    Aminoglycosides.</td></tr>
</table>

Signs and Symptoms (Table 18.3)
The most common symptoms are due to neuromuscular irritability.

<table>
<tr><td colspan="2" align="center">Table 18.3
Signs and Symptoms of Hypocalcemia</td></tr>
<tr><th>Cardiovascular Effects</th><th>Neuromuscular Effects (increase in neuromuscular excitability)</th></tr>
<tr><td>
◆ Decreased contractility
◆ Hypotension
◆ Prolonged QT (ST-segment hugging baseline for extended period)
◆ Torsades de pointes
◆ Bradycardia/heart block
◆ Heart failure
◆ Digitalis insensitivity
◆ Cardiac arrest.
</td><td>
◆ Parathesias (common)
◆ Hyperreflexia
◆ Muscle cramps
◆ Tetany (spasms of face, hands, and feet)
◆ Chvostek's sign
  ❖ Tapping of face over facial nerve located below the temple.
  ❖ Positive sign results in spasm of lip, nose or face.
◆ Trousseau's sign
  ❖ Inflate blood pressure above systolic BP and hold for 3 minutes.
  ❖ Positive sign results in contraction of fingers or hand.
◆ Stridor/wheezing/bronchospasm
◆ Laryngeal spasm
◆ Change in mental status
◆ Seizures.
</td></tr>
</table>

Chronic hypocalcemia results in dry skin and hair, brittle nails, and bone pain with risk for fractures.

Treatment
Mild hypocalcemia is well tolerated. When correcting calcium levels, the goal is to keep calcium in the low/normal range so the parathyroid gland is not suppressed.

◆ High calcium, low phosphorous diet.
◆ Vitamin D supplements if vitamin D deficiency.
◆ Phosphate binding antacids (aluminum containing).
  ❖ Giving calcium in a high phosphate state will produce calcium salt formation.

Non Cardiac Issues in the Cardiac Patient: Pulmonary Pathophysiology, Electrolytes and Renal, Sepsis

- Magnesium for concurrent hypomagnesemia.
- Correct alkalosis to increased ionized calcium.
- Thiazide diuretics to increase tubular calcium reabsorption.
- IV calcium chloride or calcium glucanate for cardiovascular or neuromuscular symptoms.
  - ❖ 100mg of calcium is given over 5-10 minutes.
    - ☆ 3 to 4 ml of calcium chloride or 10 ml of calcium gluconate.
    - ☆ Calcium glucanate: 10 ml contains 4.5 mEq of calcium, or 90 mg of calcium.
    - ☆ Calcium chloride: 10 ml contains 13.6 mEq of calcium, 272 mg of calcium.
    - ☆ Slow infusion of calcium gluconate preferred.
    - ☆ Central vein preferred – can cause chemical phlebitis or tissue necrosis.

Linking Knowledge to Practice

✔ *Critically ill and chronically ill patients commonly have hypocalcemia secondary to poor nutritional status. It is important to focus on improving the patient's overall nutritional status rather than only focusing on calcium supplementation.*

Hypercalcemia

Definition: Calcium > 10.4 mg/dL or ionized calcium > 5.26 mg/dL (Fischbach, 2004).

Causes

- Increased mobilization of calcium from the bone (increased bone resorption). This is the most common cause of hypercalcemia with neoplasms and hyperparathyroidism accounting for 80-90% of all cases of hypercalcemia. Most cases of severe hypercalcemia result from malignant neoplasms. (Society of Critical Care Medicine, 2001; Marini & Wheeler, 2006).
  - ❖ Hyperparathyroidism.
  - ❖ Neoplasms.
    - ☆ Metastatic cancer with osteolytic lesions.
    - ☆ Multiple myeloma.
  - ❖ Thyroidtoxicosis.
  - ❖ Vitamin D excess.
  - ❖ Immobility (calcium is mobilized from bones, teeth, and intestines).
- Increased calcium intake (supplement or antacids).
- Increased calcium absorption.
  - ❖ Hypophosphatemia.
  - ❖ Excessive vitamin D intake.
- Acidosis: Increased ionized calcium.
- Decreased calcium excretion.
  - ❖ Thiazide diuretics.

Chapter 18

Signs and Symptoms (Box 18.1)

Box 18.1
Signs and Symptoms of Hypercalcemia

- ◆ Hypophosphatemia.
- ◆ Signs and symptoms related to dehydration – hypercalcemia induces osmotic diuresis.
- ◆ Gastrointestinal symptoms related to slowing of the GI tract: Nausea, vomiting, anorexia, abdominal pain, constipation.
- ◆ Bone and flank pain/osteoporosis/pathological fractures.
- ◆ Muscular symptoms: Hypotonicity/weakness/fatigue.
- ◆ Neurogical symptoms: Decreased mentation, agitation, comma, seizures.
- ◆ Cardiac symptoms: Hypertension (may be offset by co-existing dehydration), cardiac ischemia, shortened QT segments , arrhythmias (conduction abnormalities), digitalis toxicity.
- ◆ Calcium salts form at high levels.
  - ❖ Pruritis from skin deposits.
  - ❖ Renal calculi and potential renal insufficiency/failure.
  - ❖ Deposits on the aorta, cardiac valves, and coronary arteries.
- ◆ Life threatening signs and symptoms are rare unless calcium levels reach > 14 mg/dL. (Marini & Wheeler, 2006; Society of Critical Medicine, 2001; Porth, 2004)

Treatment

- ◆ The primary treatment of hypercalcemia involves rehydration with 0.9NS.
- ◆ Control underlying disease process.
- ◆ Decrease calcium absorption.
  - ❖ Low calcium, high phosphorous diet. (Phosphate binds to calcium in gut, making it insoluable; therefore, there is decreased calcium absorption.)
  - ❖ Glucocorticoids.
    - ☆ Decreases calcitriol, therefore inhibiting absorption in the gut.
    - ☆ Steroids are also effective with vitamin D intoxication (Marini & Wheeler, 2006).
- ◆ Increase calcium excretion.
  - ❖ Rehydration with 0.9NS.
  - ❖ Loop diuretics.
    - ☆ Administered with 0.9NS to increase urine output.
    - ☆ Block calcium reabsorption by the kidney.
  - ❖ Dialysis if life threatening or if renal failure.
  - ❖ Inhibit bone resorption.
    - ☆ Calcitonin.
      - ✳ Inhibits osteoclasts.
      - ✳ Promotes incorporation of calcium into the bone.
      - ✳ Inhibits bone resorption.
    - ☆ Mithramycin.
      - ✳ Stimulates bone uptake of calcium.

840

Non Cardiac Issues in the Cardiac Patient: Pulmonary Pathophysiology, Electrolytes and Renal, Sepsis

☆ Biphosphonates.
  ✱ Inhibit calcium release from bone.
  ✱ More potent than calcitonin.
  ✱ Preferred treatment in patients with cancer.
◆ Prevent cardiac effects.
  ❖ Calcium channel blockers.
◆ Prevent renal calculi.
  ❖ Acidify urine.

Magnesium

Magnesium is an important intracellular cation for the electrical stability of cells and for cellular processes requiring energy. Magnesium regulates nerve and muscle tone. Magnesium is also required for many enzymes to function properly, and alteration in magnesium levels can disrupt many metabolic processes. The gut and kidneys work closely together to regulate serum magnesium levels. Magnesium is absorbed in the small bowel and excreted by the kidney.

Hypomagnesemia

Definition: Magnesium < 1.8 mg/dL or < 1.5 mEq/dL.

Hypomagnesemia is a common electrolyte disorder in hospitalized patients.

Causes
The most common causes of hypomagnesmia are renal and GI losses.

◆ Renal loss
  ❖ Renal tubular dysfunction.
  ❖ Diuretics (loop, osmotic, thiazides).
  ❖ Aminoglycosides, cyclosporine, amphotericin, and alcohol (Mirini & Wheeler, 2006).
◆ GI loss
  ❖ Malabsorption (magnesium is absorbed in the small bowel).
  ❖ Inflammatory bowel disease.
  ❖ Diarrhea.
  ❖ Nasogastric suction.
◆ Decreased intake
  ❖ Malnutrition.
  ❖ Parental nutrition without magnesium replacement.
  ❖ Alcoholism.
◆ Transcellular shift
  ❖ Refeeding.
  ❖ Recovery from hypothermia.

Low magnesium may also induce low potassium and low calcium.

Signs and Symptoms (Table 18.4)
Many signs and symptoms overlap with hypokalemia and hypocalcemia. Hypokalemia and hypocalcemia are often concurrent. Low magnesium levels cause neuromuscular irritability and decreased ability to relax neuromuscular tone.

Chapter 18

<table>
<tr><td colspan="2" align="center">**Table 18.4**
Signs and Symptoms of Hypomagnesaemia</td></tr>
<tr><td>**Cardiac**</td><td>**Neuromuscular**</td></tr>
<tr><td>◆ QT prolongation/long ST segment, flat or inverted T waves</td><td>◆ Weakness</td></tr>
<tr><td>◆ Arrhythmias (torsades de pointes)</td><td>◆ Tremor</td></tr>
<tr><td>◆ Vasospasm</td><td>◆ Tetany</td></tr>
<tr><td>◆ Ischemia</td><td>◆ Seizure</td></tr>
<tr><td>◆ Increased digitalis effect</td><td>◆ Coma</td></tr>
<tr><td colspan="2">(Society of Critical Care Medicine, 2003; Marini & Wheeler 2006)</td></tr>
</table>

Treatment

Oral magnesium can be used to treat if the patient is asymptomatic. Oral magnesium can, however, cause diarrhea, which may further decrease magnesium levels.

One to two grams of magnesium sulfate IV over 5-10 minutes if an emergency. Rapid administration can result in hypotension. Administer 1 to 2 grams over 10-60 minutes if not life threatening (Society of Critical Care Medicine, 2003). Dosage needs to be decreased if renal failure is present.

Assess for hypermagnesemia during replacement with use of deep tendon reflexes. Deep tendon reflexes are diminished when magnesium levels reach 4 to 5 mg/dL.

Hypermagnesemia

Definition: Magnesium level > 2.5 mEq/L.

Causes

Hypermagnesemia is an uncommon disorder unless renal dysfunction is present or unless IV doses of magnesium are given. Adrenal insufficiency, magnesium containing antacids or laxatives, and acidotic states can also contribute to high magnesium levels.

Signs and Symptoms
◆ Hyporeflexia.
◆ Hypotension.
◆ Heart block/bradycardia.
◆ Muscle weakness.
◆ Change in mental status.
◆ Lethargy/coma.
◆ Cardiopulmonary arrest.

Treatment
◆ Treat with fluids (0.9NS) and diuretics if normal renal function.
◆ Dialysis if renal failure or life threatening symptoms.
◆ Calcium can be used to counter cardiac and neuromuscular effects.

___

Linking Knowledge to Practice

✔ *Magnesium based laxatives should not be used in patients with renal failure due to the risk of hypermagnesemia. Osmotic agents are preferred instead.*

842

Phosphate

Phosphate is a major intracellular anion. Phosphate plays a major role in phospholipids, phosphoprotein, and phosphosugar metabolism.

Hypophosphatemia

Definition: Phosphate < 2.5 to 3.0 mg/dL.

Phosphate is important in cellular energy metabolism.

Causes
- Renal loss
  - Loss of proximal tubular function.
  - Hyperparathyroidism.
  - Diuretic use.
  - Hypokalemia.
  - Hypomagnesemia.
  - Steroids.
- GI loss
  - Malabsorption.
  - Diarrhea.
  - Antacids (phosphate binding gels).
  - Intestinal fistulas.
- Inadequate intake
  - Malnutrition.
  - Parental nutrition without phosphate replacement.
  - Alcoholism.
- Transcellular shift (increase cell uptake to form sugar phosphates)
  - Acute respiratory alkalosis (correction of metabolic acidosis).
  - Carbohydrate administration/anabolism.
  - Insulin.
  - Epinephrine.

Phosphate is easily lost from red blood cells and skeletal muscle, but stores are well preserved in cardiac muscle.

Signs and Symptoms
Low phosphate levels result in various neuromuscular and central nervous system effects. Symptoms are related to a depletion in intracellular stores.

- Parathesias.
- Muscle weakness (contributes to ventilator dependence).
- Dyspnea/respiratory failure.
- Hypotension.
- Malaise.
- Lethargy.
- Disorientation.
- Seizures.
- Coma.

Chapter 18

Treatment

Phosphate levels < 1mg/dL with symptoms are life threatening. Phosphate is predominantly intracellular so replacement is done with caution.

◆ Parenteral sodium phosphate, or potassium phosphate if severe.
  ❖ Dose 0.6mg/kg/hr to 0.9mg/kg/hr.
  ❖ Observe for signs of hypocalcemia.
  ❖ Observe for hyperkalemia or hypernatremia based on preparation used.
◆ Enteral replacement is preferred if levels are not life threatening.

Hyperphosphatemia

Definition: Phosphate > 4.5 mg/dL.

Causes

◆ Impaired renal excretion.
◆ Increased intake of phosphate containing laxatives.
◆ Hypoparathyroidism (hypocalcemia).
◆ Increased cellular release.
  ❖ Rhabdomyolysis.
  ❖ Sepsis.
  ❖ Chemotherapy/tumor lysis.

Signs and Symptoms

Same clinical signs as hypocalcemia.

Treatment

◆ Treat hypocalcemia.
◆ Aluminum antacids bind with phosphate.
◆ Acetazolamide to increase urinary excretion.
◆ Dialysis if due to renal failure or if emergency.

RENAL ISSUES IN CARDIAC AND CRITICAL CARE

Renal Anatomy and Physiology

Overview of Kidneys (Figure 18.5)

◆ Two kidneys located in extra peritoneal cavity.
◆ Size and shape of each kidney.
  ❖ 10-12 cm long.
  ❖ 5-6 cm wide.
  ❖ 2.5 cm in depth.
  ❖ Lobular in structure.
◆ Surrounded by mass of fatty connective tissue for protection.
◆ Blood vessels, nerves, and ureters connected via the hilum, a depressed area in the medial aspect of each kidney.
◆ Renal artery branches into 5 smaller arteries that enter hilus of kidney; smaller branches then give rise to afferent arterioles that enter the glomerulus.
◆ Nephron is functional unit of kidney; over 1 million nephrons per kidney.

Non Cardiac Issues in the Cardiac Patient: Pulmonary Pathophysiology, Electrolytes and Renal, Sepsis

- Longitudinal view: Outer aspect of kidney is the cortex; inner aspect is the medulla.
  - Cortex
    - Cortical area.
    - Juxtamedullary area (next to medulla).
    - Contains:
      - Glomeruli.
      - Proximal tubules.
      - Cortical loops of Henle.
      - Distal tubules.
      - Cortical collecting ducts.
  - Medulla
    - Contains renal pyramids.
      - Medullary loops of Henle.
      - Medullary portions of collecting ducts (join to form calyces, which further join to become the conduit for urine to enter the ureter).

Nephron (Figure 18.6)

- Functional unit of kidney.
- Consists of glomerulus and a tubular structure.
  - Glomerulus
    - Tuft of capillaries emerging from afferent arterioles.
    - Contained within Bowman's capsule.
    - Blood flows out of glomerular capillaries via the efferent arterioles.
    - Space within Bowman's capsule for the filtrate: Bowman's space.
    - Basement membrane of the glomerular capillary membrane determines permeability; permeable to water but not to plasma proteins.
  - Tubular structure
    - Proximal convoluted tubule.
      - The majority of all reabsorptive and secretory processes occur here (Figure 18.7).
    - Loop of Henle.
      - Descending limb (thin walled).
      - Ascending limb (thick walled).
        - Impermeable to water.
        - Solutes are reabsorbed (approximately 20% of sodium, chloride, and potassium).
        - Loop diuretics work here and block reabsorption of sodium.
        - Filtrate is diluted to allow for excretion of free water.
      - Medullary loops of Henle dip into the medulla.
    - Distal convoluted tubule.
      - More reabsorption of sodium and more dilute filtrate.
      - Thiazide diuretics work here to inhibit sodium reabsorption.

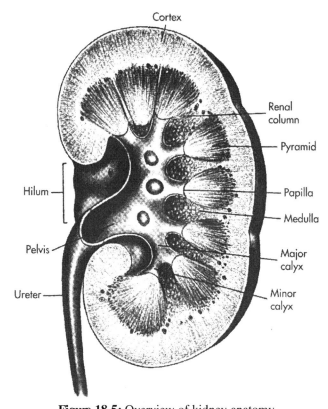

Figure 18.5: Overview of kidney anatomy.
From *Pass CCRN* (2nd ed.), by R.D. Dennison, 2000, St. Louis: Mosby. Reprinted with permission from Elsevier.

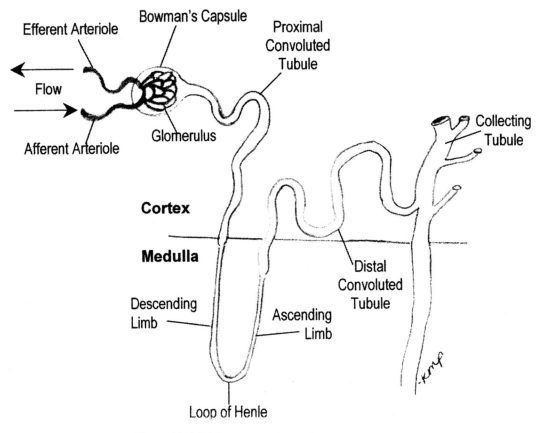

Figure 18.6: Major components of nephron.

* Hydrogen and potassium added to urine via secretion.
* Aldosterone works on late distal tubule and cortical collecting tubule (below).
★ Collecting tubule or duct
  * Several distal tubules drain into the collecting tubule.
  * Single layer of epithelial cells.
  * No further electrolyte absorption or secretion.
  * Cortical collecting tubule.
    – Aldosterone works here.
  * Medullary collecting tubule.
    – ADH (vasopressin) works here.
    – Responsible for determining concentration and acidity of urine.
◆ 85% of nephrons originate in superficial part of cortex (cortical nephrons).
◆ 15% of nephrons originate deeper in the cortex (juxtamedullary nephrons).
  ❖ Longer, thinner loops of Henle.
  ❖ Responsible for urine concentration.
◆ Capillary systems in nephron.
  ❖ Glomerular high pressure capillary system between afferent and efferent arterioles.

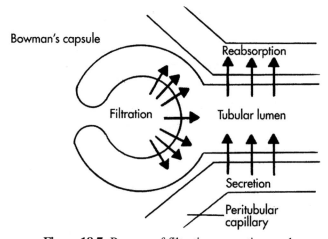

Figure 18.7: Process of filtration, secretion, and reabsorption in the formation of urine.
From *Pass CCRN* (2nd ed.), by R.D. Dennison, 2000, St. Louis: Mosby. Reprinted with permission from Elsevier.

Non Cardiac Issues in the Cardiac Patient: Pulmonary Pathophysiology, Electrolytes and Renal, Sepsis

❖ Peritubular capillary system – a low pressure system originating from the efferent arterioles.
  ☆ Surround loop of Henle.
  ☆ Most water and electrolytes reabsorbed into the blood here.
❖ Medullary nephrons have an additional capillary system, the vas recta, consisting of long straight capillaries following the long loops of Henle.

Glomerular filtration: Filtration of protein-free plasma through the glomerular capillaries into Bowman's space. The capillary filtration pressure is approximately 60 mm Hg in the glomerular capillaries. This is a higher pressure than that in other capillary beds. Both hydrostatic pressure and osmotic pressure influence glomerular filtration. Glomerular capillaries are permeable to water, but not to protein.

Glomerular filtration produces 125 mL of filtrate each minute.

Glomerular filtration remains stable with a wide range of systemic blood pressures due to autoregulation. When blood pressure decreases, afferent arterioles dilate to maintain glomerular filtration at a constant. In turn, when blood pressure is high, afferent arterioles constrict. However, when mean arterial pressure falls below 80 mm Hg, or is greater than 180 mm Hg, then the glomerular filtration rate becomes proportional to systemic perfusion pressure.

Constriction of the afferent arterioles decreases glomerular pressure and filtration. Constriction of the efferent arterioles increases glomerular pressure and filtration (Figure 18.6). Both the afferent and efferent arterioles are innervated by the sympathetic nervous system. They are also sensitive to vasoactive hormones, such as angiotensin II.

Linking Knowledge to Practice

✔ *In shock, afferent arterioles constrict (in response to SNS stimulation), and glomerular filtration and urine output can fall to near zero.*

Definitions

Azotemia: Accumulation of nitrogenous wastes in the blood.

Renal insufficiency: Reduction in glomerular filtration to 20 to 50% of normal.

Acute kidney injury: A sudden loss of the kidneys' ability to excrete wastes, concentrate urine, and conserve electrolytes.

◆ Occurs as complication in critically ill patients.
◆ Mortality ranges from 42-88% (Porth, 2004). (Note: Variations exist due to differences in definitions for renal failure, used historically in the literature.)

Oliguria: Urine output < 400 ml/24 hours.

Anuria: Urine output < 50 ml/24 hours.

Chapter 18

Diagnostics (Table 18.5)

Table 18.5 (1 of 2) Diagnostic Parameters for Assessment of Renal Function	
Urine Volume	◆ Urine output is a less specific indicator. ◆ Urine volume usually reflects kidney perfusion. Renal blood flow is adequate in non-oliguric patients. Urine output falls when there is renal hypoperfusion.
Urine Specific Gravity Urine Osmolalitty	◆ One of earliest manifestations of renal dysfunction is inability to concentrate urine. ◆ Urine concentrating represents tubular function.
BUN	◆ BUN is <u>not</u> the most specific indicator of renal function. ❖ Variations exist in the urea load. ☆ Rhabdomyolysis, increased protein intake, and corticosteroids can increase BUN levels. ☆ Liver disease and diminished muscle mass can decrease BUN levels. ❖ The proximal tubule is able to absorb filtered urea. ☆ BUN rises in disproportion to renal function when there is intravascular volume depletion. BUN is reabsorbed, along with sodium and water.
Serum Creatinine	◆ Measurement of serum creatinine ❖ Specific for renal function; creatinine is produced in a steady state. ❖ Effective in evaluating if renal function is stable, better, or worse. ❖ Increased level indicates that rate of production is exceeding clearance through GFR; a rise in serum creatinine may not be evident until 50% of GFR is lost. ❖ Renal dysfunction and GFR cannot be accurately assessed until serum creatinine stabilizes. ❖ Stable increase in creatinine implies a new steady state with a decrease in GFR; creatinine level needs to stabilize before an accurate assessment of renal function can be made. ❖ In total loss of renal function, there is a rise in creatinine of 1-2 mg/dL per day. ❖ Creatinine will stabilize at 12-15 mg/dL if there is continued complete renal shutdown.
Creatinine Clearance	◆ Limitations of creatinine clearance ❖ As GFR falls, creatinine excretion is increased and the rise in serum creatinine is less. Creatinine excretion is much greater than the filtered load, resulting in a potentially large overestimation of GFR.

848

Non Cardiac Issues in the Cardiac Patient: Pulmonary Pathophysiology, Electrolytes and Renal, Sepsis

<table>
<tr><td colspan="2" align="center">Table 18.5 (2 of 2)
Diagnostic Parameters for Assessment of Renal Function</td></tr>
<tr>
<td>Glomerular Filtration</td>
<td>

◆ Glomerular filtration rate (GFR)

   ❖ GFR is the volume of fluid filtered from the renal glomerular capillaries into Bowman's capsule per unit of time.

   ❖ Glomerular filtration determined by estimation of creatinine clearance.

   ❖ Glomerular filtration rate is best measured via a 24-hour urine. However, this method is not practical in clinical practice.

   ❖ GFR is usually estimated with the Cockroft-Gault equation:

     (140-age) x weight (kg) / plasma creatinine x 72
     (value is multiplied by 0.85 in females).

   ❖ The GFR can also be estimated using the MDRD formula. The MDRD formula estimates GFR using serum creatinine and age. A multiplier is used to adjust for race and gender.

</td>
</tr>
<tr>
<td>Kidney Size</td>
<td>◆ Small kidneys indicate a chronic component to renal failure.</td>
</tr>
</table>

Acute Kidney Injury (AKI)

Due to inconsistent definitions of acute renal failure, a new classification system has been proposed. The new term, which will include what has previously been known as acute renal failure, is acute kidney injury. The definition of acute injury includes one or more of the following that occurs abruptly (within 48 hours):

◆ An absolute increase in serum creatinine of more than or equal to 0.3 mg/dL.

◆ A percentage increase in serum creatinine of more than or equal to 50%.

◆ A reduction in urine output of less than 0.5 ml/kg per hour for more than six hours.

Acute kidney injury can be further classified into 3 stages, as defined in Table 18.6. This new staging system has been modified from the previous RIFLE classification system, which included the categories of risk, injury, failure, loss, and end-stage kidney disease. Acute kidney injury may be superimposed on chronic kidney disease or may lead to the development of chronic kidney disease.

Approximately 20% of critically ill patients develop acute kidney injury (Marini & Wheeler, 2006; Stark, 2006). Acute kidney injury in critically ill patients increases mortality; however, it is not always fatal because the excretory function of the kidneys can be performed through dialysis and filtration. In addition, the lungs, liver, and drug replacement therapy help to compensate for the metabolic functions of the failing kidney.

The term "acute kidney injury" is a newly proposed term. The term acute renal failure is still prevalent in the literature. The term "acute kidney injury" is used in this chapter synonymously with the older term, acute renal failure.

849

Chapter 18

<table>
<tr><td colspan="3" align="center">**Table 18.6**
Stages of Acute Kidney Injury</td></tr>
<tr><td>**Stage**</td><td>**Creatinine Criteria**</td><td>**Urine Output Criteria**</td></tr>
<tr><td>1</td><td>Increase in serum creatinine of more than or equal to 0.3 mg/dL or increase to more than or equal to 150% to 200%.</td><td>Less than 0.5 ml/kg per hour for more than 6 hours.</td></tr>
<tr><td>2</td><td>Increase in serum creatinine to more than 200% to 300%.</td><td>Less than 0.5 ml/kg per hour for more than 12 hours.</td></tr>
<tr><td>3</td><td>Increase in serum creatinine to more than 300% or serum creatinine of more than or equal to 4.0 mg/dL with an acute increase of at least 0.5 mg/dL.</td><td>Less than 0.3 ml/kg per hour for 24 hours or anuria for 12 hours.</td></tr>
</table>

Etiology

The etiologies of acute kidney injury and chronic renal disease differ. Uncontrolled hypertension and diabetes are common etiologies of chronic renal failure. Chronic renal failure is also more likely associated with normal urine output, small kidneys, anemia, and hypocalcemia.

The etiologies of acute kidney injury differ between in-hospital and out-of-hospital acquisition. The most common causes of acute kidney injury outside the hospital are:
◆ Glomerulonephritis.
◆ Vasculitis.
◆ Obstructive uropathy.

The most common causes of acute kidney injury in the hospital setting are:
◆ Renal hypoperfusion.
◆ Drug toxicity.
◆ Combination of hypoperfusion and drug effect.

Although oliguria is diagnostic of acute kidney injury, acute kidney injury can also occur in the presence of normal urine output. Non-oliguric kidney injury is as common as oliguric kidney injury (Shapiro, 2003). The outcome is worse with oliguric acute kidney injury than with non-oliguric acute kidney injury.

Signs and Symptoms

◆ Fatigue.
◆ Confusion.
◆ Twitching or weakness related to metabolic acidosis.
◆ Dry skin.
◆ Edema.
◆ Pallor.
◆ Uremic frost/pruritis.
◆ Flank pain.
◆ Infection.
(Stark, 2006)

Non Cardiac Issues in the Cardiac Patient: Pulmonary Pathophysiology, Electrolytes and Renal, Sepsis

Classifications of Acute Kidney Injury

◆ Pre-renal: 55-60% of AKI.

◆ Intrarenal: 35-40% of AKI.

◆ Postrenal: Post renal < 5% AKI.

(Porth, 2004)

Pre-renal Acute Kidney Injury

Causes

The most common cause of pre-renal AKI is a reduction in blood flow, resulting in hypoperfusion. When renal perfusion pressure falls below the auto regulation threshold, glomerular filtration is adversely affected. A decrease in the afferent arterial pressure to < 100 mm Hg has a negative impact on filtration (Stark, 2006). A drop in mean arterial pressure to < 60-70 mm Hg for greater than 30 minutes places the kidneys at risk for injury. There is an increased risk for ischemic injury when the patient also has hypoxemia.

Causes of pre-renal AKI include:

◆ Decreased intravascular volume.

   ❖ Hemorrhage.

   ❖ Third spacing.

   ❖ Over use of diuretics.

◆ Decreased cardiac output.

◆ Vasodilation during sepsis.

◆ Bilateral renal vascular obstruction from embolus or thrombosis.

◆ Hepatorenal syndrome is a special cause of pre-renal azotemia. This syndrome exists when there is advancing renal failure in a patient with severe hepatic disease. The renal failure usually occurs in response to changes in blood volume or fluid shifts. Ascites is usually present.

Diagnostic Parameters

◆ Positive response to a fluid challenge is diagnostic of pre-renal AKI.

◆ Oliguria.

◆ Urinary Sodium < 20 mEq/L.

   ❖ Urine sodium not accurate if chronic renal failure, hypoaldosteronism, metabolic alkalosis, or diuretic therapy within 24 hours.

◆ Concentrated urine: Urine specific gravity > 1.0150 and urine osmolality > 500 mOsm/L.

◆ BUN: Creatinine Ratio > 10:1 (usually closer to 20:1). Increased proximal tubular reabsorption of BUN.

◆ Fractional excretion of sodium (FENa) < 1%

   ❖ Needs to be assessed before the initiation of diuretics

◆ Fractional excretion of urea (FEurea) < 35%

◆ Urine Protein 0 or minimal.

◆ Urine Sediment: Normal or minimally abnormal; hyaline casts, finely granular casts.

Treatment

The treatment of pre-renal AKI is aimed at the rapid reversal of the underlying cause of renal hypoperfusion in order to restore adequate renal perfusion.

Chapter 18

Intrarenal Acute Kidney Injury

Classifications

◆ Tubular: Acute Tubular Necrosis (most common cause of intrarenal AKI).

◆ Glomerular: Glomerulonephritis and small vessel vasculitis.

◆ Intersitial: Interstitial Nephritis.

◆ Vascular: Athroembolic disease, large vessel vasculitis.

Acute Tubular Necrosis (ATN) (Medullary)

Acute tubular necrosis is the most common cause of AKI in the ICU setting (Shapiro, 2003).

Causes

◆ Nephrotoxic agents (often play a role).
  ❖ Aminoglycosides.
    ☆ 1 x daily dosing reduces risk.
    ☆ Maintenance dose should be adjusted based on GFR.
  ❖ Amphotericin B.
  ❖ Chemotherapy agents (platinum based).
  ❖ Cyclosporine.
  ❖ Contrast agents.
    ☆ Risk reduced by pretreatment with oral n-acetylcysteine.
      ✶ 24 to 48 hours before contrast exposure.
      ✶ 600 mg BID.
    ☆ Risk reduced by adequate pre-procedure hydration with 0.9NS or sodium bicarbonate drip.
      ✶ 154 mEq of sodium bicarbonate/L given at 3 ml/kg for 1 hour prior to procedure, and followed by 1 ml/kg/hr for 6 hours post procedure.
      ✶ Some evidence that sodium bicarbonate is superior to sodium chloride in preventing contrast induced nephropathy. There may be an associated antioxidant effect, in addition to volume expansion.
  ❖ ACE Inhibitors
    ☆ May induce renal failure in presence of bilateral renal artery stenosis or single kidney renal artery stenosis.
    ☆ In most patients, the benefit of increased cardiac output from afterload reduction outweighs the risk.
  ❖ Non-steroidal anti-inflammatory agents (NSAIDS).
    ☆ Patients with high renin angiotensin states depend on prostaglandin E2 (PGE2), which is a vasodilator released from the endothelium. In these patients, NSAIDS can block PGE2 formation.
    ☆ NSAIDS also promote sodium, potassium, and fluid retention.
  ❖ Other medications
    ☆ Antibiotics in addition to aminoglycosides (tetracyclines, penicillins, cephalosporins, pentamidine).
    ☆ Antivirals.
    ☆ Carbon tetrachloride.
    ☆ Heavy metals.
    ☆ Pesticides/fungicides.
    (Stark, 2006)

♦ Prolonged ischemic injury.

♦ Release of hemoglobin or myoglobin during hemolysis or rhabdomyolysis.

♦ Endotoxin release in sepsis.

♦ Hypercalcemia.

♦ Any cause of pre-renal AKI that is prolonged. The clinical challenge is to differentiate pre-renal AKI from intrarenal AKI caused by ATN.

Risk Factors

♦ Elderly.

♦ Dehydration.

♦ Hypertension.

♦ Diabetes.

♦ Underlying renal dysfunction.

♦ Myeloma.

Diagnostic Parameters

♦ Urine Sodium > 20 mEq/L.

♦ Urine osmolality < 400 mOsmol/L (loss of tubular concentrating ability).

♦ Bun:Creatinine Ratio 10:1.

♦ Fractional excretion of sodium (FENa) > 2-3%.

   ❖ Needs to be assessed before the initiation of diuretics.

♦ Fractional excretion of urea (FEurea) > 50%.

♦ Minimal to moderate proteinuria.

♦ Urine Sediment: Muddy brown casts, tubular casts, renal epithelial cells.

Pathophysiology

ATN results in the destruction of the tubular epithelial layer of cells. The injury is often reversible if treatment is promptly initiated. If the tubular basement membrane is damaged from prolonged injury and ischemia, it cannot be regenerated.

Oliguric AKI can develop when tubules become obstructed due to tissue swelling or cellular debris. There can be a reabsorption into circulation of urine filtrate through the damaged tubular epithelium. Damaged tubular cells can leak ATP and potassium, and calcium can leak into the cell. Scar tissue can form over necrotic areas (Stark, 2006).

Treatment

♦ Optimizing volume status and keeping a high volume of urine helps minimize the risk of ATN.

♦ Avoid all nephrotoxic agents; avoid or dose adjust all medications requiring renal clearance.

♦ A loop diuretic such as furosemide can be used to correct volume overload if the patient is still responsive to it. It is a positive prognostic sign when a patient is responsive to a loop diuretic (Agraharkar, 2007). Diuretics are controversial in the treatment of acute kidney injury because there is limited evidence of their benefit regarding improved mortality or improved kidney function (Agraharkar, 2007).

♦ Dopamine, fenoldopam, and mannitol are not indicated (Agraharkar, 2007).

♦ Treatment is supportive with a focus on managing fluid and acid/base balance, electrolytes, and hematologic abnormalities.

Chapter 18

Glomerulonephritis (Cortical)
Causes
Common cause of acute kidney injury outside the hospital.
◆ Subacute bacterial endocarditis.
◆ Post streptococcal infection.
◆ Systemic lupus erythematous.
◆ Drug induced vasculitis.
◆ Malignant hypertension.

Pathophysiology
Cortical involvement from the above causes renal capillary swelling. Edema and cellular debris obstruct the glomeruli, resulting in a decrease the GFR and oliguria.

Diagnostic Parameters
Urinalysis will have RBC casts, protein, and leukocytes. BUN to creatinine ratio 10:1 and elevated.

Treatment
◆ Immunosuppressant medications.
◆ Plasmapheresis.

Interstitial Nephritis (Cortical)
Causes
◆ Drug induced: Allergic nephritis.
  ❖ Common but often unrecognized allergic event in the interstiium of the kidney.
  ❖ Usually in response to a specific drug.
  ❖ May have associated fever, rash, eosinophilia.
◆ Bacterial, viral, and other infections.
◆ Immune and neoplasitc disorders.

Diagnostic Parameters
◆ WBC casts with eosinophils.
◆ BUN to creatinine ratio 10:1 and elevated.

Treatment
◆ Remove the drug that is the causative agent.
◆ Steroids may be used.

Postrenal Acute Kidney Injury

Postrenal AKI is the cause of acute kidney injury in only 1-10% of the cases (Marini & Wheeler, 2006). However, it is important to rule out because the causes are reversible. Bilateral uretal obstruction will result in acute kidney injury.

Classifications and Causes
◆ Mechanical (bladder outlet or urtethral obstruction)
  ❖ Urinary calculi.
  ❖ Tumor.
  ❖ Prostatic hypertrophy.

854

Non Cardiac Issues in the Cardiac Patient: Pulmonary Pathophysiology, Electrolytes and Renal, Sepsis

- ❖ Fibrosis.
- ❖ Blood clot.
- ❖ Retroperitoneal hemorrhage.
- ◆ Functional
  - ❖ Neurogenic bladder.
  - ❖ Ganglionic-blocking agents.

Pathophysiology

Obstruction can increase renal interstial pressure; this causes an increased opposing force to GFR.

Signs and Symptoms

With obstructive uropathy, there is an abrupt decrease in urine output. Renal ultrasound or CT can be used to detect obstruction within or proximal to the bladder. Urinalysis may show hematuria.

Stages of Acute Oliguric Kidney Injury

Mortality for oliguric acute kidney injury is higher than for non-oliguruc acute kidney injury. Acute kidney injury with oliguria has an approximate 50% mortality in the critical care setting (Stark, 2006). Oliguric acute kidney injury has 4 classic phases. Non-oliguric acute kidney injury does not have an oliguric/anuric phase.

- ◆ Onset Phase
  - ❖ Hours to days.
  - ❖ Renal blood flow and glomerular filtration fall.
  - ❖ Urine output falls.
  - ❖ BUN: Creatinine – Normal or slight increase.
- ◆ Oliguric – Anuric Phase (also referred to as maintenance phase)
  - ❖ 8-14 days.
  - ❖ Decreased GFR.
  - ❖ Urine output < 15 ml/hr (400 cc/24 hours).
  - ❖ BUN and creatinine increased.
  - ❖ Metabolic acidosis.
  - ❖ Increased potassium.
  - ❖ Water gain with hypertension, dilutional hyponatremia, and pulmonary congestion.
  - ❖ Uremia can develop: Neuromuscular irritability, seizures, coma, death.
  - ❖ High mortality rate.
- ◆ Diuretic Phase
  - ❖ 3 to 4 weeks after onset.
  - ❖ Can last 1-2 weeks.
  - ❖ BUN and creatinine begin to decrease (diuresis may occur before BUN and creatinine fall).
  - ❖ Urine output may exceed 3L/24 Hr: 150-200% of normal. GFR improves and osmotic diuresis from elevated BUN occurs. Tubular function has not yet returned to normal and tubules are not yet able to concentrate urine.
  - ❖ Fluid losses can jeopardize adequate circulating volume.
  - ❖ Uremic symptoms may not completely resolve because tubular function is not yet normal.

Chapter 18

◆ Recovery
  ❖ Recovery is shorter in non-oliguric renal failure.
  ❖ Begins with stabilization of laboratory values.
  ❖ Several months to one year.
  ❖ BUN: Creatinine almost normal; residual dysfunction may remain.
  ❖ Urine output returns to normal.

Acute kidney injury has also been classified into 3 phases: Onset, maintenance, and recovery. In this system of classification, the diuretic phase is included in the recovery phase.

Linking Knowledge to Practice

✔ *Concentrated urine is a hallmark sign of pre-renal acute kidney injury, with a urine osmolality greater than 400 mOsm/kg of water.*

✔ *When urine output falls in critical care, the nurse should first consider a pre-renal cause.*

Electrolyte Abnormalities in Acute Kidney Injury

◆ Hyperkalemia – most common with oliguric AKI.
◆ Hyperphosmatemia.
◆ Hypermagnesemia.
◆ Hypocalcemia.
◆ Acidemia
  ❖ The kidneys excrete acid.
  ❖ Oral sodium bicarbonate is typically used to treat.
  ❖ Negative hemodynamic effects have been associated with IV sodium bicarbonate bolus dosing because CO_2 is generated when bicarbonate is administered in acidotic blood, and the CO_2 can diffuse into the cell and produce an intracellular acidosis (Shapiro, 2003).
  ❖ The treatment for severe metabolic acidosis remains controversial.

Uremic Syndrome

Uremic syndrome is seen in both acute kidney injury and in chronic renal failure. All organs can be affected by uremic syndrome. Signs and symptoms can include: nausea, vomiting, pruritis, bleeding, encephalopathy, and pericarditis. The symptoms of uremic syndrome are not related solely to an elevated BUN or creatinine. The presence of uremic symptoms warrants aggressive treatment with some type of dialysis therapy.

Treatment of Acute Kidney Injury

Early Oliguric Kidney Injury (less than 8 hours of oliguria)

◆ Eliminate all contributing pre-renal factors.
  ❖ Consider invasive monitoring to assess intravascular fluid volume status.
  ❖ Consider vasoactive drugs to improve blood pressure and renal perfusion when intravascular volume is adequate.
◆ Rule out postrenal obstructive causes.
◆ A loop diuretic such as furosemide can be used to correct volume overload if the patient is still responsive to it. It is a positive prognostic sign when a patient is responsive to a loop diuretic

(Agraharkar, 2007). Diuretics are controversial in the treatment of acute kidney injury because there is limited evidence of their benefit regarding improved mortality or improved kidney function (Agraharkar, 2007).

- Dopamine, fenoldopam, and mannitol are not indicated (Agraharkar, 2007).
- Avoid all nephrotoxic agents; avoid or dose adjust all medications requiring renal clearance.
- Initiate some form of extra corporeal blood therapy (renal replacement therapy) early in the course of treatment.
- Provide meticulous supportive care.
- Avoid complications.
  - Infection.
  - Fluid, electrolyte, and acid/base imbalances.
  - Hematologic abnormalities.
  - Drug toxicity from drugs metabolized or excreted from the kidney.

Established Oliguric Acute Kidney Injury

- Modify dose of drugs metabolized or excreted from kidney. Base dose adjustment on an assumed GFR of zero.
- Limit fluid intake to avoid congestion.
- Restrict potassium, phosphate, and magnesium intake. Enteral bicarbonate may be given for acidemia. Assess for hyponatremia.
  - Oral phosphate binders effective in preventing hypocalcemia.
- Prevent complications
  - Infection-related complications are the most common cause of death in acute renal failure (Marini & Wheeler, 2006).
    - Nosocomial pneumonia.
    - IV catheter infections.
    - Intra abdominal sepsis.
  - Hemorrhage
    - Uremic toxins inhibit platelets and factor VIII.
    - Factor VIII may need to be replaced.
    - Arginine vasopressin can also increase levels of factor VIII.
- Nutrition
  - Sufficient fat and carbohydrate calories to prevent protein wasting.
  - Limit protein if not on dialysis; may be more liberal if on dialysis.
  - Folate and pyridoxine are lost through dialysis; must be supplemented.
- Avoid corticosteroids (except for interstitial nephritis and some types of renal vasculitis).
  - Catabolic effect
  - Adversely affects immune function

Nursing Care Issues in Acute Kidney Injury

- Maintain skin integrity (uremic effects place patient at high risk for breakdown).
- Prevent infection (infection is major cause of mortality). BUN > 80 to 100 mg/dL is associated with a high risk of infection.

- ◆ Nutrition (patients can have accelerated protein catabolism – indicated by BUN > 100mg/dL, despite routine dialysis). These patients will need higher protein intake.
- ◆ Maintain fluid restriction.
- ◆ Replace water soluable vitamins (caution with Vitamin A if kidneys cannot excrete).
- ◆ Monitoring of electrolytes, serum protein, albumin, hematocrit, and BUN and creatinine. Low serum protein and albumin levels have an immunosuppressive effect (Stark, 2006).

Renal Replacement Therapy

Renal replacement involves the clearance of fluids and solute, and correction of electrolytes.

- ◆ Hemodialysis (intermittent)
    - ❖ Central venous access required for emergency dialysis. The internal jugular, subclavian, and femoral can be used for emergent access.
    - ❖ Chronic intermittent hemodialysis requires arteriovenous grafts or fistulas, which are accessed using needles during the treatment (Figure 18.8).
    - ❖ Anticoagulation is required to keep blood anticoagulated within the dialysis machine. Non-heparin dialysis is being done at some centers.
    - ❖ Blood is pumped through an artificial kidney on one side of the dialysis membrane, while the dialysate (electrolyte) solution flows in the opposite direction on the other side.
    - ❖ The high flow process combines adsorption, diffusion, osmosis, and ultrafiltration to remove fluid and maximal amount of solute.

    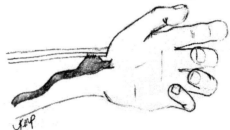

    Figure 18.8: Arteriovenous fistula.

    - ❖ Electrolytes, metabolic products, drugs, and toxins are removed. Blood is returned to systemic circulation.
    - ❖ Requires more hemodynamic stability than hemofiltration. Hypotension is the most common problem.
    - ❖ Dialysis equilibrium syndrome: complication from shifts in extracellular compartment
        - ☆ Nausea, vomiting, confusion, seizures, coma.
        - ☆ Most common in first dialysis session with high BUN.
        - ☆ Treatment.
            - ∗ Decreased dialysis time.
            - ∗ Decreased dialysis flow rates.
            - ∗ Dialyzer with smaller surface area.
            - ∗ Sodium chloride, dextrose, mannitol.
    - ❖ Intermittent sessions can be performed due to the maximal solute removal.
    - ❖ Slow efficiency daily dialysis (SLEDD) is another form of delivery of hemodialysis.
- ◆ Peritoneal Dialysis (intermittent)
    - ❖ Slow form of dialysis that involves an exchange of fluids and solutes between the peritoneal cavity and peritoneal capillaries. Utilizes diffusion.
    - ❖ Less efficient than hemodialysis in removing toxins or correcting electrolyte abnormalities.
    - ❖ No need for vascular access. No significant hemodynamic effects.

Non Cardiac Issues in the Cardiac Patient: Pulmonary Pathophysiology, Electrolytes and Renal, Sepsis

❖ 1 to 3 L of solution with dwell time of 30 to 40 minutes.

❖ Osmotic gradient for fluid removal using hyperosmolar glucose concentrations.

❖ Complications

    ☆ Abdominal distention and increased work of breathing.

    ☆ Pleural effusion if dialysate leaks.

    ☆ Hyperglycemia (dialysate solution contains high concentration of glucose).

    ☆ Peritonitis.

◆ Continuous Extracorporeal Blood Therapy (CEBT) – Previously called Continuous Renal Replacement Therapy (CRRT). Table 18.7 summarizes the differences in the types of CEBT.

❖ Ultrafiltration

    ☆ SCUF – Slow continuous ultrafiltration.

    ☆ Ultrafiltration is the movement of fluid through a semipermeable membrane. The movement of fluid is caused by a pressure gradient. A higher pressure gradient creates more fluid removal.

    ☆ Ultrafiltration therapy results in primarily fluid removal.

    ☆ Hemofiltration, hemodialysis, and hemodiafiltration all use ultrafiltration as a component of their therapy.

    ☆ Adsorption is another principle involved in all 4 therapies. Adsorption refers to the clinging of positively charged molecules to the negatively charged membrane of the filter. The filter can become clogged with these molecules. The removal of these molecules from systemic circulation via adsorption is a benefit of CEBT therapy.

❖ Hemofiltration

    ☆ CVVH – Continuous veno-venous hemofiltration.

    ☆ Hemofiltration uses convection to remove solutes. Convection is the process of solute removal by use of a solvent drag. The more fluid that moves through a semi permeable membrane, the more solute that is removed.

    ☆ Replacement solution is used to create the solvent drag. A faster rate of replacement solution creates more solvent drag.

    ☆ Convection allows the removal of medium and large molecule solutes.

    ☆ Solute removal is slow so the process must be continuous.

    ☆ In hemofiltration fluid removal still exceeds solute removal.

    ☆ Hemofiltration is less likely than hemodialysis to produce hypotension. There is a slower change in plasma osmolality.

    ☆ Some medications are cleared via hemofiltration and will require a dose adjustment. During hemofiltration medications can be dosed based on an assumed creatinine clearance of approximately 14 ml/minute (Lin, 2003).

❖ Hemodialysis

    ☆ CVVHD – Continuous veno-venous hemodialysis.

    ☆ Hemodialysis uses dialysate solution to create selective diffusion of electrolytes. Diffusion is an excellent technique for the removal of small particles.

    ☆ Hemodialysis removes both solutes and fluid.

    ☆ This form of CEBT is often used on patients who are on chronic dialysis.

    ☆ Continuous hemodialysis provides more hemodynamic stability than intermittent hemodialysis.

    ☆ Fluid overloaded critically ill patients can receive a higher caloric intake because fluid volume can be removed on a continuous basis.

Chapter 18

❖ Hemodiafiltration
  ☆ CVVHDF – Continuous veno-venous hemodiafiltration.
  ☆ This technique uses both hemodialysis and hemofiltration techniques to allow for the removal of small, medium, and large molecule solutes.

A venous to venous connection with the use of a double lumen venous catheter is preferred for CEBT. Jugular, subclavian, and femoral veins can all be used. Venous-only access avoids the risk of limb ischemia that accompanies arterial access. With venous-to-venous circuits, an extra corpeal pump is used to create flow through the system. Filtration is ineffective when MAP fall below 60 mm Hg. Equipment for CEBT involves a blood filter, blood pumps, circuit tubing, dialysate and replacement infusion tubing, anticoagulant tubing, and a collection bag.

Table 18.7
Summary of the Differences in CEBT Strategies

Therapy	Principles for fluid and solute removal	Replacement Solution Used?	Dialysate Solution Used?
SCUF	Ultrafiltration Adsorption	No	No
CVVHD	Ultrafiltration Adsorption Diffusion	No	Yes
CVVH	Ultrafiltration Adsorption Convection	Yes	No
CVVHDF	Ultrafiltration Adsorption Diffusion Convection	Yes	Yes

Criteria for Intermittent Dialysis

◆ Volume overload in presence of oliguria or anuria.
◆ Uncontrolled hyperkalemia, hyperphosphatemia, hypermagnesemia.
◆ Life threatening acidosis.
◆ Life threatening drug overdoses or toxicity requiring dialysis.
◆ Symptomatic uremia
  ❖ Nausea and vomiting.
  ❖ Bleeding.
  ❖ Pericarditis.
  ❖ Seizures, coma.
◆ BUN 80-100 mg/dL.
◆ Creatinine 10 mg/dL.

Non Cardiac Issues in the Cardiac Patient: Pulmonary Pathophysiology, Electrolytes and Renal, Sepsis

Criteria for Continuous Extracorporeal Blood Therapy (CEBT)

Patients with any of the criteria for intermittent hemodialysis who have hemodynamic instability are candidates for CEBT. Patients with hemodynamic instability do not tolerate the high flow rates used in hemodialysis. In addition, patients with an increase in intracranial pressure will not tolerate the fluid shifting associated with intermittent hemodialysis (Lin, 2003).

In addition to an alternative for intermittent hemodialysis, starting continuous extracorporeal blood therapy earlier in the course of renal dysfunction improves survival in critically ill patients. The goal is to start therapy when patients are in the risk or injury stage. Starting therapy in these stages can prevent failure, loss, and end stage renal disease. There are several proposed non-traditional uses for continuous renal replacement therapy. These indications continue to be the subject of current research. Examples of non-traditional indications include: hyperthermia, rhabdomyolysis, systemic inflammatory response syndrome, and fluid management in the hemodynamically unstable patient without renal failure (Lin, 2003).

Nursing Considerations for Extracorporeal Blood Therapy (CEBT)

Hypothermia is a side effect of CEBT. Hypothermia occurs because the patient's blood travels through an extracorporeal circuit and because dialysate solution and replacement solution are given at room temperature. Options for managing hypothermia include patient warming blankets or the use of warmers as part of the CEBT equipment.

Coagulation is another major nursing challenge in CEBT. There are two primary goals regarding coagulation: 1) maintaining a patent extracorporeal circuit, 2) avoiding patient complications related to anti-coagulation therapy. Heparin remains the most commonly used anticoagulant during CEBT. An alternative to anticoagulation is to use a technique that includes the use of a replacement solution. The use of a replacement solution creates a continuous dilution of the hematocrit.

Patients receiving CEBT are at risk for cardiac arrhythmias due to potential problems with fluid and electrolyte imbalance. However, there is also the possibility of the equipment used in CEBT causing ECG artifact that mimics cardiac arrhythmias. Prior to treating any arrhythmia, the CEBT equipment should be temporarily stopped so the patient's rhythm can be reassessed.

Linking Knowledge to Practice

✔ *Clotting of the filter is a complication of CEBT and requires replacement of the filter. Clotting is sometimes confused with clogging of the filter. Clogging of the filter is caused by adsorption, where molecules cling to the membrane of the filter. Although both conditions require replacement of the filter, clogging represents a positive benefit of therapy by removing solutes from systemic circulation.*

Chapter 18

SEPSIS

Definitions (Table 18.8)

Table 18.8
Definitions and Criteria Related to Sepsis and Septic Shock

Term	Definition
Infection	Inflammatory response to micro organisms, or invasion of normally sterile tissues.
Systemic Inflammatory Response Syndrome (SIRS)	SIRS results as a systemic response to inflammation. The inflammatory response may or may not be due to infection. Two or more of the following: ◆ Core temp > 100.4°F (38C) or < 96.8°F (36C) ◆ Elevated heart rate (>90 to 100 BMP) ◆ Respiratory rate > 20 breaths/min, PaCO₂ <32 mm Hg, or mechanical ventilation for acute respiratory process ◆ WBC count > 10,000-12,000/mm³, <4000/mm³ or >10% immature neutrophils. (Marini & Wheeler, 2006; Sharma & Mink, 2006).
Severe SIRS	Severe SIRS exists when there is a disturbance of a major organ system as a result of SIRS.
Sepsis or Sepsis Syndrome	Sepsis is diagnosed when there is a known or suspected infection, plus ≥ 2 SIRS criteria. Sepsis presents with evidence of hypoperfusion as evidenced by: ◆ Altered mental status ◆ Hypoxemia ◆ Increased plasma lactate ◆ Oliguria. (Sharma & Mink, 2006)
Severe Sepsis	Sepsis plus ≥ 1 organ dysfunction, or hypotension. Severity is determined by the host response to the initial trigger event.
Septic Shock	Sepsis with hypotension despite fluid resuscitation, and perfusion abnormalities.
Multi-Organ Dysfunction Syndrome (MODS)	MODS is the presence of altered organ function in an acutely ill patient, such that homeostasis cannot be maintained without intervention. Systems commonly affected in MODS include: pulmonary, renal, cardiovascular, and hematologic.

The above definitions regarding SIRS, sepsis, severe sepsis, and septic shock do not always fit perfectly with the clinical presentation of patients. Firstly, SIRS criteria were found not to clearly differentiate patients at risk of sepsis from those other critically ill patients with a non-specific inflammatory response. In addition, not all patients with sepsis meet the criteria for SIRS, as SIRS criteria are not specific criteria for infection or sepsis (Martin, 2006).

Biomarkers have been added to augment the above definitions and classification system. These biomarkers are used to help differentiate SIRS with infection from SIRS without infection.

862

Non Cardiac Issues in the Cardiac Patient: Pulmonary Pathophysiology, Electrolytes and Renal, Sepsis

- ◆ C-reactive protein.
- ◆ Procalcitonin.
- ◆ sTREM-I (new potential biomarker to replace C-reactive protein and procalcitonin).

C-reactive protein and procalcitonin do not consistently differentiate sepsis from other critical illnesses. For this reason the diagnosis of sepsis remains a clinical diagnosis.

In addition, refinement of the above definitions has lead to a newly developed classification system for sepsis.

Incidence and Mortality

The mortality associated with severe sepsis ranges from 30-40% (Marini & Wheeler, 2006). There is a higher incidence of sepsis and septic shock, as well as a higher mortality, in the elderly population as compared with younger patients. Patients with 3 to 4 criteria for SIRS have a similar mortality to those with sepsis. Hypothermia and/or acute renal failure in the presence of sepsis increases mortality (Widrich & Gropper, 2003; Marini & Wheeler, 2006). The more organ systems involved in sepsis, the higher the mortality. Renal failure, respiratory failure and circulatory failure are the most common organ failures in sepsis.

Etiology

Common sources of infection in sepsis include the lungs, blood, abdomen, urinary tract, and skin. The lungs are the most common site for infection (Marini & Wheeler, 2006). Organisms responsible for sepsis include gram negative and gram positive bacteria, fungi, and viruses. Bacteria is the most common cause of infection in sepsis, with gram negative bacteria playing a key role. Intravascular devices are a common cause of nosocomial infection.

Hospitalized patients at highest risk for sepsis include the following:
- ◆ Trauma patients.
- ◆ Patients having complicated surgery.
- ◆ Patients with major chronic medical conditions.
- ◆ Immunocompromised patients.

(Marini & Wheeler, 2006)

Fungal and viral infections are more commonly suspected in immunosuppressed patients. These patients may also be difficult to diagnose because they may not develop fever or leukocytosis (Widrich & Gropper, 2003).

Linking Knowledge to Practice

✔ *The lungs are both a likely source of initial infection and also the first organ to fail in MODS. For this reason, meticulous nursing care, including oral care and ventilator-acquired pneumonia prevention, is critical to impacting patient outcomes.*

Pathophysiology

There are 3 key processes involved in the pathophysiology of sepsis:
- ◆ Inflammation.
- ◆ Coagulation.
- ◆ Impaired fibrinolysis.

Inflammation and coagulation responses have a beneficial effect in keeping infection localized. When these processes become diffused, they become detrimental rather than helpful.

Chapter 18

The pathophysiology of sepsis can be explained by a sequence of events that occurs in response to an infectious process:

1. The initial trigger of sepsis is usually a substance that has come from a microbe (other substances can also trigger sepsis) that is released into the blood stream. A common potent trigger of sepsis is endotoxin, a compound found in the cell wall of gram-negative bacteria. Other substances found in the cell wall of gram positive bacteria can also be triggers. Toxins can be released into the bloodstream with bacteremia or from localized sites of infection.

2. The trigger released from the membrane of bacteria binds to receptors on the surface of monocytes and causes the release of cytokines, which are mediators of inflammation. There are 2 cytokines primarily responsible for initiating the inflammatory response: Tumor necrosis factor alpha and interleukin 1 (IL-1).

3. Tumor necrosis factor alpha and IL-1 have a direct toxic effect on tissues.

4. These inflammatory cytokines also lead to:
   a. Increased platelet activating factor.
   b. Promotion of nitric oxide.
   c. Promotion of neutrophil activity and the infiltration of tissues by neutrophils.
   d. Release of IL-6 and IL-8.

5. As a result of the proinflammatory cytokines, tissue factor is expressed on the surface of the endothelium and monocytes. Tissue factor is the first step in the extrinsic clotting cascade. This leads to the formation of thrombin, resulting in fibrin clots in microvasculature. Thrombin is also proinflammatory and promotes leukocyte adhesion to the endothelial cells, causing vessel wall damage.

6. As a defense mechanism, the fibrinolytic system is activated to break down microemboli. However, fibrinolysis is also impaired during the septic process. Tumor necrosis factor alpha and IL-1 result in the production of plasminogen activator inhibitor-1, which inhibits fibrinolysis.

7. The proinflammatory cytokines are also responsible for interfering with the body's own natural modulators of inflammation and infection. These modulators are activated protein C and antithrombin. Activated protein C has many functions including the inhibition of thrombin production and the inhibition of thrombin mediated inflammation. The proinflammatory cytokines interfere with the proper functioning of activated protein C and antithrombin, and therefore their levels are low in sepsis.

8. Tumor necrosis factor alpha also has a cardiodepressant effect.
(LaRosa, 2002; & Wheeler, 2006)

The end result of the pathophysiology of sepsis is an imbalance among inflammation, coagulation, and fibrinolysis. This imbalance leads to microvascular thrombosis with suppressed fibrinolysis. The end result is organ damage and ultimate death if the process is not reversed.

The endothelium is damaged in sepsis, which causes important clinical consequences.

Important features of the normal endothelium include:
◆ Being the largest organ in the body.
◆ Controlling vasomotor tone.
◆ Promoting movement of cells and nutrients.
◆ Maintaining blood fluidity.

Non Cardiac Issues in the Cardiac Patient: Pulmonary Pathophysiology, Electrolytes and Renal, Sepsis

The following chain of events can occur in response to endothelial damage:

◆ Increased vascular permeability.

◆ Inflammatory fluids and cells move from the blood into interstitial spaces and result in edema.

◆ Alterations in vasomotor tone, abnormal endothelium-dependent vascular relaxation, vasodilation, and hypotension.

◆ Impaired microcirculatory blood flow.

◆ Impaired gas exchange and cellular hypoxia.

Damage to the microcirculatory system (from edema) is a key end result of sepsis pathology. A decrease in the number of functional capillaries results in an inability of the tissues to extract oxygen.

Risk Factors

◆ Malignancy.

◆ Diabetes mellitus.

◆ Chronic liver disease.

◆ Chronic kidney disease.

◆ Immunosuppressed state.

◆ Surgery.

◆ Trauma.

◆ Burns.

(Sharma & Mink, 2006)

Diagnosis

Tachypnea is an early warning sign of sepsis. Greater than 90% of patients with sepsis develop hypoxemia, with approximately 3 out of 4 patients with severe sepsis requiring mechanical ventilation (Marini and Wheeler, 2006). Tachycardia is expected in all patients with sepsis unless there is a conduction defect or medication responsible for slowing heart rate.

Leukocytosis or leucopenia exists in the majority of patients with sepsis. Fever is present in the vast majority of sepsis cases. However, fever may be absent in certain subsets of patients: elderly, patients with chronic renal failure, patients taking steroids or anti-inflammatory medications. Hypothermia can actually be present in a small percentage of patients and represents a poor prognosis. Hypothermia is linked with underlying chronic disease, gram-negative bacteria, and shock (Marini & Wheeler, 2006).

Localizing the site of infection is an important part of the diagnosis. Specific signs and symptoms may relate to the location of the infection. A urine culture should be done on every patient with suspicion for sepsis. Gram stain is the only immediate test that can document infection and aide in the selection of antibiotics. Blood cultures are the primary method for diagnosing infections from intravascular devices.

Organ Dysfunction

Pulmonary dysfunction is usually the first recognized organ system failure. This may be because the lungs are the only organ that receive 100% of the cardiac output, and are therefore exposed to all toxins and mediators circulating in the blood. The lungs also contain an extensive capillary structure. In addition, sepsis requires the pulmonary system to compensate for metabolic acidosis by increasing minute ventilation. Approximately 50% of patients will develop lung injury or ARDS as a result of sepsis (Marini & Wheeler, 2006).

Chapter 18

Hypotension and kidney injury are common in sepsis. Kidney injury usually develops as a result of hypotension and shock and usually resolves if hypovolemia is quickly treated. The severity of organ failure is as important as the number of organs involved. For example, patients who require vasopressors in addition to fluid for the treatment of hypotension have a higher mortality than patients who respond to fluids alone. Higher doses of vasopressors are also associated with higher mortality (Marini & Wheeler, 2006).

Hemodynamic Response

Arterial vasodilation occurs in sepsis and septic shock; therefore, blood pressure becomes dependent on cardiac output. This is the reason for the critical importance of achieving and maintaining an adequate preload. Adequate preload is difficult to achieve because there is widespread venous as well as arterial vasodilation. Low circulating volume limits the compensatory increase in cardiac output. Although there is a compensatory increase in cardiac output, myocardial performance is actually depressed due to the effects of tumor necrosis factor alpha.

Linking Knowledge to Practice

✔ *Blood pressure is a product of cardiac output and systemic vascular resistance. In sepsis there is a decrease in systemic vascular resistance, and this is the reason why the optimal delivery of cardiac output is critical to maintain blood pressure. Cardiac output is dependent on adequate preload, which is compromised in sepsis due to venous vasodilation. This is the reason why early fluid resuscitation is the hallmark of sepsis treatment.*

Lactic acidosis develops in late septic shock. A decrease in the delivery of oxygen contributes to the development of lactic acidosis. However, other factors also contribute, including the cellular dysfunction at the mitochondrial level, resulting in decreased extraction of oxygen in some areas. In sepsis there is also a maldistribution of the cardiac output to assure deliver to the most vital organs (Marini & Wheeler, 2006). The pathology of sepsis leads to the regional changes in oxygen demand and regional changes in blood flow (Sharma & Mink, 2006). When lactate levels increase in sepsis, oxygen consumption is no longer independent of oxygen delivery; instead, consumption becomes dependent on increased oxygen delivery.

Treatment
Prevention

Meticulous hand hygiene and protocols for the prevention of ventilator-acquired pneumonia are important nursing interventions in the prevention of sepsis. Antibiotic coated central line catheters are available as an option in high-risk patients.

Antibiotics

The two important factors in antibiotic therapy are timing and appropriate coverage. Patients who are critically ill require empiric antibiotic therapy, with a broad spectrum antibiotic covering gram positive, gram negative, and anaerobic bacteria. Antipseudomonal coverage is indicated in patients with neutropenia and in those with hospital-acquired sepsis (Sharma & Mink, 2006). In addition, patients who are immunocompromised usually require two antibiotics with overlapping coverage (Sharma & Mink, 2006). Individual hospital patterns of antibiotic resistance are used in making antibiotic choices. In addition, patients who have received frequent or recent antibiotics may need their coverage adjusted. Mortality increases when antibiotics are administered after the first hour of presentation or diagnosis (Martin, 2006). Patients with abscesses or other localized infections need source control. Drainage and debridement are used to achieve source control.

Treatment Goal

Maximize the delivery of oxygen to the tissue. Remember: CI, Hemoglobin, SaO_2.

- ◆ CI
  - ❖ Volume replacement (this is the most important initial therapy).
    - ☆ Crystalloid volume resuscitation usually ranges from 4 to 8 liters.
    - ☆ An iso-oncotic colloid, such as 5% albumin, is also an option for fluid resuscitation.
  - ❖ Vasopressors (norepinephrine is the preferred vasopressor) (Widrich & Gropper, 2003).
  - ❖ May need inotropes.
- ◆ Hemoglobin
  - ❖ Transfuse when hemoglobin not adequate for tissue oxygenation.
- ◆ SaO_2
  - ❖ Oxygen.
  - ❖ Intubation.
  - ❖ Mechanical ventilation.

Early Goal Directed Therapy

In early goal directed therapy, fluid is administered early until clinical endpoints are met.

- ◆ Goals
  - ❖ CVP 8-13 mm Hg.
  - ❖ PAOP 12-18 mm Hg.
  - ❖ MAP > 65 mm Hg.
  - ❖ Cardiac index > 2.5 $L/min/mm^2$.
  - ❖ U.O. > 0.5 cc/kg/hr.
  - ❖ Central venous oxygen saturation > 70%.
  - ❖ SaO_2 > 90%.

  (Widrich & Gropper, 2003)
- ◆ Treatment components used to meet goals
  - ❖ More fluid.
  - ❖ Blood transfusions.
  - ❖ Inotropes may be used if cardiac output is very low.
  - ❖ Vasopressors may be used if patient is not responsive to fluids. Norepinephrine is often a preferred vasopressor in sepsis.
  - ❖ Outcomes are significantly improved when these goals are met.

Drotrecogin Alfa (Activated) or Xigris (trade name)

Recombinant human activated protein C, drotrecogin alfa (activated) or Xigris, decreases mortality in sepsis by regulating the clotting cascade and by also decreasing inflammation.

- ◆ Actions
  - ❖ Anticoagulation effect
    - ☆ Works as vitamin K dependent anticoagulant.
    - ☆ Activated by thrombin.
    - ☆ Inactivates coagulation factors Va–VIIIa (with the help of protein S).

Chapter 18

- ❖ Profibrinolytic effect
  - ☆ Inhibits plasminogen activating inhibitor 1.
- ❖ Anti-inflammtiory effect
  - ☆ Decreases inflammatory cytokines.
  - ☆ Decreases tumor necrosing factor alpha.
  - ☆ Decreases endothelial adhesion of leukocytes.
- ◆ Contraindications
  - ❖ Recent CVA (3 months).
  - ❖ Recent gastrointestinal bleeding (6 weeks).
  - ❖ Recent surgery (12 hours).
  - ❖ Thrombocytopenia (< 80,000).
  - ❖ Can be used with ASA.
  - ❖ Should not be used with anticoagulants or glycoprotein II b/III a inhibitors.
  - ❖ Not used in the following septic patients: pediatric patients, patients with low risk of death from sepsis, and patients with surgical sepsis with only one organ dysfunction (Martin, 2006).
- ◆ Adverse Effects: Bleeding occurs as a complication 3-5% of the time (Widrich & Gropper, 2003).

Corticosteroids

Combined hydrocortisone and fludrocortisone in modest doses may improve outcomes in septic shock in patients with documented adrenal insufficiency. Patients with an adequate adrenal response do not benefit from the therapy (Martin, 2006). Modest dose corticosteroids should be considered in patients with vasopressor dependent shock who have documented adrenal insufficiency (Sharma & Mink, 2006).

Other Options to Modify Mediators

- ◆ Antihistamines: Modify/block histamine.
- ◆ Naloxone (Narcan): Modify/block endorphins.
- ◆ Ibuprofen/Indomethacin: Modify/block prostaglandin.
- ◆ ACE Inhibitors: Inhibits production of angiotensin II.
- ◆ Anticoagulants (Heparin): Modify the clotting cascade.
  * Blocking mediators is controversial/mediators are important.

Nutrition

Enteral feedings in sepsis can improve not only the nutritional status of a patient, but also improve the immune function. Jejunal feedings are preferred to prevent aspiration. Enteral feedings help decrease stress ulcers and the translocation of bacteria. Septic patients have high energy requirements.

Other Treatment Considerations

CEBT has been considered as a potential treatment option in sepsis. The theory is that the substances responsible for inflammation can be filtered and cleared during CEBT. However, CEBT is currently not indicated in the treatment of sepsis unless accompanied by renal failure.

In addition, drugs aimed at blocking the proinflammatory cytokines have also not been found successful in reducing mortality in sepsis. One thought is that these cytokines may also play an important role in the overall immune system (Widrich & Gropper, 2003).

Nitric oxide inhibitors are being evaluated as a potential future agent for refractory shock not responsive to catecholamines.

Non Cardiac Issues in the Cardiac Patient: Pulmonary Pathophysiology, Electrolytes and Renal, Sepsis

Tight glycemic control has only been found effective in treating sepsis in the surgical population (Martin, 2006).

Lactic acidosis in septic shock typically causes an anion gap metabolic acidosis. Treatment with bicarbonate therapy, however, actually has the potential to worsen intracellular acidosis. Bicarbonate therapy is generally reserved for bicarbonate levels < 9 mEql/L (Sharma & Mink, 2006).

CONCLUSION

The lungs, kidney, and entire endothelium are intricately related to the heart. Cardiac nurses need to understand the implications of poor myocardial performance on other body organs, as well as understand the impact of other organ dysfunction on cardiac function. The human body is a delicate system in which all components are designed to work in perfect harmony. The alteration in one component can have far-reaching implications. The holistic view of nursing practice is critical to the optimum delivery of total patient care.

TEST YOUR KNOWLEDGE

1. A patient with no previous medical history presents to the emergency department in severe respiratory distress with hypoxemia evident on pulse oximetry. There is no identified immediately reversible cause of the patient's distress. An initial blood gas reveals respiratory acidosis with a $PaCO_2$ of 55 mm Hg. The nurse will anticipate which therapy?

   a. Hyperbaric oxygen chamber

   b. Sedation to decrease hyperventilation state

   c. Intubation and mechanical ventilation

   d. Stat echocardiogram to rule out acute mitral regurgitation

2. The appropriate care of a patient in respiratory distress who demonstrates an increased work of breathing includes:

   a. Referring to respiratory therapy for exercises that strengthen the muscles of inspiration.

   b. Maintaining a supine position for patient comfort.

   c. Immediate assessment for the need for intubation and mechanical intubation.

   d. a and b.

3. When caring for a patient with COPD and a history of $PaCO_2$ retention, the nurse knows the following to be true about delivering oxygen therapy:

   a. The patient should never be given more than 2 L via nasal cannula, regardless of degree of hypoxemia.

   b. The patient can tolerate oxygen therapy that achieves or maintains a SaO_2 between 90-92% because the patient uses a hypoxic drive to breathe.

   c. It is safe to place the patient on a 100% non-rebreather in an acute crisis as long as you check a pulse oximeter reading within the next 8 hours.

   d. Delivering oxygen decreases the $PaCO_2$, and a high $PaCO_2$ is the patient's drive to breathe.

Chapter 18

4. Patients with COPD who meet criteria for home oxygen therapy should wear oxygen no more than 4 hours out of each 24 hour period.

   a. True.

   b. False.

5. Risk factors for the development of pulmonary emboli include:

   a. Immobility after surgery.

   b. Malignancy.

   c. Presence of central venous catheter.

   d. a and c.

   e. All of the above.

6. A nurse is caring for an obese patient who has been on bed rest for several days. The patient develops dyspnea and pleuritic chest pain. The admitting physician is on her way to evaluate the patient when the patient develops sudden hypotension and distended jugular veins. The nurse anticipates

   a. the potential need to administer fibrinolytics for pulmonary embolus with hemodynamic compromise.

   b. the need to treat right-ventricular failure with fluids and inotropes.

   c. the need to insert an intra aortic balloon pump for left-ventricular failure.

   d. a and b.

   e. All of the above.

7. The nurse has just received an admission from the emergency department. The patient is an elderly female who lives with her daughter. She is an insulin dependent diabetic with renal failure, requiring peritoneal dialysis at home. She is admitted with a new onset confusion, flu-like symptoms, temperature of 104 degrees F, pleuritic chest pain, and productive cough. The priority intervention in her care will most likely be

   a. checking a blood glucose level and initiating treatment for HHNK.

   b. calling dialysis to set up peritoneal dialysis in the hospital.

   c. initiating a cooling blanket per hyperthermia protocol.

   d. starting antibiotics for pneumonia.

8. A patient is three weeks post trauma. Ventilator weaning has been unsuccessful. The patient continues to have hypoxemia, even with high levels of FIO_2 and mechanical ventilation. Her chest x-ray shows a fibrotic appearance bilaterally and she has decreasing lung compliance. What is the most likely cause of her inability to be weaned?

   a. ARDS

   b. Nosocomial pneumonia

   c. Unresolved hemothorax from trauma

   d. Psychological dependence on the ventilator

Non Cardiac Issues in the Cardiac Patient: Pulmonary Pathophysiology, Electrolytes and Renal, Sepsis

9. In treating a patient with ARDS, the nurse knows the following are considered lung protective strategies:
   a. Lower tidal volume $\leq$ 6 ml/kg, plateau pressures $\geq$ 30 cm H_2O
   b. Lower tidal volume $\leq$ 6 ml/kg, plateau pressures < 30 cm H_2O
   c. Higher tidal volume > 6 ml/kg, plateau pressures < 30 cm H_2O
   d. Higher tidal volume > 6 ml/kg, plateau pressures $\geq$ 30 cm H_2O

10. Chest tubes should always be clamped when transporting a patient for diagnostic procedures.
    a. True.
    b. False.

11. A patient who is hyponatremic as a result of loss in circulating volume (hypovolemia) will most likely have the following in his/her treatment plan:
    a. Administration of isotonic saline to restore circulating volume
    b. Administration of loop diuretics to eliminate free water
    c. Fluid restriction
    d. All of the above.

12. The primary effects of hyponatremia are
    a. inversely related to the calcium level.
    b. seen in the gastrointestinal and genitourinary system.
    c. central nervous system related.
    d. directly related to the body mass index.

13. Hypernatremia almost always results in a hyperosmolar state and causes cellular dehydration.
    a. True.
    b. False.

14. In caring for a patient with hypokalemia, the nurse knows the following to be true:
    a. Hypermagnesemia frequently predisposes the patient to hypokalemia, and diuretics may be necessary to lower magnesium levels prior to replacing potassium.
    b. Hypokalemia is common in patients with chronic renal failure.
    c. Hypokalemia places the patient at risk for digitalis toxicity.
    d. All of the above.

Chapter 18

15. A patient with history of heart failure on an ACE inhibitor and aldosterone antagonist presents to the emergency department with lower extremity weakness. An initial routine ECG shows tall peaked T waves throughout multiple leads. The nurse should anticipate the following interventions:

    a. Administration of calcium to stabilize the cardiac membrane.

    b. Administration of insulin along with 50% dextrose to shift potassium into the cell.

    c. Administration of IV potassium supplement with a central line.

    d. a and b.

    e. a and c.

16. When assessing a patient's calcium level in critical care, the nurse knows the following to be true:

    a. Ionized calcium refers to the calcium that is bound to albumin.

    b. Hypocalcemia is a very rare but life threatening disorder found in critically ill patients.

    c. The majority of the body's calcium is found in bone.

    d. Serum calcium and magnesium share an inverse relationship with each other.

17. When administering IV magnesium emergently to a patient with hypomagnesemia, the nurse should assess for the following anticipated side effect:

    a. Hypotension

    b. Hypertension

    c. New onset atrial fibrillation

    d. Thrombocytopenia

18. The creatinine level rises immediately in response to even a slight decrease in the glomerular filtration rate.

    a. True.

    b. False.

19. Common causes of acute kidney injury in patients in the hospital include:

    a. Exposure to nephrotoxic drugs or agents

    b. Renal hypoperfusion

    c. Post streptococcal infection

    d. a and b.

    e. All of the above.

Non Cardiac Issues in the Cardiac Patient: Pulmonary Pathophysiology, Electrolytes and Renal, Sepsis

20. A nurse is caring for a patient who develops acute kidney injury as a result of left-ventricular failure with hypotension. Knowing the etiology of the acute kidney injury, the nurse expects the following diagnostic parameters when reviewing the patient's medical record:

   a. BUN to creatine ratio of 10:1

   b. Tubular casts in the urine

   c. Fractional excretion of sodium (FENa) < 1%

   d. Urine sodium > 20 mEq/L

21. In caring for a patient with acute kidney injury, the nurse knows that oliguria represents

   a. an increase in mortality compared to non-oliguric acute kidney injury.

   b. urine with high glucose seen in Type I diabetes.

   c. complete recovery from the acute kidney injury.

   d. the last phase in acute kidney injury.

22. When caring for a patient receiving continuous veno-venous hemodiafiltration (CVVHDF), the nurse knows the patient is at risk for the following as a complication of the therapy:

   a. Hyperthermia

   b. Hypothermia

   c. Clotting of the filter

   d. a and c

   e. b and c

23. Which of the following is not a key process in the pathophysiology of sepsis?

   a. Inflammation

   b. Coagulation

   c. CO_2 retention

   d. Impaired fibrinolysis

24. Early goal directed therapy in sepsis is best described as:

   a. Starting anticoagulants at first contact with EMS to minimize clotting.

   b. Utilizing fluids (and possibly inotropes or vasopressors) early in the course of treatment until established clinical endpoints are met.

   c. Developing goals for the patient plan of care, utilizing an interdisciplinary team conference within the first 2 hours of admission.

   d. Obtaining positive cultures within the first 6 hours of admission.

Chapter 18

25. When caring for a patient with severe sepsis who is ordered *Drotrecogin Alfa (Activated) Xigris,* the nurse knows the following to be true:

   a. Bleeding is key complication of therapy

   b. This medication is indicated in all patients with suspected sepsis

   c. Aspirin administration within the last 24 hours is a contraindication

   d. All of the above.

ANSWERS

1.	C	14.	C
2.	C	15.	D
3.	B	16.	C
4.	B	17.	A
5.	E	18.	B
6.	D	19.	D
7.	D	20.	C
8.	A	21.	A
9.	B	22.	E
10.	B	23.	C
11.	A	24.	B
12.	C	25.	A
13.	A			

REFERENCES

Pulmonary

Allen, G. & Kaminsky, D.A. (2003). Asthma. In P.E. Parsons & J.P. Wiener-Kronish (Eds.), *Critical care secrets* (3rd ed., pp. 86-91). Philadelphia: Hanley & Belfus, Inc.

Burns, S.M. (2005). Mechanical ventilation of patients with acute respiratory distress syndrome and patients requiring weaning: The evidence guiding practice. *Critical Care Nurse, 25*(4), 14-23.

Cunha, B.A. (2007). Pneumonia, community acquired. Retrieved on July 10, 2007 from http://www.emedicine.com/MED/topic3162.htm

Ellstrom, K. (2006). The pulmonary system. In J.G. Alspach (Ed.), *Core curriculum for critical care nursing* (pp. 45-184). St. Louis: Saunders Elsevier.

Feied, C. & Handler, J.A. (2006). Pulmonary embolism. Retrieved on July 14, 2007, from http://www.emedicine.com/emerg/topic490.htm

Fernandez, E. (2003). Chronic obstructive pulmonary disease. In P.E. Parsons & J.P. Wiener-Kronish (Eds.), *Critical care secrets* (3rd ed., pp. 92-98). Philadelphia: Hanley & Belfus, Inc.

Fernandez, E. & Yanakakis, M.J. (2003). Cor pulmonale. In P.E. Parsons & J.P. Wiener-Kronish (Eds.), *Critical care secrets* (3rd ed., pp. 99-102). Philadelphia: Hanley & Belfus, Inc.

Halow, K.D. & Bower, M.W. (2003). Chest tubes. In P.E. Parsons & J.P. Wiener-Kronish (Eds.), *Critical care secrets* (3rd ed., pp. 61-66). Philadelphia: Hanley & Belfus, Inc.

Harris, Colonel J.R. & Tenhet, Lieutenant Colonel M.E. (2005). Common respiratory disorders. In P.G. Morton, D.K. Fontaine, C.M. Hudak, & B.M. Gallo (Eds.), *Critical care nursing: A holistic approach* (8th ed., pp. 566-607). Philadelphia: Lippincott, Williams and Wilkins.

Horlander, K.T. & Leeper, K.V. (2003). Troponin levels as a guide to treatment of pulmonary embolism. *Current Opinions in Pulmonary Medicine, 9*(5), 374-377.

Kumar, V., Abbas. A.K., & Fausto, N. (2005). *Pathologic basis of disease* (7th ed.). Philadelphia: Elsevier Saunders.

Levitzky, M.G. (2003). *Pulmonary physiology* (6th ed.). New York: McGraw-Hill.

MacIntyre, N. (2006). Fluid management in patients with ALI from the NIH ARDS network fluid management trial. *Medscape Critical Care, 7*(2). Retrieved September 24, 2006, from http://www.medscape.com/viewarticle/543504_print

MacIntyre, N. (2004). Lung recruitment in ARDS: Physiologic concepts and practical strategies. *Medscape CME.* Retrieved on September 25, 2006, from http://medscape.com/viewarticle/466521

Marini, J.J. & Wheeler A.P. (2006). *Critical care medicine the essentials* (3rd ed.). Philadelphia: Lippincott, Williams and Wilkins.

Raoof, S. &. Khan, F.A. (1998). *Mechanical ventilation manual.* Philadelphia, PA: American College of Physicians.

Schwarz, M.I. (2003). Acute pneumonia. In P.E. Parsons & J.P. Wiener-Kronish (Eds.), *Critical care secrets* (3rd ed., pp. 83-85). Philadelphia: Hanley & Belfus, Inc.

Slutsky, A.S. (July 1999). Lung injury caused by mechanical ventilation. *Chest*, 116: 9-15.

Sharma, S. (2006). Pulmonary embolism. Retrieved on July 14, 2007, from http://www.emedicine.com/med/topic1958.htm

Soeren, M.V. (2005). Acute respiratory distress syndrome. In P.G. Morton, D.K. Fontaine, C.M. Hudak, & B.M. Gallo (Eds.), *Critical care nursing: A holistic approach* (8th ed., pp. 608-626). Philadelphia: Lippincott, Williams and Wilkins.

St. John, R.E. (2003). End tidal carbon dioxide monitoring. *Critical Care Nurse, 23*(4), 83-88.

Steinberg, K.P., Hudson, L.D., Goodman, R.B., Hough C.L., Lanken, P.N., et al. (2006). Efficacy and safety of cortocosteroids for persistent respiratory distress syndrome. *New England Journal of Medicine, 354*(16), 1671-1684.

Turki, M. & Parsons, P.E. (2003). Acute respiratory distress syndrome. In P.E. Parsons & J.P. Wiener-Kronish (Eds.), *Critical care secrets* (3rd ed., pp. 106-110). Philadelphia: Hanley & Belfus, Inc.

Chapter 18

Villar, J., Kacmarek, R.M., Perez-Mendez, L. & Aguirre-Jaime, A. (2006). A high positive end-expiratory pressure, low tidal volume ventilator strategy improves outcome in persistent acute respiratory distress syndrome: A randomized controlled trial. *Critical Care Medicine, 34*(5), 1311-1318.

West, J.B. (2001). *Pulmonary physiology and pathophysiology: An integrated, case-based approach.* Philadelphia: Lippincott, Williams and Wilkins.

Zamora, M.R. & Burkhardt, D. (2003). Acute respiratory failure. In P.E. Parsons & J.P. Wiener-Kronish (Eds.), *Critical care secrets* (3rd ed., pp. 103-105). Philadelphia: Hanley & Belfus, Inc.

Renal
Acute Dialysis Quality Initiative. www.ADQI.net

Adams, K.L. (2005). Anatomy and physiology of the renal system. In P.G. Morton, D.K. Fontaine, C.M. Hudak & B.M. Gallo (Eds.), *Critical care nursing: A holistic approach* (8th ed., pp. 629-639). Philadelphia: Lippincott, Williams and Wilkins.

Adams, K.L. (2005). Patient management: renal system. In P.G. Morton, D.K. Fontaine, C.M. Hudak & B.M. Gallo (Eds.), *Critical care nursing: A holistic approach* (8th ed., pp. 658-687). Philadelphia: Lippincott, Williams and Wilkins.

Agraharkar, M. (2007). Acute renal failure. Retrieved on July 14, 2007, from http://www.emedicine.com/med/topic1595.htm

Holcombe, D., Feeley, N.K. (2005). Renal failure. In P.G. Morton, D.K. Fontaine, C.M. Hudak & B.M. Gallo (Eds.), *Critical care nursing: A holistic approach* (8th ed., pp. 688-714). Philadelphia: Lippincott, Williams and Wilkins.

Kumar, S.P., & Sorrell, V.L. (2003). Renal-dose dopamine: Myth or ally in the treatment of acute renal failure. *Cardiovascular Reviews and Reports, 24*, 413-415.

Kumar, V., Abbas. A.K., & Fausto, N. (2005). *Pathologic basis of disease* (7th ed.). Philadelphia: Elsevier Saunders.

Linas, S.L. (2003). Hypokalemia and hyperkalemia. In P.E. Parsons & J.P. Wiener-Kronish (Eds.), *Critical care secrets* (3rd ed., pp. 243-247). Philadelphia: Hanley & Belfus, Inc.

Marini, J.J. & Wheeler A.P. (2006). *Critical care medicine the essentials* (3rd Ed.). Philadelphia: Lippincott, Williams and Wilkins.

Medscape Drug Reference (2006). Drug Monograph Albumin. Retrieved July 16, 2006, from http://www.medscape.com/druginfo/monograph?cid=med&drugid=60462&drugname=Albumin+IV&monotype=monograph&secid=2

Mehta, R.L., Kellum, J.A., Shah, S.V., Molitoris, B.A., Ronco, C. Warnock, D.G., & Levin, A. (2007). Acute kidney injury network: Report of an initiative to improve outcomes in acute kidney injury. *Critical Care, 11*(2), retrieved on July 11, 2007 from http://www.medscape.com/viewarticle/557627_1

Porth, C. M. (2004). Alterations in fluids, electrolytes, and acid-base balance. In C.M. Porth (Ed.) *Essentials of altered pathophysiology: Concepts of altered health states* (pp. 84-120). Philadelphia: Lippincott, Williams & Wilkins.

Porth, C. M. (2004). Control of kidney function. In C.M. Porth (Ed.), *Essentials of altered pathophysiology: Concepts of altered health states* (pp. 410-414). Philadelphia: Lippincott, Williams & Wilkins.

Porth, C. M. (2004). Renal failure. In C.M. Porth (Ed.), *Essentials of altered pathophysiology: Concepts of altered health states* (pp. 433-445). Philadelphia: Lippincott, Williams & Wilkins.

Senkfor, S., Berl, T. & Liu, K.D. (2003). Hyponatremia and hypernatremia. In P.E. Parsons & J.P. Wiener-Kronish (Ed.), *Critical care secrets* (3rd ed. pp. 247-250). Philadelphia: Hanley and Belfus, Inc.

Speakman, E. & Weldy, N.J. (2002). *Body fluids and electrolytes* (8th ed.). St. Louis: Mosby.

Stark, J.L. (2006). The renal system. In J.G. Alspach (Ed.), *Core curriculum for critical care nursing* (pp. 525-610). St. Louis: Saunders Elsevier.

Sepsis

LaRosa, S. P. (2002). Sepsis. *The Cleveland Clinical Journal of Medicine.* Retrieved on May 26, 2007, from http://www.clevelandclinicmeded.com/diseasemanagement/infectiousdisease/sepsis/sepsis.htm#pathophysiology

Martin, G.S. (2006). New developments in sepsis. American Thoracic Society 2006 International Conference. Retrieved on March 3 2007, from http://www.medscape.com/viewarticle/540989

Sharma, S. & Mink, S. (2006). Septic shock. Retrieved on July 11, 2006, from http://www.emedicine.com/MD/topic2101.htm

GLOSSARY

Note: Pacemaker terminology for both single and dual chamber pacemakers is defined in separate glossaries in Chapter 17: Electrical Management of Arrhythmias.

2,3-Diphosphoglycerate (2,3-DPG): A substance produced by erythrocytes during their normal glycolysis, which binds to hemoglobin and decreases the affinity of hemoglobin for oxygen.

Accessory Pathway: Tract of tissue between atria and ventricles that is capable of conducting electrical impulses from atria to ventricles or from ventricles to atria, bypassing the normal AV node. These pathways can be located anywhere around the tricuspid or mitral valve rings, and are responsible for preexcitation of the ventricle in Wolff-Parkinson-White Syndrome.

ACE Inhibitor: Angiotensin Converting Enzyme Inhibitor. Medication that prevents the conversion of angiotensin I to angiotensin II. Used to treat hypertension and heart failure.

Acetylcholine: The neurotransmitter of the parasympathetic nervous system.

Acid: A substance that can give a H+ ion.

Acidemia: A blood pH below 7.35.

Acidosis: The condition that causes acidemia.

Action Potential: Depolarization and repolarization of a cardiac cell due to the exchange of ions across the cell membrane.

Acute Coronary Syndrome (ACS): The presentation of coronary artery disease in the form of unstable angina, non ST segment elevation MI (NSTEMI) and ST-segment elevation MI (STEMI).

Acute Renal Failure: A sudden loss of the kidneys' ability to excrete wastes, concentrate urine, and conserve electrolytes.

Addison's Disease: Damage to the adrenal cortex resulting in a deficiency of glucocorticoid hormones, mineralocorticoid hormones, and the sex hormones.

Adenosine Triphosphate (ATP): An enzyme in muscle cells that stores energy and produces energy when split.

Adenosine: Coronary vasodilator used in chemical stress testing. Also used as an antiarrhythmic to slow conduction through the AV node during some supraventricular tachycardias.

Adrenal cortex: Outer layer of the adrenal gland; produced mineralocorticoids, glucocorticoids, and androgens.

Adrenergic Receptors: Receptors of the sympathetic nervous system – alpha and beta receptors.

Adsorption: Refers to the clinging of positively charged molecules to the negatively charged membrane of the filter used in CRRT or CEBT.

Adventitia: The fibrous outer layer of the artery designed to protect the vessel and provide connection to other internal structures.

Afferent arterioles: Arterioles that enter the glomerulus.

Glossary

Afterload: Amount of work a ventricle must do to eject its contents; usually considered to be the resistance to ejection of blood. Right ventricular afterload measured by pulmonary vascular resistance and left ventricular afterload, measured by systemic vascular resistance.

A-H Interval: Measured from onset of atrial activation to the His bundle deflection in intracardiac signals obtained during EPS; approximates AV node conduction time.

Aldosterone antagonists: Medications that block the effects of aldosterone. Used to treat hypertension and heart failure.

Aldosterone: A mineralocorticoid hormone produced by the adrenal cortex that increases sodium and water reabsorption.

Alkalemia: A blood pH above 7.45.

Alkalosis: A condition that causes alkalemia.

Alpha1 Adrenergic Receptors: Sympathetic nervous system receptors located in the vessels of vascular smooth muscle. Stimulation results in vasoconstriction.

Alveolar membrane: Membrane of alveoli in lung tissue where gas exchange occurs.

Alveolar ventilation (V_A): The amount of ventilation that participates in gas exchange. This is tidal volume minus anatomical dead space.

Alveoli: Terminal unit of the respiratory tree. Serve as the primary unit for gas exchange.

Aminophylline: Pulmonary vasodilator used as an antidote for adenosine or dipyridamole during chemical stress testing.

Amiodarone: A class III antiarrhythmic with vasodilatory properties generally well tolerated in patients with left ventricular dysfunction; used to treat atrial and ventricular arrhythmias.

Amyloidosis: Deposition of protein fibrils (amyloid) in tissues of the body that impairs the functioning of the organ.

Anaphylactic Shock: Shock caused by an allergic reaction.

Anemia: Reduced hemoglobin or red blood cell count.

Angina Pectoris: Chest pain resulting from a decreased blood flow to the myocardium or from an increase in myocardial O_2 demands above the available O_2 supply.

Angioedema: Allergic response where skin, mucous membranes and viscera become edematous. Often occurs around eyes or lips. Swelling is deep – extending beneath the skin and can involve the airway.

Angiogenesis: A physiological process of the growth of new blood vessels from pre-existing vessels.

Angiography: the radiographic visualization of blood vessels after injection of a radiopaque substance. Used to determine the size and shape of vessels. Coronary angiogram is also called coronary arteriography.

Angiojet Thrombectomy: Atherectomy procedure used for the extraction of visible thrombi within a coronary artery or saphenous vein bypass graft.

Angiontensin I: Precursor to angiotensin II.

Angiotensin Converting Enzyme: An enzyme responsible for the conversion of angiotensin I to angiotensin II.

Angiotensin II Receptor Blockers (ARB): Medications that block the effects of angiotensin II.

Angiotensin II: Potent vasoconstrictor and stimulator of aldosterone secretion.

Anion Gap: $Na^+ - [Cl- + HCO_3-]$.

Glossary

Ankle Brachial Index (ABI): A diagnostic test for lower peripheral arterial disease where ankle pressures are divided by brachial pressures to determine a ratio. Ankle pressures are normally higher than brachial pressures; however, a ratio of > 0.9 is considered normal.

Annulus: Fibrous ring at the top of the valves.

Anterior MI: MI involving the anterior or front wall of the left ventricle.

Anterolateral MI: MI involving the anterior and lateral walls of the left ventricle.

Anteroseptal MI: MI involving the anterior wall of the left ventricle and the septum.

Antianginal Medications: Medications effective in preventing or decreasing angina.

Antibody: A protein substance developed in response to an antigen.

Anticoagulants: Medications that interfere with clot formation by interfering with the instrinsic, extrinisic, or common pathway of the coagulation cascade.

Antigen: A molecule that stimulates an immune response.

Antioxidant: An agent that protects against oxidation.

Antiplatelet: Interfering with the action of platelets in clot formation.

Antiproliferative: Inhibiting cell growth.

Antitachycardia Pacing (Overdrive Pacing): Delivery of pacing stimuli at a rapid rate into the atria or ventricles to terminate tachycardia.

Antithrombin III: Opposes the action of thrombin and inhibits the coagulation of blood; inactivates several clotting factors.

Antithrombotic: Counteracting clot formation.

Aorta: The main trunk of the arterial system originating from the left ventricle.

Aortic Dissection: The separation of the layers of the aorta.

Aortic Regurgitation: Failure of aortic valve cusps to close tightly, allowing blood to travel backward through the valve during ventricular diastole.

Aortic Root: Beginning of the aorta where the aorta attaches to the aortic valve.

Aortic Stenosis: Narrowing of the aortic valve orifice, resulting in obstruction of flow from the left ventricle to the aorta during ventricular systole.

Aortic Valve: Valve between the left ventricle and the aorta.

Apex: Bottom of the heart located at approximately the fifth intercostal space, mid-clavicular line.

Aphasia: Loss of the ability to produce and/or comprehend language due to injury to the brain. It does not necessarily affect intelligence.

Apical Impulse: The area near the apex of the heart where ventricular contraction can be palpated.

Apoptosis: Programmed cell death.

aPTT (Activated Partial Thromboplastin Time): Coagulation test used to monitor the therapeutic effectiveness and safety range of heparin.

Arginine Vasopressin: Antidiuretic hormone.

Arrhythmia: Abnormal heart rhythm. Also called dysrhythmia.

Glossary

Arrhythmogenic Right Ventricular Cardiomyopathy: Replacement of muscle tissue in the right ventricle by fibrofatty material, resulting in RV dilation and ventricular arrhythmias. Also called arrhythmogenic right ventricular dysplasia.

Arterioles: Small arteries with thick muscular walls.

Arteritis (Temporal arteritis, Giant Cell Arteritis): An inflammatory condition affecting the medium-sized blood vessels that supply the head, eyes, and optic nerves.

Ascites: Accumulation of serous fluid in the peritoneal cavity.

Atelectasis: An unexpanded or collapsed portion of the lung.

Atherectomy: Interventional procedure used to remove atheromatous plaque from within a blood vessel. Accomplished by threading a catheter with a rotating cutting blade through blood vessels to the site of the atheromatous lesion and using the blade to shave away the plaque.

Atherosclerosis: The deposit of lipids, calcium, fibrin and other cellular substances within the lining of the artery and initiating a progressive inflammatory response in the effort to heal the endothelium.

Atherosclerotic Plaque: The end result of atherosclerosis.

Atrial Fibrillation: Rapid chaotic electrical activity in the atria, resulting in loss of atrial contraction and uncoordinated quivering of atrial muscle. Recognized on the ECG as chaotic fibrillation waves (or "f" waves) instead of P waves, and an irregular ventricular response.

Atrial Kick: Atrial contraction or systole, which contributes an additional 20-30% more volume into the ventricle just prior to ventricular systole.

Atrial Myxoma: A benign tumor located in the upper chamber of the heart on the wall that separates the left chamber from the right (the atrial septum).

Atrial Natriuretic Peptide (ANP): A peptide hormone secreted by cardiac atrial cells in response to atrial stretch. Promotes salt and water excretion.

Atrioventricular (AV) Block: Failure of the electrical impulse to conduct from atria to ventricles. Block can occur in the AV node or below the AV node in the His bundle or bundle branches.

Atrioventricular (AV) Junction: Tissue surrounding the atrioventricular (AV) node and His bundle that contains pacemaker cells capable of firing at a rate of 40 to 60 beats per minute.

Atrioventricular (AV) Node: Group of cells located in the low right atrium that is responsible for conducting the electrical impulse from the atria to the ventricles. The AV node has three main functions: 1) slows transmission of the impulse from atria to ventricles to allow time for the atria to contract before the ventricles contract, 2) functions as a backup pacemaker if the sinus node fails, 3) screens out rapid atrial impulses to protect the ventricles from dangerously fast rates when the atria go too fast.

Atrioventricular (AV) Valves: The valves located between the atria and ventricles; tricuspid and mitral valves.

Atrophic / Atrophy: Related to the general physiological process of reabsorption and breakdown of tissues involving apoptosis at the cellular level. Results in complete or partial wasting away of tissue.

Autoimmune Response: Antibodies are produced against the body's own tissues.

Automatic External Defibrillators: Defibrillators designed to be used by trained lay persons in the event of cardiac arrest due to ventricular fibrillation. Rhythm recognition and defibrillation are done automatically via a hands-off approach.

Automaticity: An intrinsic ability of certain cardiac cells to depolarize spontaneously.

Glossary

Autonomic Nervous System: Nervous system concerned with involuntary bodily functions. Contains the sympathetic and parasympathetic nervous systems.

Autoregulation: Ability of certain organs, such the brain and kidneys, to maintain a consistent perfusion pressure despite changes in systemic pressures. Autoregulation remains intact when the mean arterial pressure is between 60 mm Hg and 100mm Hg.

AV Node Ablation: Use of radio frequency energy to cause permanent damage to the AV node and prevent it from conducting impulses from the atria to the ventricles. Used to treat atrial fibrillation that is refractory to medical therapy; requires implantation of a permanent pacemaker to control the ventricle.

A(a) Wave: Wave on RA and PAOP waveforms, correlating with atrial contraction.

Azotemia: Accumulation of nitrogen containing compounds (such as urea and nitrogen) in the blood.

Bachman's Bundle: Conduction pathway allowing depolarization of the left atrial tissue as conduction travels from the sinoatrial (SA) node to the atrioventircular (AV) node.

Baroreceptors: Sensory nerve endings in the carotid sinus and arch of the aorta that are sensitive to changes in blood pressure. Responsible for reflex blood pressure control.

Base: A substance that can accept a H+ ion.

Base (of the heart): Top of the heart, located at approximately the second intercostal space.

Beta$_1$ Adrenergic Receptors: Sympathetic nervous system receptors located in the heart.

Beta$_2$ Adrenergic Receptors: Sympathetic nervous system receptors located in lungs and peripheral blood vessels.

Beta-Blockers: Medications that block either beta$_1$ or beta$_2$ receptors.

Bezold-Jarisch Reflex: Reflex that, when triggered, causes a vasovagal response.

Bicarbonate (HCO$_3$): Anion that aids in elimination of hydrogen ions. Most important buffer system in the body.

Bifascicular Block: Block of two of the three major fascicles responsible for conducting the electrical impulse through the ventricles: right bundle branch block with block of either the left anterior fascicle or the left posterior fascicle.

Bile Acid Sequestrants: Lipid lowering drugs that combine with bile acids in the intestine and form an insoluble complex that is excreted in the feces. Also called resins.

Bioprosthetic Valve: Tissue valve from a human or pig donor.

Biphasic Waveform: Delivery of electrical energy in two directions through the myocardium. The initial energy is delivered in one direction, and the last portion is delivered in the opposite direction. Newer generation defibrillators use biphasic waveforms that are more efficient and require lower doses for cardioversion and defibrillation.

Bisferiens Carotid Pulse: Characteristic of a patient with HOCM. The initial upstroke of the carotid pulse is brisk; however, as systole progresses left ventricular outflow, tract obstruction may occur. This obstruction results in a collapse of the pulse and then a secondary rise.

Biventricular Pacing: Pacing of both ventricles simultaneously. See Cardiac Resynchronization Therapy.

Body mass index (BMI): A measure of body fat that is the ratio of the weight of the body in kilograms to the square of its height in meters. To calculate: Weight (Kg) ÷ Height (M^2). Estimate using pounds and inches: weight (lbs) ÷ height (inches)^2 x 704.5. Normal = 18.5 – 24.9; overweight = 25 – 29.9; obese = 30 – 34.9; extremely obese = > 40.

Glossary

Brachiocephalic Artery: Also called innominate artery, and is the largest branch off the aortic arch. Divides into the right common carotid and right subclavian arteries.

Bradycardia: Heart rate below 50 beats per minute.

Brain Natriuretic Peptide (BNP): A peptide hormone released from myocytes in the cardiac ventricle in response to volume overload and stretch during heart failure. Produces vasodilation. Serum BNP levels are used in the diagnosis of heart failure.

Brain Stem: The lower part of the brain, continuous with the spinal cord. Contains the pons, medulla oblongata, and mid-brain.

Bronchi: Trachea divides into right and left main stem bronchi. No gas exchange occurs in bronchi. Bronchi then further divide into branches to complete the respiratory tree.

Bronchioles: Branches of the bronchi that no longer contain cartilidge. Terminal bronchioles give rise to alveoli.

Bruit: An adventitious sound heard on auscultation of a vessel.

Bundle Branch Block: Block of either the right or left bundle branch of the ventricular conduction system.

Bundle of His: Conduction pathway at the bottom of the AV node that divides into the right and left bundle branches; also called the His bundle.

Calcium Channel Blockers: Medications that decrease the flux of calcium across the cell membrane.

Cannulation: The placement of tubes inside the vessels to allow the escape of blood and other fluids from the body; used in placing patient on cardiopulmonary bypass.

Capillaries: The very smallest vessels connecting the smallest arteries and veins. Also the location where the oxygen and nutrients are exchanged.

Carbon Dioxide (CO_2): Gas produced during aerobic metabolism during the oxidation of carbohydrates, fatty acids and proteins in the mitochondria of cells. $PaCO_2$ is used to measure the effectivness of alvoelar ventilation.

Carbonic Acid (H_2CO_3): A volatile acid that is formed as a result of the hydration of carbon dioxide. Can dissociate into a hydrogen ion and a bicarbonate ion.

Carbon Monoxide (CO): Colorless, odorless, and tasteless gas that is toxic due to its affinity for hemoglobin.

Cardiac Biomarkers: Substances released into the blood when necrosis occurs as a result of membrane rupture of cardiac myocytes.

Cardiac Catheterization: An invasive diagnostic procedure involving insertion of a catheter through an artery or vein and advancing it into the heart.

Cardiac Output: The amount of blood ejected by the left ventricle every minute.

Cardiac Resynchronization Therapy (CRT): Atrial synchronized biventricular pacing utilizing an atrial lead, a right ventricular lead, and a coronary sinus lead placed in a left lateral or posterior cardiac vein for left ventricular pacing. CRT is aimed at eliminating the dyssynchrony in the contraction of the right and left ventricles and septum that occurs in severe heart failure by pacing both ventricles simultaneously.

Cardiac Tamponade: Mechanical compression of the heart by large amounts of fluid or blood within the pericardial space, resulting in decreased ventricular filling that limits stroke volume and cardiac output.

Cardiogenic Shock: Failure of tissues to receive an adequate blood supply due to severely decreased cardiac output caused by left ventricular failure.

Cardiomyopathy: Primary disease of the heart muscle characterized by ventricular dilation, myocyte and wall thickening (hypertrophy), interstitial fibrosis, decreased contractility, and conduction disturbances.

Glossary

Cardioplegia: Temporary cardiac arrest induced by drugs during heart surgery.

Cardiopulmonary Bypass: Process of bringing the blood outside of the body and bypassing the heart and lungs with use of the cardiopulmonary (heart and lung) bypass machine. Used during the administration of cardioplegia during CABG.

Cardioversion: The termination of a tachyarrhythmia (atrial fibrillation, supraventricular tachycardia, ventricular tachycardia) using electrical energy or pharmacotherapy. Electrical cardioversion is the delivery of electrical energy that is synchronized on the QRS complex in order to avoid shocking on the T wave during the vulnerable period of the cardiac cycle.

Carotid Endarterectomy: The surgical removal of plaque for the prevention of ischemic events.

Carotid Sinus Massage: Manual pressure applied to the carotid sinus (just under the angle of the jaw) in order to initiate the reflex stimulation of the vagus nerve to slow AV conduction and diagnose or terminate SVTs.

Carotid Sinus: Pressure sensitive cells located at the bifurcation of the common carotid artery into the internal and external carotid arteries. When stimulated, the carotid sinus initiates reflex stimulation of the vagus nerve, which slows heart rate and AV conduction and inhibition of the cardioregulatory center in the medulla, causing peripheral vasodilation and resulting in lowering of the blood pressure.

Catabolic: Metabolic process of breaking down molecules into smaller units.

Catecholamines: The sympathetic nervous system neurotransmitters epinephrine and norepinephrine.

Caval Opening: A break in the diaphragm through which the inferior vena cava passes.

Central Venous Pressure (CVP): Pressure in the central venous system; typically measured by a catheter placed in the superior vena cava or right atrium and used as indicator of right ventricular end diastolic pressure (RV preload).

Cerebral Perfusion Pressure (CPP): Mean arterial pressure minus intracranial pressure.

Chemoreceptors: Receptors located in the aortic arch and in the carotid arteries that respond to changes in blood chemistry, including arterial oxygen content, arterial carbon dioxide levels and arterial pH.

Cholinergic: Resembling the physiological action of acetylcholine.

Chordae Tendineae: Delicate strands of fibrous material that attach valve leaflets of the AV valves to the papillary muscles.

Chronotropic: Affecting the heart rate. Chronotropic incompetence refers to the inability of the sinus node to function adequately as the primary pacemaker of the heart.

Chvostek's Sign: Spasm of lip, nose or face in response to tapping over facial nerve. Seen with hypocalcemia.

Circle of Willis: An anatomical ring of vessels joining the carotid artery system and the vertebrobasilar system.

CK (creatinine kinase): Biomarker present in the heart, brain and skeletal muscle.

CK MB: The subunit of CK found in the heart muscle; rapidly rises in the presence of myocardial damage.

CMT: Abbreviation for circus movement tachycardia. A tachycardia occurring in the presence of an accessory pathway in patients with WPW syndrome that involves re-entry of an impulse through a circuit that consists of the atria, AV node, ventricle, and accessory pathway.

Coagulapathy: Pathology of the coagulation system.

Coarctation of the Aorta: Malformation resulting in narrowing of the aorta.

Glossary

Chelation: Process of using chelating agents (complexes that bind to metals) to remove heavy metals from the body.

Colloid Solutions: Colloid solutions contain substances that do not pass through a semipermeable membrane. These solutions stay in the intravascular compartment for longer than crystalloids, and, therefore, less volume is needed in fluid resuscitation. Colloids also increase oncotic pressure.

Commissures: Point where the cardiac valve leaflets connect.

Commissurotomy: Procedure during which the valve commissures are cut apart to allow for increased movement of the leaflets.

Compartment Syndrome: An emergency following injury or surgery whereby, due to inflammation, there is an increased pressure within the confined space called the fascial compartment. This impedes blood flow and can lead to nerve and tissue damage if not promptly treated.

Complete Heart Block: Complete failure of all atrial impulses to conduct to the ventricles; also called third degree block.

Concentric Hypertrophy: Ventricular muscle wall thickening resulting from chronic pressure overload.

Conduit: Vessels available to use as graft material.

Contractility: Ability of the ventricular muscle fibers to shorten and eject blood, independent of preload or afterload.

Contrast Induced Nephropathy: Renal dysfunction caused by the administration of contrast agents during invasive or interventional cardiac procedures.

Convection: Another term used for the process of ultrafiltration.

Cor Pulmonale: Cor pulmonale is enlargement of right ventricle (either dilation or hypertrophy) as a result of pulmonary pathology or the abnormalities in the pulmonary circulation.

Coronary Artery Disease: Presence of atherosclerosis or atherosclerotic plaque in the epicardial coronary arteries.

Coronary Sinus: The vessel that receives blood from the cardiac veins and empties into the right atrium.

Cortex (Cerebral): The outer layer of the cerebrum.

Cortex (Renal): Outer portion of the kidney between the renal capsule and the renal medulla. Contains the glomeruli.

Counterpulsation Therapy: Reference to intra-aortic balloon pump therapy whereby the balloon is inflated during diastole and deflated during systole.

Creatinine Clearance: Volume of blood plasma that is cleared of creatinine per unit of time. Used to estimate the glomerular filtration rate.

Cryptogenic Stroke: Stroke of unknown cause.

Crystalloid Solutions: Clear intravenous solutions with dissolved substances that can diffuse across cell membranes. Example: Normal saline.

Cushing's Syndrome: Rare endocrine disorder caused by high levels of cortisol in the blood.

Cutting Balloon: Interventional cardiology balloon with longitudinal blades mounted on its surface. Used to make incisions into the plaque with balloon inflation during PTCA.

Cyanosis: Bluish discoloration of the skin due to deoxygenated hemoglobin in vessels near the skin surface.

Cyclooxygenase: Chemical substance that performs the first step in the creation of prostaglandins.

Glossary

Cytokines: Proteins secreted by cells of the immune system that serve to regulate the system.

DASH Diet: Dietary Approaches to Stop Hypertension. The diet manipulates potassium, calcium and magnesium while holding sodium constant.

DDD Pacemaker: Dual chamber pacemaker that paces in the right atrium and right ventricle; senses both atrial and ventricular activity and has a dual response to sensing, either triggering or inhibiting pacemaker output, depending on whether atrial or ventricular activity is sensed.

Dead Space: Air that is inhaled but does not participate in gas exchange.

Decortication: A surgical procedure involving the removal of fibrous tissue from the visceral pleural peel, allowing pus to be drained from the pleural space.

Defibrillation Threshold: Minimum amount of electrical energy that will consistently terminate ventricular fibrillation; typically used to describe minimum defibrillating energy in an ICD.

Defibrillation: Unsynchronized shock delivered to patients in ventricular fibrillation.

Delta Wave: Initial slurred portion of the QRS that occurs when the ventricle is pre-excited via an accessory pathway, as in WPW Syndrome.

De Musset's Sign: The patient's head bobs with each heart beat; commonly occurs with aortic regurgitation.

Deoxyhemoglobin: Hemoglobin that is not saturated (or bound) with oxygen.

Depolarization: Electrical activation of the cardiac muscle cell.

Diabetes Mellitus: Insulin deficit (Type I) or inappropriate response to insulin (Type II), resulting in a random glucose of > 200 mg/dL or a fasting glucose of > 126 mg/dL.

Diastole: The relaxation of the heart muscle allowing for filling of the chamber.

Diastolic Dysfunction: Left ventricular dysfunction in which the ventricle has impaired relaxation and does not fill properly.

Diencephalon: Neurological components of thalamus, hypothalamus, and limbic system.

Diffusion: Movement of particles (solute) from an area of high concentration to an area of lower concentration.

Dilated Cardiomyopathy: Cardiomyopathy in which the ventricular walls thin and the cavity dilates in response to chronic volume overload, resulting in systolic dysfunction.

Dipyridamole: A coronary vasodilator used in chemical stress testing.

Directional Atherectomy: Interventional cardiology procedure in which a cutting blade is directed toward plaque in a coronary vessel and used to cut and remove the plaque from the vessel wall.

Dobutamine: Inotropic agent used for chemical stress testing. Also used to increase contractility in cardiogenic shock or heart failure.

Dopaminergic Receptors: Sympathetic nervous system receptors located in the renal, mesenteric, and coronary blood vessels.

Dressler's syndrome: Pericarditis occurring several weeks after an infarction.

Dromotropic: Affecting cardiac conduction.

Drug Eluting Stents: Stents coated with pharmacological agents aimed at decreasing restenosis.

Dual Chamber Pacemaker: Pacemaker that has an electrode for pacing in two chambers of the heart, traditionally the right atrium and the right ventricle.

Glossary

Durozier's Sign: Systolic murmur heard over femoral artery when compressed proximally, and diastolic murmur heard over femoral artery when compressed distally; associated with high arterial pressure or aortic insufficiency.

Dyslipidemia: Abnormal concentrations of lipids or lipoproteins in the blood.

Dysphagia: Difficulty swallowing.

Dysrhythmia: Abnormal heart rhythm. Also called arrhythmia.

Eccentric Hypertrophy: Hypertrophy caused by volume overload, resulting in ventricular wall thinning and chamber dilation.

Echocardiogram: Cardiac ultrasound procedure used to aid in diagnosis of heart disease.

Ectopic Beat: Electrical impulse originating outside the sinus node; can be from the atria, AV junction, or ventricle.

Efferent Arterioles: Arterioles that exit the glomerulus.

Ejection Fraction: The percent of the end-diastolic volume in the left ventricle ejected with each beat.

Ejection: Second phase of systole when blood is ejected.

Electromechanical Interference: Electrical signals external to a pacemaker or ICD that may be sensed by the device and result in device malfunction.

Electrophysiology Study (EPS): An invasive procedure involving placement of multiple pacing and recording catheters in various places in the heart to evaluate and treat cardiac arrhythmias.

Embolus: A particle of undissolved matter in the blood (solid, liquid or gas). Can be a piece of clot or fat or an air bubble.

Empyema: Collection of pus within the pleural space.

Endocarditis: Inflammation of endocardium (inner lining of heart), including heart valves.

Endocardium: Thin serous membrane lining the cavities of the heart.

Endografts: Stent grafts used to treat abdominal aortic aneurysms. A transfemoral approach can be used instead of an open surgical repair.

Endomyocardial Biopsy: Tissue biopsy obtained from the heart muscle using an invasive catheter-based approach; used in the diagnosis of restrictive cardiomyopathy and following heart transplant.

Endomyocardial Fibrosis: Fibrosis of the ventricular endocardium and subendocardium that extends to the mitral and tricuspid valves, greatly decreasing the functioning of the ventricular chambers.

Endothelin: Endogenous hormonal vasoconstrictor released by the endothelium.

Endothelium: A layer of specialized epithelium that lines the inner surface of blood vessels. Endothelial cells line the entire circulatory system, from the heart to the smallest capillary. The endothelium of the inner surface of the heart is called the endocardium.

Endotoxins: Substances released from the cell wall of gram negative bacteria.

Epiaortic Imaging: Ultrasound imaging directly over (upon) the aorta; used in CABG.

Epicardium: The smooth outer layer of the heart that contains the network of coronary arteries and veins, the autonomic nerves, the lymphatic system and fat tissue.

Epiglottis: A flap tissue attached to the root of the tongue that protects the entrance to the glottis, the opening between the vocal folds. During swallowing the epiglottis prevents food from going into the trachea. The epiglottis is one of three cartilaginous structures that make up the larynx.

Glossary

Epinephrine: A neurotransmitter of the sympathetic nervous system; also called adrenalin.

Epithelium: Tissue composed of a layer of cells which lines both the outside (skin) and the inside cavities of bodies.

Ergonovine Maleate: Arterial vasoconstrictor that can be given during cardiac catheterization to assist in the diagnosis of vasospastic angina.

Erythropoietin: A hormone that regulates red blood cell production.

External Counterpulsation: Non-pharmacological treatment option for debilitating angina. Series of cuffs are wrapped around the patient's legs and compressed air is used to apply pressure in the cuffs during ventricular diastole, resulting in increased arterial pressure to increase retrograde aortic blood flow into the coronary arteries during diastole.

Extracorpeal: Outside the body.

Extrinsic Pathway (coagulation cascade): Pathway in the clotting cascade activated by injured tissue.

Fabry Disease: A lipid storage disorder caused by the deficiency of an enzyme involved in the biodegradation of fats.

Fascicular Block: Block in one of the two divisions of the left bundle branch: left anterior fascicular block or left posterior fascicular block. Also called hemiblock.

Fibric Acids or Fibrates: A group of lipid lowering medications most noted for their ability to lower triglycerides.

Fibrin: Fine protein filaments which entangle red and white blood cells and platelets and form a clot; formed by the action of thrombin on fibrinogen.

Fibrinogen: A protein that is converted to fibrin through the action of thrombin in the presence of calcium ions.

Fibrinolytics: Fibrin specific medications used to break down clots.

Fibrous Cap: Fibrous tissue, mainly collagen, covering the lipid core of an atheromatous plaque.

Fibrous Pericardium: The external covering of the pericardium.

Fistula: Abnormal connection or passageway between organs or vessels that normally do not connect.

Flow Cycled Breath: A flow cycled breath is a pressure support breath. It allows a constant pressure during inspiration. There is no set time in a flow cycled breath. Once a set amount of the peak flow has been delivered, exhalation begins.

Foam Cells: Macrophages (scavenger cells) that are engorged with lipids.

Free Graft: Graft where both ends of the vessel are removed from their original location and re-attached elsewhere.

Gangrene: Necrosis followed by decay of tissue caused by infection or lack of blood flow.

Glomerular Filtration Rate (GFR): A calculation that determines how well the blood is filtered by the kidneys; calculated using a mathematical formula that compares a person's age, sex, and race to serum creatinine, albumin, and blood urea nitrogen (BUN) levels. Normal GFR in both kidneys in adults is 120 to 125 milliliters per minute (mL/min).

Glomerulus: A tuft of capillaries, surrounded by Bowman's capsule, that serve as the functional unit of kidney.

Glycoprotein IIb / IIIa Receptors: The end result of platelet activation. Receptor site on platelet surface to which fibrinogen binds, allowing platelets to bind and aggregate.

Glossary

Graft: Portions of vessel taken from another part of the body used to bypass coronary artery blockage during CABG.

Great Vessels: The aorta, the pulmonary artery, the inferior vena cava and the superior vena cava.

HDL Cholesterol (HDL-C): High density lipoprotein cholesterol.

Heart Block: Varying degrees of conduction failure in the cardiac conduction system, ranging from benign to life threatening.

Heart Failure: Syndrome where the heart is unable to pump enough oxygenated blood to meet the metabolic needs of the body.

Hematoma: Mass of blood within the tissue caused by bleeding from a blood vessel.

Hemochromatosis: Condition where the body stores too much iron and the excess iron causes organ damage.

Hemodynamics: The forces influencing the circulation of blood throughout the body.

Hemoglobin A$_{1c}$ (Hb A$_{1c}$): Glycosylated hemoglobin reflecting the average blood sugar level for 2 to 3 months prior to the test.

Hemoptysis: Coughing or spitting up blood that is the result of bleeding from the respiratory system.

Hemostasis: Cessation of bleeding.

Hemothorax: Collection of blood in the pleural cavity.

Hepatojugular Reflux: Elevation of jugular venous pressure when firm pressure is applied to the mid-epigastric region; response is exaggerated in right-sided heart failure.

Hepatomegaly: Enlargement of the liver.

Hexaxial Reference System: The diagram used to calculate the QRS axis; all six frontal plane leads intersect in the middle of the diagram. Also called the "axis wheel."

High Grade Atrioventricular Block: Failure of two or more consecutive atrial impulses to conduct to the ventricles when the atrial rate is reasonable (<135 bpm). Also called advanced AV block.

Hilum: Depressed area in the medial aspect of each kidney.

Hirudin: Direct thrombin inhibitor.

HMG-CoA Reductase Inhibitors (Statins): Most widely used lipid lowering medications in the treatment of cardiovascular disease. Work by inhibiting HMG-CoA reductase during cholesterol synthesis.

HMG-CoA Reductase: Enzyme that catalyzes an early step in cholesterol synthesis.

Holosystolic Murmur: A murmur that can be heard throughout systole.

Homocysteine: An amino acid with toxic effects on the endothelium when elevated.

Homologous: Similar in both structure and in source.

hs – CRP (High Sensitivity C-Reactive Protein): A marker of inflammation; elevated levels increase cardiovascular risk.

H-V Interval: Measured from His deflection to onset of ventricular activation in intracardiac signals obtained during EPS. Reflects conduction time through the distal His-Purkinje system.

Hydrostatic Pressure: The pushing pressure inside a vessel forcing fluids and nutrients across the membrane.

Hypercalcemia: Serum calcium > 10.4 mg/dL or ionized calcium > 5.26 mg/dL.

Hypercholesterolemia: Elevated serum cholesterol.

Glossary

Hyperdynamic: An increase in contractility and ejection fraction (when referring to left ventricle).

Hyperhomocysteinemia: Elevated serum homocysteine.

Hyperkalemia: Serum potassium > 5.0 mEq/L.

Hyperlipidemia: Any of the following: elevated total cholesterol (hypercholesterolemia), elevated LDL-C, or elevated triglycerides.

Hypermagnesemia: Serum magnesium > 2.5 mEq/L.

Hypernatremia: Serum sodium > 145 mEq/L.

Hyperphosphatemia: Serum phosphate > 4.5 mg/dL.

Hyperplasia: Excessive proliferation of normal cells.

Hypertension: A systolic or diastolic blood pressure above the normal range. Pre-hypertension is systolic 120-139 or diastolic 80-89; stage 1 hypertension is systolic 140-159 or diastolic 90-99; stage 2 hypertension is systolic ≥ 160 or diastolic ≥ 100.

Hyperthyroidism: Excessive secretion of the thyroid gland, resulting in an increase in basal metabolic rate.

Hypertonic solution: Solution containing higher concentration of solutes than what is found inside the cell. Draws water out of the cell.

Hypertriglyceridemia: Elevated serum triglycerides.

Hypertrophic Cardiomyopathy (HCM): Cardiomyopathy characterized by hypertrophy and stiffening of the myocardial wall and resulting in a decrease in both ventricular filling and a decrease in cardiac output.

Hypertrophic Obstructive Cardiomyopathy (HOCM): Hypertrophic cardiomyopathy that involves hypertrophy of the high part of the interventricular septum. Results in obstruction of the left ventricular outflow tract during systole.

Hypertrophy: Increased size. Generally used to denote thickening of the ventricular muscle wall as a result of chronic pressure overload.

Hypocalcemia: Serum calcium < 8.8 mg/dL or < 4.65 mg/dL.

Hypokalemia: Serum potassium < 3.5 mEq/L.

Hypomagnesemia: Serum magnesium < 1.8 mg/dL or < 1.5 mEq/L.

Hyponatremia: Serum sodium < 135 mEq/L.

Hypophosphatemia: Serum phosphate < 2.5 to 3.0 mg/dL.

Hypoperfusion: Decreased perfusion to end organs.

Hypotension: Significantly reduced blood pressure or low blood pressure.

Hypotonic solution: Solution containing lower concentration of solutes than what is found inside the cell. Causes water to move into the cell.

Hypoventilation: Decreased ventilation (amount of inhaled oxygen).

Hypovolemia: Diminished blood volume.

Hypoxemia: Low level of oxygen in the blood.

Hypoxia: Decreased oxygenation of the tissues.

Idiopathic: No known cause

Glossary

Implantable Cardioverter Defibrillator (ICD): Implantable device similar to a pacemaker that provides a defibrillating shock and other therapies (antitachycardia pacing, low and high energy cardioverting shocks) to terminate ventricular tachycardia or ventricular fibrillation.

Incentive Spirometry: Designed to mimic natural sighing. Encourages the patient to take long, slow, deep breaths by using a device that provides him or her with visual or other positive feedback when inhaling at a predetermined volume and sustaining the inflation for a minimum of 3 seconds.

Indicative ECG Changes: Signs of myocardial ischemia or injury recorded in leads facing the damaged area: Q waves indicate necrosis, ST-segment elevation indicates injury, T wave inversion indicates ischemia.

Inferior MI: MI involving the inferior or bottom wall of the left ventricle.

Inferior Posterior MI: MI involving the inferior and posterior walls of the left ventricle.

Inferior Vena Cava: Principal vein that receives blood from below the level of the diaphragm, including the abdomen, pelvis and lower extremities. Empties into the right atrium.

Inotrope: Medication used to increase contractility.

Inotropic: Influencing the force of ventricular contractility. Positive inotropic substances increase contractility; negative inotropic substances decrease contractility.

INR (International Normalized Ratio): Developed to correct problems with standardization of the PT; relates the patient's PT to the intensity of actual coagulation.

In Situ: Having not been removed from its original place. In CABG, an in situ graft has one end left in its original location, such as is frequently done with the internal mammary artery grafts.

Inspiratory Plateau Pressure (IPP): Pressure measured by holding inspiration after delivered tidal volume is complete and reflective of the pressure in the alveoli at the end of inspiration. Pressure is independent of resistance and reflects only compliance.

Interatrial Septum: Muscle tissue separating the right and left atria.

Intercalated Disks: Disks that form a tight junction, allowing cardiac muscle cells to function as integrated units.

Intermittent Claudication: Severe pain in calf muscles with walking that is relieved by rest.

Internal Iliac Arteries: Arise from abdominal aorta and supply the lower trunk, including the reproductive organs and the legs.

Internal Mammary Artery Grafts: Most common arterial grafts used in CABG. Have improved long-term patency rates over vein grafts.

Internodal Pathways: Conduction pathways in the right atrium, allowing conduction between the sinoatrial (SA) node and atrioventricular (AV) node.

Interstitial Pneumonitis: Characterized by marked interstitial fibrosis. Has an insidious onset with slow, but severe progression and a poor prognosis, with most patients dying of their disease.

Interventricular Septum: Thick muscle mass separating the right and left ventricles; contracts and functions as part of the left ventricle during systole.

Intima: The inner layer of an artery containing a thin layer of endothelium.

Intra-aortic Balloon Pump: Invasive catheter-based assist device using counter pulsation therapy. Balloon in descending aorta is inflated during diastole and deflated during systole. Balloon deflation just before systole reduces afterload and balloon inflation during diastole increase myocardial perfusion.

Glossary

Intracoronary (Intravascular) Ultrasound: A tiny ultrasound device threaded into an artery inside a millimeter-thick catheter. Ultrasound waves measure changes in vessel wall thickness and proovide a detailed cross section of the coronary artery wall anatomy.

Intracoronary Stent: Metal scaffold type structure inserted into a coronary artery to help prevent elastic recoil and keep open the lumen of the vessel.

Intracranial Hemorrhage: Bleeding inside the skull that encloses the brain.

Intracranial Pressure (ICP): Pressure exerted by the cranium on the brain tissue. Determined by cerebrospinal fluid (CSF), brain mass, and the brain's circulating blood volume.

Intrinsic Pathway (coagulation cascade): Pathway in clotting cascade activated by damage to red blood cells or platelets; monitored by the aPTT.

Intrinsicoid deflection: Measured from beginning of QRS to peak of R wave and is a measure of ventricular activation time. Reflects the time required for peak voltage to develop under a lead.

Ionized Calcium: Calcium that is free to leave the extracellular fluid and participate in intracellular function.

Ischemia: Temporary lack of oxygen to the myocardium.

Isolated Systolic Hypertension: A systolic blood pressure greater than 160 mm Hg with a normal diastolic blood pressure.

Isovolumic or Isovolumetric Contraction: Contraction of the ventricle during the first phase of systole in which the volume of blood in the ventricle does not change.

J Point: Place on the ECG where the ST segment takes off from the end of the QRS complex.

Jugular Venous Pressure: Pressure in the jugular vein that increases or decreases in response to fluid status.

Juxtarenal: Just below the renal arteries.

Lactic acidosis: A type of metabolic acidosis caused by the buildup of lactic acid. Caused by anaerobic metabolism.

Lacunar Stroke: Stroke affecting the deeper non-cortical areas of the brain caused by small or penetrating vessel occlusive disease.

Larynx: Contains the vocal folds, and is located just below the area where the pharynx splits into the trachea and the esophagus.

Lateral MI: MI involving the lateral wall of the left ventricle.

LDL Cholesterol (LDL-C): Low density lipoprotein cholesterol.

Left Anterior Descending (LAD) Artery: Coronary artery arising from the left main coronary artery; responsible for supplying the anterior wall of the left ventricle.

Left Anterior Hemiblock: Block of the anterior fascicle of the left bundle branch.

Left Atrial Appendage: Appendage off the left atrium that is frequently the source of clot formation in atrial fibrillation.

Left Atrium: Chamber of the heart that receives oxygenated blood from the pulmonary veins.

Left Bundle Branch: Group of specialized conduction fibers that carry the electrical impulse into the left ventricle. The left bundle branch has two divisions: left anterior fascicle and left posterior fascicle.

Left Circumflex (LCX) Artery: Coronary artery arising from the left main coronary artery; responsible for supplying the lateral wall of the left ventricle.

893

Glossary

Left Common Carotid Artery: Branches directly off the aortic arch that carry blood up the left neck into the head.

Left Main Coronary Artery: Major coronary artery arising from the left side of the aortic root; divides into the left anterior descending artery and the circumflex artery.

Left Posterior Hemiblock: Block of the posterior fascicle of the left bundle branch.

Left Subclavian Artery: Arises from the aortic arch and carries blood into the left arm.

Left Ventricle: A thick-walled, high-pressure pump that receives oxygenated blood from the left atrium and pumps blood into the aorta.

Left ventricular reduction surgery (Batista procedure): Surgery involving cutting out part of the left ventricle and sewing the remaining walls together to decrease the size of the ventricle.

Lipoprotein a (Lp-a): A lipoprotein similar to LDL-C.

Loffler's Endocarditis: Endomyocardial disease characterized by endomyocardial fibrosis. An unusually large number of eosinophils in the blood with infiltration of the heart.

Lone Atrial Fibrillation: Atrial fibrillation in patients with normal cardiac and pulmonary function, as well as no known predisposing factors.

Long QT Syndrome: A hereditary syndrome with a prolonged QT interval on the ECG that predisposes people to torsade de pointes.

Loop Diuretics: Work at the loop of Henle and increase sodium and water excretion.

Low Molecular Weight Heparin (LMWH): Heparin that is lower in molecular weight and smaller in size than unfractionated heparin.

Lysis: Dissolution or decomposition of (as in clot lysis).

Macrovascular Complications (of diabetes): Coronary artery disease and stroke.

Mapping: Refers to the precise placement and movement of an intracardiac catheter around an area of the heart in an attempt to find a focus or electrical pathway responsible for an arrhythmia and locate the area where ablation might abolish the arrhythmia.

Marfan's Syndrome: Hereditary disorder of connective tissue characterized by abnormal elongation of bones, resulting in long extremities, fingers, toes, and other musculoskeletal abnormalities. Also associated with cardiovascular abnormalities, including aortic aneurysm and aortic insufficiency in addition to ocular abnormalities.

Mast Cells: Located in the tissues and contain mediators of inflammation; key role in initiation of inflammation.

Maze Procedure: Surgical procedure involving a series of incisions in the atria to prevent atrial fibrillation. Incisions are made to create scar tissue which prevents re-entrant pathways from forming in the atria and causing atrial fibrillation. The incisions are placed to channel conduction from the sinus node to the AV node while still allowing both atria to depolarize in a sequential fashion. Similar scars can be created using radiofrequency ablation techniques in the EP lab.

Media: The middle layer of an artery comprised of smooth muscle and elastic connective tissue.

Mediastinitus: Inflammation of the tissue of the mediastinum.

Mediastinum: Middle of the thoracic cavity.

Glossary

Medulla oblongata: Vital part of the brain just above the spinal cord that contains the cardiac, vasomotor, and respiratory centers. Causes peripheral vasodilation or vasoconstriction in response to signals received from the baroreceptors and chemoreceptors.

Medulla (Renal): Innermost portion of kidney divided into sections called renal pyramids.

MET: A unit of metabolic equivalent, which is defined as the number of calories consumed per minute of an activity. A single unit (1 MET) is the caloric consumption of an individual at complete rest.

Metabolic Syndrome: A grouping of cardiovascular risk factors; also called Syndrome X, insulin resistance syndrome, and "the deadly quartet." Any three of the following constitute increased risk for cardiovascular disease and Type 2 diabetes: *abdominal obesity* (waist circumference > 40 inches in men or > 35 inches in women); *triglycerides* > 150 mg/dL; HDL-C < 40 mg/dL in men or < 50 mg/dL in women; *blood pressure* ≥ 130/ ≥ 85 mm Hg; *fasting glucose* > 110-125 mg/dL.

Metformin: Oral hypoglycemic agent with potential for being nephrotoxic.

Methemoglobin: A form of hemoglobin in which the iron component is not normal and the hemoglobin is unable to carry oxygen.

Microalbuminuria: Small amounts of *albumin* in the urine that cannot be detected by urine dipstick.

Microvascular Complications (of diabetes): Vision loss, nephropathy, neuropathy, and amputation.

MIDCAB: Minimally invasive coronary artery bypass that is performed on a beating heart (no cardiopulmonary bypass) and without the use of a median sternotomy.

Minute ventilation (V$_E$): Volume of air entering the nose or mouth each minute.

Mitral Facies: Pinkish-purple discoloration of the cheeks that is common in patients with severe mitral stenosis.

Mitral Regurgitation (Insufficiency): Failure of the mitral valve to close, resulting in backwards flow of blood from the left ventricle into the left atrium during ventricular systole.

Mitral Stenosis: Mitral valve is unable to open normally, causing an obstruction of blood flow from the left atrium to the left ventricle during ventricular diastole.

Mitral Valve Prolapse: One or both of the mitral valve leaflets evert or bulge into the atrium, sometimes allowing small amounts of blood to flow back into the atrium.

Mitral Valve: Valve located between the left atrium and left ventricle.

Monophasic Waveform: Delivery of electrical energy in one direction through the myocardium, used by first generation defibrillators. Monophasic defibrillators require higher doses or escalating doses of electrical energy for cardioversion and defibrillation and are less efficient than newer biphasic machines.

Monounsaturated Fats: Beneficial fat in a heart healthy diet; plant source and liquid at room temperature. Examples: canola oil and olive oil.

Murmur: Sound made from vibrations as blood travels through a partially open valve.

Mycotic Aneurysms: Term used to describe extracardiac or intracardiac aneurysms caused by infections.

Myeloma (also known as multiple myeloma) is a type of cancer of plasma cells. Plasma cells are produced in the bone marrow and are an important part of the immune system because they produce antibodies.

Myocardial Imaging: The noninvasive studies of cardiac echocardiography or radionuclide imaging. Can be done alone or is combination with stress testing.

Myocardial Infarction (MI): Death or necrosis of myocardial tissue.

Myocarditis: Inflammation of the myocardium.

895

Glossary

Myocardium: The thick middle layer of heart containing cardiac muscle fibers.

Myocytes: Contractile cardiac muscle cells.

Myofibril: Contractile element of cardiac muscle cell that runs the length of the cell and contains contractile proteins (actin and myosin) that cause the myofibril to shorten and the muscle to contract.

Myoglobin: Cardiac biomarker that rises the earliest with myocardial damage. Not specific to myocardial damage because it is also contained in skeletal muscle.

Natriuretic Peptides (atrial natriuretic peptide and brain natriuretic peptide): Beneficial neurohormones in heart failure producing systemic and pulmonary vasodilation and enhancing sodium and water excretion.

Necrosis: Localized tissue death due to disease or injury (such as prolonged ischemia).

Nephron: Functional unit of kidney; over 1 million nephrons per kidney.

Nephrotoxic: Toxic to the kidneys.

Nesiritide (Natrecor): Synthetic brain natriuretic peptide (BNP).

Neurocardiogenic Syncope: Fainting associated with hypotension, peripheral vasodilation, and bradycardia, resulting from increased vagal stimulation. Also called vasovagal syncope or vasodepressor syncope.

Neurogenic Bladder: Term to describe a malfunctioning bladder due to neurologic dysfunction. May be from trauma, injury, or disease.

Neurohormonal Responses: Various hormonal and neurological responses that occur in heart failure to attempt to compensate for a decrease in cardiac output. Examples: sympathetic nervous system stimulation, renin-angiotensin-aldosterone stimulation.

Neuropathy: Usually short for peripheral neuropathy, a disease of the peripheral nervous system.

Niacin or Nicotinic Acid: A "B" complex vitamin with additional dose-related pharmacological positive effects on lipid levels.

Nicotine: The physically addictive substance in tobacco.

Non-compliant Ventricle: A ventricle that is unable to relax and fill properly during diastole.

Non-homologous Grafts: Grafts from another species.

Non-ST Elevation MI (NSTEMI): Myocardial infarction that does not present with ST elevation on the ECG; usually presents with ST depression or T wave inversion, but cardiac biomarkers are elevated.

Norepinephrine: Neurotransmitter of the sympathetic nervous system. Also called noradrenalin.

Nosocomial Pneumonia: Pneumonia acquired in the hospital.

Oliguria: Urine output < 400 ml/24 hours.

Omega-3 Fatty Acids: Non-essential fatty acids contained in oily fish, such as salmon, lake trout, tuna and herring.

Oncotic Pressure: The pulling pressure inside a vessel drawing fluid and substances into the vessel.

OPCAB: Off pump coronary artery bypass; done off cardiopulmonary bypass, but involves a median sternotomy.

Opening Snap: A sound made by the opening of a stenotic mitral or tricuspid valve. The opening of these valves is normally silent.

Orthopnea: Shortness of breath when in a supine position.

Orthostatic hypotension: Abnormally low blood pressure that occurs with standing.

Glossary

Osmolality: Measurement of the concentration of solutes. Calculated as the osmoles of solute per kilogram of solvent.

Ostia: Small openings in the aorta giving rise to the right and left coronary artery systems.

Oxidation: The process of a substance combining with oxygen.

Oxyhemoglobin: Hemoglobin that is loaded or combined with oxygen.

P Mitrale: Wide, M-shaped P waves that occur in left atrial enlargement.

P Pulmonale: Tall, narrow P waves that occur in right atrial enlargement.

P Wave: Wave on the ECG representing atrial depolarization.

Pacemaker Electrode: Metal tip located at the end of the pacemaker lead wire that is in contact with myocardium and delivers the electrical stimulus from the pacemaker to the heart muscle to make it depolarize.

Paclitaxel: An antiproliferative or antineoplastic agent used on drug eluting stents. Also used as a chemotherapeutic agent.

PAd: pulmonary artery diastolic pressure.

PAOP (pulmonary artery occlusive pressure): Pressure obtained by inflating the balloon on a pulmonary artery catheter; measures left ventricular end diastolic pressure and is used as clinical indicator of LV preload. Also called PWP (pulmonary wedge pressure).

Papillary Muscles: Muscle projections from the inner surface of the ventricles that attach to the chordae tendineae of the AV valves.

Parasympathetic Nervous System (PNS): Branch of the autonomic nervous system that helps the body conserve and restore resources. Cardiovascular effects include slowing of heart rate and dilation of peripheral and visceral blood vessels.

Paresthesia: A sensation of tingling, pricking, or numbness of the skin.

Parietal Pericardium: The inner lining of the fibrous pericardium.

Paroxysmal Atrial Fibrillation: Atrial fibrillation that occurs spontaneously and terminates itself; does not last longer than 7 days, and usually lasts less than 24 hours.

Paroxysmal Nocturnal Dyspnea: Awakening from a sleep state with sudden and intense shortness of breath.

Paroxysmal: Sudden onset and termination; used to describe tachyarrhythmias.

PAs: pulmonary artery systolic pressure.

Pathological Q Wave: An abnormally deep or wide Q wave on the ECG; indicates necrosis of myocardial tissue.

Peak Inspiratory Pressure (PIP): Pressure needed to get air through airways and distend the lung. Accounts for both airway resistance and lung and chest wall compliance.

Pedicle Graft: Graft, such as internal mammary artery, where one end of the artery is left in its original position. Also referred to as *in situ*.

Penumbra: The area in an acute ischemic stroke surrounding the core area of injury. Contains cells with potential for recovery.

Glossary

Percutaneous Alcohol Septal Ablation (PASA): Catheter-based interventional cardiac procedure in which alcohol is injected into septal perforator blood vessels. Used in hypertrophic cardiomyopathy with outflow tract obstruction to produce septal infarction, so the septum does not contract and contribute to outflow tract obstruction.

Percutaneous Left Atrial Appendage Transcatheter Occlusion (PLAATO): A right cardiac catheterization procedure with trans-septal puncture done to place an occlusive device into the left atrial appendage to prevent embolization of thrombus. Most commonly done in chronic atrial fibrillation to prevent embolization.

Pericardial Knock: High-frequency heart sound heard in restrictive pericarditis.

Pericardiocentesis: Perforation of the pericardium with a needle to remove fluid from the pericardial space.

Pericarditis: Inflammation of the pericardium.

Pericardium: The thin fibrous sac surrounding the heart.

Percutaneous Coronary Intervention: Umbrella term used for all catheter-based coronary artery interventional procedures, including angioplasty, atherectomy, stent insertion, rotablation.

Peripartum Cardiomyopathy: Cardiomyopathy associated with the last trimester of pregnancy or the postpartum period.

Permanent Pacemaker: Implantable electronic device consisting of a pulse generator, lead wire, and electrode that delivers an electrical stimulus to the heart to maintain a normal heart rate.

Pharynx: Part of both respiratory and digestive systems. Located immediately posterior to the mouth and nasal cavity, and superior to the esophagus, larynx, and trachea.

Phlebostatic Axis: Approximates the level of the left atrium. Located at 4th intercostal space, mid-anterior-posterior chest.

Phrenic Nerve: A motor nerve to the diaphragm with sensory fibers to the pericardium.

Plasmin: Fibrinolytic enzyme derived from plasminogen.

Plasminogen: A protein important in preventing fibrin clot formation; the precursor to plasmin.

Pleura: Membrane surrounding the lungs. The visceral pleura lines the lungs; the parietal pleura is attached to the chest wall.

Pleura Space: Also called pleural cavity; the space between the visceral and parietal pleura. Contains a small amount of serous fluid.

Pneumothorax: Collection of air in the pleural cavity from a perforation through the chest wall or visceral pleura covering the lung.

Polycythemia Vera (Primary Polycythemia): A condition in which excess red blood cells are produced due to an abnormality of the bone marrow.

Post Pericardiotomy Syndrome: Inflammation of the pericardium late after CABG due to autoimmune response.

Posterior Descending Artery (PDA): Coronary artery arising from the right coronary artery in most people; supplies the posterior wall of the left ventricle.

Posterior MI: MI involving the posterior or back wall of the left ventricle.

PR Interval: Measurement on the ECG that reflects the time it takes the electrical impulse to travel through the atria, through the AV node, and into the ventricle where ventricular depolarization begins; A-V conduction time. Measured from beginning of P wave to beginning of QRS complex.

Glossary

Precordial Leads: Chest leads on the 12-lead ECG; $V_1 - V_6$ or $V_{1R} - V_{6R}$.

Preexcitation: Early activation of the ventricular myocardium by a supraventricular impulse, entering the ventricles through an accessory pathway, as occurs in WPW Syndrome.

Preload: Stretch on the ventricular myocardial fibers caused by the volume of blood in the ventricle at the end of ventricular diastole.

Pressure Gradient (Valve): Difference in pressure from one side of a valve to the other side of that valve.

Primary Prevention: Reducing risk in persons without known coronary heart disease to prevent the development of the disease in the future.

Proarrhythmic: Causing arrhythmias.

Procalcitonin: Precursor of the hormone calcitonin, which is involved with calcium homeostasis. Produced by the thyroid gland. It is not released into the blood stream of healthy individuals. With severe infection, the blood levels of procalcitonin may rise.

Programmed Electrical Stimulation (PES): Pacing according to pre-established protocols in the atria and ventricles during an electrophysiology study. Used to evaluate conduction properties of cardiac tissue and to induce the patient's clinical tachycardias.

Prostaglandin I2: A chemical substance that produces vasodilation and inhibits platelet aggregation.

Prothrombin: A circulating chemical substance that interacts with calcium salts to produce thrombin.

Pruritis: Intense itching.

Pseudoaneurysm: An outpouching of a blood vessel involving a defect in the intima and media of artery. The adventitia may be intact, or may be damaged, with bleeding contained by a blood clot or surrounding structures.

Psychogenic Polydipsia: Excessive consumption of free water due to psychiatric causes.

PT (Prothrombin Time): Coagulation test used to monitor the safety and effectiveness of warfarin.

PTCA: Percutaneous transluminal coronary angioplasty. Catheter-based interventional procedure in which a balloon is inflated at the site of coronary stenosis to increase the vessel lumen diameter.

Pulmonary Edema: Fluid in the pulmonary alveoli that interferes with gas exchange.

Pulmonary Embolus: Embolus in the pulmonary artery system. Increases pulmonary pressures and can cause pulmonary infarction.

Pulmonary Vascular Resistance: Resistance in the pulmonary system that the right ventricle must pump against; right ventricular afterload.

Pulmonary Vein Ectopic Foci Ablation: Catheter-based procedure in which radio frequency energy is used to create a line of scar tissue around the ostia of the pulmonary veins to prevent atrial fibrillation.

Pulmonary Veins: Veins carrying oxygenated blood from the lungs to the left atrium.

Pulmonary Wedge Pressure (PWP): see Pulmonary Artery Occlusive Pressure.

Pulmonic Valve: Valve between the right ventricle and the pulmonary artery.

Pulse Pressure: Difference between systolic and diastolic blood pressure.

Pulsus Alternans: Regular rhythm with alternating strong and weak pulses; suggests severe left ventricular dysfunction.

Glossary

Purkinje Fibers: Terminal fibers of the ventricular conduction system responsible for the rapid spread of the electrical impulse through both ventricles simultaneously. May also contain pacemaker activity at a rate of 20-40 beats per minute to maintain ventricular rate when all other pacemakers fail or when third degree block is present.

Pyridoxine: One of the compounds called vitamin B6.

Q Wave: First negative deflection from baseline of the QRS complex.

QRS axis: The average direction of all electrical forces traveling through the ventricles.

QRS Complex: Complex on the ECG representing ventricular depolarization. Width of the QRS complex represents intraventricular conduction time, or how long it takes the electrical impulse to travel through the ventricles.

QT Interval: Measurement on the ECG from the beginning of the QRS complex to the end of the T wave; is a rough reflection of ventricular repolarization time. A long QT interval predisposed to torsades de pointes.

R Wave Progression: Refers to the size of the R wave as it progresses from lead V_1 to lead V_6 on the ECG. Normal R-wave progression means that the R wave starts out small in lead V_1 and progressively enlarges across the precordium where it is the dominant part of the QRS complex in V_6.

R Wave: The upright portion of the QRS complex.

Radial Artery: Artery along thumb side of wrist; used as conduit for CABG.

Reciprocal ECG Changes: The mirror image of indicative changes, recorded in leads not directly facing damaged myocardium.

Reentry: Ability of an electrical impulse to reactivate an area of myocardium more than once. Re-entry is the arrhythmogenic mechanism responsible for many clinically significant arrhythmias.

Reflex Tachycardia: Tachycardia that occurs in response to a lowered blood pressure.

Remodeling: A change in shape and function of the ventricle in response to chronic pressure and volume overload in heart failure.

Renal Insufficiency: Reduction in glomerular filtration to 20-50% of normal.

Renin: An enzyme produced by the kidney in response to decreased renal blood flow; initiates the activation of the renin-angiotensin-aldosterone system.

Renin-Angiotensin-Aldosterone System: Neurohormonal system that is activated in response to low renal blood flow, such as occurs with heart failure. The end result is production of angiotensin II, a potent vasoconstrictor, and aldosterone which causes sodium and water reabsorption.

Renovascular Disease: Disease of the renal arteries.

Reperfusion: Restoration of blood flow to ischemic tissue.

Repolarization: Return of the cardiac cell to its electrical resting state.

Resistant Hypertension: Continued hypertension on full dose therapy, including a diuretic.

Resorption: Process by which osteoclasts break down bone and release minerals (calcium) into the blood.

Respiration (Cellular Respiration): The process whereby chemical bonds of molecules such as glucose are converted into energy.

Restenosis: Re-narrowing of the vessel lumen after a PCI.

Glossary

Restrictive Cardiomyopathy: Cardiac muscle disease characterized by rigidity of the myocardial wall with a decreased ability of the chamber walls to expand during cardiac filling.

Retroperitoneal Bleed: Bleeding into the space behind the peritoneum (membrane lining the abdominal cavity).

Revascularization: Restoration, to the extent possible, of normal blood flow to the myocardium or other organ or tissues, by surgical or percutaneous means.

Rhabdomyolysis: The breakdown of muscle fibers with leakage of potentially toxic cellular contents into the systemic circulation.

Rheumatic Heart Disease: Damage to the heart that is the result of rheumatic fever, which is a hemolytic streptococcal infection of the body. Normal heart complications include bacterial endocarditis with damage to the cardiac valves.

Right Atrium: Chamber of the heart that receives deoxygenated blood from the venous system.

Right Bundle Branch: Conduction pathway carrying the electrical impulse into the right ventricle.

Right Coronary Artery (RCA): Major coronary artery arising from the right side of the aorta; supplies the inferior and posterior wall of the left ventricle in most people.

Right Gastroepiploic Artery: Artery supplying blood to the greater curvature of the stomach; can be used as conduit in CABG.

Right Precordial Leads: Leads V_1, V_2, and V_3.

Right Ventricle: A thin-walled, low-pressure pump that receives deoxygenated blood from the right atrium and pumps blood into the pulmonary artery.

Risk Equivalent: Risk factors that place the patient at the same risk as if he/she already has CAD. Includes diabetes, symptomatic carotid artery disease, peripheral arterial disease, abdominal aortic aneurysm, chronic renal insufficiency.

Risk Factor: A characteristic found in a healthy person independently related to the future development of coronary artery disease.

Ross Procedure: Placing the pulmonic valve in the aortic valve position and a tissue valve in the pulmonic valve location.

Rotational Atherectomy: Use of high speed rotating blades or burrs to remove components of the atherosclerotic plaque.

S wave: A negative deflection following an R wave in the QRS complex.

S3 (the third heart sound): Heard immediately after the second heart sound; an indication of fluid overload.

S4 (the fourth heart sound): Heard just before the first heart sound; can be heard with a non-compliant ventricle.

Saphenous Vein Graft: Most common vein graft material used in CABG; taken from the greater saphenous vein of the leg.

Sarcoidosis: Chronic disease that involves development of granulomatous lesions in many tissues, including the myocardium; can result in heart failure.

Sarcolemma: Thin membrane that covers cardiac muscle cells and separates intracellular and extracellular spaces.

Sarcomere: The functional unit of the myofibril containing the contractile proteins, actin and myosin.

Saturated Fats: Fats that are usually solid at room temperature and typically come from animals.

Glossary

Sciatica: A set of symptoms caused by compression or irritation of one of the nerve roots that are branches of the sciatic nerve. The symptoms are in the lower back, buttock, and/or various parts of the leg and foot. In addition to pain, there may be numbness, muscular weakness, and difficulty moving or controlling the leg. Typically, the symptoms are only felt on one side of the body.

SCD: Abbreviation for Sudden Cardiac Death. Cardiac arrest with cessation of cardiac function, most often due to VF or pulseless VT.

Second Degree Heart Block (second degree AV block): Failure of some atrial impulses to conduct to the ventricles; one P wave at a time fails to conduct.

Secondary Prevention: Reducing risk in persons with known coronary artery disease to prevent a future event.

Selective Serotonin Reuptake Inhibitors (SSRIs): Class of antidepressant medications commonly used to treat depression in cardiac patients. SSRIs increase the extracellular level of the neurotransmitter serotonin by inhibiting its re-uptake, increasing the level of serotonin available to bind to the postsynaptic receptor.

Semilunar Valves: The valves located between the ventricles and great vessels: pulmonic and aortic valves.

Senile Degenerative Calcification: Progressive calcification of the valve leaflets.

Sepsis: Known or suspected infection with two or more signs of SIRS.

Septic Shock: Sepsis with hypotension despite fluid resuscitation.

Sheath: Small flexible catheter inserted into an artery or vein in interventional procedures. Guidewires and catheters are thread through the sheath during interventional procedures.

Sick Sinus Syndrome: Rhythm in which there is marked sinus node dysfunction (bradycardia or sinus arrest), alternating with periods of rapid atrial arrhythmias. Also called brady-tachy syndrome.

Sickle Cell Disease: An autosomal dominant genetic disorder in which patients suffer from severe hemolytic anemia with episodes of vaso occlusive crises.

Single Chamber Pacemaker: A pacemaker that has an electrode for pacing in one chamber of the heart, traditionally a ventricular pacemaker.

Sinoatrial (SA) Node: Small group of cells located in the right atrium near the junction of the superior vena cava that functions as the normal pacemaker of the heart; automatic rate of 60-100 beats per minute.

Sirolimus: An immunosuppressive agent used on drug eluting stents. Also used to prevent organ rejection during kidney transplant.

ST Elevation MI (STEMI): Myocardial infarction that presents with ST elevation on the ECG.

ST Segment: Segment on the ECG that represents early repolarization phase and extends from the end of the QRS to beginning of T wave. The ST segment should be at the isoelectric line (baseline). ST-segment elevation or depression can represent myocardial injury or ischemia.

Stable Angina Pectoris: Angina with a stable pattern, usually brought on by exertion and relieved with rest or sublingual nitroglycerin.

Statins (HMG-CoA Reductase Inhibitors): Most widely used lipid lowering medications in the treatment of cardiovascular disease. Work by inhibiting HMG-CoA reductase during cholesterol synthesis.

Stenosis: Narrowing of a passage.

Sternotomy: Cutting through the sternum.

Stress Testing: A noninvasive assessment tool for coronary artery diseases. Uses exercise or chemicals to stress the heart and may be done with or without myocardial imaging.

Stroke volume: The volume of blood ejected by the left ventricle with each beat.

Glossary

Subendocardium: Innermost layer of the myocardium.

Superior Vena Cava: A principal vein receiving venous blood returning from the head, neck, upper extremities and the thorax; empties into the right atrium.

Supraventricular Arrhythmias: Arrhythmias originating above the ventricles; includes sinus, atrial, and junctional arrhythmias.

Surfactant: A phospholipid responsible for decreasing surface tension in the alveoli.

SVT: Abbreviation for supraventricular tachycardia. Any tachycardia that originates above the AV node, but usually used to describe atrial tachycardia, AV nodal re-entry tachycardia, or circus movement tachycardia involving an accessory pathway.

Sympathetic Nervous System (SNS): Branch of autonomic nervous system allowing the body to function under stress. Cardiovascular effects are increased heart rate and contractility, as well as peripheral vasoconstriction.

Sympathomimetic: A medication that mimics the sympathetic nervous system.

Syncope: A transient lack of consciousness due to inadequate blood flow to the brain; fainting.

Systemic Inflammatory Response Syndrome (SIRS): A systemic response to inflammation. May or may not be due to infection.

Systemic Vascular Resistance: Resistance to ventricular ejection of blood; determined by amount of vasoconstriction or dilation in peripheral arterial system.

Systole: The contraction of the heart muscle that results in ejection of blood from the chamber.

Systolic Dysfunction: Ventricular dysfunction resulting in decreased ejection of blood from the ventricle.

Systolic Ejection Murmur: Murmur that occurs as blood is ejected across stenotic aortic or pulmonic valve during ventricular systole.

T Wave: Wave on the ECG representing ventricular repolarization.

Tachyarrhythmias: Cardiac arrhythmias with ventricular rates > 100 beats per minute.

Tachycardia: Heart rate greater than 100 beats per minute.

Tachyphylactic (tachyphylaxis): Rapidly decreasing response (rapid development of immunity) after initial doses of a medication.

Tachypnea: Increased respiratory rate.

Tako Tsubo Syndrome (also known as Tako Tsubo Cardiomyopathy): Syndrome with transient LV apical ballooning in the absence of myocardial infarction. LV contractility recovers in several days.

Tetany: Combination of signs and symptoms usually related to hypocalcemia, including hyperreflexia and spasms of hands and feet.

Thiazide Diuretics: Diuretics that inhibit sodium and water reabsorption; work in ascending loop of Henle and early distal tubule.

Thiocyanate: Is formed by combining with cyanide contained in nitroprusside. Can accumulate to toxic levels if renal function is impaired.

Thoracic Aorta: Portion of aorta located in the thoracic cavity containing the ascending aorta, the aortic arch, and the descending thoracic aorta.

Thoracoscopy: An insertion of an endoscope through a very small incision in the chest wall.

Thoracotomy: An incision into the chest typically to gain access to the lungs.

Thrombin: An enzyme formed from prothrombin which converts fibrinogen to fibrin.

Glossary

Thrombocytopenia: Abnormal decrease in the number of platelets.

Thromboembolic: Emboli coming from the source of a thrombus.

Thrombolytics: Medications used to break down blood clots.

Thrombophlebitis: Inflammation of a vein in conjunction with the formation of thrombus.

Thrombosis: The formation or existence of a blood clot.

Thrombotic Stroke: Ischemic stroke caused by thrombus or embolus from thrombus.

Thromboxane A2: Substance produced by platelets in response to vascular injury; causes further platelet activation, vasoconstriction, and smooth muscle proliferation.

Thrombus: A blood clot causing obstruction.

Tidal Volume: Volume of air entering or leaving the nose or mouth per breath. Normal is 500 ml for 70 kg adult.

Time Cycled Breath: A pressure control breath is delivered at a constant pressure (i.e. 20 cm H2O) for a preset time (i.e. 2 seconds).

Torsade de pointes: Literally "twisting of the points" (French). Refers to polymorphic ventricular tachycardia associated with prolonged QT interval.

Trabe's sign (Pistol-shot sounds): Booming systolic and diastolic sounds heard over the femoral artery.

Trachea: Airway that allows oxygen and carbon dioxide to move from the throat to the lungs.

Tracheostomy (Tracheotomy): A surgical procedure performed to open a direct airway through an incision in the trachea.

Transesophageal Echocardiogram: Placement of an ultrasound probe into the esophagus to view the aorta and cardiac structures; eliminates the need to image through the chest wall.

Transluminal Extraction Atherectomy: Interventional cardiac procedure used to extract visible thrombi from a coronary artery.

Transmural: Full thickness of myocardium.

Transverse or T Tubules: Invaginations of the sarcolemma into the interior of the cardiac muscle cell. Forms a network of tubes that tunnel into the cell and carries electrical excitation to the interior of the cell.

Tricuspid Valve: Valve located between the right atrium and right ventricle.

Trifascicular Block: Block in the cardiac conduction system that involves all three fascicles that carry the impulse into the ventricle: right bundle branch, left anterior fascicle, and left posterior fascicle. Complete trifascicular block results in third degree AV block.

Triglycerides: Compound consisting of glycerol and a fatty acid; component of most animal and vegetable fats.

Troponin I: Biomarker found only in cardiac muscle; the most sensitive indicator for myocardial damage.

Trousseau's Sign: Contraction of fingers or hands in response to inflating blood pressure cuff above systolic pressure and holding for 3 minutes. Seen with hypocalcemia.

Type I Neurological Complications (post CABG): Major focal deficits and coma.

Type II Neurological Complications (post CABG): Various degrees of intellectual deterioration or memory loss.

U Wave: Small wave on the ECG that follows the T wave in some patients. Probably represents repolarization of some portion of the ventricle or Purkinje system.

Ultrafiltration: The movement of fluid through a semi-permeable membrane caused by a pressure gradient.

Glossary

Unfractionated heparin (UFH, heparin): The anticoagulant of choice in many conditions, including acute myocardial infarction, pulmonary emboli and deep vein thrombosis.

Unstable Angina Pectoris: A change in a previously stable pattern of angina: angina at rest or with minimal exertion, requiring more nitroglycerin for relief, worse pain or pain that lasts longer than usual.

Uremia (Uremic Syndrome): A toxic syndrome (multiple signs and symptoms) seen in acute and chronic renal failure associated with an accumulation of nitrogenous wastes. Condition warrants dialysis.

V (v) Wave: Wave on RA and PAOP waveforms correlating with atrial filling.

V/Q Ratio (Ventilation/Perfusion Ratio): The ratio of alveolar ventilation (air flow) to blood flow in the capillaries around the alveoli.

Vagal: Pertaining to the vagus nerve. Used to describe the cardiovascular response to parasympathetic stimulation: bradycardia, peripheral vasodilation.

Valsalva Maneuver: Forced expiratory effort against a closed glottis, such as holding of breath and straining. Results in increased intrathoracic pressure and stimulates the vagus nerve; used to slow conduction through the AV node and terminate some SVTs.

Valvuloplasty: A balloon inflated in the cardiac valve orifice to fracture the calcium deposits in the leaflets and stretch the annulus to return the valve to normal functioning.

Vasoconstriction: Constriction of vessels.

Vasodilation: Dilatation of vessels.

Vasoplegia: Profound hypotension, often seen after open heart surgery, that does not respond to standard catecholamine therapy.

Vasopressor: Medication used to increase blood pressure by causing peripheral vasoconstriction. Used to obtain acceptable mean arterial pressure to perfuse end organs.

Vasospastic Angina: Angina caused by spasm of a coronary artery; also called Prizmetal's angina or variant angina.

Vasovagal Response: Response of parasympathetic nervous system producing hypotension, bradycardia, diaphoresis, nausea and vomiting.

Venous Oxygen Saturation: The percent of oxygen saturation of venous blood (after the tissues have extracted oxygen from the arterial blood). Normal is 60-80%.

Ventilation: The process of moving air between the atmosphere and alveoli. Process occurs through inspiration and expiration.

Ventricular Aneurysm: Localized dilatation of the left ventricle at the site of infarction.

Ventricular Arrhythmias: Arrhythmias originating from the ventricles. Includes PVCs, idioventricular rhythm, accelerated ventricular rhythm, monomorphic VT, polymorphic VT and VF.

Ventricular Fibrillation: A quivering of ventricles resulting in a pulseless rhythm and cardiac arrest; treated with immediate defibrillation.

Ventricular Outflow Tract: The path the blood in the ventricle must follow when ejected from the ventricle.

Ventricular Pacemaker: Pacemaker with a lead in the right ventricle; used for ventricular pacing.

Ventricular Septal Myectomy: Surgical removal of a portion of the hypertrophied septum that is contributing to outflow tract obstruction.

Visceral Pericardium: The same as the epicardium; the inner lining of the pericardium and the outer lining of the heart and great vessels.

Glossary

Vital Capacity: Volume of air expelled from the lungs during maximal forced expiration after maximal forced inspiration.

Volume Cycled Breath: Breath is delivered at a preset tidal volume. Exhalation begins after the set volume has been delivered.

Vulnerable Plaque: Atherosclerotic plaque that is vulnerable to ulceration and rupture.

Wall Motion Abnormality: Abnormal movement of a part of the ventricular wall seen on echocardiography.

Warfarin: An oral anticoagulant agent that works indirectly through the liver by altering vitamin K dependent clotting factors.

Water-Hammer Pulse (Corrigan's pulse): When palpating peripheral pulse there is a rapid rise and collapse of the pulse.

Watershed (Border Zone) Stroke: An area of focal ischemia from decreased perfusion pressure. Bilateral watershed infarcts are usually caused by systemic hypotension.

Wolff-Parkinson-White Syndrome (WPW): Syndrome where one or more accessory pathways exist connecting the atria to the ventricles. Conduction over the accessory pathway causes pre-excitation of the ventricles and can predispose the patient to tachyarrhythmias.

ABBREVIATIONS

A

AAA: abdominal aortic aneurysm

ABI: ankle brachial index

AC: assist control

ACC: American College of Cardiology

ACE: angiotensin converting enzyme

ACEI: angiotensin converting enzyme inhibitor

ACLS: advanced cardiac life support

AED: automatic external defibrillator

AF: atrial fibrillation

AHA: American Heart Association

AIVR: accelerated idioventricular rhythm

AKI: acute kidney injury

AMI: acute myocardial infarction

ANP: atrial natriuretic peptide

ANS: autonomic nervous system

AP: used for accessory pathway, for action potential, and for anteroposterior

APCD: arterial puncture closure device

APRV: airway pressure release ventilation

APSP: assisted patient systole

AR: aortic regurgitation

ARDS: acute respiratory distress syndrome

ARF: acute renal failure

ARVD: arrhythmogenic right ventricular dysplasia

AS: aortic stenosis

ASA: aspirin

ASD: atrial septal defect

AT: atrial tachycardia

ATP: adenosine triphosphate. Also used for anti-tachycardia pacing

AV: atrioventricular

AVB: atrioventricular block

AVNRT: AV nodal reentry tachycardia

AVR: aortic valve replacement

AVRT: atrioventricular re-entry (or reciprocating) tachycardia

AWMI: anterior wall myocardial infarction

B

BAEDP: balloon-assisted end diastolic pressure

BBB: bundle branch block

BiPAP: biphasic positive airway pressure

BMI: body mass index

BNP: brain natriuretic peptide

C

CABG: coronary artery bypass graft surgery

CAD: coronary artery disease

CaO$_2$: arterial oxygen content

CEBT: continuous extracorporeal blood therapy

CHD: coronary heart disease

CHF: congestive heart failure

CI: cardiac index

CLI: critical limb ischemia

CMT: circus movement tachycardia

CMV: controlled mandatory ventilation

CPAP: continuous positive airway pressure

CPB: cardiopulmonary bypass

CO: cardiac output

CO$_2$: carbon dioxide

COPD: chronic obstructive pulmonary disease

CPB: cardiopulmonary bypass

CPP: cerebral perfusion pressure

CPR: cardiopulmonary resuscitation

CRRT: continuous renal replacement therapy

CRT: cardiac resynchronization therapy

CS: coronary sinus

CSM: carotid sinus massage

CT: computed tomography

CTA: computed tomography angiography

CVA: cerebral vascular accident; stroke.

CvO$_2$: venous oxygen content

CVP: central venous pressure

CVVH: continuous venovenous hemofiltration

CVVHD: continuous venovenous hemodialysis

CVVHDF: continuous venovenous hemodiafiltration

Abbreviations

D

DCA: directional coronary atherectomy
DES: drug eluting stent
DFT: defibrillation threshold
DKA: diabetic ketoacidosis
DN: dicrotic notch
DO$_2$: delivery of oxygen
DVT: deep vein thrombosis

E

ECF: extracellular fluid
ECG: electrocardiogram
ECMO: extracorporeal membrane oxygenation
EF: ejection fraction
EMS: emergency medical system
EP: electrophysiology
EPO: erythropoietin
EPS: electrophysiology study
ERV: expiratory reserve volume

F

FENa: fractional excretion of sodium
FEurea: fractional excretion of urea
FEV: expiratory airflow
FEV$_1$: expiratory airflow in one second
FIO$_2$: fraction of inspired oxygen
FRC: functional residual capacity

G

GFR: glomerular filtration rate

H

HCO$_3$: bicarbonate ion
H$_2$CO$_3$: carbonic acid
HB: His bundle (bundle of His)
HBG: hemoglobin (also abbreviated Hb)
HDL-C: high-density lipoprotein cholesterol
HF: heart failure
HHNK: hyperosmolar hyperglycaemic nonketotic coma
HIT: heparin induced thrombocytopenia
HOCM: hypertrophic obstructive cardiomyopathy
HR: heart rate
HRA: high right atrium

I

IAB: intra-aortic balloon
IABP: intra-aortic balloon pump
IC: inspiratory capacity
ICD: implantable cardioverter defibrillator
ICP: intracranial pressure
ID: intrinsicoid deflection
IMA: internal mammary artery
INR: International Normalized Ratio
IRV: inspiratory reserve volume
IVC: inferior vena cava
IWMI: inferior wall myocardial infarction

J

J: joules
JVD: jugular vein distention

L

LAD: used for left axis deviation and for left anterior descending (coronary artery)
LAE: left atrial enlargement
LAFB: left anterior fascicular block
LBBB: left bundle branch block
LCX: left circumflex coronary artery
LDL-C: low-density lipoprotein cholesterol
LIMA: left internal mammary artery
LMWH: low molecular weight heparin
LPFB: left posterior fascicular block
LV: left ventricle
LVH: left ventricular hypertrophy
LVSWI: left ventricular stroke work index
LWMI: lateral wall myocardial infarction

M

mA: milliamp
MAP: mean arterial pressure
MAT: multifocal atrial tachycardia
MDRD: GFR equation from Modification of Diet in Renal Disease (MDRD) study
MET: Unit of metabolic equivalent
MI: myocardial infarction
MIDCAB: minimally invasive direct coronary artery bypass
MODS: multi-organ dysfunction syndrome
MR: mitral regurgitation
MRA: magnetic resonance angiography
MRI: magnetic resonance imaging
MS: mitral stenosis
mV: millivolt
MVO$_2$: myocardial oxygen consumption

Abbreviations

N

NG: nasogastric
NSR: normal sinus rhythm
NSTEMI: non ST-elevation myocardial infarction
NYHA: New York Heart Association

O

OPCAB: off-pump coronary artery bypass

P

PA: pulmonary artery
PAC: premature atrial complex
PAD: peripheral arterial disease
PAEDP: patient's end diastolic pressure
PaO₂: arterial partial pressure of oxygen
PAO₂: alveolar partial pressure of oxygen
PAP: pulmonary artery pressure
PAOP: pulmonary artery occlusive pressure
PASA: percutaneous alcohol septal ablation
PASP: peak aortic systolic pressure
PAT: paroxysmal atrial tachycardia
PCI: percutaneous coronary intervention
PDA: used for posterior descending artery (coronary artery) and for patent ductus arteriosus
PDP: peak diastolic augmented pressure
PE: pulmonary embolus
PEEP: positive end expiratory pressure
PES: programmed electrical stimulation
PIP: peak inspiratory pressure
PJC: premature junctional complex
PLVP: peak left ventricular pressure
PMBV: percutaneous mitral balloon valvotomy
PND: paroxysmal nocturnal dyspnea
PNS: parasympathetic nervous system
PSP: patient systolic pressure
PSV: pressure support ventilation
PSVT: paroxysmal supraventricular tachycardia
PTCA: percutaneous transluminal coronary angioplasty
PVC: premature ventricular complex
PVR: pulmonary vascular resistance
pVT: pulseless ventricular tachycardia
PWMI: posterior wall myocardial infarction
PWP: pulmonary wedge pressure

Q

Q: symbol for blood flow (perfusion)

R

RA: used for right atrium and for rotational atherectomy
RAD: right axis deviation
RAAS: renin-angiotensin-aldosterone-system
RAE: right atrial enlargement
RAS: renal artery stenosis
RBBB: right bundle branch block
RCA: right coronary artery
RF: radio frequency
RFA: radio frequency ablation
RIMA: right internal mammary artery
RIND: reversible ischemic neurological deficit
RV: right ventricle (residual volume – in pulmonary)
RVEDV: right ventricular end diastolic volume
RVH: right ventricular hypertrophy
RVSWI: right ventricular stroke work index

S

SCD: sudden cardiac death
SCUF: slow continuous ultrafiltration
ScvO₂: central venous oxygen saturation
SIADH: Syndrome of inappropriate antidiuretic hormone secretion
SIMV: synchronized intermittent mandatory ventilation
SmvO₂: mixed venous oxygen saturation
SNS: sympathetic nervous system
SOB: short of breath
SSTREM-1: soluble triggering receptor expressed on myeloid cells –1.
STEMI: ST-elevation myocardial infarction
SV: stroke volume
SVC: superior vena cava
SVG: saphenous vein graft
SVI: stroke volume index
SvO₂: venous oxygen saturation
SVR: systemic vascular resistance
SVT: supraventricular tachycardia

Abbreviations

T

TCD: transcranial doppler
TCP: transcutaneous pacing
TdP: torsades de pointes
TEC: transluminal extraction catheter
TEE: transesophageal echocardiogram
TIA: transient ischemic attack
TLC: total lung capacity
tPA: tissue plasminogen activator

U

UA: unstable angina
UFH: unfractionated heparin

V

V: symbol for ventilation
VC: vital capacity
VF: ventricular fibrillation
VLDL: very low-density lipoproteins
VO_2: oxygen consumption
VSD: ventricular septal defect
V_t: tidal volume
VT: ventricular tachycardia

W

WAP: wandering atrial pacemaker
WBC: white blood cell or white blood cell count
WCT: wide complex tachycardia
WPW: Wolff-Parkinson-White

INDEX

A

abdominal aortic aneurisms (AAA), 552-66
abdominojugular reflux, 44
aberrancy, 209-11
ablation procedure, 793-95
accelerated ventricular rhythm, 195
access site management, 680-81
accessory pathway conduction (AP), 215-16
ACE inhibitors (ACEI), 596-600
acid-base balance, 103-7
acidosis, 105, 106
action potential (AP), 11-14
active transport, 26
acute coronary syndrome (ACS), 259, 325, 335-66,
acute kidney injury (AKI), 849-61
acute limb ischemia, 549-50
acute respiratory distress syndrome (ARDS), 732-33, 820-24
afterload, 18-19, 119-21, 591-92
airway resistance, 72-73
alcohol, 311
aldosterone blockers, 602
alkalosis, 105-7
alpha and beta stimulation, 613-16
alpha stimulation, 617-18
alveolar dead space, 78
amputation, 556
anaphylactic shock, 156
anemia, 396
aneurisms, 562-68
angina pectoris, 327-29, 333-34, 456, 595, 692, 734
angioplasty, 671-72
angiotensin receptor blockers (ARBs), 601
anion gap, 105
ankle brachial index (ABI), 546-47
antiarrhythmic drugs, 640-42
antibiotic prophylaxis, 533-34, 460, 466
anticoagulation, 467, 631-67, 680, 702-3
antidiuretic hormone, 618-19
anti-lipid drugs, 653-55
antiplatelet therapy, 627-31, 677-78, 726-27
antithrombin therapy, 624-40, 678
aortic recoil, 9, 453-54
aortic regurgitation (AR), 146, 468-78
aortic stenosis (AS), 146, 454-68
aortic valve disease, 353-78
aortorenal bypass, 546
apoprotein B, 312

arrhythmias, 177-216, 726
arrhythmogenic cardiomyopathy, 442-45
arterial blood gas (ABG) analysis, 105-6
arterial grafts, 711-12
arterial line monitoring, 143-44
arterial system, 4-5
arteriography, 675
arterioles, 5
atrial fibrillation, 188-89, 258, 729-30
aspiration, 820
assessment, cardiac, 35-62
asynchronous (fixed rate) pacing mode, 753
asystole, 205
atherectomy, 673-74
atherosclerosis, 313
atria, 1
atrial capture, 766
atrial line, left, PA catheter and, 716
atrial rhythms, 184-91, 729-30
atrial sensing, 766
atrioventricular blocks, 199-205
atrioventricular junction, 16
atrioventricular node, 16, 177
atrioventricular rhythms, 192-93
atrioventricular valves, 3
auscultation, 4, 49-59

B

B_1 and B_2 stimulation, 616
B_1 stimulation, 613
balloon pericardiotomy, 515
balloon pump, 157-65
baroreceptors, 22-23
Beck's triad, 518
beta blockers, 603-6, 610
bipolor pacing system, 752
biventricular pacing, 751, 774-76
bleeding, 703-4, 722-24, 733-34
blood clots, 625-27
blood gases, 78-80, 82-84, 105-6
blood pressure, 45-46, 292, 701, 713-14
blood sugar, 702, 714, 735
bradycardia, sinus, 182
breathing. *See* oxygen; oxygenation; pulmonary system
bronchitis, chronic, 807
bundle branch block, 206-8, 243-45
bundle branches, 16, 177
bundle of Kent, 256

Index

C

calcium channel (CA^{++}) blockers, 606-10
cannulation, 697
capillary system, 5
capture beats, 213
capture, 759-60, 766-67
cardiac assessment, 35-62
cardiac biomarkers, 338
cardiac chambers, 1-2
cardiac computed tomography (CT), 333
cardiac cycle, 49-50
cardiac output (CO), 17-19, 115, 590-94
    measurement, 139
cardiac resynchronization therapy (CRT), 775-76
cardiac veins, 11
cardiogenic shock, 153-55
cardiomyopathy, 413-45
    arrhythmogenic, 442-45
    dilated, 415-24
    hypertrophic, 430-42
    restrictive, 424-30
cardioplegia, 698-700
cardiopulmonary bypass (CPB), 695-98, 701-8
cardiopulmonary circuit, 19-21
cardioversion, 746-48
carotid artery stenting, 583
carotid endarterectomy, 582-83
catheterization, 322-33, 663-68, 675, 678, 679, 789-95
    monitoring, 127-28, 141-42
cellular respiration, 89
cerebral blood flow, CPB, 702
chamber enlargement, 250-53
chemoreceptors, 23
chest tubes, 826-27
cholesterol, 297-306
chronic obstructive pulmonary disease (COPD), 806-10
circulatory system, 4-11
claudication, 544, 547-48, 550-55
coagulation cascade, 625-26
cocaine, 357
collateral circulation, 9-10
compliance, 71-72
conducting airways, 69-70
conduction system, 16-17
constrictive pericarditis, 518-22
continuous extracorporeal blood therapy (CEBT), 859-61
continuous wave Doppler ultrasound, 546
contractility, 19, 122-23, 592-93
contrast agents, 676
COPD, 806-10
cor pulminale, 814-15
coronary artery bypass grafting (CABG), 689-737
    minimally invasive (MIDCAB), 709-10
    off-pump (OPCAB), 708-9
    transmyocardial laser revasulcarization (TMLR), 710-11

coronary artery disease (CAD), 285-315, 325-35
coronary ischemia, 679-80
critical limb ischemia, 548-49
cutting balloon angioplasty, 672
cyanosis, 44, 84

D

decompensation, 397-99
deep vein thrombosis (DVT) prophylactics, 726
defibrillation, 745-46
delta wave, 256
demand pacing, 753
depolarization, 232
diabetes, 307-8, 329, 705
diastole, 7-8. *See also* auscultation; valve function
diastolic dysfunction, 378-79
diffusion, 26, 78-82
dihydropyridines (DHP), 607
dilated cardiomyopathy, 415-24
directional coronary atherectomy (DCA), 674
dissections, aortic, 568-71, 679
distributive shock, 155
diuretics, 610-12
dizziness, 39, 456
dobutamine (Dobutrex), 613
dominance, 11
dopamine, 613-14
drug eluting stents (DES), 673
dual chamber pacemakers, 763-73
duplex ultrasound, 546
dye. *See* contrast agents
dynamic response testing. *See* square wave testing
dyslipidemia, 296-306
dyssynchrony, 774-75

E

edema, 59-61, 815-16
electrocardiogram (ECG), 178-80, 225-53
    in ventricular pacing, 776
electrolyte abnormalities, 827-44
electrophysiology study (EPS), 787-89, 794-95
embolism, pulmonary (PE), 810-14
emphysema, 807
endocardial disease, 534-34
endocarditis, 525-34
endocardium, 2
endomyocardial biopsy, 523
endothelin, 382
endothelium, 6
enlargement, chamber, 250-54
epiaortic imaging, 694-95
epicardial pacing, 721-22, 754-55
epicardium, 2
epinephrine (adrenalin), 614-15
escape beats, ventricular, 194
excitation-contraction coupling, 15
exercise, 310-11, 361-64

Index

F

fascicular blocks, 247-49
femoral artery pseudoaneurism, 567
fibrillation
  atrial, 188-89, 258, 729-30
  ventricular, 198-99, 258
fibrinolysis, 626-27
fibrinolytics, 347-48, 637-40
fluid balance, 25-28, 385, 714-15
flutter, atrial, 187-88, 258
frontal plane axis, 235-40
function curves, 123-24
functional capacity, 384-85
fusion beats, 213-14

G

gas exchange airways, 70
graft material, 711-12

H

heart failure, 373-404, 456
heart rate, 18, 123, 642-43
heart sounds. *See* auscultation
heart/lung machine, 695-98
hemiblocks, 247-49
hemodiafiltration, 859
hemodialysis, 858, 859
hemofiltration, 859
hemoglobin structure, 82-84
heparin reversal, 704-5
hepatojugular reflux (HJR), 48
His bundle, 16, 177
hormonal control, 25
hormone replacement therapy (HRT), 314
hydrostatic pressure (pushing pressure), 26
hypercalcemia, 839-41
hypercholesterolemia, 297
hypercoagulability, 312
hyperdynamic perfusion, 471-72
hyperhomocysteinemia, 311-12
hyperkalemia, 833-36
hyperlipidemia, 297-306
hypermagnesemia, 842
hypernatremia, 830
hyperphosphatemia, 844
hypertension, 291-96
hypertriglyceridemia, 298
hypertrophic cardiomyopathy, 430-42
hypertrophy, left ventricular, 313
hypocalcemia, 837-39
hypokalemia, 831-33
hypomagnesemia, 841-42
hyponatremia, 828-30
hypophosphatemia, 843-44
hypothermia, management of in CPB, 715-16
hypovolemic shock, 149-52

hypoxemia, 85
hypoxia, 85
hypoxic pulmonary vasoconstriction, 77

I

idioventricular rhythm, 195
implantable cardioverter defibrillator (ICD), 780-87
infarction, 259-62, 259-71
infective endocarditis (IE), 525-34
inflammation, 313
inflammatory response, 382
inflow, surgical, 554-55
influenza, 360
inotropes, 612-17
intestinal absorption inhibitors, 306
intima, 5
intra-aortic balloon pump (IABP), 157-65, 700
intracoronary stents, 672-73
intrarenal acute kidney injury, 852-54
intravascular ultrasound (IVUS), 675-76
intrinsicoid deflection, 252
ischemia, 259-63, 333, 549-50, 679-80, 692
ischemic stroke, 572-84
isoproterenol (Isuprel), 616

J

James fibers. *See* His bundle
jugular vein, 46-48

K

kidney injuries, 851-57

L

leads, 230-32, 270
left anterior fascicular block (LAFB), 248
left atrial enlargement (P mitrale), 251
left bundle branch block (LBBB), 207-8, 245
left posterior fascicular block (LPFB), 249
left-side infective endocarditis, 527
left-ventricular aneurisms, 353
left-ventricular remodeling, 383
lipoprotein a level, 312
loop diuretics, 610
low cardiac output state, 738
lower extremity aneurisms, 566

M

mean QRS axis, 232
median sternotomy, 695
mediastinitis, 730-31
medication compliance, 402
medications, 589-653
  acute coronary syndrome, 358-59
  angina, 334-35
  antiarrhythmic, 640-42
  anticoagulation, 702-3
  antifibrinolytic, 703-4

Index

anti-lipid, 301-6, 653-55
aortic regurgitation, 473-74, 477
cardiac tamponade, 521
COPD, 808-9
dilated cardiomyopathy, 420-22
claudication, 552-53
cor palminale, 815
coronary artery bypass grafting, 691-92
electrolyte abnormalities, 850, 835-36, 838-42, 844
endocarditis, 531, 532
heart failure, 388-94
hypertrophic cardiomyopathy, 437-39
heparin reversal, 704-5
ischemia, 556-57
ischemic stroke, 579-80
kidney injury, 856-57
mitral regurgitation, 483-84, 487
mitral stenoisis, 492-94
myocardial infarction, 350, 356
myocarditis, 524
pericardial effusion, 513
pericarditis, 510-11
percutaneous coronary intervention, 677-78
peripheral artery disease, 550
postoperative care, 724-27
pulmonary embolism, 812-13
renal replacement, 858
restrictive cardiomyopathy, 428-29
sepsis, 866
sympathomimetic, 612
valve disease, 459-61, 466-67
metabolic syndrome, 309-10
milrinone (Primacor), 616-17
mitral regurgitation (MR), 145, 478-88
mitral stenosis, 145, 488-98
mitral valve disease, 478-88
monitoring systems, 127-44
monomorphic VT, 197
multifocal atrial tachycardia (MAT), 186
murmurs, 54-58
muscles, cardiac, 14-15, 67-68
myocardial infarction, 33, 335-65, 734-35
    STEMI, 335-55
    non-STEMI, 355-58
myocardial oxygenation, 20-21, 595
myocardial protection, 698-700
myocarditis, 522-24
myocardium, 2
myofibrils, 14-15

N

native valve infective endocarditis, 525-26
necrosis, 383-84
nesiritide (Natrecor), 621,22
neuro anatomy and physiology, 574-77
neurogenic shock, 156-57

neurohormonal responses, 380-84
neurological complications, CABG and, 728-29
nitrates, 620-21
nitroprusside (Niprise), 622
nondihydropyridines, 607
norepinephrine (Levophed), 615-16
nosocomial infective endocarditis, 526

O

obesity, 308-9
obstructive shock, 157
obstructive sleep apnea, 313, 810
occlusion, 349
oligaric acute kidney injury, 855-57
osmolality, 27
osmosis, 26
osmotic pressure (pulling Pressure), 27
outflow, surgical procedures, 555
output, cardiac (CO), 17-19, 115, 590-94
    measurement, 139
oversensing, 761-62
oxidative stress, 312-13
oxygen therapy, 89-90
oxygenation, 19-21, 79-103, 124-27, 396, 595, 702, 717-21
oxyhemoglobin dissociation curve, 83-85

P

P wave, 178, 227
pacemaker mediated tachycardia (PMT), 772-73
pacemakers, 186, 749-80
    dual chambered, 763-73
pacing, 721-22, 750-56, 774-76
palpation, 48-49
palpitations, 39
papillary muscle dysfunction, 352
parasympathetic nervous system (PSN), 22
paroxysmal atrial tachycardia (PAT), 187
percutaneous balloon valvotomy, 465
percutaneous coronary intervention (PCI), 668-82
percutaneous transluminal coronary angioplasty, 671-72
perforation, coronary artery, 679
perfusion, 9, 74-78, 453-54
    hyperdynamic, 471-72
pericardial diseases, 505-22
pericardiocentesis, 513-14
pericarditis, 353, 505-11
pericardium, 2-3
peripheral arterial disease (PAD), 543-84
peritoneal dialysis, 858-59
Perkinje fibers, 17, 177
phenylephrine (Neosynephrine), 617-18
plaque, 325-27, 624
platelets, 624-25
pleural effusions, 733
pneumonia, 816-19
pneumothorax, 733, 824-27

polymorphic VT, 197
posterior hemiblock, 249
postoperative complications, 727-34
postpericardiotomy syndrome, 734
postrenal acute kidney injury, 854-55
potassium sparing diuretics, 610
PR interval, 178
preexcitation syndrome, 256-58
preload, 18, 116-19, 590-91
premature atrial complexes (PACs), 184-85
premature ventricular complexes (PVCs), 193-94
pre-renal acute kidney injury, 851
pressure monitoring, pulmonary artery, 129-32
prophylactics, 725
prophylaxis, 533-34
prosthetic valve infective endocarditis, 526
pulmonary artery catheter, 127-28
pulmonary embolism (PE), 810-14
pulmonary system, 67-107
pulmonary vascular resistance (PVR), 76-78
pulses, 60-61
pulsus paradoxis, 516-17

Q

QRS axis, 235-40
QRS beats, 208-16
QRS complex, 178, 228, 233
QT interval, 178, 230

R

radio frequency (RF) ablation, 789-95
rate adaptive pacing, 751
recoil, 9, 453-54
refractory periods, 14, 767
regurgitation, aortic, 146, 468-78
remodeling, ventricular, 383-84
renal anatomy, 104, 844-47
renal artery disease, 557-61
renal dysfunction, 731-32
renal replacement therapy, 858-61
renin-angeotensin-aldosterone system (RAAS), 23-24, 381-82,
      596-97
reperfusion, 346-49
respiratory failure, acute, 805-6
resternotomy, 724
restrictive cardiomyopathy, 424-30
resynchronization therapy, 394-95
revascularization, 553, 560-61. *See also* coronary artery
      bypass grafting
rhythms, atrial, 184-89
            AV junction, 192-93
            sinus, 181-84
            supraventricular, 189-91
right atrial enlargement (P pulmonale), 250
right bundle branch block, (RBBB), 206-8
right-sided infective endocarditis, 526-27

Ross procedure, 465
rotational atherectomy, (RA), 674
rupture, 352

S

sapheneous vein graft, 711
sarcoplasmic reticulum, 15
saturation of mixed venous blood (ScVO2) monitoring, 88-89,
      140
semilunar valves, 4
sensing, 760, 766-67
sensitivity threshold testing, 761
sepsis, 862-69
septal rupture, 352
septum, ventricular, 10
shock states, 147-57
single-chamber pacing, 750
sinus (SA) node, 16, 177
sinus rhythms, 181-84
sleep apnea, obstructive, 313, 810
smoking, 287-91
SmvO2 monitoring, 140
sodium restriction, 403
soy, 313-14
specific gravity, 27
square wave testing, 130-32
ST segment, 178, 228
STEMI, 335-55
stenosis
            aortic, 146, 454-68
            mitral, 488-97
stent thrombosis, 679
stimulation threshold testing, 761
stimulus release, 758
stress resting, 330-32
stress ulcer prophylactics, 725
stress, 311, 364-65
stroke cycle, 116
ST-T "strain" pattern, 252
subxiphoid pericardiostomy, 514
supraventricular tachycardia, 189-91
SVO2 monitoring, 88, 140
sympathetic nervous system (SNS), 21-22, 380-81, 595-96
sympathomimetic drugs, 612
synchrony, ventricular, 19
syncope, 39, 456
syndrome X, 358
synergy, ventricular, 19
systemic flow, during CPB, 701-2
systole, 8. *See also* auscultation; valve function
systolic dysfunction, 377-78

T

T wave, 178, 229
tachycardias, 181-82, 192-93, 208-16, 258
            multifocal atrial (MAT), 186

Index

pacemaker mediated (PMT), 772-73
paroxysmal atrial (PAT), 187
supraventricular, 189-91
ventricular (VT), 196-98
tako tsubo syndrome, 358
tamponade, 146-47, 352, 515-18
temporary pacing, 750
termination therapies, 782-83
thiazide diuretics, 610
thoracic aortic aneurism, 567-68
thorascopic pericardiostomy, 515
threshold potential (TP), 12
thrombolytics, 347-48, 637-40
timing cycles, pacemakers and, 763-64
toe brachial index, 546
Torsades de Pointes (TdP), 197-98
transcutaneous pacing (TCP), 756
transesophogeal echocardiography (TEE), 694-95
transfusion, 722-24
transluminal extraction catheter (TEC), 675
transmembrane resting potential (TRP), 12
transmyocardial laser revascularization (TMLR), 710-11
transplantation, 400-1
transvenous pacing, 753-54

U

U wave, 229
ultrafiltration, 859
ultrasound, 546, 675
undersensing, 760-61
unipolor pacing system, 753
uremic syndrome, 856

V

vagal response, 22
valves, 3-4, 451-53
atrioventricular, 3
diseases of, 145, 453-98
function of, 451-52
semilunar, 4
valvular heart disease, 145-46
variant angina, 357-58
vasodilators, 77-78, 619-22
vasopressin (Pitressin), 25, 382, 618-19
vasopressors, 617-19
vein grafts, 711
venous system, 5-6
ventilation, 71-74, 91-103, 717-21
ventricles, 1-2, 19, 123-24
dysfunction of, 387
failure of, 379-80
remodeling of, 383-84
ventricular enlargement, 252
ventricular fibrillation, 198-99, 258
ventricular rhythms, 193-99
ventricular tachycardia (VT), 196-98

ventricular, 193-99
ventriculography, 675

W

waveform analysis, 132-39
Wolff-Parkinson-White syndrome (WPW), 256-59